Adult-Gerontology Acute Care Practice Guidelines

Catherine Harris, PhD, MBA, AGACNP, is an associate professor of graduate programs and a faculty in the Acute Care Nurse Practitioner Program at Thomas Jefferson University in Philadelphia. She earned her PhD in nursing at the University of Pennsylvania and an MBA from Drexel University before becoming credentialed as an acute care nurse practitioner at Thomas Jefferson University in Philadelphia. Dr. Harris specializes in neurocritical care, having presented extensively on ischemic and hemorrhagic stroke. She has been a mentee for the Fellows of the American Association of Nurse Practitioner Mentorship Program and has won numerous research grants in neurocritical care and global health.

Adult-Gerontology Acute Care Practice Guidelines

Catherine Harris, PhD, MBA, AGACNP

Editor

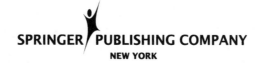

SPRINGER PUBLISHING COMPANY
NEW YORK

Springer Publishing Company, LLC
11 West 42nd Street
New York, NY 10036
www.springerpub.com

Acquisitions Editor: Suzanne Toppy
Compositor: diacriTech, Chennai

ISBN: 978-0-8261-7004-0
e-book ISBN: 978-0-8261-7005-7

19 20 21 22 / 5 4 3 2

The author and the publisher of this Work have made every effort to use sources believed to be reliable to provide information that is accurate and compatible with the standards generally accepted at the time of publication. Because medical science is continually advancing, our knowledge base continues to expand. Therefore, as new information becomes available, changes in procedures become necessary. We recommend that the reader always consult current research and specific institutional policies before performing any clinical procedure. The author and publisher shall not be liable for any special, consequential, or exemplary damages resulting, in whole or in part, from the readers' use of, or reliance on, the information contained in this book. The publisher has no responsibility for the persistence or accuracy of URLs for external or third-party Internet websites referred to in this publication and does not guarantee that any content on such websites is, or will remain, accurate or appropriate.

Library of Congress Cataloging-in-Publication Data

Names: Harris, Catherine AGACNP, editor.
Title: Adult-gerontology acute care practice guidelines / [edited by]
    Catherine Harris, PhD, MBA, AGACNP.
Description: New York, NY : Springer Publishing Company, LLC, [2019] |
    Includes bibliographical references and index.
Identifiers: LCCN 2019015624| ISBN 9780826170040 | ISBN 9780826170057 (ebook)
Subjects: LCSH: Geriatric nursing. | Intensive care nursing | Older
    people–Medical care. | Nurse practitioners.
Classification: LCC RC954 .A38 2019 | DDC 618.97/0231–dc23 LC record available at https://lccn.loc.gov/2019015624

Contact us to receive discount rates on bulk purchases.
We can also customize our books to meet your needs.
For more information please contact: sales@springerpub.com

Publisher's Note: New and used products purchased from third-party sellers are not guaranteed for quality, authenticity, or access to any included digital components.

Printed in the United States of America.

To Matthew,

My beautiful little boy, you are always in my heart, and I am so proud of you!

Mom and Dad,

Thank you for your encouragement and always being there for me.

Contents

I. ACUTE CARE GUIDELINES BY SYSTEM

1. ENT Guidelines

2. Pulmonary Guidelines

3. Cardiac Guidelines

4. Gastrointestinal Guidelines

5. Nephrology Guidelines

6. Neurology Guidelines

II. PERIOPERATIVE CONSIDERATIONS

III. PROCEDURES

IV. SPECIAL TOPICS

APPENDIX

Contributors

Dana A. Albinson, MSN, BSN, AGACNP
Adult-Gerontology Acute Care Nurse Practitioner
Thomas Jefferson University Hospital
Philadelphia, Pennsylvania

Frank O. Amanze, MSN, AGACNP-BC, CFRN, CCRN, PHRN, NRP
Nurse Practitioner
Thomas Jefferson University
Philadelphia, Pennsylvania

M. Kamran Athar, MD
Assistant Professor of Medicine and Neurological Surgery
Thomas Jefferson University Hospital
Philadelphia, Pennsylvania

Ponrathi Athilingam, PhD, RN, ACNP, FAANP, FHFSA
Associate Professor, College of Nursing
University of South Florida
Tampa, Florida

Asha Avirachen, MSN, BSN, AG, ACNP
Adult-Gerontology Acute Care Nurse Practitioner
Department of Neurosurgery, Hospital of University of Pennsylvania
Philadelphia, Pennsylvania

Suzanne Barron, MSN, RN, CRNP, FNP
Adult and Gerontology Acute Care Nurse Practitioner
Thomas Jefferson University
Philadelphia, Pennsylvania

Karen A. Beaty, MPAS, PA-C
Physician Assistant
MD Anderson Cancer Center
Houston, Texas

David Bergamo, MSPAS, PA-C, AAHIVS
Physician Assistant
Infectious Disease Associates and Christiana Care Health System
Christiana, Delaware

Amy Blake, MSN, FNP-BC
Family Nurse Practitioner
TeamHealth Hospitalist & Post Acute Care
Wilmington, Delaware

Ann E. Burke, MSN, CRNP, FNP-BC
Nurse Practitioner

Thomas Jefferson University Hospital
Philadelphia, Pennsylvania

Dana Cafaro, MS, PA-C
Associate Program Director & Assistant Professor
Thomas Jefferson University Physician Assistant Program
Atlantic City, New Jersey

E. Moneé Carter-Griffin, DNP, RN, ACNP-BC
Associate Chair for Advanced Practice Nursing
University of Texas at Arlington
Arlington, Texas

Alexis Chettiar, PhD, MSN, RN
Director of Quality Improvement
Center for Elders' Independence
Oakland, California

Christine M. Chmielewski, MS, CRNP, ANP-BC, CNN-NP
Nephrology Nurse Practitioner
Thomas Jefferson University Hospital
Philadelphia, Pennsylvania

Kelly Cimino, MSN, RN, CRNP, AG ACNP-BC
Nurse Practitioner
Thomas Jefferson University
Philadelphia, Pennsylvania

Jennifer Coates, DNP, MBA, ACNP-BC, ACNPC
Critical Care Nurse Practitioner
Drexel University
Philadelphia, Pennsylvania

Lisa Coco, MSN, CRNP, CDE
Nurse Practitioner
Thomas Jefferson University
Philadelphia, Pennsylvania

Courtney Connolley, MSN
Nurse Practitioner
Thomas Jefferson University
Philadelphia, Pennsylvania

Heather Warren Cook, MSN, RN, AGACNP-BC
Acute Care Nurse Practitioner
Hospital of the University of Pennsylvania
Philadelphia, Pennsylvania

Jane S. Davis, DNP, MSN, BSN, CRNP
University of Alabama at Birmingham
Birmingham, Alabama

Erin Michelle Dean, MS, PA-C, RD
Physician Assistant
Department of Surgical Oncology, MD Anderson Cancer Center
Houston, Texas

Michele DeCastro, MSN, CRNP
Nurse Practitioner
Division of Hospital Medicine, Thomas Jefferson University
Philadelphia, Pennsylvania

Jingyi Deng, MSN, RN-BC, AGACNP-BC
Cardiac Surgery Nurse Practitioner
Lankenau Medical Center
Philadelphia, Pennsylvania

Jessica S. Everitt, Pharm D
Assistant Professor
University of Mississippi Medical Center
Jackson, Mississippi

Susan F. Galiczynski, MSN, RN, CRNP, CEN
Nurse Practitioner
Crozer-Chester Medical Center
Philadelphia, Pennsylvania

Alexis C. Geppner, MLS (ASCP), PA-C
Physician Assistant
MD Anderson Cancer Center
Houston, Texas

Bridget Gibson, CRNP, Adult Acute Care, MSN, BSN
Neurocritical Care Nurse Practitioner
Thomas Jefferson University
Philadelphia, Pennsylvania

Debra Hain, PhD, APRN, AGPCNP-BC, FAANP, FNKF
Professor/Nurse Practitioner
Florida Atlantic University, Chrisitne E. Lynn College of Nursing and Cleveland Clinic Florida, Department of Nephrology
Boca Raton, Florida

Catherine Harris, PhD, MBA, AGACNP
Associate Professor
Thomas Jefferson University College of Nursing
Philadelphia, Pennsylvania

Carey Heck, PhD, CRNP, AGACNP-BC, CCRN, CNRN
Assistant Professor, Director, AGACNP Program
Thomas Jefferson University, College of Nursing
Philadelphia, Pennsylvania

Shannon B. Holloway, MHS, PA-C
Physician Assistant
MD Anderson Cancer Center
Houston, Texas

John Hurt, MPAS, PA-C
Director of Clinical Education
Samford University Physician Assistant Program
Birmingham, Alabama

Alicia John, MSN, RN, CNS
Advanced Practice Provider
Kingwood Medical Center
Houston, Texas

Cynae Johnson, DNP, MSN, WHNP-BC
Advanced Practice Provider
MD Anderson Cancer Center
Houston, Texas

Swetha Rani Kanduri, MD
Assistant Professor of Medicine
University of Mississippi Medical Center
Jackson, Mississippi

Kiffon M. Keigher, MSN, APN, ACNP-BC
Program Manager, Acute Care Nurse Practitioner
Advocate Aurora Health
Park Ridge, Illinois

Alison M. Kelley, MSN, AGACNP-BC
Critical Care Nurse Practitioner
Emory University Hospital
Atlanta, Georgia

Karthik Kovvuru, MD
Assistant Professor of Medicine
University of Mississippi Medical Center
Jackson, Mississippi

Kathryn Evans Kreider, DNP, APRN, FNP-BC, BC-ADM
Assistant Professor of Nursing
Duke University
Durham, North Carolina

Megan Krug, MHS, PA-C
Physician Assistant
Dana Farber Cancer Institute
Boston, Massachusetts

Monique Lambert, DNP, APN, ACNP-BC, FAANP
Anesthesia Critical Care
Northshoure University Health Care System
Skokie, Illinois

Sarah L. Livesay, DNP, RN, ACNP-BC, ACNS-BC, FNCS, FAHA
Associate Professor
Rush University, Department of Adult Health and Gerontological Nursing
Chicago, Illinois

Kristopher R. Maday, MS, PA-C
Program Director, Associate Professor
University of Tennessee Health Science Center Physician Assistant Program
Memphis, Tennessee

Shawn Mangan, MSN, RNFA, ANP-C, AGACNP-BC
Acute Care Surgery/Trauma Intensive Care Unit Nurse Practitioner
Thomas Jefferson University Hospital
Philadelphia, Pennsylvania

Amelita B. Marzan, MS, APRN, FNP-C, OCN
Advanced Practice Provider
MD Anderson Cancer Center
Houston, Texas

Sijimol Mathew, MSN, ACNP-BC
Advanced Practice Provider
MD Anderson Cancer Center
Houston, Texas

Juan A. Medaura, MD
Assistant Professor of Medicine
University of Maryland Medical Center
Baltimore, Maryland

Heather H. Meissen, MSN, ACNP, CCRN, FCCM, FAANP
Program Director NPPA Critical Care Residency
Emory Healthcare
Atlanta, Georgia

Rose Milano, DNP, MS, BSN, RN, ACNP-BC
Assistant Professor
Rush University College of Nursing
Chicago, Illinois

Robin Miller, DNP, MPH, ACNP-BC
Assistant Professor of Clinical Nursing
Oregon Health & Science University
Portland, Oregon

Robin Miller, MSN, FNP-BC, AGACNP-BC
Nurse Practitioner
Thomas Jefferson University Hospital
Philadelphia, Pennsylvania

Divya Monga, MD
Division of Nephrology
University of Mississippi Medical Center
Jackson, Mississippi

Madeleine Nguyen-Cao, PA-C
Physician Assistant
MD Anderson Cancer Center
Houston, Texas

Karen Sheffield O'Brien, PhD, RN, ACNP-BC
Assistant Professor
University of St. Thomas and Memorial Hermann Sugar
    Land Nurse Practitioner
Houston, Texas

Dominick Osipowicz, MSN, CRNP, AGACNP-BC
Nurse Practitioner
Christiana Care Health System
Newark, Delaware

Jennifer W. Parker, PhD, MSN, BSN
Acute Care Nurse Practitioner
University of Pennsylvania Health System
West Chester, Pennsylvania

Joanne Elaine Pechar, MSN, ANP-BC, AGACNP-BC
Acute Care Nurse Practitioner
Department of Penn Orthopedics, Pennsylvania Hospital
Philadelphia, Pennsylvania

Cheryl Pfennig, MSN, RN, NP-C, AOCNP
Advanced Practice Registered Nurse, Surgical Oncology
MD Anderson Cancer Center
Houston, Texas

Allyson Price, MPAS, PA-C
Physician Assistant
MD Anderson Cancer Center
Houston, Texas

Rae Brana Reynolds, PhD, RN, ACNP-BC
Manager, Advanced Practice Providers
MD Anderson Cancer Center
Houston, Texas

Monica Richey, MSN, ANP-BC
Nurse Practitioner
Northwell Health
New York, New York

Courtney Robb, MS, RN, CRNFA, FNP-C
Nurse Practitioner
MD Anderson Cancer Center
Houston, Texas

Allison Rusgo, MHS, MPH, PA-C
Assistant Clinical Professor
Drexel University
Philadelphia, Pennsylvania

Annamma Sam, PhD, WHNP-BC
Advanced Practice Provider
MD Anderson Cancer Center
Houston, Texas

Leigh A. Samp, MPAS, PA-C
Physician Assistant
MD Anderson Cancer Center
Houston, Texas

Laura A. Santanna Lonergan, MHS, PA-C
Physician Assistant
Pennsylvania Hospital
Philadelphia, Pennsylvania

Syed Omar Shah, MD, MBA
Assistant Professor of Neurology and Neurological Surgery
Thomas Jefferson University Hospital
Philadelphia, Pennsylvania

Christina Shin, PA-C
Physician Assistant
Rush University
Chicago, Illinois

RuthAnne Skinner, DNP, ACNP-BC, C-NP, CNRN
ACNP Lead Faculty
College of Nursing & Health Care Professions, Grand
Canyon University
Phoenix, Arizona

Mary Rogers Sorey, MSN, RN, ACNP
Assistant Professor
Division of Nephrology, Vanderbilt University Medical
    Center
Nashville, Tennessee

Cara M. Staley, MSN, RN-BC, AGACNP-BC
Vascular Surgery Nurse Practitioner
Thomas Jefferson University Hospital
Philadelphia, Pennsylvania

Jerrad M. Stoddard, MS, MA, PA-C
Physician Assistant
Texas Oncology
Round Rock, Texas

Frances M. Stokes, DNP, RN, ACNP-BC, CMNL
Nurse Practitioner
Intensivist
Austin, Texas

Julie Stone, MSN, RN, ACNP-BC, BC-ADM
Endocrinology Nurse Practitioner
Ascension St. Vincent Heart Center
Indianapolis, Indiana

Siji Thomas, ACNP, OCN
Acute Care Nurse Practitioner
MD Anderson Cancer Center
Houston, Texas

Nicole Thomer, MSN, AG-ACNP
Nurse Practitioner, Neuro Critcal Care
Thomas Jefferson University Hospital
Philadelphia, Pennsylvania

Melissa Timmons, PA-C
Physician Assistant
MD Anderson Cancer Center
Houston, Texas

Amber Tran, MSN, CRNP, FNP-BC
Family Nurse Practitioner
Department of Dermatology and Cutaneous Biology, TJU
Philadelphia, Pennsylvania

Fiona Unac, MN, NP, GDipAL&T
Nurse Practitioner
Radiology Department, Soldiers' Memorial Hospital
Hastings, New Zealand

Dawn Vanderhoef, PhD, DNP, PMHNP, FAANP
Assistant Professor and Academic Director
Vanderbilt University School of Nursing
Nashville, Tennessee

Susan Varghese, MSN, RN, ANP-C
Adult Nurse Practitioner
MD Anderson Cancer Center
Houston, Texas

Valerie F. Villanueva, MSN, RN, FNP-BC
Supervisor, Advanced Practice Providers
MD Anderson Cancer Center GYNONC and Reproductive
    Medicine
Houston, Texas

Catherine Wells, DNP, ACNP, CNN-NP, FNKF
Assistant Professor
Division of Nephrology, University of Mississippi Medical
    Center
Jackson, Mississippi

Mary L. Wilby, PhD, MSN, MPH, RN, CRNP, ANP-BC
Assistant Professor, Nurse Practitioner Track Coordinator
La Salle University
Philadelphia, Pennsylvania

Joseph Willmitch, MSPAS, PA-C, DFAAPA
Director of Clinical Education
University of Tennessee Health Science Center Physician
    Assistant Program
Memphis, Tennessee

Danielle Zielinski, MSN, BSN, RN, ACNP-BC
Acute Care Nurse Practitioner
Northwestern Medicine, Neurosurgery
Chicago, Illinois

Kim Zuber, MS, PAC
Executive Director
American Academy of Nephrology Pas
Oceanside, California

Reviewers

M. Kamran Athar, MD
Assistant Professor of Medicine and Neurological Surgery
Thomas Jefferson University
Philadelphia, Pennsylvania

Ashley L. Barba, DNP, ANP
Acute Care Nurse Practitioner
Duke University Medical Center
Durham, North Carolina

Mark E. Baus, MSN, CRNP, RNFA
Lead Orthopaedic Nurse Practitioner
Thomas Jefferson University Hospital
Philadelphia, Pennsylvania

Brennan Bowker, MHS, PA-C, CPAAPA
Physician Assistant; Part-Time Clinical Assistant Professor of
    Physician Assistant Studies
Yale New Haven Hospital Department of Surgery;
    Quinnipiac University Department of Physician
    Assistant Studies
New Haven, Connecticut

Theresa M. Campo, DNP, FNP-C, ENP-C, FAANP, FAAN
Director of the Emergency Nurse Practitioner and Co-
    Director of the Family Nurse Practitioner Tracks,
    Associate Clinical Professor for the College of Nursing
    and Health Professions
Drexel University College of Nursing and Health Professions
Philadelphia, Pennsylvania

Shawnna Cannaday, MSN, AGACNP, FNP-BC
Acute Care Nurse Practitioner Department of Surgery,
    Surgical Oncology
Jefferson University Physicians Department of Surgery,
    Hepato-Biliary-Pancreatic Surgery
Philadelphia, Pennsylvania

Dawn Carpenter, DNP, ACNP-BC, CCRN
Coordinator, Adult-Gerontology Acute Care Nurse
    Practitioner Program
University of Massachusetts Medical School
Worcester, Massachusetts

Nicole Cavaliere, MSN, AGACNP-BC
Acute Care Nurse Practitioner Department of Surgery,
    Cardiothoracic Surgery
Thomas Jefferson University Hospital
Philadelphia, Pennsylvania

Kathleen O. Chennell, MS, CNS, ACNP-BC, CCRN
Adult-Gerontology Acute Care Nurse Practitioner
Division of Nephrology, University of Cincinnati
Cincinnati, Ohio

Carolina Dimsdale Tennyson, DNP, ACNP-BC, AACC
Nurse Practitioner, Clinical Associate Faculty
Duke University School of Nursing
Durham, North Carolina

Patricia Galanis, MSN, CRNP
Oncology Nurse Practitioner
Thomas Jefferson University
Philadelphia, Pennsylvania

Carey Heck, PhD, CRNP, AGACNP-BC, CCRN, CNRN
Assistant Professor, Director, AGACNP Program
Thomas Jefferson University, College of Nursing
Philadelphia, Pennsylvania

Heather Hobbs, MSN, CRNP, AGACNP-BC
Adult-Gerontology Acute Care Nurse Practitoner
Department of Otolaryngology/Head & Neck Surgery,
    Thomas Jefferson University Hospital
Philadelphia, Pennsylvania

Robert Kirk, MSN, PMHNP-BC
Psychiatric Nurse Practitioner
University of Pennsylvania School of Nursing
Philadelphia, Pennsylvania

Stefanie La Manna, PhD, MPH, APRN, FNP-C, AGACNP-BC
Program Director for the PhD/DNP/AGACNP Programs
Nova Southeastern University
Palm Beach Gardens, Florida

Johannah Lebow, MSN, CRNP
Oncology Nurse Practitioner
University of Pennsylvania Health System
Philadelphia, Pennsylvania

Gail Ann Lis, DNP, ACNP-BC
Professor, Graduate Chair
Madonna University
Livonia, Michigan

Karen Bradley Lodge, MSN, CRNP
Nurse Practitioner

Northwest Internal Medicine
Wydnmoor, Pennsylvania

Mary Anne McCoy, PhD, RN, ACNS, ACNP-BC
Assistant Professor; Graduate Coordinator, AGACNP
    Specialty
Wayne State University College of Nursing
Detroit, Michigan

Anne Bradley Mitchell, PhD, MN, ANP-BC
Assistant Professor of Nursing
Jefferson University College of Nursing
Philadelphia, Pennsylvania

Dominick Osipowicz, MSN, CRNP, AGACNP-BC
Nurse Practitioner
Christiana Care Health System
Newark, Delaware

Jennifer W. Parker, PhD, MSN, BSN
Acute Care Nurse Practitioner
University of Pennsylvania Health System
West Chester, Pennsylvania

Belbina Pereira, MSN
Nephrology Nurse Practitioner
Brooklyn Hospital
Brooklyn, New York

Marilyn Riley, PhD, MSN, RN, APRN-BC, FNP
NP Intensivist, Chief Nursing Officer
Indiana University Health
Indianapolis, Indiana

Fred Rincon, MD, FACP
Associate Professor of Medicine
Thomas Jefferson University
Philadelphia, Pennsylvania

Tracy Setji, MD
Associate Professor of Medicine
Duke University
Durham, North Carolina

Jennifer Sheehan, MSN, CRNP, RNFA
Nurse Practitioner

Philadelphia VA Medical Center
Philadelphia, Pennsylvania

Benjamin Smallheer, PhD, RN, ACNP-BC, FNP-BC, CCRN, CNE
Assistant Professor of Nursing; Lead Faculty, Adult-
    Gerontology Acute Care NP Program
Duke University School of Nursing
Durham, North Carolina

R. Shane Smith, MS, PA-C, EMT-P(NREMT), SFC (RET), US Army
Trauma Surgery, Critical Care
Ballad Health Systems, Milligan College Adjunct Faculty
Johnson City, Tennessee

Frances Stokes, DNP, RN, ACNP-BC, CMNL
NP Intensivist
St. Davids Medical Center
Austin, Texas

Kevin Tipton, MSN, CRNP
Nurse Practitioner
Lehigh Valley Hospital
East Stroudsburg, Pennsylvania

Mark Ubbens, MSN, CRNP, AG-ACNP-BC, PHRN
Advanced Practice Chief, Trauma Surgery; Aquarium
    Medical Advisor, Ski Patroller
Geisinger Medical Center, National Aquarium, Big Boulder
    Ski Patrol
Danville, Pennsylvania; Baltimore, Maryland; Lake
    Harmony, Pennsylvania

Karen L. Visich, MSN, RN, ANP-BC, AOCNP
Nurse Practitioner, Genitourinary Oncology; Acting
    Associate Director of Nursing and Patient Education
Rutgers Cancer Institute of New Jersey
New Brunswick, New Jersey

Michael Zychowicz, DNP, ANP, ONP, FAAN, FAANP
MSN Program Director
Duke University School of Nursing
Durham, North Carolina

Foreword

There is no blueprint for acute care.

The term itself is as broad and nebulous as the field it describes. Our patients reserve the right to present with any configuration of symptoms, to respond to our treatments when—and if—their bodies deem appropriate, and to decompensate without warning. Unlike the neat black and white lines of our textbooks, the reality of acute medicine is a messy gray.

Of course, the geriatric population adds yet another wrinkle to that hazy clinical landscape. The aging body owes no guarantees. Every tent pole of our didactic education—the classic triads and notorious eponyms—fades with the march of time.

As a young clinician thrust into the halls of famous hospitals, surrounded by brilliant clinicians and the sickest patients, these lessons often landed with a painful thud. But over time I began to appreciate the subconscious calculations that registered as subtle sensations. The flutter in my chest that told me to double-check a detail, the tickle deep in my skull that said to investigate further, the lead weight in my gut that meant something was wrong.

Of course, you cannot buy those instincts in any store. They are earned over the course of a career. In the meantime, you can insulate yourself with as much raw knowledge as possible. And the book you are holding is a great start.

The following pages provide a skeleton on which to build that knowledge. They are not a replacement for clinical acumen but a guide to help you find a deeper understanding of acute care. They are the concepts that should flash through your mind when your patients are at their most vulnerable, when time is precious, and when mistakes are costly.

This book is authored by a coalition of talented physician assistants and nurse practitioners who have collaborated as we so often do in the clinical setting. They bring decades of collective experience and use it to distill the cloudy concoction of acute care into clear, manageable parts. They have fortified the material with threads of relevant wisdom for the geriatric patient. This is not the dense tome that will collect dust on your bookshelf. It is designed for utility, sleek and practical. It is the book I wish I would have had as a new clinician.

So, while there is no blueprint for acute care, do not worry. You may have found the next best thing.

Harrison Reed, MMS, PA-C

Assistant Professor
School of Medicine and Health Sciences
George Washington University
Washington, DC

Preface

The need for an acute care textbook has been growing. Although outpatient practices have long seen the value of utilizing advanced practice providers (APPs), the surge in acute care providers has been relatively recent. I remember when I was a registered nurse back in the 1990s, I had no idea there was such a role as a nurse practitioner or a physician assistant in the hospital, despite the fact they have been around since the 1960s!

I was immediately fascinated and intrigued by the role of APPs. It was not long before I found myself enrolled in a nurse practitioner program. When I graduated, I was one of the first nurse practitioners on the neurosurgery service in the facility where I practiced. The service appreciated the help, but they did not really know what to do with me. It took many months for me to garner the trust of the surgeons, and to show them the true capacity of what APPs could do and how we could really become essential parts of the team.

APPs have come a long way over the years. I have seen the role of nurse practitioners and physician assistants expand tremendously since I first began practicing in this role. I have seen the negative terms to describe us, such as midlevels, physician extenders, and helpers, evolve into advance practice providers.

I have also seen collaborative growth and mutual respect grow between nurse practitioners and physician assistants, a relationship that was previously more isolated. I respect my physician assistant colleagues, and, as a nurse practitioner, I have learned quite a bit from their struggles with role and identity. I find that I personally relate to these struggles in how I practice and how I see my own role on the healthcare team. I have also learned the value of combining resources and focusing on how we are similar, rather than different.

It was important to write this textbook with physician assistants and nurse practitioners together. Both groups have immense value to provide each other in terms of knowledge, resources, and experience.

Finally, it was essential to write this textbook because it fills a void in the marketplace. Countless times my students have asked if there were an acute care textbook that they could use. I have tried many different textbooks, but either I found them to be too cumbersome or the information provided was just too scant.

This final iteration of the textbook came about as a result of those experiences and discussions with students about what they needed and they wanted. We all suffer from information overload and overwhelm, so the focus of this textbook was to provide the minimum of what new graduate students need to know in order to be competent when they start practice.

Catherine Harris

Organization

This book is organized into four major sections.

Part I: Acute Care Guidelines by System—In Part I, the advanced practice provider (APP) is exposed to the most common medical conditions organized by system. Although it is by no means comprehensive or inclusive of every medical condition, the section is meant to provide APP students with an overview of very common medical conditions that they should focus on during their studies. In my teachings, I have found students tend to gravitate toward understanding the "zebras" in medicine, or those conditions that are unusual, instead of diagnosing common problems or unusual variants of common problems. This phenomenon might have to do with the common practice of testing on zebras or the student perception that we (as academic institutions) are out to trick them on a test. By not introducing zebras into the context of this book, the students can maintain focus on the most common disease states.

Part II: Perioperative Considerations—Part II contains an operative overview. Again, this section is not a comprehensive review of the operating room, but it does provide APP students an overview of what they should know regardless of where they work. In the acute care setting, operative procedures are very common. It does not matter if acute care practitioners work directly or indirectly with patients in the perioperative period. A review of the common issues is mandatory.

Part III: Procedures—Not all APPs will perform procedures, but students frequently feel a sense of accomplishment in being able to do something tangible. It is difficult to measure the progress of one's own critical thinking, but if a student can perform a procedure, his or her confidence level goes up quickly. In this section, some of the more common procedures are listed.

Part IV: Special Topics—There are many issues that we will deal with as APPs; however, these issues do not all fall neatly into predefined categories. This section was created for select topics that could not be defined by systems but were equally important to address. These topics include end-of-life issues, health promotion, hemodynamic monitoring devices, telemedicine, and transitions of care. All APPs will deal with these issues during the course of their careers. These topics will also continue to evolve as we conduct more research and clinical studies and as technology improves.

What Is Different About This Book

This book was created for advanced practice provider (APP) students in the acute care setting. In talking to students about their wants and needs in a textbook, I found students were not able to absorb and assimilate information in heavy, dense textbooks that we had been using. I also found myself telling my students not to bother with a large portion of the textbook because it was not immediately relevant to their basic knowledge. Students struggled to understand what to focus on and what they needed to know versus what was nice to know.

No one can memorize everything they need to know about medicine. As students specialize in various fields, they will learn in-depth information about their specialties that is beyond the scope of this book. However, there is a body of knowledge that every APP should know, and I have done my best to include those topics in this book.

Acknowledgments

I have so many people to acknowledge in the creation of this textbook, particularly Dr. Ksenia Zukowsky, Dr. Carey Heck, and Dr. Jack Jallo. Dr. Zukowsky saw so much potential in my plans. She pushed me to do things I was scared to do, and she made them seem possible. Her incredible stories have inspired me over the years, and she remains a powerful influence in my life.

Dr. Heck has been an incredible colleague. As the director of the Acute Care Nurse Practitioner Program at Thomas Jefferson University, she has entertained my "big" ideas and helped me implement them. She has been a rock of support and has contributed massively to the publication of this book as well as the profession.

Dr. Jallo has been my main physician support over the years in neurocritical care and neurosurgery. He never told me something could not be done, and he has made me believe that more was always possible.

I want to acknowledge all the people who contributed to my growth as a nurse and an academic, especially Dr. Bob Hess. Dr. Hess knew me as a little girl. He was my neighbor across the street. Then, he was my teacher when I went to undergraduate nursing school at the University of Pennsylvania. Then he became my employer when I picked up extra time doing some editing work at the nursing magazine that he edited. Finally, he became my colleague and friend who encouraged me to keep rising through the ranks.

Of course, I would not be the clinician, academic, and nurse I am today without my students, fellow faculty, friends, and family. I want to express my gratitude to so many people, but it is not possible to list them all here. From my first nursing job to where I am today, I am thankful for everyone in my life who has taught me so much.

It has been an absolute pleasure to work with Springer Publishing Company. I worked most closely with Suzanne Toppy. Her talent, expertise, and encouragement were the guiding light for me through this entire process.

I need to acknowledge all the work done by the editing team. What you produced is absolutely amazing. I really appreciate everything you have done in the editorial process.

Introduction

Information Overload

No book can serve all the needs of students, nor should that be the goal. This book was specifically designed to provide a foundation of basic information about acute care that students or any advanced practice provider (APP) should know about a body system. Acute care is defined as treatment that is received in the short term for an injury, emergency, or episode of illness. Acute care can be delivered in the hospital setting, EDs, or even outpatient clinics and includes a vast array of conditions and issues. However, patients come to the acute care setting with chronic problems as well that APPs need to address, and the table of contents was developed with this in mind. The table of contents is divided into four parts to accommodate the large scope of acute care. In Part I, the contents are arranged by body system and include the most commonly encountered diseases and conditions that are seen in acute care. In Part II, perioperative considerations are included because surgery is often the main reason for hospitalization in the acute care setting. In Part III, procedures that are commonly performed by APPs are included, as well as videos for certain procedures when a visual demonstration can be particularly helpful.

Part IV is designed to address special issues that are unique to the acute care setting. The topics addressed are transitional care, end-of-life issues, health promotion, hemodynamic monitoring devices, and telemedicine. When a patient comes into the acute care setting, it is an opportunity for all healthcare providers to address health promotion. Not everyone sees healthcare providers on a regular basis or gets evaluated for routine screening. Therefore, it is essential for all acute care providers to be well versed on the types of health promotion that are necessary based on a patient's age and other demographic factors.

Telemedicine is also addressed because it is becoming increasingly prevalent. The ICUs in rural areas can now be monitored by intensivists and APPs in central regions. There is a burgeoning role for APPs in this area. Transitional care is the point where a patient either comes into the acute care setting or returns to the outpatient community. This period of transition is the most vulnerable time for patients. Careful attention must be devoted to updating and informing the accepting provider on patient status and the management plan. Finally, end-of-life issues often are addressed in the hospital system after an acute episode. Knowledge of these issues is essential to practice.

The appendix provides normal lab values as a reference tool for APPs. There may be slight variations from institution to institution that may be attributed to different vendors. Please use these values as guides for quick reference, but defer to your institutional normal reference range.

Medicine is clearly and overwhelmingly a vast body of knowledge. Students who try to take it all on at once make learning seem like an unsurmountable task. The brain can only absorb so much information at once. When students pick up a dense textbook and see there are hundreds of conditions that could exist with just one body system, it makes it difficult for them to focus on the relatively few conditions that we treat commonly. The goal of this book is to deconstruct large topics into focused, core conditions. Students will not learn everything they need to know about a topic by using this book, but they will get what they need to know as a new graduate. Practicing APPs can refer to this resource as a quick review of what they need to know. Continuing to strive for more learning is a lifelong duty as an APP. Furthering the learning process far beyond graduate school and continuing to search out information that is unfamiliar is essential.

In this day and age, the Internet is a quick and easy resource to utilize. Patients will be using it as well. While no one expects any one person to know everything at all times, there is an expectation that the providers are resourceful and will know how to find the information.

Imposter Syndrome

At the end of the day, students will never feel like they know enough to get started, and much of this anxiety can be attributed to what we know about *imposter syndrome*. Going from the role of an expert in one area to a novice is extremely challenging and creates feelings of uneasiness. This is a completely natural transition mode. In fact, I would be more concerned about a student who thinks he or she knows everything than a student who feels like his or her peers just have not "figured out" that they do not belong.

This unease and uncertainty of feeling like an imposter will help students be cautious and humble when they enter the healthcare system as an acute care provider. Developing clinical judgment is an art that is guided by science and occurs over time and through experiential learning. Being unsure will motivate new graduates to consult evidence-based materials to search for answers.

Frequently textbooks, articles, and case studies provide classic presentations that are useful for learning a concept. However, in practice, the APP quickly discovers that didactic content in a lecture or a book does not account for the number of variables that are present in real clinical situations.

Hence, textbook learning has limitations that can only be remedied with practice. A student in the novice stage of a new role would be best advised to spend as much time as possible with patients, practicing active, focused listening and asking questions. This practice will help the new graduate APP gain confidence quickly.

Role of APPs

The role of APPs continues to evolve and expand in the healthcare system. New opportunities open up as the healthcare system begins to depend heavily on the utilization of APPs, particularly in the acute care system. It was not too long ago that most nurse practitioners (NPs) and physician assistants (PAs) worked primarily in primary care settings. Now, NPs and PAs work in primary care, all aspects of the acute care system, and beyond.

More and more collaborative efforts are being established between NPs and PAs as we move away from contrasting how we are different and focus on achieving the same goals.

Both NPs and PAs struggle with practice issues, prescribing issues, and levels of autonomy. However, many legislative advancements have been achieved over the past 10 years that have created a growing demand for APPs. As the roles and responsibilities of APPs continue to expand, the stronger the collaboration between them needs to be. This book is one step forward in developing and creating these collaborative efforts for NPs and PAs.

Future Opportunities

There are many opportunities for APPs. One of the major next steps I see for APPs is acute care billing. Billing provides visibility of the extent of work that is truly being done by APPs. Billing can also be leveraged for improved working conditions and better pay. In the current system where APP billing is absorbed by physician groups, APPs are left with basically nothing to show for their efforts. How can a hospital administration effectively determine if more or fewer APPs are needed in a particular department? How can a practice group determine if an APP is exceeding expectations in his or her work or even underperforming? How can an APP justify a raise for himself or herself when there is nothing quantifiable to show the value of what has been done?

Billing is more than just sending off charges to insurance companies to get paid. Billing provides visibility, which in turn comes with responsibilities and challenges. At the time of the writing of this book, there were no models (or too few to use) of acute care billing for APPs to devote an entire section to the issue; however, it is definitely coming. Insurance companies and compliance programs are taking steps to implement a structure that recognizes the contribution of the APP to the patient's care.

Acute care billing is going to be a controversial issue in the years to come, and APPs would be well advised to keep on top of how it is implemented and to participate in any committees that are designated to discuss such planning.

Final Note

Being an APP is an exciting and excellent career choice that has countless opportunities. Learning about disease states and management of patients is one aspect of the role of the APP. There is so much to learn, and it can be incredibly overwhelming. My advice to students, new graduates, and even seasoned APPs would be this: Acknowledge that there is a massive amount of information to be learned . . . *over time.* Accept that you have roles and responsibilities to the healthcare system and your community that extend beyond treating disease states. And accelerate your learning curve by being present with your patients, collaborating with your team, and staying involved in your profession.

Best of luck in this amazing profession as an APP.

I

Acute Care Guidelines by System

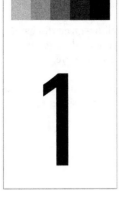

1 ENT Guidelines

Carey Heck

Conjunctivitis

Carey Heck

Definition
A. Inflammation of the conjunctiva, a thin transparent membrane that lines the inside of the eyelids and covers the sclera.
B. Commonly called "pink eye."

Incidence
A. Allergic conjunctivitis.
  1. Most common cause of conjunctivitis (15%–40% of population).
  2. Most frequently occurs in spring and summer.
B. Viral conjunctivitis.
  1. Most common cause of infectious conjunctivitis.
  2. Most common type in adults.
  3. More frequently occurs in the summer months.
C. Bacterial conjunctivitis.
  1. Most common cause of infectious conjunctivitis in children.
  2. Most frequently occurs in the winter and early spring months.

Pathogenesis
A. Allergic.
  1. Not contagious.
  2. Common in individuals with other signs of allergic disease.
  3. Reaction to allergic triggers.
B. Infectious.
  1. Bacterial.
    a. Highly contagious.
    b. Most common causative agents.
      i. *Staphylococcus aureus.*
      ii. *Haemophilus influenzae.*
      iii. *Streptococcus pneumoniae.*
      iv. *Moraxella catarrhalis.*
  2. Viral.
    a. Highly contagious.
    b. Most common causative agent.
      i. Adenoviruses.
      ii. Rubella virus.
      iii. Rubeola virus.
      iv. Herpes viruses.
C. Noninfectious.
D. Other causes.
  1. Environmental irritants.
  2. Medications.
  3. Toxins.
  4. Chemicals.

Predisposing Factors
A. Exposure to allergens.
B. Exposure to environmental irritants.
C. Contact lens wearers.
D. Use of ophthalmic drops.
E. Old makeup products.
F. Occupational exposure to chemicals.

Subjective Data
A. Common complaints/symptoms.
  1. Redness.
  2. Discharge.
    a. From the eye.
    b. Crusts over the eyelid, especially after sleep.
  3. Itching, burning.
  4. Increased tearing.
  5. Blurred vision.
  6. Painless.
  7. Feeling of foreign body in the eye.
B. Common/typical scenario.
  1. Specific presentation varies dependent on type of conjunctivitis.
  2. Symptoms of eye redness and discharge are common regardless of specific cause.
  3. Contributing history and appearance of discharge often determines diagnosis.
C. Family and social history.
  1. Review of symptoms.
    a. Elicit the onset and duration of symptoms.
    b. Determine if the patient or close contacts have any systemic illnesses.
    c. Assess the patient for any risk factors.
    d. Associated symptoms.
      i. Rhinorrhea.
      ii. Earache.
      iii. Sore throat.
      iv. Rash.
    e. Single or both eyes.
  2. Past medical history.
    a. Recent illnesses.
    b. Sick contacts.
    c. Allergies.
    d. Possible occupational exposure history.
    e. Sexual history.
    f. Contact lens use.

D. Review of systems.

1. Recent illnesses. Determine the onset and duration of symptoms.
   a. Abrupt or gradual onset.
   b. Determine if the patient or close contacts have any systemic illnesses.
2. Allergies.
3. Possible occupational exposure history.
4. Sexual history.
5. Pertinent systems review.
   a. Head, ear, eyes, nose, and throat (HEENT).
      i. Headache.
      ii. Vision loss.
      iii. Eye pain.
      iv. Eye discharge.
      v. Ear pain.
      vi. Rhinorrhea.
      vii. Nasal congestion.
      viii. Cough.
   b. Integumentary.
      i. Rash.
      ii. Lesions.

Physical Examination

A. Perform an eye examination, assessing for vision loss and eye discharge.

1. Appearance of eyes.
   a. Allergic: Typically both eyes are infected.
   b. Bacterial: Typically one eye is infected but may spread to other eye.
   c. Viral: Typically both eyes are infected.
2. Discharge.
   a. Allergic: Stringy.
   b. Bacterial: Mucopurulent.
      i. Copious yellow–green discharge is consistent with gonorrheal infection.
   c. Viral: Watery.
3. Visual acuity.
4. Corneal opacity.
5. Pupil size and shape.
6. Eyelid swelling.
7. Presence of proptosis.

B. Red flags.

1. Reduction of visual acuity.
2. Ciliary flush.
3. Photophobia.
4. Severe foreign body sensation.
5. Corneal opacity.
6. Fixed pupil.
7. Severe headache with nausea.
8. Dendriform lesion indicative of herpes simplex virus (HSV).

Diagnostic Tests

A. Diagnosis is made with history and physical examination.
B. Imaging studies are not indicated unless underlying condition is suspected.
C. Culture should be considered.

1. In severe cases.
2. In patients who wear contact lenses.
3. In patient unresponsive to initial treatment.
4. If sexually transmitted disease (STD) is suspected.

Differential Diagnosis

A. Conjunctivitis.

1. Allergic: Likely with accompanying allergic symptoms and contributing history.
2. Bacterial: Likely with thick, yellow–green discharge.
3. Viral: Likely with accompanying cold or respiratory symptoms and watery discharge from the eye.

B. Corneal abrasion.

1. Different from conjunctivitis in that there is a subjective complaint of severe pain that worsens over time.

C. Foreign body in the eye.
D. Keratitis.
E. Varicella zoster ophthalmicus.
F. Glaucoma.

Evaluation and Management Plan

A. General plan.

1. Symptomatic relief is adequate for all forms of conjunctivitis.
   a. Most symptoms: Resolve without treatment.
   b. Supportive care.
      i. Over-the-counter (OTC) products.
         1) Topical OTC medications are of limited efficacy for allergic conjunctivitis.
         2) Systemic antihistamines may be useful for allergic conjunctivitis.
      ii. Moist cold compresses to eyes.
      iii. Avoidance of allergic triggers.
2. Antibiotics are not indicated in most cases of bacterial conjunctivitis.
   a. Return to work or school requirements. These may necessitate initiation of antibiotic for confirmed cases of bacterial conjunctivitis.
      i. Antibiotics initiated within the first 2 to 5 days can hasten the resolution of symptoms.
      ii. Initiation of antibiotics after 5 days of the start of symptoms has a minimal effect, and use is not recommended.
   b. Indications for antibiotic therapy.
      i. Cases caused by gonorrhea infection.
      ii. Cases caused by chlamydia infection.
      iii. Contact lens wearers.
         1) Consider pseudomonas infection.

B. Patient/family teaching points.

1. Use handwashing to prevent spread.
2. Avoid touching eyes.
3. Instruct patients to dispose of current contact lenses and to avoid wearing contact lenses until irritation/infection is cleared.
4. Instruct patients to dispose of all eye makeup.

C. Pharmacotherapy.

1. Allergic.
   a. Artificial tears.
   b. Antihistamine/decongestant drops (OTC).
   c. Mast cell stabilizer/antihistamine drops (OTC).
2. Viral.
   a. Antibiotics not indicated.
   b. Antihistamine/decongestant drops (OTC).
   c. Artificial tears (OTC).
   d. Viral therapy for HSV infection.
3. Bacterial conjunctivitis.
   a. Topical (eye drops or ointment) antibiotic therapy.
      i. Erythromycin 5 mg/g ophthalmic ointment: One-half inch (1.25 cm) four times daily for 5 to 7 days.
      ii. Ciprofloxacin 0.3% ophthalmic drops (preferred agent in contact lens wearer): 1 to 2 drops four times daily for 5 to 7 days.
   b. Systemic antibiotics indicated for gonorrhea and chlamydia infections.
      i. 1 gm ceftriaxone IM plus azithromycin 1 gm PO for one dose.

D. Discharge instructions.
 1. Symptoms should resolve in 5 to 7 days.
 2. If symptoms continue or different symptoms appear, then follow-up is recommended.

Follow-Up

A. Instruct patients with acute bacterial conjunctivitis to follow-up in 1 to 2 days if symptoms worsen or do not improve.
B. Instruct patients with other forms of conjunctivitis to follow-up within 2 weeks if symptoms worsen or do not improve.

Consultation/Referral

A. Consider referral to allergy specialist for allergen testing in severe cases of allergic conjunctivitis.
B. Referral to ophthalmologist for cases that are resistant to initial treatment.
C. Urgent referral to ophthalmologist due to increased risk of vision loss.
 1. Hyperacute bacterial conjunctivitis.
 2. Keratitis.
 3. Varicella zoster ophthalmicus.

Special/Geriatric Considerations

A. Infants (highly susceptible to conjunctivitis).
 1. At risk for more serious complications.
 2. Prophylactically treated with optic antibiotics at birth.
B. Contact lens wearers.
 1. Higher risk for keratitis: Careful evaluation to rule out keratitis is essential before diagnosis of conjunctivitis is made.
 2. Discontinue use until eye has healed. Use can begin again when eye is white and patient has no discharge for 24 hours after completion of antibiotics.
C. Returning to school or work. This is appropriate 24 hours after antibiotics have been initiated or there is no discharge.
D. Awareness of local board of health reporting laws for STDs. This is essential when the diagnosis of conjunctivitis is made in the setting of gonorrhea and chlamydia.

Bibliography

Alfonso, S. A., Fawley, J. D., & Lu, X. A. (2015). Conjunctivitis. *Primary Care: Clinics in Office Practice, 42*(3), 325–345. doi:10.1016/j.pop.2015.05.001
Azari, A., & Barney, N. (2013). Conjunctivitis: A systematic review of diagnosis and treatment. *Journal of the American Medical Association, 310*(16), 1721–1729. doi:10.1001/jama.2013.280318
Bielory, B. P., O'Brien, T. P., & Bielory, L. (2012). Management of seasonal allergic conjunctivitis: Guide to therapy. *Acta Ophthalmologica, 90*(5), 399–407. doi:10.1111/j.1755-3768.2011.02272.x
Gore, J. (2013). Conjunctivitis. *Journal of the American Academy of Physician Assistants, 26*(3), 60.
McAnena, L., Knowles, S. J., Curry, A. S., & Cassidy, L. (2015). Prevalence of gonococcal conjunctivitis in adults and neonates. *Eye, 29*(7), 875–880. doi:10.1038/eye.2015.57
Segal, K., Lai, L., & Starr, E. (2014). Management of acute conjunctivitis. *Current Ophthalmology Reports, 2*(3), 116–123. doi:10.1007/s40135-014-0046-4

Pharyngitis

Carey Heck

Definition

A. Inflammation of the pharynx.
B. Commonly referred to as a "sore throat."

Incidence

A. Acute pharyngitis accounts for more than 12 million office and emergency/urgent care visits in the United States annually.
B. Viral pharyngitis occurs most frequently; increased incidence in adult population.
C. Bacterial pharyngitis occurs more frequently in children and adolescents.
 1. Particularly the Group A beta-hemolytic *streptococci* (GAS).
  a. Peak incidence occurs in 5 to 15 year age group.
  b. Only 5% to 15% of adults present with GAS.
 2. Bacterial pharyngitis occurs most frequently in winter and early spring months.

Pathogenesis

A. Infectious.
 1. Viral.
  a. Adenoviruses and rhinoviruses responsible for most cases of viral pharyngitis.
  b. Other causes include.
   i. Herpes simplex virus (HSV) 1 and 2.
   ii. Coxsackievirus.
   iii. Human herpes virus 4 (Epstein–Barr virus [EBV]).
   iv. Human herpes virus 5 (cytomegalovirus).
   v. HIV.
 2. Bacterial.
  a. The most important causative agent is the GAS.
   i. Severe complications of GAS warrant prompt identification and treatment.
  b. Other causes include.
   i. Group C streptococci.
   ii. *Neisseria gonorrhoeae*.
   iii. *Corynebacterium diphtheriae*.
   iv. *Treponema pallidum*.
   v. Mixed anaerobes.
B. Noninfectious.
 1. Allergy.
 2. Irritants.
 3. Gastrointestinal reflux.

Predisposing Factors

A. Exposure to infectious agents.
 1. Bacteria.
 2. Viruses.
B. Exposure to allergens.
C. Exposure to environmental irritants.
D. History of gastrointestinal reflux.
E. History of immunosuppression.

Subjective Data

A. Common complaints/symptoms.
 1. "Sore throat."
 2. Difficulty swallowing.
 3. Nasal congestion.
 4. Sinus tenderness.
 5. Cough.
 6. Malaise.
 7. Headache.
 8. Distinguishing features of pharyngitis associated with GAS.
  a. Absent cough.
  b. Fever.

c. Tonsillar exudates.
d. Anterior cervical lymphadenopathy.
B. Common/typical scenario.
   1. Patients typically complain of sore or scratchy throat, fever, and general malaise.
C. Review of systems.
   1. Past medical history.
      a. Recent illnesses. Determine the onset and duration of symptoms.
         i. Abrupt or gradual onset.
         ii. Duration longer than 3 weeks unlikely to be pharyngitis.
      b. Sick contacts. Determine if the patient or close contacts have any systemic illnesses.
      c. Assess the patient for any risk factors.
   2. Allergies.
   3. Possible occupational exposure history.
   4. Travel history.
   5. Sexual history.
   6. Pertinent systems review.
      a. Constitutional.
         i. Fever.
         ii. Malaise.
      b. Head, ear, eyes, nose, and throat (HEENT).
         i. Sore throat.
         ii. Cough.
         iii. Rhinorrhea.
         iv. Nasal congestion.
         v. Headache.
         vi. Sinus tenderness/pain.
      c. Integumentary.
         i. Rash.
         ii. Lesions.

Physical Examination

A. Appearance of pharynx.
   1. Pale to red.
   2. Mild erythema to profound edema.
   3. Vesicular lesions.
      a. HSV.
      b. Coxsackievirus.
B. Appearance of tonsils.
   1. Redness.
   2. Edema.
   3. Exudates.
      a. White (oropharyngeal candidiasis, GAS).
      b. Grayish membrane (diphtheria).
C. Lymph nodes.
   1. Cervical lymphadenopathy.
   2. Tonsillar lymphadenopathy.
D. Integumentary.
   1. Scarlatiniform rash may be present in GAS infections.
   2. Palatine petechiae may be present in GAS infection.
E. Red flags.
   1. "Hot potato" voice.
      a. Garbled speech due to pharyngeal edema.
      b. Suggestive of peritonsillar abscess.
   2. Unilateral neck swelling.
   3. Difficulties with secretion management.
      a. Drooling.
      b. Compromised airway.
         i. Tonsillar pillars touching.
         ii. "Kissing tonsils."
   4. Uvula deviation.
      a. Indicative of peritonsillar abscess.

TABLE 1.1 **Modified Centor Criteria**

Clinical Finding	Score
Fever	+1
Absence of cough	+1
Anterior cervical lymphadenopathy	+1
Tonsillar exudates	+1
Age (years)	
2–14	+1
15–44	0
45+	−1

Source: Fine, A. M., Nizet, V., & Mandl, K. D. (2012, June 11). Large-scale validation of the Centor and McIsaac scores to predict group A streptococcal pharyngitis. Archives of Internal Medicine, 172(11), 847–852.

Diagnostic Tests

A. Clinical examination: Modified Centor criteria.
   1. Scoring system developed to quickly diagnose the likelihood of GAS.
   2. One point assigned for each of the following clinical findings: History of fever, tonsillar exudates, anterior cervical lymphadenopathy, and absence of cough (see Table 1.1).
   3. Empiric treatment based on symptoms and higher Centor score is no longer recommended by the Infectious Disease Society of America.
B. Rapid antigen detection testing (RADT).
   1. Indicated because clinical examination alone cannot differentiate between viral and bacterial pharyngitis.

Modified Centor Score	Guidelines for Treatment
0–1	No further evaluation necessary Provide supportive care Antibiotics not recommended
2–3	Assess for GAS pharyngitis Consider throat cultures and RADT Treat if cultures positive
≥4	Assess for GAS pharyngitis Throat cultures and RADT indicated Empiric treatment controversial IDSA does not recommend empiric treatment Treat if cultures positive

GAS, group A beta-hemolytic streptococci; IDSA, Infectious Disease Society of America; RADT, rapid antigen detection testing.

   2. May not be necessary if overt viral symptoms are present (i.e., cough, rhinorrhea).
      a. Throat culture.
   3. Pediatric: Indicated in children with negative RADT and clinical symptoms supportive of bacterial pharyngitis.
   4. Adults.
      a. Not necessary in adults with negative RADT due to low incidence of GAS in adults.

b. Possibly indicated.
    i. In adults with negative RADT if high suspicion of GAS.
    ii. In adults at high risk for infection (immunocompromised or other comorbidities).
    iii. Those who are in close contact with high risk populations.

Differential Diagnosis
A. Viral pharyngitis.
B. Bacterial pharyngitis.
C. Oropharyngeal candidiasis (thrush).
  1. Immunocompromised patients.
  2. Patients receiving broad spectrum antibiotics or corticosteroids.
D. Gonococci.
Possible in patients engaging in orogenital sex.
E. Diphtheria.
F. Mononucleosis.

Evaluation and Management Plan
A. General plan.
  1. Pain relief.
    a. Over-the-counter (OTC) oral analgesics.
      i. Nonsteroidal anti-inflammatory drugs.
      ii. Acetaminophen.
      iii. Aspirin.
    b. Topical therapies.
      i. Lozenges.
      ii. Sprays.
      iii. Fluids (i.e., tea, honey).
    c. Environmental measures.
      i. Humidified air.
      ii. Avoidance of irritants.
    d. Glucocorticoid.
      i. Not recommended for routine use.
      ii. Limited role in the patient with extreme sore throat and inability to swallow.
  2. Antibiotics for confirmed bacterial infection.
B. Patient/family teaching points.
  1. Handwashing to prevent spread.
C. Pharmacotherapy.
  1. Avoidance of empiric antibiotics.
    a. Overprescribing contributes to antibiotic resistance.
    b. Antimicrobial therapy generally does not benefit bacterial pharyngitis caused by infection other than streptococcal bacteria.
    c. Infections due to other organisms are possible but tend to be the exception.
      i. *N. gonorrhoeae.*
      ii. *C. diphtheriae.*
  2. Bacterial pharyngitis.
    a. Penicillin is antibiotic of choice for GAS pharyngitis.
      i. 10-day course recommended.
    b. First generation cephalosporin for penicillin allergies.
    c. Alternatively 5-day course of azithromycin is acceptable.
      i. Local and regional resistance has been reported.

  3. Viral pharyngitis.
    a. Supportive care.
D. Discharge instructions.
  1. Follow-up is recommended if symptoms do not improve in 3 to 4 days.

Follow-Up
A. Instruct patients to follow-up if pharyngitis does not improve in 5 to 7 days.
B. Further evaluation indicated if no improvement or worsening of symptoms.
  1. Possible suppurative complication.
  2. Alternative diagnosis.

Consultation/Referral
A. Urgent referral to otolaryngologist for suppurative complications.
  1. Peritonsillar abscess.
  2. Retropharyngeal abscess.
  3. Epiglottitis.

Special/Geriatric Considerations
A. Suppurative complications.
  1. Rare but potentially life threatening complications of GAS pharyngitis.
  2. Early recognition and appropriate treatment essential to avoid associated morbidity and mortality.
  3. Complications include:
    a. Peritonsillar abscess.
    b. Retropharyngeal abscess.
    c. Streptococcal bacteremia.
    d. Epiglottitis.
B. Nonsuppurative complications.
  1. Rheumatic fever.
    a. Rare in developed countries.
  2. Poststreptococcal glomerulonephritis.
C. Other considerations.
  1. Morbilliform rash may develop in patients with pharyngitis caused by EBV who have been treated with penicillin or amoxicillin.

Bibliography
Fine, A. M., Nizet, V., & Mandl, K. D. (2012, june 11). Large-scale validation of the Centor and McIsaac scores to predict group a streptococcal pharyngitis. *Archives of Internal Medicine, 172*(11), 847–852.
Gore, J. (2013). Acute pharyngitis. *Official Journal of the American Academy of Physician Assistants, 26*(2), 57–58. doi:10.1097/01720610-201302000-00012
McIsaac, W. J., White, D., Tannenbaum, D., & Low, D. E. (1998). A clinical score to reduce unnecessary antibiotic use in patients with sore throat. *Canadian Medical Association Journal, 158*(1), 75–83.
Nicoteri, J. (2013). Adolescent pharyngitis: A common complaint with potentially lethal complications. *Journal for Nurse Practitioners, 9*(5), 295–300. doi:10.1016/j.nurpra.2013.02.023
Shapiro, D., Lindgren, C., Neuman, M., & Fine, A. (2017). Viral features and testing for streptococcal pharyngitis. *Pediatrics, 139*(5), e20163403. doi:10.1542/peds.2016-3403
Shulman, S., Bisno, A., Clegg, H., Gerber, M., Kaplan, E., Lee, G., & Van Beneden, C. (2012). Executive summary: Clinical practice guideline for the diagnosis and management of group A streptococcal pharyngitis: 2012 update by the Infectious Diseases Society of America. *Clinical Infectious Diseases, 55*(10), 1279–1282. doi:10.1093/cid/cis847
Weber, R. (2014). Pharyngitis. *Primary Care: Clinics in Office Practice, 41*, 91–98. doi:10.1016/j.pop.2013.10.010

Rhinosinusitis

Carey Heck

Definition

A. Inflammation of the nasal cavity and paranasal sinuses.
B. Preferred terminology: "Rhinosinusitis" rather than "sinusitis" since inflammation of the sinuses rarely occurs without inflammation of the nasal mucosa as well.
C. Classification.
    1. Acute rhinosinusitis (ARS): Symptoms lasting less than 4 weeks.
    2. Acute bacterial rhinosinusitis (ABRS): ARS with bacterial etiology.
    3. Chronic rhinosinusitis (CRS): Symptoms lasting greater than 12 weeks.

Incidence

A. Viral infection due to rhinopharyngitis (common cold) is the most common cause of ARS.
B. Annually, 1 in 7-8 persons in the United States will experience an episode of ARS.
C. More frequent in women.
D. Higher in 45- to 64-year -ld age group.
E. ABRS accounts for less than 2% of the cases of ARS.

Pathogenesis

A. Viral.
    1. Rhinovirus.
    2. Influenza virus.
    3. Parainfluenza virus.
B. Bacterial.
    a. *Streptococcus pneumoniae.*
    b. *Haemophilus influenzae.*
    c. *Moraxella catarrhalis.*

Predisposing Factors

A. Older age.
B. Smoking.
C. Air travel.
D. Exposure to changes in atmospheric pressure.
E. Asthma and allergies.
F. Swimming.
G. Dental disease.
H. Immunodeficiency.

Subjective Data

A. Common complaints/symptoms.
    1. Nasal congestion.
    2. Nasal discharge.
    3. Facial pressure or feeling of fullness.
    4. Reduced sense of smell.
B. Other complaints.
    1. Fatigue.
    2. Headache.
    3. Difficulty sleeping.
    4. Toothache.
    5. Ear pain or fullness.
C. Family and social history.
    1. Family and social history is noncontributory.
D. Common/typical scenario.
    1. Common complaints are:
        a. Fever.
        b. Sore throat.
        c. Nasal discharge.
        d. Facial pain.
        e. Frontal pain or pressure that worsens when patient bends forward.
    2. Patients frequently complain of headaches.
E. Review of systems.
    1. Past medical history.
        a. Recent illnesses. Elicit onset and duration of symptoms.
        b. Sick contacts. Determine if patient or close contacts have any systemic illnesses.
        c. Asthma.
    2. Allergies.
    3. Possible occupational exposure history.
    4. Travel history.
    5. Pertinent systems review.
        a. Constitutional.
            i. Fever.
            ii. Malaise.
        b. Head, ear, eyes, nose, and throat (HEENT).
            i. Sinus pain/tenderness.
            ii. Headache.
            iii. Nasal congestion.
            iv. Cough.
            v. Rhinorrhea.
            vi. Purulent discharge with bacterial infection.

Physical Examination

A. Appearance.
    1. Erythema and/or edema of involved cheek.
    2. Erythema and/or edema of periorbital area.
B. Drainage.
    1. Mucopurulent more likely ABRS.
    2. Clear more likely viral ARS.
C. Percussion.
    1. Increased pain or tenderness of sinuses.
    2. Not specific or sensitive test for diagnosis of rhinosinusitis.
D. Transillumination of frontal and maxillary sinuses.
    1. Limited diagnostic value.
    2. Not specific or sensitive test for diagnosis of rhinosinusitis.
E. Nasal examination.
    1. Diffuse mucosal edema.
    2. Narrowing of middle meatus.
    3. Inferior turbinate hypertrophy.
    4. Presence or absence of polyps.
        a. Presence may indicate anatomic risk for development of ABRS.

Diagnostic Tests

A. Generally not indicated for uncomplicated cases of rhinosinusitis.
B. Nasal cultures are not useful in the diagnosis of ABRS.
C. Gold standard for culture identification: Sinus aspiration.
    1. Reserved for complicated cases.
    2. Referral to otolaryngologist.
D. CT.
    1. Persistent symptoms.
    2. Recurrent symptoms.
    3. Complicated ABRS.
    4. Planning for sinus surgery.

Differential Diagnosis

A. Rhinosinusitis.
B. Allergic rhinitis.

C. Rhinopharyngitis.

D. Headache.

Evaluation and Management Plan

A. General plan.

1. Use pain relief: Over-the-counter (OTC) analgesics and antipyretics.

2. Reduce mucosal inflammation: Topical nasal corticosteroids.

3. Enhance sinus drainage: Saline irrigation.

4. Modulate environmental triggers.

    a. Treat concurrent allergic rhinitis symptoms if present with OTC antihistamines and allergy therapy as needed.

5. Eradicate infection indicated for ABRS.

B. Patient/family teaching points.

1. Use handwashing to prevent spread.

C. Pharmacotherapy.

1. Acute sinusitis.

    a. Most cases of acute sinusitis are viral and pharmacotherapy is targeted to symptomatic relief.

        i. OTC analgesics and antipyretics.

        ii. Saline nasal irrigation.

        iii. Possibly topical corticosteroids.

            1) Literature suggests that high-volume corticosteroid irrigations are more effective than low-volume corticosteroid sprays.

        iv. Topical decongestants.

            1) Use not to exceed 3 to 5 days to avoid rebound congestion.

        v. Antihistamines.

            1) No clinical studies support use in viral sinusitis.

        vi. Expectorants and cough suppressants.

            1) Clinical studies do not support efficacy in use for viral sinusitis.

    b. Suspected bacterial sinusitis.

        i. Classic progression is mild symptoms that begin to resolve and then suddenly become worse.

        ii. Watchful waiting: Plan to follow-up if symptoms worsen or do not improve in 7 days.

        iii. Nonmacrolide therapy.

            1) Amoxicillin/clavulanate 875/125 mg orally twice daily × 5 to 7 days.

            2) Doxycycline 200 mg orally daily × 5 to 7 days for PCN allergies.

        iv. OTC analgesics and antipyretics.

        v. Saline irrigation.

            1) Use as adjuvant to corticosteroids in chronic sinusitis.

        vi. Topical corticosteroids.

            1) Literature suggests that high-volume corticosteroid irrigations are more effective than low-volume corticosteroid sprays.

2. Chronic sinusitis.

    a. Initial management is high-volume saline irrigation with topical corticosteroid therapy.

    b. Consider short course of nonmacrolide therapy if active mucopurulence is present on examination.

    c. For patients with persistent symptoms.

        i. Consider systemic corticosteroids.

        ii. Use long-term macrolide therapy for patients without nasal polyps.

    d. Topical antibiotics and antifungals are not recommended in the treatment of chronic sinusitis.

D. Discharge instructions.

1. Follow-up is recommended in 3 to 4 days if no improvement in symptoms.

Follow-Up

A. Patients should be instructed to follow-up if symptoms do not improve in 7 days.

B. Further evaluation is indicated if no improvement or worsening of symptoms.

Consultation/Referral

A. Persistent cases should be referred to otolaryngology.

1. Endoscopic nasal evaluation.

2. Endoscopic nasal surgery.

Special/Geriatric Considerations

A. Long-term use of nasogastric tubes can put patients at risk for developing sinusitis.

Bibliography

Bird, J., Biggs, T., Thomas, M., & Salib, R. (2013). Adult acute rhinosinusitis. *British Medical Journal, 346*, f2687. doi:10.1136/bmj.f2687

Cevc, G. (2017). Differential diagnosis and proper treatment of acute rhinosinusitis: Guidance based on historical data analysis. *Allergy & Rhinology, 8*(2), e45–e52. Advance online publication. doi:10.2500/ar.2017.8.0206

Cho, S. H., Kim, D. W., & Gevaert, P. (2016). Chronic rhinosinusitis without nasal polyps. *Journal of Allergy and Clinical Immunology: In Practice, 4*(4), 575–582. doi:10.1016/j.jaip.2016.04.015

Rosenfeld, R., Piccirillo, J., Chandrasekhar, S., Brook, I., Kumar, K., Kramper, M., . . . Corrigan, M. (2015). Clinical practice guideline (Update): Adult sinusitis. *Otolaryngology–Head and Neck Surgery, 152*(2 Suppl.), S1–S39. doi:10.1177/0194599815572097

Rudmik, L., & Soler, Z. (2015). Medical therapies for adult chronic sinusitis: A systematic review. *Journal of the American Medical Association, 314*(9), 926–939. doi:10.1001/jama.2015.7544

2 Pulmonary Guidelines

E. Moneé Carter-Griffin

Acute Respiratory Distress Syndrome

E. Moneé Carter-Griffin

Definition

A. Acute respiratory distress syndrome (ARDS) is defined by three variables.

    1. Bilateral opacities on imaging.

    2. Onset within 7 days of a clinical event or worsening respiratory symptoms.

    3. Origin of pulmonary edema not fully explained by cardiac failure or volume overload.

B. ARDS is identified as mild, moderate, or severe based on the PF ratio (PaO_2/FiO_2).

C. Acute lung injury does not exist in the new definition of ARDS.

D. Exclusion of heart failure is not required in the new definition of ARDS.

Incidence

A. It is difficult to obtain an accurate incidence due to variations in the definition used to identify or describe ARDS.

B. An estimated 200,000 cases of ARDS occur each year in the United States.

C. The incidence increases with advancing age.

D. ARDS has not been shown to occur more in one sex than the other.

E. Mortality and morbidity are associated with worsening of the PF ratio.

Pathogenesis

A. An indirect or direct insult causes an inflammatory response and accumulation of pro-inflammatory mediators in the lung microcirculation. Injury occurs to the microvascular endothelium and alveolar epithelium. Endothelium injury leads to capillary permeability and migration of protein-rich fluid into the alveolar space. Due to injury of the alveolar epithelium, pulmonary edema forms and damage occurs to the cells lining the alveoli.

B. Damage to type I and II cells leads to decreased clearance of fluid in the pleural space, increased fluid entry into the alveoli, and decreased surfactant production resulting in decreased alveolar compliance and alveoli collapse.

C. An influx of fibroblasts leads to collagen deposition and possibly fibrosis.

Predisposing Factors

A. Aspiration, including gastric content and drowning.

B. Sepsis.

C. Pneumonia.

D. Massive transfusions.

E. Pancreatitis.

F. Burns.

G. Trauma, including cases with and without pulmonary injury.

H. Underlying interstitial lung disease.

Subjective Data

A. Common complaints/symptoms.

    1. Severe dyspnea.

    2. Chest discomfort.

    3. Tachypnea.

B. Common/typical scenario.

    1. Onset is typically 12 to 48 hours after the insult.

    2. History shows progressive worsening symptoms.

    3. Extrapulmonary complaints may have led to the development of ARDS.

Physical Examination

A. Dyspnea (see Figure 2.1).

B. Tachypnea.

C. **Abdominal retractions; obvious respiratory distress**.

D. Hypoxia and possibly cyanosis.

E. Tachycardia.

F. Altered mental status, agitation, or confusion.

G. Rales during auscultation.

H. Additional findings that may relate to the underlying etiology of ARDS (e.g., febrile, hypotension, an acute abdomen, or nausea and vomiting seen in pancreatitis).

Diagnostic Tests

A. Chest x-ray (CXR).

    1. Patchy infiltrates rapidly evolve and progress to diffuse, bilateral infiltrates.

    2. Daily CXRs may be required, especially for patients on mechanical ventilation.

B. Arterial blood gas (ABG).

    1. Regular ABGs are required to evaluate management.

    2. Development of respiratory acidosis (decreased pH and rising CO_2).

    3. Hypoxemia is defined by the PF ratio.

        a. Less than 300: As mild ARDS.

        b. Less than 200: Moderate ARDS.

        c. Less than 100: Severe ARDS.

C. Complete blood count (CBC).

    1. Evaluate the white blood cell count and platelets.

D. Comprehensive metabolic panel.

    1. Evaluate renal and liver function.

Obtain the History
Quality/sensation, timing, precipitating factors, alleviating factors, any associated factors.
- Gradual or sudden onset?
- Continuous or episodic?
- Occur with exertion or at rest?
- Positional?

Physical Examination
General: Positioning? Accessory muscle use? Paradoxical abdominal movement? Overt distress? Able to speak in full sentences? Audible stridor?
Vital Signs: Tachycardia? Tachypnea? Pulsus paradoxus? Oxygen desaturations?
Cardiac: Elevated JVD? Murmur? S3 or S4 gallop? Edema?
Respiratory: Adventitious breath sounds such as crackles/rales, wheezes, or diminished? Chest shape? Dullness or hyperresonance on percussion? Respiratory pattern? Symmetrical chest movement?
Extremities: Cyanosis? Edema? Clubbing?

The physical exam should always focus on airway, breathing, circulation first. Proceed with a full exam in the stable patient

Initial Diagnostics
Chest x-ray: Evidence of pulmonary edema? Pneumonia? Pleural effusion? Hyperinflation of the lungs suggestive of obstructive disease? Heart size? Lung volumes? Elevation of hemidiaphragm?
ECG: To assess for myocardial injury or ischemia.

Respiratory
ABG: Assess for hypercapnia or hypoxemia
D-dimer, age-adjusted: Can aid in ruling out a pulmonary embolus.
Chest CT/Angiography: Assess for pneumonia, emphysematous changes, fluid, honeycombing suggestive of fibrosis, pulmonary embolus.
Pulmonary function testing: Assess for obstructive or restrictive disease.

Cardiovascular
Echocardiogram: Assess heart size, function, valves, pulmonary pressures, pericardial effusion, and so forth.
NT-proBNP: Can aid in the diagnosis of heart failure in the appropriate clinical context.

Additional Testing
Thyroid studies: Assess for hyperthyroidism (high cardiac output state).
Hemoglobin/Hematocrit: Assess for anemia.
Cardiopulmonary exercise test: Can help distinguish between the two by indicating ischemic changes on ECG (cardiac), bronchospasm during exercise (respiratory), and so forth.

FIGURE 2.1 Algorithm for the evaluation of dyspnea.
JVD, jugular venous distention; NT-proBNP, N-Terminal pro brain natriuretic peptide.

2. Magnesium and phosphorus. Strict electrolyte repletion is necessary for cardiac stability and prevention of arrhythmias, especially in the setting of profound tissue hypoxia and/or septic shock, which is often concomitant.
E. Coagulation studies.
  1. Prothrombin time and international normalized ratio.
  2. Fibrinogen level.
  3. Fibrin degradation products.
F. N-Terminal pro brain natriuretic peptide level.
  1. This is used to assess for heart failure causing or contributing to the bilateral infiltrates and hypoxemia.
  2. It is important for the clinician to note that this value may be elevated secondary to etiologies other than heart failure, such as sepsis and renal failure.
G. Blood cultures.
  1. Evaluate infective etiology as a source for ARDS development.
H. Systemic infection markers.

  1. Lactic acid. Measure level of end-organ tissue hypoxia and consider trend.
  2. Procalcitonin. Consider trend every 24 hours and monitor for effectiveness of treatment of the primarily offending process.
I. Urinalysis and urine culture.
  1. Evaluate infective etiology as source for ARDS development.
J. Sputum culture.
  1. Evaluate infective etiology as source for ARDS development.

Differential Diagnosis
A. Asthma.
B. Chronic obstructive pulmonary disease (COPD).
C. Congestive heart failure (CHF).
D. Acute lung injury.
E. Pleural effusions.
F. Pneumonia.

Evaluation and Management Plan

A. Treatment is dependent on the severity of ARDS.

   1. Oxygen therapy (e.g., high flow nasal cannula, noninvasive positive pressure ventilation, invasive mechanical ventilation).

   a. In acute hypoxemic respiratory failure, high flow nasal cannula may be necessary. It resulted in improved mortality at 90 days compared to noninvasive and invasive mechanical ventilation.

   b. Invasive mechanical ventilation: Recommended tidal volume of 6 to 8 mL/kg and maintaining plateau pressures less than 30 cm H_2O.

   i. It may be necessary to reduce the tidal volume to 4 to 5 mL/kg if one is unable to obtain a plateau pressure less than 30 cm H_2O.

   ii. Plateau pressures less than 30 cm H_2O may not be attainable in obese patients.

   iii. Low tidal volumes usually result in hypoventilation. Permissive hypercapnia is typically accepted to a pH of 7.20.

   c. The use of lung recruitment measures and titrated positive end-expiratory pressure (PEEP) is controversial in patients with moderate to severe forms of ARDS due to recent studies indicating negative consequences. Recent recommendations are conditional for use of higher levels of PEEP.

   d. Weaning from mechanical ventilation is typically initiated once the patient requires 50% or less FiO_2, physiologic levels of PEEP, hemodynamically stable, assessed neurological status, and so forth.

   2. Positioning.

   a. Studies have shown that prone positioning results in decreased mortality.

   i. Recommended to start in early and severe ARDS.

   b. Prone positioning requires the patient to be hemodynamically stable while proning, adequate sedation and paralytics, well-trained staff to care for the patient, and adequate space for the equipment.

   3. Conservative fluid management.

   a. Increased ventilator-free days but no difference in mortality.

   b. Initial fluid resuscitation depends on the underlying etiology for the development of ARDS. Conditions such as hemorrhagic shock and pancreatitis initially require more aggressive fluid management.

   c. Guidelines for fluid resuscitation should be followed for certain diagnoses such as sepsis, pancreatitis, and so forth.

B. Pharmacotherapy.

   1. Paralytics and sedatives.

   a. Paralytics should be administered in combination with sedatives.

   i. Minimal sedation to achieve compliance with ventilation and early mobilization show improved outcomes in the ICU setting when clinically appropriate in mild–moderate ARDS.

   ii. Daily sedation vacation and ventilator liberation procedures should be initiated when oxygen requirements are compatible with extubation.

   b. Paralytics should be considered with ventilatory dyssynchrony and difficulty with ventilation such as poor airway compliance.

   c. Early administration in severe ARDS has not been associated with increased muscle weakness.

   d. A commonly used paralytic is cisatracurium.

   2. Corticosteroids: Evidence is lacking to recommend for or against steroid use in ARDS.

   3. Antibiotics are indicated in patients with an infective etiology.

   4. Nitric oxide has not shown to improve outcomes.

   5. Deep vein thrombosis (DVT) and stress ulcer prophylaxis is required.

   a. DVT prophylaxis is held in patients with significant coagulopathies using subcutaneous heparin or lovenox.

   b. Proton pump inhibitors and fluoroquinolones are used with caution due to increasing incidence of renal complications and *Clostridium difficile* colitis with concurrent use.

C. Other treatment methods.

   1. High frequency ventilation: Has not shown to improve outcomes and some evidence suggests it may increase mortality.

   2. Extracorporeal membrane oxygenation.

   a. Limited evidence to support regular use and no guidelines for widespread use.

   b. Limited to certain institutions.

Follow-Up

A. This is dependent on the patient's clinical course, outcomes, and length of hospital stay.

Consultation/Referral

A. Consultation with a pulmonologist and/or intensivist would be required for management of mechanical ventilation and critical care needs.

B. Additional consultation may be required depending on the underlying etiology for ARDS (e.g., trauma, infectious disease).

Special/Geriatric Considerations

A. Open communication with the family is required.

B. Nutritional support is recommended. The preferred route is enteral.

C. Patients with prolonged mechanical ventilation—typically greater than 14 days—should undergo tracheostomy placement.

Bibliography

Adhikari, N. K., Dellinger, R. P., Lundin, S., Payen, D., Vallet, B., Gerlack, H., . . . Friedrich, J. O. (2014). Inhaled nitric oxide does not reduce mortality in patients with acute respiratory distress syndrome regardless of severity: Systematic review and meta-analysis. *Critical Care Medicine, 42*, 404–412. doi:10.1097/CCM.0b013e3182a27909

Cavalcanti, A. B., Suzumura, R. A., Laranjeira, L. N., de Mores Paisani, D., Damiani, L. P., Guimaraes, H. P., . . . Ribeiro de Carvalho, C. R. (2017). Effect of lung recruitment and titrated positive end-expiratory-pressure (peep) vs low peep on mortality in patients with acute respiratory distress syndrome: A randomized clinical trial. *Journal of American Medical Association, 318*, 1335–1345. doi:10.1001/jama.2017.14171

Fan, E., Del Sorbo, L., Goligher, E. C., Hodgson, C. L., Munshi, L., Walkey, A. J., . . . Brochard, L. J. (2017). An official American Thoracic Society/European Society of Intensive Care Medicine/Society of Critical Care Medicine clinical practice guideline: Mechanical ventilation in adult patients with acute respiratory distress syndrome. *American Journal of Respiratory and Critical Care Medicine, 195*, 1253–1263. doi:10.1164/rccm.201703-0548ST

Ferguson, N. D., Fan, E., Camporota, L., Antonelli, M., Anzueto, A., Beale, R., & Ranieri, V. M. (2012). The Berlin definition of ARDS: An expanded rationale, justification, and supplementary material. *Intensive Care Medicine, 38*, 1573–1582. doi:10.1007/s00134-012-2682-1

Frat, J. P., Thille, A. W., Mercat, A., Girault, C., Ragot, S., Perbet, S., & Robert, R. (2015). High-flow oxygen through nasal cannula in acute hypoxemic respiratory failure. *New England Journal of Medicine, 372*, 2185–2196. doi:10.1056/NEJMoa1503326

Guerin, C., Reignier, J., Richard, J. C., Beuret, P., Gacouin, A., Boulain, T., . . . Ayzac, L. (2013). Prone positioning in severe acute respiratory distress syndrome. *New England Journal of Medicine, 368*, 2159–2168. doi:10.1056/NEJMoa1214103

Papazian, L., Forel, J.-M., Gacouin, A., Penot-Ragon, C., Perrin, G., Loundou, A., . . . Roch, A. (2010). Neuromuscular blockers in early acute respiratory distress syndrome. *New England Journal of Medicine, 363*, 1107–1116. doi:10.1056/NEJMoa1005372

Rhodes, A., Evans, L. E., Alhazzani, W., Levy, M. M., Antonelli, M., Ferrer, R., . . . Dellinger, R. (2017). Surviving sepsis campaign: International guidelines for management of sepsis and septic shock: 2016. *Critical Care Medicine, 45*, 486–552. doi:10.1097/CCM.0000000000002255

Tenner, S., Baillie, J., DeWitt, J., & Vege, S. S. (2013). American College of Gastroenterology Guideline: Management of acute pancreatitis. *American Journal of Gastroenterology, 108*, 1400–1415. doi:10.1038/ajg.2013.218

Asthma

E. Moneé Carter-Griffin

Definition

A. A chronic airway inflammatory disease defined by a variation of expiratory airflow limitation and history of respiratory symptoms that vary in intensity over time. There are various asthma phenotypes, such as allergic asthma and late-onset asthma.

Incidence

A. Approximately 39.5 million people in the United States have been diagnosed with asthma in their lifetime.
B. It is estimated that 18.9 million adults still have asthma.
C. Asthma accounts for greater than 400,000 hospitalizations, 1.8 million ED visits, and 14.2 million office visits.
D. The prevalence in adults is highest in women and African Americans.

Pathogenesis

A. Interplay among host factors and environmental exposures, resulting in airway inflammation, airflow obstruction, and bronchial hyperresponsiveness.
   1. Immune response to antigen, causing activation of T-lymphocytes.
   2. Release of cytokines and interleukins, leading to a release of mast cells, eosinophils, and basophils.
   3. Subsequent release of inflammatory mediators (e.g., histamine, prostaglandins) that cause airway inflammation and mucus secretion.
B. Resulting development of airway hyperplasia, airway obstruction, and bronchial hyperresponsiveness.

Predisposing Factors

A. Direct and indirect exposure to tobacco smoke.
B. Allergens (e.g., animals such as cats and dogs, dust mites, pollen).
C. Occupational exposures or irritants (e.g., paint, sprays).
D. Pollution.
E. Respiratory infections.
F. Exercise.
G. Stress.
H. Gastroesophageal reflux disease.
I. Obesity.
J. Sex (more likely in female adults).
K. Viral infections.

Subjective Data

A. Common complaints/symptoms.
   1. Respiratory symptoms (e.g., wheezing, dyspnea, chest tightness, and cough).
   2. Possible extrapulmonary manifestations (e.g., allergic skin conditions or conjunctival irritation).
B. History of the present illness.
   1. Onset of asthma and/or symptoms.
   2. Precipitating factors.
   3. Asthma severity such as frequency of rescue inhaler use.
   4. Comorbid conditions that may predispose the patient to developing asthma.
   5. Number of exacerbations in the past year.
   6. History of ED visits, hospitalizations, and intubations related to asthma.
C. Family and social history.
   1. Family history of asthma.
   2. Social history such as smoking and inhaled illicit drug use.
   3. Employment/environmental factors (e.g., working outside, mining operations, military service).

Physical Examination

A. The physical examination may vary depending on the severity of the asthma and if the patient is having an exacerbation.
B. Expiratory wheezing on auscultation may be audible (see Figure 2.2).
C. Dyspnea may be evident (see Figure 2.1).
D. Changes in mentation (e.g., confusion, lethargy) may be apparent.
E. Patients with moderate to severe asthma exacerbations may be in a tripod position and have tachypnea, absent breath sounds (silent chest) on auscultation, accessory muscle use (e.g., intercostal), and tachycardia.
F. As previously stated, some patients may have extrapulmonary symptoms such as dermatitis, conjunctival irritation, and a swollen nasal mucosa.

Diagnostic Tests

A. Lung function. Initial diagnosis is based on a history of variable symptoms and confirmed variation in expiratory airflow limitation. Lung function is typically normal between symptoms.
   1. Evidence of obstruction with reduction in the forced expiratory volume in 1 second/forced vital capacity (FEV_1/FVC) and at least one low FEV_1.
   2. One or more tests documented with excessive variability in lung function.
      a. Positive bronchodilator reversibility test with a greater than 12% and 200 mL increase from baseline in the FEV_1.
      b. Excessive variability of greater than 10% in twice-daily peak expiratory flow (PEF) over 2 weeks.
      c. Positive exercise challenge test with decrease in FEV_1 of greater than 10% and 200 mL from baseline.
      d. Positive bronchial challenge test.
      e. Increase in the FEV_1 by greater than 12% and 200 mL OR a greater than 20% increase in the PEF from baseline after 4 weeks of treatment.
      f. Variation of lung function between office visits.
B. PEF.
   1. Can be routinely monitored in the outpatient setting.
   2. Repeat values compared with personal best or predicted value by patients.
   3. Typically, severe symptoms: At or less than 50% predicted.

Obtain the history.
Onset, quality, precipitating factors, alleviating factors, any associated factors.
- Acute or gradual onset?
- Associated with other symptoms such as dyspnea, cough, hoarseness, flushing, pruritus, chest discomfort/tightness, and so forth?
- Triggers such as exercise, fumes/smoke, allergens, and so forth?
- Medication or food allergies? Initiation of new medications?
- Comorbid conditions such as asthma, COPD, heart failure, myocardial infarction, GERD, and so forth?
- Recent respiratory infections?
- Current or history of smoking?
- Prior intubations? History of throat or neck cancer, surgeries, and so forth?
- Aspiration?

Completed in the stable patient with wheezing

Physical Examination
General: Accessory muscle use? Diaphoresis? Flushing?
Vital Signs: Febrile? Tachypnea? Tachycardia? Oxygen desaturations?
HEENT: Facial or lip/oropharynx swelling? Central cyanosis? Rhinorrhea? Redness and/or watery eyes? Assessment of voice quality?
Neck: Surgical scars? Old tracheostomy sites? Swelling? Goiter? Tracheal deviation? High pitched noises or stridor on auscultation?
Cardiac: Elevated JVD? Murmur? S3 or S4 gallop? Edema?
Respiratory: Inspiratory or expiratory wheezing? Other adventitious breath sounds such as crackles? Diminished breath sounds? Chest shape? Respiratory pattern? Retractions? Dullness or hyperresonance on percussion?
Extremities: Cyanosis? Edema? Clubbing?
Skin: Rash? Hives? Noted insect stings or bites?

Diagnostics
Pulse oximetry: Assess oxygen saturations
ABG: Assess oxygenation and ventilation
Chest x-ray: Assess for lung mass, consolidation/infiltrate, pulmonary edema, or hyperinfiation
Pulmonary function testing: Assess for obstructive or restrictive disease
Chest CT/Angiography: Assess for pneumonia, changes associated with obstructive disease, fluid, fibrosis, pulmonary embolus, mass, tracheal narrowing/stenosis, and so forth
Allergy testing
Respiratory viral testing: Such as RSV
Bronchoscopy: Assess for tracheomalacia, tracheal narrowing/stenosis, foreign objects, masses/tumors
Echocardiogram: To evaluate for heart failure
Esophagram/barium swallow: Assess for reflux disease or aspiration

FIGURE 2.2 Algorithm for the evaluation of wheezing. ABG, arterial blood gas; COPD, chronic obstructive pulmonary disease. GERD, gastroesophageal reflux disease; JVD, jugular venous distention; RSV, respiratory syncytial virus

---

C. Allergy skin testing.
   1. Positive allergen test: Allergen not necessarily causing asthma symptoms.
   2. Essential to account for the timing of symptoms in relation to allergen exposure and the patient's history.
D. Chest x-ray.
   1. Usually normal in patients with asthma but may reveal hyperinflation.
   2. If a patient has a fever in conjunction with respiratory symptoms: May be diagnostic for pneumonia.
E. Pulse oximetry and arterial blood gas (ABG).
   1. Used to evaluate for hypoxemia.
   2. ABG: Can also be used to evaluate for hypercapnia and respiratory acidosis, especially in those patients presenting with an acute exacerbation.

Differential Diagnosis
A. Chronic obstructive pulmonary disease (COPD).
B. Pulmonary embolism.
C. Congestive heart failure (CHF).
D. Chronic rhinosinusitis.
E. Alpha-1 antitrypsin deficiency.

Evaluation and Management Plan
A. General plan.
   1. The goal is to control symptoms and minimize the risk of asthma exacerbations.
   2. Treatment includes assessment, adjustment of medications, and response review.
   3. Emergency treatment: Patients with progressively worsening symptoms may present to the ED.
      a. Evaluation of ABCs, physical assessment, and PEF is necessary.
      b. Medication management consists of a short-acting beta$_2$ agonist (SABA) via continuous nebulizer or a metered-dose inhaler, corticosteroids, oxygen therapy, and ipratropium bromide.
      c. Patients with a more severe exacerbation as demonstrated by a PEF less than 50% will receive

intravenous instead of oral corticosteroids (OCS) and possibly intravenous magnesium sulfate.

d. Posttreatment, the PEF should be reassessed.

e. Patients with an alteration in mental status (e.g., somnolence, confusion), absent breath sounds, worsening hypoxemia or hypercapnia, and hemodynamic instability should be placed on invasive mechanical ventilation and admitted to the ICU.

B. Patient/family teaching points.

1. Nonpharmacological interventions should be addressed such as smoking cessation, engagement in regular physical activity, and avoidance of known occupational exposures and allergen triggers.

2. Patients should be provided with self-management education to reduce morbidity. Essential components included in self-management are:

a. Self-monitoring of symptoms and/or PEF.

b. A written action plan that includes recognition and response to worsening asthma symptoms.

c. Regular review of asthma control and treatment by a healthcare provider.

C. Pharmacotherapy.

1. A daily controller treatment is recommended once an asthma diagnosis has been confirmed.

2. Early treatment with an inhaled corticosteroid (ICS) has been shown to improve lung function.

a. A controller treatment is not indicated in patients with rare asthma symptoms, no night awakenings, no exacerbations in the past year, and a normal FEV_1.

b. An ICS (controller treatment) is recommended in patients with two or more asthma symptoms monthly, waking from asthma more than one night per month, and asthma symptoms plus risk factors for exacerbations.

3. A stepwise approach is used for treatment adjustment. See Table 2.1 for commonly used medications in asthma management.

a. Step 1: SABA as needed with consideration of a controller treatment with an ICS.

b. Step 2: Low dose ICS plus a SABA as needed.

i. The provider can consider a leukotriene receptor antagonist (LTRA) but research has shown it to be less effective.

ii. An ICS and long-acting beta$_2$ agonist (LABA) combination leads to improvement in symptoms but is more expensive and has similar exacerbation rates compared to an ICS alone.

c. Step 3: Low dose ICS/LABA plus a SABA as needed **OR** ICS/formoterol and reliever therapy.

d. Step 4: Low dose ICS/formoterol plus a reliever therapy **OR** medium dose ICS/LABA plus a SABA as needed. The provider can add on tiotropium in patients with a history of exacerbations.

e. Step 5: Patients should be referred to an expert. Additional medication management includes changing the patient to a high dose ICS/LABA plus oral corticosteroids OCS.

4. With the stepwise approach, the treatment regimen can be adjusted up or down by the provider based on frequency and severity of asthma symptoms.

5. Asthma exacerbations are characterized by an increase or worsening in respiratory symptoms and lung function compared to the patient's baseline.

6. Patients with acute exacerbations and an asthma action plan in place can increase their SABA or usual reliever, as well as maintenance controller. OCS can be

TABLE 2.1	Asthma Medications
Beta$_2$ agonists	
SABA	
Levalbuterol	
Salbutamol (albuterol)	
Terbutaline	
Anticholinergics/Antimuscarinics	
SAMA	
Ipratropium bromide (reduces risk of admissions in acute asthma; less effective in the long term)	
LAMA	
Tiotropium (add-on option in patients with history of exacerbations on controller medications)	
ICSs	
Beclometasone	
Budesonide	
Fluticasone furoate	
Fluticasone propionate	
Mometasone	
Triamcinolone acetonide	
Combination ICS plus LABA	
ICS/LABA	
Beclometasone/formoterol	
Budesonide/formoterol	
Fluticasone furoate/vilanterol	
Fluticasone propionate/formoterol	
Fluticasone propionate/salmeterol	
Mometasone/formoterol	
Systemic corticosteroids	
Prednisone (oral)	
Methylprednisolone (intravenous)	
LTRA	
Montelukast	
Pranlukast	
Zafirlukast	
Zileuton	

ICS, inhaled corticosteroid; LABA, long-acting beta$_2$ agonist; LAMA, long-acting muscarinic antagonist; LTRA, leukotriene receptor antagonist; SABA, short-acting beta$_2$ agonist; SAMA, short-acting muscarinic antagonist.

added for patients who fail to respond to treatment or severe exacerbations with a PEF or FEV_1 less than 60% predicted or their personal best (see Exhibit 2.1).

D. Discharge instructions.

1. Discharge criteria. Patients should

a. Show improvement in symptoms such as resolution of accessory muscle use and dyspnea, improved respiratory rate, and O_2 saturation greater than 94% on room air.

b. Improved PEF of greater than 60% predicted or personal best.

c. Have adequate home resources.

2. Diet.

    a. Restrictions: Specific diet based on whether the patient has underlying comorbid conditions such as diabetes or renal disease.

    b. No restrictions: Patient can resume a regular diet.

3. Medications.

    a. OCS: Usually prescribed for 5 to 7 days.

    b. Reliever medications such as SABA: Can be resumed on an as-needed basis.

    c. ICS prior to discharge.

        i. ICS/LABA **OR** ICS/formoterol.

        ii. If the patient is already on an ICS: Increase the dose for 2 to 4 weeks.

    d. Medication reconciliation and continuation of appropriate medications for comorbid conditions.

4. Treatment plan.

    a. Identification of risk factors that contribute to exacerbations.

    b. Individualized written asthma action plan.

    c. Evaluation of maintenance therapy understanding.

    d. Assessment of inhaler technique.

    e. Assessment of PEF meter technique if applicable outside of an acute exacerbation.

    f. Smoking cessation counseling.

    g. Immunizations such as influenza. Influenza can trigger acute and severe asthma exacerbations that could potentially result in necessitating ventilatory support.

    h. Management of comorbid conditions.

5. Discuss with patient.

    a. Importance of medication compliance and proper inhaler technique to reduce symptoms and exacerbations.

    b. As previously stated, avoidance of known risk factors that worsen asthma symptoms or lead to exacerbations such as smoking or other known allergens.

    c. Signs and symptoms of an impending exacerbation such as increasing reliever inhaler use, frequent awakening at night with coughing or dyspnea, and PEF less than 60% of predicted or personal best.

Follow-Up

A. Regular follow-up is dependent on symptom control and exacerbation risk but should last for 1 to 3 months after treatment initiation and every 3 to 12 months once stabilized.

B. Patients should see their primary care provider or pulmonologist 1 to 2 weeks after self-management of an exacerbation.

C. Patients should see their primary care provider or asthma specialist/pulmonologist within 2 to 7 days of discharge from the ED or hospital.

Consultation/Referral

A. Patients with progressively worsening asthma despite increasing treatment may require a referral to a pulmonologist or allergist.

B. A pulmonologist and/or intensivist consultation is indicated for patients with a moderate to severe exacerbation necessitating ICU admission and/or noninvasive and invasive mechanical ventilation.

Special/Geriatric Considerations

A. Poor inhaler technique needs to be considered in patients with persistent symptoms.

B. Comorbid conditions may contribute and complicate asthma management.

C. Routine chest x-rays and antibiotic therapy are not indicated in asthma management.

D. In the elderly population, asthma can be underdiagnosed or overdiagnosed due to varying assumptions and perceptions over dyspnea.

Bibliography

Centers for Disease Control and Prevention. (2013). *Asthma facts: CDC's National Asthma Control Program Grantees.* Atlanta, GA: U.S. Department of Health and Human Services. Retrieved from https://www.cdc.gov/asthma/pdfs/asthma_facts_program_grantees.pdf

Global Initiative for Asthma. (2017). *Global strategy for asthma management and prevention.* Retrieved from https://ginasthma.org/wp-content/uploads/2016/01/wms-GINA-2017-main-report-tracked-changes-for-archive.pdf

Chronic Obstructive Pulmonary Disease

E. Moneé Carter-Griffin

Definition

A. A chronic and progressive respiratory disease characterized by expiratory airflow limitation.

Incidence

A. Chronic obstructive pulmonary disease (COPD) is the third leading cause of death in the United States and fourth leading cause of death worldwide.

B. The incidence is much higher in smokers and ex-smokers compared to nonsmokers.

C. It is more prevalent in individuals greater than 40 years with the greatest prevalence in those greater than 65 years.

D. Traditionally, prevalence has been higher in men but recent literature suggests the occurrence may be rising in women, and women may be more susceptible to poorer outcomes.

Pathogenesis

A. The lungs are exposed to a stimulus (e.g., smoking, fumes) that causes inflammation of the airways. Neutrophils and various other immune cells are recruited to the airways leading to breakdown of elastin fibers and increasing oxidative stress.

B. Ultimately, there is destruction of alveolar walls, decreased repair of the alveoli, fibrosis, and bronchiolar wall thickening leading to narrowed airways, impaired gas exchange, and enlarged air spaces.

Predisposing Factors

A. Tobacco smoke: Leading environmental risk factor.

B. Individuals greater than 40 years.

C. Occupational exposures to lung irritants (e.g., dust, chemical agents, fumes).

D. Alpha-1 antitrypsin is a genetic condition leading to COPD that should be tested in a new diagnosis of COPD.

E. Airway hyperresponsiveness (e.g., asthma).

F. Allergies.

G. Recurrent respiratory infections.

Subjective Data

A. Common complaints/symptoms.

    1. Dyspnea (see Figure 2.1): Chronic and progressive. This is a cardinal symptom.

Obtain the history.

Onset, timing, description of cough, alleviating factors, any associated factors.
- Acute (<3 weeks), subacute (3–8 weeks), or chronic (>8 weeks)?
- Associated with other symptoms such as dyspnea, wheezing, chest tightness, or hemoptysis?
- Recent respiratory infection?
- Occupational or environmental exposures?
- Medications such as ACE inhibitors?
- Known comorbid conditions such as asthma, COPD, GERD, and so forth?
- Current or history of smoking?
- Occurrence of cough? Upon awakening? Lying down? During exercise?

Physical Examination

The initial physical exam focuses on clues suggestive of cardiopulmonary disease. A thorough full exam should follow because a cough may be a manifestation of a more systemic disease process.
General: Weight loss? Fatigue?
Vital Signs: Usually normal unless associated with another disease process. May have tachypnea, tachycardia, oxygen desaturations, and/or fever.
HEENT: Red and/or watery eyes? Fluid behind eardrum? Boggy, swollen, and/or pale mucus membranes? Nasal polyps? Thin, watery, or purulent secretions? Congestion? Throat redness? Hoarseness?
Respiratory: Adventitious breath sounds such as crackles or wheezing? Chest shape? Respiratory pattern? Dullness or hyperresonance on percussion?
Extremities: Clubbing? Edema?

Initial Diagnostic

Chest x-ray:
- All individuals with a chronic cough.
- All individuals with an acute cough AND dyspnea, chest pain, fever, hemoptysis, or weight loss

Acute/Subacute	Chronic
Usually does not require further testing. Additional testing focuses on a suspected etiology. - Allergy testing - **Chest CT/Angiography:** Assess for pneumonia, changes associated with obstructive disease, fluid, fibrosis, pulmonary embolus - **Pulmonary function testing:** Assess for obstructive or restrictive disease - **Tuberculosis skin testing** - **Pertussis testing**	**Pulmonary function testing:** Assess for obstructive or restrictive disease <u>Additional work-up may follow after empirical treatment for disorders such as GERD.</u> **Bronchoscopy:** To evaluate for chronic inflammation **Sinus Imaging** **High-resolution Chest CT:** Used in cough with atypical presentations and concern for chronic pulmonary disease **Esophagram or swallow evaluation:** Assess for reflux disease or aspiration **Echocardigram:** To evaluate for heart failure or elevated pulmonary pressures

FIGURE 2.3 Algorithm for the evaluation of cough.
ACE, angiotensin-converting enzyme; COPD, chronic obstructive pulmonary disease; GERD, gastroesophageal reflux disease; HEENT, head, ear, eyes, nose, and throat.

2. Cough (see Figure 2.3) with or without sputum production.

    a. Not uncommon for individuals to produce small amounts of sputum.

    b. Increasing sputum production, especially with change in color: May indicate bacterial infection.

3. Wheezing (see Figure 2.2) and/or chest tightness.

4. Severe COPD: Possible fatigue, weight loss, and anorexia.

B. Family and social history.

    1. Inquire about environmental risk factors and family history.

    2. Inquire about smoking because it can accelerate or exacerbate COPD symptoms.

C. Review of symptoms.

    1. Evaluate for symptom onset, duration, severity, associated symptoms (e.g., increased wheezing or sputum), and aggravating and alleviating factors.

2. Inquire about early onset of COPD.

3. Assess for risk factors such as a history of allergies, asthma, or recurrent respiratory infections.

Physical Examination

A. The physical examination for COPD is rarely diagnostic. Physical signs of COPD may or may not be present, depending on the severity of disease. However, it is still important to assess for the respiratory and systemic symptoms that may be associated with COPD.

B. General examination.

    1. Assess the respiratory rate. It may be normal or increased.

    2. Assess the patient's posture. Leaning forward with outstretched palms is associated with an attempt to relieve dyspnea.

    3. Check breathing. In advanced disease or severe dyspnea, pursed-lip breathing is possible.

4. Inspect for clubbing.

5. In more severe disease, cyanosis, elevated jugular venous pressure, and peripheral edema may be present.

C. Respiratory examination.

    1. Inspect the chest.

        a. Check for an increased anteroposterior chest diameter due to hyperinflation of the lungs, giving a barrel chest shape.

        b. Assess for use of accessory muscles (e.g., sternocleidomastoids, scalenes, intercostals).

    2. Percuss the chest wall.

        a. Observe for hyperresonance due to overinflation of the lungs.

    3. Auscultate bilaterally.

        a. Diminished breath sounds throughout.

        b. Occasional expiratory wheezing.

        c. Prolonged expiratory phase.

        d. Coarse rhonchi throughout the respiratory phase, especially during times of increased sputum production.

Diagnostic Tests

A. Pulmonary function test: Spirometry.

    1. Objective measurement of airflow limitation.

    2. Ratio between the volume of air forcibly exhaled after maximal inspiration (forced vital capacity [FVC]) and the volume of air forcibly exhaled during the first second (forced expiratory volume [FEV_1]). A ratio less than 0.7 after bronchodilator testing indicates obstruction.

    3. Reduced FEV_1 (reduction in expiratory flow rates).

    4. Possibly reduced FVC, usually to a lesser extent than the FEV_1.

B. Chest x-ray (see Figure 2.3).

    1. Hyperinflation, as evidenced by a flattened diaphragm and increased retrosternal air space.

    2. Hyperlucency of the lungs.

    3. Rapid tapering of the vascular markings.

C. Arterial blood gas (ABG).

    1. May reveal hypercapnia and/or hypoxemia.

        a. Early or mild COPD: Typically normal.

        b. Worsening as COPD progresses. Individuals with moderate to severe disease may have a chronic respiratory acidosis often with metabolic compensation as evidenced by increased serum bicarbonate.

    2. Can provide clues to the acuteness and severity of COPD in those individuals with an exacerbation.

D. Pulse oximetry.

    1. Used to assess arterial oxygen saturation. If the pulse oximetry is less than 92%, then an ABG is warranted.

E. Exercise testing (e.g., 6-minute walking distance).

    1. Objectively measures functional capacity by evaluating whether the individual has a reduction in walking distance.

    2. Useful for disability assessment, risk of mortality, and indicator of impairment of health status.

F. Laboratory evaluation.

    1. Alpha-1 antitrypsin screening: This should be assessed in those individuals with a family history of COPD at an early age and less than 45 years.

Differential Diagnosis

A. Bronchitis.

B. Chronic cough.

C. Congestive heart failure (CHF).

D. Emphysema.

E. Asthma.

Evaluation and Management Plan

A. General plan.

    1. The interventions listed in the following are part of the general plan for a COPD patient. We should incorporate these interventions in all COPD patients who meet criteria.

    2. Specific interventions.

        a. Smoking cessation.

            i. Literature has indicated that counseling from healthcare professionals increases cessation rates compared to self-initiated strategies.

            ii. A five-step program initiated by healthcare providers offers a helpful framework for cessation.

            iii. Nicotine replacement (e.g., gum, lozenge, transdermal patch) can increase long-term cessation rates.

            iv. Pharmacologic agents, such as varenicline and bupropion, can increase long-term cessation rates but should be used as an adjunct to an intervention program.

        b. Individuals should receive the influenza and pneumococcal.

        c. Reduction of risk factors such as avoidance of occupational irritants can help.

        d. Pulmonary rehabilitation lasting from 6 to 8 weeks has been shown to improve dyspnea, health status, exercise intolerance, and hospitalizations in patients with a recent exacerbation. This requires collaboration among multiple healthcare professionals.

        e. Treatment recommendations should consider the symptomatic assessment (ABCD group) and the individual's spirometric classification (GOLD 1–4). In addition, they should consider comorbid conditions and other medications.

        f. The GOLD categories one through four (spirometric grade) are used to classify the degree or severity of airflow limitation, which is identified using:

            i. GOLD 1: Mild, FEV_1 80% or greater than the predicted.

            ii. GOLD 2: Moderate, FEV_1 greater than or equal to 50% predicted but less than 80% predicted.

            iii. GOLD 3: Severe, FEV_1 greater than or equal to 30% predicted but less than 50% predicted.

            iv. GOLD 4: Very severe, FEV_1 is less than 30% predicted.

        g. Symptom assessment can be evaluated using the COPD Assessment Test (CAT) or the COPD Control Questionnaire (CCQ). The CAT is commonly used in the clinical setting and a score greater than t10 is associated with symptoms.

        h. The ABCD Assessment Tool (Groups A–D) is a measure of the individual's symptoms and history of exacerbations.

            i. Groups A and B indicate the individual has no more than one exacerbation with no hospitalizations and a CAT score less than 10 or greater than 10, respectively.

            ii. Groups C and D indicate the individual has more than two exacerbations or more than one exacerbation leading to hospitalization and a CAT score less than 10 or greater than 10, respectively.

    3. Management of stable COPD.

        a. Treatment should be individualized based on symptoms and risk for exacerbations.

    4. Goals of treatment.

        a. Symptom relief.

b. Increased exercise tolerance.

c. Improved health status.

d. Reduction of mortality.

e. Prevention of disease progression and exacerbations.

f. Management should include pharmacological and nonpharmacological interventions.

g. Smoking cessation and avoidance of occupational irritants are important.

h. The GOLD guidelines suggest treatment escalation or de-escalation in those with persistent symptoms or resolution of symptoms, respectively. Trials are needed to investigate treatment escalation and de-escalation.

5. Management of exacerbations.

a. Acute worsening in symptoms from baseline occurs.

i. Increased sputum, including purulence, increased dyspnea, and increased cough and/or wheezing.

b. Can be classified as:

i. Mild: Treatment with short-acting bronchodilators.

ii. Moderate: Treatment with short-acting bronchodilators plus antibiotics and/or oral steroids.

iii. Severe: Requires hospitalization or ED visits.

c. Symptoms can last 7 to 10 days and contribute to disease progression.

d. Severity of exacerbation is based on the individual's symptoms and whether respiratory failure is present.

i. No respiratory failure to respiratory rate 20 to 30/minute; no accessory muscle use, mental status change, or elevation in $PaCO_2$; hypoxemia improved with less than 35% of inspired oxygen.

ii. Respiratory failure, nonlife threatening to respiratory rate greater than 30/minute; use of accessory muscles, no change in mental status, $PaCO_2$ above baseline or 50 to 60 mmHg; hypoxemia improved with less than 30% of inspired oxygen.

iii. Respiratory failure, life threatening to respiratory rate greater than 30/minute; accessory muscle use, mental status changes, $PaCO_2$ above baseline or greater than 60 mmHg or presence of a respiratory acidosis with a pH less than 7.25; hypoxemia requiring greater than 40% of inspired oxygen or not improving with supplemental oxygen.

B. Pharmacotherapy.

1. See Table 2.2.

2. Adequate pharmacotherapy can reduce symptoms and severity of exacerbations, and improve overall health status.

3. Most medications are inhaled. It is essential that individuals receive education on proper technique.

4. Bronchodilators.

a. Often prescribed in COPD to prevent or reduce symptoms.

b. Central to symptom management.

c. Inhaled beta$_2$ agonists.

i. Functional antagonism to bronchoconstriction by relaxing airway smooth muscle.

ii. Short-acting (SABA) and long-acting (LABA) beta$_2$ agonists.

iii. SABAs: Typically last 4 to 6 hours; shown with regular use to improve symptoms and FEV_1 in COPD.

TABLE 2.2 COPD Medications
Beta₂ agonists (inhaled)
SABA
Fenoterol
Levalbuterol
Salbutamol (albuterol)
Terbutaline
LABA
Arformoterol
Formoterol
Salmeterol
Anticholinergics/Antimuscarinics (inhaled)
SAMA
Ipratropium bromide
Oxitropium bromide
LAMA
Aclidinium bromide
Glycopyrronium bromide
Tiotropium
Combination SABA plus short-acting anticholinergic (inhaled)
SABA/SAMA
Fenoterol/ipratropium
Salbutamol/ipratropium
Combination LABA plus long-acting anticholinergic (inhaled)
LABA/LAMA
Formoterol/aclidinium
Formoterol/glycopyrronium
Combination LABA plus ICS (inhaled)
LABA/ICS
Formoterol/budesonide
Formoterol/mometasone
Salmeterol/fluticasone
Vilanterol/fluticasone furoate
Methylxanthines (oral and intravenous)
Theophylline (SR)
Systemic Corticosteroids
Prednisone (oral)
Methylprednisolone (intravenous)
Phosphodiesterase-4 inhibitors (oral)
Roflumilast
Antibiotics (oral)
Azithromycin
Erythromycin

COPD, chronic obstructive pulmonary disease; ICS, inhaled corticosteroid; LABA, long-acting beta₂ agonist; LAMA, long-acting antimuscarinics; SABA, short-acting beta₂ agonist; SAMA, short-acting antimuscarinics.

iv. LABAs: Duration of 12 hours or more; shown to improve lung function, dyspnea, and reduce exacerbations.

d. Anticholinergics/antimuscarinics.

i. Blockage of acetylcholine on muscarinic receptors leading to relaxation of airway smooth muscle.

ii. Short-acting (SAMA) and long-acting (LAMA) antimuscarinics.

iii. SAMAs: Shown to improve symptoms and FEV_1 with regular or as needed use.

iv. LAMAs: Shown to improve lung function, dyspnea, and health status. Literature has shown that LAMAs compared to LABAs reduce exacerbations and decrease hospitalizations.

e. Methylxanthines.

i. Need to monitor therapeutic drug levels and for signs and symptoms of toxicity.

f. Inhaled corticosteroids (ICS).

i. No mortality benefit or modification in the long-term decline of the FEV_1 with ICS monotherapy.

ii. Severe COPD and regular use of ICS: Increased risk for pneumonia.

g. Combination inhaled therapy.

i. Combination of a SABA and SAMA: Superior in improving symptoms compared to either medication used alone.

ii. Combination of an LABA and LAMA: Improves FEV_1 and reduces symptoms and exacerbations compared to either medication used alone or compared to those individuals treated with a combination of ICS and LABA.

iii. Combination therapy with an ICS and LABA compared to monotherapy with either medication: Improves lung function and health status as well as reduces exacerbations.

h. Oral glucocorticoids.

i. Long-term risks: Preclude use in stable COPD.

ii. In acute exacerbations in hospitalized patients: Decreased treatment failure and relapse as well as improved lung function.

i. Phosphodiesterase$_4$ inhibitors.

i. Only one approved drug, roflumilast: Used for patients with a history of exacerbations and severe to very severe COPD.

ii. Has been shown to improve lung function and decrease moderate to severe exacerbations.

iii. Requires caution in those with depression and those who are underweight.

j. Antibiotics.

i. Reduced exacerbations: Azithromycin 250 mg daily or 500 mg three times a week OR erythromycin 500 mg twice daily for 1 year.

1) Use of azithromycin: Association with increased antibiotic resistance.

ii. No data indicating efficacy of chronic antibiotic therapy beyond 1 year.

k. Mucolytics.

i. Reduced risk of exacerbation in select populations.

5. Pharmacologic treatment using the ABCD Assessment Tool.

a. Utilization of an algorithm based on the ABCD Assessment Tool Groups A–D.

b. Group A.

i. Should be placed on a bronchodilator.

ii. The provider should evaluate drug effectiveness and decide to continue, stop, or try an alternative bronchodilator class.

c. Group B.

i. Should be initiated on a long-acting bronchodilator. Choice of long-acting bronchodilator should be based on symptom relief.

ii. Two bronchodilators: Recommended for individuals with persistent dyspnea.

d. Group C.

i. Should be initiated on a bronchodilator; preferred choice is a LAMA secondary to superior exacerbation prevention.

ii. Individuals with persistent dyspnea: Two long-acting bronchodilators (LABA/LAMA) OR combination of long-acting bronchodilator and ICS (LABA/ICS). The primary choice is LABA/LAMA secondary to the increased risk of pneumonia in certain individuals on ICS.

e. Group D.

i. LABA/LAMA combination for certain patients. In individuals with findings suggestive of asthma–COPD overlap, initiation of LABA/ICS may be the first choice.

ii. Individuals with persistent exacerbations despite being on LABA/LAMA triple inhaled therapy with a LABA/LAMA/ICS OR switch to a LABA/ICS. However, there is no clinical evidence that switching to a LABA/ICS from LABA/LAMA will improve symptoms.

iii. For continued exacerbations despite triple inhaled therapy, possible:

1) Addition of roflumilast.

2) Addition of a macrolide, specifically azithromycin.

3) Stopping the ICS.

6. Hospital medication management and medical therapy of COPD exacerbations.

a. Combination of SABA and anticholinergics.

b. Possible systemic steroids.

i. Have been shown to shorten recovery time, improve oxygenation, and improve the risk of early relapse and treatment failure.

ii. Oral prednisone recommended at 40 mg daily for 5 days.

c. Consideration of oral antibiotics when signs of bacterial infection are present.

d. Possible O_2 therapy and noninvasive ventilation.

i. Noninvasive ventilation: Shown to reduce intubation rates, mortality, and hospital length of stay.

7. Invasive mechanical ventilation: Warranted in patients who are unable to undergo or fail noninvasive ventilation, are hemodynamically unstable, have status postarrest, have profound hypoxemia in patients not able to tolerate noninvasive ventilation, massive aspiration, and encounter significant changes in levels of consciousness.

C. Discharge instructions.

1. Be aware that these vary based on the severity of the underlying COPD and exacerbation.

2. Review all clinical (e.g., improved dyspnea, sputum production, cognition) and laboratory data.

3. Assess continual need for oxygen therapy. Patients on chronic home O_2 should resume their baseline O_2 requirements.
4. Check functional status.
5. Ensure adequate home resources.
6. Activity.
   a. Pulmonary rehabilitation.
      i. Shown to reduce hospitalizations, as well as improve dyspnea and health status.
      ii. Indicated in all patients with symptoms and/or high risk for exacerbation.
      iii. Early rehabilitation has been associated with improved mortality.
   b. Regular physical activity.
      i. Combination interval training with strength training.
      ii. Strong predictor of mortality.
7. Diet.
   a. May vary depending on underlying comorbid conditions such as diabetes, heart failure, or renal disease.
   b. Nutritional supplementation: Recommended; should be considered in malnourished COPD patients.
8. Medications (see section "Pharmacotherapy").
   a. Bronchodilators.
      i. Most patients are likely to receive two long-acting bronchodilators (LABA/LAMA) or a long-acting bronchodilator and ICS (LABA/ICS).
   b. Additional agent: The provider may choose to initiate a long-term macrolide or roflumilast in patients who meet criteria and continue to have exacerbations despite multimedication inhaled therapy.
   c. Other drugs: Medication reconciliation and continuation of medications for comorbid conditions are necessary.
9. Treatment plan.
   a. Evaluation of psychosocial needs and home resources such as availability of home O_2.
   b. Inclusion of family in the treatment and education plan.
   c. Evaluation maintenance therapy understanding.
   d. Ensuring of understanding of withdrawal medications prescribed for an acute exacerbation such as steroids.
   e. Assessment of inhaler technique.
   f. Pulmonary hygiene (e.g., deep breathing).
   g. Smoking cessation counseling.
   h. Encouragement of pneumococcal and influenza vaccinations.
   i. Setting up of pulmonary rehabilitation.
   j. Management of comorbid conditions such as gastroesophageal reflux disease (GERD) and heart failure.
10. Discuss with patient.
    a. Discuss signs and symptoms associated with infection and/or exacerbations such as fever, chills, increased dyspnea, and increasing sputum production or change in sputum color.
    b. Instruct patients on the importance of medication compliance and physical activity to reduce the occurrence of exacerbations, reduce symptoms, and improve quality of life.

Follow-Up

A. Follow-up with a primary care physician or pulmonologist, ideally within 1 to 4 weeks of discharge.
   1. Especially during initiation, escalation, and de-escalation in therapy.
   2. With new or worsening symptoms.
   3. Posthospitalization.
B. Association of early follow-up with fewer readmissions.

Consultation/Referral

A. Consultation with a pulmonologist: In patients with progressively worsening symptoms, severe or very severe COPD, frequent exacerbations, and respiratory failure.

Special/Geriatric Considerations

A. Chronic use of oxygen is indicated for patients with severe hypoxemia at rest and chronic respiratory failure.
B. Patients should be evaluated and treated for comorbid conditions such as heart failure, obstructive sleep apnea, obesity, hypoventilation syndrome, and so forth.
C. Education alone has not been shown to change behaviors; however, education and self-management with a case manager may prevent exacerbation complications.
D. Physical activity is highly encouraged given its strong mortality prediction.
E. Nutritional supplements may be indicated in malnourished patients.
F. Patients should be considered for lung volume reduction surgery if they have upper-lobe predominance emphysema.
G. Patients with very severe COPD and advanced systemic symptoms may be considered for lung transplantation.
H. Discussions with patients and families regarding palliative and end-of-life care should take place in the event the patient becomes critically ill.

Bibliography

American Lung Association. (2013). *Taking her breath away: The rise of COPD in women.* Chicago, IL: Author. Retrieved from https://www.lung.org/assets/documents/research/rise-of-copd-in-women-full.pdf

Decramer, M. L., Chapman, K. R., Dahl, R., Frith, P., Devouassoux, G., Fritscher, C., & McBryan, D. (2013). Once-daily indacaterol versus tiotropium for patients with severe chronic obstructive pulmonary disease (INVIGORATE): A randomized, blinded, parallel-group study. *The Lancet Respiratory Medicine, 1,* 524–533. doi:10.1016/S2213-2600(13)70158-9

Global Initiative for Chronic Obstructive Lung Disease. (2017). Global strategy for the diagnosis, management, and prevention of chronic obstructive pulmonary disease. Retrieved from https://www.goldcopd.org

Karner, C., Chong, J., & Poole, P. (2012). Tiotropium versus placebo for chronic obstructive pulmonary disease. *Cochrane Database of Systematic Reviews, 2014*(7), CD009285. doi:10.1002/14651858.CD009285.pub3

Vogelmeier, C., Hederer, B., Glaab, T., Schmidt, H., Rutten-van Molken, M., Beeh, K., . . . Fabbri, L. M. (2011). Tiotropium versus salmeterol for the prevention of exacerbations of COPD. *New England Journal of Medicine, 364,* 1093–1103. doi:10.1056/NEJMoa1008378

Pleural Effusions

E. Moneé Carter-Griffin

Definition

A. Result of excess fluid production or decreased absorption of fluid in the pleural space.

Incidence

A. There are an estimated 1 to 1.5 million cases annually.
B. In general, the incidence is similar in both males and females. However, certain causes are more likely in males or females.

Pathogenesis

A. Pleural effusions are a manifestation of an underlying disease process.
B. Effusions can be transudative or exudative.
  1. Transudative effusions are typically due to imbalance that occurs between the hydrostatic pressure and oncotic pressure.
  2. Exudative effusions are the result of an alteration of the pleural surface such as pleural or lung inflammation, impairment of lymphatic drainage, and so forth.

Predisposing Factors

A. Any disease that may lead to accumulation of pleural fluid. The most common causes of pleural effusions are heart failure, malignancy, and pneumonia.
B. Diseases that can predispose a patient to a transudative effusion.
  1. Heart failure.
  2. Cirrhosis.
  3. Nephrotic syndrome.
C. Diseases that can predispose a patient to an exudative effusion.
  1. Pneumonia (parapneumonic effusion or empyema).
  2. Malignancy.
  3. Pancreatitis/pancreatic disease.
  4. Trauma.

Subjective Data

A. Common complaints/symptoms.
  1. Patients may have complaints of cough, pleuritic chest pain, and dyspnea.
  2. Patients may have additional symptoms or clinical manifestations secondary to the underlying etiology for the pleural effusion.
B. Review of systems.
  1. Depending on the suspected etiology of the effusion, the provider may want to inquire about heart failure, known liver disease or chronic alcoholism, recent trauma, history of cancer, occupational exposures, recent signs and symptoms of respiratory infection, and so on.

Physical Examination

A. Typically, no physical findings when the pleural effusion is less than 300 mL.
B. Other findings.
  1. Diminished breath sounds.
  2. Dullness on percussion.
  3. Pleural friction rub.
  4. Decreased tactile fremitus.
C. Possible other findings such as fever and edema, depending on the etiology.

Diagnostic Tests

A. Chest x-ray (see Figure 2.4).
  1. Blunting of costophrenic angle in upright posteroanterior x-ray when 175 mL or more is present.
B. Smaller pleural effusions observed in lateral decubitus x-rays.

C. Failure of a pleural effusion to layer on a lateral decubitus x-ray. This may indicate a loculated pleural effusion.
D. Chest CT: Possible for evaluation of a loculated pleural effusion.
E. Ultrasonography: Can be used to evaluate the size of the pleural effusion and location.
F. Diagnostic thoracentesis.
  1. Should be performed in patients whose etiology is unclear and who fail to respond to therapy.
  2. Pleural fluid for diagnosis. Send for glucose, lactate dehydrogenase (LDH), pH, cell count, protein, and culture to aid with a possible diagnosis. Serum blood levels of LDH, total protein, and glucose are needed for comparison.
  3. Light's criteria: Used to differentiate between transudative and exudative pleural effusions.
    a. Exudative if one of the following is present.
      i. Ratio of pleural fluid to serum protein is greater than 0.5.
      ii. Ratio of pleural fluid to serum LDH is greater than 0.6.
      iii. Pleural fluid LDH is greater than two-thirds the normal serum LDH.
  4. Additional testing may be indicated when trying to identify the etiology.

Differential Diagnosis

A. First, it is important to determine if the pleural effusion is transudate or exudate using Light's criteria in order to establish a differential diagnosis.
B. Transudate pleural effusion.
C. Congestive heart failure (CHF).
D. Cirrhosis.
E. Exudate pleural effusion.
F. Pneumonia.
G. Cancer.
H. Tuberculosis.
I. Pulmonary embolism.

Evaluation and Management Plan

A. General plan.
  1. For transudative effusions, manage the underlying disease process such as diuretics for patients with effusions due to heart failure.
  2. Specific interventions.
    a. Monitoring of chest x-rays: As needed pending the size, symptoms associated with the effusion, and following treatment to evaluate for reaccumulating fluid.
    b. Therapeutic thoracentesis: Used for patients with refractory, large pleural effusions and/or severe respiratory compromise to relieve symptoms. Diagnostic evaluation may be required if concerned for malignancy, infectious process, and so forth.
      i. Patients with malignant pleural effusions may require more than one thoracentesis due to reaccumulating fluid.
      ii. Patients who need frequent thoracentesis may require a pleurodesis or indwelling tunneled pleural catheter for home drainage. The patient and family will require teaching about home use of the tunneled pleural catheter.
    c. Chest tube.
      i. Required for a parapneumonic effusion or an empyema, but ultimately the patient will need to be treated with antibiotics and possible surgical intervention.

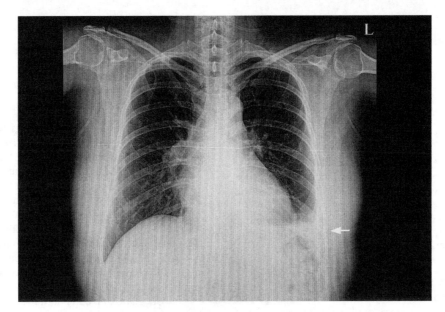

FIGURE 2.4 Chest x-ray of left pleural effusion.
Source: By Tomatheart/Shutterstock.

ii. Required for patients with a hemothorax (bloody pleural effusion).

B. Patient/family teaching points.

1. Teach patients that it may help to cough or take a deep breath by holding a pillow against your chest to prevent pain.

2. Practice smoking cessation and avoid secondhand smoke.

3. Keep hydrated.

4. Use an incentive spirometer for frequent deep breathing and coughing exercises.

C. Pharmacotherapy—depends on the etiology of pleural effusion.

1. Antibiotics.

a. For use in parapneumonic effusions, empyemas, and abscesses.

b. Use empiric coverage and consider the patient's age, comorbidities, and clinical picture before tailoring the final selection of antibiotics.

c. In general, the antimicrobial coverage should cover anaerobic organisms.

2. Vasodilators and diuretics: For use in pleural effusions related to CHF and pulmonary edema.

3. Anticoagulants: For use in pleural effusions due to pulmonary emboli.

D. Discharge instructions.

1. Instruct patients to report any increased work in breathing, fevers, and pain that does not go away or gets worse. Take medications as prescribed.

Follow-Up

A. Patients in the hospital: Monitor with serial chest x-rays and/or based on their symptoms.

B. Etiology of the effusion: Determines the course and frequency of outpatient follow-up.

Consultation/Referral

A. Thoracentesis: This can be completed by a hospitalist, pulmonologist, or interventional radiologist. If a more invasive procedure such as a surgical intervention is indicated, then a cardiothoracic surgeon will need to be consulted.

B. Further referrals may be indicated depending on the etiology of the effusion. If the effusion is malignant, then oncology will need to be consulted.

Bibliography

Bhatnagar, R., & Maskell, N. (2015). The modern diagnosis and management of pleural effusions. *British Medical Journal, 351*, 26–30. doi:10.1136/bmj.h4520

Kummerfeldt, C. E., Pastis, N. J., & Huggins, J. T. (2017). Pleural diseases. In S. C. McKean, J. J. Ross, D. D. Dressler, & D. B. Scheurer (Eds.), *Principles and practice of hospital medicine* (2nd ed., pp. 1923–1932). New York, NY: McGraw-Hill.

Saguil, A., Wyrick, K., & Hallgren, J. (2014). Diagnostic approach to pleural effusion. *American Family Physician, 90*, 99–104. Retrieved from https://www.aafp.org/afp/2014/0715/p99.html

Pneumonia

E. Moneè Carter-Griffin

Definition

A. An infection of the lungs that can have varying degrees of severity.

B. Caused by bacteria, viruses, or fungi.

C. Can be further divided into four types: Community, hospital, ventilator acquired, and aspiration.

Incidence

A. Pneumonia (combined with influenza) is the eighth leading cause of mortality in the United States, accounting for approximately 50,000 deaths annually.

B. Thirty-day mortality is higher in elderly patients treated for hospital-acquired pneumonia (HAP) compared to community-acquired pneumonia (CAP).

C. Pneumonia is the third leading cause of ED visits that led to a hospitalization, with the highest prevalence in patients 65 to 84 years.

D. It is the most common cause of readmissions for the elderly population.

E. It accounts for the top 10 most costly hospitalizations in the United States, with approximately $10.6 billion spent for 1.1 million hospital stays.

F. Most common cause of sepsis and septic shock.

Pathogenesis

A. A pathogenic microorganism invades the lung parenchyma. Neutrophils aggregate to the site of invasion and begin to phagocytize the microorganisms and release an extracellular trap.

B. The immune response is activated. Inflammatory mediators are released, causing the capillaries to become permeable and an exudative fluid to be formed. The protein rich fluid containing neutrophils, bacteria, fibrin, and so forth, fills the alveoli, leading to a lung consolidation.

Predisposing Factors

A. An impaired immune response and/or dysfunction of the body's defense mechanism, HIV.

B. Advanced age.

C. Smoking.

D. Chronic lung disease (e.g., chronic obstructive pulmonary disease [COPD] and asthma).

E. Other chronic comorbid conditions (e.g., heart failure, diabetes).

F. Recent respiratory viral infection.

G. Excessive alcohol consumption.

Subjective Data

A. Common complaints/symptoms.
  1. Cough with sputum production (see Figure 2.3).
  2. Fever.
  3. Chills.
  4. Altered mental status or confusion, especially in the elderly.
  5. Pleuritic chest pain.

B. Common/typical scenario.
  1. Patients typically present with sudden onset of symptoms such as shortness of breath, productive cough, and fever. They may also complain of chills and malaise.

C. Family and social history.
  May be more prevalent in smokers, among the elderly, and in the chronically ill.

D. Review of symptoms.
  1. Symptoms may vary depending on the age, activity level, and underlying comorbid conditions. Elderly people typically present differently than younger adults.
  2. The provider should inquire about onset, severity, and associated symptoms.
  3. Assessment of recent respiratory viral illnesses is important, especially given the correlation of pneumonia following influenza.
  4. It may help to enquire about recent sick contacts.

Physical Examination

A. General: Vital signs.
  1. Fever, which may occur. Note that approximately 30% of patients are afebrile on presentation.
  2. Tachycardia, which may or may not be present.
  3. Possibly high respiratory rate; this may be normal or increased.

B. Neurological.
  1. More likely to see changes in the elderly. Patients can be described as having confusion, decreased interactions, and/or "acting differently."

C. Respiratory.
  1. Rales/crackles on auscultation in the affected area. Patients may also have rhonchi.
  2. Dullness on percussion in the affected area.
  3. Increased tactile fremitus in the affected area.
  4. Possible pleural friction rub.
  5. Decreased breath sounds.

D. Possible other findings.
  1. Cyanosis, respiratory failure, and septic shock in patients with a more virulent type of pneumonia, multilobar pneumonia, age, and/or comorbid conditions.

Diagnostic Tests

A. Chest x-ray.
  1. Evidence of an infiltrate, which can be patchy or a dense consolidation of a lobe(s) or segment.

B. Sputum culture and gram stain.
  1. Used to identify the microorganism responsible for the pneumonia.
  2. Most sensitive if the patient can provide an adequate specimen and has not recently been treated or is not currently receiving treatment with antibiotics.
  3. Intubated patient: Obtain an endotracheal aspirate.

C. Blood cultures.
  1. Usually indicated for patients with more severe forms of pneumonia, specifically CAP.
  2. Most common pathogen isolated in patients with CAP: *Streptococcus pneumoniae*. However, in more severe infections, other microorganisms may be present.

D. Urinary antigen testing.
  1. Used to assess for pneumococcal pneumonia, mycoplasma pneumonia, and Legionnaire's disease.
  2. Rapid and simple; however, do not provide information for narrowing of antibiotics.

E. Serum procalcitonin.
  1. Can assist the provider with antibiotic duration in conjunction with the patient's clinical presentation.
  2. No recommended use of procalcitonin in patients with hospital or ventilator-acquired pneumonia according to Infectious Diseases Society of America and the American Thoracic Society guidelines.

F. Comprehensive metabolic panel.
  1. Can assist with risk stratification and sequela of pneumonia.

G. Complete blood count.
  1. Assessment of a leukocytosis or leukopenia.

H. Arterial blood gas (ABG).
  1. May be indicated in more severe presentations such as cyanosis or respiratory failure to evaluate for hypoxemia and/or hypercapnia.

I. Chest CT scan.
  1. Not typically indicated, especially if one is able to obtain a good-quality chest x-ray.

Differential Diagnosis

A. COPD.

B. Asthma.

C. Pulmonary edema.

D. Bronchiectasis.

E. Lung cancer.

F. Pulmonary embolism.

G. Bronchitis.

H. Viral or bacterial pneumonia.

I. Pneumocystis pneumonia (PCP).

Evaluation and Management Plan

A. General plan.
  1. Management of pneumonia: Dependent on the severity of the disease, classification or type of pneumonia (e.g., community vs. hospital acquired), and pathogens involved.
  2. Supportive care, such as oxygen therapy or other methods of respiratory support (e.g., noninvasive

ventilation, invasive mechanical ventilation); this should be considered in those patients with hypoxemia and/or respiratory failure.

3. Patients presenting with sepsis due to pneumonia. These patients should receive care in accordance with the sepsis guidelines.

4. Guidelines suggest that antimicrobial therapy be de-escalated rather than fixed therapy.

5. Transitioning to oral therapy. Oral therapy is appropriate once patients' clinical status has improved, and they are hemodynamically stable.

6. Patients with coexisting Influenza A. Early treatment with oseltamivir or zanamivir is appropriate.

7. Systematic corticosteroids: May be appropriate in certain patient populations who present with severe CAP.

B. CAP.

1. Evaluation of patients for hospital admission. Use the CURB-65 criteria, which evaluates/looks at confusion, uremia, respiratory rate, low blood pressure, and age 65 years or greater, or pneumonia severity index (PSI) to identify patients who can be treated as outpatient versus inpatient.

2. Duration of treatment. Patients should receive a minimum of 5 days of treatment and literature suggests that more than 7 days is typically not needed.

3. Antibiotic therapy, which focuses on the likely pathogen and severity.

    a. The most common outpatient pathogens are *S. pneumoniae, Haemophilus influenzae, Mycoplasma pneumoniae, Chlamydia pneumoniae, Legionella*, and respiratory viruses.

        i. Previously healthy patients with no exposure to antibiotics within the past 3 months should be started on a macrolide. If they are unable to tolerate a macrolide, then doxycycline may be used.

        ii. Patients with chronic comorbid conditions (e.g., heart failure, liver or renal disease, diabetes) or antibiotic therapy within the past 3 months should be started on a respiratory fluoroquinolone (e.g., moxifloxacin, levofloxacin, or gemifloxacin) **OR** beta-lactam plus a macrolide. Remember, a beta-lactam alone will not work for atypical pneumonia because of the lack of a beta-lactam ring.

    b. The most common inpatient, non-ICU pathogens are *S. pneumoniae, M. pneumoniae, C. pneumoniae, H. influenzae, Legionella* species, aspiration, and respiratory viruses.

        i. Patients should be treated with a respiratory fluoroquinolone **OR** a beta-lactam plus a macrolide.

    c. The most common inpatient, ICU pathogens are *S. pneumoniae, Staphylococcus aureus, Legionella* species, gram-negative bacilli, and *H. influenzae*.

        i. Patients should be started on a beta-lactam (e.g., cefotaxime, ceftriaxone, or ampicillin–sulbactam) plus either azithromycin or a respiratory fluoroquinolone.

        ii. If the patient has a penicillin allergy, then a respiratory fluoroquinolone and aztreonam are recommended.

        iii. Gram-negative organisms are selectively responsive to aztreonam treatment.

    d. If a pseudomonal infection is suspected, then providers should prescribe one of the following.

        i. Antipneumococcal, antipseudomonal beta-lactam plus levofloxacin **OR,**

        ii. Beta-lactam plus an aminoglycoside and azithromycin **OR,**

        iii. Beta-lactam plus an aminoglycoside and antipneumococcal fluoroquinolone.

    e. If methicillin-resistant *Staphylococcus aureus* (MRSA) is suspected, then intravenous vancomycin or linezolid is indicated.

C. HAP.

1. Develops 2 or more days after admission to the hospital.

2. Use of a local antibiogram tailored to HAP pathogens and susceptibilities for empiric coverage as recommended by guidelines.

3. Antibiotic treatment: Recommended 7-day course.

    a. Empiric coverage depends on the patient's mortality risk and suspicion for multidrug resistant (MDR) pathogens.

    b. Patients not at high risk for mortality or likelihood of MDR pathogens can be placed on piperacillin-tazobactam (Zosyn) **OR** cefepime **OR** levofloxacin.

    c. Patients not at high risk for mortality but who have factors that may increase their likelihood of MRSA should be placed on cefepime **OR** levofloxacin **OR** meropenem **OR** aztreonam plus vancomycin or linezolid (second line due to toxic effects if vancomycin cannot be used).

    d. Patients with a high mortality risk, coverage for pseudomonas, or who have received intravenous antibiotics in 3 months should be started on:

        i. Piperacillin-tazobactam (Zosyn) **OR** cefepime **OR** levofloxacin **OR** meropenem **OR** amikacin/gentamicin/tobramycin **OR** aztreonam plus vancomycin or linezolid.

        ii. Providers should cover for MRSA and pick two additional medications while avoiding prescribing two beta-lactams.

D. Ventilator-acquired pneumonia (VAP).

1. A pneumonia that develops more than 2 days after intubation and mechanical ventilation.

2. Use of a local antibiogram tailored to the ICU population, VAP pathogens, and susceptibilities for adequate coverage as recommended per guidelines.

3. Antibiotic treatment: Recommended 7-day course.

    a. *S. aureus, Pseudomonas*, and other gram-negative bacilli coverage should be included in all empiric regimens.

    b. Patients with risk factors for MRSA should receive empiric coverage with vancomycin or linezolid.

    c. Patients with no known risk factors for MRSA and suspected of methicillin-susceptible *Staphylococcus aureus* (MSSA), then the suggested regimen includes piperacillin-tazobactam, cefepime, levofloxacin, or meropenem. If the patient has proven MSSA, then the preferred agents are cefazolin or nafcillin.

    d. Patients with risk factors for gram-negative infection, including pseudomonas and resistant microorganisms, should receive treatment with two antipseudomonal drugs.

        i. Piperacillin-tazobactam **OR,**

        ii. Cefepime **OR,**

        iii. Meropenem **OR,**

        iv. Aztreonam **OR,**

        v. Ciprofloxacin.

    e. Guidelines recommend against the routine use of aminoglycosides and colistin if adequate coverage is available with alternative antibiotics.

E. Discharge instructions.

1. Discharge criteria. These primarily focus on improvement in the clinical status/condition.

a. Resolution of fever (e.g., <38°C).

b. Improving symptoms (e.g., dyspnea, cough, sputum production).

c. Heart rate less than 100 bpm.

d. Respiratory rate less than 24/minute.

e. Oxygen saturations greater than 90%.

f. Diminishing leukocytosis.

g. Maintaining oral intake.

h. Systolic blood pressure greater than 90 mmHg.

i. Return to baseline mentation.

2. Activity.

a. Regular or baseline activity as tolerated.

3. Diet.

a. Comorbid conditions such as diabetes, heart failure, or renal disease: May vary.

b. No underlying comorbid conditions: Resumption of regular diet.

4. Medications.

a. Antibiotics: Duration of 7 days. This includes the days the patient received antibiotics while hospitalized.

b. Other drugs. Medication reconciliation and continuation of medications for comorbid conditions.

5. Treatment plan.

a. Important for patient to complete the full course of antibiotics even if feeling better.

b. Coughing with sputum production: Normal. This should improve over time.

c. Vaccinations such as influenza annually and pneumococcal disease necessary for those at risk.

d. Pulmonary hygiene (e.g., deep breathing).

e. Smoking cessation counseling.

f. Remaining hydrated.

g. Managing comorbid conditions.

6. Discuss with patient.

a. Stress that patients should contact their provider if they develop fever or worsening symptoms such as increased cough and dyspnea despite antibiotic therapy, decreased appetite, nausea, and mentation changes.

b. Reemphasize the importance of completing antibiotic therapy to reduce reoccurrence and avoid resistance emergence.

Follow-Up

A. Follow-up is highly dependent on the type and severity of pneumonia as well as functional status and comorbid conditions.

B. Patients in the outpatient setting typically see improvement in symptoms within 3 to 7 days, so failure to see improvement or clinical deterioration should be dealt with immediately.

C. Patients discharged from the hospital should be seen 1 to 2 weeks after discharge.

Consultation/Referral

A. Outpatient management typically does not require a referral unless the patient's clinical status worsens, in which case the patient should be sent to the hospital.

B. Inpatient management may include a pulmonologist and infectious disease pending the severity of the pneumonia and the patient's condition.

Special/Geriatric Considerations

A. The elderly should be instructed to receive pneumococcal and influenza vaccinations.

B. All patients should be counseled regarding smoking cessation.

Bibliography

American Thoracic Society. (2018). Top 20 pneumonia facts. Retrieved from https://www.thoracic.org/patients/patient-resources/resources/top-pneumonia-facts.pdf

Hines, A. L., Barrett, M. L., Jiang, J., & Steiner, C. A. (2014). *Conditions with the largest number of adult hospital readmissions by payer, 2011.* Retrieved from https://www.hcup-us.ahrq.gov/reports/statbriefs/sb172-Conditions-Readmissions-Payer.pdf

Kalil, A. C., Metersky, M. L., Klompas, M., Muscedere, J., Sweeney, D. A., Palmer, L. B., & Brozek, J. L. (2016). Management of adults with hospital-acquired and ventilator-associated pneumonia: 2016 clinical practice guidelines by the Infectious Diseases Society of America and the American Thoracic Society. *Clinical Infectious Diseases, 63,* e61–e111. doi:10.1093/cid/ciw353

Klompas, M. (2017). Health care and hospital-acquired pneumonia. In S. C. McKean, J. J. Ross, D. D. Dressler, & D. B. Scheuer (Eds.), *Principles and practice of hospital medicine* (2nd ed., pp. 1514–1518). New York, NY: McGraw-Hill.

Kochanek, K. D., Murphy, S. L., Xu, J., & Tejada-Vera, B. (2016). Deaths: Final data for 2014. *National Vital Statistics Reports, 65,* 1–122. Retrieved from https://www.cdc.gov/nchs/data/nvsr/nvsr65/nvsr65_04.pdf

Mandell, L. A., Wunderlink, R. G., Anzueto, A., Bartlett, J. G., Campbell, G. D., Dean, N. C., & Whitney, C. G. (2007). Infectious Diseases Society of America/American Thoracic Society consensus guidelines on the management of community-acquired pneumonia in adults. *Clinical Infectious Diseases, 44,* S27–S72. doi:10.1086/511159

Musher, D. M. (2017). Community-acquired pneumonia. In S. C. McKean, J. J. Ross, D. D. Dressler, & D. B. Scheurer (Eds.), *Principles and practice of hospital medicine* (2nd ed., pp. 1503–1513). New York, NY: McGraw-Hill.

Musher, D. M., & Thorner, A. R. (2014). Community-acquired pneumonia. *New England Journal of Medicine, 371,* 1619–1628. doi:10.1056/NEJMra1312885

Wunderlink, R. G., & Waterer, G. W. (2014). Community-acquired pneumonia. *New England Journal of Medicine, 370,* 543–541. doi:10.1056/NEJMcp1214869

Pulmonary Embolism

E. Moneé Carter-Griffin

Definition

A. A blockage of a pulmonary artery or one of the smaller branches. Most commonly, pulmonary embolism (PE) is the result of an embolic thrombus formation elsewhere in the body (e.g., lower extremity).

Incidence

A. PE is more common in patients with deep vein thrombosis (DVT).

B. It affects more than 600,000 people annually.

C. An estimated 60,000 to 100,000 people die annually.

D. Approximately one-third of patients will have a recurrence within 10 years.

Pathogenesis

A. A thrombus forms secondary to a hypercoagulable state, injury to the vascular endothelium, and venostasis, which concentrates blood clotting factors at the site of vessel injury. Clot formation occurs as a result of blood pooling.

B. The clot can dislodge from the extremity, travel through the venous system, move through the right side of the heart, and obstruct a pulmonary artery or the smaller branches.

Large enough obstructions can prevent blood flow to the affected area, creating a ventilation/perfusion mismatch leading to respiratory failure and/or increase the pulmonary artery pressure, resulting in right-sided heart failure.

Predisposing Factors

A. Factor V mutation.
B. Protein C or S deficiency.
C. Malignancy.
D. Immobility.
E. Trauma.
F. Surgery.
G. Smoking.
H. Obesity.
I. Prior PE.
J. Chronic diseases such as heart failure and chronic obstructive pulmonary disease (COPD).
K. Prolonged travel.

Subjective Data

A. Common complaints/symptoms.
  1. These can vary depending on the degree of clot burden.
  2. Patients may be asymptomatic, especially in the setting of a small segmental branch PE. The condition is usually found incidentally in these cases.
  3. Symptoms may include:
    a. Pleuritic chest pain.
    b. Dyspnea/Tachypnea.
    c. Hypoxia.
    d. Cough with possible blood-tinged sputum production.
    e. Tachycardia.
    f. Dizziness or syncope.
    g. Hypotension/shock with a massive PE.
    h. Recent symptoms associated with a DVT (e.g., extremity pain, warmth, erythema, edema).
B. Family and social history.
C. The provider should assess symptom onset and any associated risk factors for PE development such as history or current malignancy, decreased mobility, travel, recent surgeries, and so forth.
D. It is important for the provider to assess for family history of clot formation or known factor deficiencies.

Physical Examination

A. Findings depend on the degree of clot burden.
B. Perform a general examination, which may reveal diaphoresis, fever, and tachycardia. On presentation, most patients are hemodynamically stable.
C. Assess neurological status. Patients may present with syncope, altered mentation, or agitation.
D. Assess the respiratory rate. In more significant PEs, the rate will be increased. Auscultation of breath sounds may reveal rales or crackles.
E. Perform a cardiac examination. Patients may have a murmur, accentuated second heart sound, or S3/S4 gallop.
F. Extremities may reveal signs of a deep vein thrombosis such as pain, edema, or erythema.

Diagnostic Tests

A. D-dimer (age adjusted).
  1. High sensitivity: With negative results and a low probability of a PE.

  2. Most reliable in young patients with no comorbid conditions and short symptom onset.
  3. Can have nonspecific elevations in the elderly and those with other acute illnesses requiring hospitalization.
B. Chest CT Angiography (CTA).
  1. Allows for direct visualization of the emboli.
  2. Considered the standard of care for diagnosing patients with high probability of a PE or low/intermediate probability but positive D-dimer.
  3. Right ventricular (RV) dilation: Associated with short-term adverse outcomes.
C. Ventilation/Perfusion (V/Q) Lung Scan.
  1. An alternative to the chest CTA, especially in the setting of contraindications such as renal failure.
  2. Evaluates for perfusion defects, which are nonspecific and only present in one-third of patients with PE.
  3. Increased likelihood of nonconclusive results in patients older than 75 years.
D. Echocardiography.
  1. Often indirectly helps diagnose PE in conjunction with the patient's clinical presentation.
  2. Can also be utilized as a prognostic factor in PE.
  3. Possible findings consistent with a PE: Acute RV enlargement and in some cases dysfunction, evidence of pulmonary hypertension with elevated RV systolic pressures, and possible flattening of the septum.
  4. May be able to visualize an intracardiac thrombi.
  5. RV dilation: Associated with an increased risk for adverse outcomes.
E. Ultrasonography.
  1. Can assist in the diagnosis of PE.
F. Additional diagnostics for acute risk stratification.
  1. Pulmonary embolism severity index (PESI).
    a. Used to predict the 30-day outcomes/mortality in patients with acute PE.
    b. Score greater than 106 on the original PESI: High risk for morbidity and mortality.
    c. Score greater than 1 on the simplified PESI: High risk for morbidity and mortality.
  2. Troponin.
    a. Elevated troponin levels in patients presenting or receiving treatment for PE: Associated with adverse outcomes.
  3. N-Terminal pro brain natriuretic peptide (NT-proBNP).
  4. Elevated levels: Associated with adverse outcomes (in literature).

Differential Diagnosis

A. Pericarditis.
B. Pleuritis.
C. Musculoskeletal pain.

Evaluation and Management Plan

A. General plan.
  1. Diagnosis of a PE requires the provider to account for the patient's clinical presentation as well as evaluating diagnostic tests.
  2. Treatment recommendations are highly dependent on the patient's clinical status including respiratory and hemodynamic stability at the time of presentation.
  3. In the clinical setting and literature, PEs have been described as low risk, submassive, and massive.
    a. Low risk PEs: Patients with hemodynamic stability, no elevation in biomarkers, and no evidence of RV dysfunction on imaging.

b. Submassive PEs: Patients with hemodynamic stability but evidence of RV dysfunction on imaging and/or biomarker elevation.

c. Massive PEs: Patient with hemodynamic instability, elevation in biomarkers, and evidence of RV dysfunction.

4. Ideally, patients should have pretest clinical assessment, diagnostics with consideration of risk stratification, and initiation of treatment.

5. Low to intermediate probability of PE.

a. Pretest clinical assessment.

i. Wells Clinical Prediction Rule for PE. Patients are evaluated using seven variables in which they can receive 1 to 3 points. A score of 2 to 6 points indicates a moderate risk and a score greater than 6 indicates high risk.

ii. Revised Geneva Score. Patients are evaluated using eight variables in which they can receive 1 to 5 points. A score of 4 to 10 points indicates an intermediate risk and a score greater than 11 indicates high risk.

iii. Appropriate for patients who are hemodynamically stable. Patients with a high probability of PE should proceed immediately to diagnostic testing.

b. Age-adjusted D-dimer.

i. If negative: No further imaging needed.

ii. If positive: Further imaging needed.

iii. It is important that the provider use an age-adjusted scale due to decreased specificity in the elderly population. Using the appropriate scale can reduce the number of false-positive results.

c. Chest CTA versus V/Q Lung Scan.

i. If no contraindications to CTA: Chest CTA is preferred.

d. Treatment: Anticoagulation therapy.

6. High probability of PE.

a. Patients likely to be hemodynamically unstable; pretest clinical assessment not appropriate.

b. Immediate chest CTA. If unable to obtain a chest CTA due to hemodynamic instability/uncontrolled hypotension, then findings consistent with a PE on echocardiography may be a suitable alternative.

B. Pharmacotherapy.

1. Decision about medication management should consider whether the PE was provoked (caused by an identifiable risk factor such as cancer) and duration of therapy.

2. Patients should be routinely reevaluated for anticoagulation needs if receiving extended therapy.

3. Treatment with dabigatran, rivaroxaban, apixaban, or edoxaban is recommended over a vitamin K antagonist in patients with a PE.

4. A vitamin K antagonist is recommended for patients with an unprovoked PE if not receiving treatment with dabigatran, rivaroxaban, apixaban, or edoxaban.

5. It is suggested that a provider treating a patient with a PE and cancer use a low molecular weight heparin (LMWH). It is also recommended that patients receive extended therapy (e.g., no stop date) depending on their bleeding risk.

6. Anticoagulation is recommended for 3 months in patients with a PE provoked by surgery or transient risk factors.

7. For patients with an unprovoked PE at a low or moderate bleeding risk, initiation of extended anticoagulation therapy (e.g., no stop date) is suggested. For patients with a high bleeding risk, it is recommended to initiate anticoagulation for 3 months.

8. Surveillance is suggested in patients with a distal (subsegmental) PE who have no proximal DVTs and a low risk for recurrent venous thromboembolism (VTE).

9. Systemic thrombolytic therapy is suggested for hemodynamically unstable patients.

10. Additional management: Catheter-directed thrombolysis.

C. Patient/family teaching.

1. Prevent more blood clots from forming by taking the medication as prescribed.

2. Be sure to follow-up with lab tests as directed.

3. Encourage patients to get up and be active.

4. Smoking cessation.

5. On long trips, make frequent stops to get out and move about.

6. On airplane rides, perform exercises that keep your legs, feet, and toes moving.

D. Discharge.

1. Call your healthcare provider if there is any increase in symptoms.

Follow-Up

A. Patient follow-up is variable in the literature primarily due to the type of medication, cause of PE, and severity of illness due to the PE.

B. A vitamin K antagonist requires that the patient follow-up 2 to 3 days postdischarge for international normalized ratio (INR) evaluation.

Consultation/Referral

A. Pulmonologist may be consulted due to the pulmonary symptoms associated with a PE.

B. Hematologist may be warranted especially if concerned for a procoagulant defect.

C. An interventional radiologist or interventional cardiologist may be consulted for catheter-directed thrombolysis.

D. Critical care may be needed if the patient is admitted to the ICU or becomes hemodynamically unstable.

Special/Geriatric Considerations

A. Inferior vena cava (IVC) filters are not recommended for patients treated with anticoagulation.

B. IV anticoagulation therapy should be started prior to administering dabigatran and edoxaban.

Bibliography

Beckman, M. G., Hooper, W. C., Critchley, S. E., & Ortel, T. L. (2010). Venous thromboembolism: A public health concern. *American Journal of Preventive Medicine, 38*, S495–S501. doi:10.1016/j.amepre.2009.12 017

Jaff, M. R., McMurtry, S., Archer, S. L., Cushman, M., Goldenberg, N., Goldhaber, S. Z., & Zierler, B. K. (2011). Management of massive and submassive pulmonary embolism, iliofemoral deep vein thrombosis, and chronic thromboembolic pulmonary hypertension. *Circulation, 123*, 1788–1830. doi:10.1161/CIR.0b013e318214914f

Kearon, C., Akl, E. A., Ornelas, J., Blaivas, A., Jimenez, D., Bounameaux, H., Huisman, M., & Moores, C. L. (2016). Antithrombotic therapy for VTE disease: CHEST guideline and expert panel report. *Chest, 149*, 315–352. doi:10.1016/j.chest.2015.11.026

Konstantinides, S. V., Barco, S., Lankeit, M., & Meyer, G. (2016). Management of pulmonary embolism: An update. *Journal of the American College of Cardiology, 67*, 976–990. doi:10.1016/j.jacc.2015.11.061

Meyer, N. J., & Schmidt, G. A. (2015). Pulmonary embolic disorders: Thrombus, air, and fat. In J. B. Hall, G. A. Schmidt, & J. P. Kress

(Eds.), *Hall, Schmidt, and Wood's principles of critical care* (4th ed., pp. 318–336). New York, NY: McGraw-Hill.

Raja, A. S., Greenberg, J. O., Qaseem, A., Denberg, T. D., Fitterman, N., & Schuur, J. D. (2015). Evaluation of patients with suspected acute pulmonary embolism: Best practice advice from the clinical guidelines committee of the American College of Physicians. *Annals of Internal Medicine, 163,* 701–711. doi:10.7326/M14-1772

Restrictive Lung Disease

E. Moneé Carter-Griffin

Definition

A. A reduction in the total lung capacity secondary to a decrease in lung elasticity or disease of the chest wall, pleura, or neuromuscular etiology. Disorders can be classified as intrinsic or extrinsic.

Incidence

A. The incidence is highly variable and dependent on the etiology of restriction.

B. The incidence of some disorders is not well known.

C. Interstitial lung diseases (ILDs), although rare, are a cause of restrictive lung disease affecting approximately 500,000 individuals each year and resulting in 40,000 deaths.

D. Nonidiopathic and idiopathic pulmonary fibrosis (type of ILD) are a common cause of restrictive lung disease.

E. Approximately 30 cases per 100,000 of restrictive lung disease are due to idiopathic pulmonary fibrosis.

F. The prevalence of disease increases with age.

G. Frequency of occurrence is typically higher in men.

Pathogenesis

A. An exogenous or endogenous stimulus causes repetitive injury to the lung parenchyma, leading to epithelial and endothelial damage. Activation of local and systemic factors (e.g., fibroblasts, growth factors, clotting, factors, cytokines) occurs.

B. A provisional matrix is formed. There is a dysregulation of the intricate network and lack of matrix degradation, leading to aberrant wound healing and progressive lung remodeling, ultimately causing pulmonary fibrosis.

Predisposing Factors

A. Predisposing factors depend on the etiology of the restrictive lung disease.

B. Risk factors include:
  1. Obesity.
  2. Kyphoscoliosis.
  3. Myasthenia gravis.
  4. Chronic pleural disease (e.g., trapped lung).
  5. Autoimmune disease (e.g., scleroderma, systemic lupus erythematosus).
  6. Occupational exposures.
  7. Medications such as amiodarone, bleomycin, and methotrexate.
  8. Idiopathic lung disease such as pulmonary fibrosis, more common in the elderly and men.
  9. Sarcoidosis.

Subjective Data

A. Common complaints/symptoms.
  1. Symptoms and complaints may vary depending on the underlying cause of the restrictive lung disease.
  2. Dyspnea (see Figure 2.1): Most common complaint. It can be present with exercise or at rest as the disease progresses.
  3. Possible chronic cough (see Figure 2.3), wheezing (see Figure 2.2), or chest discomfort.
  4. Possible hemoptysis.
  5. Fatigue.

B. Common/typical scenario.
  1. Duration of illness (e.g., acute onset, chronic).

C. Family and social history.
  1. Smoking history.
  2. Occupational history or exposures.
  3. Family history of fibrotic lung disease.

D. Review of symptoms.
  1. Neurologic—any confusion, fatigue, muscle weakness.
  2. Respiratory—shortness of breath at rest, upon exertion, or that is progressive; dry cough; bloody sputum; pain on inspiration; recent or frequent colds.
  3. Use of medications such as nitrofurantoin, amiodarone, or others that have the potential to cause lung disease.

Physical Examination

A. Dyspnea, which may be more evident with activity.

B. Tachypnea.

C. Cyanosis or oxygen desaturation with activity.

D. Possible bibasilar inspiratory crackles, scattered inspiratory rhonchi, or wheezing.

E. Digital clubbing.

F. Obese.

G. Other disease-specific signs and symptoms (e.g., rash, Raynaud's, muscle weakness), depending on the underlying etiology.

Diagnostic Tests

A. Laboratory studies.
  1. Usually nonspecific.
  2. Serologic testing. This may be appropriate in patients suspected of having an underlying disorder causing restrictive disease such as rheumatoid arthritis.

B. Chest x-ray.
  1. Typically nonspecific findings, which may vary with the type of restrictive disease.
  2. Possible evidence of increased interstitial markings, bibasilar reticular pattern, or a nodular pattern.
  3. Honeycombing, which is typically noted as a late or advanced finding.
  4. If an extrinsic factor is suspected, then imaging may reveal a trapped lung, pleural effusion, etc.

C. Chest CT
  1. More sensitive and better assessment of the extent of disease compared to a chest x-ray.
  2. May reveal findings characteristic of specific restrictive diseases. Some restrictive diseases such as idiopathic pulmonary fibrosis can be diagnosed solely with a chest CT.
  3. If an extrinsic factor is suspected, then imaging may reveal a trapped lung, pleural effusion, etc.

D. Pulmonary Function Testing
  1. Valuable for assessing the response to therapy and monitoring disease progression.
  2. Does not diagnosis a specific disease.
  3. Characteristic findings include a reduced total lung capacity (TLC), functional residual capacity (FRC), and residual volume (RV).

4. The forced expiratory volume in one second (FEV1) and forced vital capacity ratio is usually normal or increased.

5. The diffusing capacity of carbon monoxide is reduced in patients with an intrinsic etiology of restrictive disease. If the diffusing capacity is normal, then the etiology of restrictive disease is an extrinsic factor such as neuromuscular disease.

E. Arterial blood gas

  1. May be normal or indicate hypoxemia and a respiratory alkalosis.

  2. May reveal an increased alveolar-arterial gradient.

F. Bronchoscopy and/or lung biopsy

  1. Beneficial for identifying diseases associated with intrinsic factors or the lung parenchyma.

  2. A bronchoalveolar lavage (BAL) may be useful in narrowing the differential diagnoses.

    a. The clinical usefulness of the BAL has not been well established.

  3. A lung biopsy can confirm the diagnosis, evaluate disease activity, and exclude other diagnoses.

    a. Open thoracotomy

    b. Video-assisted thoracoscopic lung biopsy

    c. Transbronchial lung biopsy via bronchoscopy

G. Additional imaging or testing may be warranted to assess for complications resulting from restrictive diseases such as an echocardiogram to evaluate for pulmonary hypertension or right-sided heart failure.

Evaluation and Management Plan

A. Treatment may vary depending on the underlying etiology for restrictive disease.

B. Intrinsic etiologies are defined as diseases of the lung parenchyma. Extrinsic etiologies are extra-pulmonary causes including neuromuscular disorders, the chest wall, etc.

C. Patients should receive smoking cessation counseling.

D. Avoidance of environmental and/or occupational exposures.

E. Medications suspected of causing restrictive disease should be stopped immediately.

F. Supplemental oxygen therapy should be administered for all patients with oxygen saturations less than 88% on room air at rest or upon exertion.

G. Pulmonary rehabilitation or regular activity/exercise should be encouraged because it has been shown to improve endurance and quality of life.

H. Patients should receive vaccinations for influenza and pneumococcal.

I. Treatment regimens for intrinsic causes usually includes:

  1. Corticosteroid therapy

    a. Use of corticosteroids is generally accepted; however, timing, dosing, and continuation versus discontinuation of treatment is highly variable and dependent on the intrinsic cause for restrictive disease as well as patient responsiveness.

    b. The long-term effects of corticosteroid therapy must be considered.

    c. Pulse high dose corticosteroids are typically used for acute exacerbations.

  2. Immunosuppressive agents (e.g. cyclosporine, azathioprine) may be used in certain diagnoses. These medications should not be routinely or empirically used without a definitive diagnosis.

  3. If worsening respiratory symptoms, patients may require invasive mechanical ventilation.

  4. Patients with refractory disease to treatment and progressive worsening, may be a candidate for lung transplantation and should be referred to lung transplant specialist and center.

J. Treatment for extrinsic causes include:

  1. Weight loss counseling and plan for obese patients

  2. Non-invasive positive pressure ventilation for patients who have impaired gas exchange

  3. Identification of the extrinsic disorder and treatment accordingly.

  4. For patients with a trapped lung, chronic effusion, or empyema, a decortication may be required.

Follow Up

A. Follow-up is variable and dependent on the patient's symptoms and medical management. It should be individualized.

B. Post-hospital discharge, patients will follow-up with their provider in one week.

Consultation/Referral

A. Patients with restrictive lung disease should be referred to a pulmonologist for diagnosis and management.

B. Patients with an extrinsic etiology for restrictive disease such as myasthenia gravis should be referred to a neurologist or the appropriate consultant for the disorder.

Individual/Special/Geriatric Considerations

A. To adequately assess responsiveness to immunosuppressive medications, the provider should note it may not be evident until eight to twelve weeks after therapy initiation.

B. Patients with parenchymal restrictive disease (e.g. idiopathic or non-idiopathic pulmonary fibrosis) receiving treatment with high dose steroids should receive prophylactic treatment for pneumocystis jiroveci pneumonia (PJP).

C. Patients with progressive disease are typically discharged on home oxygen therapy. Increased oxygen requirements may be necessary to maintain a goal saturation greater than 88%. The patient and family is instructed that oxygen therapy may be tailored to maintain oxygen saturations at rest and with exertion. If the patient is requiring increased oxygen therapy from baseline, then an immediate follow-up appointment with their pulmonologist or hospital admission may be warranted.

| EXHIBIT 2.1 | Stepwise Approach for Managing Asthma Long Term |

The stepwise approach tailors the selection of medication to the level of asthma severity or asthma control. The stepwise approach is meant to help, not replace, the clinical decision making needed to meet individual patient needs.

ASSESS CONTROL:

STEP UP IF NEEDED (first, check medication adherence, inhaler technique, environmental control, and comorbidities)

STEP DOWN IF POSSIBLE (and asthma is well controlled for at least 3 months)

| STEP 1 | STEP 2 | STEP 3 | STEP 4 | STEP 5 | STEP 6 |

At each step: Patient education, environmental control, and management of comorbidities

0–4 years of age

		Intermittent Asthma	Persistent Asthma: Daily Medication. Consult with asthma specialist if step 3 care or higher is required. Consider consultation at step 2.				
	Preferred Treatment[b]	SABA[a] as needed	Low-dose ICS[a]	Medium-dose ICS[a]	Medium-dose ICS[a] + either LABA[a] or montelukast	High-dose ICS[a] + either LABA[a] or montelukast	High-dose ICS[a] + either LABA or montelukast + oral corticosteroids
	Alternative Treatment[b,c]		Cromolyn or montelukast				

If clear benefit is not observed in 4–6 weeks, and medication technique and adherence are satisfactory, consider adjusting therapy or alternate diagnoses.

	Quick-Relief Medication	■ SABA[a] as needed for symptoms; intensity of treatment depends on severity of symptoms. ■ With viral respiratory symptoms: SABA every 4–6 hours up to 24 hours (longer with physician consult). Consider short course of oral systemic corticosteroids if asthma exacerbation is severe or patient has history of severe exacerbations. ■ Caution: Frequent use of SABA may indicate the need to step up treatment.

5–11 years of age

		Intermittent Asthma	Persistent Asthma: Daily Medication. Consult with asthma specialist if step 4 care or higher is required. Consider consultation at step 3.				
	Preferred Treatment[b]	SABA[a] as needed	Low-dose ICS[a]	Low-dose ICS[a] + either LABA[a], LABA[a], theophylline[b] or medium-dose ICS	Medium-dose ICS[a] + LABA[a]	High-dose ICS[a] + LABA[a]	High-dose ICS[a] + LABA[a] + OCS
	Alternative Treatment[b,c]		Cromolyn, LTRA[a], or theophylline[d]		Medium-dose ICS[a] + either LTRA[a] or theophylline[d]	High-dose ICS[a] + either LTRA[a] or theophylline[d]	High-dose ICS[a] + either LTRA[a] or theophylline[d] + OCS
			Consider subcutaneous allergen immunotherapy for patients who have persistent, allergic asthma.[e]				

	Quick-Relief Medication	■ SABA[a] as needed for symptoms. The intensity of treatment depends on severity of symptoms: Up to three treatments every 20 minutes as needed. Short course of oral systemic corticosteroids may be needed. ■ Caution: Increasing use of SABA or use >2 days/week for symptom relief (not to prevent EIB) generally indicates inadequate control and the need to step up treatment.

(continued)

EXHIBIT 2.1   **Stepwise Approach for Managing Asthma Long Term (*continued*)**

ASSESS CONTROL:

STEP UP IF NEEDED (first, check medication adherence, inhaler technique, environmental control, and comorbidities)

STEP DOWN IF POSSIBLE (and asthma is well controlled for at least 3 months)

STEP 1	STEP 2	STEP 3	STEP 4	STEP 5	STEP 6

		At each step: Patient education, environmental control, and management of comorbidities					
≥ 12 years of age		**Intermittent asthma**	**Persistent asthma: Daily medication.** Consult with asthma specialist if step 4 care or higher is required. Consider consultation at step 3.				
	Preferred Treatment[b]	SABA[a] as needed	Low-dose ICS[a]	Low-dose ICS[a] + LABA[a] OR medium-dose ICS[a]	Medium-dose ICS[a] + LABA[a]	High-dose ICS[a] + LABA[a] **AND** consider omalizumab for patients who have allergies[f]	High-dose ICS[a] + LABA[a] + OCS[h] **AND** consider omalizumab for patients who have allergies[f]
	Alternative Treatment[b,c]		Cromolyn, LTRA[a], or theophylline[d]	Low-dose ICS[a] + either LTRA[a], theophylline[d], or zileuton[g]		Medium-dose ICS[a] + either LTRA[a], theophylline[d], or zileuton[g]	
			Consider subcutaneous allergen immunotherapy for patients who have persistent, allergic asthma.[e]				
	Quick-Relief Medication	■ SABA[a] as needed for symptoms. The intensity of treatment depends on severity of symptoms: Up to three treatments every 20 minutes as needed. Short course of oral systemic corticosteroids may be needed. ■ Caution: Use of SABA >2 days/week for symptom relief (not to prevent EIB[a]) generally indicates inadequate control and the need to step up treatment.					

[a]*EIB, exercise-induced bronchospasm; ICS, inhaled corticosteroid; LABA, long-acting beta₂ agonist; LTRA, leukotriene receptor antagonist; OCS, oral corticosteroids; SABA, short-acting beta₂ agonist.*

[b]Treatment options are listed in alphabetical order, if more than one.

[c]If alternative treatment is used and response is inadequate, discontinue and use preferred treatment before stepping up.

[d]Theophylline is a less desirable alternative because of the need to monitor serum concentration levels.

[e]Based on evidence for dust mites, animal dander, and pollen; evidence is weak or lacking for molds and cockroaches. Evidence is strongest for immunotherapy with single allergens. The role of allergy in asthma is greater in children than in adults.

[f]Clinicians who administer immunotherapy or omalizumab should be prepared to treat anaphylaxis that may occur.

[g]Zileuton is less desirable because of limited studies as adjunctive therapy and the need to monitor liver function.

[h]Before oral corticosteroids are introduced, a trial of high-dose ICS + LABA + either LTRA, theophylline, or zileuton, may be considered, although this approach has not been studied in clinical trials.
SABA, short-acting beta

Source: U.S. Department of Health and Human Services. (2012). *Asthma care quick reference: Diagnosing and managing asthma.* Retrieved from https://www.nhlbi.nih.gov/files/docs/guidelines/asthma_qrg.pdf

3 Cardiac Guidelines

Allison Rusgo

Acute Coronary Syndromes

Allison Rusgo

Definition

A. Umbrella term encompassing unstable angina (UA), non-ST-segment elevation myocardial infarction (NSTEMI), and ST-segment elevation myocardial infarction (STEMI).
B. UA: No cardiac damage, no elevation in cardiac laboratory biomarkers, and no ST-segment elevation on ECG, but may show ST-segment depression.
    1. Indicates narrowing of coronary arteries secondary to thrombosis, hemorrhage, or plaque rupture. In variant angina (Prinzmetal) cause is vasospasms.
    2. Myocardial oxygen demand: Unchanged but available blood supply is decreased because of overall reduced coronary blood flow.
C. NSTEMI: Evidence of cardiac damage, evidence of elevation in cardiac laboratory biomarkers, and no ST-segment elevation on ECG (but may show ST-segment depression and other ECG abnormalities; T wave inversion, or peaked T waves).
    1. Indicates partial blockage of coronary artery secondary to atherosclerotic narrowing.
    2. Cardiac damage at the area of the heart supplied by the partially blocked artery.
D. STEMI: Evidence of cardiac damage, evidence of elevation in cardiac biomarkers, and positive ST-segment elevation on ECG. Infarction may produce Q waves (pathologic).
    1. Indicates complete blockage of an artery, damaging the area of the heart supplied by the completely occluded vessel.
E. Important note: Patients with stable coronary artery disease (CAD) can have acute coronary syndrome (ACS) without atherosclerotic plaque rupture where physiologic stress (i.e., trauma, anemia, infection, acute blood loss) increases the myocardial oxygen demand of the heart.

Incidence

A. Ischemic heart disease is the leading cause of death among U.S. adults, estimated to be 405,000/annually.
B. Approximately 1.4 million individuals are hospitalized for ACS; of these, 810,000 experience an myocardial infarction (MI).
C. STEMI is more common in middle-aged patients, and NSTEMI is more common in elderly patients.

Pathogenesis

A. Mismatch between myocardial oxygen supply and demand, where supply is affected by coronary blood flow and oxygen-carrying capacity of the blood.
B. Overall oxygen-carrying capacity determined by hemoglobin level and oxygen saturation.
C. Coronary artery blood flow: Interplay between peripheral vascular resistance and ability of the heart to relax during diastole.
D. Primary cardiac ischemia caused by atherosclerotic narrowing of the coronary vasculature.
E. Secondary cardiac ischemia (less common) secondary to causes unrelated to atherosclerotic narrowing of the coronary vasculature.
    1. Increased myocardial oxygen demand (i.e., infection, tachyarrhythmias, thyrotoxicosis).
    2. Decreased blood flow (i.e., hypotension).
    3. Decreased oxygen availability (i.e., anemia).
F. Atherosclerotic-related ACS: Coronary arteries undergo a cascade of reactions leading to increased plaque accumulation, resulting in plaque rupture, and finally artery blockage.
    1. Vascular injury: Triggered by factors such as tobacco by-products, elevated blood pressure (BP), elevated glucose, and oxidized low-density lipoproteins.
    2. Results in increased vascular permeability and inflammation.
    3. Inflammatory mediators (macrophages and smooth muscle cells) activated: Create "fatty streaks" in vasculature.
    4. "Fatty streaks": Transformed into foam cells (i.e., plaque), which form fibrous caps.
    5. When the top layer of the fibrous cap ruptures, platelets are activated.
    6. Platelet response: Consists of adhesion, aggregation, and activation; potentiates further damage to affected artery via platelet-laden thrombi, hemorrhage, and inflammation (overall blood flow decreased).
    7. Immediate onset of the artery blockage created by ischemia secondary to rapid decrease in blood flow.
    8. Amount and duration of the myocardial oxygen supply and demand mismatch related to whether person experiences reversible ischemia (UA) or irreversible damage with cell death (STEMI or NSTEMI).

Predisposing Factors

A. Hypertension (HTN).
B. Hyperlipidemia.
C. Diabetes mellitus (DM).
D. Metabolic syndrome.
E. Obesity and sedentary lifestyle.
F. Tobacco use.
G. Family history of cardiovascular disease.
H. Medications/toxins (cocaine, ergonovine, serotonin).

Subjective Data

A. Common complaints/symptoms.

    1. Chest discomfort (vise-like or crushing, aching, pressure, tightness, or burning); less likely sharp/stabbing or knife-like.

        a. Reproducible chest tenderness in some cases.

        b. Classic: Left-sided or substernal chest discomfort that radiates to the jaw or left arm.

        c. Can also radiate to the upper abdomen, back, or shoulders.

    2. Nausea/vomiting.

    3. Diaphoresis.

    4. Palpitations.

    5. Dyspnea.

    6. Lightheadedness or syncope.

    7. Feelings of anxiety.

    8. Women, elderly persons, and those with DM: More likely to experience atypical ACS presentations.

        a. Fatigue.

        b. Weakness.

        c. Generalized malaise.

        d. Nonspecific chest or back discomfort.

        e. Decreased exercise tolerance.

        f. Altered mental status (elders).

        g. Gastrointestinal symptoms radiating the back (women).

        h. No pain (elders and DM persons).

B. History of the present illness.

    1. Information regarding onset, provoking and alleviating factors, duration, quality, severity, and timing of chest discomfort.

        a. Compared to stable angina or UA, MIs cause more severe chest discomfort that is prolonged (>20 minutes) and unrelieved by nitroglycerin.

        b. Can be potentiated by exposure to cold, physical activity, or emotional stress.

        c. Possible previous history of angina and any recent changes in anginal symptoms over the past several months.

        d. Possible recent decrease in activity level due to decreased tolerance.

    2. More likely to experience associated symptoms with MIs as opposed to angina (i.e., nausea, dyspnea, fatigue, diaphoresis).

C. Family and social history.

    1. Family history of premature CAD or MI in first-degree relative (males <45 years and females <55 years).

    2. Tobacco or illegal substance use, especially cocaine.

    3. Lifestyle factors, including level of exercise and dietary habits.

D. Review of systems.

    1. General: Fatigue and diaphoresis.

    2. Cardiovascular: Chest pain/discomfort (with radiation) and palpitations.

    3. Pulmonary: Dyspnea on exertion and shortness of breath.

    4. Abdominal: Epigastric discomfort, indigestion, nausea, and vomiting.

    5. Neurological: Dizziness, lightheadedness, near-syncope/syncope, and mental status changes.

Physical Examination

A. General appearance (one of the following).

    1. Unremarkable and appearing well without any signs of distress, resting calmly.

    2. Insignificant clinical/respiratory distress and instability.

    3. Cyanotic, in respiratory distress.

B. Vital signs: Assess pulse, BP, respirations, oxygen saturation, and temperature.

    1. Pulse: Can be regular, irregular, tachycardic, or bradycardic (bradycardia can occur with anterior or inferior wall MIs).

    2. BP: Can be elevated (due to anxiety, pain, underlying HTN, catecholamine surge) or decreased (indicates ventricular dysfunction).

C. Skin: Diaphoresis, cool/clammy skin (concern for cardiogenic shock), and peripheral edema.

D. Neck: Possible jugular venous distention (JVD).

E. Cardiac.

    1. Inspect for lifts, heaves, and pulsations.

    2. Palpate for possible chest wall tenderness.

    3. Auscultate.

        a. Extra heart sounds. S3 is present in approximately 15% of cases and indicates acute MI with heart failure.

        b. A new systolic murmur. This is concerning for papillary muscle dysfunction, ventricular septal defect, or new mitral regurgitation from a flail segment of the valve.

F. Pulmonary: Auscultate lung sounds for evidence of rales/crackles; concern for pulmonary edema or congestive heart failure.

G. Abdominal: Inspect, auscultate for bruits, and palpate for tenderness and evidence of pulsatile abdominal mass (concern for abdominal aortic aneurysm).

Diagnostic Tests

A. ECG: Should be performed within 10 minutes of presentation to healthcare provider. Note that a normal ECG or one unchanged from the patient's baseline does not rule out the possibility of ischemic cardiac damage.

    1. Fixed ST-segment elevations (STEMI).

    2. Fixed ST-segment depressions (shows ischemia).

    3. T-wave changes (can indicate ischemia).

    4. Transient ST-segment elevations (consider pericarditis, Prinzmetal angina, left ventricular aneurysm).

B. Cardiac biomarkers.

    1. Serial troponins (cTnI or cTnT): Sensitive and specific for ACS diagnosis (biomarker of choice); recommended as set of three drawn approximately 4 to 6 hours apart.

    2. Complete blood count: Useful for baseline information and ruling out anemia as cause of ACS.

C. Basic metabolic panel.

    1. To assess electrolytes, especially magnesium and potassium (causes of cardiac arrhythmias).

    2. To assess renal function: Important if going to use angiotensin-converting enzyme (ACE) inhibitors for future therapy and/or contrast dye during catheterization (want to avoid contrast-induced nephropathy).

D. Chest radiography: To assess for pulmonary edema and cardiomegaly, and rule out other causes of chest pain such as pneumonia or thoracic aneurysm.

E. Cardiac echocardiography: Can be especially helpful if diagnosis is questionable. It is used to:

    1. Assess left ventricular function.

    2. Evaluate for regional wall motion abnormalities.

    3. Check for pericardial effusions or valvular abnormalities (i.e., acute mitral regurgitation).

F. Computed tomography coronary angiography (CTCA)/CT coronary artery calcium (CAC) scoring.

    1. Noninvasive diagnostic studies: Aid in early CAD diagnosis.

    2. CTCA: Uses contrast dye to evaluate the integrity of coronary arteries (can also evaluate previously implanted stents and bypass grafts for patency).

    3. CT CAC: Useful for low-risk ACS patients (no contrast dye and low radiation levels; evaluation of calcium in coronary arteries, which is related to atherosclerotic burden.

Differential Diagnosis

A. Myocardial infarctions (STEMI, NSTEMI).

B. Stable or unstable angina.

C. Pericarditis.

D. Myocarditis.

E. Esophagitis/gastritis/ruptured peptic ulcer.

F. Hypertensive emergency.

G. Anxiety/panic attack.

H. Ruptured thoracic or abdominal aortic aneurysm.

I. Pulmonary embolus.

J. Pneumonia.

Evaluation and Management Plan

A. General plan.

    1. Management based on patient presentations, characteristics of symptoms, past medical history, physical examination findings, and diagnostic results.

    2. Goal: To limit necrosis and overall cardiac damage.

    3. Risk stratification: Imperative when designing treatment plan. One option is the Thrombosis in Myocardial Infarction (TIMI) Score (see Table 3.1).

        a. Instrument for determining risk of all-cause morbidity, new or recurrent MI, or need for emergent revascularization within 14 to 30 days of presentation of NSTEMI or UA.

        b. Each of the seven items on the checklist is equivalent to 1 point; the higher the score, the higher the patient's risk.

B. Management of STEMI.

    1. Aspirin 324 mg in ED (or prehospital).

    2. Loading dose of antiplatelet agent (i.e., clopidogrel, 300–600 mg).

    3. Supplemental oxygen if hypoxemia.

TABLE 3.1	Thrombosis in Myocardial Infarction Score
Age >65 y	1 point
≥ CAD risk factors (HTN, hyperlipidemia, DM, tobacco use, family history of CAD)	1 point
Known CAD with stenosis ≥50%	1 point
Acetylsalicylic use in past 7 d	1 point
At least two episodes of severe angina in past 24 hr	1 point
ST changes on ECG 0.5 mm above baseline	1 point
Positive cardiac biomarkers	1 point

CAD, coronary artery disease; DM, diabetes mellitus; HTN, hypertension.
Source: Agabegi, S. S., & Agabegi, E. D. (2008). *Step-up to medicine* (2nd ed.). Philadelphia, PA: Wolters Kluwer.

4. Antithrombolytic agent (unfractionated or low-molecular weight heparin).

5. Nitrates: Provide symptomatic relief; do not improve mortality.

    a. Strong risk of hypotension: Causes decreased coronary perfusion.

    b. Should not be given if patient has hypotension, known right ventricular infarction, large pericardial effusion, recent use of 5-phosphodiesterase inhibitor, or severe aortic stenosis.

6. Beta-blockers.

    a. Caution if decreased systolic BP, cardiogenic shock, severe asthma, decompensated congestive heart failure, or severe bradycardia.

7. Goal: Reperfusion therapy.

    a. Obtained via percutaneous coronary intervention (PCI) with or without stent placement.

        i. Should be achieved within 90 minutes of patient arrival at PCI-capable hospital.

        ii. If hospital is without PCI capabilities, goal is patient transfer to PCI center within 120 minutes of patient arrival.

    b. PCI options.

        i. Coronary angioplasty with or without stent placement.

        ii. Balloon angioplasty stretches inner layer of the coronary artery.

        iii. Drug eluting stents (DES) or bare metal stents (BMS): Wire mesh cage implanted in the blocked vessel for structure and patency.

        iv. BMS preferable if unable to utilize dual antiplatelet therapy (DAPT) for at least a year or upcoming invasive surgical procedure.

    c. If PCI is not achievable in these time parameters, fibrinolytics should be administered within 30 minutes of patient arrival to hospital.

        i. Indicated if symptom onset is within 6 to 12 hours; 1 mm ST-segment elevation in more than 2 ECG leads.

        ii. Aims to dissolve existing clot, improve left ventricular function, and decrease mortality.

        iii. Examples: Tissue plasminogen factor, streptokinase, or tenecteplase.

        iv. Major risk: Bleeding such as intracranial hemorrhage (ICH).

    d. At discretion of cardiothoracic surgeon and interventional cardiologist, consider coronary artery bypass grafting (CABG) if cardiac catheterization yields extensive stenosis and/or stenosis not amenable to stenting/balloon options.

    e. For unconscious STEMI patients with prehospital cardiac arrest caused by ventricular fibrillation or pulseless ventricular tachycardia, obtain immediate cardiology consultation regarding the usage of therapeutic hypothermia prior to cardiac intervention.

C. Management of NSTEMI and/or UA.

    1. Monitoring during inpatient hospitalization for serial ECGs, biomarker elevation, and symptom evolution.

    2. Early invasive therapy (PCI) in NSTEMI or UA: Recommended only if refractory angina; high risk for cardiac events or hemodynamic instability.

    3. American Heart Association (AHA) and American College of Cardiology (ACC) recommendations for early (within 48 hours) PCI intervention in NSTEMI/UA if: Refractory angina, elevated biomarkers, new ST-changes, positive stress test results, decreased left ventricular function, or hemodynamic instability.

4. NSTEMI/UA patients requiring PCI should receive similar medications to STEMI management.

    a. Aspirin 324 mg initially followed by daily dose of 81 mg.

    b. Antiplatelet agent (clopidogrel).

    c. Supplemental oxygen if evidence of hypoxemia.

    d. Nitrates.

    e. Antithrombolytic agent (unfractionated or low-molecular weight heparin).

    f. Beta-blockers if not contraindicated.

5. Patients admitted for ACS evaluations with normal serial ECGs, normal biomarkers, and complete resolution of symptoms can undergo stress testing or CTCA prior to discharge or within 72 hours of discharge if deemed appropriate by cardiologist. The following is for patients discharged prior to definitive diagnostic testing.

    a. Prescribe aspirin, short-acting nitroglycerin, and beta-blockers (if appropriate).

    b. Provide instructions regarding lifestyle modification (i.e., no physical activity until evaluated by cardiologist), tobacco cessation, and cardiac healthy diet.

6. Helpful flow chart for evaluation of patients with ACS (see Figure 3.1).

D. Patient/family teaching points.

1. Knowledge of ACS/angina symptoms: Decreases time before presenting for medical care (decreases door to PCI time, if STEMI).

2. Tobacco cessation.

3. Importance of regular physical activity.

4. Use of heart-healthy (low fat, low cholesterol, low salt) diet.

5. Compliance with all medications (especially aspirin and antiplatelet agent) and clinic follow-up visits.

E. Pharmacotherapy.

1. Antiplatelet drugs.

    a. Aspirin: To prevent platelet aggregation.

      i. Immediate administration of 324 mg aspirin if STEMI, NSTEMI, or UA.

      ii. Daily use of aspirin to reduce cardiac mortality; for patients with high risk for ICH, a lower ASA dose of 81 to 160 mg should be considered.

      iii. Can be combined with other antiplatelets for DAPT.

      iv. Consider use of proton pump inhibitor or H2 receptor block to prevent gastrointestinal irritation.

    b. Adenosine diphosphate receptor antagonists.

      i. Examples: Prasugrel, clopidogrel, or ticagrelor.

      ii. Overall function: Platelet inhibition via complex pharmacologic mechanisms.

      iii. Major risk: Bleeding—Food and Drug Administration issued Black Box Warning for prasugrel (not for use in those with prior cerebrovascular accident [CVA]/transient ischemic attack [TIA] or bleeding disorders).

      iv. Can be combined with aspirin for DAPT.

      v. If elective CABG planned: Recommended to hold clopidogrel for 5 days to reduce risk of bleeding and improve morbidity/mortality.

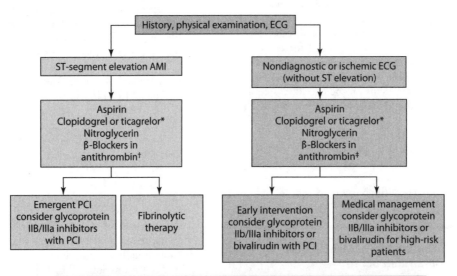

FIGURE 3.1 Algorithm for evaluation of patients with ACS. ACS, acute coronary syndrome; AMI, acute myocardial infarction; PCI, percutaneous coronary intervention; PR, progesterone.

Source: Hollander, J. E., & Diercks, D. B. (2016). Acute coronary syndromes. In J. E. Tintinalli, J. Stapczynski, O. Ma, D. M. Yealy, G. D. Meckler, & D. M. Cline. *Tintinalli's emergency medicine: A comprehensive study guide* (8th ed., pp. 332–348). New York, NY: McGraw-Hill.

vi. Specific agent chosen by cardiologist/interventional cardiologist and continued for at least several months post-PCI.

   c. Glycoprotein IIB/IIIA inhibitors.

     i. Examples: Abciximab and tirofiban.

     ii. Routine administration in ED not recommended due to timing of PCI and risk of bleeding.

     iii. During hospitalization, can be used in combination with aspirin for high-risk ACS patients and those likely to undergo PCI.

  2. Thrombolytics.

   a. Examples: Low-molecular weight (enoxaparin) or unfractionated heparin.

   b. Used in STEMI and NSTEMI management.

   c. Combining aspirin with heparin should be done in ACS.

  3. Beta-blockers.

   a. Examples: Metoprolol, bisoprolol.

   b. Very useful in patients with STEMI/NSTEMI (if no known contraindications) because of anti-ischemic characteristics (decreases infarct size and mortality).

   c. Maintains anti-arrhythmic and antihypertensive properties.

   d. Reduces cardiac afterload and overall cardiac stress (helps to equalize myocardial oxygen supply and demand levels).

  4. Additional medication options.

   a. ACE inhibitors: For those with left ventricular ejection fraction less than 40% and/or HTN, DM, or stable chronic kidney disease (can consider angiotensin receptor blockers if ACE intolerant).

   b. High-intensity statin (if no contraindications; as tolerated) with ongoing lipid panel and side effect monitoring.

   c. Nondihydropyridine calcium channel blockers: Can be used if intolerance or contraindication to beta-blockers as long as there is no left ventricular dysfunction, known prolonged PR interval on ECG, or second- or third-degree heart block.

F. Discharge instructions.

  1. Prior to hospital discharge.

   a. Ensure all required prescriptions have been given based on cardiac status and interventions performed during hospitalization.

   b. Emphasize lifestyle modifications via teach-back method regarding tobacco cessation, cardiac rehabilitation for exercise program, and eating heart-healthy diet.

  2. Verify that patient has appropriate follow-up with cardiologist/interventional cardiologist, primary care provider, and cardiac rehabilitation.

  3. For patients discharged with instructions to follow-up with cardiologist for stress testing, ensure appointment occurs within 72 hours after discharge with instructions for no physical activity prior to appointment.

  4. Ensure patients understand all reasons to return to ED regarding cardiac-related symptoms.

Follow-Up

A. Patients should have regular monitoring by their primary care provider and/or cardiologist to address medication compliance; adherence to lifestyle changes; and monitoring laboratory markers, including lipid and metabolic panels.

B. Cardiologist may consider follow-up echocardiogram to assess left ventricular function ([EF] percentage) at 40 days post-MI; this will help determine the need for further interventions such as an implantable cardiac defibrillator (ICD).

Consultation/Referral

A. Consult with cardiologist for all ACSs.

B. Consult with interventional cardiologist for cardiac catheterization.

C. Consult with cardiothoracic surgeon for CABG and/or acute valvular complications.

D. Referral to cardiac rehabilitation recommended for patients with ACS.

Special/Geriatric Considerations

A. Chest pain following PCI or CABG.

  1. Patients presenting with chest pain immediately after PCI or angioplasty warrant consideration for sudden vessel closure (i.e., in-stent stenosis, in-stent thrombosis, or stent failure).

   a. Treat aggressively for ACS and immediately consult cardiologist.

   b. Use of BMS is more likely to lead to restenosis in the short term while the use of DES is more likely to lead to restenosis within 9 to 12 months (after cessation of daily antiplatelet such as clopidogrel).

  2. Chest pain after CABG may indicate possible graft failure; immediate consultation with cardiologist and cardiothoracic surgeon is necessary.

  3. Consider other etiologies such as post-MI pericarditis.

B. Chest pain secondary to cocaine intoxication.

  1. MI occurs in approximately 6% of patients after cocaine use.

  2. Use of cardiac biomarkers is imperative for diagnosis.

  3. Treatment involves aspirin, nitrates, and benzodiazepines (no beta-blockers for first 24 hours).

  4. For STEMI secondary to cocaine, patients typically undergo PCI with antithrombolytic and antiplatelet agents per cardiologist and interventional cardiologist.

C. Geriatric considerations.

  1. Recognize that atypical symptoms are common (confusion, malaise, weakness, fatigue).

  2. Considerations must be made regarding the use of the most beneficial diagnostic testing.

   a. Age-related cardiac changes (specifically, if unable to reach target heart rate during stress testing) can mask diagnosis.

   b. Elderly patients may be unable to walk on treadmill due to orthopedic comorbidities (nuclear or pharmacologic stress testing is often preferred).

   c. Coronary atherosclerosis is more diffuse and more calcified combined with decreased diastolic filling.

   d. Risk versus benefit analysis should be done with regard to the use of multiple antiplatelet and anticoagulant agents due to increased risk of bleeding.

   e. Overall health status, cognitive abilities, and comorbidities should be considered before utilizing invasive clinical or surgical interventions.

Bibliography

Agabegi, S. S., & Agabegi, E. D. (2008). *Step-up to medicine* (2nd ed.). Philadelphia, PA: Wolters Kluwer.

Amsterdam, E. A., Wenger, N. K., Brindis, R. G., Casey, D. E., Jr., Ganiats, T. G., Holmes, D. R., Jr., & Zieman, S. J. (2014). 2014 AHA/ACC guideline for the management of patients with non–ST-elevation acute coronary syndromes. *Circulation, 130*, e344–e426. doi:10.1161/CIR. 0000000000000134

Coven, D., Shirani, J., & Kalyanasundaram, A. (2018, Septermber 5). Acute coronary syndrome. In E. Yang (Ed.), *Medscape*. Retrieved from http://emedicine.medscape.com/article/1910735-overview

Hollander, J. E., & Diercks, D. B. (2016). Acute coronary syndromes. In J. E. Tintinalli, J. Stapczynski, O. Ma, D. M. Yealy, G. D. Meckler, & D. M. Cline. *Tintinalli's emergency medicine: A comprehensive study guide* (8th ed., pp. 332–348). New York, NY: McGraw-Hill.

Angina

Allison Rusgo

Definition

A. Most common symptom of coronary artery disease (CAD) secondary to coronary vascular obstruction from atherosclerosis.
B. Three types.
  1. Stable angina.
    a. Secondary to fixed atherosclerotic plaques that narrow coronary vasculature.
    b. Occurs because of an imbalance between myocardial blood supply and oxygen demand.
  2. Unstable angina (UA).
    a. Progression from stable angina, leading to total vessel occlusion.
    b. Indication that narrowing of coronary vasculature has increased via thrombosis, hemorrhage, or plaque rupture.
    c. Myocardial oxygen demand unchanged, but blood supply decreased because of reduced coronary flow.
  3. Prinzmetal angina: Transient coronary vasospasms in the setting of fixed atherosclerosis (75% of cases) or healthy coronary arteries.

Incidence

A. Estimated 9.8 million Americans experience angina yearly.
B. Age-adjusted prevalence of angina is higher in females than males.
C. Annual incidence rates are highest in African Americans as compared to other ethnicities.
D. Incidence and prevalence of angina and CAD increase with age.

Pathogenesis

A. Coronary atherosclerosis causes narrowing of the coronary arteries, thereby reducing blood flow through the system.
B. Myocardial ischemia (damage) results when the amount of blood flow through the coronary arteries is insufficient to meet myocardial oxygen demand.
C. Sensation of angina is caused by the stimulation of the sensory nerve fibers in the coronary vessels.
  1. The nerve fibers extend from the spinal nerves (via the spinal cord) to the thalamus to the cerebral cortex to convey pain.
  2. Adenosine is thought to be the chemical mediator of angina by stimulating the afferent cardiac nerve fibers.

Predisposing Factors

A. Diabetes mellitus.
B. Hyperlipidemia (elevated low-density lipoprotein [LDL], low high-density lipoprotein [HDL], or elevated triglycerides [TGs]).
C. Hypertension (HTN).
D. Tobacco use.
E. Increased age (males >45 years and females >55 years).
F. Family history of premature CAD or MI in first-degree relative (males <45 years and females <55 years).
G. Obesity or metabolic syndrome.
H. Sedentary lifestyle.
I. Underlying valvular heart disease such as aortic stenosis.

Subjective Data

A. Common complaints/symptoms.
  1. Stable angina.
    a. Retrosternal chest discomfort: Described as pressure, heaviness, burning, squeezing.
    b. Can be located in central chest, epigastrium, neck, back, or shoulders (pain below mandible and below epigastrium is rarely angina).
    c. Can radiate to jaw, left arm, or shoulders.
    d. Typically preceded by exertion, eating, cold exposure, or emotional upset.
    e. Usually does not change with positions or respiration.
    f. Typically lasts 1 to 5 minutes and relieved by rest or use of nitroglycerin.
  2. Differentiating features of UA.
    a. Symptoms occur at rest.
    b. Any new-onset angina or change in usual stable anginal symptoms.
    c. Angina unrelieved by rest or nitroglycerin.
    d. Typically lasts longer than stable angina.
B. History of the present illness.
  1. Obtain information regarding onset, provoking and alleviating factors, duration, quality, severity, and timing of the anginal-type discomfort.
  2. Assess for associated symptoms, including:
    a. Fatigue.
    b. Diaphoresis.
    c. Shortness of breath.
    d. Decreased exercise tolerance.
    e. Nausea/vomiting.
C. Family and social history.
  1. Family history of premature CAD or MI in first-degree relative (males <45 and females <55 years).
  2. Tobacco use, alcohol consumption, and illegal substance use (especially cocaine).
  3. Lifestyle, including exercise and dietary habits.
D. Review of systems.
  1. General: Fatigue or diaphoresis.
  2. Cardiovascular: Chest pain or palpitations.
  3. Pulmonary: Dyspnea on exertion or shortness of breath.
  4. Abdominal: Epigastric discomfort, nausea, or vomiting.
  5. Peripheral vascular: Claudication or skin changes related to venous stasis and HTN.

Physical Examination

A. Unremarkable in most patients with stable angina.
B. Vital signs: Assess heart rate and rhythm, blood pressure, oxygen saturation, and respiration rate.
C. General: Observe patient's level of distress.
  1. Levine sign: Fist clenched over sternum is suggestive of angina.
D. Skin: Diaphoresis and evidence of poor lipid metabolism (xanthoma) are possible.
E. Neck: Carotid bruits and increased jugular venous pressure are possible.

F. Cardiovascular: Inspect, palpate (pain on chest wall palpation is not usually cardiac in nature), and auscultate (partially audible S3, S4 due to left ventricular dysfunction and/or murmur of mitral regurgitation as sign of papillary muscle dysfunction).
G. Pulmonary: Auscultate lungs for evidence of rales/crackles (concern for congestive heart failure and pulmonary edema).
H. Abdomen: Auscultate for bruits, palpate for discomfort, assess for a pulsatile abdominal mass.
I. Peripheral vascular: Assess peripheral pulses, possible venous stasis changes, and peripheral edema.

Diagnostic Tests

A. ECG: Usually normal in patients with stable angina (if prior MI, could see Q-waves).
B. Chest radiograph: Usually normal but evaluate for cardiomegaly, pulmonary edema, pericardial effusion.
C. Cardiac biomarkers: Serial troponins, troponin T (cTnT), and troponin I (cTnI) to rule out MI.
D. Lipid panel to assess for risk of atherosclerosis.
E. Complete blood count to assess for underlying exacerbating cardiac factors such as evidence of anemia.
F. Complete metabolic panel to assess electrolytes (metabolic dysfunction can lead to arrhythmias) and kidney function (important if cardiac catheterization with contrast dye is needed).
G. Stress testing.
  1. For a positive stress test and when deemed appropriate by the cardiologist and interventional cardiologist, a cardiac catheterization with coronary angiography is performed. During this intervention, contrast dye is injected into the coronary vasculature to aid in the visualization and revascularization of the affected vessel(s).
  2. Exercise stress testing.
    a. Stress ECG: An ECG is performed before, during, and after treadmill exercise. The test is 75% sensitive if heart rate reaches 85% of maximum predicted value for age. Exercise-induced ischemia results in subendocardial ischemia (ST-segment depression on ECG); can also see hypotension or ventricular arrhythmias.
    b. Stress echocardiography: Cardiac echocardiography is performed before and after exercise.
      i. Exercise-induced ischemia is detected by cardiac wall-motion abnormalities not present at rest.
      ii. It is more sensitive for detecting ischemia than stress ECG and beneficial for determining left ventricular function.
  3. Pharmacologic stress testing (for patients unable to walk on treadmill).
    a. Intravenous adenosine or dobutamine can be used to replace treadmill activity.
    b. These agents create cardiac stress, and they can be combined with an ECG, echocardiogram, or nuclear imaging.
  4. Nuclear stress testing.
    a. Thallium or technetium 99m Tc sestamibi are used in patients with baseline ECG abnormalities to localize ischemia.
    b. Areas of damage will be ill-perfused on imaging.
H. Other cardiac diagnostic testing.
  1. Computed tomography coronary angiography (CTCA).
    a. Relatively new test.
    b. Utilizes electron-beam or multidetector CT imaging to evaluate the coronary arteries for level of calcium (coronary artery calcium [CAC] score).
    c. Useful in detecting the amount of atherosclerosis within the coronary arteries.
I. The flow chart in Figure 3.2 can help with diagnosis and risk stratification in angina.

Differential Diagnosis

A. MI.
B. Coronary vasospasm.
C. Pulmonary embolus.
D. Pericarditis.
E. Congestive heart failure.
F. Acute gastritis.
G. Cholecystitis.
H. Ruptured abdominal or thoracic aortic aneurysm.
I. Anxiety/panic attack disorders.
J. Gastroesophageal reflux/peptic ulcer disease.
K. Cocaine toxicity.
L. Hypertensive urgency or emergency.
M. Valvular abnormalities.
N. Hiatal hernia.
O. Costochondritis.

Evaluation and Management Plan

A. General plan.
  1. Prevention of MIs and reduction of angina-type symptoms; can consider the **ABCDE** mnemonic.
    A: Aspirin and antianginal agents.
    B: Beta-blockers and blood pressure management.
    C: Cholesterol management and cigarette smoking abstinence.
    D: Diet and diabetic management.
    E: Education and exercise.
  2. Treatment using risk stratification considerations.
    a. Mild disease (normal cardiac function and mild angina): Aspirin, nitrates, and beta-blockers (possibly calcium channel blockers).
    b. Moderate disease (moderate angina, normal cardiac function, two-vessel coronary disease): Use of medications for mild disease and cardiac catheterization for revascularization.
    c. Severe disease (decreased cardiac function, three-vessel/left main/left anterior artery disease with severe angina): Pharmacologic and consideration of coronary artery bypass grafting (CABG).
  3. Evaluation of patients with anginal symptoms for acute cardiac ischemia (ST-elevation MI or non-ST-segment elevation MI).
  4. For patients with UA, hospitalization for monitoring, stabilization, and possible cardiac catheterization (or stress testing if determined safe by cardiologist).
B. Patient/family teaching points.
  1. Compliance with medications and primary care provider appointments.
  2. HTN: Tight blood pressure (BP) control decreases CAD risk, especially in those with diabetes mellitus.
  3. Diabetes mellitus: Strict control of blood sugars to reduce macrovascular (CAD) disease.
  4. Hyperlipidemia: Using lifestyle modifications and the enzyme hydroxymethylglutaryl-coenzyme A (HMG-CoA) reductase inhibitors to reduce cholesterol.
  5. Obesity: Weight loss, which is imperative for cardiovascular health.

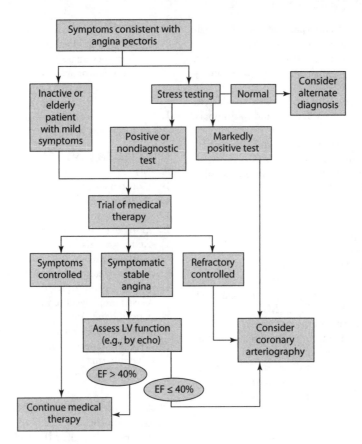

FIGURE 3.2 Diagnosis and risk stratification in angina.
EF, ejection fraction
Source: Kasper, D. L., Fauci, A. S., Hauser, S. L., Longo, D. L., Jameson, J. L., & Loscalzo, J. (Eds.). (2015). Chronic stable angina. *Harrison's principles of internal medicine* (19th ed.). New York, NY: McGraw-Hill.

6. Diet: Reducing saturated fat (<7% of total calories) and total cholesterol (<200 mg/d).

7. Physical activity: Imperative for cardiovascular health; recommend aerobic exercise for 30 minutes/day for 5 to 7 days/week.

8. Tobacco cessation to decrease risk of CAD.

C. Pharmacotherapy.

  1. Aspirin: Antiplatelet that decreases risk of MI.

  2. Beta-blockers: Decrease cardiac work (decrease pulse, BP, contractility), thus lowering myocardial oxygen demand.

  3. Nitrates: Work via vasodilation.

    a. Alleviate angina via reduction of cardiac preload and myocardial oxygen demand.

    b. Can be administered sublingually, orally, transdermally, or intravenously.

    c. Side effects: Flushing, headache, dizziness, and/or hypotension.

  4. Phosphodiesterase inhibitors: Caution necessary with medications such as sildenafil, tadalafil, and vardenafil; risk of hypotension.

  5. Calcium channel blockers: Decrease cardiac afterload and cause coronary vasodilation to increase coronary blood flow.

  6. Lipid lowering agents: HMG-CoA reductase inhibitors to decrease atherosclerosis and risk of MIs.

Follow-Up

A. Important issues during follow-up visits for patients with angina.

  1. Increased or decreased exercise tolerance.

  2. Any change in anginal symptoms.

  3. Problems with medication compliance.

  4. Any changes in modifiable risk factors (diet, activity level, tobacco cessation).

  5. Monitoring of management of comorbid conditions that contribute to CAD.

B. Additional recommendations.

  1. Annual treadmill stress testing for patients with stable CAD.

  2. Stress imaging in patients with change in CAD status or who underwent initial stress imaging due to known risk factors.

  3. Use of echocardiography to evaluate left ventricular function and wall motion in CAD patients with worsening congestive heart failure or recent MI.

Consultation/Referral

A. Consult with a cardiologist in patients with angina/CAD for proper risk stratification, diagnostic testing, treatment regimen planning, and ongoing monitoring.

B. Consult with an interventional cardiologist for patients requiring cardiac catheterization.

C. Consult with a cardiothoracic surgeon for patients requiring CABG or those with severe valvular disease requiring repair/replacement.

Special/Geriatric Considerations

A. Prinzmetal angina.

  1. Also known as variant angina caused by coronary vasospasms.

2. Rare diagnosis: Usually occurs in patients 40 to 60 years of age.

3. Can be provoked by factors such as cold exposure, tobacco use, cocaine use, emotional stress, thyrotoxicosis, excessive alcohol use, and medications (histamine, serotonin).

4. Underlying atherosclerosis in 75% of patients.

5. Chest pain episodes: Very painful; last approximately 15 minutes and usually occur at rest.

6. Can mimic symptoms of MIs; very difficult to differentiate on history and physical examination.

7. Hallmark: Transient ST elevation on ECG during chest pain episodes.

8. Coronary angiography is test of choice: Will see evidence of coronary vasospasm when IV ergonovine is administered (to stimulate chest pain).

9. Can be relieved by antianginal medications.

10. Use of calcium channel blockers and nitrates can be helpful for treatment.

B. Geriatric considerations.

1. Age: Not a limitation for evaluation and treatment of CAD.

2. Presentation: Possibly atypical symptoms.

3. Higher incidence of multivessel coronary disease.

4. Greater prevalence of renal impairment (concern for use of contrast dye during catheterization).

5. Higher incidence of polypharmacy: Potential drug interactions and medication compliance.

6. Possibly too risky for surgical intervention, thus requiring only conservative (medical) management.

7. Important to assess baseline cognitive status and comorbidities when discussing treatment plan and to involve family when necessary.

Bibliography

Agabegi, S. S., & Agabegi, E. D. (2008). *Step-up to medicine* (2nd ed.). Philadelphia, PA: Wolters Kluwer.

Alaeddini, J., & Shirani, J. (2018, July 19). Angina pectoris. In E. Yang (Ed.), *Medscape*. Retrieved from http://emedicine.medscape.com/article/150215-overview

Kasper, D. L., Fauci, A. S., Hauser, S. L., Longo, D. L., Jameson, J., & Loscalzo, J. (Eds.). (2015). Chronic stable angina. In *Harrison's manual of medicine* (19th ed.). New York, NY: McGraw-Hill.

Arrhythmias

Allison Rusgo

Definition

A. Any change from the normal electrical cardiac conduction: Can result in impulses that occur too quickly, too slowly or erratically.

B. Divided into two categories: Ventricular and supraventricular.

1. Ventricular abnormalities begin in the ventricles.

2. Supraventricular disorders originate above the ventricles (in the atria).

C. Can result in tachycardias or bradycardias.

1. With respect to bradycardia: Typically defined as a pulse less than 60 beats/minute and clinically significant when pulse is less than 45 beats/minute.

2. Possible causes of bradycardia: Sick sinus syndrome (SSS) or heart block (first-degree atrioventricular [AV] block, second-degree AV block types 1 and 2, and third-degree AV block).

Incidence

A. Atrial fibrillation (AF) is the most common sustained cardiac arrhythmia where prevalence increases with age. It affects 2.7 to 6.1 million U.S. adults.

1. Median age of AF presentation is 75 years; 84% of patients are older than 65 years of age at time of diagnosis.

2. AF affects 4% of patients younger than 60 years of age and 8% of patients younger than 80 years of age.

3. The incidence of AF is greater in males than in females and more common in Caucasians than in African Americans.

B. Approximately 50% of patients experience sudden cardiac death as an initial clinical presentation of a cardiac arrhythmia.

1. The arrhythmias most likely to cause sudden cardiac death are ventricular fibrillation (VF) or ventricular tachycardia (VT), with approximately 300,000 deaths per year.

2. VT is more commonly seen in males secondary to underlying CAD.

C. Supraventricular tachycardias: Specifically, paroxysmal supraventricular tachycardia (PSVT) maintains a prevalence of approximately 0.2% of U.S. population; noted to also increase with age.

Pathogenesis

A. The pathophysiology of arrhythmias can be complex and vary based on type of abnormality.

B. Overall, there is an abnormality in the normal activation sequence of the cardiac fibers within the myocardium. There are three primary mechanisms.

1. Increased or decreased automaticity: Increased automaticity can result in atrial or ventricular arrhythmia.

2. Triggered activity.

3. Dysfunction in circulatory pathways: Specifically notable for reentry conduction pathways.

C. The pathogenesis of AF occurs because of three underlying factors: Electrical, structural, and contractile dysfunction.

1. In the simplest terms, AF's irregularly irregular tachycardic rhythm arises because of multiple foci within the atria (principally around orifices of the pulmonary arteries) that send chaotic impulses through the heart's electrical system.

2. This causes the atria to quiver or "fibrillate" instead of contract normally.

3. Typically, the atrial rate is greater than 400 beats/minute, but some impulses are successfully blocked by the AV node. Thus, a ventricular (or calculated pulse) rate of 75 to 175 beats/minutes is appreciated.

D. Atrial flutter is a variation of AF where there is one primary automatic focus in the atria that fires between 250 and 350 beats/minute. The ventricular rate is typically one-half to one-third the atrial rate due to a refractory period of the AV node.

E. PSVT occurs because of AV nodal reentry tachycardia.

1. Two pathways within the AV node: Fast and slow.

2. Reentrant circuit revolving around the AV node.

F. Ventricular arrhythmias.

1. VT originates below the bundle of His and occurs because of quick and constant firing of three or more premature ventricular contractions (PVCs) at a rate of 100 to 250 beats/minute.

2. PVCs are defined as a heartbeat that fires on its own accord from a specific focus in one ventricle and proceeds to simulate the other ventricle.

3. VF occurs when there are multiple foci within the ventricles that are functioning on overdrive. This leads to irregular quivering of the ventricles and results in no cardiac output.

G. Bradycardias.

1. SSS: Typically occurs because of spontaneous persistent bradycardia.

2. First-degree AV block: Noted to have a conduction delay at the AV node that results in decreased pulse.

3. Second-degree AV block.

a. Type 1: Occurs because of a block within the AV node to cause bradycardia.

b. Type 2: Occurs because of a block within the bundle of His-Purkinje fibers to cause bradycardia (this can also progress to third-degree AV block).

4. Third-degree AV block: Complete dissociation between the atria and ventricles. There is no continuation of cardiac impulses between the two structures; results in significant bradycardia, typically 25 to 40 beats/minutes.

Predisposing Factors

A. AF.

1. Underlying CAD/previous MI.

2. HTN.

3. Mitral valve dysfunction.

4. History of pulmonary embolus.

5. Endocrine and adrenal disorders: Hypothyroidism or hyperthyroidism, pheochromocytoma.

6. Postoperative physiologic stress.

7. SSS.

8. Systemic illnesses such as sepsis or cancers.

9. Excess alcohol consumption (known as "holiday heart syndrome").

10. Age.

B. Atrial flutter.

1. Chronic obstructive pulmonary disease (most common cause).

2. Comorbid CAD.

3. Congestive heart failure (CHF).

4. Atrial septal defects or rheumatic heart disease.

C. PSVT.

1. Acute cardiac ischemia.

2. Medications: Most common is digoxin toxicity (causes paroxysmal atrial tachycardia with 2:1 block).

3. Atrial flutter with rapid ventricular response.

4. Excess caffeine, stimulant, or alcohol consumption.

D. VT.

1. Comorbid MI and CAD (most common causes).

2. Acute cardiac ischemia or hypotension.

3. Cardiomyopathy.

4. Congenital heart defects.

5. History of prolonged QT syndrome.

E. VF.

1. Ischemic cardiac damage (most common cause).

2. Medications: Antiarrhythmic drugs that prolong the QT interval and combination of drugs, particularly antidepressive agents (SSRIs and Tricyclics).

Subjective Data

A. Common complaints/symptoms.

1. Fatigue.

2. Dyspnea on exertion (or at rest).

3. Chest discomfort.

4. Palpitations or "heart fluttering."

5. Dizziness, lightheadedness, syncope, or near-syncope.

6. Diaphoresis.

B. History of the present illness.

1. Recognize that patient presentation varies based on type and degree of arrhythmia.

a. For example, SSS can present with dizziness, fatigue, and change in mental status while VT can present asymptomatically as sudden cardiac death (if rate is slow enough).

2. Understand onset, provoking/palliative factors, quality, severity, and timing of symptoms.

3. Obtain information regarding a patient's past medical history, specifically regarding the aforementioned conditions, that can predispose patients for abnormal heart rhythms.

C. Family and social history.

1. Determine any family history of CAD, HTN, hyperlipidemia, valvular heart disease (VHD), congenital heart defects, or arrhythmias.

2. Obtain information on tobacco use, alcohol/caffeine consumption, and illegal substance use (especially stimulants).

D. Review of systems.

1. General: Fatigue, malaise, fevers, and chills.

2. Cardiac: Angina, racing heartbeat, palpitations, decreased exercise tolerance, and peripheral edema.

3. Pulmonary: Shortness of breath and dyspnea on exertion.

4. Neurological: Lightheadedness, dizziness, syncope, and near-syncope.

Physical Examination

A. Vital signs: Assess heart rate, blood pressure, respiration, temperature, and oxygen saturation.

1. Important to note temperature, as an underlying febrile illness can exacerbate underlying AF.

2. In VF, it is likely that the patient will be unconscious with no pulse and unmeasurable BP.

B. Neck: Jugular venous distention (JVD; concern for CHF).

C. Pulmonary: Possible rales or crackles (sign of increased fluid accumulation as related to underlying CHF).

D. Cardiac: Inspection and palpation for thrills and auscultation.

1. Auscultation.

a. Assess rate (tachycardic or bradycardic).

b. Rhythm (regular, irregularly irregular, or irregularly regular).

c. Extra heart sounds (S3 and S4).

d. Murmurs consistent with underlying VHD.

E. Peripheral vascular: Assess peripheral pulses, possible peripheral edema (sign of fluid overload and concomitant CHF).

F. Neurology: Mental status examination (if mental status changes) or complete neurological examination if concern for associated syncope/near-syncope.

Diagnostic Tests

A. ECG.

1. AF: Tachycardia rate (110–180 beats/minute), irregularly irregular rhythm (irregularly spaced R-R intervals) with no discernable P-waves.

2. Atrial flutter: Tachycardic rate with a "saw-tooth" (F-wave) baseline pattern; best seen in leads VI, II, III and aVF where the QRS complex appears after several "saw-tooth" P-waves (number of F waves can vary depending on atrioventricular node [AVN] blockade).

3. VF: Irregular rhythm, no identifiable P-waves, or QRS complexes.

4. VT: Tachycardic rate (150–250 beats/minute) and wide QRS complexes (can have identical morphologies in monomorphic VT or different ones in polymorphic VT).

5. PSVT (most common etiology of reentry conduction): Tachycardic rate, narrow QRS complexes with no discernable P-waves (P-waves are buried within the QRS complexes secondary to simultaneous rapid firing of the atria and ventricles).

6. First-degree heart block: Hallmark is a PR interval greater than 0.20 seconds where a QRS complex follows each P-wave.

7. Second-degree heart block.

    a. Type 1 (Mobitz Type I or Wenckebach): Hallmark is progressive prolongation of the PR interval with a nonconducted P-wave. The longest PR interval preceding the dropped QRS and the shortest immediately after.

    b. Type 2 (Mobitz Type II): Hallmark is an intermittent nonconducted P-wave without progressive prolongation, but immediate PR interval to dropped QRS is prolonged.

8. Third-degree heart block: Bradycardic rate, with no discernable pattern or connection between P-waves and QRS complexes.

B. Laboratory tests.

1. Complete blood count with differential: Determine if an anemia is contributing to the arrhythmia.

2. Complete metabolic panel: Determine if an electrolyte disturbance or renal dysfunction is contributing to the arrhythmia.

3. Thyroid panel: Hypothyroidism or hyperthyroidism can be an underlying etiology for arrhythmias (i.e., thyrotoxicosis can trigger AF).

4. Cardiac biomarkers: These should be obtained in any patient with chest discomfort or evidence of an arrhythmia; they evaluate for the possibility of underlying myocardial infarction.

5. Digitalis level (if clinically indicated): Supratherapeutic levels can lead to various arrhythmias, including PSVT and AF with rapid ventricular response.

6. Toxicology screening (if clinically indicated): Illegal substances, especially stimulants, can precipitate arrhythmias.

7. D-dimer: This can help rule out a pulmonary embolus, which can occur in the setting of AF.

C. Chest x-ray: Checks for underlying cardiomegaly, pulmonary edema, or pulmonary infections such as pneumonia, or pneumothorax, which can exacerbate or precipitate arrhythmias.

D. Exercise stress testing: Helps provide an overall understanding of one's cardiovascular health and evaluate for underlying ischemia.

E. Holter monitor or loop recorder: Can be helpful for monitoring patients on a continuous basis when an arrhythmia is suspected but unable to be captured via ECG; can also be helpful for patients with vague or nonspecific cardiac symptoms.

F. Transesophageal echocardiogram (TEE): Especially important for new-onset arrhythmias to evaluate overall cardiac function (ejection fraction [EF]), identify VHD, and measure atria and ventricle sizes.

1. With AF, if there is concern for a thrombus, particularly within the left atrial appendage, the test of choice is a TEE.

Differential Diagnosis

A. AF.

B. Atrial flutter.

C. VF.

D. Ventricular flutter.

E. Atrial tachycardia.

F. PSVT.

G. SSS.

H. First-degree heart block.

I. Second-degree heart block types 1 and 2.

J. Third-degree heart block.

Evaluation and Management Plan

A. General plan.

1. Determine type of arrhythmia.

2. Stabilize heart rate and rhythm based on clinical scenario using pharmacologic or procedural methods such as electrocardioversion or transcutaneous/transvenous pacing.

3. Evaluate underlying cardiac status and comorbidities to guide treatment plan.

4. Determine if arrhythmia is secondary to an underlying etiology that requires additional management (i.e., sepsis, thyrotoxicosis, myocardial infarction).

5. Consult with cardiologist (and electrophysiologist) if device implantation or ablation procedures are required.

6. For arrhythmias requiring anticoagulation (AC) for thromboembolic prophylaxis, such as AF, complete risk stratification assessment, and discuss risks and benefits of these medications with patients and families.

    a. Utilize the CHA_2DS_2-VASc score, which is a risk stratification tool to determine the chance of thromboembolic strokes (see Table 3.2).

    b. For patients with a score of 2+, oral AC is recommended using a vitamin K antagonist (i.e., warfarin with international normalized ratio [INR] goal 2.0–3.0) or a novel anticoagulant (i.e., dabigatran, rivaroxaban, edoxaban, or apixaban).

    c. For patients with a score of "0" in males or "1" in females, no therapy is recommended.

B. Patient/family teaching points.

1. Educate regarding specific arrhythmia and symptoms that can precipitate recurrence (if clinically relevant).

2. Educate on reasons to return to the ED, specifically those that signal worsening cardiac status or development of a life-threatening arrhythmia.

3. Educate on the importance of medication compliance and regular follow-up appointments with cardiologist/electrophysiologist.

4. For patients utilizing warfarin for AC, it is important to discuss dietary restrictions. It is also essential to educate patients on any anticoagulant regarding risk of bleeding.

5. For implantable devices—ensure patients understand the purpose of their device, importance of device maintenance, who to contact if there is an equipment malfunction, and how device monitoring will occur.

C. Pharmacotherapy.

1. Acute AF/atrial flutter.

    a. Rate control: Target rate is 60 to 100 beats/minute.

i. Calcium channel blockers are preferred (can use beta-blockers).

ii. If there is significant left ventricular dysfunction, consider digoxin or amiodarone.

iii. For patients with chronic AF: Can utilize calcium channel blockers or beta-blockers for long-term rate control.

b. Rhythm control.

i. Can utilize electrical or pharmacological methods (electrical cardioversion is preferred).

ii. If pharmacologic conversion, consider options such as sotalol, flecainide, amiodarone, dofetilide.

c. AC: Assess need based on risk stratification tools and comorbidities.

i. If a patient is hemodynamically unstable, initiate immediate electrical cardioversion to convert to normal sinus rhythm regardless of AC considerations.

ii. If a patient is hemodynamically stable and AF is under hypothermic conditions, gradual slow rewarming via a warming blanket is recommended.

iii. AF present for greater than 48 hours (or unknown period of time), there is high risk of stroke if electrical cardioversion is performed immediately; recommend AC for 3 weeks before and at least 4 weeks after successful cardioversion (INR goal 2.0–3.0 if using warfarin).

iv. To expedite cardioversion timing: Obtain TEE to rule out thrombus in left atrial appendage, administer IV heparin, cardiovert within 24 hours, and then utilize oral AC agent for 1 month.

v. If a patient is hemodynamically stable and AF is present for less than 48 hours, electrical cardioversion without prior AC or TEE can occur at the discretion of the cardiologist and must take into account a patient's CHA_2DS_2VASc Score. If the procedure is completed, postprocedure AC is also utilized for 1 month.

2. PSVT.

a. If hemodynamically stable, first attempt vagal maneuvers such as Valsalva, breath holding, or immersion of head in cold water.

b. If nonpharmacological maneuvers are unsuccessful, administer intravenous adenosine (drug of choice) to reduce sinoatrial (SA) and AV node activity using a short-acting medication.

c. If adenosine is unsuccessful in converting acute PSVT to normal sinus rhythm, the most common intravenous alternatives are beta-blockers (i.e., metoprolol, propranolol, esmolol) or calcium channel blockers (i.e., verapamil, diltiazem) for patients without left ventricular dysfunction; for individuals with heart failure or structural heart disease, intravenous amiodarone can be used.

d. If pharmacologic methods are unsuccessful or the patient is hemodynamically unstable, perform electrical cardioversion (almost always successful).

e. For long-term rate control, beta-blockers and calcium channel blockers are used. Digoxin can also be used in the setting of heart failure; if symptoms are recurrent and persistent, refer to electrophysiologist for ablation.

3. VT.

a. If sustained VT (lasts longer than 30 seconds, usually symptomatic and with hemodynamic instability), initiate immediate electrical cardioversion and then intravenous amiodarone to maintain sinus rhythm.

i. If sustained VT without hemodynamic compromise and mild symptoms, consider intravenous medications such as sotalol, procainamide, or lidocaine.

ii. If sustained VT and abnormal EF, placement of ICD for long-term management will likely be required.

b. If nonsustained VT (brief asymptomatic episodes of VT) without cardiac comorbidities, do not treat (no increased risk of morbidity).

i. If nonsustained VT with underlying cardiac disease, consider ICD as first-line long-term management.

4. VF.

a. Medical emergency that requires immediate CPR and defibrillation.

b. Imperative to follow Advanced Cardiac Life Support (ACLS) algorithm for pharmacologic recommendations.

5. Bradycardic rhythms.

a. For several types of bradycardias, including SSS, second degree heart block type 2, and third degree heart block, pacemaker implantation is the most effective long-term monitoring strategy.

b. Pharmacologic interventions.

i. Atropine: Can utilize for acute symptomatic bradycardia (if reversible cause not identified).

ii. Dopamine: Second-line drug for symptomatic bradycardia if atropine is ineffective.

iii. Epinephrine: Can utilize as an infusion for symptomatic bradycardia if atropine or pacing methods are unsuccessful.

D. Discharge instructions.

1. Ensure patients receive all appropriate prescriptions prior to discharge.

2. Ensure patients have prearranged follow-up appointments with cardiologist/electrophysiologist.

3. For patients with newly implanted devices, ensure information is provided regarding the device, clinic follow-up, and home monitoring systems (if indicated).

TABLE 3.2	CHA_2DS_2VASc Score for Risk Assessment in AF

	Criteria	Score
C	Congestive heart failure	1
H	Hypertension: Blood pressure consistently above 140/90 mmHg (or treated hypertension on medication)	1
A2	Age ≥75 y	2
D	Diabetes mellitus	1
S2	Prior stroke or transient ischemic attack	2
V	Vascular disease (e.g., peripheral artery disease, myocardial infarction, aortic plaque)	1
A	Age 65–74 y	1
Sc	Sex (i.e., female gender)	1

AF, atrial fibrillation.

a. Educate on proper wound care of incision site for a newly implanted device and reasons to return to a healthcare provider for signs of infection (i.e., erythema, edema, worsening pain, drainage, dehiscence, systemic symptoms).

4. Understand that it is important that patients understand limitations regarding physical activity, depending on their type and degree of arrhythmia and cardiac status.

Follow-Up

A. Ensure patient compliance with all medications, particularly with respect to antiarrhythmic or AC therapy.

1. Patients on antiarrhythmic therapy should have close follow-up with a cardiologist or electrophysiologist to minimize adverse effects.

    a. Patients utilizing amiodarone should have a clear understanding of its side effects and monitor closely for amiodarone-induced liver, lung, thyroid, and other organ toxicities.

2. Patients on AC therapy with warfarin should understand their follow-up plan with regard to frequency of INR monitoring and how dosing adjustments will be communicated.

B. Outpatient oral medication choices for arrhythmias depend on degree of ventricular dysfunction, type of arrhythmia, and comorbidities.

C. Patients should have close monitoring of their electrolytes to reduce the risk of arrhythmias secondary to electrolyte imbalances.

D. Patients with ICDs and pacemakers require regular outpatient device follow-up at electrophysiology clinics where their devices are monitored for lead integrity and battery-life.

Consultation/Referral

A. Consult with cardiologist to further evaluate arrhythmia and underlying cardiac status.

B. Consult with electrophysiologist for in-depth electrophysiologic diagnostics and ablative procedures.

Special/Geriatric Considerations

A. Additional device considerations.

1. Temporary pacemakers.

    a. Transcutaneous pacing.

        i. Used for symptomatic bradycardias if the patient fails to respond to atropine, dopamine, or epinephrine (can also be utilized in setting of tachyarrhythmias to break the conduction disturbance).

        ii. Should be started immediately if patient is hemodynamically unstable, especially in those with second degree heart block type II or third degree heart block.

        iii. Can be painful; use analgesia and sedation for pain control.

        iv. Use transvenous pacing if transcutaneous pacing is unsuccessful (cardiologist or electrophysiologist should be consulted prior to initiation).

2. Permanent pacemakers.

    a. Single-chamber pacemakers: Stimulate either the atria or (more commonly) the ventricle.

    b. Dual-chamber pacemakers: Send electrical impulses to both the atrium and the ventricle; provides synchronization that closely mimics the natural heartbeat (commonly used for bradycardias).

    c. Biventricular pacemakers: Pace the rhythm of the ventricles so that the chambers contract simultaneously; used in patients with heart failure and conduction abnormalities.

    d. Combination pacemaker: Have pacemaker and defibrillation functions.

3. Implantable cardiac defibrillator: Surgically placed and functions by detecting lethal cardiac arrhythmias and delivering electrical shocks until the rhythm normalizes; indicated in VF and/or VT that is uncontrolled with medication (important prevention for sudden cardiac death).

B. Geriatric considerations.

1. Aging process is associated with the development of arrhythmias, particularly AF.

2. Degenerative changes of the cardiac conduction system (i.e., SA and AV nodes) are more common in elderly patients, who are more likely to experience heart blocks due to conduction delays.

3. Elderly patients are more likely to have ventricular heart disease and thus a higher risk of arrhythmias secondary to structural abnormalities (especially within the aortic and mitral valves).

4. During the physiologic aging process, the PR interval can be prolonged.

5. Geriatric patients can report vague complaints (i.e., weakness, fatigue, malaise) as presenting symptoms for an arrhythmia. It can be difficult to separate these from the normal aging process.

6. The frequency of PVCs also increases with age.

7. If considering a device for geriatric patients, it is important to address comorbidities, life span, impact on quality of life, maintenance of device, and occurrence of unnecessary shocks during end-of-life care.

8. The use of anticoagulants in the geriatric population should be carefully reviewed with patients (and family members, if necessary) to ensure that risks versus benefits of these medications are evaluated.

    a. Cognitive status (important for medication compliance).

    b. Comorbidities (e.g., is patient already utilizing other antiplatelet or anticoagulant agents, thus increasing the risk of bleeding events?).

    c. Overall functional status—important to address risk of falls and bleeding complications.

Bibliography

Agabegi, S. S., & Agabegi, E. D. (2008). *Step-up to medicine* (2nd ed.). Philadelphia, PA: Wolters Kluwer.

Bashore, T. M., Granger, C. B., Jackson, K. P., & Patel, M. R., Heart disease. In M. A. Papadakis, S. J. McPhee, & M. W. Rabow (Eds.), *Current medical diagnosis & treatment 2018* (57th ed., pp. 328–446). New York, NY: McGraw-Hill.

Gugneja, M., & Kraft, P. L. (2017, April 5). Paroxysmal supraventricular tachycardia. In M. F. El-Chami (Ed.), *Medscape*. Retrieved from http://emedicine.medscape.com/article/156670-overview

MedCalc 3000. (2011). Atrial fibrillation CHA$_2$DS$_2$-VASc score for stroke risk. Retrieved from https://reference.medscape.com/calculator/chads-vasc-af-stroke

Rosenthal, L., McManus, D. D., & Sardana, M. (2018, July 18). Atrial fibrillation. In J. N. Rottman (Ed.), *Medscape*. Retrieved from http://emedicine.medscape.com/article/151066-overview

Sohinki, D., & Obel, O. A. (2014). Current trends in supraventricular tachycardia management. *The Ochsner Journal*, 14(4), 586–595. Retrieved from https://www.ncbi.nlm.nih.gov/pmc/articles/PMC4295736

Dyslipidemia

Allison Rusgo

Definition

A. Hyperlipidemia: Elevation of total cholesterol (TC), phospholipids, or triglycerides (TG).
B. Hyperlipidemia can be inherited or caused by secondary diagnoses.
C. It increases the risk of atherosclerosis, leading to stroke and heart disease.
D. Dyslipidemia: Elevation of plasma cholesterol, TGs, or both, or a decreased high-density lipoprotein level (HDL) that augments atherosclerosis.

Incidence

A. Framingham Heart Study noted an epidemiological link between elevated cholesterol and atherosclerotic cardiovascular disease (ASCVD).
B. Current statistics also show that elevated cholesterol is responsible for an estimated 2.6 million deaths per year worldwide.
C. An estimated 31% of U.S. adults have elevated TG (>150 mg/dL).

Pathogenesis

A. Disease process starts in gastrointestinal tract with hydroxymethylglutaryl-coenzyme A (HMG-CoA).
B. HMG-CoA is a precursor that undergoes complex biochemical reactions to produce cholesterol.
C. Once synthesized, cholesterol travels through the plasma.
D. The liver also plays a role, converting very low-density lipoprotein (VLDL) to low-density lipoprotein (LDL), which moves through the plasma.
E. Also, dietary cholesterol that moves from the small intestines to the liver through the serum with LDLs must be considered.
F. Cholesterol is an important organic molecule for cell membrane integrity and serves as precursor to steroid hormones, vitamin D, and bile acid. However, with increased levels of cholesterol, concern is for atherosclerosis.
G. Atherosclerosis is an inflammatory process where various cells and mediators undergo a cascade of reactions to form plaques in the vasculature.
  1. Various factors trigger inflammation, such as elevated glucose, tobacco by-products, elevated blood pressure (BP), and oxidized LDLs.
  2. With increased inflammation, there is increased permeability and injury to vessel walls. The result is increased accumulation of LDLs within the tunica intima layer of the vasculature.
  3. The inflammation causes increased activation of inflammatory mediators (i.e., monocytes and macrophages).
  4. Inflammatory mediators uptake the oxidized LDLs, leading to transformation of macrophages into foam cells, also known as "fatty streaks" within the vasculature.
  5. Foam cells eventually result in plaque formation with fibrous caps; when the thin top layer of these caps dislodges, exposing highly thrombotic necrotic contents, platelet aggregation and cardiac ischemia can result.

Predisposing Factors

A. Hereditary: Genetic component for the metabolism of LDL.

1. Familial hypercholesterolemia (FH): A type of hyperlipidemia (HLD) caused by genetic mutation (chromosome 19) where those affected have TC greater than 300 mg/dL and LDL greater than 200 mg/dL (other variations exist with TC >1,000 mg/dL).
B. Diet: Foods high in saturated fat and cholesterol.
C. Lifestyle: Physical inactivity, which can lead to increased cholesterol levels.
D. Comorbidities.
  1. Secondary causes of hyperlipidemia: Hypothyroidism, diabetes mellitus (DM), nephrotic syndrome, Cushing disease, chronic kidney disease (CKD), and medications (oral contraceptives, diuretics).
  2. Secondary causes of elevated TGs: Obesity, DM, alcohol use, CKD, and medications (estrogen).
  3. Concern for metabolic syndrome: Large waist circumference, elevated TGs, low HDL level, elevated BP, elevated glucose levels.

Subjective Data

A. Common complaints/symptoms.
  1. Rarely any complaints from hyperlipidemia alone.
  2. Concern exists from its sequelae, such as cardiovascular disease, peripheral vascular disease (PVD) secondary to claudication, and neurological diseases (i.e., transient ischemic attack [TIA] and cerebrovascular accident [CVA]).
B. Common history of present illness (HPI).
  1. Determine the duration of a patient's hyperlipidemia diagnosis and how the diagnosis occurred (i.e., detected during routine screening versus after an acute event such as an myocardial infarction [MI] or CVA/TIA).
  2. Assess a patient's routine monitoring of his or her cholesterol—when levels were last checked and how they have evolved over time.
  3. Assess a patient's past medical history for associated comorbidities such as hypertension (HTN), MI, peripheral artery disease (PAD)/PVD, coronary artery disease (CAD), carotid artery stenosis, or DM II. It is also important to assess for any underlying liver disease, which is a contraindication to statin use.
  4. If a patient is utilizing lipid-lowering medication, assess for side effects, such as myopathies that are commonly appreciated in statin use. If a patient is utilizing nonpharmacological interventions, such as diet and exercise, those interventions should also be reviewed.
  5. Determine if a patient is experiencing any cardiovascular or neurological complaints as a result of the hyperlipidemia.
C. Family and social history.
  1. Assess for family history of hyperlipidemia, dyslipidemia, CAD, DM type 2, PVD, PAD, and neurological complications (CVA, TIA).
  2. Understand dietary routine, exercise/activity levels, and use of tobacco and alcohol consumption.
D. Review of systems.
  1. Evidence of weight gain.
  2. Skin changes: Yellow deposits (xanthomas).
  3. Cardiac symptoms: Chest pain, palpitations, decreased exercise tolerance, shortness of breath, and dyspnea on exertion.
  4. Peripheral vascular status: Claudication.
  5. Neurological (if concern for CVA or TIA): Changes in mental status, vision, speech, sensation, and strength.

Physical Examination

A. Vital signs: Determine body mass index (BMI) and consider comorbid HTN.

B. Skin: Check for xanthomas.

C. Ophthalmologic: Perform funduscopic examination and check for possible corneal arcus.

D. Neck: Auscultate carotid arteries and evaluate for carotid bruits.

E. Cardiovascular: Inspect for lifts/heaves/visible pulsations, assess point of maximum impulse (PMI), palpate for thrills, and auscultate using diaphragm and bell for murmurs and extra heart sounds.

F. If concern for CVA/TIA—consider complete neurological examination.

Diagnostic Tests

A. For the evaluation of dyslipidemia, the U.S. Preventive Services Task Force (USPSTF) strongly recommends (level A evidence) the routine screening of males 35 years old and older and females 45 years old and older for lipid disorders.

B. Evaluation should consist of fasting (9–12 hours fast) lipid panel for TC, LDL, and HDL (see Table 3.3).

C. For secondary causes of dyslipidemia, workup should include a complete blood count, complete metabolic panel, fasting glucose, thyroid-stimulating hormone (TSH), and urinary protein.

D. Lipid measurement should be accompanied by evaluation for other cardiovascular risk factors, including an ECG, stress testing, and echocardiogram.

Differential Diagnosis

A. The focus of the differential diagnosis in dyslipidemia is on primary versus secondary causes.

    1. Primary causes—inherited disorder.

    2. Secondary causes.

        a. Hypothyroidism.

        b. Corticosteroids.

        c. Alcoholism.

        d. Smoking.

        e. Obstructive liver disease.

TABLE 3.3   **Diagnostic Interpretation of Lipid Panel**

LDL Cholesterol (mg/dL)	
<100	Optimal
100–129	Near optimal
130–159	Borderline high
160–189	High
>190	Very high
HDL Cholesterol (mg/dL)	
<40	Low
>60	High
TC (mg/dL)	
<200	Preferable
200–239	Borderline high
>240	High

HDL, high-density lipoprotein; LDL, low-density lipoprotein; TC, total cholesterol.

    f. Renal failure.

    g. Uncontrolled diabetes.

    h. Nephrotic syndrome.

Evaluation and Management Plan

A. General plan.

    1. The National Cholesterol Education Program (NCEP) and Adult Treatment Panel (ATP) III have created a process for the management of elevated cholesterol.

    2. Determine LDL, TC, and HDL levels.

    3. Identify any comorbidities, including cardiovascular disease or its equivalents (DM, PAD, abdominal aortic aneurysm).

    4. Identify modifiable and unmodifiable risk factors: Low HDL, tobacco use, HTN, age (males >45 years and females >55 years), and family history of CAD.

    5. Assess overall cardiovascular risk and determine goal LDL.

    6. Initiate therapeutic lifestyle changes (TLC) plan if LDL is higher than goal: Consists of increased physical activity, weight management, and low trans fat and low cholesterol diet.

    7. Utilize medications if LDL remains above goal.

    8. Assess for metabolic syndrome and evaluate TGs.

    9. Treat elevated HDL and TGs if required.

B. Patient/family teaching points.

    1. Emphasize medication compliance, use of TLC plan, and elimination of modifiable risk factors (i.e., tobacco cessation).

    2. Stress importance of compliance with clinician appointments.

C. Pharmacotherapy.

    1. Lipid management.

        a. Statins (HMG-CoA reductase inhibitor).

            i. Important considerations regarding side effects of statins.

            ii. Elevation in liver enzymes (usually alanine aminotransferase [ALT]).

            iii. Myalgias: Occurs in approximately 10% of patients, can be dose dependent; switching to different statin can help relieve symptoms.

            iv. Rhabdomyolysis: Myalgias plus creatine kinase (CK) levels greater than 10,000 U/L can result in renal failure.

            v. Myositis: Myalgias with CK less than 10,000 U/L.

        b. Bile acid sequestrants.

        c. Cholesterol absorption inhibitors.

        d. Injectable medications (monoclonal antibodies); works by allowing liver to absorb increased level of cholesterol, thus decreasing circulating plasma cholesterol).

    2. Medications for high TG.

        a. Fibrates.

        b. Niacin.

        c. Omega-3 fatty acids supplements.

Follow-Up

A. Check lipid levels per American College of Cardiology (ACC) and American Heart Association (AHA) recommendations, which stipulate checking levels at 4 to 12 weeks after initiating (or changing) statin therapy and then every 3 to 12 months thereafter.

B. Obtain baseline liver and CK levels before initiating statin therapy (routine monitoring not required).

Consultation/Referral

A. Consult with lipidologist in the following situations.

1. Suspicion for primary genetic disorder.

2. Unsuccessful treatment plans despite optimal therapy and patient compliance.

3. Comorbid liver disease if limiting therapeutic options.

4. Young adults in whom long-term therapy and monitoring is a consideration.

Special/Geriatric Considerations

A. Patients with statin intolerance. Use the following.

1. Lower intensity statin or nondaily moderate intensity statin.

2. Low-dose statin with selective cholesterol-absorption therapy (ezetimibe), bile acid sequestrants, or niacin.

3. Nonstatin monotherapy with goal of 30% reduction in LDL levels.

B. Geriatric considerations.

1. Patients *at least* 65 to younger than 80 years of age with ASCVD or DM: Consider moderate or high intensity statin (once risks/benefits assessed by provider and patient).

2. For secondary cardiovascular prevention in patients 80 years of age or older: Consider moderate intensity statin once risks/benefits assessed by provider and patient.

Bibliography

Lloyd-Jones, D. M., Morris, P. B., Ballantyne, C. M., Birtcher, K. K., Daly, D. D., Jr., DePalma, S. M., & Smith, S. C., Jr. (2017, October). 2017 focused update of the 2016 ACC expert consensus decision pathway on the role of non-statin therapies for LDL-cholesterol lowering in the management of atherosclerotic cardiovascular disease risk. *Journal of the American College of Cardiology, 70*(14), 1785–1822. doi:10.1016/j.jacc.2017.07.745

National Cholesterol Education Program, National Heart, Lung, and Blood Institute, National Institutes of Health. (2001, May). NIH Publication No. 01-3670. Retrieved from https://www.nhlbi.nih.gov/files/docs/guidelines/atp3xsum.pdf.

Prabhakaran, D., Anand, S., Gaziano, T. A., Mbanya, J.-C., Wu, Y., & Nugent, R. (2017). *Disease control priorities: Cardiovascular, respiratory, and related disorders* (3rd ed., Vol. 5). Washington, DC: World Bank. Retrieved from https://openknowledge.worldbank.org/handle/10986/28875. License: CC BY 3.0 IGO

Reamy, B. V. (2011). Dyslipidemias. In J. E. South-Paul, S. C. Matheny, & E. L. Lewis (Eds.), *CURRENT diagnosis & treatment in family medicine* (3rd ed., pp. 224–228). New York, NY: McGraw-Hill.

Tsai, S. A., Ravenell, J., Fernandez, S., Schoenthaler, A., Kenny, K., & Ogedegbe, G. (2014). Cardiovascular disease prevention. In S. S. Gorin (Ed.), *Prevention practice in primary care.* (pp. 120–149). New York, NY: Oxford University Press.

Tsao, C. W., & Vasan, R. S. (2015, December 1). Cohort profile: The Framingham Heart Study (FHS): Overview of milestones in cardiovascular epidemiology. *International Journal of Epidemiology, 44*(6), 1800–1813. doi:10.1093/ije/dyv337

Heart Failure

Allison Rusgo

Definition

A. Inability of the heart to meet the metabolic demands of the body.

B. Left-sided heart failure (HF): Further classified by the functional capacity of the left ventricle via ejection fraction (EF).

1. Heart failure with preserved ejection fraction (HFpEF).

a. EF at least 40%.

b. Occurs when the ventricle is unable to properly fill during diastole (muscle has stiffened).

c. Amount of available blood for circulation is decreased.

2. Heart failure with reduced ejection fraction (HFrEF).

a. EF less than 40%.

b. Occurs when ventricle has lost its normal contractile ability.

c. Force/amount of blood pumped during systole is decreased.

C. Right-sided HF: An additional subtype of HF; usually occurs secondary to HFrEF, but also seen in HFpEF, idiopathic pulmonary arterial hypertension (IPAH), and chronic obstructive pulmonary disease (COPD).

1. Left ventricular dysfunction causes an increase in fluid pressure that travels into the lungs and affects the right ventricle (RV).

2. This results in fluid accumulation in the peripheral system.

D. High-output HF: A subtype of HF where there is an increase in the body's oxygen demands (i.e., chronic anemia, pregnancy, hyperthyroidism).

1. Increased demand forces the heart to work harder to meet these needs.

2. This eventually results in decreased cardiac function.

E. HF can be defined by the New York Heart Association (NYHA) classification, which is a method to categorize severity of HF based on patient symptoms (see Table 3.4).

Incidence

A. HF affects approximately 5.7 million Americans, with 850,000 new cases diagnosed per year.

B. Prevalence of HF increases with age, doubling with each decade of life and exceeding 10% in males and females older than 80 years.

C. HF is the leading cause of hospital admissions for patients older than 65 years of age.

D. HF is the second most common cardiovascular diagnosis evaluated during outpatient primary care visits.

E. Overall, the United States spends more than 30 billion dollars per year on HF.

TABLE 3.4	NYHA Classification of HF
Class I	Nearly asymptomatic; can experience HF symptoms (angina, palpitations, dyspnea) with very vigorous sporting activities
Class II	Slight limitation of physical activity where ordinary activities (i.e., climbing steps) causes HF symptoms; no symptoms at rest
Class III	Marked limitation of physical activity where very basic activity (i.e., walking on a flat surface) causes HF symptoms; no symptoms at rest
Class IV	Unable to perform any activity without symptoms of HF; symptoms also present at rest, disease is Incapacitating

HF, heart failure; NYHA, New York Heart Association.

Pathogenesis

A. During the aging process, the heart develops a decreased ability to respond appropriately to normal stressors (i.e., physical activity) or disease states (i.e., hypertension [HTN] or myocardial infarctions [MIs]).

B. Four major pathophysiologic changes have been identified.

    1. Decreased ability to reach maximum heart rate and contractility under stressful conditions (secondary to impaired beta-adrenergic activity).

    2. Increased stiffness of coronary and peripheral vasculature: This affects EF and causes increased afterload.

    3. Altered diastolic filling ability.

    4. Insufficient amount of energy production (on a cellular level) to meet the needs of the heart under stressful physiologic and/or pathophysiologic conditions.

Predisposing Factors

A. Coronary artery disease (CAD; MI/ischemic cardiomyopathy).

B. HTN/hyperlipidemia.

C. Valvular heart disease (VHD; atrial stenosis [AS], atrial regurgitation [AR], mitral stenosis [MS], mitral regurgitation [MR]).

D. Peripheral vascular disease.

E. Connective tissue diseases (i.e., sarcoidosis).

F. Arrhythmias (new onset/persistent atrial fibrillation, ventricular arrhythmias, bradyarrhythmias).

G. Cardiomyopathies (alcohol related; nonischemic, restrictive, or hypertrophic; medication related).

H. Infectious (myocarditis, pericarditis, endocarditis).

I. High-output HF (anemia of chronic disease, pregnancy, hyperthyroidism, thiamine deficiency, atrioventricular [AV] shunting).

J. Noncardiac etiologies: Pulmonary embolus, pneumonia, exacerbation of COPD.

Subjective Data

A. Common complaints/symptoms.

    1. Shortness of breath (SOB) or dyspnea (during activity or rest).

    2. Fatigue or generalized weakness.

    3. Decreased exercise tolerance.

    4. Orthopnea: Manifests as difficulty breathing while supine; relieved with head elevation using pillows.

    5. Paroxysmal nocturnal dyspnea (PND): Sudden awakening during sleep secondary to acute SOB.

    6. Nonproductive cough (worse at night).

    7. Confusion/change in mental status: Due to inadequate cerebral perfusion in late stages of HF.

    8. Swelling of extremities: Secondary to volume overload.

B. History of the present illness.

    1. Determine chief complaint that is associated with HF and evaluate the onset, provoking factors, palliative factors, quality, and severity and timing of the symptoms.

    2. Determine if this is an initial presentation or exacerbation of a previously diagnosed HF.

    3. Evaluate the past medical history for known HF, previous MI, HTN, HLD, diabetes mellitus (DM), cardiomyopathies, congenital heart defects, sleep apnea, renal disease, or collagen vascular diseases.

    4. Determine if a previous cardiac evaluation was performed (i.e., ECG, stress test, echocardiogram, cardiac catheterization).

C. Family and social history.

    1. Determine past and present tobacco use, alcohol consumption, and use of illegal substances.

    2. Review daily diet and nutrition information.

    3. Determine frequency and degree of physical activity routines.

    4. Evaluate family history for cardiac diseases such as HF, MI, HTN, hyperlipidemia, CAD, and cardiovascular equivalents (i.e., DM).

        a. If there is evidence of cardiomyopathy, the Heart Failure Society of America recommends an in-depth three-generation family history evaluation for cardiovascular diseases, especially those related to cardiomyopathies.

D. Review of systems.

    1. General: Fatigue, malaise, weight changes, appetite changes, and generalized weakness.

    2. Skin/nails: Changes in nail shape (i.e., clubbing).

    3. Cardiac: Chest discomfort, palpitations, decreased exercise tolerance, and peripheral edema.

    4. Pulmonary: Nonproductive cough, SOB, dyspnea on exertion, orthopnea, PND.

    5. Gastrointestinal: Bloating, nausea, changes in bowel habits.

    6. Genitourinary: Oliguria, nocturia.

    7. Neurological: Syncope, near-syncope, confusion, memory impairment, sleep disturbances, headaches.

    8. Psychological: Anxiety, irritability.

Physical Examination

A. Assessment of HF patients can vary based on stage of disease and underlying comorbidities.

B. The most common physical examination findings are based on severity (see Table 3.5).

Diagnostic Tests

A. The American Heart Association (AHA), American College of Cardiology (ACC), and Heart Failure Society of America recommend the following tests in the evaluation of HF.

    1. Complete blood count: Identify anemias or infections as underlying factors of HF.

    2. Complete metabolic panel: Identify electrolyte imbalances (especially important for patients using diuretics).

    3. Renal function: Identification of underlying kidney dysfunction (decreased renal perfusion) as a marker for HF.

    4. Fasting glucose: Helps identify underlying DM as a contributing factor to overall cardiovascular health.

    5. Natriuretic peptides (brain natriuretic peptide [BNP] or pro-BNP): Help evaluate ventricular pressure and volume status.

    6. Liver function panel: Evaluate aspartate aminotransferase (AST) and alanine aminotransferase (ALT), which can be elevated in cardiac cirrhosis or congestive hepatomegaly as a result of long-standing HF.

    7. Urinalysis: Evaluates for proteinuria, which is a marker of cardiovascular disease.

    8. ECG: Somewhat nonspecific but can be useful to detect left ventricular hypertrophy (LVH) or underlying cardiac ischemia or arrhythmias.

    9. Chest x-ray: Important evaluation tool for size and shape of the cardiac silhouette and presence of effusions.

        a. Can appreciate cardiomegaly.

b. May show Kerley B Lines: Short, thin horizontal lines that are noted near the border of the lung and extend outward as a marker of increased interstitial pulmonary fluid.

c. Can appreciate pleural effusions or pulmonary edema.

10. Echocardiogram: **Diagnostic test of choice for suspected HF.**

   a. Utilized to determine type of HF (i.e., HFpEF or HFrEF).

   b. Useful for determining the EF, where a value less than 40% can help delineate between HF with preserved versus reduced EF.

   c. Evaluates for VHD, overall dilatation, and/or hypertrophy: In addition, can consider a stress echocardiogram as a measure of underlying cardiac ischemia/CAD.

11. Cardiac catheterization/coronary angiography.

   a. Useful in the following scenarios.

      i. For refractory HF in patients without CAD.

      ii. For HFrEF with concomitant angina, wall-motion abnormalities on echocardiogram, nuclear evidence of reversible ischemia, or if percutaneous revascularization is considered.

      iii. If there is a high suspicion of ischemic cardiomyopathy and surgical procedures are a consideration.

      iv. If cardiac transplant or device implantation is being considered.

TABLE 3.5	Common Physical Findings in HF (Grouped by Severity)
Mild	• Crackles in lung bases • S3 gallop (best heard at apex with bell) • S4 gallop (best heard at left sternal border with bell) • Jugular vein distention • Generalized weakness • Peripheral pitting edema • Weight gain/increased abdominal girth • Displaced point of maximal impulse (usually leftward)
Moderate	In addition to the earlier findings: • Nonproductive cough • Right ventricular heave • Loud pulmonic component of second heart sound (best heard at left sternal border due to pulmonary HTN) • Crackles in lung bases • Dullness to percussion of lung bases and decreased tactile fremitus (secondary to pleural effusions) • Tachypnea (especially at rest) • Tachycardia • Hepatomegaly/ascites/hepatojugular reflex • Edema (extremities, sacral, and scrotal)
Severe	• Ascites • Central and peripheral cyanosis • Decreased level of consciousness • Frothy sputum and/or pink sputum • Hypotension

HF, heart failure; HTN, hypertension.

b. Patients can undergo unilateral (right-sided) catheterizations, which provide detailed information regarding cardiac hemodynamics, including cardiac output, ventricular filling pressures, and vascular resistance.

Differential Diagnosis

A. Acute respiratory distress syndrome (ARDS).
B. COPD.
C. Pulmonary edema.
D. Cirrhosis.
E. Idiopathic pulmonary fibrosis.
F. Viral pneumonia.
G. Bacterial pneumonia.
H. Pulmonary embolus.
I. MI.
J. Nephrotic syndrome.
K. Acute kidney injury/insufficiency.
L. Acute bronchitis.

Evaluation and Management Plan

A. General plan: Utilize pharmacologic and nonpharmacologic mechanisms to achieve the following goals.

   1. Improve overall quality of life.

   2. Decrease frequency of HF exacerbations and need for hospitalizations.

   3. Extend patient survival.

   4. Increase exercise/functional capacity and enhance overall patient well-being.

   5. Treat underlying comorbidities that may contribute to HF (i.e., cardiac revascularization for ischemia, valvular replacement for compromising VHD, and treatment of HTN).

B. Patient/family teaching points.

   1. Strong focus on nonpharmacologic modalities.

      a. Emphasize importance of medication and clinic appointment compliance.

      b. Discuss signs and symptoms of worsening HF and when to seek medical care.

      c. Design daily weight chart for patients with specific instructions regarding weight parameters and when to seek medical care.

      d. Educate on dietary guidelines.

         i. Sodium: Less than 2.3 g/d.

         ii. Fluid restriction: Less than 2.0 L/d.

         iii. Low fat and low cholesterol diet.

      e. Ensure patients have close follow-up via in-person and phone contact with providers.

      f. Educate on tobacco cessation and decreased alcohol intake (if indicated).

      g. Collaborate with cardiac rehabilitation specialist to design HF-focused exercise program.

         i. Should contain flexibility, strengthening, and aerobic activities.

         ii. Encourage daily low to moderate activity with gradual increased intensity over weeks to months with heart monitoring (for most patients).

C. Pharmacotherapy.

   1. Angiotensin-converting enzyme (ACE) inhibitors: Work by increasing preload and afterload via vascular dilatation; known to decrease morbidity and hospitalizations while alleviating HF-related symptoms and improving quality of life.

      a. Recommended that all patients regardless of symptoms receive an ACE inhibitor.

b. Important to monitor blood pressure, renal function, and electrolytes.

c. Advised to start at low dose and titrate.

d. Caution to avoid nonsteroidal anti-inflammatory drugs (NSAIDs) in combination with ACE inhibitors because NSAIDs are ACE inhibitor antagonists and will decrease ACE inhibitor effectiveness; in addition, NSAIDs promote sodium and water retention.

e. Typically, combination of an ACE inhibitor and diuretic: First-line therapy for most HF patients.

   i. Patients who cannot tolerate ACE inhibitors should use angiotensin II receptor blockers (ARBs).

   ii. Patients are intolerant to ACE and ARB therapy can utilize a combination of hydralazine and oral or topical nitrates for similar benefits.

2. Beta-blockers: Proven to decrease mortality in post-MI HF patients.

   a. In the United States, carvedilol and metoprolol succinate are approved for treatment of NYHA HF classes I, II, and III.

   b. Several contraindications to beta-blocker therapy include NYHA class IV HF, significant pulmonary disease, marked bradycardia, baseline hypotension, and all heart blocks except first degree.

3. Mineralocorticoid antagonists.

   a. Most commonly used: Spironolactone.

   b. Function as a potassium-sparing diuretic that affects aldosterone.

   c. Recommended in NYHA HF classes II to IV HF with EF less than 35% or an EF less than 40% in post-MI HF.

   d. Contraindicated in patients with renal dysfunction (Cr >2.5 mg/dL) or known hyperkalemia.

   e. Caution: In the geriatric population, many patients with underlying renal dysfunction are predisposed to electrolyte abnormalities.

4. Diuretics.

   a. Diuretics are the most effective pharmacologic treatment for fluid balance and decreasing symptoms of edema; however, no proven morbidity/mortality benefits.

   b. Either thiazide (less potent) or loop diuretics (more potent) can be used.

   c. If the patient is unresponsive to loop or thiazide diuretics, consider the addition of metolazone for enhanced results (caution with metolazone in the elderly, as small doses can result in life-threatening hyponatremia).

   d. The most important side effect of diuretics is electrolyte imbalance, particularly hypokalemia, hyponatremia, hypomagnesemia, and increased bicarbonate.

   e. All patients, but especially geriatric individuals, utilizing these medications should have routine electrolyte monitoring.

5. Digoxin.

   a. Has a positive ionotropic effect.

   b. Beneficial in HF patients with EF less than 30%, NYHA HF class IV, or concomitant AF.

   c. Has not been shown to decrease morbidity/mortality.

   d. Careful monitoring of digoxin levels necessary.

   e. Can be added to preexisting therapy with diuretics, ACE inhibitors, or ARBs in patients with severe disease.

D. Additional treatment options.

1. Implantable cardiac defibrillator (ICD) placement: Reduces mortality rate from sudden cardiac death in patients with NYHA class II and III HF and an EF less than 35% (primary prevention) or following cardiac arrest secondary to ventricular arrhythmias (secondary prevention).

   a. Note that ICDs help prevent sudden cardiac death but do not improve quality of life.

2. Cardiac resynchronization therapy (CRT): Used in patients with systolic (decreased EF) HF to improve clinical symptoms, exercise tolerance, and overall survival.

   a. Procedure requires placement of a biventricular pacemaker (one lead in RV and one lead in the left ventricle via the coronary sinus vein) to assist in pacing the left ventricle: Helps by improving cardiac contractile ability.

   b. Works by increasing stroke volume, EF, and cardiac output.

   c. Indicated in patients with NYHA HF classes II to IV, EF less than 35%, and QRS duration greater than 150 ms on ECG.

3. Considerations for refractory HF: Defined as advanced structural heart disease and marked HF symptoms at rest or repeated exacerbations despite optimal medical therapy.

   a. Consider additional supportive devices such as left ventricular assistive devices (LVADs), right ventricular supportive devices (RVADs), or biventricular assistive devices (BIVADs).

   b. Can also consider advanced intravenous ionotropic therapy to increase cardiac output and strength of contractility (i.e., dobutamine or milrinone).

   c. Use extracorporeal membrane oxygenation (ECMO) in settings of worsening cardiomyopathy or HF; indicated in persistent NYHA class IV HF as potential bridge to transplantation.

4. Cardiac transplantation: Can be a consideration in patients with refractory cardiogenic shock, constant dependency on intravenous ionotropic therapy, or persistent NYHA class IV HF with oxygen consumption less than 10 mL/kg/min.

   a. However, many contraindications to transplant exist.

   b. In-depth evaluation and dedicated cardiac transplant treatment team are necessary.

E. Discharge instructions.

1. Ensure proper transition from inpatient to outpatient management of underlying comorbidities that can exacerbate HF (DM, HTN, and hyperlipidemia).

2. Ensure adequate understanding of modifiable cardiovascular risk factors (i.e., smoking cessation, weight loss, and diet/activity restrictions).

3. Prior to discharge:

   a. Ensure that the patient is at optimal volume status with proper transition from intravenous to oral diuretic therapy.

   b. Ensure that the patient has had echocardiogram with documented EF.

   c. Ensure that the patient has been stable on all oral cardiac medications for 24 hours.

   d. Ensure that the patient is receiving optimal oral pharmacologic therapy including an ACE inhibitor and beta-blocker (if decreased EF); if optimal therapy is not prescribed, must document reasoning for deviation from accepted practice guidelines.

e. Consult with physical therapy (and occupational therapy) to ensure patient is stable with ambulation and activities of daily living prior to discharge.

f. Ensure that the patient has follow-up with outpatient cardiologist scheduled for 7 to 10 days postdischarge.

g. Based on the patient's functional status and degree of HF, consider home health nursing or short-term rehabilitation facilities (or long-term care).

Follow-Up

A. Ensure effective coordination of care between primary care physician and cardiologist. If recent hospitalization:

   1. Follow-up within 7 days of discharge, then 1 to 2 weeks until patient is asymptomatic and then every 3 to 6 months thereafter.

   2. All providers should ensure efficient communication regarding a patient's current clinical status, medication regimen, diagnostic test results, and goals of care.

B. Ensure medication compliance and importance of all clinic visits.

C. Create patient-centered exercise plan: Consider referral to cardiac rehabilitation.

D. Provide instruction about daily home weight monitoring.

   1. If weight gain is more than 2 lb. in 24 hours or 5 lb. above target in 1 week, notify healthcare provider.

   2. Discuss weight loss if indicated (body mass index [BMI] $\geq$30 kg/m^2).

E. Educate on proper dietary habits including low fat, low cholesterol, and low salt (<2,300 mg/daily).

   1. Consider possibility of fluid restriction.

F. Provide smoking cessation and decreased alcohol consumption information, if necessary.

G. Ensure patient understanding regarding symptoms of worsening HF (cough, weight gain, worsening or rest dyspnea, orthopnea, and edema) and importance of seeking early medical care.

Consultation/Referral

A. Recommend consultation with cardiologist and HF specialist.

B. Refer to interventional cardiologist and cardiothoracic surgeon for device implantation or if cardiac catheterization/revascularization is needed. Consider referral to transplant surgeon in special cases where cardiac transplantation is a consideration.

C. Recommend consultation with nutritionist to assist with dietary restrictions of HF.

D. Recommend referral to cardiac rehabilitation for assistance with physical activity plan (newly approved for NYHA classes II to IV, EF less than 35%, and on optimal medical therapy for at least 6 weeks).

E. Consider consultation with physical therapy, occupational therapy, and case manager during hospitalization to evaluate patients' functional capacity and assist with discharge planning.

F. Refer to palliative/hospice care for end-stage HF.

Special/Geriatric Considerations

A. Additional considerations for HF.

   1. Considerations for hospitalization.

     a. Hypotension or other hemodynamic instability.

     b. Worsening renal function or significant electrolyte disturbance.

     c. Change in mental status.

     d. Dyspnea at rest (resting tachypnea) or oxygen saturation less than 90%.

     e. New-onset or worsening arrhythmia such as atrial fibrillation or a ventricular arrhythmia.

     f. HF with concomitant ACS.

     g. Evidence of worsening pulmonary congestion on physical examination (rales, jugular venous distention [JVD]).

B. Geriatric considerations.

   1. HF in the geriatric population can manifest with nondescript symptoms.

     a. Malaise.

     b. Weight loss.

     c. Decreased exercise tolerance.

     d. Changes in mental status (confusion, changes in mood/irritability, sleep disturbances).

     e. Gastrointestinal dysfunction (nausea, abdominal pain, anorexia, alterations in bowel habits).

   2. Note that geriatric patients also experience typical HF symptoms, especially orthopnea; inquire about sleeping in a recliner (to alleviate SOB) and elevated JVD (noted on physical examination).

   3. The mnemonic **DEFEAT** (**D**iagnosis, **E**tiology, **F**luid volume status, **E**jection fr**A**ction, and **T**reatment) may be useful in the geriatric population.

     a. General principle for the treatment of HF in older adults is similar to that of younger adults: Divided between symptom-relieving and disease-modifying treatment.

     b. All geriatric HF patients should receive an ACE inhibitor or an ARB; can also utilize a low dose beta-blocker such as metoprolol.

     c. Can also utilize an aldosterone antagonist (i.e., spironolactone) in advanced HF; however, use caution in those with impaired renal function (common in geriatric population) due to risk of hyperkalemia.

     d. Recommend to avoid digoxin in geriatric patients but could consider in low doses if patient remains symptomatic despite maximal medical therapy with other pharmacologic classes.

     e. Diuretics should be used to achieve euvolemia using lowest dose possible with careful monitoring of electrolytes.

     f. Realize that HF is a debilitating condition in the geriatric population: Fewer than 25% will survive greater than 5 years. It is important to:

       i. Have comprehensive discussions with patients and families regarding end-of-life wishes and ensure that appropriate referrals to palliative care and hospice are made when the patient's condition declines.

       ii. Understand patients and family members' wishes regarding aggressiveness of clinical interventions before designing treatment plans.

         1) Recommend that risk versus benefit analysis for geriatric patients be considered with regard to device implantation.

         2) Understand that patients with low life expectancies (12–18 months) are unlikely to benefit from ICDs and patients older than 80 years of age are likely to experience major complications following device placement.

Bibliography

Agabegi, S. S., & Agabegi, E. D. (2008). *Step-up to medicine* (2nd ed.). Philadelphia, PA: Wolters Kluwer.

Dumitru, I., & Baker, M. M. (2018, May 7). Heart failure. In G. K. Sharma (Ed.), *Medscape*. Retrieved from http://emedicine.medscape.com/article/163062-overview

Rich, M. W. (2016). Heart failure. In J. B. Halter, J. G. Ouslander, S. Studenski, K. P. High, S. Asthana, M. A. Supiano, & C. Ritchie (Eds.), *Hazzard's geriatric medicine and gerontology* (7th ed.). New York, NY: McGraw-Hill. Retrieved from http://accessmedicine.mhmedical.com/book.aspx?bookid=1923

Yancy, C. W., Jessup, M., Bozkurt, B., Butler, J., Casey, D. E., Jr., Colvin, M. M., & Westlake, C. (2017a). 2017 ACC/AHA/HFSA focused update of the 2013 ACCF/AHA guideline for the management of heart failure: A report of the American College of Cardiology/American Heart Association Task Force on Clinical Practice Guidelines and the Heart Failure Society of America. *Circulation, 136*, e137–e161. doi:10.1161/CIR.0000000000000509

Yancy, C. W., Jessup, M., Bozkurt, B., Butler, J., Casey, D. E., Jr., Colvin, M. M., & Westlake, C. (2017b). 2017 ACC/AHA/HFSA focused update of the 2013 ACCF/AHA guideline for the management of heart failure. *Journal of the American College of Cardiology, 70*(6), 776–803. doi:10.1016/j.jacc.2017.04.025

Hypertension

Allison Rusgo

Definition

A. According to 2017 guidelines from the American College of Cardiology and American Heart Association, normal blood pressure (BP) is defined as a systolic blood pressure (SBP) less than 120 mmHg and diastolic blood pressure (DBP) less than 80 mmHg. An elevated BP is now defined as a SBP between 120 and 129 mmHg *and* a DBP less than 80 mmHg; Stage I hypertension (HTN) is now defined as an SBP between 130 and 139 mmHg *or* a DBP between 80 and 90 mmHg. Stage II HTN is any SBP of 140 mmHg or more *or* a DBP of 90 mmHg or more.

B. Condition applies to anyone taking antihypertensive medication or a person who is told by a clinician on two separate occasions that his or her BP is greater than or equal to 140 mmHg/90 mmHg.

Incidence

A. According to the National Health and Nutrition Examination Survey (NHANES), HTN affects 86 million U.S. adults (age ≥20 years) with a prevalence of 34%.

B. Majority of patients (90%–95%) are diagnosed with primary (idiopathic) HTN.

C. Global prevalence of approximately 972 million individuals (26% of world's population).

D. Globally, African Americans maintain the highest prevalence rate of HTN and experience the highest mortality rates from associated complications including cardiovascular disease, end-stage renal disease, and cerebrovascular accidents (CVAs).

Pathogenesis

A. Believed to be multifactorial, with many sites of target organ damage.

  1. Cardiac: Left ventricular hypertrophy (LVH), myocardial infarctions (MIs), congestive heart failure (CHF), and acceleration of atherosclerosis.

  2. Central nervous system (CNS): CVAs, transient ischemic attacks (TIA).

  3. Renal: Chronic kidney disease (CKD).

  4. Vascular: Peripheral vascular disease (PVD).

  5. Ophthalmological: Retinopathy.

B. In increased systemic vascular resistance (cardiac afterload), concentric LVH, and decreased left ventricular function secondary to left ventricular dilatation: Leads to a weakened heart muscle and eventual CHF.

C. Decreased stroke volume and cardiac output.

D. Endothelial cell dysfunction due to altered renin–aldosterone–angiotensin cascade.

Predisposing Factors

A. Nonmodifiable risk factors.

  1. Age: Both SBP and DBP increase with age.

  2. Gender.

    a. Until age 45, more males are affected than females.

    b. From ages 45 to 64, males and females are affected equally.

    c. After age 65, more females are affected than males.

  3. Race and ethnicity: Most common in African Americans.

  4. Hereditary: Heritable component between 33% and 57% according to Framingham Heart Study.

B. Modifiable risk factors.

  1. Sedentary lifestyle; obesity (BMI ≥30 kg/m^2).

  2. Increased sodium intake.

  3. Increased alcohol consumption (8 oz. wine or 24 oz. beer per day).

  4. Tobacco use.

  5. Hyperlipidemia: Elevated low-density lipoprotein (LDL) cholesterol (or total cholesterol ≥240 mg/dL) or low HDL cholesterol.

  6. Diabetes mellitus as a component of metabolic syndrome.

Subjective Data

A. Common complaints/symptoms.

  1. Headache (particularly headache upon awakening) and dizziness.

  2. Visual changes; subconjunctival hemorrhages.

  3. Epistaxis.

B. History of the present illness.

  1. Documented elevated BP on three separate occasions (three clinic visits required for HTN diagnosis).

    a. Based on average of two or more readings at each follow-up visit after initial screening.

  2. HTN-related comorbidities and evidence of target end-organ damage.

  3. Possible evaluation for secondary causes of HTN based on patients' symptomatology.

    a. Pheochromocytoma: Facial flushing, labile HTN, and palpitations.

    b. Hypothyroidism: Cold intolerance, lethargy, and bradycardia.

    c. Hyperthyroidism: Heat intolerance, tachycardia, and diaphoresis.

    d. Obstructive sleep apnea: Snoring and daytime sleepiness.

    e. Hyperparathyroidism: Nephrolithiasis, gastrointestinal symptoms, osteitis fibrosa cystica.

    f. Cushing disease: Weight gain, hirsutism, abdominal striae.

C. Family and social history.

  1. Family history of HTN and premature history of cardiovascular disease (males <55 years and females <65 years).

  2. Use of alcohol, tobacco, anabolic steroids, and illicit drugs, particularly cocaine and amphetamines.

3. Diet (salt, fat, caloric intake), exercise, and life stressors.

D. Review of systems (focus should be on target organ damage).

    1. General: Weight gain/obesity.

    2. Integumentary: Edema and ulcerations.

    3. Neurological: Headache, dizziness, lightheadedness, syncope/near-syncope, and weakness.

    4. Ophthalmological: Visual changes.

    5. Cardiovascular and respiratory: Chest pain, palpitations, tachycardia, shortness of breath, and dyspnea on exertion.

    6. Gastrointestinal/genitourinary: Abdominal pain and changes in urinary habits.

Physical Examination

A. Measure accurate BP: Average of three readings taken 2 minutes apart; on first visit, BP should be taken in both arms and one leg to evaluate for coarctation of aorta and subclavian artery stenosis.

B. Evaluate pulse, oxygen saturation, respiratory rate, and temperature.

C. Assess skin for changes related to venous stasis: Brawny appearance with red/blue discoloration and possible venous stasis ulcerations.

D. Check the following body systems.

    1. Ophthalmological: Perform visual acuity; funduscopic examination for arteriovenous nicking, copper/silver wiring, cotton wool spots, retinal hemorrhages, and papilledema.

    2. Neck: Evaluate thyroid, carotid bruits, and jugular venous distention.

    3. Respiratory: Auscultate all lung fields.

    4. Cardiac: Assess for point of maximum impulse (PMI) displacement, sustained/enlarged apical impulse, presence of S3 or S4, evidence of murmurs, rubs or gallops, femoral pulse abnormalities, and peripheral edema.

    5. Abdomen: Evaluate for pulsatile abdominal mass over aorta, presence of bruits (aortic, renal, femoral, and iliac), and assess radial–femoral delay.

    6. Neurological: Perform complete mental status examination.

Diagnostic Tests

A. BP measurement (diagnostic criteria): Two or more diastolic BP measurements on at least two subsequent visits (after initial screening) of greater than or equal to 90 mmHg or when the average of systolic BP readings on two or more subsequent visits is consistently greater than or equal to 140 mmHg.

B. Initial laboratory evaluation.

    1. Complete blood count.

    2. Complete metabolic panel, including renal function and glomerular filtration rate (GFR).

    3. Fasting lipid panel.

    4. Hemoglobin A1C.

    5. Urinalysis (microalbumin levels correlate with clinical BP readings).

    6. Can also consider ECG, echocardiogram, and stress testing to further evaluate cardiac status.

C. Additional diagnostic tests for secondary causes of HTN.

    1. Pheochromocytoma: 20-hour urinary metanephrine level.

    2. Primary aldosteronism: Plasma aldosterone-to-renin activity ratio.

    3. Renal artery stenosis (RAS): Doppler flow ultrasound or computed tomographic angiography (CTA).

    4. Obstructive sleep apnea: Sleep study with oxygen saturation measurements.

    5. Thyroid and parathyroid disease: Thyroid and parathyroid hormone levels.

    6. Cushing disease: Dexamethasone suppression test.

    7. Coarctation of the aorta: CTA.

Differential Diagnosis

A. Primary idiopathic HTN.

B. Secondary HTN.

    1. Drug/toxin: Nicotine, alcohol, cocaine, amphetamines, ephedrine-containing decongestants, herbal supplements containing licorice, nonsteroidal anti-inflammatory drugs (NSAIDs), and oral contraceptives.

    2. Cardiovascular: MI, CHF.

    3. Endocrine: Primary hyperaldosteronism, Cushing disease, pheochromocytoma, hyperthyroidism or hypothyroidism, and hyperparathyroidism.

    4. Neurological: CVA, TIA, obstructive sleep apnea, intracranial HTN, brain tumor, and serotonin syndrome.

    5. Vascular: Coarctation of aorta, vasculitis, collagen vascular diseases, and subclavian artery stenosis.

    6. Renal: CKD, polycystic kidney disease (PCKD), and RAS.

Evaluation and Management Plan

A. General plan.

    1. Lifestyle modification.

        a. Diet modification: Dietary approaches to stop hypertension (DASH) diet; no-added-salt diet (4 g/d) or low-sodium diet (2 g/d).

        b. Limit alcohol and encourage tobacco cessation.

        c. Exercise regularly (30 minutes/day for 5–7 days/week).

        d. Engage in stress-reduction activities.

        e. Discontinue unnecessary medications that can raise BP.

B. Patient/family teaching points.

    1. Encourage family support with regard to lifestyle modifications and medication compliance.

C. Pharmacotherapy.

    1. Appropriate medications.

        a. Thiazide diuretics: Initial medication of choice (especially important to use in African Americans).

        b. Angiotensin-converting enzyme (ACE) inhibitors: Preferred in patients with diabetes mellitus because of its renal protective properties (can use angiotensin II receptor blocker [ARB] if patient intolerant to ACE inhibitor).

        c. Beta-blockers: Decrease heart rate, cardiac output, and renin release.

        d. Calcium channel blockers: Work by vasodilatation of atrial vasculature.

    2. Patients with HTN and diabetes mellitus often require two medications for control.

    3. If BP is greater than 20/10 mmHg above goal, consider use of two agents—one of which is usually a thiazide diuretic.

    4. Often a combination drug of a thiazide with either an ACE inhibitor or ARB is used because thiazides increase the effectiveness of other antihypertensive medications.

    5. Note that if the patient has poor response to one medication, experts recommend changing to another first-line agent in an alternative class before adding a second agent.

6. Medications such as hydralazine and minoxidil are not commonly used; if initiated, it is typically done with beta-blockers or diuretics for resistant HTN.

7. Caution: With clonidine, it is important to educate about not stopping abruptly due to risk of rebound HTN.

Follow-Up

A. Encourage patients to monitor BP at home and keep a log.

B. Emphasize medication compliance and clinic appointment follow-up with cardiologist or primary care provider.

Consultation/Referral

A. Consider consultation with a cardiologist for patients with multiple cardiovascular risk factors and/or comorbidities.

B. Consider consultation with a nephrologist for patients with resistant HTN and/or comorbid renal disease.

C. Based on etiology of secondary HTN, consultation with an appropriate specialist is advised.

Special/Geriatric Considerations

A. BP goals for special populations.
  1. Renal insufficiency: Less than 130/80 mmHg.
  2. Diabetes mellitus: Less than 130/80 mmHg.
  3. Age 65 years or older and high burden comorbidities; provider judgment and patient preferences.
  4. HTN/CHF: Less than 130/80 mmHg.
B. Complications
  1. Thoracic and abdominal aortic aneurysms.
  2. MI.
  3. Hypertensive urgency and emergency.
  4. CVA, TIA.
  5. Target end-organ damage (eyes, kidneys, nervous system).
C. Urgent and emergent hypertensive situations.
  1. Hypertensive urgency: BP of 180/110 mmHg or greater without end-organ damage.
    a. Patients should seek immediate evaluation and treatment.
    b. Avoid rapid lowering of BP to prevent neurological complications; initiate treatment of BP using oral agents for gradual reduction of BP over 24 to 48 hours.
    c. Ensure close follow-up and BP monitoring in addition to regulation of antihypertensive medications to prevent future recurrence.
  2. Hypertensive emergency: BP greater than 180/120mmHg with symptoms of end-organ damage.
    a. Goal is to reduce BP safely to reverse target organ damage without iatrogenic malperfusion. Maintained to less than 180/105 mmHg for the first 24 hours.
    b. Hypertensive emergency in pregnancy is defined as acute onset, with BP greater than 160/110 mmHg persisting more than 15 minutes.
    c. Patients should be monitored in the ICU with use of intravenous antihypertensive medications until stabilized.
D. Geriatric considerations: Structural changes due to aging.
  1. Changes in venous system due to aging.
    a. Reflex alterations in venous vasomotor tone.
    b. Vasoconstriction.
    c. Stiffness and loss of elasticity of valves in veins.
  2. Arterial changes due to aging.
    a. Thickening of the intimal and medial layers of the vasculature.
    b. Lipid deposits.
    c. Over time, the intimal and medial layers of the arteries acquire collagen deposits that subsequently decrease their elasticity and cause hardening of the vasculature walls.

Bibliography

Agabegi, S. S., & Agabegi, E. D. (2008). *Step-up to medicine* (2nd ed.). Philadelphia, PA: Wolters Kluwer.

Benjamin, E. J., Blaha, M. J., Chiuve, S. E., Cushman, M., Das, S. R., Deo, R., . . . Muntner, P. (2017, March 7). Heart disease and stroke statistics-2017 update: A report from the American Heart Association. *Circulation, 135*(10), e146–e603. doi:10.1161/CIR.0000000000000485

Chobanian, A. V., Bakris, G. L., Black, H. R., Cushman, W. C., Green, L. A., Izzo, J. L., Jr., . . . Roccella, E. J. (2003, December). Seventh report of the Joint National Committee on Prevention, Detection, Evaluation, and Treatment of High Blood Pressure. *Hypertension, 42*(6), 1206–1252. doi:10.1161/01.HYP.0000107251.49515.c2

Institute for Clinical Systems Improvement. (2010). *Hypertension diagnosis and treatment.* Retrived from https://www.icsi.org/

James, P. A., Oparil, S., Carter, B. L., Cushman, W. C., Dennison-Himmelfarb, C., Handler, J., . . . Ortiz, E. (2014). 2014 evidence-based guideline for the management of high blood pressure in adults: Report from the panel members appointed to the Eighth Joint National Committee (JNC 8). *Journal of the American Medical Association, 311*(5), 507–520. doi:10.1001/jama.2013.284427

Jermendy, G., Horvath, T., Littvay, L., Steinbach, R., Jermendy, A. L., Tarnoki, A. D., . . . Osztovits, J. (2011, November 3). Effect of genetic and environmental influences on cardiometabolic risk factors: A twin study. *Cardiovascular Diabetology, 10*, 96. doi:10.1186/1475-2840-10-96

Levy, D., DeStefano, A. L., Larson, M. G., O'Donnell, J., Lifton, R. P., Gavras, H., . . . Myers, R. H. (2000, October). Evidence for a gene influencing blood pressure on chromosome 17. Genome scan linkage results for longitudinal blood pressure phenotypes in subjects from the Framingham Heart Study. *Hypertension, 36*(4), 477–483. doi:10.1161/01.HYP.36.4.477

Mitchell, G. F., DeStefano, A. L., Larson, M. G., Benjamin, E. J., Chen, M.-H., Vasan, R. S., . . . Levy, D. (2005, July 12). Heritability and a genome-wide linkage scan for arterial stiffness, wave reflection, and mean arterial pressure: The Framingham Heart Study. *Circulation, 112*(2), 194–199. doi:10.1161/CIRCULATIONAHA.104.530675

Mozaffarian, D., Benjamin, E. J., Go, A. S., Arnett, D. K., Blaha, M. J., Cushman, M., . . . Turner, M. B. (2015, January 27). Heart disease and stroke statistics—2015 update: A report from the American Heart Association. *Circulation, 131*(4), e29–322.

NHANES (n. d.). National health and nutrition examination survey. Retrieved from http://www.cdc.gov/nchs/nhanes.htm

Whelton, P. K., Carey, R. M., Aronow, W. S., Casey, D. E., Jr., Collins, K. J., Dennison Himmelfarb, C., . . . Wright, J. T., Jr. (2018). 2017 ACC/AHA/AAPA/ABC/ACPM/AGS/APhA/ASH/ASPC/NMA/PCNA guideline for the prevention, detection, evaluation, and management of high blood pressure in adults. *Journal of the American College of Cardiology, 71*(19), e127–e248. doi:10.1016/j.jacc.2017.11.006

Pericardial Effusions

Allison Rusgo

Definition

A. An abnormal amount or type of fluid within the pericardium of the heart secondary to various etiologies.

B. Can be acute or chronic, pathologic or idiopathic, or symptomatic or asymptomatic.

C. Arise when there is an increase in production or a decrease in drainage of pericardial fluid; both mechanisms lead to an overabundance of fluid within the pericardial space. The excess fluid leads to inflammation and irritation of the pericardium, which is termed pericarditis.

Incidence

A. Data from the Framingham Heart Study ($n = 5,652$) showed that 6.5% of adults had pericardial effusions from echocardiogram results.

B. Pericardial effusions are common after cardiac bypass and valve replacement procedures (self-limiting).

C. It is common for patients with underlying hematological/oncological malignancies to have malignant pericardial effusions (21%).

    1. Lung cancer (37%), breast cancer (22%), and leukemia/lymphoma (17%) are the most common cancers that cause pericardial effusions.

D. Evidence of HIV or AIDS increases the risk of pericardial effusions (prevalence between 5% and 43%, depending on the study's inclusion criteria).

Pathogenesis

A. The pericardium is a double-walled sac that surrounds the heart. Its two layers work together to evenly distribute pressure and volume forces across the heart, allowing for stretching of the myocardium and uniform contractions. The layers are:

    1. Visceral pericardium (closer to the heart): Composed of ultrafiltered plasma (pericardial fluid is thought to come from this layer).

    2. Parietal pericardium (farther from the heart): Contributes to diastolic pressure and pressure within the right side of the heart.

B. The pericardium normally contains 15 to 50 mL of pericardial fluid, which is used for lubrication for each of the pericardial layers.

C. Clinical manifestations of pericardial effusions differ based on the rate of accumulation of the fluid. For example:

    1. Instant accumulation of less than 80 mL of fluid can cause significant cardiac compromise.

    2. Slow accumulation (months-years) requires more than 2 L of fluid before symptoms arise.

    3. Acute pericarditis typically involves accumulation of 150 to 200 mL of fluid when symptoms occur.

D. Pericardium has an important role during inspiration.

    1. As the right atrium and ventricle fill, the pericardium prevents the left atrium and ventricle from expanding.

    2. This process stretches the atrial and ventricular septum, decreases left ventricular filling volumes, and reduces cardiac output.

    3. If there is a significant accumulation of fluid within the pericardial space, the pressure within the pericardial spaces increases, stroke volume declines, and life-threatening cardiac tamponade can result.

Predisposing Factors

A. Postprocedures (coronary artery bypass grafting [CABG] or valve replacement).

B. Post-myocardial infarctions (MIs).

C. Neoplastic status.

    1. Benign: Atrial myxoma.

    2. Primary malignancy: Mesothelioma.

    3. Metastatic malignancy: Lung cancer or breast cancer.

    4. Hematologic malignancy: Leukemia or lymphoma.

D. Congestive heart failure as a result of rheumatic heart disease, cor pulmonale, or cardiomyopathies.

E. Connective tissue disorders: Rheumatoid arthritis, systemic lupus erythematosus, or scleroderma.

F. Chronic renal disease (secondary to uremia) or nephrotic syndrome.

G. Severe hypothyroidism with myxedema coma.

H. Medications: Procainamide, hydralazine, or status post radiation therapy.

I. Infectious pericarditis (most common is viral).

    1. HIV/AIDS: Secondary bacterial infection, opportunistic infections, or Kaposi sarcomas.

    2. Viral: Coxsackievirus A and B, adenovirus, influenza, and some forms of hepatitis.

    3. Fungal: Candida, histoplasmosis, or coccidioidomycosis.

    4. Protozoal.

    5. Parasitic.

    6. Pyogenic: Streptococci, pneumococci, *Neisseria*, *Legionella*, or staphylococci.

    7. Tuberculosis.

    8. Syphilitic.

J. Trauma (blunt or penetrating).

Subjective Data

A. Common complaints/symptoms.

    1. Chest pain/discomfort: Can be relieved by leaning forward and worsened by laying supine (27% of patients).

    2. Palpitations.

    3. Syncope/lightheadedness.

    4. Cough/hoarseness (47% of patients).

    5. Dyspnea (78% of patients).

    6. Anorexia (90% of patients).

    7. Anxiety.

    8. Confusion/change in mental status.

B. History of the present illness.

    1. Inquire about onset, provoking/alleviating factors, quality, severity, and timing of symptoms.

        a. Especially important regarding chest pain and positioning for pericarditis (sitting up/leaning forward improves symptoms while lying flat worsens discomfort).

        b. Chest discomfort often described as pleuritic (worse with inspiration) and sharp/stabbing.

    2. Discuss past medical history, particularly connective tissue disorders; neoplastic diseases; cardiac comorbidities; and infectious diseases such as HIV/AIDS, tuberculosis, or hepatitis.

C. Family and social history.

    1. Review family history for connective tissue disorders, cardiac diseases, neoplastic diseases, or renal failure.

    2. Determine use of tobacco, alcohol, or illegal substances.

    3. Obtain information regarding medications, especially procainamide or hydralazine.

    4. Ensure vaccinations and screenings are current.

        a. Influenza vaccine.

        b. Tuberculosis purified protein derivative (PPD), HIV/AIDS, and sexually transmitted infection testing (i.e., gonorrhea and syphilis).

        c. Cancer screenings.

    5. Assess for recent travel to wooded areas (exposure to tick-borne illnesses).

D. Review of systems.

    1. General: Fevers, chills, weight changes, appetite changes, or malaise.

    2. Cardiac: Chest pain/discomfort, or palpitations.

    3. Pulmonary: Shortness of breath, dyspnea, cough, or hoarseness/change in voice quality.

    4. Gastrointestinal: Singultus (hiccoughs).

    5. Neurological: Syncope, lightheadedness, confusion, or change in mental status.

    6. Psychiatric: Anxiety.

Physical Examination

A. Vital signs: Pulse, blood pressure (BP), respirations, temperature, oxygen saturation, and weight.

    1. Necessary to assess; possible hypotension, pulsus paradoxus, fever, tachycardia, or tachypnea.

B. General: Variable based on patient status; could be asymptomatic or in hemodynamic compromise if positive cardiac tamponade.

C. Neck: Possible hepatojugular reflux or jugular venous distention (JVD).

D. Pulmonary: Possible tachypnea, decreased breath sounds, Ewart sign (dullness to percussion below left scapula secondary to pericardial fluid near left lung).

E. Cardiac: Possible tachycardia, S1 and S2, murmurs, rubs, extra heart sounds (i.e., S3 and S4), pericardial friction rub, and muffled heart sounds. Also assess for increased JVD, hypotension, and muffled heart sounds (Beck's Triad) which is hallmark for cardiac tamponade.

F. Peripheral vascular: Possible peripheral edema, decreased pulses, or cyanosis.

G. Gastrointestinal: Possible hepatosplenomegaly.

H. Neurological: Mental status examination (if necessitated by patient status).

Diagnostic Tests

A. ECG (abnormal in 90% of cases).

    1. Low-voltage QRS.

    2. Diffuse nonspecific ST wave changes (can see T-wave flattening) and/or electrical alternans (electrical alternans is usually a sign of a massive effusion).

B. Echocardiography (imaging test of choice): Used to assess overall cardiac function and amount of pericardial fluid present; can detect as little as 20 mL of fluid.

C. Chest x-ray.

    1. Can show a "water-bottle" shaped cardiac silhouette and/or pericardial fat stripe.

    2. Can show an associated pleural effusion.

D. CT or MRI: Can be helpful in some instances for small effusions or loculated effusions.

E. Laboratory studies.

    1. Complete metabolic panel: Assess electrolytes and renal function.

    2. Complete blood count: Assess for leukocytosis and/or underlying HIV/AIDS or malignant process.

    3. Cardiac biomarkers: Can see minimal elevation.

    4. Thyroid-stimulating hormone (TSH): Assess for hypothyroidism as a cause for pericardial effusion.

    5. Rheumatoid factor and/or antinuclear antibody (ANA): Obtain if concern for underlying rheumatologic etiology.

    6. HIV/AIDS screening: Obtain if clinically suggested.

    7. Rickettsial antibody tests: Obtain if clinically indicated.

    8. Throat swab for influenza and adenovirus virus.

    9. Blood cultures: Obtain if febrile and clinically indicated.

    10. Tuberculin skin testing: Perform if indicated.

F. Pericardial fluid analysis.

    1. Currently under debate: Usually done if poor prognosis, likelihood of purulent effusion, pericardial tamponade, or recurrent and/or large effusions (especially conditions that do not resolve with medical management).

    2. Can send fluid for a variety of laboratory studies.

        a. Cell count and differential.

        b. Protein and lactate dehydrogenase.

        c. Glucose.

        d. Gram stain.

        e. Cultures: Bacterial, fungal, acid-fast stain, and culture.

        f. Tumor cytology.

        g. Rheumatoid factor and ANA if collagen vascular disease is suspected.

Differential Diagnosis

A. Acute pericarditis.

B. Chronic pericarditis.

C. Myocardial infarction (Dressler syndrome is defined as pericarditis after an MI).

D. Pulmonary embolus.

E. Cardiac tamponade.

F. Constrictive pericarditis.

G. Cardiogenic pulmonary edema.

H. Dilated cardiomyopathy.

Evaluation and Management Plan

A. General plan.

    1. Goal is to determine underlying etiology and treat accordingly; also important to determine level of care that patient requires (intensive care, inpatient, or outpatient).

    2. If positive cardiac tamponade or significant hemodynamic compromise, ICU admission required.

    3. Pericardiocentesis is required if hemodynamically unstable; recommended for large effusions or those secondary to bacterial infections or cancerous processes.

        a. This procedure is considered to be diagnostic and therapeutic.

            i. Done via open surgical procedure or catheter drainage.

            ii. Catheter drainage via fluoroscopy, echocardiography, or CT-guidance is the most common method.

        b. Following the procedure, an in-dwelling catheter can be placed to prevent fluid reaccumulation: This is removed or replaced within 72 hours.

        c. A sclerosing agent (i.e., tetracycline or bleomycin) within the pericardium can also be used to prevent reaccumulation.

        d. Other options to prevent recurrence are surgical intervention (pericardial window, thoracotomy or video-assisted thoracic surgery, or balloon pericardiotomy).

        e. If constrictive pericarditis, surgical resection is always indicated.

    4. Pharmacologic treatments (see section "Pharmacotherapy").

B. Patient/family teaching points.

    1. Educate regarding symptoms of cardiac compromise and signs and symptoms of worsening effusions; especially important if patient is treated as outpatient.

    2. Educate regarding importance of medication compliance and follow-up visits with provider.

    3. Explain to patients that despite proper diagnostic testing, an underlying etiology remains undiscovered in 50% of cases.

C. Pharmacotherapy.

    1. Aspirin or nonsteroidal anti-inflammatory drugs (NSAIDs): Can be used for acute idiopathic or viral pericarditis.

        a. Aspirin is preferred for post-MI pericarditis.

b. NSAIDs are preferred for viral pericarditis (avoid indomethacin in those with coronary artery disease [CAD]).

2. Colchicine: Can be used for acute pericarditis in combination with aspirin or NSAIDs.

a. Avoid in asymptomatic postoperative pericarditis.

b. Discuss with patients regarding side effects: Most common is diarrhea.

3. Steroids: If used early in acute pericarditis, there is an increased risk of reoccurrence once steroids are tapered.

a. Consider in recurrent disease that is unresponsive to NSAIDs and colchicine.

b. Consider for patients with comorbid connective tissue disorder, uremic pericarditis, or autoreactive pericarditis.

c. Recommend to use for at least 1 month with slow taper.

4. Antibiotics.

a. If purulent pericardial fluid and bacterial infection, combine urgent drainage and aggressive intravenous antibiotics (e.g., vancomycin, ceftriaxone, and ciprofloxacin).

D. Discharge instructions.

1. Educate regarding pericardial effusions and pericarditis.

2. Educate on reasons to return to the ED: Specifically signs of hemodynamic instability, cardiac compromise, or worsening infection (if etiology is bacterial or viral).

3. Educate on importance of medication and clinic follow-up compliance.

Follow-Up

A. Patients will require close monitoring until pericardial effusion and symptoms resolve.

B. Patients should have repeat echocardiography to ensure effusion resolution and no evidence of constrictive pericarditis (usually within 4 weeks of diagnosis).

C. Pericardial effusions usually resolve with treatment and when underlying illness is treated; often reoccur with comorbid conditions such as neoplasms.

Consultation/Referral

A. Consult with cardiologist.

B. Consult with interventional cardiologist (if cardiac catheterization or minimally invasive pericardiocentesis is indicated).

C. Consult with cardiothoracic surgeon (if invasive procedure is required or patient is status post cardiothoracic surgery).

D. Consult with infectious disease specialist (if indicated).

E. Consult with rheumatologist (if indicated).

F. Consult with interventional radiologist (if pericardial drainage procedure via fluoroscopy is indicated).

G. Consult with hematologist/oncologist (if indicated).

Special/Geriatric Considerations

A. It is important to assess the cognitive status and comorbidities of geriatric patients, especially if invasive procedures may be required.

B. Studies have shown that in elderly patients undergoing echocardiography for other purposes, those with incidental small asymptomatic pericardial effusions had a higher mortality than those without effusions.

C. Elderly patients may present with more vague symptoms (generalized malaise, confusion).

D. As with many other diagnoses, elderly patients with pericarditis and pericardial effusions have poorer outcomes as compared to younger patients with the same disease process.

Bibliography

Agabegi, S. S., & Agabegi, E. D. (2008). *Step-up to medicine* (2nd ed.). Philadelphia, PA: Wolters Kluwer.

Olshaker, J. S. (2014). Cardiovascular emergencies in the elderly. In J. H. Khan, B. G. Magauran Jr., & J. S. Olshaker (Eds.), *Geriatric emergency medicine: Principles and practice* (pp. 199–206). New York, NY: Cambridge University Press.

Strimel, W. J., Ayub, B., & Contractor, T. (2019, November 28). Pericardial effusion. In T. X. O'Brien (Ed.), *Medscape*. Retrieved from http://emedicine.medscape.com/article/157325-overview

Usatine, R. P., Smith, M. A., Chumley, H. S., & Mayeaux, E. J., Jr. (2013). Pericardial effusion. In A. Jawaid & J. Delzell, *The color atlas of family medicine* (2nd ed., pp. 292–296). New York, NY: McGraw-Hill. Retrieved from http://accessmedicine.mhmedical.com/book.aspx?bookID=685

Valvular Heart Disease

Allison Rusgo

Definition

A. Damage or defect in one of the four heart valves: Mitral, aortic, tricuspid, or pulmonary.

B. Two most common abnormalities: Regurgitation and stenosis of the aortic and mitral valves.

1. Regurgitation or insufficiency: Occurs when the valve leaflets do not close tightly; blood leaks backward into the respective chamber instead of flowing forward through the proper circulatory path.

2. Stenosis: Occurs because of stiffening and narrowing of the valve leaflets.

a. This prevents the valve from opening properly; the result is not enough blood flowing through the valve and circulatory path, which leads to an outflow-type obstruction during systole.

b. Mitral stenosis (MS) results in an increase in left atrial, pulmonary artery, and right ventricular pressures.

c. Mitral regurgitation (MR) leads to a backflow (or reversal) of blood from the left ventricle to the left atrium during systole; it can be primary or secondary and acute or chronic.

i. Acute MR: Typically occurs because of endocarditis or myocardial infarction (MI) with structural cardiac damage (papillary muscle rupture, chordae rupture).

ii. Chronic MR: Can be primary or secondary.

iii. Causes of primary MR: Mitral valve prolapse (MVP; subtype of MR where the mitral valve leaflets close improperly and bulge into the left atrium during systole), rheumatic heart disease, MI with resultant structural cardiac damage, or endocarditis.

iv. Causes of secondary MR: Left ventricular dysfunction.

Incidence

A. Globally, the prevalence of valvular heart disease (VHD) is estimated at 2.5%.

B. Prevalence of VHD increases in individuals older than 65 years of age, particularly in those with aortic stenosis (AS) or MR. More than 33% of those older than age 75 have moderate to severe VHD.

C. AS is the leading cause of clinically significant VHD in geriatric patients (prevalence of 2%–9%).

D. Acute aortic regurgitation (AR) is a rare and life-threatening condition. Chronic AR is common in geriatric patients (prevalence of 20%–30% in geriatric patients).

E. MS is more common in females as compared to males and usually occurs because of rheumatic heart disease (97%).

1. MS caused by rheumatic heart disease typically presents in the fourth or fifth decade but can occur in individuals older than age 65 years.

2. Only 60% of patients with MS secondary to rheumatic heart disease can recall a previous history of the infection.

3. Among geriatric patients with non-rheumatic heart disease-related MS, the etiology is typically because of age-related calcifications that narrow the valve.

F. MR occurs equally in males and females, with a prevalence of 2%.

1. Most common cause of MR is MVP.

2. MVP can be spontaneous or genetically linked.

Pathogenesis

A. Stenosis.

1. Senile AS or MS.

a. Exact mechanism is still not entirely understood; it is thought to be secondary to a buildup of calcifications within the valve.

b. Very similar to the process of atherosclerosis.

c. Increase in lipids, inflammation, and calcification of the valve.

2. Bicuspid AS: Secondary to an inherited congenital condition where two (of the normally structured three) leaflets of the aortic valve are fused together.

a. This improper fusion of the two valve leaflets results in a bicuspid aortic valve instead of a tricuspid-shaped valve.

b. Result is an increase in calcification formation and outflow obstruction.

3. Rheumatic heart disease-related AS or MS: Can affect the aortic or mitral valves via fusion of the leaflets to create narrowing and outflow obstruction.

B. Regurgitation.

1. Acute MR: Results in increase in preload and decrease in afterload.

a. This causes an increase in end-diastolic volume (EDV) and decrease in end-systolic volume (ESV).

b. Thus, stroke volume and left atrial pressures are increased.

2. Chronic MR: Slow deterioration of the valve allows the left atrium and left ventricle to adjust (dilate) to the increased backflow of blood.

a. Left atrial pressure is usually normal or slightly elevated; end-diastolic pressure is also within an acceptable range.

b. Over time, the left ventricle will continue to dilate, further damaging the mitral valve leaflets and worsening the MR.

3. Acute AR: Increased volume in the left ventricle during diastole; the ventricle does not have sufficient time to dilate appropriately to accommodate the sudden increase in fluid.

a. EDV increases quickly, which this causes an elevation in pulmonary artery pressures, affecting coronary and pulmonary circulation.

b. With this increase in volume and pressures, patients develop symptoms consistent with pulmonary congestion (i.e., dyspnea).

4. Chronic AR: Results in slow progressing fluid overload within the left ventricle.

a. This condition causes the left ventricle to dilate over time, resulting in left ventricular hypertrophy.

b. Initially, the hypertrophy helps mitigate the increased pressure and volume that occurs within the left ventricle.

c. In early phase, cardiac contractility (or ejection fraction [EF]) remains normal via compensation mechanisms.

d. As the disease progresses and the ventricle continues to dilate, it reaches maximal stretch capacity; beyond this threshold there is an increase in end-diastolic pressures and decrease in perfusion of the coronary system.

e. As the left ventricle structure and function worsens, the EF decreases and symptoms (i.e., dyspnea) ensue.

Predisposing Factors

A. Recent MI with resultant structural damage of valve leaflets, chordae, and papillary muscles.

B. Most common risk factors for MR: MVP, rheumatic heart disease, infective endocarditis, known coronary artery disease (CAD), and cardiomyopathies. Note the following:

1. Rheumatic heart disease most commonly causes regurgitation of the mitral valve followed by the aortic valve (rarely affects tricuspid or pulmonary valves).

2. Infective endocarditis can technically affect any valve—it most commonly targets the tricuspid but also affects the aortic and mitral valves.

C. Possible cause of MS: Age-related degenerative changes or more rare etiologies, including congenital malformations and intracardiac tumors (myxoma).

D. AS: Age-related changes, bicuspid aortic valves, and rheumatic heart disease.

E. Advanced hypertension (HTN) and atherosclerosis, which can affect valvular function.

F. Conditions that can lead to VHD: Autoimmune and connective tissue processes such as systemic lupus erythematous and Marfan's syndrome.

G. Other conditions that increase risk: Tobacco use, insulin resistance/diabetes mellitus (DM), obesity, and a family history of VHD.

H. Acute aortic dissection, which can result in acute life-threatening AR.

Subjective Data

A. Common complaints/symptoms.

1. AS: Angina, syncope, and findings associated with heart failure (i.e., fatigue, orthopnea, paroxysmal nocturnal dyspnea, shortness of breath, decreased exercise tolerance, dyspnea on exertion).

2. AR.

a. Acute AR: Dramatic presentation of cardiogenic shock (secondary to infective endocarditis or aortic dissection).

b. Chronic AR: Palpitations, angina, heart failure presentation (dyspnea on exertion, peripheral edema, fatigue, paroxysmal nocturnal dyspnea).

3. MS.

    a. Often presents with new-onset atrial fibrillation (i.e., fatigue, chest discomfort, palpitations, light-headedness, dizziness).

    b. Rarely presents with Ortner's syndrome: Occurs with MS where there is compression of the left recurrent laryngeal nerve due to an enlarged left atrium; results in hoarseness.

4. MR: New-onset atrial fibrillation (similar to MS), anxiety, chest discomfort, dyspnea, fatigue, and/or signs of volume overload consistent with heart failure.

B. History of the present illness.

    1. Obtain information regarding specific symptom: Onset, provoking/palliative, quality, severity, radiation (if applicable), and timing.

    2. Review patient's past medical history: Particularly, recent MIs, known CAD, HTN, or HLD; congenital cardiac abnormalities, previous rheumatic fever, connective tissue disorders, cardiomyopathies, or congestive heart failure (CHF).

    3. Determine if the patient ever had a previous cardiac evaluation, especially an echocardiogram, or learned about a heart murmur.

    4. Understand that patient scenarios will vary based on the valve affected, type of dysfunction (stenosis or regurgitation), and underlying etiology.

C. Family and social history.

    1. Gather information regarding family history of VHD (especially bicuspid aortic valves or MVP), HTN, hyperlipidemia, CHF, arrhythmias (i.e., atrial fibrillation), or connective tissue disorders.

    2. Obtain social history information, especially regarding tobacco use, alcohol use, and illegal substance use (very important to document any intravenous drug use due to high risk of infective endocarditis).

D. Review of systems.

    1. General: Fatigue, malaise, fevers, chills, weight changes, and appetite changes.

    2. Skin/Nails: Painful red-purple nodules on hands/feet (Osler nodes of infective endocarditis) and painless red areas on palms/soles (Janeway lesions of infective endocarditis).

    3. Head, ear, eyes, nose, and throat (HEENT): Hoarseness.

    4. Cardiac: Chest discomfort, palpitations, racing heartbeat, decreased exercise tolerance, peripheral edema, and uncomfortable awareness of heartbeat (associated with AR).

    5. Pulmonary: Cough, shortness of breath, dyspnea on exertion, orthopnea, paroxysmal nocturnal dyspnea, and hemoptysis (rare but associated with MS).

    6. Gastrointestinal: Increasing abdominal girth.

    7. Neurological: Lightheadedness, dizziness, syncope, and near-syncope.

    8. Psychological: Anxiety.

Physical Examination

A. Vital signs: Assess pulse rate and rhythm, blood pressure (BP), respirations, temperature, and oxygen saturation.

    1. Possible tachycardia or bradycardia.

    2. Possible irregularly irregular pulse (consistent with atrial fibrillation).

    3. Possible hyperthermia (concern for infection) or hypothermia (in geriatric patients with infections who cannot mount fevers).

    4. Decreased oxygen saturation (concern for signs of CHF).

    5. Possible HTN (acute or long-standing) or hypotension (concern for cardiogenic shock).

    6. Widened pulse pressure (associated with AR).

    7. Mayne sign: Decrease in BP with arm elevation (associated with AR).

    8. Hill sign: Higher BP in lower as compared to upper extremity (associated with AR).

B. General survey: Determine if patient is in acute distress, or asymptomatic.

C. Skin/Nails: Assess for Osler nodes and Janeway lesions.

D. Head: Possible evidence of head bobbing with each heartbeat (de Musset sign of AR).

E. Neck.

    1. Consider possible jugular venous distention (JVD; concern for CHF).

    2. Evaluate carotids.

        a. "Pulsus parvus et tardus" (associated with AS) where there is a weakened and delayed pulse with late carotid upstroke.

        b. Brisk carotid upstroke (associated with MR).

F. Pulmonary: Possible rales or crackles (sign of increased fluid accumulation).

G. Gastrointestinal: Possible ascites or hepatomegaly (concern for worsening heart failure).

H. Cardiac.

    1. Inspect for lifts/heaves (concern for ventricular enlargement).

    2. Palpate for thrills (grade IV to VI murmurs) and the point of maximum impulse (PMI; if displaced, concern for ventricular hypertrophy).

    3. Auscultate for S1, S2, and evidence of extra heart sounds (S3 and S4) and murmurs.

        a. AS: Harsh late-peaking crescendo-decrescendo systolic murmur that radiates to carotids and best heard over right second intercostal space (ICS), can also have paradoxical splitting of second heart sound.

        b. Aortic regurgitation: PMI often displaced toward axilla, possible S3, diastolic low-pitched rumbling murmur best heard at left sternal border; can also hear an Austin Flint murmur (severe AR: Low-pitched, rumbling, mid-diastolic murmur; heard best at apex).

        c. MS: Loud first heart sound, positive high-pitched opening snap after A2 heart sound; nonradiating mid-diastolic murmur best heard at apex.

        d. MR: Decreased S1, wide splitting of S2, high-pitched holosystolic (can be early systole in acute MR) best heard at cardiac apex and radiates to left axilla.

            i. MVP: If concern for MVP (associated with MR): Murmur is usually in late systole and associated with the hallmark mid-systolic click that precedes that MR murmur.

I. Peripheral vascular: Possible bounding peripheral pulses (water hammer pulse associated with AR), possible peripheral edema.

J. Neurological: Mental status examination (if positive mental status changes) and complete neurological examination if concern for associated syncope/near-syncope.

Diagnostic Tests

A. MS.

    1. Routine laboratory studies: Complete blood count, electrolytes, renal function, and liver function.

2. Chest x-ray: Can see left atrial enlargement, prominent pulmonary vasculature, and interstitial edema (Kerley A and B lines).

3. ECG: If severe MS, signs of left atrial enlargement, atrial fibrillation, and right ventricular hypertrophy.

4. Transthoracic echocardiogram (TTE) to assess overall cardiac function, left ventricular dysfunction, and degree of stenosis.

   a. Mild: Valve area greater than 1.5 cm^2.

   b. Moderate: Valve area of 1.0 to 1.5 cm^2.

   c. Severe: Valve area less than 1.0 cm^2.

   d. Consider transesophageal echocardiogram (TEE) if TTE does not produce quality images; there is question of a left atrial thrombus or prior to surgical intervention.

5. Cardiac catheterization is not routine, but can be considered in several circumstances.

   a. If discrepancy between physical examination and echocardiogram results.

   b. Patients with severe underlying lung disease and pulmonary HTN who require further evaluation.

   c. Geriatric patients with severe MS to rule out comorbid CAD.

B. AS.

1. Routine laboratory studies: Complete blood count, electrolytes, cardiac biomarkers, renal function, and liver function.

2. ECG: Could be normal, possible left ventricular hypertrophy pattern, and possible atrial fibrillation.

3. TTE.

   a. Follow recommendations of American Heart Association (AHA) for evaluation of grade 3 AS murmurs via TTE.

   b. Consider stress echocardiogram in asymptomatic patients with severe AS to determine need for clinical intervention.

   c. Perhaps consider TEE if concern for bicuspid aortic valve.

4. Cardiac catheterization.

   a. Use if discrepancy between patient presentation and echocardiogram results.

   b. Consider in patients older than 35 years of age with AS requiring surgical intervention to evaluate for CAD.

5. Exercise stress testing: Absolutely contraindicated in severe symptomatic AS (can be considered in those with asymptomatic severe AS under strict surveillance of cardiologist).

6. CT angiography: Can be used in patients for whom transcatheter aortic valve replacement (TAVR) is being considered.

7. Chest x-ray: Findings vary based on severity of AS.

   a. In severe AS: May appreciate aortic valve calcifications, left atrial enlargement, right-sided heart enlargement, and pulmonary congestion.

C. AR: Evaluation is based on clinical scenario and suspected underlying etiology.

1. Laboratory studies.

   a. For infective endocarditis: Complete blood count, electrolytes, renal function, kidney function, blood cultures, lactate levels, prothrombin time (PT)/partial thromboplastin time (PTT), and international normalized ratio (INR).

   b. For connective tissue disorders: Consider serologic tests (antinuclear antibody [ANA], Anti-dsDNA).

2. TTE: Assess valve structure and degree of dysfunction, overall left ventricular function, EF percentage, size of aortic root, and presence of vegetations (TEE may be required if + vegetation on TTE).

3. Cardiac catheterization: Obtain if surgical intervention is a consideration, especially if concern for underlying CAD.

D. MR.

1. Chest x-ray: Possible left ventricular enlargement and increased pulmonary venous congestion (if concomitant CHF).

2. TTE.

   a. The American College of Cardiology (ACC) and American Heart Association (AHA) recommend TTEs for several reasons.

      i. Evaluate left ventricular size and function.

      ii. Determine right ventricle and left atrial size, pulmonary artery pressure, and severity of MR.

      iii. Monitor EF of symptomatic patients with moderate-to-severe MR.

      iv. Determine etiology of MR.

      v. Monitor EF and left ventricular size and function if patient has change in clinical status.

      vi. Evaluate MR integrity and left ventricular function in patients with mitral valve repair or replacement.

   b. Consider TEE if TTE is nondiagnostic or prior to surgical repair/replacement.

Differential Diagnosis

A. MS.

B. MR.

C. MVP.

D. AS.

E. AR.

F. Pulmonic stenosis.

G. Acute coronary syndrome.

H. Tricuspid stenosis.

I. Tricuspid regurgitation.

J. Infective endocarditis.

Evaluation and Management Plan

A. General plan.

1. Determine etiology of given VHD and treat accordingly.

2. Monitor patients for symptoms of worsening VHD.

3. Evaluate patients for determination of management: Medical versus surgical (open approach vs. percutaneous approach, such as TAVR).

4. Manage symptoms associated with given VHD (i.e., CHF).

5. Treat underlying comorbidities that contribute to worsen VHD (i.e., HTN, HLD, DM).

B. Patient/family teaching points.

1. Explain underlying etiology and specific type of VHD.

2. Discuss course of therapy: Medical versus surgical and importance of ongoing monitoring.

3. Emphasize importance of compliance with follow-up appointments and medications.

   a. If utilizing anticoagulation agents: Ensure patients understand not to discontinue drugs prior to any procedures without consulting cardiologist.

b. If clinically indicated: Educate regarding preinvasive procedure prophylactic antibiotics.

4. Geriatric patients: Consider involving family members to help determine best course of treatment.

5. For patients at high risk for endocarditis, discuss use of preprocedure prophylactic antibiotics.

6. Ensure understanding regarding reasons for urgent return to ED such as hemodynamic instability, new or worsening chest discomfort, palpitations, new or worsening difficulty breathing, syncope/near-syncope, or mental status changes.

C. Management of specific valvular diseases.

1. AR.

a. Surgical intervention via valve replacement: If angina, evidence of CHF, or ventricular failure.

b. Medical management: Typically reserved for patients who are not surgical candidates (due to comorbidities) because conservative management of symptomatic patients is rarely successful.

i. There is conflicting evidence with regard to use of medical management for asymptomatic patients with AR.

ii. With medications: Goal is to reduce afterload via vasodilators such as calcium channel blockers or ACE inhibitors); beta-blockers are not first-line drugs (due to bradycardia) but could benefit patients with significant left ventricular dysfunction.

2. AS.

a. According to AHA, there is no acceptable medical management to alleviate AS.

b. Available medical therapy is only used to alleviate symptoms and manage comorbidities (diuretics are not indicated due to the possibility of a decrease in cardiac output).

i. Beta-blockers (help with HTN and CAD).

ii. ACE inhibitors (help with HTN, DM, and left ventricular fibrosis).

c. Once patients are symptomatic, considerations should be made for surgery.

i. If patient is not a candidate for open (traditional) aortic valve replacement (AVR), consider TAVR.

3. MS.

a. Medical management may be useful, although it cannot ameliorate the narrowing of the mitral valve.

b. Several classes of medications can be used to assist with symptoms.

i. Beta-blockers: Decrease heart rate and improve dyspnea on exertion.

ii. Diuretics: Decrease pulmonary edema.

c. Symptomatic patients will require surgical intervention. There are several options.

i. Percutaneous mitral valvuloplasty: Typically used in younger patients and those with mild MS (contraindicated in moderate to severe disease).

ii. Surgical procedures: Open repair with commissurotomy or valve replacement with mechanical or bioprosthetic valve (considered high-risk procedures; mortality >20% in geriatric population with multiple comorbidities).

4. MR.

a. Asymptomatic patients with normal BPs and no left ventricular dysfunction do not require treatment.

b. Medical therapy can be used for symptom management (i.e., vasodilators and diuretics to manage BP).

c. Symptomatic patients should be considered for surgical repair/replacement.

i. If possible, valve repair is preferred to replacement: Eliminates requirement of long-term anticoagulation, improves symptoms, and increases postoperative survival rates.

ii. Surgical management indicated if NYHA class II to IV CHF, severe MR regardless of cardiac size and function, or asymptomatic patients with MR and atrial fibrillation, pulmonary HTN, or left ventricular dysfunction.

iii. Various percutaneous options are in the development process.

D. Additional pharmacologic considerations.

1. Outpatient anticoagulation.

a. INR monitoring is recommended in patients with mechanical prosthetic valves.

b. Goal is INR of 2.0 to 3.0 in patients with mechanical AVR and no other risk of thromboembolism.

c. Goal is INR 2.5 to 3.5 in patients with a mechanical AVR, MVR, and additional risk factors for thromboembolisms (i.e., atrial fibrillation, previous thromboembolism).

d. Low-dose daily aspirin is recommended in addition to anticoagulation in patients with a mechanical valve prosthesis.

e. Low-dose daily aspirin can be used in patients with a bioprosthetic aortic or mitral valve.

f. Anticoagulation can be used for the first 3 months after bioprosthetic MVR or AVR or repair to achieve an INR of 2.5.

g. Can consider clopidogrel 75 mg daily for the first 6 months after TAVR in addition to daily lifelong aspirin.

2. Anticoagulation with bridging.

a. Continuation of anticoagulation with a therapeutic INR is recommended in patients with mechanical heart valves undergoing minor procedures (i.e., dental extractions or cataract removal) where bleeding is easily controlled.

b. Bridging anticoagulation with heparin is recommended for invasive procedures when the INR is subtherapeutic preoperatively in those with a mechanical AVR, any thromboembolism risk factor, older generation mechanical AVRs, or a mechanical MVR.

E. Discharge instructions.

1. Ensure patient receives all prescriptions prior to discharge.

2. Arrange timely follow-up appointments with cardiologist.

3. Educate patients about reasons to return to ED with regard to worsening symptoms of VHD.

4. Based on clinical scenario and degree of VHD, provide patients with information regarding physical activity restrictions.

Follow-Up

A. Patients require monitoring via history/physical examinations and echocardiography based on clinical scenario, degree of VHD, and overall cardiac status (i.e., EF and left ventricular function). In AS, for example:

1. If mild disease, echocardiograms every 3 to 5 years.

2. If moderate disease, echocardiograms every 1 to 2 years.

3. If severe disease, echocardiograms every 6 months to 1 year.

Consultation/Referral

A. Consult with cardiologist for VHD.

B. Consult with infectious disease specialist (if concern for underlying infective endocarditis).

C. Consult with rheumatologist (if concern for underlying connective tissue disorder).

D. Consult with cardiothoracic surgeon (if surgical repair is a consideration).

E. Consult with interventional cardiologist (if consideration for TAVR).

F. Refer to cardiac rehabilitation following invasive valve repair/replacement procedure.

Special/Geriatric Considerations

A. Antibiotic prophylaxis.

  1. According to AHA, preinvasive procedure prophylactic antibiotics (against *Streptococcus viridans*) should be used in certain populations and scenarios with risk of infective endocarditis.

    a. Prosthetic heart valve.

    b. History of previous infective endocarditis.

    c. Congenital heart disease (CHD) that is unrepaired and cyanotic, repaired CHD using prosthetic material/device for 6 months, or repaired CHD with a residual defect.

    d. Cardiac transplant patients with VHD.

    e. Recommended for patients with MVP or moderate to severe primary MR.

    f. Procedures: Dental (if manipulation of gingiva, perforation of oral mucosa, or significant teeth manipulation) or respiratory (i.e., tonsillectomy, adenoidectomy). Amoxicillin (2 g 1-hour preprocedure), clindamycin (600 mg 1-hour preprocedure), or cephalexin (2 g 1-hour preprocedure) may be used.

B. Geriatric considerations.

  1. Aortic valve disease is the most common type of VHD in this demographic.

  2. If surgical intervention is a consideration, it is important to assess underlying CAD risk, cognitive status, and overall health status.

  3. For elderly patients with severe AS who are not surgical candidates, consultation should be obtained for TAVR, which is minimally invasive.

  4. If valve replacement procedure is indicated, it is necessary to assess risk versus benefit regarding use of anticoagulation.

  5. It is important to remember that VHD symptoms in this population can be vague (i.e., fatigue and dyspnea) and difficult to differentiate from normal aging.

Bibliography

Christensen, B. (2018, December 4). Endocarditis prophalaxis, adults. In B. Christensen (Ed.), *Medscape*. Retrieved from http://emedicine.medscape.com/article/2172262-overview

Dima, C. (2018, February 2). Mitral stenosis. In T. X. O'Brien (Ed.), *Medscape*. Retrieved from http://emedicine.medscape.com/article/155724-overview

Hanson, I., & Alfanso, L. C. (2018, November 28). Mitral regurgitation. In T. X. O'Brien (Ed.), *Medscape*. Retrieved from http://emedicine.medscape.com/article/155618-overview

Karavas, A. N., & Edwards, N. M. (2016). Valvular heart disease. In J. B. Halter, J. G. Ouslander, S. Studenski, K. P. High, S. Asthana, M. A. Supiano, & C. Ritchie (Eds.), *Hazzard's geriatric medicine and gerontology* (7th ed.). New York, NY: McGraw-Hill. Retrieved from http://accessmedicine.mhmedical.com.ezproxy2.library.drexel.edu/content.aspx?bookid=1923&sectionid=144524931

Ren, X. (2017, March 23). Aortic stenosis. In T. X. O'Brien (Ed.), *Medscape*. Retrieved from http://emedicine.medscape.com/article/150638-overview

Wang, S. S. (2018, November 19). Aortic regurgitation. In T. X. O'Brien (Ed.), *Medscape*. Retrieved from http://emedicine.medscape.com/article/150490-overview

4 Gastrointestinal Guidelines

Catherine Harris

Acute Abdomen

Shawn Mangan

Definition

A. Acute abdomen is defined as pain, which arises suddenly and is usually less than 48 hours duration. Acute abdomen sometimes requires urgent surgical intervention, but not always.

B. Nontraumatic pain in the abdominal region with an onset of less than a few days and has worsened progressively until presentation.

C. Conditions categorized under acute abdomen.
   1. Abdominal aortic aneurysm (AAA).
   2. Acute cholecystitis.
   3. Acute mesenteric ischemia.
   4. Acute pancreatitis.
   5. Appendicitis.
   6. Diverticulitis.
   7. Ectopic pregnancy/ovarian torsion.
   8. Intestinal obstruction.
   9. Perforated duodenal ulcer.

Incidence

A. Acute abdomen accounts for approximately 5% to 10% of all ED visits.

B. Approximately 20% of these patients will have small bowel obstruction, 14% will be diagnosed with appendicitis, 5% with cholecystitis, and less than 1% with perforated peptic ulcer. Another 25% will not be able to be diagnosed and will be discharged from the ED.

Pathogenesis

A. Acute abdomen depends on the origin of the pain: Ischemia, distension, obstruction, ulceration, or inflammation in the affected area.

Predisposing Factors

A. Previous abdominal surgery.
B. Diverticulitis.
C. Constipation.
D. History of gallstones.
E. Abdominal cancers.
F. Peptic/duodenal ulcers.
G. Crohn's disease or ulcerative colitis.
H. Severe endometriosis or ectopic pregnancy.
I. Medications including nonsteroidal anti-inflammatory drugs (NSAIDS), steroids.
J. Alcohol abuse.
   1. Age greater than 50.

Subjective Data

A. Common complaints/symptoms.
   1. Right upper quadrant (RUQ).
      a. Cholecystitis: Colicky, intermittent waves of pain that come and go. The pain may radiate to back, cause nausea, and worsen after a fatty meal. Pain improves with rest.
      b. Peptic ulcer disease: Pain worsens after a meal.
      c. Pancreatitis: Diffuse, burrowing, stabbing pain radiates to mid back.
   2. Right lower quadrant (RLQ).
      a. Appendicitis: Starts in mid abdomen, becoming more acute in RLQ. Sometimes nausea and vomiting occur.
   3. Left lower quadrant (LLQ).
      a. Diverticulitis.
B. Common/typical scenario.
   1. AAA: If ruptured, patients who do not die immediately present with abdominal or back pain, hypotension, and tachycardia. They may have a recent history of straining (such as lifting a heavy object), and most will also have a history of hypertension.
   2. Acute cholecystitis: Abrupt, severe, constant, aching pain in RUQ with radiation to the back and right shoulder lasting 24 hours or more, associated with nausea and vomiting.
   3. Acute mesenteric ischemia: Patients are usually greater than 50 years old.
      a. Arterial: Sudden onset of severe pain out of proportion to physical findings (abdomen soft; little or no tenderness) in patients at risk (coronary artery disease, atrial fibrillation, generalized atherosclerosis, low flow states). Patients may have a history of post prandial pain suggesting intestinal angina. However, many patients have no identifiable risk factors.
      b. Venous: Similar symptoms to arterial, but with a more gradual onset.
   4. Acute pancreatitis: Steady, piercing, upper abdominal pain, severe enough to require intravenous (IV) opioid pain management. Pain radiates to the back in some patients. Patients may find pain reduction by sitting up and leaning forward. Nausea and vomiting may be present. The pain develops suddenly in gallstone pancreatitis. In alcoholic pancreatitis, pain usually develops over several days.
   5. Appendicitis: In about 50% of patients, epigastric or periumbilical pain is followed by nausea, vomiting, then

pain shifting to the RLQ. Direct and rebound tenderness at McBurney's point is present. In other patients, pain may not be localized or may be diffuse.

6. Diverticulitis: Pain or tenderness in the LLQ with fever. Rebound or guarding, nausea, vomiting, and abdominal distention occur if concurrent bowel obstruction is present.

7. Ectopic pregnancy: Sudden, severe pelvic pain and/or vaginal bleeding followed by syncope and signs of hemorrhagic shock in females of reproductive age.

8. Intestinal obstruction.

    a. Small bowel: Cramping near epigastrium, vomiting (with some relief in pain), and, if complete obstruction, obstipation. Range of bowel sounds on auscultation from high pitched peristalsis in early presentation to no BS in later presentations.

    b. Large bowel: Gradual development of constipation, then abdominal distention, lower abdominal cramps, and borborygmi (loud prolonged bowel sounds).

9. Perforated duodenal ulcer—sudden agonizing pain usually in patients with history of peptic ulcer disease or NSAID therapy. Frequently occurs in the elderly (60 to 70 year age group). Pain occurs initially in the upper abdomen then becomes diffuse. Patients lay still, in a knee to chest position, breathe shallowly, and are tachycardic. Hypotension and fever are late findings. Abdomen appears nondistended with board-like rigidity.

C. Family and social history.

    1. Smoking.

    2. Alcohol abuse.

    3. Low fiber or fatty diet.

    4. Obesity.

    5. Family history may increase risk.

D. Review of systems.

    1. SOCRATES acronym.

        a. Site: Ask about location of pain.

        b. Onset: Inquire about exact time and mode of pain. Did it occur suddenly or gradually?

        c. Character: How is the pain characterized? Is it confined to one area or all around? Is the pain dull or sharp?

        d. Radiation or referral of pain: Does the pain stay in one place or does it move around?

        e. Associated symptoms: Is there any weight loss, nausea, vomiting, diarrhea, constipation, pain on urinating, skin discoloration, vaginal bleeding?

        f. Time course: Is the pain continuous or intermittent?

        g. Exacerbating/relieving factors: Does it hurt to cough, eat, or does it feel better to vomit?

        h. Severity: Can the pain be measured on a scale from 1 to 10, 10 being the worst pain ever felt?

Physical Examination

A. Vital signs: Check postural VS to assess for hypovolemia or bleeding.

B. Inspection: From nipples to knees.

    1. Distention.

    2. Scars.

    3. Ecchymosis such as Grey Turner sign.

C. Auscultation.

    1. Bowel sounds (hyperactive/hypoactive/absent?).

    2. Bruit.

D. Palpation.

    1. Rebound tenderness.

    2. Ask patient to cough to ascertain peritonitis.

    3. Guarding.

    4. Organomegaly.

    5. Hernia.

    6. Rectal, pelvic, testicular examination.

E. Diagnosis: Specific findings.

    1. AAA.

        a. Abdomen rigid or distended, very tender.

        b. Shock-like symptoms (pallor, diaphoresis, tachycardia).

    2. Ectopic pregnancy.

        a. Appears toxic and shock-like symptoms.

        b. Lower abdominal tenderness.

    3. Appendicitis: Guarding and rebound tenderness, prefers fetal position.

    4. Diverticulitis: LLQ pain.

    5. Biliary colic cholecystitis: RUQ pain with Murphy's sign.

    6. Renal colic: Severe pain, costovertebral angle tenderness on affected side.

    7. Pancreatitis.

        a. Epigastric tenderness, abdominal distention, fever, and tachycardia.

        b. Signs of jaundice.

        c. May develop Cullen or Grey Turner sign.

    8. Special abdominal examination maneuvers: Prior to the advent of radiologic imaging, several clinical maneuvers were utilized to differentiate abdominal pain diagnoses. While most of these tests will be followed by imaging studies today to confirm findings, they are still utilized.

        a. Iliopsoas sign: Have the patient roll on his/her left side and hyperextend the right hip joint. If pain is present, the test is positive and suggests irritation of the iliopsoas muscle by appendicitis.

        b. Obturator sign: With the patient supine, passively flex the thigh and rotate inward. If pain is elicited, the obturator muscle is inflamed because of pathology such as appendicitis, diverticulitis, pelvic inflammatory disease, or ectopic pregnancy.

        c. Rovsing sign: Apply pressure to the LLQ. If pain is referred to McBurney's Point (RLQ), the test is positive and appendicitis is suspected.

        d. Murphy's sign: Ask the patient to take a deep breath while palpating the RUQ. If the patient abruptly stops inspiration, the sign is positive and suggests acute cholecystitis.

        e. Cullen and Grey Turner signs: Both Cullen and Grey Turner signs are associated with ecchymosis on the abdomen.

            i. Cullen sign is superficial edema and bruising in the subcutaneous tissue around the umbilicus. This is associated with ruptured ectopic pregnancies but can be seen in other conditions as well such as pancreatitis or trauma.

            ii. Grey Turner sign is bruising along the flank associated with retroperitoneal bleeding or intraabdominal bleeding.

Diagnostic Tests

A. Ordered based on differential diagnosis, but can include:

    1. In all women of childbearing age, assume the woman is pregnant unless proven otherwise; use HCG test, or possibly transvaginal ultrasound (US).

    2. Complete blood count (CBC) with differential.

    3. Metabolic panel.

    4. Electrolytes.

    5. Amylase and lipase.

6. Consider blood culture in elderly with fever or hypothermia for suspected sepsis.

7. Urinalysis.

8. Abdominal x-ray.

9. Chest x-ray.

10. EKG to rule out cardiac cause of pain.

11. Consider abdominal US.

12. Consider CT abdomen with PO and IV contrast.

13. Consider endoscopic retrograde cholangiopancreatography (ERCP) to visualize distal common bile duct.

14. *Helicobacter pylori* testing.

15. Endoscopy.

16. Stool guaiac.

17. Colonoscopy.

Differential Diagnosis

A. Location and duration of abdominal pain can often help in narrowing.

    1. RUQ pain.

        a. Acute cholecystitis and biliary colic.

            i. Biliary tract—Increased serum amylase.

            ii. Ascending cholangitis presents with fever and jaundice.

            iii. In acute cholecystitis, pain radiates to scapula associated with nausea, vomiting, and fever. Murphy's sign (inspiratory arrest in response to deep RUQ palpation) may be seen.

        b. Perforated duodenal ulcer: Accompanied by increased serum amylase.

        c. Acute pancreatitis.

            i. Bilateral right and left upper quadrant pain.

            ii. Accompanied by increased serum amylase.

        d. Myocardial infarction.

        e. Pulmonary pathology.

    2. RLQ pain.

        a. Appendicitis: Dull, steady periumbilical pain and nausea, which then localizes to the RLQ at McBurney's point.

        b. Abdominal aneurysm.

        c. Ruptured ectopic pregnancy/ovarian cyst.

        d. Incarcerated inguinal hernia.

        e. Diverticulitis.

    3. LUQ pain.

        a. Acute pancreatitis: Epigastric pain which radiates to the back and is associated with nausea.

        b. Splenic enlargement infarction or aneurysm.

        c. Myocardial ischemia.

        d. Left lower lobe pneumonia.

    4. LLQ pain.

        a. Diverticulitis.

        b. Aortic aneurysm.

        c. Ruptured ectopic pregnancy/ovarian cyst.

    5. Must not miss diagnoses.

        a. Small bowel obstruction.

        b. Large bowel obstruction.

        c. Nonspecific bowel pain.

            i. Appendicitis.

            ii. Perforated ulcer.

            iii. Acute cholecystitis.

    6. Common abdominal pain culprits.

        a. Acute pancreatitis.

        b. Diverticulitis.

        c. Acute pyelonephritis.

Evaluation and Management Plan

A. General plan.

1. Determine if patient is hemodynamically stable and if peritoneal signs are present.

2. Obtain imaging studies and treat based on suspected condition.

    a. AAA.

        i. If rupture is suspected, attempts at hemodynamic stability are begun as the patient is optimized for surgery. An US provides bedside results to assist in diagnosis (without treatment, mortality rate approaches 100%).

        ii. Patients who present in shock will need fluid resuscitation but mean arterial pressure should not exceed 65 mmHg to prevent further bleeding.

        iii. If the patient is stable, abdominal CT or computed tomography angiography (CTA) can more precisely characterize aneurysm size and anatomy to assist with surgical intervention if necessary.

            1) Surgical options include endovascular stent grafting VS open repair.

            2) Medical management if AAA less than 5 mm includes repeat imaging every 6 to 12 months to monitor for size increase greater than 5 mm or to assess for rapid growth. Both are indications for elective surgical repair.

    b. Acute cholecystitis.

        i. On examination, RUQ pain to palpation with inspiratory arrest (+ Murphy's sign).

        ii. US (showing presence of stones, gallbladder wall thickening, or enlargement) is the study of choice and can often establish the diagnosis.

        iii. Management.

            1) Medical—single episode may not warrant surgery. Counsel patient to avoid fatty foods, fasting, or starvation diets and to see provider for recurrent pain. Tylenol PRN for pain. Actigall decreases amount of cholesterol produced by the liver and absorbed by intestines and may be helpful.

            2) Surgical management—laparoscopic cholecystectomy. Conversion to open procedure occurs approximately 5% of the time.

            3) Surgical cases a need liver and pancreatic enzyme levels assessed, as elevated levels may show common duct stones.

    c. Acute mesenteric ischemia.

        i. Clinical diagnosis is more important than testing due to time delay. Increased mortality is observed once intestinal infarction occurs. Intestinal infarction can occur as soon as 10 hours after the onset of symptoms. Untreated, mortality approaches 90%.

        ii. Proceed directly to surgery for diagnosis and treatment in patients with peritoneal signs. CTA is used if diagnosis is unclear.

        iii. Support blood pressure (BP) with IV fluids (avoid vasopressors), adequate oxygenation, broad spectrum antibiotics, and adequate pain control. Consider anticoagulation.

        iv. Treatment involves surgical embolectomy and revascularization with possible bowel resection. Angiographic vasodilators (papaverine) or thrombolytics may be used.

        v. Depending on the severity of bowel ischemia, the patient may require a long inpatient hospital stay, maintaining *nil per os* (NPO) status, and supporting nutrition with total parenteral nutrition.

    vi. Find and treat predisposing causes.

    vii. Plan for long-term anticoagulation.

d. Acute pancreatitis: Condition ranges from mild abdominal pain and vomiting to severe with systemic inflammatory response syndrome (SIRS) response, shock, and multiorgan failure.

e. Mortality rates are as high as 40% to 50% of cases. Important to assess the severity of illness on admission utilizing tools (Ranson criteria, others) that predict mortality risk. Early recognition of severe pancreatitis improves outcomes by risk stratification and correct admission placement of the patient.

    i. Diagnose based on clinical suspicion, especially in patients with a history of gallstones or chronic heavy alcohol abuse and noting elevated amylase and lipase.

    ii. Urine dipstick for trypsinogen-2 has sensitivity and specificity of greater than 90%. WBC elevation range is 12 to 20,000. Imaging with plain abdominal film shows calcifications within pancreatic ducts and gallstones. Obtain US if gallstone pancreatitis is suspected. CT abdomen with contrast is usually done to identify necrosis, fluid collection, or cysts once condition is diagnosed.

    iii. Treatment includes fluid resuscitation (up to 8 L/day), maintaining NPO status (until tenderness subsides, amylase WNL), pain control, antibiotic therapy if pancreatic necrosis, and drainage of collections.

f. Appendicitis.

    i. Surgical management: Appendectomy.

    ii. Medical management: Antibiotics may be used to treat uncomplicated, nonsurgical appendicitis; however, there are recurrences. More studies need to be done in order to determine the efficacy of antibiotic therapy alone.

g. Diverticulitis.

    i. Typical presentation is with LLQ pain with or without peritonitic findings; an absence of vomiting; fever; and leukocytosis with left shift. May also complain of back pain, flatulence, borborygmi (loud prolonged bowel sounds), diarrhea, or constipation.

    ii. A C-reactive protein greater than 50 mg/L, along with LLQ pain and absence of vomiting, is highly predictive of acute colonic diverticulosis.

    iii. CT scan of abdomen and pelvis is the current gold standard in confirming the diagnosis of acute diverticulitis if the clinical picture is unclear.

    iv. US is fast becoming an additional modality in diagnosis of the disease.

    v. Management.

        1) Medical: Bowel rest. *nil per os* (NPO). NG tube placement to low suction, IV fluid replacement therapy. Antimicrobial therapy covering gram negative organisms and anaerobes should be initiated when associated with systemic manifestations of infection. If relapse, same regimen × 1 month.

        2) Surgical resection for abscess, peritonitis, obstruction, fistula, failure to improve after several days, or recurrence.

        3) Nonsurgical cases should be referred for a colonoscopy 4 to 6 weeks after the event.

h. Ectopic pregnancy.

    i. Urine pregnancy test (beta-hcg) is 99% sensitive for ectopic and uterine pregnancy. If positive, follow with serum beta-hcg and transvaginal pelvic US. Diagnostic laparoscopy may be necessary for confirmation.

    ii. Surgical resection is usually necessary to treat. If possible, salpingotomy is done to conserve the tube. Salpingectomy indicates when ectopic pregnancies are greater than 5 cm, when tubes are severely damaged, or when no future childbearing is planned.

    iii. Resuscitate if hemodynamically unstable or in hemorrhagic shock and prepare for immediate surgery.

    iv. Methotrexate may be an option if unruptured tubal pregnancy is less than 3 cm, no fetal heart activity is heard, and beta-hcg level is less than 5,000. Follow-up within 1 week for repeat beta-hcg level.

i. Intestinal obstruction.

    i. Supine and, if possible, upright abdominal x-rays are usually adequate to diagnose obstruction, showing a "coiled spring" sign in a series of distended small bowel loops or right colon. Large bowel obstruction shows distention of the colon proximal to the obstruction.

    ii. Treatment for both small and large bowel obstruction includes NG decompression and resuscitation with IV crystalloid fluid administration and IV antibiotics covering gram negative and anaerobes if bowel ischemia is suspected.

    iii. Complete obstruction of small bowel is treated with early laparotomy.

    iv. Obstructing colon cancers can be treated with resection and anastomosis, with or without a colostomy or ileostomy.

j. Perforated duodenal ulcer.

    i. Upright chest x-ray reveals free air. Upper GI film with water-soluble contrast is also helpful to diagnose perforation and if it has healed spontaneously.

    ii. Leukocytosis and elevated amylase usually present.

    iii. In approximately 50% of cases, the perforation self-heals. Those who are poor surgical candidates or who present more than 24 hours after perforation and who are stable may be admitted. Provide careful observation for clinical deterioration, IV fluids, NG suction, and broad spectrum antibiotics. Low threshold for surgical repair if condition deteriorates.

        1) *H. pylori* infection is implicated in 70% to 90% of all perforated ulcers. Medical therapy for peptic ulcer disease includes the combination of omeprazole 20 mg BID, plus clarithromycin 500 mg BID, plus metronidazole 500 mg TID × 14 days; for non-PCN allergic patients.

B. Patient/family teaching points.

1. Do not take laxatives, use enemas, or take medications, food, or liquids until consulting a healthcare provider for suspected abdominal pain and the following:

    a. Increased or unusual looking vomit or stool.

    b. Hard, swollen abdomen.

    c. Lump in scrotum, groin, or lower abdomen.

    d. Missed period or suspected pregnancy.

2. Engage in activity as tolerated. Abdominal pain with nausea and vomiting, fever, or pain that lasts more than

3 hours which halts daily activities should be reported to a healthcare provider.

3. Eat regular foods as tolerated. Do not eat food or drink liquids until a healthcare provider is consulted if pain occurs with nausea and vomiting, fever is present, or pain lasts longer than 3 hours.

C. Pharmacotherapy.

1. Regardless of the cause, early use of analgesia before diagnosis is associated with improved diagnosis and treatment.

   a. Acetaminophen 1,000 g IV recommended regardless of pain severity.

   b. IV narcotic analgesics can be added depending on the severity of pain. Morphine and opioids such as fentanyl can be considered in cases of acute abdomen.

   c. NSAIDs are effective for colic of biliary tract and ureteral stones.

2. If abdominal infections are suspected, blood cultures should be obtained and antimicrobial agents administered (within 1 hour in cases of suspected septic shock). Coverage of gram negative organisms is prudent. Broad antibiotic coverage is used if concern for sepsis.

3. When surgery is necessary, antimicrobial agents should be given just prior to the start of surgery (ideally within 30 minutes), which significantly reduces the risk of surgical site infection.

D. Discharge instructions.

1. Surgery instructions depend on the procedure and surgeon preference, if applicable.

2. Stress the importance of follow-up, adherence to prescription instructions, and to call the healthcare provider with questions.

Follow-Up

A. If surgical intervention, perform as per surgeon instructions.

Consultation/Referral

A. Consultation/referral depends on the underlying cause of acute abdomen.

1. Surgery.

2. Medicine (anticoagulation, antibiotic therapy management).

3. Nutrition.

4. Oncology.

5. Gynecology.

6. Counseling.

7. Geriatric medicine.

Special/Geriatric Considerations

A. Consider that obesity distorts the abdominal examination, making organ palpation or pelvic examination difficult.

B. Men over 40 and women over 50 should warrant a high suspicion of cardiac origin of pain when epigastric.

C. Geriatric patients have a higher incidence of:

1. Biliary disease.

2. Ischemic disease.

3. Mortality.

4. Hospital admission and complication rates.

5. Reliable history and physical can be difficult as findings in other age groups are often absent in the elderly.

6. Elderly individuals may have a vague or atypical presentation

of pain, varying in location, severity, and presentation of fever or nonspecific findings. Classical presentation of peritonitis rebound tenderness and local rigidity occur

less often. Urinary tract infection (UTI) symptoms are more likely to be frequency, dysuria, or urgency. Abdominal pathology may advance to a dangerous point prior to symptom development, and altered mental status may play a role in assessment.

7. Aortic abdominal aneurysm (AAA) occurs most often in the elderly. Maintain a high level of suspicion in patients presenting with symptoms suggestive of renal colic or musculoskeletal back pain (approximately 65% of men older than 65 years have AAA).

8. Patients older than 65 have a 30% to 50% risk of gallstones and may not present with significant pain.

9. Fever and elevated white blood cell (WBC) count occur in less than half of elderly patients with diverticulitis.

10. Presence of peptic ulcer disease (PUD) is more common in the elderly due to NSAIDs. The most common presenting symptom of PUD in the elderly is melena.

Bibliography

Banks, P. A., & Freeman, M. L. (2006). Practice guidelines in acute pancreatitis. *The American Journal of Gastroenterology, 101*, 2379–2400. Retrieved from https://journals.lww.com/ajg/Citation/2006/10000/Practice_Guidelines_in_Acute_Pancreatitis.31.aspx

Barkley, T. W., & Meyers, C. M. (2015). *Practice considerations for adult-gerontology acute care nurse practitioners* (Vol. 1, 2nd ed.). West Hollywood, CA: Barkley & Associates.

Cartwright, S. L., & Knudson, M. P. (2008). Evaluation of acute abdominal pain in adults. *American Family Physician, 77*(7), 971–978.

Cash, J. C., Glass, C. A. (2017). *Family practice guidelines* (4th ed.). New York, NY: Springer Publishing Company.

Cervellin, G., Mora, R., Ticinesi, A., Meschi, T., Comelli, I., Catena, F., & Lippi, G. (2016). Epidemiology and outcomes of acute abdominal pain in a large urban emergency department: Retrospective analysis of 5,340 cases. *Annals of Translational Medicine, 4*(19), 362. doi:10.21037/atm.2016.09.10

Chey, W. D., Leontiadis, G. I., Howden, C. W., & Moss, S. F. (2017). ACG clinical guideline: Treatment of *Helicobacter pylori* infection. *American Journal of Gastroenterology, 112*, 212–239. Retrieved from https://journals.lww.com/ajg/Abstract/2017/02000/ACT_Clinical_Guideline__Treatment_of_Helicobacter.12.aspx

DeStigter, K. K., & Keating, D. P. (2009). Imaging update: Acute colonic diverticulitis. *Clinics in Colon and Rectal Surgery, 22*(3), 147–155. doi:10.1055/s-0029-1236158

El-Garem, H., Hamdy, E., Hamdy, S., El-Sayed, M., Elsharkawy, A., & Saleh, A. (2013). Use of the urinary trypsinogen-2 dipstick test in early diagnosis of pancreatitis after endoscopic retrograde cholangiopancreatography (ERCP). *Open Journal of Gastroenterology, 3*, 289–294. doi:10.4236/ojgas.2013.36049

Hardy, A., Butler, B., & Crandall, M. (2013). The evaluation of the acute abdomen. In L. Moore, K. Turner, & S. Todd (Eds.), *Common problems in acute care surgery* (pp. 17–30). New York, NY: Springer Publishing Company.

Kendal, J. L., & Moreira, M. (2018). Evaluation of the adult with abdominal pain in the emergency department. In J. Grayzel (Ed.), *UpToDate*. Retrieved from https://www.uptodate.com/contents/evaluation-of-the-adult-with-abdominal-pain-in-the-emergency-department

Macaluso, C. R., & McNamara, R. M. (2012). Evaluation and management of acute abdominal pain in the emergency department. *International Journal of General Medicine, 5*, 789–797. doi:10.2147/IJGM.S25936

Malbrain, M. L., Chiumello, D., Pelosi, P., Bihari, D., Innes, R., Ranieri, V. M., . . . , Gattinoni, L. (2005). Incidence and prognosis of intraabdominal hypertension in a mixed population of critically ill patients: A multiple-center epidemiological study. *Critical Care Medicine, 33*(2), 315–322. doi:10.1097/01.CCM.0000153408.09806.1B

Mayumi, T., Yoshida, M., Tazuma, S., Furukawa, A., Nishii, O., Shigematsu, K., & Hirata, K. (2016). The practice guidelines for primary care of acute abdomen 2015. *Japanese Journal of Radiology, 34*, 80–115. doi:10.1007/s11604-015-0489-z

Murray, H., Baakdah, H., Bardell, T., & Tulandi, T. (2005, October 11). Diagnosis and treatment of ectopic pregnancy. *Canadian Medical Association Journal, 173*(8), 905–912. doi:10.1503/cmaj.050222

Musson, R. E., Bickle, I., & Vijay, R. (2011). Gas patterns on plain abdominal radiographs: A pictorial review. *Journal of Postgraduate Medicine, 87*, 274–287. doi:10.1136/pgmj.2009.082396

Saccomano, S. J., & Ferrara, L. R. (2011). Evaluation acute abdominal pain. *The Nurse Practitioner, 38*(11), 46–53. doi:10.1097/01.NPR.0000433077.14775.f1

Stollman, N., Smalley, W., & Hirano, I. (2015, December). American Gastroenterological Association Institute guideline on the management of acute diverticulitis. *Gastroenterology, 149*(7), 1944–1949. doi:10.1053/j.gastro.2015.10.003

Vaidyanathan, S., Wadhawan, H., Welch, P., & El-Salamani, M. (2008). Ruptured abdominal aortic aneurysm masquerading as isolated hip pain: An unusual presentation. *Canadian Journal of Emergency Medicine, 10*(3), 251–254. doi:10.1017/S1481803500010186

Cirrhosis

Robin Miller and Ann E. Burke

Definition

A. Cirrhosis: Chronic inflammation leading to fibrosis/scarring of the liver. Causes of injury may be viral, autoimmune, metabolic, drug induced, or due to alcohol and/or fat.

    1. Compensated: Mild portal hypertension but normal synthetic function (bilirubin, prothrombin time [PT], albumin, creatinine).

    2. Decompensated: Progression of disease due to complications of portal hypertension which include variceal hemorrhage, hepatic encephalopathy, ascites, spontaneous bacterial peritonitis (SBP).

        a. Median survival in decompensated cirrhosis is 6 months or less.

        b. MELD score—model to predict prognosis in patients with cirrhosis using the bilirubin, creatinine, and international normalized ratio (INR).

Incidence

A. Centers for Disease Control and Prevention (CDC) data from 2015 reports 3.9 million people in the United States with cirrhosis (see Figure 4.1).

B. National Institutes of Health (NIH)—cirrhosis is the 12th leading cause of death in the United States.

Pathogenesis

A. Most common causes of cirrhosis in the United States include: Hepatitis C, alcoholic liver disease, and nonalcoholic fatty liver disease (NAFLD). These three causes account for 80% of patients on the liver transplant list during the years 2004 to 2013.

B. Other less common causes include: Viral hepatitis B, hemochromatosis, autoimmune disease, primary biliary cholangitis, primary sclerosing cholangitis, drug-induced liver injury (DILI), Wilson's disease, Alpha 1 antitrypsin deficiency, celiac disease, polycystic liver disease, sarcoidosis, and right-sided heart failure.

Predisposing Factors

A. Combination of more than one factor may lead to an accelerated progression to fibrosis.

    1. Heavy alcohol use.

    2. Viral hepatitis.

    3. Fatty liver disease.

    4. Genetic or metabolic disorder—that is, Wilson's, Alpha 1 antitrypsin, hemochromatosis.

    5. Autoimmune disease.

    6. Hepatic congestion, that is, heart failure.

Subjective Data

A. Common complaints/symptoms.

    1. Nonspecific—anorexia, weight loss, fatigue.

    2. Decompensated—jaundice, abdominal distension, confusion, gastrointestinal (GI) bleeding.

B. Common/typical scenario.

    1. May be incidental finding on lab tests or imaging without any symptoms.

    2. There may be an acute presentation with hepatic decompensation.

C. Family and social history.

    1. Detailed history of alcohol use, drug use, sex partners, body piercings, tattoos.

    2. Inquire about family history of autoimmune disease, liver disease, and liver cancer.

    3. Living situation—household contacts with infected individuals with viral hepatitis.

    4. Occupation—potential exposure to viral hepatitis.

    5. Travel—recent travel or country of origin.

D. Review of systems.

    1. May present with jaundice, pruritus, easy bruising, hematemesis, melena, hematochezia, ascites, lower extremity edema, confusion, or sleep disturbances.

Physical Examination

A. May have no physical findings.

B. In cirrhosis, one may see:

    1. Jaundice.

    2. Spider angiomata on the neck or chest.

    3. Gynecomastia.

    4. Ascites—associated with edema in the scrotum and/or lower extremities.

    5. Firm nodular liver.

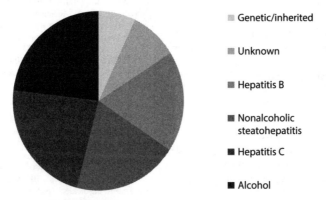

■ Genetic/inherited

■ Unknown

■ Hepatitis B

■ Nonalcoholic steatohepatitis

■ Hepatitis C

■ Alcohol

FIGURE 4.1 Common causes of cirrhosis.
Source: Chaney, A. (2017). *Fast Facts about GI and Liver Diseases for Nurses: What APRNs need to know in a nutshell.* New York, NY: Springer Publishing Company.

6. Splenomegaly.
7. Palmar erythema.
8. Digital clubbing.
9. Asterixis: Bilateral flapping of dorsiflexed hands.
10. Low blood pressure.

Diagnostic Tests

A. Labs: Complete blood count (CBC), comprehensive metabolic panel (CMP), PT, INR.

   1. All liver tests may be abnormal. In decompensated disease, rising bilirubin, low albumin, elevated INR, and creatinine indicate synthetic dysfunction and progression of cirrhosis.

   2. Thrombocytopenia: Related to portal hypertension and splenomegaly; platelets less than 150/L.

   3. Anemia: Due to GI blood loss, chronic disease, renal disease, bone marrow suppression, or hemolysis.

   4. Leukopenia: Secondary to hypersplenism.

   5. Hyponatremia: Inability to excrete free water.

B. Imaging.

   1. Ultrasound (US): Shrunken nodular liver with or without splenomegaly/ascites.

   2. US with Doppler: Portal hypertension, portal vein thrombosis, or collateral flow may be present.

   3. MRI: Can identify cirrhosis, hepatocellular carcinoma, or other liver masses. It is the preferred study for cancer surveillance and staging.

C. Liver biopsy.

   1. It is the gold standard to diagnose or identify the cause of cirrhosis.

   2. Fibroscan is a noninvasive tool to stage fibrosis.

Differential Diagnosis

A. Cirrhosis related to chronic hepatic inflammation due to:

   1. Viral: Hepatitis A, B, C.

   2. Alcohol.

   3. Fatty liver.

   4. Autoimmune: Autoimmune hepatitis, celiac, primary biliary cholangitis (PBC), primary sclerosing cholangitis (PSC).

   5. Genetic/metabolic: Wilson's, hemochromatosis, Alpha 1 antitrypsin, polycystic liver disease.

B. Extrahepatic causes of cirrhosis.

   1. Congestive heart failure.

   2. Sarcoidosis.

   3. Budd Chiari.

   4. Portal and splenic vein thrombosis.

Evaluation and Management Plan

A. General plan.

   1. See Figure 4.2.

   2. Ascites and SBP.

   a. Ascites: Abdominal accumulation of fluid due to high portal pressures. It is typically treated with sodium restriction and diuretics. Refractory cases require paracentesis or transjugular intrahepatic portosystemic shunt (TIPS).

   b. SBP is an infection of the ascitic fluid unrelated to perforated viscus. Patients with high MELD scores are at most risk, and failure to identify the diagnosis can lead to refractory sepsis. Cultures will show high absolute polymorphonuclear leukocyte counts greater than 250 cells/mm.

   3. Encephalopathy.

   a. Impairment in cognitive and neuromuscular function associated with decompensated cirrhosis.

   b. Disturbance in sleep pattern, insomnia, and hypersomnia are common early features before more typical levels of consciousness alterations.

   c. Manifestations range from mild confusion to severe somnolence and coma.

   d. Treatment is based on underlying cause/trigger (e.g., GI bleeding, infection, dehydration, medication noncompliance).

   4. GI bleeding.

   a. Acute variceal hemorrhage is the result of portal hypertension and usually occurs in the upper GI tracts. Other causes of GI bleeding in patients with liver disease include peptic ulcers, portal hypertensive gastropathy, and gastric antral vascular ectasias (GAVE).

   b. Bleeding presents as hematemesis and/or melena.

   c. Plan: Stabilization of patient.

   i. Blood and blood products: Goal hemoglobin of 7 to 9 g/dL.

   ii. Restoration of intravascular volume: Intravenous (IV) fluids.

   iii. Treatment with endoscopic evaluation and interventions to stop the bleeding. Epinephrine, banding, Argon plasma coagulation, and clipping may be used alone or in combination.

   iv. Patients at high risk of rebleeding may be considered a candidate for TIPS.

   v. Bleeding that is refractory to traditional measures may require esophageal tamponade. Short-term only.

   vi. Prevention and management of complications (e.g., sepsis, renal failure, aspiration pneumonia) desired.

   5. Hepatorenal syndrome (HRS).

   a. Chronic or acute kidney injury related to advanced hepatic failure and portal hypertension. Must exclude other causes (e.g., shock, nephrotoxic drugs, dehydration). Can be precipitated by an acute insult such as SBP or GI bleeding. Without therapy, most patients with HRS die within weeks of the onset of renal impairment.

   i. Type I HRS: More severe with rapid onset and poor prognosis. May reverse if cause of hepatic disease is treatable, that is, alcohol cessation, antiviral therapy.

   ii. Type II HRS: Less rapid progression.

   b. Plan.

   i. Correction of underlying hepatic cause, if able.

   ii. Medications to raise the mean arterial pressure and improve renal perfusion.

   iii. Monitor fluid status closely.

   iv. Dialysis as a bridge to transplant or renal recovery.

   v. May need dual renal/liver transplant.

B. Patient/family teaching points.

   1. Ascites and SBP.

   a. Ascitic fluid may reaccumulate despite diuretic therapy and will likely require multiple paracenteses to manage fluids and mitigate side effects such as shortness of breath and edema.

   b. Daily weights.

   c. 2,000 mg sodium restricted diet.

   d. Laboratory monitoring of electrolytes and renal function for safe dosing of diuretics.

   e. Report any fever, abdominal pain, or altered mental status that may indicate SBP.

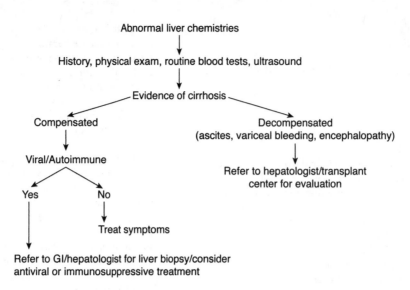

FIGURE 4.2 Comprehensive management of patients with cirrhosis.

f. Prophylactic antibiotics for SBP is lifelong therapy or until transplant.

2. Encephalopathy.

a. Review with family/caregiver to be alert for confusion, memory lapses, mood changes, speech abnormalities, slowed movements, gait disturbance, or day/night reversal.

b. Clearance of neurotoxins such as ammonia is important. This is primarily achieved through the stool. Medications for treatment target that means of clearance through promotion of several bowel movements daily.

3. GI bleeding.

a. High risk of recurrent bleeding within 6 weeks of initial episode.

b. If banding was performed, expect a sore throat for a few days. Soft diet recommended.

c. Review signs of bleeding: Vomiting blood or coffee ground emesis, black tarry or maroon-colored stools, weakness, lightheadedness.

d. If TIPS was placed, may see worsening encephalopathy.

e. Avoid NSAIDs.

4. HRS.

a. Avoid nephrotoxic drugs.

b. Stop diuretic therapy.

c. May require dialysis while awaiting transplant.

d. Teach SQ injections for home therapy (e.g., octreotide).

C. Pharmacotherapy.

1. Ascites and SBP.

a. Combination diuretics, usually Lasix and Aldactone, to balance potassium. Diuretic starting dose is 20 mg Lasix with 50 mg Aldactone, which then increases using the same ratio.

b. SBP is typically treated with third generation cephalosporin such as ceftriaxone or cefotaxime, typically for 5 days. At discharge, switch to long-term prophylaxis using Cipro 500 mg po daily or Bactrim DS one tablet daily.

2. Encephalopathy.

a. Lactulose: Synthetic disaccharide that is a mainstay of therapy and causes a purging of ammonia through the bowels. This has been shown to improve symptoms in 70% to 80% of patients. Typical dose is 30 to 45 mL orally, two to four times per day. Dose is titrated to achieve two to three bowel movements per day. If comatose, it may be given as an enema.

b. Xifaxan: Also known as rifaximin. A nonabsorbable antibiotic that reduces the risk of hepatic encephalopathy recurrence. This is usually added to lactulose therapy or for patients who are intolerant of lactulose side effects. Dose is usually 550 mg orally twice daily.

c. Benzodiazepines are contraindicated with cirrhotic patients who have encephalopathy.

3. GI bleeding.

a. Vasoactive medication: Initiated at the time of presentation to decrease portal blood flow, that is, octreotide. Usually given 2 to 5 days.

b. Proton pump inhibitor.

c. Prophylactic antibiotics: Broad spectrum antibiotics such as ceftriaxone 1 g IV daily for 7 days to prevent bacterial infections, which can occur in 20% of hospitalized cirrhotic patients (e.g., urinary tract infection [UTI], bacteremia, respiratory infections).

d. A nonselective beta blocker is often prescribed to reduce portal pressures for prevention of rebleeding after vasoactive medication has been discontinued. Titrate dose to a heart rate of 60 bpm. Propranolol or nadolol are commonly used.

4. HRS.

a. Combined therapy with the goal to improve renal and systemic hemodynamics.

b. Midodrine: Selective Alpha 1 adrenergic agonist; 7.5 to 15 mg orally three times a day.

c. Octreotide: Somatostatin analog; IV infusion: 50 mcg/hr or SQ 100 mcg three times a day.

d. Albumin: Volume expander; IV bolus: 1 g per kg of body weight per day.

D. Discharge instructions.

1. Ascites and SBP.

a. Low sodium diet.

b. Take diuretics as prescribed.

c. Lab testing as recommended.

d. Follow-up with hepatologist.

e. Call office or report to emergency department (ED) with abdominal pain, distension, shortness of breath, fever, or altered mental status.

2. Encephalopathy.

    a. Medication compliance is reinforced.

    b. Encourage two to three bowel movements daily for control of encephalopathy.

    c. Call the office or report to the ER with worsening confusion, fever, slurred speech, or lethargy.

    d. Follow-up with hepatologist.

3. GI bleeding.

    a. If esophageal band ligation was performed, will need a repeat esophagogastroduodenoscopy (EGD) every 4 weeks until eradicated.

    b. Medication compliance with beta blockers.

    c. Monitor CBC.

    d. Follow-up visit with hepatology.

4. HRS.

    a. Compliance with medical regimen of dialysis and medications.

    b. Close monitoring of electrolytes and renal function.

    c. Follow-up with hepatology.

Follow-Up

A. Follow-up with hepatology.

B. Patients will need hepatocellular carcinoma and esophageal varices screening.

    1. Imaging every 6 months: Alternating US and MRI of the abdomen.

    2. Variceal surveillance: EGD every 2 to 3 years.

C. Labs every 3 months: CBC, CMP, INR, alpha fetoprotein (AFP).

D. Will need vaccination for hepatitis A and B if not immune.

Consultation/Referral

A. MELD score of 10 or higher will be referred to a transplant center.

B. If alcohol-related cirrhosis, must complete a substance abuse program.

C. Social services may need to help with insurance coverage if transplant is indicated.

Special/Geriatric Considerations

A. Transplant eligibility varies between centers, but usually age greater than 70 is contraindicated.

B. Cirrhosis is considered a high risk for abdominal, cardiac, or orthopedic surgeries due to high portal pressures and coagulopathies. It is usually determined by the surgeon on a case-by-case basis.

Bibliography

Bajaj, J. S., & Sanyal, A. J. (2017, May 5). Methods to achieve hemostasis in patients with acute variceal hemorrhage. In A. C. Travis (Ed.), *UpToDate*. Retrieved from https://www.uptodate.com/contents/methods-to-achieve-hemostasis-in-patients-with-acute-variceal-hemorrhage

Centers for Disease Control and Prevention. (2016, October 6). Chronic liver disease and cirrhosis. Retrieved from https://www.cdc.gov/nchs/fastats/liver-disease.htm

Chaney, A. (2016). *Fast facts about GI and liver diseases for nurses: What APRNs need to know in a nutshell,* New York, NY: Springer Publishing Company.

Ferenci, P. (2019, February 5). Hepatic encephalopathy in adults: Treatment. In K. M. Robson (Ed.), *UpToDate*. Retrieved from https://www.uptodate.com/contents/hepatic-encephalopathy-in-adults-treatment.

Garcia-Tsao, G., Abraldes, J. G., Berzigotti, A., & Bosch, J. (2017). Portal hypertensive bleeding in cirrhosis: Risk stratification, diagnosis, and management: 2016 practice guidance by the American Association for the study of liver diseases. *Hepatology, 65*(1), 310–335. doi:10.1002/hep.28906

Goldberg, E., & Chopra, S. (2018, September 5). Cirrhosis in adults: Etiologies, clinical manifestations, and diagnosis. In K. M. Robson (Ed.), *UpToDate*. Retrieved from https://www.uptodate.com/contents/cirrhosis-in-adults-etiologies-clinical-manifestations-and-diagnosis

Goldberg, E., & Chopra, S. (2018, June 14). Cirrhosis in adults: Overview of complications, general management, and complications. In K. M. Robson (Ed.), *UpToDate*. Retrieved from https://www.uptodate.com/contents/cirrhosis-in-adults-overview-of-complications-general-management-and-prognosis

Runyon, B. A. (2018, September 21). Spontaneous bacterial peritonitis in adults: Treatment and prophylaxis. In K. M. Robson (Ed.), *UpToDate*. Retrieved from https://www.uptodate.com/contents/spontaneous-bacterial-peritonitis-in-adults-treatment-and-prophylaxis

Runyon, B. A. (2018, February 13). Hepatorenal syndrome. In J. P. Forman (Ed.), *UpToDate*. Retrieved from https://www.uptodate.com/contents/hepatorenal-syndrome

Sanyal, A. J. (2019, February 4). General principles of the management of variceal hemorrhage. In K. M. Robson (Ed.), *UpToDate*. Retrieved from https://www.uptodate.com/contents/general-principles-of-the-management-of-variceal-hemorrhage

Singleton, J. K., DiGregorio, R. D., Green-Hernandez, C., Holzemer, S. P., Faber, E. S., Ferrara, L. R., & Slyer, J. T. (2015). *Primary care: An interprofessional perspective* (2nd ed.). New York, NY: Springer Publishing Company.

Such, J., & Runyon, B. A. (2018, August 13). Ascites in adults with cirrhosis: Initial therapy. In K. M. Robson (Ed.), *UpToDate*. Retrieved from https://www.uptodate.com/contents/ascites-in-adults-with-cirrhosis-initial-therapy

Drug-Induced Liver Injury

Catherine Harris

Definition

A. Liver injury due to prescription medications, over-the-counter (OTC) medications, and herbal supplements.

Incidence

A. Estimated annual incidence is 10% of all cases of acute hepatitis; the most common cause of acute liver failure in the United States.

Pathogenesis

A. Over 1,000 medications and herbal products have been implicated in the development of drug-induced liver injury (DILI).

B. Most common drug in acute DILI in the United States is acetaminophen.

Predisposing Factors

A. Women—more susceptible due to smaller size.

B. Alcohol abuse.

C. Malnutrition.

Subjective Data

A. Common complaints/symptoms.

    1. Itching.

    2. Jaundice.

    3. Malaise.

    4. Low grade fever.

    5. Nausea and vomiting.

    6. Right upper quadrant (RUQ) pain.

    7. Dark urine.

    8. Clay-colored stools.

B. Common/typical scenario.

    1. Patients may be asymptomatic with incidental finding of elevated liver tests.

2. Ask patients about recent antibiotic use, herbal supplements, weight loss products, or OTC medications.
3. Thorough medication reconciliation.
C. Family and social history.
  1. Be culturally sensitive to nontraditional medicine and the patient's use of herbal products.
  2. Alcohol use.
D. Review of systems.
  1. Same as common complaints.
  2. Rash.
  3. Pruritus.
  4. Weight loss.

Physical Examination

A. Depending on the severity, no physical findings or the following:
B. Scleral icterus.
C. Generalized jaundice.
D. Skin excoriations from scratching.
E. RUQ tenderness.
F. Hepatomegaly.

Diagnostic Tests

A. Lab workup includes: Complete blood count (CBC), comprehensive metabolic panel (CMP), international normalized ratio (INR), hepatitis A, B, and C serologies, antinuclear antibody (ANA), antimitochondrial antibody (AMA), anti smooth muscle antibody (ASMA), liver kidney microsomal type 1 (LKM1), ceruloplasmin (Wilson's disease), iron, ferritin (hemochromatosis), Alpha 1 antitrypsin.
B. Hepatic function panel will show cholestatic, hepatocellular, or mixed pattern of injury.
C. Imaging: Ultrasound (US), MRI.
D. Liver biopsy: If labs and imaging are nondiagnostic, biopsy may be considered.

Differential Diagnosis

A. Acute viral hepatitis.
B. Alcoholic liver disease.
C. Nonalcoholic fatty liver disease.
D. Autoimmune hepatitis.
E. Wilson's disease.
F. Biliary obstruction: Primary biliary cholangitis (PBC) or primary sclerosing cholangitis (PSC).

Evaluation and Management Plan

A. General plan.
  1. Obtaining a careful drug history and ruling out other causes.
  2. Monitoring for improvement of symptoms and serologic markers after stopping the offending drug.
B. Patient/family teaching points.
  1. Regular liver tests at recommended interval to monitor for improvement.
  2. Avoid alcohol.
  3. Normalization of liver tests may take several months.
  4. Do not start any new medications or OTC supplements.
  5. Teach signs and symptoms associated with hepatic injury.
  6. Follow-up with gastrointestinal (GI)/hepatology.
C. Pharmacotherapy.
  1. Primary treatment is withdrawal of the offending drug.
  2. Recovery will occur in the majority of patients once the medication is stopped.

3. In acetaminophen toxicity, treatment is N-acetylcysteine.
D. Discharge instructions.
  1. Monitor labs.
  2. Follow-up with gastroenterologist or hepatologist.

Follow-Up

A. Gastroenterologist/hepatologist should be monitoring labs and seeing the patient on a regular basis.

Consultation/Referral

A. May refer for liver transplant if there is no recovery of liver function.

Special/Geriatric Considerations

A. Treatment of older patients with liver disease may require different or longer interventions.
B. Maintain pharmacokinetic precautions in geriatric patients.

Bibliography

Goldberg, E., & Chopra, S. (2018, June 14). Cirrhosis in adults: Overview of complications, general management, and complications. In K. M. Robson (Ed.), *UpToDate*. Retrieved from https://www.uptodate.com/contents/cirrhosis-in-adults-overview-of-complicationsgeneral-management-and-prognosis
Larson, A. M. (2017, July 10). Drug-induced liver injury. Retrieved from https://www.uptodate.com/contents/drug-induced-liver-injury

Gastroesophageal Reflux Disease

Catherine Harris

Definition

A. Gastric reflux that irritates and erodes the lining of the esophagus.

Incidence

A. 60% of adult population experience gastroesophageal reflux disease (GERD) of some type.
B. Affects up to 10 million adults in the United States on a daily basis.
C. Many people experience heartburn two to three times per week.

Pathogenesis

A. The esophagus contracts to propel food into the stomach via peristalsis.
B. A circular ring of muscle called the lower esophageal sphincter (LES) relaxes to allow food to enter the stomach, then contracts to avoid regurgitation of food or acid into the esophagus.
C. When the LES is weak due to stomach distention, acid can wash up into the esophagus.
D. Most episodes of heartburn occur shortly after meals.
E. Functional or mechanical problem of LES is the most common cause of GERD.
F. Transient relaxation of LES can be caused by food (coffee, alcohol, chocolate, meals heavy in fat), medications (beta agonists, nitrates, calcium channel blockers, anticholinergics), hormones, and nicotine.

Predisposing Factors

A. Obesity.
B. Smoking.
C. Pregnancy.

D. Certain medications.
E. Peptic ulcers.
F. Hiatal hernia.
G. Diabetes (due to associated gastroparesis).
H. Asthma (chronic, continuous coughing may contribute).
I. Connective tissue disorders.
J. Zollinger–Ellison syndrome.

Subjective Data

A. Common complaints/symptoms.
1. Heartburn or burning sensation after eating.
2. Nausea or vomiting.
3. Difficulty or pain when swallowing.
4. Regurgitation.
5. Hoarseness from irritation of the vocal cords.
6. Difficulty breathing.
B. Common/typical scenario.
1. Most patients will complain of burning sensation or discomfort that occurs after eating or when lying supine or bending over.
C. Family and social history.
1. Smoking.
2. Lifestyle.
3. Diet.
D. Review of systems.
1. Head, ear, eyes, nose, and throat (HEENT): Laryngitis, dysphagia, hoarseness, teeth decay, ear infections.
2. Respiratory: Chronic cough, new or worsening asthma.
3. Cardiac: Burning sensations behind breastbone.

Physical Examination

A. HEENT: Evaluate throat for redness or irritation, look for enamel decay of the teeth, evaluate ears for possible infections if warranted.
B. Respiratory: Listen for wheezing or decreased lung sounds.
C. Cardiac: Evaluate for palpitations, murmurs, or a rapidor slow heart rate.

Diagnostic Tests

A. Diagnosis of GERD can be made upon symptoms and response to treatment alone.
B. If a patient presents with chest pain or the diagnosis of GERD is not clear, then one or more of the following tests may be ordered.
1. Endoscopy: Evaluate for damage to the lining of the esophagus, stomach, and small intestine.
2. 24-hour esophageal pH study: Measure frequency of acid reflux.
3. Esophageal manometry: Evaluate functioning of LES.

Differential Diagnosis

A. Gastritis.
B. Esophagitis.
C. Irritable bowel syndrome.
D. Peptic ulcer disease.
E. Hiatal hernia.
F. Gallstones.
G. Coronary atherosclerosis.

Evaluation and Management Plan

A. General plan.
1. Stepwise approach.
   a. Control symptoms.
   b. Heal esophagitis.
   c. Prevent recurrence and complications of GERD.
2. Start with lifestyle modification and control of gastric acid secretion with medical therapy.
   a. Weight loss.
   b. Eat small, frequent meals.
   c. Avoid foods that trigger reflux such as alcohol, chocolate, tomato-based products, caffeine.
   d. Avoid lying down for 3 hours after a meal.
   e. Avoid bending or stooping for 3 hours after a meal.
3. Surgery may be indicated in the following cases.
   a. Symptoms not controlled with proton pump inhibitor (PPI) therapy.
   b. Presence of Barrett esophagus.
   c. Extraesophageal symptoms.
   d. Young patients.
   e. Poor compliance.
   f. Patients with cardiac conduction defects.
B. Patient/family teaching points.
1. Stop smoking.
2. Reduce or eliminate alcohol intake.
3. Weight loss will improve symptoms.
4. Avoid tight fitting clothing.
5. Chew gum or use oral lozenges to increase saliva production.
6. If your symptoms are not controlled or last a long time, report this to your provider.
7. Chest pain can also be cardiac in nature; if the pain radiates to the jaw, left shoulder, or arm, be sure to seek medical attention immediately.
C. Pharmacotherapy.
1. Antacids can be taken after each meal and before bedtime.
2. H2 Receptor antagonists: First-line agent for mild to moderate symptoms.
3. Proton pump inhibitors.
   a. Most powerful medications.
   b. Most commonly reported adverse reactions.
      i. Sore throat.
      ii. Flatulence.
      iii. Constipation.
   c. Superior to H2 receptor antagonists.
4. Prokinetics.
   a. Improve motility of esophagus.
   b. Somewhat effective in patients only with mild symptoms.
   c. May have long-term serious or potentially fatal complications.
D. Discharge instructions.
1. Follow patient teaching points upon discharge for best results.
2. Lifestyle changes and medical therapy should resolve GERD symptoms within 4 weeks and esophagitis in 8 weeks.
3. Complications of untreated GERD include:
   a. Ulcers that can cause bleeding.
   b. Strictures of esophagus.
   c. Lung and throat problems.
   d. Barrett's esophagus.
   e. Esophageal cancer.

Follow-Up

A. As per your provider or if symptoms are not controlled.

Consultation/Referral

A. If symptoms are not controlled with one PPI.
B. If symptoms do not confirm diagnosis or another problem is potentially causing symptoms.

Special/Geriatric Considerations

A. GERD can occur in pregnancy because of normal weight gain and hormone changes that allow muscles in the esophagus to relax more easily and frequently.

B. As the uterus expands, particularly in the third trimester, pressure builds up in the stomach, which may cause food and acid to regurgitate into the esophagus.

    1. Antacids are first-line agents in pregnancy but may not be sufficient.

    2. Histamine blockers and proton pump inhibitors are also approved for treatment of GERD during pregnancy.

Bibliography

El-Serag, H. B. (2007). Time trends of gastroesophageal reflux disease: A systematic review. *Clinical Gastroenterology and Hepatology, 5*(1), 17–26. doi:10.1016/j.cgh.2006.09.016

Giannini, E. G., Zentilin, P., Dulbecco, P., Vigneri, S., Scarlata, P., & Savarino, V. (2008). Management strategy for patients with gastroesophageal reflux disease: A comparison between empirical treatment with esomeprazole and endoscopy-oriented treatment. *American Journal of Gastroenterology, 103*(2), 267–275. Retrieved from https://journals.lww.com/ajg/Abstract/2008/02000/Management_Strategy_for_Patients_With.4.aspx

Grant, A. M., Cotton, S. C., Boachie, C., Ramsay, C. R., Krukowski, Z. H., Heading, R. C., & Campbell, M. K. (2013). Minimal access surgery compared with medical management for gastro-oesophageal reflux disease: Five year follow-up of a randomised controlled trial (REFLUX). *BMJ, 346*, f1908. doi:10.1136/bmj.f1908

Hampel, H., Abraham, N. S., & El-Serag, H. B. (2005). Meta-analysis: Obesity and the risk for gastroesophageal reflux disease and its complications. *Annals of Internal Medicine, 143*(3), 199–211. doi:10.7326/0003-4819-143-3-200508020-00006

Oor, J. E., Roks, D. J., Ünlü, C., & Hazebroek, E. J. (2016). Laparoscopic sleeve gastrectomy and gastroesophageal reflux disease: A systematic review and meta-analysis. *American Journal of Surgery, 211*(1), 250–267. doi:10.1016/j.amjsurg.2015.05.031

Gastrointestinal Bleeding

Catherine Harris

Definition

A. Gastrointestinal bleeding (GIB) is a symptom of a disease process or condition in the gastrointestinal (GI) tract.

B. Bleeding that occurs in any part of the GI tract.

C. Upper GI tract includes esophagus and stomach.

D. Lower GI tract includes structures distal to the ligament of Treitz including small and large intestines, rectum, and anus.

Incidence

A. Upper gastrointestinal bleeding (UGIB).

    1. Most common with approximately 100 cases per 100,000 population.

    2. Mortality rates 6% to 10%.

    3. Associated with comorbid illness.

        a. Peptic ulcer disease is most common cause of UGIB in up to 40% of cases.

        b. Mallory–Weiss tears account for 15% of UGIB cases.

        c. Caused by forceful vomiting, retching, coughing, or straining.

        d. Gastritis.

        e. Caused by acute stress, acute renal failure, and sepsis.

B. Lower gastrointestinal bleeding (LGIB).

    1. Annual incidence 20 to 27 cases per 100,000 population.

    2. May be significantly underreported.

    3. Four main types of LGIB.

        a. Anatomic (diverticulosis, hemorrhoids)—most common type, accounting for approximately 60% of cases.

        b. Vascular (ischemia, radiation-induced).

        c. Neoplasms account for approximately 12.7% of cases.

        d. Inflammatory (infectious versus noninfectious such as Crohn's disease).

    4. Segmented into significance of bleeding.

        a. Occult bleeding.

        b. Moderate bleeding.

        c. Massive bleeding.

Pathogenesis

A. UGIB.

    1. Variceal hemorrhage—increases in blood pressure in portal vein system, usually from cirrhosis, can create enlarged veins (varices) which are prone to bleeding.

    2. Nonvariceal hemorrhage—process occurs from either arterial hemorrhage, typically from ulcers, deep mucosal tears, or from low pressure venous hemorrhage from telangiectasias or arteriovenous malformations.

B. LGIB.

    1. The most common cause of LGIB is diverticulosis. Bleeding can occur in the absence of diverticulitis. Bleeding occurs when segmental weakness of the lumen of the bowel predisposes the artery to rupture. Bleeding can be massive and life-threatening.

    2. Other forms of LGIB occur from ulceration or erosion of the mucosa, inflammatory changes that predispose the GI tract to mucosal friability, fissures, and fistulas that develop from infectious processes, radiation exposure, and vascular malformations.

Predisposing Factors

A. Occurs more frequently in men.

B. Older age.

C. Nonsteroidal anti-inflammatory drug (NSAID) use.

D. Admission to ICU for sepsis, trauma, or ventilatory support.

Subjective Data

A. Common complaints/symptoms.

    1. UGIB: Presence of bleeding from vomiting, black tarry stools, dyspepsia.

    2. LGIB: Presence of bright red blood in stool, may present with or without abdominal pain.

B. Common/typical scenario.

    1. UGIB: Patients typically complain of presence of vomiting blood or passing black malodorous stool. They may present with weakness, dizziness, and possibly syncope.

    2. LGIB: Depends on the amount of bleeding.

        a. Minor bleeding—may complain of some rectal bleeding, diarrhea, and abdominal pain.

        b. Moderate and massive bleeding—may present with signs and symptoms of shock including dehydration, hypotension, tachycardia, and fever.

C. Family and social history.

    1. Ask about family history of colon cancer.

    2. Smoking or alcohol use.

    3. NSAID use.

D. Review of systems.

    1. Constitutional: Dizziness or episodes of lightheadedness, may appear exhausted.

    2. GI: Ask about color and consistency of stools, any pain during defecation, any associated nausea or vomiting, red streaking on toilet paper, abdominal pain severity and location, presence of heartburn, or unintentional weight loss.

Physical Examination

A. Head, ear, eyes, nose, and throat (HEENT): Assess oropharynx and nasopharynx for sources of bleeding.

B. GI: May have benign abdominal examination; check for hematemesis and melena, or rectal exam for bleeding.

C. Cardiovascular: Hemodynamic instability in massive hemorrhage; assess for signs and symptoms of shock, or orthostatic hypotension.

Diagnostic Tests

A. Lab studies.

    1. Complete blood count (CBC), basic metabolic panel (BMP), coagulation studies.

    2. In suspected UGIB, check calcium level for increased levels, which can be associated with excessive acid secretion.

    3. Test for *Helicobacter pylori* in UGIB.

B. Imaging studies.

    1. UGIB.

        a. Endoscopy to find source of bleeding.

        b. Chest radiography to exclude other causes of symptoms.

        c. CT may be used to find unusual causes of bleeding.

        d. Ultrasound can be useful to evaluate liver disease that may be associated with bleeding.

        e. Angiography offered when bleeding persists and a clear source has not been found or if an arterial UGIB does not respond to endoscopic management.

    2. LGIB.

        a. Colonoscopy: Initial approach starts with colonoscopy unless the patient is unstable and offers ability to treat during diagnostic stage.

        b. Esophagogastroduodenoscopy (EGD): Can rule out UGIB.

        c. CT: Useful when endoscopy is limited.

        d. Computed tomography angiography (CTA): Has high positive predictive value for LGIB and often used as a first-line diagnostic study.

        e. Angiography: Useful in active bleeding where colonoscopy cannot be done or fails to identify a source. Also can be used emergently in massive ongoing LGIB.

Differential Diagnosis

A. Determine location in UGIB.

    1. Esophagus.

        a. Barrett esophagus.

        b. Esophageal cancer.

        c. Esophageal varices.

        d. Esophagitis.

    2. Stomach.

        a. Gastric cancer.

        b. Gastric outlet obstruction.

        c. Gastric ulcers.

        d. Peptic ulcer disease.

B. Consider process in LGIB.

    1. Anatomic: Diverticulosis.

    2. Vascular.

        a. Arteriovenous malformations.

        b. Angiodysplasia.

        c. Vasculitides.

    3. Neoplasm.

        a. Colon cancer.

        b. Polyps.

    4. Inflammation.

        a. Inflammatory bowel disease.

        b. Colitis.

        c. Radiation induced.

        d. Ulceration.

        e. Abscess.

        f. Fistulas.

        g. Fissures.

Evaluation and Management Plan

A. General plan.

    1. UGIB.

        a. Stabilize and fluid resuscitate patient by correcting states of shock and bleeding abnormalities.

        b. Insert nasogastric tube for lavage to determine if GIB is upper or lower. LGIB will result in bile aspirate but no bleeding.

        c. Risk assessment using predictive models.

            i. Rockall score.

            ii. Blatchford score.

            iii. AIMS65.

        d. Perform EGD to identify and treat source of bleeding.

            i. Contraindicated in uncooperative or unstable patients.

            ii. Consider surgical intervention if:

                1) Two attempts at endoscopic control are unsuccessful.

                2) Failure of medical therapy or persistent bleeding.

                3) Bleeding from perforation, obstruction, or malignancy.

                4) Prolonged bleeding.

        e. Start proton pump inhibitors.

        f. Assess for complications of treatment with EGD.

            i. EGD can cause:

                1) Aspiration pneumonia.

                2) Perforation.

                3) Arrhythmias.

            ii. Surgery.

                1) Poor wound healing.

                2) Rebleeding.

                3) Ileus.

                4) Sepsis.

    2. LGIB.

        a. Stabilize and resuscitate patients with active bleeding and signs of hemodynamic instability.

        b. Insert nasogastric tube to rule out UGIB source.

        c. Risk assessment.

        d. Localize bleeding site.

            i. If stable colonoscopy should be performed for diagnosis and treatment.

            ii. Endoscopic hemostasis therapy can control active bleeding.

            iii. Angiography for embolization of source and to temporize bleeding with vasopressin infusion if needed.

            iv. Emergent surgery may be required if:

                1) Medical and endoscopic therapy is unsuccessful.

2) Persistent hemodynamic instability with active bleeding.

3) Persistent, recurrent bleeding.

4) Transfusion of more than four units of packed red blood cells in a 24-hour period with active or recurrent bleeding.

    e. Supportive measures.

      i. Fluid resuscitation.

      ii. Blood transfusions for hemoglobin less than 7 g/dL.

      iii. Management of coagulopathies or antiplatelet agents: Consider transfusing with fresh frozen plasma and platelets if prolonged prothrombin time with international normalized ratio greater than 1.5 or low platelet count less than 50,000/L.

    f. Assess for complications of treatment of LGIB.

      i. Reactions to multiple blood transfusion.

      ii. Bleeding from surgery.

      iii. Sepsis.

      iv. Poor wound healing from surgery.

      v. Anastomotic strictures, incisional hernias after surgery.

B. Patient/family teaching points.

  1. UGIB.

    a. Lower the risk of UGIB by avoiding NSAIDs as much as possible.

    b. Anticoagulants and antiplatelet agents must be ordered in consultation with GI provider. The risk and benefits must be weighed in deciding which medications are necessary.

    c. Advise patient to take medications as prescribed for the entire duration.

    d. Follow-up with the necessary tests as determined by provider.

    e. If *H. pylori* positive, will need eradication therapy and confirmation of eradication in 4 to 6 weeks with a stool sample.

    f. Long-term acid suppression therapy is needed.

  2. LGIB.

    a. If symptoms recur may need further workup. LGIB can be difficult to isolate in some cases.

    b. Avoid NSAIDs and aspirin use.

    c. Diet and lifestyle may prevent progression of certain causes of LGIB.

C. Pharmacotherapy.

  1. UGIB.

    a. Proton pump inhibitors (PPIs): Reduce acid secretion.

      i. Inpatient start intravenous (IV) high dose therapy.

        1) Bolus followed by twice daily injections.

        2) Continuous infusions of PPIs have failed to show a difference in clinically relevant endpoints.

    b. Prokinetics to promote gastric emptying; especially useful to improve gastric visualization prior to endoscopy.

      i. Erythromycin.

      ii. Metoclopramide.

    c. Vasoactive medications treat variceal bleeding, may be used as adjunctive therapy in select cases of nonvariceal UGIB.

      i. Octreotide: IV bolus followed by a continuous infusion.

    d. Prophylactic antibiotics are used in patients with cirrhosis due to the high rate of bacterial infections associated with hospitalized events of UGIB.

  2. LGIB.

    a. There are no medications specifically to treat LGIB. Medications used are supportive and depend heavily on identifying and treating the source of bleeding.

D. Discharge instructions.

  1. UGIB.

    a. Depending on the cause of UGIB, certain medications will be prescribed.

    b. Follow-up with gastroenterologist within 2 weeks.

    c. Endoscopy typically repeated with ulcers to document healing.

    d. If symptoms recur, patient should call the office immediately.

    e. Diet and lifestyle changes.

  2. LGIB.

    a. Will need to follow-up within 2 weeks.

    b. Start psyllium seed.

    c. Encourage fluids.

    d. Diet and lifestyle changes.

    e. May need repeat colonoscopy if recurrence of symptoms.

Follow-Up

A. Follow-up with gastroenterologist within 2 weeks of leaving the hospital.

Consultation/Referral

A. GIB is a sign of an underlying condition. Refer to gastroenterologist for full workup.

B. General surgery should be consulted as needed and emergently if there is massive bleeding.

C. Patients who are hemodynamically unstable will require monitoring in the ICU.

Special/Geriatric Considerations

A. Older patients may present with minimal symptoms typically in LGIB.

Bibliography

Cirocchi, R., Grassi, V., Cavaliere, D., Renzi, C., Tabola, R., Poli, G., . . . Fingerhut, A. (2015, November). New trends in acute management of colonic diverticular bleeding: A systematic review. *Medicine, 94*(44), e1710. doi:10.1097/MD.0000000000001710

Fujishiro, M., Iguchi, M., Kakushima, N., Kato, M., Sakata, Y., Hoteya, S., . . . Fujimoto, K. (2016, February 22). Guidelines for endoscopic management of non-variceal upper gastrointestinal bleeding. *Digestive Endoscopy, 28*(4), 363–378. doi:10.1111/den.12639

Jairath, V., & Desborough, M. J. (2015, December 28). Modern-day management of upper gastrointestinal haemorrhage. *Transfusion Medicine, 25*(6), 351–357. doi:10.1111/tme.12266

Monteiro, S., Gonçalves, T. C., Magalhães, J., & Cotter, J. (2016, February 15). Upper gastrointestinal bleeding risk scores: Who, when and why? *World Journal of Gastrointestinal Pathophysiology, 7*(1), 86–96. doi:10.4291/wjgp.v7.i1.86

Qayed, E., Dagar, G., & Nanchal, R. S. (2016, April). Lower gastrointestinal hemorrhage. *Critical Care Clinics, 32*(2), 241–254. doi:10.1016/j.ccc.2015.12.004

Strate, L. L., & Gralnek, I. M. (2016, April). ACG clinical guideline: Management of patients with acute lower gastrointestinal bleeding. *American Journal of Gastroenterology, 111*(4), 459–474. Retrieved from https://journals.lww.com/ajg/Abstract/2016/04000/ACG_Clinical_Guideline__Management_of_Patients.14.aspx

Villanueva, C., Colomo, A., Bosch, A., Concepción, M., Hernandez-Gea, V., Aracil, C., . . . Guarner, C. (2013, January 3). Transfusion strategies for acute upper gastrointestinal bleeding. *The New England Journal of Medicine, 368*(1), 11–21. doi:10.1056/NEJMoa1211801

Wilkins, T., Embry, K., & George, R. (2013, May 1). Diagnosis and management of acute diverticulitis. *American Family Physician, 87*(9), 612–620. Retrieved from https://www.aafp.org/afp/2013/0501/p612.html

Hepatitis-Alcoholic

Robin Miller and Ann E. Burke

Definition

A. Syndrome of progressive inflammatory liver injury associated with long-term heavy intake of alcohol.

B. Alcohol abuse is the most common cause of serious liver disease in Western society.

Incidence

A. In the United States, alcoholic liver disease affects more than 2 million people.

B. The true prevalence of alcoholic hepatitis is unknown as the patient may be asymptomatic or never seek medical attention.

Pathogenesis

A. Although the pathogenesis is not known, genetic, environmental, nutritional, metabolic, and immunologic factors may play a role.

Predisposing Factors

A. Majority of patients have a history of heavy alcohol use for two or more decades. Heavy is defined as greater than 100 g per day.

B. Women are more susceptible than men.

C. Peak age is 40 to 50 years old.

D. Alcoholic liver disease is more common in minority groups, particularly among Native Americans.

Subjective Data

A. Common complaints/symptoms.

  1. Anorexia.

  2. Fever.

  3. Right upper quadrant (RUQ) pain.

  4. Abdominal distension.

  5. Dark urine.

  6. Clay-colored stools.

B. Common/typical scenario.

  1. History of daily alcohol use.

  2. Stressful life events may trigger an increase in intake.

  3. It is common for patients to cease alcohol intake several weeks prior to presentation due to feeling more ill.

C. Family and social history.

  1. It is essential that the healthcare provider take a careful alcohol history.

  2. May need to elicit a more accurate history by including family members.

  3. Drinking patterns may vary. Heavy drinking can be intermittent (e.g., weekends only) or hidden from family members.

  4. A standard drink is defined as 14 g of alcohol. Examples include:

  a. 12 ounces of beer.

  b. 5 ounces of wine.

  c. 1.5 ounces of distilled spirits.

  d. 8 to 9 ounces of malt liquor.

D. Review of systems.

  1. Cognitive changes (encephalopathy).

  2. Jaundice.

  3. Anorexia.

  4. Fever.

  5. RUQ/epigastric pain.

  6. Abdominal distension.

Physical Examination

A. Temporal wasting.

B. Scleral icterus.

C. Generalized jaundice.

D. Hepatomegaly.

E. Ascites.

F. Spider angiomata, palmar erythema, and gynecomastia suggest advanced disease.

G. Lower extremity edema.

Diagnostic Tests

A. Lab tests.

  1. Hepatic function panel: Aspartate aminotransferase (AST)/alanine aminotransferase (ALT) ratio is 2:1.

  2. Complete blood count (CBC): Elevated white blood cell (WBC).

  3. International normalized ratio (INR): Elevated.

  4. Testing for hepatitis A, B, and C; autoimmune markers (antinuclear antibody [ANA], AMA, ASMA, LKM1).

B. Imaging.

  1. Abdominal ultrasound with Dopplers to rule out biliary obstruction, Budd–Chiari malformation, or cirrhosis.

C. Liver biopsy.

D. If labs and imaging are nondiagnostic, biopsy may be considered.

Differential Diagnosis

A. Acute viral hepatitis.

B. Autoimmune hepatitis.

C. Drug-induced liver injury (DILI).

D. Shock liver.

E. Ischemic hepatitis.

F. Budd–Chiari.

G. Wilson's disease.

H. Alpha 1 antitrypsin deficiency.

I. Toxin-induced hepatitis (e.g., mushroom poisoning).

Evaluation and Management Plan

A. General plan.

  1. Admission to ICU in patients that are unstable, that is, encephalopathic.

  2. Fluid management and nutritional support.

  3. Acuity of illness based on Maddrey Discriminant Function (DF) score and need for glucocorticoid therapy. DF is a calculation using bilirubin and prothrombin time (PT).

  4. Alcohol withdrawal protocol per institutional guidelines.

  5. Infectious workup to rule out other causes of mental status change.

  6. Prophylaxis against gastrointestinal (GI) bleeding.

B. Patient/family teaching points.

  1. Referral for substance abuse counseling.

  2. Length of sobriety to meet transplant candidacy requirement per institution policy.

  3. Steroid tapering schedule.

C. Pharmacotherapy.

  1. GI prophylaxis: Proton pump inhibitors (PPI) or H2 blocker.

  2. Stop nonselective beta blocker during acute crisis due to risk of acute kidney injury (AKI). May resume later.

3. Nutritional support: Adequate calories and protein; vitamins thiamine, folate.
4. Glucocorticoids.
  a. Severe cases with DF greater than 32 receive prednisone/prednisolone for 28 days.
  b. Discontinue if no improvement after 7 days. This is based on the Lille score, a predictor of response to steroid treatment.
5. Lactulose or trial of xifaxan therapy for encephalopathy.
D. Discharge instructions.
  1. Review tapering schedule of steroids if applicable.
  2. Set up outpatient substance abuse counseling or inpatient rehab.
  3. Repeat lab tests in 1 week.
  4. Close follow-up with hepatologist.

Follow-Up

A. As per discharge instructions, close follow-up with hepatologist and transplant center, if appropriate.

Consultation/Referral

A. Psychiatry: Addiction specialist.
B. Transplant center.

Special/Geriatric Considerations

A. Hemolysis, elevated liver enzymes, low platelet count in the setting of pregnancy (HELLP).

Bibliography

Friedman, S. L. (2018, August 13). Alcoholic hepatitis: Clinical manifestations and diagnosis. In K. M. Robson (Ed.), *UpToDate*. Retrieved from https://www.uptodate.com/contents/alcoholic-hepatitis-clinical-manifestations-and-diagnosis

Friedman, S. L. (2018, August 28). Management and prognosis of alcoholic hepatitis. In K. M. Robson (Ed.), *UpToDate*. Retrieved from https://www.uptodate.com/contents/management-and-prognosis-of-alcoholic-hepatitis

Heuman, D. M. (2016). Alcoholic hepatitis: Overview. In B. S. Anand (Ed.), *Medscape*. Retrieved from https://emedicine.medscape.com/article/170539-overview

National Institute on Alcohol Abuse and Alcoholism. (n.d.). What is a standard drink? Retrieved from https://www.niaaa.nih.gov/alcohol-health/overview-alcohol-consumption/what-standard-drink

Hepatitis-Autoimmune

Robin Miller and Ann E. Burke

Definition

A. Chronic: Clinical or biochemical evidence of liver disease greater than 6 months duration.
B. Chronic inflammatory condition of the liver characterized by transaminase elevation in the presence of autoantibodies.

Incidence

A. The exact prevalence in the United States is unknown but is estimated to be 1.1 per 100,000 persons per year.
B. Female predominance but occurs in both genders and all age groups.

Pathogenesis

A. Thought to result from an environmental trigger in a genetically predisposed individual.

Predisposing Factors

A. Strong genetic association with other autoimmune diseases from 26% to 49%.

Subjective Data

A. Common complaints/symptoms.
  1. Presentation can vary from asymptomatic (up to 25%) to fulminant hepatic failure (rare).
  2. May see anorexia, arthralgia, rash, or fatigue.
B. Common/typical scenario.
  1. Insidious onset with constitutional symptoms as listed earlier.
  2. Asymptomatic patients will be diagnosed incidentally with laboratory testing.
C. Family and social history.
  1. Not applicable.
D. Review of systems.
  1. Flu-like symptoms.
    a. Nausea.
    b. Anorexia.
    c. Fatigue.
    d. Lethargy.
    e. Malaise.
    f. Abdominal pain.
    g. Itching.
    h. Arthralgia.

Physical Examination

A. Ranges from a normal physical examination to evidence of advanced disease, including:
  1. Hepatomegaly.
  2. Splenomegaly.
  3. Jaundice.
  4. Temporal wasting.
  5. Spider angiomata.

Diagnostic Tests

A. Lab workup includes: Complete blood count (CBC), comprehensive metabolic panel (CMP), international normalized ratio (INR), hepatitis B and C serologies, antinuclear antibody (ANA), AMA, ASMA, LKM1, quantitative immunoglobulins, ceruloplasmin (Wilson's disease), iron, ferritin (hemochromatosis), Alpha 1 antitrypsin.
B. Lab abnormalities include: Elevated aspartate aminotransferase (AST)/alanine aminotransferase (ALT) 5 to 10X upper limit, elevated immunoglobin G (IMG), positive ANA, ASMA, or LKM1.
C. Imaging: Abdominal ultrasound (US), MRI/magnetic resonance cholangiopancreatography (MRCP) to rule out other biliary disorders.
D. Liver biopsy: Gold standard to confirm diagnosis and severity of disease.

Differential Diagnosis

A. Hepatitis A, B, and C.
B. Primary biliary cholangitis (PBC).
C. Primary sclerosing cholangitis (PSC).
D. Wilson's disease.
E. Hemochromatosis.
F. Alpha 1 antitrypsin deficiency.
G. Fatty liver disease.
H. Drug-induced liver injury.
I. Alcohol use.

Evaluation and Management Plan

A. General plan.

1. Decision to treat a patient is based on the severity of symptoms, magnitude of AST/ALT elevations, histologic findings, and the potential for side effects.

2. Supportive care.

3. Monitor liver function tests.

4. Glucocorticoid mono therapy or in combination with azathioprine.

B. Patient/family teaching points.

1. Avoid alcohol or over-the-counter (OTC) supplements.

2. Discuss side effect management of steroid therapy.

3. Discuss importance of steroid tapering schedule; do not stop abruptly.

C. Pharmacotherapy.

1. Glucocorticoids: Goal of therapy is to achieve quick remission and taper off steroids to minimize potential side effects.

    a. Moderate–severe activity: Prednisolone IV or oral prednisone starting at 60 mg daily.

    b. Mild activity: Lower dose of prednisone starting at 20 mg daily.

2. Nonsteroidal immunosuppressant: Imuran or 6 Mercaptopurine (6MP) in combination with steroids that are continued long term after steroid taper. This may also be appropriate for populations that are steroid sensitive. Thiopurine methyltransferase (TPMT) should be obtained prior to starting Imuran or 6MP. It measures the enzyme that breaks down azathioprine and helps guide dosing and risk for potential side effects.

D. Discharge instructions.

1. Teaching points as listed earlier.

2. Avoid alcohol or OTC supplements.

3. Discuss side effect management of steroid therapy.

4. Discuss importance of steroid tapering schedule; do not stop abruptly.

5. Weekly CBC, glucose, and liver tests.

6. Follow-up with gastroenterology or hepatologist.

Follow-Up

A. Get baseline bone density scan.

B. Follow-up with pneumocystis pneumonia (PCP) for lab monitoring.

C. Follow-up with gastroenterologist or hepatologist within 1 month.

Consultation/Referral

A. Refer to transplant center; 10%– to 20% of patients with autoimmune hepatitis will require a liver transplant for acute liver failure, decompensated cirrhosis, and hepatocellular carcinoma.

Special/Geriatric Considerations

A. Patients at increased risk for glucocorticoid side effects.

1. Prediabetes, diabetes.

2. Osteoporosis.

3. Emotional liability.

4. Sleep disturbance.

Bibliography

Fialho, A., Fialho, A., & Carey, W. (2015, July). Autoimmune hepatitis. Retrieved from http://www.clevelandclinicmeded.com/medicalpubs/diseasemanagement/hepatology/chronic-autoimmune-hepatitis

Heneghan, M. A. (2018, November 14). Autoimmune hepatitis: Treatment. In K. M. Robson (Ed.), *UpToDate*. Retrieved from https://www.uptodate.com/contents/autoimmune-hepatitis-treatment

Hepatitis A

Robin Miller and Ann E. Burke

Definition

A. General: Inflammation of the liver.

B. Acute: Clinical or biochemical evidence of liver disease less than 6 months.

C. Vaccine preventable, communicable disease of the liver caused by the hepatitis A virus.

D. Self-limited disease that does not result in chronic infection.

Incidence

A. Most common form of acute viral hepatitis in the world.

B. In the United States, the estimated number of new infections in 2015 was 2,800 people.

Pathogenesis

A. Transmitted person-to-person by the fecal–oral route or consumption of contaminated food or water.

Predisposing Factors

A. International travel to developing countries.

B. Day-care employees and children.

C. Poor hygiene practices at restaurants/cafeterias.

D. Living with an infected person.

E. Men who have sex with men.

Subjective Data

A. Common complaints/symptoms.

1. Fatigue.

2. Fever.

3. Malaise.

4. Headache.

5. Nausea.

6. Right upper quadrant pain.

7. Loss of appetite.

8. Itching.

9. Myalgia.

B. Common/typical scenario.

1. Onset of symptoms.

2. Vaccination history.

3. Recent travel.

4. Food history.

C. Family and social history.

1. Living situation.

2. Sexual practices/preferences.

D. Review of systems.

1. Dark urine.

2. Light-colored stool.

3. Jaundice.

Physical Examination

A. Jaundice.

B. Scleral icterus.

C. Fever up to 104°F.

D. Right upper quadrant (RUQ) tenderness.

E. Hepatomegaly.

Diagnostic Tests

A. Workup includes: Complete blood count (CBC), comprehensive metabolic panel (CMP), international normalized ratio (INR), hepatitis A IgM and IgG antibodies, hepatitis B serologies (Hep B surface antibody, Hep B surface antigen, Hep B core antibody), hepatitis C antibody screen, hepatitis E antibody.

B. Lab abnormalities include: Elevations of aspartate aminotransferase (AST)/alanine aminotransferase (ALT) often greater than 1,000 IU-L, followed by elevations of bilirubin up to 10 mg/dL.

C. Ultrasound of the abdomen.

Differential Diagnosis

A. Hepatitis E.
B. Alcoholic hepatitis.
C. Autoimmune hepatitis.
D. Acute drug-induced liver injury (DILI)
E. Acute HIV infection.
F. Cytomegalovirus (CMV) infection.
G. Epstein–Barr virus (EBV).
H. Herpes simplex virus (HSV).

Evaluation and Management Plan

A. General plan.
   1. Supportive care.
      a. Intravenous (IV) fluids.
      b. Antiemetic medications.
B. Patient/family teaching points.
   1. Vaccination of close contacts.
   2. Safe sex practices.
   3. Good hand hygiene.
C. Pharmacotherapy.
   1. Acetaminophen may be cautiously administered but limited to 2 g per day.
   2. Administration of immunoglobulin within 14 days of exposure to achieve passive immunization and reduce severity of illness.
D. Discharge instructions.
   1. Rest.
   2. Return to work should be delayed for 10 days after the onset of jaundice.
   3. Follow-up with primary care physician.

Follow-Up

A. Primary care doctor visit: Repeat liver tests.
B. Vaccination for hepatitis B, if not immune.
C. Most people have a full recovery; infection confers life-long immunity (positive hepatitis A antibody).
D. Up to 10% of patients experience a relapse of symptoms during the 6 months following acute illness.

Consultation/Referral

A. Hepatologist for chronic elevated liver tests post infection.

Special/Geriatric Considerations

A. Liver transplant should be considered in fulminant disease.
B. This occurs in less than 1% of patients and is most common in individuals over 50, or with any other chronic liver disease.

Bibliography

Centers for Disease Control and Prevention. (n.d.). Hepatitis A questions and answers for health professionals. Retrieved from https://www.cdc.gov/hepatitis/hav/havfaq.htm

Gilroy, R. K. (2017, October 16). Hepatitis A. In B. S. Anand (Ed.), *Medscape*. Retrieved from https://emedicine.medscape.com/article/177484-overview

Lai, M., & Chopra, S. (2018, December 17). Hepatitis A virus infection in adults: Epidemiology, clinical manifestations, and diagnosis. In E. L. Baron (Ed.), *UpToDate*. Retrieved from https://www.uptodate.com/contents/hepatitis-a-virus-infection-in-adults-an-overview

Mayo Clinic. (n.d.). Hepatitis A. Retrieved from https://www.mayoclinic.org/diseases-conditions/hepatitis-a/symptoms-causes/syc-20367007.

Hepatitis B

Robin Miller and Ann E. Burke

Definition

A. Vaccine preventable, communicable disease of the liver caused by the hepatitis B virus.
B. Global health problem.
C. Acute or chronic forms.

Incidence

A. More than 250 million carriers worldwide.
B. 600,000 deaths annually in the world.
C. In the United States, the rate of hepatitis B-related hospitalizations, cancer, and death has doubled in the last decade.

Pathogenesis

A. Transmission through activities that involve percutaneous or mucosal contact with infectious blood or body fluids.

Predisposing Factors

A. Intravenous (IV) drug use that involves sharing needles.
B. Birth from an infected mother (vertical transmission).
C. Needle sticks: Healthcare worker.
D. Sex with an infected partner.
E. Travel to region that has high infection rates (e.g., Asia, Pacific Islands, Africa, Eastern Europe).

Subjective Data

A. Common complaints/symptoms.
   1. Fever.
   2. Fatigue/malaise.
   3. Headache.
   4. Nausea.
   5. Vomiting.
   6. Right upper quadrant (RUQ) pain.
   7. Loss of appetite.
   8. Itching.
   9. Myalgias.
B. Common/typical scenario.
   1. Onset of symptoms.
   2. Vaccination history.
   3. Recent travel.
   4. Food history.
C. Family and social history.
   1. Sexual activity (unprotected intercourse, gender, multiple partners).
      a. IV drug use.
      b. Alcohol use.
      c. Living situation (infected roommate or partner).
      d. Family history of hepatitis B.
   2. Dialysis.
D. Review of systems.
   1. See common complaints in previous section (jaundice, dark urine, clay-colored stool).

Physical Examination

A. Acute illness.
  1. Jaundice.
  2. Scleral icterus.
  3. Fever—low grade.
  4. RUQ tenderness.
B. Chronic illness.
  1. Fatigue.
  2. Anorexia.
  3. Nausea.
  4. Mild RUQ tenderness.
C. Fulminant illness: Onset of liver failure as manifested by encephalopathy and systemic dysfunction within 8 weeks of the recognition of liver disease.
  1. Ascites.
  2. Hepatic encephalopathy.
  3. Gastrointestinal (GI) bleeding.

Diagnostic Tests

A. Lab tests.
  1. Hepatitis B surface antigen, surface antibody, core antibody, IgM antibody.
  2. Antibodies for hepatitis A, C, D, and E.
  3. HIV.
  4. Complete blood count (CBC).
  5. International normalized ratio (INR).
  6. Liver function tests.
  7. Iron studies.
  8. Alpha fetoprotein (AFP).
B. Imaging.
  1. Abdominal ultrasound (US).
  2. Abdominal MRI.
C. Liver biopsy if indicated.

Differential Diagnosis

A. Hepatitis A, C, D, or E.
B. Alcoholic hepatitis.
C. Autoimmune hepatitis.
D. Acute drug-induced liver injury (DILI).
E. Hemochromatosis.
F. Wilson's disease.

Evaluation and Management Plan

A. General plan.
  1. Supportive care.
    a. The likelihood of liver failure from acute hepatitis B is less than 1%.
    b. Likelihood of progression to chronic hepatitis B is less than 5% in an immune competent adult.
B. Patient/family teaching points.
  1. Vaccination of close contacts.
  2. Safe sex practices.
C. Pharmacotherapy.
  1. Antiviral medication—Tenofovir or entecavir for patients with acute liver failure or severe disease (elevated bilirubin, coagulopathic).
  2. Fulminant hepatitis—refer for liver transplant.
D. Discharge instructions.
  1. Follow-up with pneumocystis pneumonia (PCP) or hepatologist.
  2. Avoidance of alcohol or drugs that could harm the liver.
  3. Do not share: Toothbrush, razor, needle.
  4. Limit sexual partners, perform safe sex practices.
  5. Call for fever, vomiting, bloody or black stool, dark urine, jaundice, ascites.

Follow-Up

A. See PCP if mild course.
B. Antiviral medication as prescribed.
C. Repeat lab tests to monitor recovery.
D. Vaccination for hepatitis A if indicated.

Consultation/Referral

A. Hepatologist to manage if condition becomes chronic hepatitis B.
B. Transplant center per hepatologist.

Special/Geriatric Considerations

A. Hepatitis D coinfection: Requires the presence of hepatitis B virus for infection. Should be treated by a hepatologist with peg interferon.
B. Pregnancy: Child born to a hepatitis B mother receives immunoglobulin as well as vaccination after delivery.
C. Fulminant failure: Consider for transplant.

Bibliography

Centers for Disease Control and Prevention. (n.d.). Hepatitis B questions and answers for health professionals. Retrieved from https://www.cdc.gov/hepatitis/hbv/hbvfaq.htm

Lok, A. (2017, September 29). Hepatitis B virus: Overview of management. In J. Mitty (Ed.), *UpToDate*. Retrieved from https://www.uptodate.com/contents/hepatitis-b-virus-overview-of-management

Mayo Clinic. (n.d.). Hepatitis B. Retrieved from https://www.mayoclinic.org/diseases-conditions/hepatitis-b/symptoms-causes/syc-20366802.

Pyrsopoulos, N. T. (2018, August 1). Hepatitis B workup. In B. S. Anand (Ed.), *Medscape*. Retrieved from https://emedicine.medscape.com/article/177632-workup

Hepatitis C

Robin Miller and Ann E. Burke

Definition

A. Chronic: Clinical or biochemical evidence of liver disease greater than 6 months duration.
B. One of the most common liver diseases.
C. Blood-borne disease of the liver caused by the hepatitis C virus.
D. 70% to 85% of those infected develop chronic illness.

Incidence

A. According to the Centers for Disease Control and Prevention (CDC), estimates of new hepatitis C infections from 2015 were 33,900 in the United States.
B. Estimated prevalence is approximately 3.6 million people.
C. Accounts for 8,000 to 13,000 deaths each year in the United States.
D. Infection rates have dramatically increased among young adults in the past decade due to the opioid epidemic.

Pathogenesis

A. Transmission through blood from a contaminated individual or blood products.
B. After 1990, blood and blood products underwent screening.

Predisposing Factors

A. Intravenous (IV) drug use and needle sharing.
B. Healthcare worker.
C. Transfusion before 1990.
D. Body piercing and tattoos.

E. Shared razors.

F. Baby boomer—CDC recommendations to test those born between 1945 and 1965.

G. Dialysis patient.

H. Maternal history of hepatitis C virus (HCV)—vertical transmission rate is 5%.

Subjective Data

A. Common complaints/symptoms.

    1. Most people have no symptoms.

    2. Among those who do have symptoms, they complain of fatigue, muscle and joint pain, pruritus, nausea, loss of appetite, weakness, and weight loss.

B. Common/typical scenario.

    1. Incidental diagnosis for elevated liver tests, insurance screening, or pneumocystis pneumonia (PCP) following CDC recommendations.

C. Family and social history.

    1. Injection drug use.

    2. Sexual or household contact.

    3. Incarceration.

D. Review of systems.

    1. In chronic illness, there are very few symptoms unless advanced to cirrhosis.

Physical Examination

A. Generally there are no obvious features of chronic hepatitis C unless cirrhosis is present.

Diagnostic Tests

A. Hepatitis C antibody.

B. Hepatitis C viral RNA quantitative level and genotype.

C. Screening tests to rule out coinfection for HIV or hepatitis B.

D. Complete blood count (CBC), comprehensive metabolic panel (CMP), thyroid-stimulating hormone (TSH), drug, and alcohol screen.

E. Imaging—Ultrasound or MRI if advanced disease present.

F. Procedure to assess the degree of fibrosis: Elastography (FibroScan), liver biopsy.

Differential Diagnosis

A. Autoimmune hepatitis.

B. Cholangitis.

C. Hepatitis A, B, D, and E.

Evaluation and Management

A. General plan.

    1. Treatment with antiviral therapy is well tolerated and effective in curing the disease.

    2. The decision to treat is based on genotype, the person's overall health and comorbidities, and stage of fibrosis.

B. Patient/family teaching points.

    1. If the decision is made to pursue antiviral treatment, medication adherence is essential to achieve optimal outcomes.

    2. Skipping doses may lead to resistant strains and impact success of therapy.

    3. Alcohol is prohibited as well as herbal supplements.

    4. Successful treatment can mitigate progression to cirrhosis.

C. Pharmacotherapy.

    1. Antiviral therapy—must be ordered by specialist. Drug options include: Harvoni, Epclusa, Vosevi, Mavyret, Zepatier, Ribavirin.

    2. Common side effects: Usually mild and may include fatigue, headaches, or nausea.

D. Discharge instructions.

    1. Follow-up with gastrointestinal (GI)/hepatologist.

    2. Will need vaccinations for hepatitis A or B if indicated.

    3. Avoid alcohol or any over-the-counter (OTC) supplements.

Follow-Up

A. GI/Hepatologist to initiate treatment and monitor therapy and side effects.

B. For the cirrhotic patient, biannual imaging of the liver to screen for hepatocellular cancer.

Consultation/Referral

A. GI/Hepatologist.

B. If they have hepatocellular carcinoma (HCC), will be referred to interventional radiology or oncology.

C. Consider transplant for any patient with decompensated cirrhosis or HCC.

Special/Geriatric Considerations

A. Decision to treat any dialysis patient is undertaken on a case-by-case basis.

B. A patient with HIV/hepatitis C coinfection may require changes in his or her highly active antiretroviral therapy (HAART) due to drug interactions with hepatitis C treatment.

C. Pregnancy is contraindicated for treatment.

Bibliography

Centers for Disease Control and Prevention. (n.d.). Hepatitis C information. Retrieved from https://www.cdc.gov/hepatitis/hcv/index.htm

Chopra, S., & Pockros, P. J. (2018, June 5). Overview of the management of chronic hepatitis C virus infection. In A. Bloom (Ed.), *UpToDate*. Retrieved from https://www.uptodate.com/contents/overview-of-the-management-of-chronic-hepatitis-c-virus-infection

Dhawan, V. K. (2019, January 17). Hepatitis C clinical presentation. In B. S. Anand (Ed.), *Medscape*. Retrieved from https://emedicine.medscape.com/article/177792-clinical

Inflammatory Bowel Disease

Catherine Harris

Definition

A. Inflammatory bowel disease (IBD) is an umbrella term for a group of disorders that causes inflammation of the bowel such as ulcerative colitis (UC) and Crohn's disease (CD).

Incidence

A. Approximately 1 to 2 million people in the United States have UC or CD.

B. IBD: 396 cases per 100,000/year.

C. UC: 0.5 to 24.5 cases per 100,000.

D. CD: 0.1 to 16 cases per 100,000.

Pathogenesis

A. IBD causes inflammation of the mucosa of the intestinal tract.

1. Ulceration.
2. Edema.
3. Bleeding.
4. Fluid and electrolyte loss.

B. Inflammatory mediators and cytokines disrupt intestinal mucosa, allowing chronic inflammatory processes to occur.

C. UC: Inflammation begins in the rectum (always involved) with 25% of cases confined to the rectum.

1. Disease progresses in a contiguous manner and does not "skip" sections of bowel as common in CD.
2. Pancolitis occurs in 10%.

D. CD: Can affect any part of the gastrointestinal tract from the mouth to the anus.

1. Three patterns of involvement.
   a. Inflammatory disease.
   b. Strictures.
   c. Fistulas.
2. Involves all layers of bowel, not just mucosa and submucosa.
3. Pattern is discontinuous (unlike UC) and typically has "skip" areas of interspersed disease in two or more areas.
4. May have rectal sparing.
5. Anorectal complications common.

Predisposing Factors

A. Higher prevalence rate in Jewish populations.

B. Females have a slightly greater incidence.

C. Young adults 15 to 40 years old.

D. Living in a developed country, colder climates, and in urban areas.

E. Genetic disposition.

Subjective Data

A. Common complaints/symptoms.

1. Diarrhea.
2. Constipation.
3. Bowel movement issues such as pain or bleeding.
4. Abdominal cramping and pain.
   a. Right lower quadrant pain in CD.
   b. Left lower quadrant or periumbilical in UC.
5. Nausea and vomiting.

B. Common/typical scenario.

1. Patients typically complain of low grade fevers, sweats, malaise, or general fatigue with associated bowel movement changes that include pain or bleeding.
2. Patients may report irregular bowel patterns with either diarrhea or constipation or a combination of both.
3. Most patients report recurrent abdominal pain and diarrhea over several months to years.
4. May occur with or without blood or pus in the stool.

C. Family and social history.

1. Family history of IBD, celiac disease, or colorectal cancer.
2. Use of nonsteroidal anti-inflammatory drugs (NSAIDs).
3. History of smoking.
4. Recent travel.
5. Stress.
6. Dietary problems.

D. Review of systems.

1. Head, ear, eyes, nose, and throat (HEENT): Evidence or history of scleritis, anterior uveitis (redness, pain, itchiness), aphthous stomatitis (mouth sores).
2. Dermatology: Psoriasis, erythema nodosum.
3. Rheumatology: Inflammatory arthritis, ankylosing spondylitis.
4. Arthritis.
5. Gastrointestinal (GI): Liver disease, gallstones, blood or pus in stool, diarrhea, constipation.
6. Genitourinary (GU): History of kidney stones.
7. Fatigue, night sweats, loss of appetite, fever, or recent infection.

Physical Examination

A. Constitutional: Patients who become dehydrated may have fever or appear lethargic.

B. Gastrointestinal: Abdominal examination is often benign; a rectal examination can be done if there is concern for perianal fissures, fistulas, or evidence of rectal prolapse; occult stool may be present.

C. Cardiovascular: Tachycardia from dehydration may be present.

D. Skin: Pallor may be noted if there is anemia

Diagnostic Tests

A. Lab studies.

1. No laboratory test is specific for irritable bowel syndrome (IBS).
2. Complete blood cell (CBC) count to assess for anemia or infection.
3. Markers of nutritional status may have value if concern for significant deficiencies.
   a. Albumin.
   b. Prealbumin.
   c. Vitamin B_{12}.
   d. Folate.
   e. Transferrin.
4. Erythrocyte sedimentation rate (ESR) and C-reactive protein are useful markers for inflammation.
5. Perinuclear antineutrophil cytoplasmic antibodies (pANCA) and anti-*Saccharomyces cerevisiae* antibodies (ASCA).
   a. Positive pANCA and negative ASCA is more specific for UC.
   b. Negative pANCA and positive ASCA is more specific for CD.
6. Stool studies.
   a. Check stool culture, ova, and parasites.
   b. Check *Clostridium difficile* infection with toxin assay.

B. Imaging studies.

1. Abdominal x-ray can be used to rule out other conditions.
   a. Free air is consistent with toxic megacolon.
   b. Dilated colon is consistent with colitis.
   c. Osteoporosis may explain some pain symptoms.
2. Barium enema studies: Can be useful in diagnosing UC versus CD.
3. Ultrasound, MRI, and CT may be useful in identifying fistulas, abscesses, and stenosis.

C. Colonoscopy.

1. Most valuable tool to diagnose type of IBS.
2. Can be used to determine extent and severity.
3. Obtain tissue.
4. Document ulceration and assess inflammation.

D. Flexible sigmoidoscopy.

1. Limited length of scope can help diagnosis rectal bleeding and diagnose distal UC.

E. Esophagogastroduodenoscopy (EGD).

  1. Used to evaluate upper GI tract symptoms.

  2. Can evaluate ulceration.

Differential Diagnosis

A. Gastritis.

B. Colitis.

C. Abdominal infections.

D. Diverticulitis.

E. Appendicitis.

F. The differential diagnosis often depends on presentation.

  1. If patients present with diarrhea consider:

    a. Celiac disease.

    b. Lactose intolerance.

    c. Gastrointestinal infections.

    d. Cancer of the GI tract.

  2. If patients present with abdominal pain or gastrointestinal bleeding.

    a. Arteriovenous malformations.

    b. Cancer of the GI tract.

    c. Colitis.

Evaluation and Management Plan

A. General plan.

  1. Symptomatic therapy.

    a. Treat underlying inflammation in outpatient setting.

    b. Admit to hospital if surgical intervention required, uncontrolled pain, significant dehydration from vomiting, evidence of emergent complications such as toxic megacolon, severe colitis, or bowel obstruction.

    c. Avoid antidiarrheals in acute phase because of risk of toxic megacolon.

    d. Supportive care.

  2. Start stepwise medical therapy.

    a. Step 1: Treat with aminosalicylates +/− antibiotics (controversial for prophylactic use).

    b. Step 2: Treat with corticosteroids. which provide rapid relief of symptoms.

    c. Step 3: Treat with immune modifying agents if steroids fail or are required for prolonged periods.

    d. Step 4: Experimental agents.

      i. Thalidomide.

      ii. Nicotine patch.

      iii. Butyrate enema.

      iv. Heparin subcutaneous injections.

  3. Surgery.

    a. Not curative in CD because of the skip lesions and more diffuse nature of the disease.

      i. Performed in patients with complications such as strictures or fistulas.

      ii. Recurrent inflammation in 93% of cases at 1 year post surgery.

    b. Colectomy required in 2% to 30% of patients with UC.

      i. Intractable inflammation.

      ii. Medical therapy fails.

      iii. Precancerous changes.

      iv. Toxic megacolon.

      v. Perforation.

  4. Remission therapy.

    a. Continue medications used to achieve remission.

    b. Taper off steroids: No role in maintaining remission.

B. Patient/family teaching points.

  1. Dietary changes: Certain foods and drinks can make symptoms worse; avoid foods that cause flare ups, particularly too much fiber, spicy food, alcohol, and caffeine.

    a. Eat smaller meals more often.

    b. Drink plenty of fluids.

  2. Stress may exacerbate the condition.

  3. Quit smoking to improve remission rates.

  4. IBD may increase the risk of colon cancer. Colonoscopies should be done early and often.

  5. If taking immunosuppressant therapy, the immune system's ability to fight infection is reduced.

C. Pharmacotherapy.

  1. Corticosteroids.

    a. Treatment of choice in acute attack in intravenous form.

    b. Inhibitors of inflammation.

    c. Do not use for maintaining state of remission.

  2. Immunosuppressants.

    a. Steroid sparing agents.

    b. Great in patients refractory to steroids.

  3. 5-Aminosalicyclic acid derivatives.

    a. Reduce inflammatory reactions.

    b. Useful in mild to moderate UC.

    c. May be used to maintain remission in CD.

  4. Tumor necrosis factor alpha.

    a. Induces proinflammatory cytokines.

    b. Promotes mucosal healing.

  5. Antibiotics: Broad spectrum antibiotics to treat intestinal bacteria are controversial. Antibiotics are thought to reduce recurrence rate, particularly in CD, though therapy is not well established in UC. American College of Gastroenterology guidelines state that controlled trials have not consistently demonstrated efficacy.

    a. May be used for complications associated with IBS.

      i. Abscesses.

      ii. Fistulas.

      iii. Pouchitis.

    b. Metronidazole.

    c. Ciprofloxacin.

  6. Histamine H2 antagonists: Reduce gastric acid secretion.

  7. Proton pump inhibitors.

    a. Reduce gastric acid secretion.

    b. Used in patients who fail H2 antagonist therapy.

  8. Antidiarrheals for symptomatic relief.

  9. Anticholinergic/antispasmodic agents.

    a. Treats spastic disorders or motility disturbances.

  10. Probiotics: Certain strains (*Escherichia-coli* Nissle 1917 & VSL # 3 [Mutaflor, Ardeypharm]) have shown to be effective in mild-moderate IBD (esp. UC) comparable to Metronidazole.

  11. Supplements.

    a. Iron supplements.

    b. Nutritional supplements.

    c. Calcium and vitamin D supplements.

D. Discharge instructions.

  1. Avoid foods with caffeine, spicy foods, or milk products.

  2. Eat small meals several times a day instead of fewer big meals.

  3. Follow-up with gastroenterologist.

Follow-Up

A. Follow-up with gastroenterologist.

Consultation/Referral

A. Refer to gastroenterology for medical management.

B. Consult surgery in UC if medical therapy fails.

C. Consult surgeon if severe disease or extraluminal complications.

D. Specialty consults to manage extracolonic manifestations.

    1. Ophthalmology for uveitis.

    2. Arthritis.

    3. Dermatitis.

    4. Dietician.

Special/Geriatric Considerations

A. The elderly may experience a delay in diagnosis because of the wide possibilities in the differential diagnosis.

Bibliography

Amezaga, A. J., & Van Assche, G. (2016). Practical approaches to "top-down" therapies for Crohn's disease. *Current Gastroenterology Reports, 18*(7), 35. doi:10.1007/s11894-016-0507-z

Ha, C., & Kornbluth, A. (2010). Mucosal healing in inflammatory bowel disease: Where do we stand? *Current Gastroenterology Reports, 12*(6), 471–478. doi:10.1007/s11894-010-0146-8

Henriksen, M., Jahnsen, J., Lygren, I., Sauar, J., Kjellevold, Ø, Schulz, T., . . . Moum, B. (2006). Ulcerative colitis and clinical course: Results of a 5-year population-based follow-up study (the IBSEN study). *Inflammatory Bowel Diseases, 12*(7), 543–550. doi:10.1097/01.MIB.0000225339.91484.fc

Khan, K. J., Ullman, T. A., Ford, A. C., Abreu, M. T., Abadir, A., Marshall, J. K., . . . Moayyedi, P. (2011). Antibiotic therapy in inflammatory bowel disease: A systematic review and meta-analysis. *The American Journal of Gastroenterology, 106*(4), 661–673. Retrieved from https://journals.lww.com/ajg/Abstract/2011/04000/Antibiotic_Therapy_in_Inflammatory_Bowel_Disease_.14.aspx

Kornbluth, A., & Sachar, D. B. (2010). Ulcerative colitis practice guidelines in adults: American College of Gastroenterology, Practice Parameters Committee. *The American Journal of Gastroenterology, 105*(3), 501–523. Retrieved from https://journals.lww.com/ajg/Abstract/2010/03000/Ulcerative_Colitis_Practice_Guidelines_in_Adults_.6.aspx

Leighton, J. A., Shen, B., Baron, T. H., Adler, D. G., Davila, R., Egan, J. V., . . . Fanelli, R. D. (2006). ASGE guideline: Endoscopy in the diagnosis and treatment of inflammatory bowel disease. *Gastrointestinal Endoscopy, 63*(4), 558–565. doi:10.1016/j.gie.2006.02.005

Lichtenstein, G. R., Abreu, M. T., Cohen, R., & Tremaine, W. (2006). American Gastroenterological Association Institute medical position statement on corticosteroids, immunomodulators, and infliximab in inflammatory bowel disease. *Gastroenterology, 130*(3), 935–939. doi:10.1053/j.gastro.2006.01.047

Molodecky, N. A., Soon, I. S., Rabi, D. M., Ghali, W. A., Ferris, M., Chernoff, G., & Kaplan, G. G. (2012). Increasing incidence and prevalence of the inflammatory bowel diseases with time, based on systematic review. *Gastroenterology, 142*(1), 46–54.e42. doi:10.1053/j.gastro.2011.10.001

Saez-Lara, M. J., Gomez-Llorente, C., Plaza-Diaz, J., & Gil, A. (2015). The role of probiotic lactic acid bacteria and bifidobacteria in the prevention and treatment of inflammatory bowel disease and other related diseases: A systematic review of randomized human clinical trials. *BioMed Research International.* doi:10.1155/2015/505878

Wilkins, T., Jarvis, K., & Patel, J. (2011). Diagnosis and management of Crohn's disease. *American Family Physician, 84*(12), 1365–1375. Retrieved from https://www.aafp.org/afp/2011/1215/p1365.html

Nonalcoholic Fatty Liver Disease

Robin Miller and Ann E. Burke

Definition

A. Medical condition characterized by fatty infiltration in the liver without a history of alcohol use.

B. Two types exist based on presence of inflammation.

    1. Nonalcoholic fatty liver disease (NAFLD)—benign condition without inflammation.

    2. Nonalcoholic steatohepatitis (NASH)—Inflammation is present which leads to scarring. May progress to cirrhosis in 20% of the population.

Incidence

A. Most common liver disease in Western industrialized countries.

B. In the United States, the prevalence of NAFLD is estimated at 10% to 46%.

C. Incidence as high as 50% to 75% in obese patients.

Pathogenesis

A. Cause is not fully understood but thought to be linked to insulin resistance and oxidative stress in an individual with risk factors.

Predisposing Factors

A. Male sex.

B. Higher prevalence in Hispanics.

C. Commonly diagnosed at age 40 to 50.

D. Metabolic syndrome is present with one or more of the following.

    1. Obesity.

    2. Diabetes.

    3. Hypertension (HTN).

    4. Dyslipidemia.

E. Other disorders that may be associated: Polycystic ovarian syndrome (PCOS), sleep apnea, hypothyroidism.

Subjective Data

A. Common complaints/symptoms.

    1. Most patients are usually asymptomatic.

    2. May have fatigue, malaise, or right upper quadrant (RUQ) discomfort.

B. Common/typical scenario.

    1. Incidental findings of elevated alanine aminotransferase (ALT) on lab testing or imaging suggestive of fatty infiltration.

C. Family and social history.

    1. Take a detailed history of alcohol intake to rule out alcohol-related liver disease.

    2. Diet and weight history.

D. Review of systems.

    1. There are very few symptoms.

    2. In advanced liver disease, they may have evidence of synthetic dysfunction.

Physical Examination

A. Most patients are obese.

B. Hepatomegaly.

C. In cirrhosis, may have stigmata of chronic liver disease.

Diagnostic Tests

A. Diagnosis made after exclusion of other causes and positive findings of fatty infiltration on imaging or biopsy.

B. Labs: Complete blood count (CBC), comprehensive metabolic panel (CMP), cholesterol, iron studies, ferritin, thyroid-stimulating hormone (TSH), celiac antibody.

C. Hepatitis A, B, and C serologies.

D. Autoimmune markers antinuclear antibody (ANA), AMA, ASMA.

E. Ceruloplasmin, Alpha 1 antitrypsin, HFE gene for hemochromatosis.

F. Imaging: Ultrasound or MRI.

G. Liver biopsy.

Differential Diagnosis

A. Viral hepatitis.

B. Autoimmune disease.

C. Wilson's disease.
D. Alpha 1 antitrypsin deficiency.
E. Hemochromatosis.
F. Alcohol-related hepatitis.
G. Celiac disease.
H. Thyroid disease.
I. Medication induced: Amiodarone, methotrexate, tamoxifen, steroids, antiretrovirals.

Evaluation and Management

A. General plan.
   1. If no biopsy performed, consider noninvasive testing to assess degree of fibrosis, that is, Fibroscan.
   2. Lifestyle modifications—weight loss, diet, and exercise.
   3. Control of sugars.
   4. Treatment of hyperlipidemia and HTN.
   5. Monitor liver tests every 3 months.
   6. Bariatric surgery may be considered if appropriate.
B. Patient/family teaching points.
   1. In general, control of risk factors contributing to metabolic syndrome.
   2. Weight loss of 7% to 10% of current weight to improve fibrosis.
   3. Avoid alcohol.
   4. Good glucose control.
   5. Vitamin E is not recommended if patient has heart disease or diabetes.
   6. Reassure the patient that NAFLD is a chronic condition. Most people will not develop advanced liver disease.
C. Pharmacotherapy.
   1. Vitamin E: Improves liver histology. 800 IU per day is recommended.
   2. Statin therapy.
   3. Clinical trials: Obeticholic acid (OCA) shows promise for future therapy.
D. Discharge instructions.
   1. Follow-up with gastrointestinal (GI)/hepatologist, pneumocystis pneumonia (PCP), and/or endocrinologist.
   2. Lifestyle modifications of diet and exercise.
   3. Avoid alcohol.
   4. Do not take any new medications/supplements without consulting your doctor.

Follow-Up

A. As noted in the discharge instructions, follow-up with PCP, GI/hepatology, and/or endocrinology.
B. Patients with NASH cirrhosis will need hepatocellular carcinoma (HCC) screening and esophageal varices screening under the supervision of a hepatologist.

Consultation/Referral

A. Dietician.
B. Endocrinologist.
C. Bariatric surgeon.
D. Cardiologist.

Special/Geriatric Considerations

A. Another cause of hepatic steatosis is acute fatty liver of pregnancy.
B. This is a rare condition and typically occurs in the third trimester to mothers with multiple gestation pregnancies.
C. Early diagnosis and prompt delivery is primary treatment.

Bibliography

Chalasani, N., Younossi, Z., Lavine, J. E., Charlton, M., Cusi, K., Rinella, M., . . . Sanyal, A. J. (2018). The diagnosis and management of nonalcoholic fatty liver disease: Practice guidance from the American Association for the Study of Liver Diseases. *Hepatology, 67*(2), 328–357. doi:10.1002/hep.29367

Chopra, S., & Lai, M. (2018, December 10). Management of nonalcoholic fatty liver disease in adults. In K. M. Robson (Ed.), *UpToDate*. Retrieved from https://www.uptodate.com/contents/management-of-nonalcoholic-fatty-liver-disease-in-adults

Sheth, S. G., & Chopra, S. (2018, April 3). Epidemiology, clinical features, and diagnosis of nonalcoholic fatty liver disease in adults. In K. M. Robson (Ed.), *UpToDate*. Retrieved from https://www.uptodate.com/contents/epidemiology-clinical-features-and-diagnosis-of-nonalcoholic-fatty-liver-disease-in-adults

Tendler, D. A. (2018, September 14). Pathogenesis of nonalcoholic fatty liver disease. In K. M. Robson (Ed.), *UpToDate*. Retrieved from https://www.uptodate.com/contents/pathogenesis-of-nonalcoholic-fatty-liver-disease

Pancreatitis

Catherine Harris

Definition

A. Acute pancreatitis is a sudden inflammation of the pancreas.

Incidence

A. The incidence of acute pancreatitis ranges from 4.9 to 13/100,000 persons.
B. Leading gastrointestinal cause of hospitalization, with more than 300,000 admissions per year.
C. 16.5% to 25% of patients experience recurrent episodes in the first several years post diagnosis.
D. Acute pancreatitis is frequently an isolated event, but may develop into chronic pancreatitis, particularly in the setting of chronic alcoholism.
E. 60% to 90% of patients with pancreatitis have a history of chronic alcohol consumption; however, only a minority of alcoholics develop the disease.
F. Mortality rate for acute pancreatitis has remained the same over the past decade at 10%.
G. Optimal outcomes depend on recognition of acute pancreatitis as quickly as possible.

Pathogenesis

A. Gallstones and alcohol account for about 80% of all cases of acute pancreatitis.
B. Other causes of acute pancreatitis can be related to medications and very rarely to infections, trauma, or surgery of the abdomen. About 10% of cases are idiopathic.
   1. Gallstones.
     a. Gallstones can lodge in the common bile duct and cause obstruction of the pancreatic fluid by impinging on the main pancreatic duct.
     b. Mechanism is not completely understood.
   2. Alcohol.
     a. Alcohol is metabolized by the pancreas and is thought to have a toxic effect on key cells.
     b. Alcohol may also cause the production of excess collagen that contributes to fibrosis.
     c. Large amounts of alcohol (80 g/day; approximately 10 to 11 drinks) for 6 to 12 years is required to produce symptomatic pancreatitis.

3. Medications.

    a. Very rare and not well understood mechanism of how medications induce acute pancreatitis.

    b. Possible theories include pancreatic duct constriction, cytotoxic, and metabolic effects.

    c. Medications associated with acute pancreatitis.

        i. Angiotensin-converting enzyme inhibitors.

        ii. Statins.

        iii. Oral contraceptives.

        iv. Diuretics.

        v. Valproic acid.

        vi. Glucagon-like peptide 1 (GLP-1) hypoglycemic agents.

4. Trauma or surgery.

    a. Injury to pancreas from trauma or surgery typically occurs from hemorrhage and sepsis related to primary injury.

    b. Least commonly injured organ in abdominal trauma due in part to its location.

Predisposing Factors

A. Choledocholithiasis.

B. Chronic alcoholism.

C. Hypertriglyceridemia (greater than 1,000 mg/dL).

Subjective Data

A. Common complaints/symptoms.

    1. Severe abdominal pain.

    2. Nausea and vomiting.

    3. Diarrhea.

B. Common/typical scenario.

    1. Patients may start with sudden onset dull pain in the abdomen that becomes increasingly more severe.

    2. Pain localizes to the upper abdomen and may radiate to back.

    3. Usually associated with nausea and vomiting.

    4. Patients usually restless and bending forward to try to alleviate the constant pain.

C. Family and social history.

    1. Alcoholism.

    2. Familial history of hypertriglyceridemia.

    3. Recent abdominal surgery or trauma.

D. Review of systems.

    1. Constitutional: Ask about any fever.

    2. Cardiovascular: May have rapid heartbeat or feel lightheaded.

    3. Respiratory: Ask about any difficulty breathing or trouble getting air in.

    4. Gastrointestinal: Ask about nausea, vomiting, diarrhea, pain location and intensity, and if any radiation.

    5. Weight loss.

Physical Examination

A. Gastrointestinal—abdominal tenderness, distention, guarding, bowel sounds may be diminished or absent, may have jaundice.

B. Respiratory—dyspnea from diaphragmatic inflammation.

C. Cardiovascular—hemodynamic instability in severe acute pancreatitis; assess for signsand symptoms of shock.

D. Skin—physical findings consistent with severe necrotizing pancreatitis.

    1. Cullen sign: Periumbilical bluish discoloration.

    2. Grey Turner sign: Reddish brown discoloration along flanks consistent with extravasated pancreatic exudate.

Diagnostic Tests

A. Lab studies.

    1. Amylase and lipase are routinely ordered and will be elevated at least 3✕ above normal reference range in acute pancreatitis. The serum level of amylase or lipase does not correlate with severity.

        a. Amylase: Half-life is short (less than 12 hours) and will return to normal; not specific to acute pancreatitis.

        b. Lipase elevations support diagnosis of acute pancreatitis and is more specific than amylase to the pancreas.

    2. Liver function tests (LFTs).

        a. Alkaline phosphatase.

        b. Total bilirubin.

        c. Aspartate aminotransferase (AST).

        d. Alanine aminotransferase (ALT) greater than 150 U/L suggests gallstone pancreatitis.

    3. Basic metabolic panel, electrolytes, cholesterol, and triglycerides.

        a. Hypertriglyceridemia (greater than 1,000 mg/dL).

    4. C-reactive protein.

        a. Higher levels (greater than 10 mg/dL) associated with severe pancreatitis, but is not specific for pancreatitis.

    5. Lactic dehydrogenase (LDH) should be checked to provide prognosis based on the Ranson criteria (see section "Evaluation and Management Plan").

    6. Immunoglobulin G4 (IgG4) if concern for autoimmune pancreatitis.

B. Imaging studies.

    1. Ultrasound.

        a. Good screening test for determining the etiology of pancreatitis and standard of care for detecting gallstones.

        b. Cannot measure severity of disease.

    2. Endoscopic ultrasonography.

        a. High frequency ultrasound can provide more detailed imagery.

    3. Contrast-enhanced CT or MRI only necessary if a diagnosis is uncertain with clinical presentation and laboratory data.

C. Endoscopic retrograde cholangiopancreatography (ERCP).

    1. Endoscopic procedure used in patients with severe acute pancreatitis with suspected gallstones or biliary pancreatitis with worsening clinical examination.

    2. Not used routinely in patients with acute pancreatitis and should be used with caution and only in cases where gallstones are suspected to be the underlying etiology.

Differential Diagnosis

A. Cholecystitis.

B. Acute abdomen.

C. Pneumonia.

D. Peptic ulcer disease.

E. Hepatitis.

F. Irritable bowel syndrome.

G. Myocardial infarction.

H. Chronic pancreatitis.

I. Gastroenteritis.

J. Peritonitis.

Evaluation and Management Plan

A. General plan.

1. Stage acute pancreatitis to determine prognosis using the 11-point Ranson criteria within 48 hours. Each criteria is 1 point. Ranson score 0 to 2: Minimal mortality; Ranson score 3 to 5: 10% to 20% mortality; Ranson score greater than 5 after 48 hours has a mortality rate greater than 50%.

   a. Present on admission.

      i. Patient older than 55 years.

      ii. White blood cell (WBC) count higher than 16,000 uL.

      iii. Blood glucose higher than 200 mg/dL.

      iv. Serum LDH level higher than 350 IU/L.

      v. AST level higher than 250 IU/L.

   b. Develops within 48 hours.

      i. Drop of hematocrit more than 10%.

      ii. Blood urea nitrogen (BUN) increases more than 8 mg/dL.

      iii. Fluid retention greater than 6 L.

      iv. Base deficit greater than 4 mEq/L.

      v. PaO2 less than 60 mmHg.

      vi. Serum calcium less than 8 mg/dL.

2. Supportive medical care.

   a. Bowel rest for several days except in mild cases where there is no nausea or vomiting.

   b. Nutritional support with dextrose 5% in water for mild pancreatitis.

   c. In moderate to severe pancreatitis, start nasojejunal feeds with low fat formulation.

   d. Parenteral nutrition should be avoided except in very severe cases in order to minimize the risk of infections.

   e. Pain management.

   f. Aggressive rehydration with intravenous fluids within the first 12 to 24 hours of symptom onset—monitor patients with cardiovascular and renal comorbidities very closely.

3. Surgical therapy.

   a. ERCP within 24 hours of admission if patient has concurrent acute cholangitis.

   b. Gallstones may require surgical intervention.

   c. Resection of necrotic tissue if necrotizing pancreatitis or abscess.

   d. Sphincteroplasty may be performed if sphincter dysfunction is found.

4. Monitor for complications associated with severe acute pancreatitis.

   a. Shock.

   b. Pulmonary complications.

   c. Inflammatory changes.

      i. Kidney dysfunction.

      ii. Gastrointestinal bleeding.

      iii. Colitis.

      iv. Splenic vein thrombosis.

   d. Localized complications are more likely to occur in patients with alcoholic and biliary pancreatitis.

      i. Fluid collection.

      ii. Ascites.

      iii. Pseudocysts.

B. Patient/family teaching points.

1. Acute pancreatitis is typically relieved after a couple days but can become severe.

2. Avoid binge drinking.

3. Smoking cessation is thought to exacerbate episodes of acute pancreatitis but the studies are not conclusive.

4. Recurrence of acute pancreatitis may occur and prevention depends on the cause.

   a. If gallstones caused acute pancreatitis, you may need to have your gallbladder removed.

   b. If alcohol is the cause, you should stop drinking.

5. Diet changes may be required in people with high fat intake.

6. Medication changes may be necessary if acute pancreatitis is associated with a particular drug.

7. Some patients may develop chronic pancreatitis but acute pancreatitis is more frequently a one off event, especially if the underlying cause is treated.

C. Pharmacotherapy.

1. No specific pharmacological therapy for acute pancreatitis.

2. Supportive fluid resuscitation and management of pain.

3. Antibiotic therapy only in cases of suspected infection.

D. Discharge instructions.

1. Eliminate alcohol from diet.

2. Eat small frequent meals.

3. Reduce fat in diet.

4. Don't smoke.

5. Follow-up with the gastroenterologist.

Follow-Up

A. No guidelines established for long-term follow-up.

B. Depending on etiology, may need follow-up imaging or lab monitoring.

Consultation/Referral

A. Gastroenterology should evaluate all cases of pancreatitis.

B. Surgical consult for acute pancreatitis related to gallstones.

C. Endocrinology consult if patient has hyperparathyroidism, hypertriglyceridemia, or hypercalcemia-induced pancreatitis.

D. Refer patients to social work if alcohol abuse suspected.

Special/Geriatric Considerations

A. Gallstone pancreatitis is much more likely in elderly and pregnant persons.

B. Presenting abdominal pain may be more vague in elderly patients.

C. Acute pancreatitis is rare during pregnancy but typically occurs in the third trimester and is mostly due to gallstones, which can cause preterm labor or in utero fetal demise.

Bibliography

Balthazar, E. J. (2002). Staging of acute pancreatitis. *Radiologic Clinics, 40*(6), 1199–1209. doi:10.1016/S0033-8389(02)00047-7

Banks, P. A., Bollen, T. L., Dervenis, C., Gooszen, H. G., Johnson, C. D., Sarr, M. G., . . . Vege, S. S. (2013). Classification of acute pancreatitis—2012: Revision of the Atlanta classification and definitions by international consensus. *Gut, 62*(1), 102–111. doi:10.1136/gutjnl-2012-302779

Ducarme, G., Maire, F., Chate, P., Luton, D., & Hammel, P. (2014). Acute pancreatitis during pregnancy: A review. *Journal of Perinatology, 34*, 87–94. doi:10.1038/jp.2013.161

Imrie, C. W. (2003). Prognostic indicators in acute pancreatitis. *Canadian Journal of Gastroenterology, 17*(5), 325–358. doi:10.1155/2003/250815

Jones, M., Hall, O., Kaye, A. M., & Kaye, A. D. (2015). Drug-induced acute pancreatitis: A review. *Ochsner Journal, 15*(1), 45–51. Retrieved from http://www.ochsnerjournal.org/content/15/1/45

Strate, T., Yekebas, E., Knoefel, W., Bloechle, C., & Izbicki, J. (2002). Pathogenesis and the natural course of chronic pancreatitis. *European Journal of Gastroenterology & Hepatology, 14*(9), 929–934. Retrieved from https://journals.lww.com/eurojgh/Fulltext/2002/09000/Pathogenesis_and_the_natural_course_of_chronic.2.aspx

Tenner, S., Baillie, J., DeWitt, J., & Vege, S. S. (2013). American College of Gastroenterology guideline: Management of acute pancreatitis. *The American Journal of Gastroenterology, 108*(9), 1400–1416. Retrieved from https://journals.lww.com/ajg/Abstract/2013/09000/American_College_of_Gastroenterology_Guideline_.6.aspx

Vege, S. S., Ziring, B., Jain, R., & Moayyedi, P. (2015). American Gastroenterological Association institute guideline on the diagnosis and management of asymptomatic neoplastic pancreatic cysts. *Gastroenterology, 148*(4), 819–822. doi:10.1053/j.gastro.2015.01.015

Whitcomb, D. C. (2006). Clinical practice. Acute pancreatitis. *New England Journal of Medicine, 354*(20), 2142–2150. doi:10.1056/NEJMcp054958

Whitcomb, D. C., Yadav, D., Adam, S., Hawes, R. H., Brand, R. E., Anderson, M. A., . . . Barmada, M. M. (2008). Multicenter approach to recurrent acute and chronic pancreatitis in the United States: The North American Pancreatitis Study 2 (NAPS2). *Pancreatology, 8*(4–5), 520–531. doi:10.1159/000152001

Peptic Ulcer Disease

Catherine Harris

Definition
A. An ulcer that forms in the lining of the esophagus, stomach, or small intestine.

Incidence
A. 10% of the population is thought to have evidence of peptic ulcer disease (PUD).
B. Similar occurrence in males and females.
C. Mortality rate due to hemorrhagic ulcer is approximately 5%.

Pathogenesis
A. Defect of mucosal lining of digestive tract; frequently occurs when there is an imbalance between gastric acid secretion and degradation of the mucosal defense mechanism caused by use of anti-inflammatory drugs, *Helicobacter pylori* infection, alcohol, acid, and pepsin.
B. *H. pylori* infection can colonize the gastric mucosa and cause inflammation.
C. Nonsteroidal anti-inflammatory drug (NSAID) use can disrupt the mucosal barrier.
D. Alcohol is a gastric mucosal irritant.
E. Stress ulceration can occur and is associated with serious systemic illnesses.
F. Brain injury or tumors are associated with high gastric acid output.
G. Hypersecretory states can also cause PUD, most notably Zollinger–Ellison syndrome.
H. Three types of ulcers (location based).
    1. Gastric ulcers.
    2. Esophageal ulcers.
    3. Duodenal ulcers.
I. Major risk of perforation, which carries a mortality rate of up to 30%.

Predisposing Factors
A. Taking NSAIDs including ibuprofen, aspirin.
B. Smoking.
C. Excessive alcohol.
D. Excess stress.
E. Obesity.
F. Zollinger–Ellison disease.

Subjective Data
A. Common complaints/symptoms.

    1. Gnawing or burning sensation that occurs shortly after meals (gastric ulcers) or at 2 to 3 hours (duodenal ulcers).
    2. Heartburn.
    3. Belching.
    4. Bloating.
    5. Distention.
B. Common/typical scenario.
    1. Gastric and duodenal ulcers typically cannot be differentiated with history alone, but there are some differences.
        a. Most patients regardless of type of PUD complain of epigastric pain.
        b. Patients with gastric ulcers typically complain of pain shortly after meals.
        c. In patients with duodenal ulcers:
            i. Antacid use commonly ineffective.
            ii. Complaints of pain 2 to 3 hours after a meal.
            iii. Frequent night waking.
C. Family and social history.
    1. Ask about smoking and alcohol use.
    2. Ask about family history of any type of gastric cancer.
D. Review of systems.
    1. Evaluate for dysphagia, nausea, vomiting, or blood in stool.
    2. Evaluate pain intensity, timing, and duration.
    3. Inquire about back pain (which may indicate gallstones or pancreatitis).

Physical Examination
A. Gastrointestinal focus.
    1. Epigastric tenderness.
    2. Typically pain will be vague and nonlocalizing.
    3. Melena may be present.
B. If the ulcer perforates.
    1. Sudden onset of severe abdominal pain that is generalized and worsens with movement.
    2. Rebound abdominal tenderness.
    3. Guarding.
    4. Rigidity.
    5. May have signs of shock including:
        a. Tachycardia.
        b. Hypotension.
        c. Anuria.

Diagnostic Tests
A. Obtain complete blood count (CBC) and liver function tests (LFTs) in all suspected cases of PUD.
B. Use amylase or lipase to rule out other causes of epigastric pain.
C. Test for *H. pylori*.
D. Upper gastrointestinal (GI) endoscopy is the preferred diagnostic test in PUD.
    1. Differentiates gastric and duodenal ulcers.
    2. Allows for biopsy if indicated.
E. Angiography may be needed in cases with massive GI bleeding.
F. If Zollinger–Ellison syndrome is suspected, obtain serum gastrin level: If inconclusive, order secretin stimulation test.
G. Biopsy if concern for cancer.

Differential Diagnosis
A. Gastritis.
B. Gastroesophageal reflux disease (GERD).
C. Inflammatory bowel disease.
D. Cholecystitis.

E. Coronary artery disease.
F. Esophageal rupture.
G. Diverticulitis.
H. Pancreatitis.
I. Viral hepatitis.

Evaluation and Management Plan

A. General plan.

   1. Gastric ulcers can be staged according to Johnson classification.

      a. Type I—normal or decreased gastric acid secretion.

      b. Type II—combination of stomach and duodenal ulcers with normal or increased gastric acid secretion.

      c. Type III—prepyloric associated with normal or increased gastric acid secretion.

      d. Type IV—near gastroesophageal junction with normal or decreased gastric acid secretion.

   2. Treatment plans vary on the location of the peptic ulcer and clinical presentation.

   3. Typical treatment options include:

      a. Empiric antisecretory therapy.

      b. Triple therapy for *H. pylori* infection.

      c. Endoscopy 6 to 8 weeks after diagnosis to document healing of ulcers.

      d. Document *H. pylori* cure with noninvasive test.

         i. Urea breath test.

         ii. Fecal antigen test (complicated ulcers).

B. Patient/family teaching points.

   1. Avoid NSAIDs and aspirin.

   2. Reduce or eliminate alcohol.

   3. Smoking cessation.

   4. Reduce or eliminate caffeine from diet.

   5. Weight loss.

   6. Stress reduction.

C. Pharmacotherapy.

   1. *H. pylori* infection.

      a. Option 1—10 to 14 days of quadruple therapy.

         i. Bismuth.

         ii. Proton pump inhibitor.

         iii. Tetracycline.

         iv. Nitroimidazole.

      b. Option 2—10 to 14 days.

         i. Proton pump inhibitor.

         ii. Clarithromycin.

         iii. Amoxicillin.

         iv. Nitroimidazole.

      c. Option 3—10 to 14 days of triple therapy (no previous macrolide exposure and clarithromycin resistance low).

         i. Clarithromycin.

         ii. Proton pump inhibitor.

         iii. Amoxicillin or metronidazole.

      d. Other suggested options per guidelines.

   2. *H. pylori* infection persists.

      a. Avoid previously used antibiotics.

      b. Choose a new option from the aforementioned list.

D. Discharge instructions.

   1. Follow-up with primary care provider for long-term monitoring and further evaluation.

Follow-Up

A. Follow-up routinely with primary care provider to assure proper maintenance therapy is initiated and symptoms are controlled.
B. If *H. pylori* eradication is not achieved, antisecretory therapy should be recommended.

Consultation/Referral

A. Consult to gastroenterology for bleeding (hematemesis or melena), anemia, unexplained weight loss, associated vomiting, or family history of gastrointestinal cancer.
B. Surgical consultation for all bleeding ulcers or suspected perforations.
C. Urgent referral for sudden and severe onset of symptoms, which may indicate perforation.
D. Failure of medical management.

Special/Geriatric Considerations

A. NSAID-induced PUD may not be overtly symptomatic in elderly patients.
B. Elderly patients may also present with significantly less profound signs and symptoms of shock in the case of perforated ulcers.

Bibliography

Boparai, V., Rajagopalan, J., & Triadafilopoulos, G. (2008). Guide to the use of proton pump inhibitors in adult patients. *Drugs, 68*(7), 925–947. doi:10.2165/00003495-200868070-00004

Chey, W. D., Leontiadis, G. I., Howden, C. W., & Moss, S. F. (2017). ACG clinical guideline: Treatment of *Helicobacter pylori* infection. *The American Journal of Gastroenterology, 112*, 212–238. Retrieved from https://journals.lww.com/ajg/Abstract/2017/02000/ACG_Clinical_Guideline__Treatment_of_Helicobacter.12.aspx

Chey, W. D., & Wong, B. C. (2007). American College of Gastroenterology guideline on the management of *Helicobacter pylori* infection. *The American Journal of Gastroenterology, 102*(8), 1808–1825. Retrieved from https://journals.lww.com/ajg/Abstract/2007/08000/American_College_of_Gastroenterology_Guideline_on.36.aspx

Ford, A. C., Marwaha, A., Lim, A., & Moayyedi, P. (2010). What is the prevalence of clinically significant endoscopic findings in subjects with dyspepsia? Systematic review and meta-analysis. *Clinical Gastroenterology and Hepatology, 8*(10), 830–837.e2. doi:10.1016/j.cgh.2010.05.031

Leontiadis, G. I., Sreedharan, A., Dorward, S., Barton, P., Delaney, B., Howden, C. W., . . . Forman, D. (2007). Systematic reviews of the clinical effectiveness and cost-effectiveness of proton pump inhibitors in acute upper gastrointestinal bleeding. *Health Technology Assessment, 11*(51), 1–164. doi:10.3310/hta11510

Ramakrishnan, K., & Salinas, R. C. (2007). Peptic ulcer disease. *American Family Physician, 76*(7), 1005–1012. Retrieved from https://www.aafp.org/afp/2007/1001/p1005.html

Schubert, M. L., & Peura, D. A. (2008). Control of gastric acid secretion in health and disease. *Gastroenterology, 134*(7), 1842–1860. doi:10.1053/j.gastro.2008.05.021

Sung, J. J., Tsoi, K. K., Ma, T. K., Yung, M.-Y., Lau, J. Y., & Chiu, P. W. (2010). Causes of mortality in patients with peptic ulcer bleeding: A prospective cohort study of 10,428 cases. *The American Journal of Gastroenterology, 105*(1), 84–89. Retrieved from https://journals.lww.com/ajg/Abstract/2010/01000/Causes_of_Mortality_in_Patients_With_Peptic_Ulcer.15.aspx

5 Nephrology Guidelines

Acute Kidney Injury

Alexis Chettiar

Definition
A. Abrupt decline in renal function associated with an increase in nitrogen waste products over the course of a short time frame (hours to days).
B. Can be defined by the RIFLE criteria (also has implied staging built into the definition).
    1. Risk: Increase in serum creatinine 50% to 99% (increased SCreat ×1.5 or glomerular filtration rate [GFR] decrease >25%) OR Urine output less than 0.5 mL/kg/hr for 6 to 12 hours.
    2. Injury: Increase in serum creatinine 100% to 199% (increased SCreat ×2 or GFR decrease >50%) OR Urine output less than 0.5 mL/kg/hr for 12 to 24 hours.
    3. Failure—Increase in serum creatinine greater than 200% (increase SCreat ×3 GFR decrease >75% OR SCreat >4.0 mg/dL) OR increase in serum creatinine by 0.5 mg/dL to greater than 4.0 mg/dL OR urine output less than 0.3 mL/kg/hr for greater than 24 hours or anuria for greater than 12 hours OR Initiation of renal replacement therapy.
    4. Loss—Persistent acute renal failure (ARF) and complete loss of kidney function; need for renal replacement therapy for greater than 4 weeks.
    5. End-stage renal disease (ESRD)—End-stage kidney disease greater than 3 months; need for renal replacement therapy for greater than 3 months.

Incidence
A. The true incidence of acute kidney injury (AKI) is difficult to determine due to variation in diagnostic criteria.
B. The incidence is estimated at 1% to 25% of ICU patients.
    1. This increases the odds ratio of mortality from 2.2 to 8.8, depending on the AKI stage.
    2. Even small increases in serum creatinine are associated with a significant increase in mortality.

Pathogenesis
A. AKI is the reduction of renal blood flow and decrease of GFR typically from one of three main mechanisms.
    1. Prerenal: Decreased renal perfusion from hypotension or hypovolemia.
    2. Intrinsic: Renal failure from diseases of the kidney, with ischemic causes being the most common. May also result from medications and poorly controlled chronic kidney disease.
    3. Obstructive—build up of tubular pressure caused by an obstruction of the urinary tract.

Predisposing Factors
A. Prerenal.
    1. Hemorrhage.
    2. Diarrhea.
    3. Diuretics.
    4. Heart failure.
    5. Acute myocardial infarction (MI).
    6. Pulmonary embolus.
    7. Sepsis.
    8. Anaphylaxis.
    9. Medications, including nonsteroidal anti-inflammatory drugs (NSAIDs).
    10. Hepatorenal syndrome.
    11. Any condition that causes hypovolemia.
B. Intrinsic.
    1. Renal artery or vein obstruction.
    2. Severe hypertension.
    3. Atherosclerosis.
    4. Nephrotoxic medications (amphotericin B, NSAIDs, radiocontrast agents).
    5. Goodpasture's syndrome.
    6. Glomerulonephritis from lupus.
    7. Systemic diseases such as lymphoma, Sjögren's syndrome, leukemia.
C. Postrenal.
    1. Urinary stones.
    2. Strictures.
    3. Tumors of urinary tract.
    4. Thrombosis.

Subjective Data
A. Common complaints/symptoms.
    1. Usually asymptomatic.
        a. However, patients may experience symptoms related to the underlying cause of AKI (see section "Differential Diagnosis").
    2. If symptomatic, patients may complain of:
        a. Edema.
        b. Decreased urine output.
        c. Nausea.
        d. Anorexia.
B. Family and social history.
    1. May not be relevant; history of chronic kidney disease.
C. Review of systems.
    1. Ask patient about the presence of:

a. Any new medications, especially:
    i. Statins (rhabdomyolysis).
    ii. Antibiotics (nephrotoxicity, intrarenal AKI).
    iii. Angiotensin-converting enzyme (ACE) inhibitors or angiotensin receptor blockers (ARBs).
    iv. NSAIDs.
b. Chemotherapy treatment.
c. Exposure to toxic substances such as ethyl alcohol or ethylene glycol.
d. Changes in blood pressure or blood pressure management (prerenal AKI, vasculitis intrarenal AKI).
e. Blood loss or transfusion.
f. History of liver disease (cirrhotic prerenal AKI).
g. Recent or past history of thrombus or embolisms (prerenal AKI due to renal artery thrombosis).
h. History of renal artery stenosis.
i. Recent history of infectious disease (post infectious glomerulonephritis).
j. Recent procedures or diagnostic examinations involving the use of IV radiocontrast.
    i. Examples: Angiography or CT.
k. Extreme exercise or trauma (rhabdomyolysis).
l. History of myeloma.
    i. Bone pain.
    ii. Fractures.
    iii. Weight loss.
m. History of kidney stones or gout (acute tubular necrosis [ATN]) due to intratubular crystal deposition.
n. Rash (vasculitis).

Physical Examination

A. Skin.
    1. Livedo reticularis (systemic vasculitis).
        a. Digital ischemia.
        b. Butterfly rash.
        c. Palpable purpura.
    2. Maculopapular rash (allergic interstitial nephritis).
    3. Track marks (endocarditis).
    4. Mucosal or cartilaginous lesions (Wegener's granulomatosis).
    5. Skin turgor (hypovolemic AKI).
B. Ophthalmic examination.
    1. Conjunctival jaundice.
    2. Band keratopathy (hypercalcemia due to multiple myeloma).
    3. Symptoms of malignant hypertension.
        a. Papilledema.
        b. Flame-shaped hemorrhages.
    4. Atheroemboli (renal ischemia due to atheroemboli or renal artery thrombosis).
    5. Uveitis (interstitial nephritis/necrotizing vasculitis).
    6. Ocular palsy (ethylene glycol poisoning).
C. Ears.
        a. Hearing acuity (hearing loss related to aminoglycoside).
D. Cardiovascular system.
    1. Assessment of volume status (intra- and extra-vascular volume).
        a. Blood pressure and pulse: Sitting and standing.
        b. Jugular vein distention.
        c. S3 heart sounds (heart failure).
        d. Peripheral/dependent edema.
        e. Hourly intake and output records.
        f. Daily weight.

2. Heart rate/rhythm.
    a. Atrial fibrillation (thromboembolism, decreased cardiac output).
    b. Murmurs (endocarditis).
    c. Pericardial friction rub (endocarditis).
E. Pulmonary system.
    1. Auscultation of lung sounds.
        a. Pulmonary vascular congestion (congestive heart failure).
        b. Rales (pulmonary-renal syndromes).
    2. Hemoptysis.
    3. Respiratory rate and effort (congestive heart failure).
F. Abdomen.
    1. Pulsatile mass or bruit (atheroemboli).
    2. Abdominal or costovertebral angle tenderness (nephrolithiasis, renal artery thrombosis, renal vein thrombosis).
    3. Abdominal fluid wave (ascites, cirrhosis, or elevated intra-abdominal pressure).
    4. Symptoms of urinary obstruction.
        a. Pelvic/rectal masses.
        b. Prostatic hypertrophy.
        c. Distended bladder.

Diagnostic Tests

A. Comprehensive blood chemistry panel, with serum osmolality.
B. Complete blood count (CBC).
    1. Prolonged AKI causes nephrogenic anemia (due to reduced renal erythropoietin synthesis).
C. Renal ultrasound.
    1. Rule out hydronephrosis due to obstructive process.
    2. Assess underlying state of kidney mass and sclerosis.
D. 24-hour creatinine clearance.
    1. Gives an accurate assessment of current renal clearance. Serum creatinine is a late indicator of renal dysfunction.
E. Hourly urine output.
F. Urinalysis with microscopy.
    1. Granular, muddy casts in urine sediment suggest tubular necrosis.
    2. Oxalate crystals also observed in ATN.
    3. Eosinophils common in interstitial nephritis.
G. Urine sodium and osmolality.
H. Fractional Excretion of Sodium and Urea (FENa) helps differentiate cause of AKI in the presence of oliguria.
    1. $FENa = (U_{Na}/P_{Na})/(U_{Cr}/P_{Cr}) \times 100$.
        a. FENa less than 1% is usually prerenal azotemia.
        b. FENa greater than 1% is usually ATN caused by contrast, burns, rhabdomyolysis, or acute glomerulonephritis.
I. Further testing depends on the suspected cause of AKI.
J. Renal biopsy: May be indicated if the cause cannot be determined and renal function does not return for a prolonged period of time.

Differential Diagnosis

A. Prerenal.
    1. Hemorrhage.
    2. Volume depletion.
    3. Congestive heart failure.
    4. Cirrhosis.
    5. Renal artery.
    6. Stenosis.
    7. Thrombosis/embolism.
    8. NSAIDs.
    9. ACE inhibitor and ARB.

B. Intrarenal.
   1. ATN.
      a. Ischemic.
      b. Toxic.
         i. Exogenous.
            1) Antibiotics.
            2) Contrast.
            3) Chemotherapy.
         ii. Endogenous.
            1) Pigment (hemoglobinuria, myoglobinuria).
            2) Intratubular proteins (myeloma).
            3) Intratubular crystals (uric acid, oxalate).
   2. Acute interstitial nephritis.
      a. Drug associated.
      b. Acute glomerulonephritis.
      c. Post infectious.
      d. Vascular.
         i. Vasculitis.
         ii. Malignant hypertension.

C. Postrenal.
   1. Obstructive.
   2. Bladder outlet obstruction.
   3. Bilateral ureteral obstruction.

Evaluation and Management Plan

A. General plan.
   1. Use the ABCDE-IT mnemonic to quickly determine a treatment plan (see Box 5.1, AKI ABCDE-IT Mnemonic).
   2. Determine the stage of AKI using the RIFLE criteria and manage accordingly (see Figure 5.1, AKI Treatment Algorithm).
   3. Monitor serum creatinine.
   4. Avoid further renal insult.
   5. Ensure that blood pressure is in the target range (varies depending on the patient's age and comorbid disease status).
   6. Correct fluid overload to achieve volume homeostasis.
   7. Correct any acidosis or electrolyte abnormalities.

BOX 5.1

Acute Kidney Injury ABCDE-IT Mnemonic

- **A**ssess for acute complications (high potassium, acidosis, fluid overload).
- **B**P check (if systolic BP <110, consider fluid challenge).
- **C**atheterize (to eliminate postbladder obstructive process and monitor I/O).
- **D**rugs; stop/avoid nephrotoxins, hold ACE inhibitors.
- **E**xclude obstruction (Renal US).
- **I**nvestigations; urinalysis with micro, for stage 2/3 AKI add ANCA, AntiGBM Ab, DSDNA, ANA, immunoglobulin, electrophoresis.
- **T**reat the cause.

ACE, angiotensin-converting enzyme; AKI, acute kidney injury; ANA, antinuclear antibody; ANCA; antineutrophil cytoplasmic antibodies; BP, blood pressure; DSDNA, double stranded deoxyribonucleic acid; US, ultrasound

---

B. Patient/family teaching points.
   1. Signs/symptoms to monitor: Edema, headache, dizziness, or syncope.
   2. Common occurrences: Hypotension or hypertension.
   3. Readmission concerns.
      a. Recurrent AKI due to secondary renal insult that is often due to inappropriate resumption of medications (ACE inhibitors/ARBs, NSAIDs) or hypotension/hypertension.
      b. Patients should be clear about which medications to hold/restart after discharge and check home blood pressure. If the patient is able to check home blood pressure, provide high and low parameters for reporting readings.
      c. These parameters will vary according to the clinical context, but generally patients should call the provider to report a systolic blood pressure less than 130 mmHg, systolic blood pressure greater than 180 mmHg, and diastolic blood pressure greater than 100 mmHg.
      d. Renal vasculature is sensitive to blood pressure fluctuations in the recovery phase of AKI, and hypotension or hypertension can precipitate further renal injury.
C. Pharmacotherapy.
   1. No pharmacotherapy treatment in AKI. The primary cause must be reversed.
   2. Intravenous isotonic sodium chloride solution should be used to maintain euvolemia as clinically indicated.
   3. Medications.

   a. Hold ACE inhibitors, ARBs, NSAIDs, and any other medications associated with renal insult (e.g., nephrotoxic chemotherapy, aminoglycoside, and beta lactam antibiotics) until patient's serum creatinine has stabilized at baseline.
   b. Note that renal dose dopamine may cause some dilatation to enhance renal perfusion. However, no study has been able to demonstrate a beneficial role of vasodilator use.
D. Discharge instructions.
   1. Serum creatinine has either returned to baseline OR,
   2. It has significantly improved with a downward trend and resolution of AKI etiology.

Follow-Up

A. Monitor.
   1. Serum creatinine and electrolytes.
   2. Urine output.
   3. Volume status.
B. Pursue other follow-up as indicated specific to the underlying cause of the AKI.
C. Check creatinine within 1 to 2 weeks after discharge to confirm improvement.
D. If medications are on hold due to AKI, follow to determine when medications should be restarted.

Consultation/Referral

A. Early nephrology consultation should occur after hospitalization.

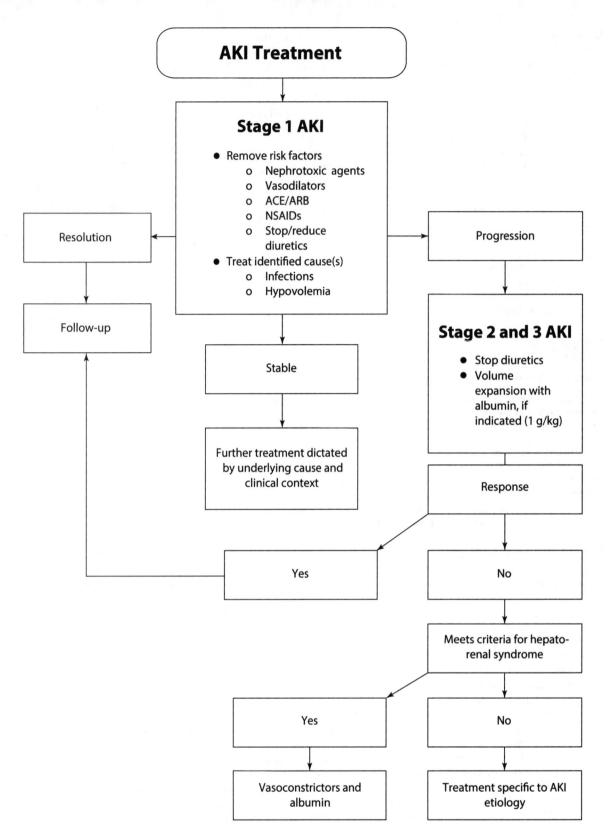

FIGURE 5.1 Acute kidney injury treatment algorithm.
ACE, angiotensin-converting enzyme; AKI, acute kidney injury; ARB, angiotensin II receptor blockers; NSAIDs, nonsteroidal anti-inflammatory drugs.

Special/Geriatric Considerations

A. Geriatric considerations.

  1. Elderly patients are at high risk for AKI, particularly those treated with diuretics, ACE inhibitors, ARBs, and NSAIDs.

  2. Serum creatinine in elderly patients with diminished muscle mass underestimates the extent of renal impairment.

Bibliography

Brivet, F. G., Kleinknecht, D. J., Loirat, P., & Landais, P. J. (1996). Acute renal failure in intensive care units–causes, outcome, and prognostic factors of hospital mortality: A prospective, multicenter study. French Study Group on Acute Renal Failure. *Critical Care Medicine, 24*(2), 192–198. doi:10.1097/00003246-199602000-00003

Hoste, E. A. J., Clermont, G., Kersten, A., Venkataraman, R., Angus, D. C., De Bacquer, D., & Kellum, J. A. (2006). RIFLE criteria for acute kidney injury are associated with hospital mortality in critically ill patients: A cohort analysis. *Critical Care, 10*(3), R73. doi:10.1186/cc4915

Kidney Disease, Improving Global Outcomes. (2012). *KDIGO clinical practice guideline for acute kidney injury.* Cranford, NJ: International Society of Nephrology. Retrieved from https://kdigo.org/wp-content/uploads/2016/10/KDIGO-2012-AKI-Guideline-English.pdf

Leblanc, M., Kellum, J. A., Gibney, R. T. N., Lieberthal, W., Tumlin, J., & Mehta, R. (2005). Risk factors for acute renal failure: Inherent and modifiable risks. *Current Opinion in Critical Care, 11*(6), 533–536. doi:10.1097/01.ccx.0000183666.54717.3d

Liaño, F., & Pascual, J. (1996). Epidemiology of acute renal failure: A prospective, multicenter, community-based study. Madrid Acute Renal Failure Study Group. *Kidney International, 50*(3), 811–818. doi:10.1038/ki.1996.380

Thakar, C. V., Christianson, A., Freyberg, R., Almenoff, P., & Render, M. L. (2009). Incidence and outcomes of acute kidney injury in intensive care units: A Veterans Administration study*. *Critical Care Medicine, 37*(9), 2552–2558. doi:10.1097/CCM.0b013e3181a5906f

Uchino, S. (2005). Acute renal failure in critically ill patients: A multinational, multicenter study. *Journal of the American Medical Association, 294*(7), 813. doi:10.1001/jama.294.7.813

Benign Prostatic Hypertrophy

Suzanne Barron

Definition

A. A histological change that develops within the prostate gland, which may lead to the presence of an enlarged prostate gland and associated lower urinary tract symptoms.

Incidence

A. 50% of men over the age of 40 develop histologic evidence of benign prostatic hypertrophy (BPH).
    1. 30%–50% of these men develop bothersome lower urinary tract symptoms (LUTS).
B. Prevalence of BPH increases with age.
    1. 60% for men in their 60s.
    2. Up to 90% for men in their 70s and 80s.

Pathogenesis

A. There is abnormal microscopic hyperplasia and macroscopic growth.
B. The detrusor muscle generates higher pressures, leading to frequency, urgency, and nocturia.
C. BPH may lead to bladder decompensation, with the bladder muscle no longer able to provide enough pressure to urinate.
D. The role of hormonal involvement in the development of BPH is still poorly understood, but there is evidence that the hormone androgen, which becomes dihydrotestosterone (DHT), plays a critical role in the growth of prostatic tissue.

Predisposing Factors

A. Advancing age.
B. Family history of BPH.
C. Ethnic background.
    1. The risk of BPH is higher in black and Hispanic men than in white men and Asian men.
D. Diabetes and heart disease: Possible increased incidence in BPH.
E. Obesity: Possible association with increased prostate volume and LUTS.

Subjective Data

A. Common complaints/symptoms: LUTS.
    1. Storage symptoms or irritative voiding symptoms: Frequency, nocturia, dysuria, decreased volume, urgency, or urge incontinence.
    2. Voiding symptoms or obstructive voiding symptoms: Weak stream, intermittent stream, hesitancy, retention, abdominal straining, incomplete emptying, or post void dribbling.
B. Common/typical scenario.
    1. Onset is gradual, with symptoms increasing over time.
    2. Symptoms are often aggravated at night with significant nocturia, which may often cause difficulty sleeping.
    3. Symptoms may be aggravated by cough/cold medications (antihistamines, pseudoephedrine).
C. Family and social history.
    1. Increased likelihood if father or brother have history of BPH.
    2. Increased physical activity: Possible protection against BPH.
D. Review of systems.
    1. Constitutional: Weight loss or insomnia.
    2. Neurological: Dizziness, weakness, tremors, or other signs that may indicate a neurological condition such as multiple sclerosis or Parkinson's disease.
    3. Genitourinary: LUTS; usually no flank pain.
        a. Possible report of suprapubic fullness/tenderness.
        b. Hematuria: Possible indication of genitourinary malignancy (bladder cancer).
    4. Cardiovascular: Lower extremity edema that may indicate heart failure or diuretic use.
    5. Endocrine: Polyuria, polyphagia, or polydipsia that may indicate diabetes mellitus or diabetes insipidus.

Physical Examination

A. Neurological.
    1. Evaluate for musculoskeletal weakness, especially lower extremity motor and sensory function.
    2. Evaluate gait.
B. Digital rectal examination (DRE).
    1. To estimate prostate size, assess for prostatitis, or evaluate prostate nodules that may indicate prostate cancer.
    2. Assess for anal sphincter tone; if absent or decreased, possible neurological disorder.
C. Abdominal.
    1. Palpate for masses that may be pressing on the bladder.
D. Genitourinary.
    1. Assess for costovertebral angle tenderness.
    2. Assess for obvious urethral strictures and phimosis.

Diagnostic Tests

A. Urinalysis to exclude hematuria or possible infection.
B. Blood work.
    1. Prostate specific antigen (PSA), especially if prostatic nodules are palpated on DRE or high concern for prostate cancer.
    2. Basic metabolic panel to assess for renal function, electrolyte abnormalities, and hyperglycemia.
C. Imaging: CT or MRI generally not indicated.
D. Uroflowmetry: Measures the volume/time of urine accumulation.
E. Post void residual: Volume of urine remaining in bladder after voiding.
    1. Obtain from bladder ultrasound/bladder scan if possible.
    2. Straight catheterization if bladder ultrasound not available.
F. Urodynamic study to differentiate between bladder outlet obstruction and hypocontractile bladder. This may be necessary prior to surgical intervention for BPH.

Differential Diagnosis

A. Foreign body in urethra/bladder (stone or retained ureteral stents)

B. Meatal stenosis.

C. Urethral stricture.

D. Detrusor sphincter dyssynergia.

E. Neurogenic bladder (e.g., multiple sclerosis, Parkinson's disease).

F. Bladder cancer.

G. Prostate cancer.

H. Overactive bladder.

I. Interstitial cystitis.

J. Infectious source: Acute cystitis, acute prostatitis/chronic prostatitis, or prostatic abscess.

K. Pelvic floor dysfunction.

L. Radiation cystitis.

M. Diabetes insipidus causing polyuria.

N. Diabetes mellitus causing polyuria.

Evaluation and Management Plan

A. General plan.

   1. Obtain urinalysis/urine culture.

   2. Obtain PSA if concern for prostate cancer.

   3. Place Foley catheter for urinary retention or teach patient how to perform clean intermittent catheterization.

   4. Observe for post obstructive diuresis with urinary retention.

   5. Advise watchful waiting, with no treatment for men with mild symptoms and good quality of life.

   6. Use pharmacotherapy: Alpha blockers or 5-alpha-reductase inhibitors (5-ARIs).

   7. Obtain prostate biopsy if elevated PSA or prostatic nodule.

   8. Order uroflowmetry/post void residual.

   9. Order urodynamic study if indicated.

   10. Advise surgery if indicated.

B. Patient/family teaching points.

   1. Have a thorough discussion with patient and family about the usefulness of PSA screening test in detecting prostate cancer.

      a. If the PSA is elevated, this will prompt prostate biopsy and possible treatment for prostate cancer, which may be a slow-growing disease.

      b. In 2010, the U.S. Preventive Task Force recommended against PSA screening, stating that the test has no net benefit and that the harms outweigh benefits. The American Urologic Association in 2013 also started to recommend against routine cancer screening.

   2. Discuss keeping a voiding diary.

   3. Discuss possible side effects of medical therapy, including orthostatic hypotension, dizziness, and retrograde ejaculation.

   4. Educate the patient with retention regarding how to perform clean intermittent catheterization because this is a better alternative to an indwelling Foley catheter.

   5. Avoid becoming constipated because this aggravates symptoms.

C. Pharmacotherapy.

   1. Alpha blockers, which rapidly relax the smooth muscles of the bladder neck and prostate without impairing bladder body contractility.

      a. Most commonly used: Tamsulosin 0.4 mg daily (max 0.8 mg daily).

   2. 5-ARIs, which block intracellular DHT conversion.

      a. Best for larger prostate glands (>40 mL).

      b. Most commonly used: Finasteride 5 mg.

   3. Antimuscarinic agents, which help with bladder over-activity.

      a. Most commonly used: Oxybutynin 5 mg TID.

   4. Phosphodiesterase-5 inhibitor, which is Food and Drug Administration (FDA) approved for LUTS secondary to BPH.

      a. Tadalafil (Cialis): 2.5 to 5 mg; contraindicated in men taking nitrates, nonselective alpha blockers, and cytochrome P 450 inhibitors.

D. Discharge instructions.

   1. Advise patients to limit caffeine, fluids, and alcohol. These may increase LUTS.

   2. Advise them to avoid cold medications, antihistamines, and pseudoephedrine.

   3. Advise them to seek medical attention if they are unable to void or have flank pain, gross hematuria, or passage of clots.

   4. Advise them to discontinue alpha blockers with dizziness, lightheadedness, or falls.

Follow-Up

A. Monitor response to treatment with uroflowmetry, post void residual, and presence of symptoms.

B. Advise that urodynamic studies may be indicated if there is no improvement of symptoms with medical therapy.

C. Advise that surgery may provide relief in the case of excessive symptoms refractory to medical management. Some of the more common options include:

   1. Transurethral resection of the prostate (TURP).

   2. Holmium laser enucleation of the prostate (HoLEP).

   3. Simple prostatectomy for large prostates greater than 100 mL.

Consultation/Referral

A. Urology.

   1. Urinary retention.

   2. Hematuria/clot retention.

   3. PSA elevation, will need prostate biopsy.

   4. Suspected genitourinary malignancy.

   5. Failed medical treatment with moderate to severe symptoms.

B. Neurology: With any concern for neurological condition that may be causing LUTS.

C. Endocrinology.

   1. For hyperglycemia.

   2. Concern for diabetes insipidus.

Special/Geriatric Considerations

A. Many patients limit fluids due to symptoms; this may lead to dehydration, especially in geriatric individuals. Assess for dehydration and provide education to maintain a normal fluid intake.

B. Monitor the geriatric population for medication side effects.

   1. Alpha-blockers: Hypotension and dizziness.

   2. Anti-muscarinic agents: Dry mouth, constipation, and mental status changes.

      a. Monitor for polypharmacy with other possible anticholinergic medications that patients may be prescribed or taking over the counter.

b. Studies have shown that transdermal oxybutynin and the newer anticholinergics may be better tolerated.

Bibliography

Deters, L. A. (2019, January 15). Benign prostatic hypertrophy (BPH) differential diagnoses. , In E. D. Kim (Ed.), *Medscape*. Retrieved from http://emedicine.medscape.com/article/437359-differential

Kim, E. H., Larson, J. A., & Andriole, G. L. (2016). Management of benign prostatic hyperplasia. *Annual Review of Medicine, 67,* 137–151. doi:10.1146/annurev-med-063014-123902.

Nicholson, T., & Ricke, W. (2011, November-December). Androgens and estrogens in benign prostatic hyperplasia, past, present and future. *National Institutes of Health, 82*(4–5), 184–189. Retrieved from https://www.ncbi.nlm.nih.gov/pmc/articles/PMC3179830

Chronic Kidney Disease

Jane S. Davis, Kim Zuber, and Christine M. Chmielewski

Definition

A. Reduction of kidney function: An estimated glomerular filtration rate (GFR) less than 60 mL/min/1.73 m^2 for greater than 3 months.

OR

B. Evidence of kidney damage, including persistent albuminuria—defined as greater than 30 mg of urine albumin per gram of urine creatinine for greater than 3 months.
   1. Anatomical abnormalities including, but not limited to, polycystic kidneys, kidney transplant, and genetic abnormalities.
   2. Chronic kidney disease (CKD) versus acute kidney injury (AKI). A 3-month time frame is used to distinguish CKD from AKI.

C. Classification.
   1. CKD stages are defined by a presence of albuminuria and the GFR (see Table 5.1).
   2. The GFR requires age, race, gender, and serum creatinine for calculation.

TABLE 5.1 Stages of CKD

Stage of CKD	GFR (mL/min/1.73 m²)	Albuminuria
1	≥90	Normal or high
2	60–89	Mildly decreased
3a	45–59	Mildly to moderately decreased
3b	30–44	Moderately to severely decreased
4	15–29	Severely decreased
5	<15	Kidney failure/ESRD
Albuminuria categories in CKD (ACR in mg/g)		
A1	<30	Normal to mildly increased
A2	30–300	Moderately increased
A3	>300	Severely increased

Notes: ACR, albumin-to-creatinine ratio; CKD, chronic kidney disease; ESRD, end-stage renal disease; GFR, glomerular filtration rate.

Incidence

A. It is estimated that approximately 14.8% of the adults in the United States have CKD.

B. Approximately 96% of those with mild to moderate reduced kidney function are unaware that they have CKD.

C. Approximately 48% of those with severely reduced kidney function are unaware that they have CKD.

D. Approximately 661,000 individuals in the United States have end-stage renal disease (ESRD); of these, 468,000 are on dialysis and 193,000 have a functioning kidney transplant.

Pathogenesis

A. Initial kidney injury or insult leads to the loss of functioning nephrons (nephron loss).

B. Hyperfiltration of the remaining intact nephrons occurs (glomerular hypertrophy).

C. Initial beneficial, adaptive response leads to ongoing damage (interstitial inflammation, fibrosis, and endothelial/vascular injury).

D. This injury eventually leads to further nephron loss (disease progression).

Predisposing Factors

A. General risk factors.
   1. Diabetes mellitus.
   2. Hypertension.
   3. Cardiovascular disease (CVD).
   4. History of kidney disease.
   5. Family history of CKD.
   6. Race/ethnicity.
      a. African Americans.
      b. Hispanics.
      c. Native Americans.
      d. Asians.
   7. AKI.
   8. Older age.
   9. Smoking.
   10. Exposure to nephrotoxins.
   11. Obesity.

B. Risk factors for progression of CKD to next stage.
   1. Male gender.
   2. African American race.
   3. Diabetes mellitus.
   4. Hypertension.
   5. Proteinuria.
   6. Prior trajectory of kidney function.

Subjective Data

A. Common complaints/symptoms.
   1. Often silent.
   2. Lethargy due to low hemoglobin.
   3. Metallic taste due to uremia.
   4. Increased incidence of confusion with uremia.
   5. Edema.

B. Medication history.
   1. Medication review.
      a. Prescription drugs.
      b. Over-the-counter drugs.
      c. Herbal supplements.
   2. Medication-associated risk.
      a. Clearance by kidney.
      b. Narrow therapeutic window.

    c. High risk in older population.

    d. Potential central nervous system (CNS) effects.

    e. Drug dosing data availability.

C. Review of systems.

  1. Constitutional: Change in activity, appetite changes.

  2. Head, ear, eyes, nose, and throat (HEENT): Changes in vision, facial swelling, nosebleeds.

  3. Cardiovascular: Any pain in chest.

  4. Respiratory: Difficulty breathing.

  5. Gastrointestinal: Nausea or vomiting, hiccups, blood in stool.

  6. Genitourinary: Difficulty urinating or pain on urination.

  7. Musculoskeletal: Back pain, muscle cramps.

  8. Neurological: Dizziness or balance problems.

  9. Integumentary: Dry skin, itching, or rash.

  10. Psychiatric: Confusion or difficulty concentrating, sleep disturbance.

  11. Endocrine: Cold intolerance.

  12. Hematologic: Bruising easily.

Physical Examination

A. Vital signs, including orthostatic signs.

B. Constitutional.

C. Eyes: Funduscopic examination.

  1. Look for retinopathy secondary to diabetes mellitus.

D. Cardiovascular: Palpitations, dysrhythmia, tachycardia, heart sounds (S3 and S4, murmurs, rubs), distal pulses, lower extremity edema, carotid bruit, jugular venous distension (JVD).

E. Pulmonary: Breath sounds, effort (use of accessory muscles), wheezing.

F. Abdominal: Abdominal palpation, bowel sounds, dysgeusia, melena.

G. Genitourinary: Dysuria, flank pain, proteinuria, hematuria, oliguria, anuria.

H. Musculoskeletal: Arthralgias, gait disturbances, myalgias.

I. Integumentary/nails: Rash, pruritus, uremia.

J. Confusion, asterixis.

K. Endocrine: Polydipsia, polyphagia, polyuria.

L. Hematologic/lymphatic: Bruising, petechiae, ecchymosis.

Diagnostic Tests

A. Renal function panel.

B. Complete blood count (CBC) with differential.

C. Serum albumin.

D. Fasting lipid panel.

E. Urinalysis.

F. Urine albumin to creatinine ratio (UACR).

G. Urine culture and sensitivity (C & S; if indicated).

H. Renal ultrasound with post void residual.

I. Specialty serologic studies if indicated: Antinuclear antibody (ANA), C3, C4, hepatitis B and C serologies.

J. CKD mineral bone disorder: Calcium, phosphorus, intact parathyroid hormone (PTH), 25(OH) vitamin D.

K. Anemia.

  1. Microcytic: Iron studies (iron, total iron-binding capacity [TIBC], ferritin).

  2. Macrocytic: Folate and B_{12} levels.

L. Multiple myeloma/paraprotein.

  1. Serum protein electrophoresis (SPEP), urine protein electrophoresis (UPEP).

  2. Serum and urine for immunoelectrophoresis.

  3. Serum for free light chains.

M. Renal biopsy: Reserved to guide management or when the cause of CKD is unclear.

Differential Diagnosis

A. AKI.

  1. Prerenal.

  2. Intrinsic.

  3. Postrenal.

B. Multiple myeloma.

C. Nephrolithiasis.

D. Diabetic nephropathy.

E. Glomerulonephritis.

Evaluation and Management Plan

A. General plan.

  1. Determine CKD stage (see Table 5.2).

    a. CKD Stage 1: Manage comorbid conditions and identify CVD risk factors.

    b. CKD Stage 2: Monitor CKD progression.

    c. CKD Stages 3a and 3b: Treat CKD complications.

    d. CKD Stage 4: Refer to nephrology.

    e. CKD Stage 5: Start kidney replacement therapy (KRT).

  2. Manage complications.

    a. Acidosis.

    b. Anemia.

    c. Hypertension.

    d. CKD mineral bone disorder.

    e. Dyslipidemia.

    f. Diabetic complications: Indications for initiation of dialysis.

      i. Hyperkalemia.

      ii. Uremic pericarditis.

      iii. Refractory metabolic acidosis.

      iv. Volume overload.

      v. Pulmonary edema.

      vi. Uremic encephalopathy.

      vii. Refractory hypertension.

      viii. Persistent nausea and vomiting.

      ix. Blood urea nitrogen (BUN) greater than 100 mg/dL.

B. Patient/family teaching points.

  1. Patient-centered educational efforts: A conceptual model.

    a. Prevent kidney disease.

      i. Awareness of risk.

      ii. Knowledge of prevention.

    b. Identify kidney disease.

      i. Awareness of diagnosis.

      ii. Knowledge of health implications.

    c. Manage kidney disease.

      i. Knowledge of management goals and how to achieve them.

    d. Comprehensive conservative care for ESRD.

      i. Knowledge of treatments, risks, benefits, and management goals.

  2. Dietary modifications.

    a. Sodium intake: Less than 2 g/day.

    b. Potassium intake: 2 g/day.

    c. Protein intake.

      i. Avoid high protein intake.

      ii. Lower protein intake to 0.8 g/kg/day in adults with diabetes or without diabetes and a GFR less than 30 mL/min/ 1.73 m^2.

    d. Phosphorus intake: 800 to 1,000 mg/day.

TABLE 5.2 **Stages of CKD With Monitoring Recommendations**

CKD classified based on: • GFR (G) • Albuminuria (A) KDIGO 2012				Albuminuria categories Description and range		
				A1	A2	A3
				Normal to mildly increased	Moderately increased	Severely increased
				<30 mg/g <3 mg/mmol	30–299 mg/g 3–29 mg/mmol	≥300 mg/g ≥30 mg/mmol
GFR categories (mL/min/1.73 m² Description and range	G1	Normal or high	≥90	Monitor 1	Monitor 1	Refer* 2
	G2	Mildly decreased	60–90	Monitor 1	Monitor 1	Refer* 2
	G3a	Mildly to moderately decreased	45–59	Monitor 1	Monitor 2	Refer 3
	G3b	Moderately to severely decreased	30–44	Monitor 2	Monitor 3	Refer 3
	G4	Severely decreased	15–29	Refer* 3	Refer* 3	Refer* 4+
	G5	Kidney failure	<15	Refer* 4+	Refer* 4+	Refer* 4+

Shades: Represents the risk for progression, morbidity, and mortality by shades, from best to worst.
White: Low risk (if no other markers of kidney disease, no CKD). **Light gray:** Moderately increased risk. **Medium gray:** High risk. **Dark gray:** Very high risk. **Black:** High risk +4 times per year.
Numbers: Represent a recommendation for the number of times per year the patient should be monitored.
Refer: Indicates that nephrology referral and services are recommended.
CKD, chronic kidney disease; GFR, glomerular filtration rate; KDIGO, Kidney Disease: Improving Global Outcomes.
*Referring clinicians may wish to discuss with their nephrology service depending on local arrangements regarding monitoring or referral.
Source: Modified with permission from KDIGO. (2012). Clinical practice guideline for the evaluation and management of chronic kidney disease. *Kidney Int, 2013*(Suppl. 3), 1–150.

e. Diabetes dietary guidelines: Target hemoglobin A1c (HbA1c) of ~7.0%.
f. Target HbA1c can be extended above 7.0% (53 mmol/mol) in individuals with comorbidities or limited life expectancy and risk of hypoglycemia.
g. Hyperlipidemia dietary modifications.
    i. Decrease intake of saturated and trans fat foods.
    ii. Substitute with monounsaturated fats and moderate intake of polyunsaturated fats.
C. Pharmacotherapy: Targeted at preventing complications.
1. Acidosis: Maintenance of carbon dioxide/bicarbonate level with sodium citrate tablets.
2. Anemia: Performance of iron studies to determine iron supplementation plan.
    a. Ferrous sulfate tablets.
    b. Folic acid replacement tablets.
    c. Cobalamin for vitamin B_{12} replacement/supplementation.
    d. Erythropoiesis stimulating agents (not recommended in patients with active malignancy or recent history of malignancy).
3. Hypertension: CKD with or without diabetes: Use an angiotensin-converting enzyme (ACE) inhibitor or an angiotensin receptor blocker (ARB).

    a. Obtain a baseline serum creatinine and serum potassium and follow.
    b. Recheck those levels 1 week after starting or increasing dose to avoid further decreases in GFR and/or hyperkalemia.
4. CKD mineral bone disorder: Follow common minerals and replace as needed.
    a. Phosphate binders: Example of calcium-based binders is calcium acetate.
    b. Vitamin D replacement.
    c. Bisphosphonates (avoid in CKD with GFR less than 30 mL/min/1.73 m²).
5. Dyslipidemia: Lipid lowering agent.
6. Diabetic complications: Keep HbA1c ~7%.
7. Malnutrition: High biologic value protein intake.
8. Proteinuria: ACE inhibitor/ARB or non dihydropyridine calcium channel blocker.

Follow-Up

A. Follow-up in CKD is important to mitigate progression of disease and to manage risk factors that may contribute to worsening of the patient's clinical health.
B. A nephrologist should be consulted if there is an increase in urine protein or abrupt decline in GFR.

C. Regular visits with a primary provider are essential for long-term health maintenance.

Consultation/Referral

A. Consult nephrology in the acute care setting for patients with the following.

1. An estimated GFR less than 30 mL/min/1.73 m^2.
2. Significant albuminuria or overt proteinuria.
3. An abrupt decrease in estimated GFR/acute rise in serum creatinine.
4. Evidence of worsening kidney function/CKD progression.
5. Persistent hematuria.
6. Resistant hypertension.

Special/Geriatric Considerations

A. The incidence of cardiovascular death increases with each stage of CKD. Individuals are more likely to die than to reach the next stage of CKD. In addition, the incidence of death related to cardiovascular procedures increases with CKD stage.

B. The incidence of hospitalization increases with CKD stage, although in the past 10 years, the number of hospitalizations has decreased.

C. It is important to identify CKD in hospitalized patients because it is an important prognostic factor for increased risk of in-hospital AKI.

D. The incidence of CKD and AKI increase with age.

1. Polypharmacy is more common in the elderly. It is important to review medications regularly to identify medications that are actual or potential nephrotoxins that require dose or schedule changes, as these should be avoided.

E. Older individuals have an increased prevalence of decreased estimated GFR and increased ACR.

1. There is a debate concerning whether decreased GFR or increased urine albumin-to-creatinine ratio in older individuals represents disease or normal aging.

Bibliography

Alleman, K., & Houle, K. (2015). Module 6. The APRN's approaches to care in nephrology. In C. S. Counts (Ed.), *Core curriculum for nephrology nursing* (6th ed., pp. 1–206). Pitman, NJ: AJ Jannetti, Inc.

Fliss, E. M., Burns, A., Moranne, O., Morton, R. L., & Naicker, S. (2016). Supportive care: Comprehensive care in end-stage kidney disease. *Clinical Journal of the American Society of Nephrology, 11*(10), 1909–1914. doi:10.2215/CJN.04840516

Jayadevappa, R., & Chhatre, S. (2011). Patient centered care—A conceptual model and review of the state of the art. *Open Health Services and Policy Journal, 4*, 15–25. doi:10.2174/1874924001104010015

Kidney Disease: Improving Global Outcomes (KDIGO) Anemia Work Group. (2012). KDIGO clinical practice guideline for anemia in chronic kidney disease. *Kidney International, 2*(Suppl.), 279–335. doi:10.1038/ki.2012.270

Kidney Disease: Improving Global Outcomes CKD-MBD Work Group. (2009). KDIGO clinical practice guideline for the diagnosis, evaluation, prevention, and treatment of chronic kidney disease—mineral and bone disorder (CKD-MBD). *Kidney International, 76*(113 Suppl), S1–S130.

Kidney Disease: Improving Global Outcomes CKD Work Group. (2013). KDIGO 2012 clinical practice guideline for the evaluation and management of chronic kidney disease. *Kidney International, 3*(1 Suppl. 3), 1–150.

Kidney Disease: Improving Global Outcomes Lipid Work Group. (2013). KDIGO clinical practice guideline for lipid management in chronic kidney disease. *Kidney International, 3*(Suppl. 3), 1–305.

National Kidney Disease Education Program. (2014, July). *Making sense of CKD a concise guide for managing chronic kidney disease in the primary care setting.* Bethesda, MD: National Institutes of Health.

Nissenson, A. R., & Fine, R. N. (2017). *Handbook of dialysis therapy* (5th ed.). Philadelphia, PA: Elsevier.

Ponnaluri, S., & King, M. J. (2016). A retrospective study of research data on end stage renal disease. *Journal of Emerging Investigators, 5.* doi:10.1177/2054358118799689

Rosenberg, M. (2018, June 29). Overview of the management of chronic kidney disease in adults. In S. Motwani (Ed.), *UpToDate.* Retrieved from https://www.uptodate.com/contents/overview-of-the-management-of-chronic-kidney-disease-in-adults

Shingarev, R., Wille, K., & Tolwani, A. (2011). Management of complications in renal replacement therapy. *Seminars in Dialysis, 24*(2), 164–168. doi:10.1111/j.1525-139X.2011.00828.x

U.S. Renal Data System. (2014). *USRDS 2014 annual data report: Atlas of chronic kidney disease and end-stage renal disease in the United States.* Bethesda, MD: National Institutes of Health, National Institute of Diabetes and Digestive and Kidney Diseases.

Weir, M. R., & Fink, J. C. (2014). Safety of medical therapy in patients with chronic kidney disease and end-stage renal disease. *Current Opinion in Nephrology Hypertension, 23*(3), 306–313. doi:10.1097/01.mnh.0000444912.40418.45

Hematuria

Suzanne Barron

Definition

A. Gross hematuria: Visible blood in the urine.

1. Visible blood in the urine may be seen with as little as 1 mL of blood in 1 L of urine.

B. Microscopic hematuria: Greater than three red blood cells (RBCs) per high power field in a single urinalysis.

Incidence

A. Population-based studies have shown prevalence rates of less than 1% to as high as 16%.

B. Older men have a higher prevalence of hematuria.

C. Associated conditions.

1. No diagnosis after workup: 60.5%.
2. Urinary tract infection (UTI): 13%.
3. Stone disease: 3.6%.
4. Cancer: 13%.
5. Glomerular disease: 9.8%.

Pathogenesis

A. Glomerular or nephronal hematuria (originates from nephron).

1. On microscopic evaluation, RBCs that are dysmorphic (irregular shapes and uneven hemoglobin distribution) often represent glomerular disease. There may be casts.
2. On urinalysis, the combination of RBCs and proteinuria most often indicates a glomerular source of hematuria.

B. Extraglomerular hematuria (originates from urologic source): Anything that disrupts the genitourinary (GU) epithelium, which may include irritation, trauma, inflammation, or invasion.

1. On microscopic evaluation, the RBCs in the urine are isomorphic; have smooth, round membranes; and display even hemoglobin distribution.
2. Associated conditions include tumors, kidney stones, trauma, infection, anatomic abnormalities of the urinary tract such as ureteropelvic junction obstruction, and benign prostatic hypertrophy (BPH).

Predisposing Factors

A. Age greater than 35.

B. Smoking history.

C. Recent trauma.
D. Recent urinary tract surgery or instrumentation.
E. BPH.
F. Family history of renal disease.
G. Personal history of nephrolithiasis.
H. Pelvic radiation.
I. Recent febrile illness.
J. Frequent UTIs.
K. Occupational exposure to chemicals and dyes (benzenes or aromatic amines).
L. Medications (abuse of analgesics such as nonsteroidal anti-inflammatory drugs [NSAIDs]).
M. Chronic indwelling catheters (Foley, suprapubic tube).

Subjective Data

A. Common complaints/symptoms.
  1. Flank pain: Possible recent trauma, stones, renal cancer, ureteral tumor, or pyelonephritis.
  2. Dysuria/lower urinary tract symptoms (LUTS) such as urgency/frequency and urinary retention: Possible UTI/prostatitis, BPH, or bladder stones.
  3. Fever: Possible UTI, prostatitis, or pyelonephritis.
  4. Worm-like (vermiform) clots: Possible origin from upper urinary tract.
B. Common/typical scenario.
  1. Visual appearance of blood in the urine or presence with microscopic hematuria.
  2. Timing of hematuria during urinary stream: May indicate the site of pathology (i.e., initiation of stream—anterior urethral pathology; termination of stream—bladder neck, prostate, or urethra inflammation/pathology; throughout stream—bladder or upper urinary tract origin).
  3. Aggravating factors.
    a. Pain, recent trauma, or recent vigorous activity/exercise.
    b. Recent upper respiratory infection (associated with glomerulonephritis).
    c. Ingestion of certain foods and drugs (pseudohematuria).
    d. Excessive use of analgesics such as NSAIDs.
C. Family and social history.
  1. Smoking (past or present).
  2. Excessive ingestion of barbecued/smoked foods (associated with link to bladder cancer).
  3. Sexual history (recent sexually transmitted infections [STIs]).
  4. Work history: Exposure to chemicals and dyes in rubber and/or petroleum industries (associated with bladder cancer).
  5. Family history.
    a. GU malignancies.
    b. Primary renal disease.
    c. Polycystic kidney disease.
    d. Nephrolithiasis.
    e. Hypertension.
D. Review of systems.
  1. Constitutional symptoms: Recent weight loss, fevers, or night sweats that may indicate malignancy.
  2. Respiratory: Cough or shortness of breath that may indicate recent upper respiratory infection or tumor invasion.
  3. Musculoskeletal: Generalized pain may indicate excessive NSAID use.
  4. GU: LUTS, flank pain, dysuria, cloudy urine, or foul smelling urine.
  5. Gynecologic: Menorrhagia.
  6. Gastrointestinal: Nausea, vomiting, or abdominal pain may indicate renal mass, or nephrolithiasis.
  7. Neurological: Confusion, dizziness, or mental status changes may indicate metastatic malignant disease (renal cancer).
  8. Skin: Rashes or pallor that may be associated with systemic lupus erythematosus.
  9. Hematologic: Excessive bruising or petechiae may indicate blood clotting disorder.
  10. Ear, nose, and throat (ENT): Frequent nosebleeds, rhinorrhea, or sinus congestion.

Physical Examination

A. Vital signs.
  1. Temperature: Measurement greater than 101.5°F may indicate UTI, pyelonephritis, or prostatitis.
  2. Blood pressure.
    a. Hypertension: Glomerular source or renal failure.
    b. Hypotension: Possible acute blood loss anemia from gross hematuria.
  3. Pulse: Tachycardia, sepsis, or hypovolemia from acute blood loss anemia.
B. Skin: Rashes, pallor, or bruising/lacerations from recent trauma.
C. Edema: Possible nephrotic syndrome; rule out deep vein thrombosis (DVT) from GU malignancy.
D. GU examination.
  1. Costovertebral angle tenderness: Nephrolithiasis; pyelonephritis.
  2. Urethral trauma: Urethral caruncle, vaginal prolapse, phimosis, obvious urethral stricture.
E. Digital rectal exam (DRE).
  1. Boggy, tender warm prostate: Acute prostatitis.
  2. Nodularity: Prostate cancer.

Diagnostic Tests

A. Urinalysis.
  1. Color: Red (recent bleeding, most likely urologic source) versus brown or tea color (old blood clots or renal disease).
  2. Proteinuria: Heavy 3 to 4+ (renal disease).
  3. Leukocyte positive and/or nitrite positive: Infection.
  4. Pyuria: Infection.
  5. Red cell casts: Glomerular bleeding.
  6. Crystalluria: Possible nephrolithiasis.
B. Phase contrast microscopy: Helps differentiate renal (presence of distorted RBCs) versus nonglomerular bleeding.
C. Urine culture: Evaluate for infectious sources.
D. Laboratory/blood work.
  1. Complete blood count (CBC): Anemia.
  2. Basic metabolic panel: Renal function.
  3. Prothrombin time (PT)/partial thromboplastin time (PTT) and international normalized ratio (INR): Bleeding disorders.
E. Urine cytology.
  1. Recommended for all patients with risk factors for GU malignancy and with LUTS and voiding symptoms.
  2. Not recommended by the American Urologic Association as part of the routine evaluation of asymptomatic microhematuria.
  3. Negative result does not rule out malignancy.
  4. False positive results can be seen with calculi or inflammation.

F. Imaging.

1. Computed tomographic urogram (CTU) with and without contrast: Gold standard.

  a. Three phase test.

  b. Used to assess for stones (non contrast image); tumors of bladder or kidneys; hydronephrosis; other anatomic abnormalities (contrast image); tumors of upper tract; and collecting system filling defects (excretory phase).

  c. Contraindicated with a serum creatinine greater than 2 mg/dL.

  d. Highest sensitivity and specificity.

2. MRI/magnetic resonance urography (MRU; MRI urogram): Alternative imaging modality when not able to perform CTU due to renal insufficiency, contrast allergy, or pregnancy.

  a. Less sensitivity at recognizing calculus of the GU tract.

3. Renal ultrasound: Not as specific or sensitive.

  a. Can be used to grossly rule out clots in bladder or to detect hydronephrosis.

G. Diagnostic procedures/surgery.

1. Cystoscopy.

  a. Indicated for all patients older than 35 years of age with microscopic hematuria or gross hematuria.

  b. Also indicated for patients younger than 35 years of age with risk factors for GU malignancies and smoking history.

2. Retrograde pyelogram with or without ureteroscopy: May be performed to evaluate the upper tract in patients who are unable to have intravenous contrast for the CTU/MRU imaging.

3. Renal biopsy: Nephrology referral if glomerulonephritis is suspected.

Differential Diagnosis

A. Pseudohematuria: Certain foods, beets/certain drugs, or phenazopyridine (Pyridium).

B. Hereditary disorders: Polycystic kidney disease, nephropathy, renal tubular acidosis, or cystinuria.

C. Hematologic abnormalities: Bleeding disorders or sickle cell disease.

D. Anatomic abnormalities: Urethral strictures, ureteral strictures, ureteropelvic junction obstruction, urethral caruncle, or phimosis.

E. Vascular malformations (hemangioma).

F. Trauma: Abdominal and pelvic injury (degree of hematuria is a poor indicator of the severity of the injury).

G. Exercise-induced hematuria.

H. Foreign bodies (catheters, ureteral stents, self-introduced foreign body into urethra).

I. Infectious (UTI, pyelonephritis, prostatitis, schistosomiasis, tuberculosis).

J. Radiation (radiation cystitis and nephritis).

K. Stones of the GU tract.

L. Malignancy (renal, bladder, ureteral, prostate, penile, urethral, vulvar).

M. Benign tumor.

N. BPH.

O. Endometriosis of urinary tract (cyclic hematuria).

P. Benign essential hematuria.

Q. Glomerulonephritis or renal disorders (IgA nephropathy, drug-induced nephropathy).

R. Overanticoagulation with medications such as warfarin.

1. Clinical caveat—patients should still be thoroughly evaluated for other possible causes.

Evaluation and Management Plan

A. General plan.

1. Urinalysis, urine culture, and laboratory tests (see section "Diagnostic Tests").

2. Urine cytology if indicated.

3. Imaging (CTU).

4. Patients with gross hematuria and/or urinary retention.

  a. Place three-way Foley catheter (22–24 French most commonly used) and irrigate clots (continuous bladder irrigation with sterile saline solution).

  b. If bleeding is not controlled, propose evaluation with urologic surgery for cystoscopy under anesthesia for clot evacuation/fulguration.

5. Patients who are voiding without clots or urine retention: Observation, with increase in oral fluid intake.

6. Patients with gross hematuria or history of trauma for acute blood loss anemia: Monitor with serial hemoglobin and hematocrit and transfuse as indicated.

B. Patient/family teaching points.

1. Provide patient education and prognosis depending on the cause of the hematuria.

2. Explain the various tests that are necessary to determine the cause of bleeding and the treatments that may be necessary for control of gross hematuria (e.g., cystoscopy, clot evacuation, Foley catheter placement for bladder irrigation).

3. Help to ease anxiety by providing appropriate analgesics (e.g., lidocaine jelly before placing a three-way catheter or narcotics/anticholinergics for painful bladder spasms due to clot retention/catheter placement).

C. Pharmacotherapy.

1. No specific medications are primarily indicated to treat hematuria.

2. Appropriate antimicrobials may be used to treat underlying infections.

3. Finasteride may be helpful in controlling bleeding from the prostate.

D. Discharge instructions.

1. Advise patients to refrain from vigorous activity for one week after gross hematuria has resolved.

2. Avoid NSAIDs and aspirin (if possible, some patients may need to continue based on history of coronary artery disease) for 3 days.

3. Advise patients that it is normal to have tea-colored urine for a few days as the hematuria is resolving.

4. Recommend that patients drink plenty of fluids.

5. Suggest that patients prevent constipation and straining by taking stool softeners such as docusate sodium.

6. Advise that patients should seek medical attention promptly if they develop bright red urine, pass clots, are unable to urinate, or have fevers or chills.

Follow-Up

A. Follow-up as indicated for the condition that is causing the hematuria.

B. Once the condition has resolved, reevaluate for microhematuria.

C. In asymptomatic microhematuria with a negative work-up, follow-up annually for repeat urinalysis/microscopy. If negative for 2 years, release from care. If positive, repeat imaging every 3 years and refer for renal evaluation.

Consultation/Referral

A. Nephrology consult for nephrogenic source of hematuria.
B. Urology consult for stones, tumors of the GU tract, BPH, anatomic evaluation, and control of bleeding.
C. Infectious disease consult for treatment of infectious sources (pyelonephritis, prostatitis, UTIs, possible tuberculosis work-up, or possible schistosomiasis).
D. Rheumatology consult for autoimmune disorders such as systemic lupus erythematosus.
E. Hematology consult for bleeding disorders.

Special/Geriatric Considerations

A. Screen elderly individuals appropriately for renal function prior to obtaining imaging studies with contrast.
B. The reduced capacity to retain salt and water increases as the kidney ages, predisposing to dehydration.
C. Older individuals are more susceptible to acute kidney injury from acute blood loss anemia and certain medications such as NSAIDs.
D. Elderly patients should be monitored closely for hypovolemia that present with gross hematuria.

Bibliography

Diagnosis, Evaluation and Follow-Up of Asymptomatic Microhematuria (AMH) in Adults. American Urologic Association. Published 2012. Reviewed and Validity Confirmed 2016.
Fatica, R., & Fowler, A. (2009, January). Hematuria. Cleveland Clinic for Continuing Education. Retrieved from https://www.auanet.org/guidelines/asymptomatic-microhematuria-(amh)-guideline#x2396
Lambert, M. (2013, May). AUA guideline addresses diagnosis, evaluation and follow-up of asymptomatic microhematuria. *American Family Physician, 87*(9), 649–653.

Hypercalcemia

Jessica S. Everitt, Divya Monga, and Catherine Wells

Definition

A. Serum total calcium greater than 10.2 mg/dL (corrected for low albumin; see Box 5.2).

Incidence

A. Hypercalcemia is a relatively common abnormality that is usually mild in presentation.
B. Approximately 90% of cases of hypercalcemia may be caused by some type of malignancy or hyperparathyroidism.
C. Other causes may be from vitamin D deficiencies or kidney transplantation.

Pathogenesis

A. Calcium is controlled by three major hormones: Parathyroid, calcitonin, and vitamin D.
B. Dysregulation in these hormones can lead to hypercalcemia.
C. Calcium is tightly regulated in the bloodstream; therefore, even mild cases of hypercalcemia are concerning and should be investigated for possible malignancy.

Predisposing Factors

A. Women over the age of 50.
B. Patients taking excessive calcium or vitamin D supplements.
C. Cancer.
D. Genetics.
E. Immobility may contribute to release of calcium.
F. Lithium.

Subjective Data

A. Common complaints/symptoms.
  1. Gastrointestinal, including nausea, vomiting, and constipation.
  2. Anorexia.
  3. Fatigue and lethargy.
  4. Confusion.
  5. Severe hypercalcemia.
    a. Cardiac effects, including bradycardia or arrhythmias with EKG changes.
    b. Volume depletion secondary to polyuria and hypercalcemia-induced natriuresis.
    c. Possible acute renal failure if severe and prolonged.
  6. Chronic hypercalcemia: Possible nephrolithiasis, systemic calcifications (e.g., vascular), and renal failure.

Physical Examination

A. Volume status.
B. Cardiac examination.
C. Neurological examination.
D. Reflexes.
E. Musculoskeletal examination.

Diagnostic Tests

A. Serum calcium and phosphorus.
B. 25-hydroxyvitamin D.
C. Intact parathyroid hormone (PTH).
D. Creatinine, blood urea nitrogen (BUN).
E. Protein electrophoresis and immunofixation (serum and urine).
F. Thyroid-stimulating hormone (TSH).
G. EKG.

Differential Diagnosis

A. Malignancy: Local osteolytic hypercalcemia, or hematological malignancies.
B. Hyperparathyroidism: Primary, secondary, and tertiary.
C. Paget's disease.
D. Milk-alkali syndrome.
E. Thyrotoxicosis.
F. Granulomatous diseases (such as sarcoidosis and tuberculosis).
G. Immobilization.
H. Medication-induced.
  1. Vitamin A and D overdose/toxicity.
  2. Parenteral nutrition.
  3. Thiazide diuretics.
  4. Lithium.
  5. Estrogens, antiestrogens, and androgens.
  6. Calcium supplements and calcium-containing phosphorus binders.
I. Impaired renal function (chronic kidney disease [CKD] or acute kidney injury [AKI])—usually due to clearance of drugs.

BOX 5.2

Calcium in Humans

- Normal total serum calcium is 8.6 to 10.2 mg/dL.
- Normal ionized serum calcium is 1.12 to 1.3 mmol/L.
- Extracellular calcium is found in three forms.
  - 40% of calcium in serum is protein-bound, primarily to albumin.
  - 50% is free (ionized or unbound) calcium.
  - 10% is complexed (i.e., calcium citrate).

- Total serum calcium underestimates active calcium.
  - Ionized or unbound calcium is the biologically active form.
  - Correct serum calcium in hypoalbuminemic patients for actual total calcium.
    - Corrected calcium = serum total calcium + (0.8 × [4 - serum albumin concentration]).

- 99% of total body calcium is found in bones.
- PTH and vitamin D regulate serum calcium.
- Physiologic functions.
  - Bone metabolism.
  - Electrophysiology of cardiac and smooth muscle.
  - Coagulation.
  - Endocrine and exocrine secretory functions.

- Phosphorus and calcium directly affect each other.
  - Elevated phosphorus binds to ionized calcium, decreasing unbound, active calcium.
  - Maintain the optimal relationship between calcium and phosphorous.
    - For bone health.
    - To prevent vascular and soft tissue calcifications.

- Calcium is an inotrope if given at accelerated doses (due to its effects on cardiac and smooth muscle).
- Calcium is critical to the coagulation cascade; thus, low calcium or blocking calcium can lead to bleeding.

PTH, parathyroid hormone.

Evaluation and Management Plan

A. Goal: To correct the underlying cause of hypercalcemia and prevent complications of hypercalcemia.

B. Step 1—Treat symptoms.

1. Use aggressive volume resuscitation with intravenous (IV) normal saline 0.9% (200–500 mL/hr) in patients with volume depletion and normal heart and kidney function.

2. Manage cardiac effects: EKG changes and hypotension or hypertension.

3. Replace phosphorus if hypophosphatemia is present.

C. Step 2—Treat hypercalcemia and identify the underlying cause.

1. Discontinue all vitamin D and calcium (oral and intravenous).

2. Acute, severe hypercalcemia.

a. Give loop diuretics (such as furosemide 40–100 mg IV), once volume resuscitation has taken place, to increase renal calcium excretion and avoid volume overload.

b. Possibly arrange for hemodialysis in patients with renal dysfunction.

3. Mild or asymptomatic hypercalcemia. Some therapies may also be beneficial in combination with severe hypercalcemia management.

a. Calcitonin.

i. Rapid onset of action but with short-term effectiveness (<48 hours) due to tachyphylaxis.

ii. Can be used in initial treatment of severe hypercalcemia along with intravenous hydration.

iii. Increases renal excretion and decreases osteoclast-mediated bone resorption of calcium.

iv. Dose: 4 to 8 units/kg IV or intramuscularly (IM) every 12 hours.

b. Glucocorticoids.

i. Useful in patients with granulomatous disorders or lymphoma.

ii. Decreases calcitriol production, which subsequently lowers intestinal calcium absorption.

iii. Sample regimens: Prednisone 20–60 mg/day PO or hydrocortisone 200 mg/day IV.

c. Bisphosphonates.

i. Examples: Pamidronate and zoledronate.

ii. Potent inhibitors of osteoclast-mediated bone resorption frequently used in hypercalcemia of malignancy.

iii. Due to delayed onset of action, limited role in severe, acute hypercalcemia.

d. Cinacalcet or etelcalcetide.

i. Indication: For outpatient management of primary hyperparathyroidism and secondary hyperparathyroidism of renal origin.

ii. Mimics the effects of calcium (calcimimetic) by binding to the calcium-sensing receptor on the parathyroid gland, thus reducing PTH and serum calcium.

iii. Dosing.

1) Cinacalcet: Initially at 30 mg one to two times daily to max of 180 mg/day.

2) Etelcalcetide: Initial dosing 5 mg three times weekly IV (after dialysis) to a maximum of 15 mg three times weekly IV (after dialysis).

e. Denosumab.

i. Indicated for hypercalcemia of malignancy.

ii. Delayed onset of action.

iii. Binds to receptor activator of nuclear factor-kappa ligand (RANKL), leading to decreased bone resorption.

iv. Given subcutaneously every 4 weeks with additional doses during the first month of treatment.

D. Step 3—Treat other electrolyte and acid–base disorders.

Follow-Up

A. Hypercalcemia can lead to osteoporosis, kidney stones or failure, nervous system disorders, and arrhythmias.

B. Follow-up of calcium levels is essential to prevent adverse outcomes.

Consultation/Referral

A. Patients should be referred to the appropriate service to treat the underlying disorder.

B. Oncology may be needed for patients with cancer.

C. Endocrine can be consulted for hormonal disorders contributing to hypercalcemia.

D. Nephrology should be consulted if there is renal involvement.

Special/Geriatric Considerations

A. Geriatric patients may be at increased risk due to immobility and dehydration.

B. Sitting or lying for long periods of time can cause calcium to leak into the bloodstream.

C. Severe dehydration can also transiently increase calcium concentration secondary to hypovolemia.

D. Hypercalcemia can contribute to arrhythmias that further put geriatric patients at risk for adverse events.

Bibliography

Kraft, M. D., Btaiche, I. F., Sacks, G. S., & Kudsk, K. A. (2005, August). Treatment of electrolyte disorders in adult patients in the intensive care unit. *American Journal of Health System Pharmacy, 62*(16), 1663–1682. doi:10.2146/ajhp040300

Moe, S. M., & Daoud, J. R. (2004). Disorders of mineral metabolism: Calcium, phosphorous, and magnesium. In D. S. Gipson, M. A. Perazella, & M. Tonelli (Eds.), *National kidney foundation's primer on kidney diseases* (6th ed., pp. 100–112). Philadelphia, PA: Elsevier Saunders.

Shane, E. (2018, August 13). Diagnostic approach to hypercalcemia. In J. E. Mulder (Ed.), *UpToDate.* Retrieved from https://www.uptodate.com/contents/diagnostic-approach-to-hypercalcemia

Shane, E., & Berenson, J. R. (2017). Treatment of hypercalcemia. In J. E. Mulder (Ed.), *UpToDate.* Retrieved from https://www.uptodate.com/contents/treatment-of-hypercalcemia

Hyperkalemia

Jessica S. Everitt, Divya Monga, and Catherine Wells

Definition

A. Serum potassium concentration of greater than 5.5 mEq/L (see Box 5.3).

Incidence

A. Most common in patients with renal disease (impaired potassium elimination).

Pathogenesis

A. Causes.

1. Redistribution (a net shift of potassium from intracellular to extracellular space).

2. Total body excess (due to increased potassium ingestion or impaired potassium elimination).

BOX 5.3

Potassium in Humans

- Normal serum potassium concentration is 3.5 to 5.5 mEq/L.
  - Serum potassium levels represent extracellular potassium.
  - The vast majority (98%) of total body potassium is intracellular.
- Kidneys excrete 90% to 95% of dietary potassium, with the remaining excreted by the gut.
- Physiologic functions.
  - Cellular metabolism.
  - Glycogen and protein synthesis.
  - Regulation of the electrical action potential across cell membranes.

Predisposing Factors

A. High potassium, low sodium diets.

B. Potassium supplements.

C. Renal insufficiency.

Subjective Data

A. Common complaints/symptoms.

1. General malaise.

2. Weakness.

3. Gastrointestinal complaints.

a. Nausea and vomiting.

b. Diarrhea.

4. Neuromuscular.

a. Muscle twitching.

b. Cramping.

c. Weakness.

d. Ascending paralysis.

e. Paresthesia.

f. Hyperreflexia.

Physical Examination

A. Inspect and assess for volume/hydration status: Skin, mucous membranes, and jugular venous distension.

B. Assess for cardiac and renal comorbidities.

1. Auscultate and evaluate heart and lung.

2. Perform neurological examination.

Diagnostic Tests

A. Initial laboratory tests.

1. Serum potassium (preferably plasma).

2. Venous or arterial CO_2 or HCO_3 and/or pH.

B. Other laboratory tests.
  1. Complete chemistry panel.
  2. Complete blood count.
  3. Drug levels (i.e., digoxin).
  4. Trans-tubular potassium gradient (TTKG).
    a. [Urine potassium/plasma potassium]/[urine osmolarity/plasma osmolarity].
    b. Assessment of the kidney's capability to appropriately conserve potassium.
    c. Valid only if the patient is not taking any diuretics or drugs to block the renin–angiotensin–aldosterone system (RAAS), the urine osmolarity is greater than 300 mOsm/kg, and the urine sodium is greater than 25 mEq/L.
    d. Should be greater than 10 during hyperkalemia, indicating that the kidneys are trying to remove potassium.
C. Cardiac function tests.
  1. EKG changes including:
    a. Peaked T-waves, prolonged PR-interval, widened QRS complex, and shortened QT-interval.
    b. Progressive worsening as potassium rises.
    c. Brady arrhythmias.
    d. Ventricular fibrillation.
    e. Asystole.

Differential Diagnosis

A. Pseudohyperkalemia.
  1. Hemolysis during blood draw.
  2. Preexisting hemolysis (e.g., sickle cell disease, transfusion reaction, drug induced).
  3. Sampling error (i.e., collected above the level of an infusion).
  4. Polycythemia.
  5. Thrombocytosis (>500,000 to 1 million/mm^3): Potassium release when clots are formed.
  6. Leukocytosis (>100–200,000/mm^3): Elevated potassium in serum but not in plasma.
  7. Familial pseudohyperkalemia.
B. Redistribution of intracellular potassium (shifts from intracellular to extracellular fluid).
  1. Metabolic acidosis or diabetic ketoacidosis: Insulin deficiency.
  2. Muscular injury (e.g., trauma and rhabdomyolysis).
  3. Succinylcholine.
  4. Digoxin overdose.
  5. Reduced effective plasma volume/hypertonic state.
    a. Severe dehydration.
    b. Heart failure.
    c. Liver failure.
  6. Hyperkalemic periodic paralysis.
  7. Medications (toxicity): Beta-blockers, succinylcholine;,and digitalis.
C. Impaired elimination.
  1. Kidney failure: Acute versus chronic.
  2. Medication-induced.
    a. Potassium-sparing diuretics.
    b. Angiotensin-converting enzyme (ACE) inhibitors.
    c. Angiotensin receptor blockers (ARBs).
    d. Aldosterone antagonists.
    e. Nonsteroidal anti-inflammatory drugs (NSAIDs).
    f. Trimethoprim.
    g. Heparin.
  3. Decreased action of aldosterone/aldosterone deficiency.
    a. Medications: ACE inhibitors; ARBs; NSAIDs; potassium-sparing diuretics; antibiotics

(trimethoprim, penicillin G potassium); clonidine; cyclosporine; heparin; and others.
    b. Type IV renal tubular acidosis.
    c. Hyporeninemic hypoaldosteronism.
    d. Addison's disease (primary adrenal insufficiency).
    e. Gordon's syndrome (Type II pseudohypoaldosteronism).
  4. Hypocalcemia.
D. Increased ingestion (requires impaired elimination).

Evaluation and Management Plan

A. Step 1—Cardiac stabilization (stabilize the action potential in the myocardium).
  1. Intravenous calcium administered as calcium gluconate or calcium chloride transiently stabilizes cardiac muscle but does not decrease serum potassium.
    a. Calcium gluconate contains 4.65 mEq Ca^{++}/g and calcium chloride contains 13.6 mEq Ca^{++}/g. Adjust doses accordingly.
  2. Transient but immediate effect.
  3. 1 to 2 g given immediately and prior to other therapies (i.e., intravenous bicarbonate), and may be repeated as needed.
  4. Central line preferred (especially for calcium or high doses of calcium gluconate).
B. Step 2—Shift potassium to intracellular space.
  1. 10 units intravenous insulin with 50 mL dextrose 50% to prevent hypoglycemia. Repeat as needed. Monitor glucose and potassium.
  2. High dose β-agonists such as nebulized albuterol.
  3. Sodium bicarbonate in acidotic patients.
    a. Note: Correcting acidosis can also lower calcium levels. Give intravenous calcium before intravenous bicarbonate.
C. Step 3—Remove excess potassium.
  1. Potassium-wasting diuretics; adequate dosing for renal function.
  2. Potassium binders.
    a. Sodium polystyrene sulfonate (Kayexalate) given as 15 to 30 g PO every 4 to 6 hours or 30 to 60 g per retention enema.
    b. Patiromer (Veltassa) as 8.4 g PO once daily.
D. Step 4—Dialysis. Consult a nephrology expert.
  1. Assess all electrolytes and acid–base balance and treat as indicated with nephrology.

Follow-Up

A. Continue to monitor potassium levels for 24 to 48 hours after the last dose of medication to account for the half-life of all medications.
B. Consider chronic treatment, which also includes potassium restriction and increased potassium elimination.
  1. Dietary potassium restriction.
  2. Discontinuation of medications associated with hyperkalemia.
  3. Potassium-wasting medications (diuretics or potassium binders).
C. Follow-up with nephrology and cardiology as needed until potassium is normalized.

Consultation/Referral

A. Consult nephrology for any refractory electrolyte disorder with or without acute kidney injury (AKI) or chronic kidney disease (CKD).
B. Consult endocrinology for any uncontrolled diabetes.

Special/Geriatric Considerations

A. Sodium polystyrene sulfonate (Kayexalate) is associated with bowel obstruction. Use with caution in all populations but especially patients at risk for slow gastrointestinal motility.

B. The high doses of β-agonists required to shift potassium intracellularly can cause tachycardia. Use with caution in patients with preexisting arrhythmias, and other at-risk populations.

C. Patients with CKD and end-stage renal disease (ESRD) as well as high risk of history of cardiac arrhythmias have a higher risk of mortality with hypokalemia than hyperkalemia. Monitor carefully.

D. Patients with chronic hyperkalemia may not require acute lowering of potassium levels for baseline potassium in the absence of EKG changes or other signs/symptoms.

Bibliography

Allon, M. (2014). Disorders of potassium metabolism. In D. S. Gipson, M. A. Perazella, & M. Tonelli (Eds.), *National Kidney Foundation's primer on kidney diseases* (6th ed., pp. 90–99). Philadelphia, PA : Elsevier Saunders.

Choi, M. J., & Ziyadeh, F. N. (2008, March). The utility of the transtubular potassium gradient in the evaluation of hyperkalemia. *Journal of the American Society of Nephrology, 19*(3), 424–426. doi:10.1681/ASN. 2007091017

Cohnm, J. N., Kowey, P. R., Whelton, P. K., & Prisant, L. M. (2000). New guidelines for potassium replacement in clinical practice. *Archives of Internal Medicine, 160,* 2429–2436. doi:10.1001/archinte.160.16.2429

Ethier, J. H., Kamel, K. S., Magner, P. O., Lemann, J., & Halperin, M. L. (1990, April). The transtubular potassium concentration in patients with hypokalemia and hyperkalemia. *American Journal of Kidney Diseases, 15*(4), 309–315. doi:10.1016/s0272-6386(12)80076-x

Kraft, M. D., Btaiche, I. F., Sacks, G. S., & Kudsk, K. A. (2005). Treatment of electrolyte disorders in adult patients in the intensive care unit. *American Journal Health System Pharmacy, 62*(16), 1663–1682. doi:10.2146/ajhp040300

Pepin, J., & Sheilds, C. (2012). Advances in diagnosis and management of hypokalemic and hyperkalemic emergencies. *Emergency Medical Practice, 14*(2), 1–20.

Sood, M. M., Sood, A. R., & Richardson, R. (2007). Emergency management and commonly encountered outpatient scenarios in patients with hyperkalemia. *Mayo Clinic Proceedings, 82*(12), 1553–1561. doi:10.1016/S0025-6196(11)61102-6

Hypermagnesemia

Jessica S. Everitt, Divya Monga, and Catherine Wells

Definition

A. See Box 5.4.

B. Mild hypermagnesemia 2.5 to 4 mg/dL.

C. Moderate hypermagnesemia 4 to 12.5 mg/dL.

D. Severe hypermagnesemia greater than 12.5 mg/dL.

BOX 5.4

Magnesium in Humans

- Normal serum range is 1.5 to 2.4 mg/dL.
- Found primarily in soft tissue, bone, and muscle.
- Approximately 1% of total body magnesium is found in the extracellular fluid.
- Homeostasis managed primarily by the kidneys, but gastrointestinal tract, parathyroid hormone, and serum magnesium concentrations also involved.
- Serves as a cofactor in many enzymatic and biochemical reactions, including reactions involving adenosine triphosphate.

Incidence

A. Hypermagnesemia is rare in patients with normal renal function.

Pathogenesis

A. Magnesium is the second most abundant intracellular cation in the body after potassium.

B. It is critical in the functioning of neuromuscular, cardiac, and nervous system functions.

C. Magnesium is vital to vascular tone, heart rhythm, bone formation, and muscle contraction among many other critical functions.

Predisposing Factors

A. Excessive intake of magnesium.

B. Lithium.

C. Hypothyroidism.

D. End-stage renal disease.

Subjective Data

A. Common complaints/symptoms.

   1. Typically asymptomatic until serum concentrations exceed 4 mg/dL.

   2. Mild hypermagnesemia.

      a. Nausea and vomiting.

      b. Loss of deep tendon reflexes.

      c. Hypotension.

      d. Bradycardia.

      e. EKG changes such as increased PR interval, and increased QRS interval.

   3. Severe hypermagnesemia.

      a. Respiratory paralysis.

      b. Refractory hypotension.

      c. Atrioventricular block.

      d. Cardiac arrest.

Physical Examination

A. Check reflexes.

B. Check blood pressure.

C. Perform cardiac examination.

Diagnostic Tests

A. Serum magnesium.

B. Serum creatinine/blood urea nitrogen (BUN).

C. EKG.

D. Evaluation for pregnancy.

Differential Diagnosis

A. Ingestion.

   1. Magnesium-containing laxatives or antacids.

2. Accidental ingestion of Epsom salts (magnesium sulfate).
B. Intravenous magnesium infusion (intentional overdose).
  1. Therapy for preeclampsia and eclampsia.
  2. Parenteral nutrition or magnesium supplementation.
C. Reduced excretion.
  1. Reduced renal function due to chronic kidney disease or acute kidney injury.
D. Theophylline intoxication.
E. Acromegaly.
F. Tumor lysis syndrome.
G. Familial hypocalciuric hypercalcemia.
H. Adrenal insufficiency.

Evaluation and Management Plan

A. Step 1—If severe cardiac symptoms exist, give intravenous calcium immediately. It can transiently stabilize the cardiac effects of severe, symptomatic hypermagnesemia.
  1. Calcium chloride 1 gm or calcium gluconate 3 gm (see section "Hypocalcemia" for safety details regarding intravenous calcium).
B. Step 2—Determine the cause.
  1. Intentional overdose for medical reasons should not be corrected.
  2. If indicated, restrict or discontinue all magnesium-containing agents.
C. Step 3—Treat other electrolyte and acid–base disorders.
D. Step 4—Accelerate renal magnesium clearance.
  1. Loop diuretics, which can increase urinary excretion of magnesium.
  2. Hemodialysis, which can remove excess magnesium.

Follow-Up

A. Hypermagnesemia is a rare occurrence. Follow-up with nephrology if persistent.

Consultation/Referral

A. Nephrology should be consulted if hypermagnesemia cannot be explained or requires intervention such as dialysis.

Special/Geriatric Considerations

A. This is a rare condition that is typically caused by ingestion of excessive magnesium.

Bibliography

Kraft, M. D., Btaiche, I. F., Sacks, G. S., & Kudsk, K. A. (2005, August). Treatment of electrolyte disorders in adult patients in the intensive care unit. *American Journal of Health System Pharmacy, 62*(16), 1663–1682. doi:10.2146/ajhp040300

Moe, S. M., & Daoud, J. R. (2014). Disorders of mineral metabolism: Calcium, phosphorous, and magnesium. In D. S. Gipson, M. A. Perazella, & M. Tonelli (Eds.), *National Kidney Foundation's primer on kidney diseases* (6th ed., pp. 100–112). Philadelphia, PA: Elsevier Saunders.

Hypernatremia

Jessica S. Everitt, Divya Monga, and Catherine Wells

Definition

A. Serum sodium greater than 145 mEq/L (see Box 5.5).

Incidence

A. Up to 80% of hypernatremia is hospital acquired. Only 0.1% to 1.4% of hypernatremia is present on admission.
B. Overall inpatient incidence is 1% to 5%, and incidence in critically ill patients is 9% to 26%.
C. Hypernatremia is associated with increased length of stay and is an independent predictor of mortality (increased >40%).
D. Populations at increased risk.
  1. Extremes of age (infants and elderly), especially patients with pulmonary or urinary tract infections.
  2. Restricted access to water.
  3. Altered mental status/neurological illness.
  4. Chronic debilitating illnesses associated with impaired thirst/dehydration.

Pathogenesis

A. Reflects a water deficit relative to total body sodium.
B. Can occur in hypovolemic, euvolemic, and hypervolemic patients.
C. Causes plasma hypertonicity (effect of plasma on cells that causes cells to shrink).
D. Almost always requires reduced intake of water with or without loss of the normal thirst response. Otherwise, individuals' normal thirst would encourage them to drink a sufficient amount to correct plasma hypertonicity.

BOX 5.5

Sodium in Humans

- Normal serum concentration 135 to 145 mEq/L.
- Most abundant extracellular cation.
- The majority of total body sodium is found in cells and plasma water. Additional bound sodium is found (and can accumulate) in bone, cartilage, and connective tissue.
- Plasma sodium is approximately the same as interstitial sodium.
- Sodium does not cross the blood–brain barrier, but plasma sodium levels and tonicity of plasma affect brain cells.
- Changes in serum sodium concentration typically reflect changes in water balance rather than actual changes in total body sodium.

E. Hypovolemic hypernatremia: Represents a pronounced water deficit with a mild sodium deficit and requires impaired thirst or decreased intake of water in addition to losses.
F. Euvolemic hypernatremia: Represents a pure body water deficit.

G. Hypervolemic hypernatremia: Represents minimal decrease or no change in total body water (TBW) with an increase in total body sodium.
H. Acute salt poisoning: Large intake of sodium (whether accidental or intentional), resulting in a rapid rise in sodium and subsequent severe hypertonicity.

Predisposing Factors

A. Alterations in thirst.

B. Volume depletion.

C. Hyperglycemia.

D. Certain brain tumors such as pituitary tumors.

Subjective Data

A. Common complaints/symptoms.

1. Vary depending on cause, severity, and rate of development of hypernatremia.

a. Altered skin turgor commonly found in hypovolemic or euvolemic hypernatremia.

b. Signs of volume overload: Hypervolemic hypernatremia.

2. Spectrum of neurological symptoms: Beginning with irritability, dizziness, fatigue, lethargy, and confusion; can progress to seizures and coma.

3. Other symptoms: Nausea, vomiting, and generalized muscle weakness.

4. Polyuria.

a. Definition: 3 L or more per day.

b. Urine output exceeding 5 to 10 L per day indicates antidiuretic hormone (ADH) deficiency (as in diabetes insipidus [DI]); these affected patients often crave ice.

5. Acute salt poisoning: High fever, intracranial hemorrhage, seizures, and coma.

Physical Examination

A. Physical examination to assess volume status.

1. Check skin, mucous membranes, heart, lungs, jugular venous distension (JVD), edema.

2. Assess blood pressure and orthostatic changes.

3. Determine weight changes.

B. Neurological assessment (initial and ongoing).

Diagnostic Tests

A. Serum sodium.

B. Complete chemistry panel to assess causes.

C. Serum osmolality.

D. Spot urine osmolality (measured).

1. Greater than 300 mOsm/kg: Urine is concentrated and hypertonic but not necessarily because of sodium. This indicates a relative increase in solute compared to water.

2. Less than 100 mOsm/kg: Urine is dilute and hypotonic. This indicates a relative increase in water and/or decrease in solute.

E. Spot urine sodium.

1. Less than 20 mEq/L: Renal sodium retention as in low effective arterial blood volume.

a. Common with extra-renal volume losses.

2. Greater than 20 to 30 mEq/L: Renal-related losses of electrolytes (sodium).

a. Common with loop diuretics, osmotic diuresis, or hyperglycemia.

b. Post-AKI diuresis and post obstructive diuresis.

F. Determination of patient volume status.

1. Consider volume assessment to be unreliable initial diagnostic criteria but is necessary when interpreting hypernatremia-related lab tests.

2. Review and calculate history of fluid intake and output.

Differential Diagnosis

A. Hypovolemic hypernatremia.

1. Water and salt deficit.

2. Renal losses (Urine sodium >20 mEq/L).

a. Loop diuretics (spot urine osmolality <100 mOsm/kg [hypotonic]).

b. Post-obstructive or post-acute kidney injury (AKI) diuresis.

c. Osmotic diuresis: Hyperglycemia, mannitol, urea (enteral tube feedings; spot urine osmolality >300 mOsm/kg or 24-hour urine osmolality >1,200 mOsm/kg).

3. Extrarenal losses: Urine sodium less than 20 mEq/L; urine osmolality greater than 300 mOsm/kg (hypertonic).

a. Gastrointestinal losses such as vomiting, diarrhea (i.e., acute infectious, osmotic [enteral tube feedings]), nasogastric suctioning, or enterocutaneous fistula.

b. Skin losses: Perspiration, burns, or severe wounds.

B. Euvolemic hypernatremia.

1. Pure water deficit; body sodium preserved.

2. Renal losses: Hypotonic urine (urine osmolality/plasma osmolality <1).

a. DI: Inadequate ADH release (spot urine osmolality <100 mOsm/kg).

i. Central DI: Congenital, head trauma, post neurosurgical surgery, neoplasms, infiltrative disorders (i.e., sarcoidosis), hypoxic encephalopathy, bleeding, infection, aneurysm, meningitis/encephalitis.

b. Gestational DI: Peripheral degradation of ADH.

c. Nephrogenic DI (hereditary): Inadequate renal response to ADH.

i. X-linked nephrogenic DI.

ii. Autosomal recessive nephrogenic DI.

d. Acquired nephrogenic DI: ADH independent urine concentrating defect.

i. Hypercalcemia or hypokalemia.

ii. Medication-induced: Lithium, vasopressin V_2 receptor antagonists, demeclocycline, amphotericin B, methoxyflurane, or foscarnet.

iii. Chronic kidney diseases (i.e., medullary cyst disease, sickle cell disease, amyloidosis, Sjögren's syndrome).

iv. Bartter's syndrome.

v. Malnutrition.

3. Extrarenal losses: Hypertonic urine (urine osmolality/plasma osmolality >1).

a. Insensible losses.

i. Cutaneous: Fever, sweating, burns, or increased ambient temperature.

ii. Respiratory: Tachypnea or mechanical ventilation.

b. Decreased water intake.

i. Primary hypodipsia.

ii. Reset osmostat.

iii. Decreased access to water (i.e., altered mental status, iatrogenic).

iv. Water loss intracellular (i.e., seizures, extreme exercise).

C. Hypervolemic hypernatremia.

1. Increased sodium intake (TBW and sodium can be variable).

2. Iatrogenic causes.

a. Sodium administration (e.g., normal saline, 3% saline, or sodium bicarbonate) via intravenous or oral routes.

b. Hyperalimentation.

3. Mineralocorticoid excess.

4. Medications: Lithium, demeclocycline, glyburide, amphotericin, colchicine, vinblastine, and others.

5. Hypertonic dialysis.

6. Salt ingestion.

Evaluation and Management Plan

A. Initial goal: To replace free water deficit and prevent ongoing water loss.

1. Assess volume status.

2. Calculate water losses and exact replacement necessary to avoid overcorrection.

a. TBW for lean men is usually 60% of weight in kilogram, and for lean women is usually 50% of weight in kilogram. TBW is lower (approximated to 45%) in obese patients because of adipose tissue. Elderly patients also have a lower TBW (commonly estimated around 50%).

b. Free water deficit (L) = Normal TBW × [140 mEq/l / (Current NA $_{Plasma}$) – 1].

3. Choose appropriate replacement fluid and initial rate of repletion based on acuity and degree of hypovolemia.

4. Estimate ongoing water losses: Renal and extrarenal.

5. Choose an appropriate replacement fluid based on sodium level and underlying cause/diagnosis.

6. Choose replacement rate based on water losses.

B. Hypovolemic hypernatremia.

1. Step 1—Replace intravascular volume deficit (plasma volume deficit) with isotonic crystalloids within the first several hours. The goal is stable hemodynamics.

2. Step 2—Replace total free water deficit/loss over 3 to 4 days (include ongoing losses).

a. Calculate free water deficit (as previously noted).

b. Choose hypotonic replacement fluid.

i. 0.45% NaCl IV (1/2 of the volume given is water).

ii. Water (D$_5$NS, D$_5$W, oral/gastric tube water).

c. Replacement rate.

i. Acute rise in sodium (hypernatremia developed over <48 hours).

1) Rapid water replacement/correction over 24 hours.

ii. Chronic rise in sodium (hypernatremia developed over >48 hours; NOTE: If unknown whether hypernatremia is acute or chronic—treat as chronic).

1) Maximum rate for sodium correction = 10 mEq/l per day over 2 to 3 days.

2) Less than 6 mEq/L per day in elderly patients.

d. Monitor fluid intake and output closely.

e. With low sodium intake, do not allow sodium intake to exceed output as this will exacerbate hypernatremia.

f. Determine and treat the underlying cause.

g. Perform neurological checks frequently.

h. Monitor sodium levels every 4 hours, then daily.

i. Monitor all electrolytes and replace as indicated.

j. Initially monitor closely in an intensive care setting.

3. Step 3—Replace ongoing water losses.

a. Choose fluid with less sodium than current urine concentration.

b. Monitor sodium at least daily.

c. Monitor fluid intake and output closely.

d. Give a low salt diet.

4. Step 4—Monitor/replace other electrolyte losses due to polyuria (e.g., hypokalemia, bicarbonate).

C. Euvolemic and hypervolemic hypernatremia.

1. Step 1—If necessary, correct water deficit (as previously noted).

2. Step 2—Monitor fluid intake and output closely. Low salt diet. Do not allow sodium intake to exceed output as this will exacerbate hypernatremia.

3. Step 3—Define/treat underlying cause.

a. Review medications.

b. Consider desmopressin (dDAVP) for central DI (synthetic ADH analog; also increases factor VIII and von Willebrand factor levels—monitor for clotting) at ONE of the following doses.

i. 0.05–0.6 mg BID PO.

ii. 1–2 mcg BID IV.

iii. 10–20 mcg BID intranasal.

c. Perform neurological checks frequently.

d. Monitor sodium levels every 4 hours then daily.

e. Monitor all electrolytes and replace as indicated.

f. Initially monitor closely in an intensive care setting.

4. Step 4—Treat other electrolyte and acid–base disorders.

D. Acute salt poisoning—rapid rise in sodium.

1. Give a rapid infusion of water to correct at a rate of 1 mEq/L per hour.

2. Consider hemodialysis for sodium correction.

3. Closely monitor and avoid overcorrection.

Follow-Up

A. Follow-up depends on the nature of the underlying condition.

B. Hypernatremia needs to be corrected and maintained.

Consultation/Referral

A. Consult nephrology to help regulate hypernatremia.

B. Consult neurosurgery if central DI is responsible for hypernatremia.

Special/Geriatric Considerations

A. Increased age: Decline in TBW, decreased urinary concentrating ability, and impaired thirst; thus, elderly patients lack the same defenses against hypernatremia as younger patients.

Bibliography

Kraft, M. D., Btaiche, I. F., Sacks, G. S., & Kudsk, K. A. (2005, August). Treatment of electrolyte disorders in adult patients in the intensive care unit. *American Journal of Health System Pharmacy, 62*(16), 1663–1682. doi:10.2146/ajhp040300

Lindner, G., Funk, G. C., & Schwarz, C. (2007). Hypernatremia in the critically ill is an independent risk factor for mortality. *American Journal of Kidney Diseases, 50*, 952. doi:10.1053/j.ajkd.2007.08.016

Sterns, R. H. (2015). Disorders of plasma sodium. *The New England Journal of Medicine, 372*(1), 55–65. doi:10.1056/NEJMc1501342

Hyperphosphatemia

Jessica S. Everitt, Divya Monga, and Catherine Wells

Definition
A. Serum phosphorus greater than 4.5 mg/dL (see Box 5.6).

Incidence
A. Hyperphosphatemia is most common in renal impairment (acute or chronic).

BOX 5.6

Phosphorus in Humans

- 85% of total body phosphorus is located in bones.
  - ○ Approximately 14% is intracellular.
  - ○ Remaining 1% is extracellular.
- Two-thirds of ingested phosphorus is excreted in the urine with the remainder excreted in stool.
- Normal serum phosphorus is 2.5 to 4.5 mg/dL.
- Many physiological functions.
  - ○ Bone and cell membrane composition.
  - ○ Nerve conduction.
  - ○ Muscle function.
  - ○ Energy-rich bonds of adenosine triphosphate.

Subjective Data
A. Common complaints/symptoms.

1. Most common and significant manifestations are signs/symptoms of hypocalcemia due to calcium-phosphate precipitation with decrease in ionized calcium.

2. Can lead to soft-tissue calcification due to precipitation of calcium-phosphate crystals in soft tissues producing symptoms of pruritus, dermatologic changes, and (in severe cases) calciphylaxis.

Physical Examination
A. Respiratory examination.
B. Musculoskeletal examination.
C. Dermatological examination.

Diagnostic Tests
A. Serum phosphorus.
B. Serum total calcium, ionized calcium.
C. Venous CO_2.
D. Renal function evaluation (blood urea nitrogen [BUN] and serum creatinine).

Differential Diagnosis
A. Renal failure or decreased renal excretion.

1. In chronic dialysis patients, poor compliance with phosphorus binding medications.

B. Increased intestinal absorption: Rapid shifts from intracellular to extracellular.

1. Acidosis (respiratory or metabolic).
2. Hemolysis.
3. Rhabdomyolysis.
4. Tumor lysis syndrome.

C. Hypoparathyroidism.
D. Vitamin D toxicity.
E. Phosphorus containing laxatives or enemas.

B. Sustained hyperphosphatemia is rare in the absence of renal disease.

Pathogenesis
A. Homeostasis of phosphate is maintained through gastrointestinal (GI) absorption and renal excretion. Imbalances in either of these mechanisms can result in hyperphosphatemia.

Predisposing Factors
A. Excessive intake is rare, but potential cause.
B. Patients with renal failure.

F. Hypocalcemia (reciprocal rise).
G. Thyrotoxicosis, acromegaly (rare).

Evaluation and Management Plan
A. Step 1—Volume expansion despite fluid volume status.

1. Initial bolus resuscitation.
2. Continue isotonic intravenous hydration.

B. Step 2—Emergency treatment for acute and severe hyperphosphatemia due to risk of renal failure.

1. Calcium replacement (see section "Hypocalcemia"). Acute, severe hyperphosphatemia can cause reciprocal hypocalcemia.

2. Emergency treatment: Continuous renal replacement therapy. Consult nephrology.

3. Additional management.

  a. Phosphorus binders (as noted in the text that follows) at large doses with three meals, snacks, plus a dose at bedtime.

  b. Consultation with a renal dietician for dietary counseling.

    i. Tightly restrict unnecessary sources of phosphorus in the diet such as food preservatives and higher phosphorus grains and vegetables.

    ii. Choose an individualized target for protein intake that will not place the patient at risk for nutrition deficiencies or allow excessive phosphorus intake from protein sources.

  c. Continuation of isotonic intravenous hydration. Consider loop diuretics if needed to increase urine output.

C. Step 3—If nonemergent, assess for cause of hyperphosphatemia.

1. Hyperphosphatemia management is oral phosphate binders and dietary restriction in patients with chronic renal disease.

a. Give phosphate binders with food in order to bind dietary phosphorus in the intestinal tract and prevent absorption.

b. Avoid magnesium- and aluminum-based binders because of risk of accumulation in renal disease.

2. Phosphorus binders should not be given to patients with acute kidney injury (AKI) due to risk for overcorrection (hypophosphatemia) during recovery.

3. Current available formulations.

a. Calcium-based (calcium acetate or calcium carbonate).

b. Sevelamer.

c. Lanthanum.

d. Iron-based (ferric citrate or sucroferric oxyhydroxide).

e. Dose is specific to formulation used.

D. Step 4—Treat underlying cause if possible.

E. Step 5—Treat other electrolyte and acid–base disorders.

Follow-Up

A. Calcium levels, phosphate levels, and renal function should be monitored at intervals consonant with the severity of the underlying disorder.

Consultation/Referral

A. Nephrology may be consulted if the hyperphosphatemia is associated with renal failure.

Endocrinology may be consulted if the patient has hypoparathyroidism.

Special/Geriatric Considerations

A. Elderly patients with chronic kidney disease (CKD) are at risk for hyperphosphatemia.

Bibliography

Kraft, M. D., Btaiche, I. F., Sacks, G. S., & Kudsk, K. A. (2005, August). Treatment of electrolyte disorders in adult patients in the intensive care unit. *American Journal of Health System Pharmacy, 62*(16), 1663–1682. doi:10.2146/ajhp040300

Moe, S. M., & Daoud, J. R. (2014). Disorders of mineral metabolism: Calcium, phosphorous, and magnesium. In D. D. Gipson, M. A. Perazella, & M. Tonelli (Eds.), *National Kidney Foundation's primer on kidney diseases* (6th ed., pp. 100–112). Philadelphia, PA: Elsevier Saunders.

Stubbs, J. R., & Yu, A. S. L. (2017). Overview of the causes and treatment of hyperphosphatemia. In S. Goldfarb & A. Q. Lam (Eds.), *UpToDate,* Waltham, MA: Retrieved from https://www.uptodate.com/contents/overview-of-the-causes-and-treatment-of-hyperphosphatemia

Hypocalcemia

Jessica S. Everitt, Divya Monga, and Catherine Wells

Definition

A. Total serum calcium less than 8.6 mg/dL or ionized calcium less than 1.1 mmol/L (see Box 5.2).

Incidence

A. The incidence of hypocalcemia is difficult to quantify.

B. In intensive care patients, hypocalcemia is estimated between 15% and 88% of all patients.

Pathogenesis

A. Calcium is necessary for bone mineralization, nerve conduction, muscle relaxation, and cardiac conduction.

Predisposing Factors

A. Renal failure.

B. Advancing age.

C. Volume depletion.

D. Hepatic insufficiency.

E. Chronic heart failure.

Subjective Data

A. Common complaints/symptoms.

1. Most specific symptoms are perioral numbness and spasms of upper and lower extremities.

2. Severe hypocalcemia can lead to tetany and seizures.

3. Other neuromuscular, central nervous system (CNS), and cardiovascular symptoms may be present, even with mild to moderate hypocalcemia.

a. Prolonged QT interval.

b. Paresthesia.

4. Chronic hypocalcemia may present with skin manifestations such as brittle and grooved nails, hair loss, dermatitis, and eczema.

Physical Examination

A. Cardiac examination.

B. Neurological examination (reflexes).

C. Possible bleeding.

D. Chvostek's sign or Trousseau's sign: Increased neuromuscular activity can be demonstrated by tapping over the facial nerve.

Diagnostic Tests

A. Total and ionized serum calcium.

B. Serum phosphorus.

C. Serum magnesium.

D. 25-hydroxyvitamin D.

E. Intact parathyroid hormone (PTH).

Differential Diagnosis

A. Hypoparathyroidism.

B. Pseudohypoparathyroidism (low calcium with low phosphorus also known as iPTH resistance).

C. Hypomagnesemia.

D. Vitamin D deficiency.

1. Poor intestinal absorption (e.g., short bowel, poor nutritional intake).

2. Lack of sun exposure.

3. Decreased activation of vitamin D (e.g., cirrhosis).

E. Tissue consumption of calcium.

1. Acute severe pancreatitis.

2. Sepsis.

3. Acute malignancies/blastic bone metastases (excess bone formation).

4. "Hungry bone syndrome" post parathyroidectomy in chronic kidney disease (CKD) or end-stage renal disease (ESRD) patients with history of hyperparathyroidism.

5. Acute hyperphosphatemia (i.e., rhabdomyolysis, tumor lysis syndrome).

6. Citrate infusion (citrate binds to ionized calcium decreasing unbound, active calcium).

a. Transfusion of blood products preserved with citrate.

b. Circuit anticoagulation for dialysis/apheresis.

Evaluation and Management Plan

A. Step 1—Replace acute calcium needs.

1. Intravenous administration used when rapid correction is required.

2. Initial dose: 1 g calcium chloride or 3 g calcium gluconate.

    a. Repeat dose as needed.

    b. Calcium chloride contains three times more elemental calcium than calcium gluconate.

3. Caution: Intravenous calcium can cause vascular and tissue necrosis if extravasation occurs as both calcium chloride and calcium gluconate. A central intravenous line is recommended for all calcium infusions.

B. Step 2—Assess for ongoing calcium replacement needs and replace as indicated.

1. Use intravenous or oral calcium replacement.

2. Oral calcium supplements used in asymptomatic patients and patients with chronic hypocalcemia.

    a. Calcium carbonate contains maximum elemental calcium compared to other formulations.

    b. Typical dose is calcium carbonate 1,250 mg (equivalent to 500 mg elemental calcium) twice daily.

    c. Take on empty stomach to maximize absorption of calcium.

3. Administer vitamin D to increase intestinal absorption of calcium if vitamin is deficient.

    a. NOTE: Patients with renal failure need activated formulas of vitamin D replacement. Consult nephrology for assistance.

C. Step 3—Treat other electrolyte and acid–base disorders (i.e., hypomagnesemia).

Follow-Up

A. Follow-up with an outpatient provider to monitor labs would be advised.

Consultation/Referral

A. Consider consults based on the underlying cause of hypocalcemia and the severity of the condition.

Special/Geriatric Considerations

A. Severe hypocalcemia may result in seizures, tetany, refractory hypotension, or arrhythmias that require a more aggressive approach.

Bibliography

Goltzman, D. (2000, updated 2016). Approach to hypercalcemia. In K. R., Feingold, B. Anawalt, & B, A. Boyce et al(Eds.), *Endotext*, South Dartmouth, MA: MDText.com. Retrieved from https://www.ncbi.nlm.nih.gov/books/NBK279129/

Kraft, M. D., Btaiche, I. F., Sacks, G. S., & Kudsk, K. A. (2005, August). Treatment of electrolyte disorders in adult patients in the intensive care unit. *American Journal of Health System Pharmacy, 62*(16), 1663–1682. doi:10.2146/ajhp040300

Moe, S. M., & Daoud, J. R. (2014). Disorders of mineral metabolism: Calcium, phosphorous, and magnesium. In D. S. Gipson, M. A. Perazella, & M. Tonelli (Eds.), *National Kidney Foundation's primer on kidney diseases* (6th ed., pp. 100–112). Philadelphia, PA: Elsevier Saunders.

Hypokalemia

Jessica S. Everitt, Divya Monga, and Catherine Wells

Definition

A. Serum potassium concentration of less than 3.5 mEq/L (see Box 5.3).

Incidence

A. Hypokalemia occurs in 20% of hospitalized patients.

Pathogenesis

A. Causes.

1. Total body deficiency (increased losses or decreased intake). This condition may develop as a result of:

    a. Gastrointestinal losses.

    b. Renal losses with or without metabolic abnormalities.

    c. Decreases in intake that surpass the kidneys' ability to compensate.

2. Redistribution (a net shift of potassium from extracellular to intracellular space).

3. Hypomagnesemia. This causes the kidneys to secrete potassium into the urine at a higher rate than they would with the same potassium levels and higher magnesium levels, leading to hypokalemia or accelerating it.

4. Elevated plasma sodium levels (due to a high salt diet). These cause the kidneys to lose potassium while making an effort to balance ion neutrality via available ion exchange transporter.

Predisposing Factors

A. Nonpotassium sparing diuretics.

B. Eating disorders.

C. Alcoholism.

Subjective Data

A. Common complaints/symptoms.

1. Palpitations or arrhythmias.

2. Gastrointestinal.

    a. Nausea and vomiting.

    b. Constipation, ileus.

3. Muscle weakness (severe hypokalemia).

    a. Skeletal muscle weakness and paralysis.

    b. Respiratory compromise due to diaphragmatic paralysis.

    c. Rarely, rhabdomyolysis.

4. Cramping (lower legs).

B. Postural hypotension.

Physical Examination

A. EKG changes include ST-segment depression, T-wave flattening, T-wave inversion, and the presence of U-waves.

B. Can progress to life-threatening and/or fatal arrhythmias and sudden cardiac death.

1. Check gastrointestinal system: Abdominal pain and bowel sounds.

2. Inspect musculoskeletal system: Strength.

3. Perform neurological examination.

Diagnostic Tests

A. Initial lab tests.

1. Serum potassium (preferably plasma).

2. Venous or arterial CO_2 or HCO_3 and/or pH.

B. Other lab tests.

1. Complete chemistry panel.

2. Blood urea nitrogen (BUN) and creatinine to assess kidney function.

C. Estimate of total body extracellular potassium and potassium deficit.

1. Total body potassium (mEq/L) = Extracellular fluid volume (ECFV) × Serum potassium (mEq/L).

    a. ECFV = Total body water [0.6 × weight (kg)] × 1/3.

2. Potassium deficit (mEq/L) =

a. ECFV × ***Desired*** serum potassium (4.0 or 4.5 mEq/L) - ECFV × Serum potassium (mEq/L).

b. NOTE: This calculation does not account for ongoing losses or intracellular deficits.

D. Assessment for cause of potassium losses.

1. Trans-tubular potassium gradient (TTKG): Assessment of the kidney's capability to appropriately conserve potassium.

a. Valid only if the patient is not taking any diuretics or drugs to block the renin–angiotensin–aldosterone system (RAAS).

b. During hypokalemia, TTKG should be less than 3, indicating the kidneys are conserving potassium.

2. Urine potassium concentration—24-hour collection.

E. Cardiac function.

1. EKG changes including peaked T-waves, prolonged PR-interval, widened QRS complex, shortened QT-interval.

2. Bradyarrhythmias.

3. Ventricular fibrillation.

4. Asystole.

Differential Diagnosis

A. Spurious hypokalemia or pseudohypokalemia.

1. Leukocytosis greater than $100,000/mm^3$.

2. Insulin dosing/timing of lab draw.

B. Redistribution.

1. Metabolic alkalosis.

2. Catecholamine excess.

a. Alkalemia.

b. Familial hypokalemic periodic paralysis.

c. Thyrotoxicosis.

d. Factor replacement in megaloblastic anemia.

e. Medications: Insulin, theophylline toxicity, β-adrenergic activity/agents (epinephrine), bronchodilators, caffeine-containing drugs.

C. Increased potassium losses.

1. Gastrointestinal losses: Prolonged vomiting or diarrhea.

2. Extra-renal potassium loss (urine potassium < 20 mEq/24 hours).

a. Prolonged diarrhea.

b. Nasogastric suctioning.

c. Intestinal potassium binders (e.g., sodium polystyrene sulfonate or patiromer).

d. Poor intake/malnutrition.

e. Laxative abuse.

f. Excessive sweating.

g. Villous adenoma recto-sigmoid colon.

3. Renal potassium loss (urine potassium >20 mEq/24 hours): Non anion gap metabolic acidosis.

a. Renal tubular acidosis Type I (distal) and Type II (proximal).

b. Liddle's syndrome (decreased aldosterone secretion; normal renin level).

c. Diabetic ketoacidosis, lactic acidosis.

d. Ureterosigmoidostomy.

e. Medications: Carbonic anhydrase inhibitors, laxative overuse, topiramate.

4. Renal potassium loss (urine potassium >20 mEq/24 hours): Metabolic alkalosis.

a. Vomiting or nasogastric suction.

b. Mineralocorticoid excess syndromes (normotensive primary hyperaldosteronism).

c. Bartter's syndrome.

d. Gitelman's syndrome.

e. Medications: Diuretics (loop, thiazide), especially in the setting of high salt intake.

5. Renal potassium loss (urine potassium >20 mEq/24 hours): No acid–base disorder.

a. Elevated renin levels: Malignant hypertension, renovascular disease, renin-secreting tumor.

b. Low renin levels: Elevated aldosterone levels (primary hyperaldosteronism, bilateral adrenal hyperplasia, dexamethasone suppression).

c. Low aldosterone levels.

i. Mineralocorticoid ingestion.

ii. Congenital adrenal hyperplasia.

iii. Cushing's syndrome.

iv. Ectopic ACTH.

v. Tobacco.

vi. Black licorice.

d. Hypomagnesemia.

e. Enuresis/polyuria: Hypercalcemia, acute kidney injury recovery, postobstructive diuresis, osmotic diuresis (e.g., hyperglycemia).

f. Medications: Aminoglycosides, amphotericin B, high dose corticosteroids, mineralocorticoids.

6. Other.

a. Leukemia.

b. Any disorder causing severe or progressive weakness: Myasthenia gravis, polyneuropathy.

Evaluation and Management Plan

A. Goal: To avoid or resolve the cause of the hypokalemia and treat the condition and its related symptoms.

B. **Step 1**—Immediate treatment: Potassium supplementation. The total dose is at least equal to the calculated potassium deficit. The calculated dose to replace potassium in extracellular fluid is:

1. [Ideal plasma potassium mmol/L − Actual plasma potassium] × [TBW (L) × Extracellular fluid (%)].

a. TBW = Weight (kg) × 0.5 (women), 0.6 (men), 0.45 (elderly).

b. ECFV is 26% to 30% of TBW.

2. $[4.0 \text{ mmol/L}–2.5] \times [(80 \text{ kg} \times 0.5) \times 0.26] = 1.5 \times [40 \times 0.26] = 1.5 \times 10.4 = 15.6$ mmol/L or 16.

a. 16 mmol/L–16 mEq/L

b. Deliver intravenously. Oral doses will be higher due to poor absorption.

C. **Step 2**—Repeated calculations and doses for ongoing potassium losses.

1. Intravenous supplementation.

a. Initial dose of 20 to −40 mEq: Common, but in severe hypokalemia will likely need to be repeated.

b. Dose: 10 to 20 mEq/hr.

c. Reserved for severe and/or symptomatic hypokalemia or for patients unable to tolerate oral supplementation.

2. Oral supplementation.

a. Available in tablet, capsule, or liquid formulations.

b. Total daily doses: 40 to 100 mEq; sufficient replacement in most cases.

c. Divided into two to four doses to reduce gastrointestinal side effects.

d. Patients with renal dysfunction: Decrease dose by 50% and avoid repeating doses.

D. **Step 3**—Treatment of underlying disorder.

1. Correct hypomagnesemia as it can result in refractory hypokalemia.

2. Decrease or discontinue medications associated with hypokalemia if possible.

3. Decrease sodium intake (especially with diuretic use).

E. Step 4—Treatment of other electrolyte and acid–base disorders.

F. Step 5—Assessment of need for chronic management.

1. Some patients will require chronic oral potassium supplements or high potassium diets.

2. Consider potassium-sparing diuretics (e.g., spironolactone, amiloride, triamterene) in patients on potassium-depleting medications.

3. All patients on potassium-depleting medications need a low-salt diet.

Follow-Up

A. For hypokalemia related to acute episodes, such as severe diarrhea, no follow-up is necessary.

B. However, patients on long-term diuretic therapy should have periodic monitoring of serum potassium levels.

Consultation/Referral

A. Consult nephrology for any refractory electrolyte disorder with or without acute kidney injury or chronic kidney disease (CKD).

B. Consult endocrinology for any uncontrolled diabetes or other hormone disorders.

C. Consult gastroenterology for refractory symptoms and suspected villous adenoma.

Special/Geriatric Considerations

A. Monitor patients with CKD, congestive heart failure, or medications associated with hypokalemia carefully to avoid overcorrecting.

Bibliography

Allon, M. (2014). Disorders of potassium metabolism. In D. S. Gipson, M. A. Perazella, & M. Tonelli (Eds.), *National Kidney Foundation's primer on kidney diseases* (6th ed., pp. 90–99). Philadelphia, PA: Elsevier Saunders.

Cohnm, J. N., Kowey, P. R., Whelton, P. K., & Prisant, L. M. (2000). New guidelines for potassium replacement in clinical practice. *Archives of Internal Medicine, 160*, 2429–2436. doi:10.1001/archinte.160.16.2429

Kraft, M. D., Btaiche, I. F., Sacks, G. S., & Kudsk, K. A. (2005, August). Treatment of electrolyte disorders in adult patients in the intensive care unit. *American Journal of Health System Pharmacy, 62*(16), 1663–1682. doi:10.2146/ajhp040300

Pepin, J., & Shields, C. (2012). Advances in diagnosis and management of hypokalemic and hyperkalemic emergencies. *Emergency Medical Practice, 14*(2), 1–20.

Hypomagnesemia

Jessica S. Everitt, Divya Monga, and Catherine Wells

Definition

A. Serum magnesium less than 1.5 mg/dL (see Box 5.4).

Incidence

A. 2% of general population.

B. 10% to 20% hospitalized patients.

Pathogenesis

A. Magnesium is the second most abundant intracellular cation in the body after potassium.

B. It is critical in the functioning of neuromuscular, cardiac, and nervous system functions. Magnesium is vital to vascular tone, heart rhythm, bone formation, and muscle contraction, among many other critical functions.

Predisposing Factors

A. Starvation.

B. Alcohol use.

C. Diarrhea.

D. Vomiting.

E. Gastrointestinal fistulas.

Subjective Data

A. Common complaints/symptoms.

1. Neuromuscular symptoms similar to hypocalcemia.

a. Hyperreflexia.

b. Carpopedal spasm.

c. Tetany.

d. Seizures.

e. Positive Chvostek's and Trousseau's signs.

2. Severe hypomagnesemia: Possible EKG changes and life-threatening arrhythmias (including torsades de pointes).

Physical Examination

A. Reflexes.

B. EKG.

C. Blood pressure.

D. Cardiac examination.

Diagnostic Tests

A. Serum magnesium.

B. Total calcium and ionized calcium (hypomagnesemia is often accompanied by hypokalemia and/or hypocalcemia).

C. Potassium.

D. Serum creatinine and blood urea nitrogen (BUN).

Differential Diagnosis

A. Decreased intake.

1. Chronic alcoholism.

2. Prolonged fasting.

3. Protein-calorie malnutrition.

4. Inadequate supplementation in parenteral nutrition-dependent patients.

B. Gastrointestinal losses.

1. Inflammatory bowel disease.

2. Chronic diarrhea.

3. Laxative abuse.

4. Malabsorption syndromes.

5. Surgical bowel resection or small intestinal bypass surgery.

C. Renal losses.

1. Drugs.

a. Diuretics.

b. Amphotericin B.

c. Aminoglycosides.

d. Cyclosporine.

e. Tacrolimus.

f. Pentamidine.

g. Proton pump inhibitors.

h. Foscarnet.

i. Cetuximab.

j. Cisplatin.

2. High urinary output.

a. Post-obstructive or resolving acute tubular necrosis (ATN) diuresis.

b. Post-transplant polyuria.
  c. Hypercalcemia.
3. Inherited hypomagnesemia.
  a. Gitelman's syndrome.
  b. Bartter's syndrome.
  c. Phosphate depletion.
4. Primary hyperaldosteronism.
5. Chronic metabolic acidosis.
6. Idiopathic renal wasting.

Evaluation and Management Plan

A. Step 1—Initiate intravenous (IV) magnesium replacement 4 g for all patients with severe symptoms or eclampsia/preeclampsia.
  1. Deliver first dose quickly (over 4–5 minutes) if followed by an infusion or repeat slow IV bolus (over 6–12 hours).
  2. Infuse 4 to 6 g over 8 to 12 hours.
    a. Magnesium distributes into tissues slowly, but is rapidly eliminated by the kidney.
B. Step 2—Replace magnesium.
  1. Available in IV and oral forms.
    a. Use IV replacement for patients with severe depletion, those who cannot tolerate oral replacement, those who have eclampsia/preeclampsia, and those who are symptomatic.
    b. Use oral supplements for chronic hypomagnesemia and asymptomatic states.
      i. Absorption is unpredictable with oral supplements, and diarrhea is common.
      ii. Repletion of total body stores takes several days.
  2. Recommended IV doses of magnesium sulfate (dose should be decreased by 50% in patients with renal impairment).
    a. 1 to 4 g if serum magnesium 1 to 1.5 mg/dL.
    b. 4 to 8 g if serum magnesium less than 1 mg/dL.
  3. Oral supplements.
    a. Magnesium oxide 400 mg BID.
C. Step 3—Treat other electrolyte and acid–base disorders.
D. Step 4—Assess cause and initiate a plan for prevention.
  1. Potassium-sparing diuretics can reduce renal magnesium wasting.

Follow-Up

A. Follow-up depends on underlying cause.
B. Patients who have cardiac arrhythmias should be closely followed until magnesium levels are restored.

Consultation/Referral

A. Consult cardiology as needed for cardiac arrhythmias.
B. Consult nephrology for management of renal impairment.

Special/Geriatric Considerations

A. Geriatric patients are at high risk for cardiac arrhythmias and renal impairment.
B. Caution should be used to assure magnesium levels are optimized in this patient population.

Bibliography

Kraft, M. D., Btaiche, I. F., Sacks, G. S., & Kudsk, K. A. (2005, August). Treatment of electrolyte disorders in adult patients in the intensive care unit. *American Journal of Health System Pharmacy, 62*(16), 1663–1682. doi:10.2146/ajhp040300

Moe, S. M., & Daoud, J. R. (2014). Disorders of mineral metabolism: Calcium, phosphorous, and magnesium. In D. S. Gipson, M. A. Perazella, & M. Tonelli (Eds.), *National Kidney Foundation's primer on kidney diseases* (6th ed., pp. 100–112). Philadelphia, PA: Elsevier Saunders.

Hyponatremia

Jessica S. Everitt, Divya Monga, and Catherine Wells

Definition

A. See Box 5.5 for further details.
B. Serum sodium less than 135 mEq/L (measured by ion-specific electrode; see Box 5.5).
  a. Mild: 130 to 135 mEq/L.
  b. Moderate: 125 to 129 mEq/L.
  c. Severe or profound: Less than 125 mEq/L.
C. Acute hyponatremia: Low serum sodium documented for 48 or fewer hours.
D. Chronic hyponatremia: Low serum sodium that is either documented for greater than 48 hours or onset is unknown.

Incidence

A. The incidence is 15% to 38% in hospitalized patients, with only ~7% incidence in ambulatory settings.
B. In institutionalized geriatric patients, an incidence as high as 53% has been reported.
C. The incidence of moderate and severe hyponatremia (serum sodium <130 mEq/L) is 1%, with a prevalence of 2.5%.
  1. 67% of cases are hospital acquired, and 30% occur in the ICU.
D. Admission of patients with hyponatremia is directly associated with inpatient mortality.

Pathogenesis

A. Pseudohyponatremia.
  1. Apparent low sodium with plasma and urine osmolality and tonicity, as well as hyperlipidemia or hyperproteinemia.
  2. Normal serum sodium that appears falsely low when using indirect ion-selective electrode (ISE) method to assess plasma for sodium.
    a. The original sample is diluted to 1:10 ratio, measuring whole plasma sodium, assuming the sample contains 93% water and 7% proteins/lipids.
    b. But increased proteins or lipids decrease the ratio of total water, causing a perceived lower than actual sodium level.
  3. Solution: Measurement of sodium via direct ion-sensitive electrode and serum sample (undiluted blood).
    a. This is usually a point of care test.
B. Dilutional hyponatremia (↑ total body water [TBW] +/− ↓ Solutes).
  1. Due to transcellular water shifts—hypertonicity.
    a. Hyperglycemia (>250 mg/dL).
    b. Hypertonic solutions (e.g., mannitol, intravenous immunoglobulin [IVIG]).
C. Solute depletion hyponatremia (↓ Solutes + ↑ TBW; requires water intake).
  1. Loss of solute while maintaining water intake.
D. Potassium and sodium.
  1. Potassium is an active cation; Sodium is an anion. To maintain electroneutrality, potassium + chloride exchange across cell membranes for sodium.

2. As a result, when infusing potassium, some potassium ions become intracellular, and some sodium ions become extracellular, thus raising sodium levels.

Predisposing Factors
A. Elderly patients.
B. Taking psychiatric medications.
C. Cardiac disease.
D. Chronic kidney disease.
E. Malignancy.
F. Alcoholism.

Subjective Data
A. Common complaints/symptoms.
  1. Neurological symptoms: Range from mild and nonspecific to severe and potentially fatal.
    a. Severity of symptoms increases with acuity of onset.
      i. Chronic hyponatremia often presents with relatively mild symptoms.
      ii. Acute, severe hyponatremia is associated with marked neurological deficits.
  2. Neurological and other symptoms grouped by severity.
    a. Mild symptoms (nonspecific and rarely progress to herniation).
      i. Headache.
      ii. Nausea and vomiting.
      iii. Mild confusion.
    b. Moderate (sometimes known as moderately severe): Most often seen in chronic hyponatremia, and thus not associated with impending herniation.
      i. Anorexia.
      ii. Fatigue/malaise.
      iii. Confusion, agitation, disorientation, or forgetfulness.
      iv. Gait disturbance.
      v. Abnormal sensorium (i.e., dizziness).
    c. Severe.
      i. Vomiting.
      ii. Cardiopulmonary distress.
        1) Pulmonary edema.
        2) Acute respiratory failure secondary to tentorial herniation with subsequent brainstem compression.
        3) Cheyne–Stokes respiration.
      iii. Delirium.
      iv. Somnolence/obtundation.
      v. Seizures (10% incidence with severe hyponatremia).
      vi. Pathologic or depressed reflexes.
      vii. Pseudobulbar palsy.
      viii. Coma (Glasgow Scale ≤ 8).
    d. Other signs (e.g., falls).
  3. Possible hypovolemia or hypervolemia depending on the etiology of the hyponatremia.

Physical Examination
A. Physical examination to assess volume status.
  1. Check skin, mucous membranes, heart, lungs, jugular venous distension (JVD), edema.
  2. Assess blood pressure and orthostatic changes.
  3. Determine weight changes.
B. Neurological assessment (initial and ongoing).

Diagnostic Tests
A. Serum sodium.
B. Serum osmolality.
C. Complete chemistry panel including potassium.
D. Spot urine osmolality.
  1. Greater than 300 mOsm/kg: Urine is concentrated/hypertonic but not necessarily because of sodium. This indicates a relative increase in solute compared to water.
  2. Less than 150 mOsm/kg: Urine is dilute/hypotonic. This indicates a relative increase in water and/or decrease in solute.
E. Spot urine sodium.
  1. Less than 20 mEq/L: Renal sodium retention as in low effective arterial blood volume.
  2. 20 mEq/L or more: Diuretics will induce increased urine sodium.
F. Determination of patient volume status.
  1. Volume assessment is known to be unreliable as initial diagnostic criteria in hyponatremia but is necessary when interpreting hyponatremia-related lab tests.
  2. Physical examination to include assessments.
    a. Skin, mucous membranes, heart, lungs, JVD, edema, and weight changes.
    b. Blood pressure and orthostatic changes (especially in patients using diuretics).
G. Other lab tests to consider.
  1. Fractional excretion of uric acid (FE_{UA} %) or chloride (FE_{CL} %).
    a. These have better specificity and sensitivity than fractional excretion of sodium (FE_{NA} %) to help determine volume status and renal clearance of solutes.
  2. Vasopressin levels.
  3. Thyroid-stimulating hormone (TSH).
  4. Glucose and glycosylated hemoglobin.
  5. Cortisol.

Differential Diagnosis
A. Pseudohyponatremia.
  1. Hypertriglyceridemia greater than 1,000 mg/dL.
  2. Familial hypercholesterolemia.
  3. Proteinemia greater than 10 gm/dL (i.e., multiple myeloma).
B. Dilutional hyponatremia ($\uparrow$ TBW $+/- \downarrow$ Solutes).
  1. Impaired free water excretion: Renal tubular water losses.
    a. Endocrine: Hypothyroidism or adrenal/ glucocorticoid insufficiency.
    b. Physical/emotional stress.
    c. Syndrome of inappropriate antidiuretic hormone (SIADH).
      i. Central nervous system (CNS) etiologies: Tumor, meningitis, intracranial hemorrhage/ hematoma, stroke, or trauma.
      ii. Pulmonary disease: Pneumonia, acute respiratory failure, tuberculosis, or aspergillosis.
      iii. Neoplasm: Small cell carcinoma lung, pancreatic cancer, or duodenal cancer.
      iv. HIV/AIDS.
      v. Postoperative.
    d. Edema syndromes: Nephrotic syndrome, cirrhosis, or heart failure.
    e. Drugs: Amitriptyline, carbamazepine, chlorpropamide, clofibrate, cyclophosphamide, haloperidol, narcotics, nicotine, nonsteroidal

anti-inflammatory drugs (NSAIDs), serotonin reuptake inhibitors, thiothixene, thioridazine, vincristine, ecstasy, or oxytocin.

    f. Thiazide diuretics.

    g. Diminished solute intake with ongoing water intake: "Tea and toast" diet or beer potomania.

  2. Excess water intake.

    a. Primary polydipsia.

    b. Dilute infant formula.

    c. Hypotonic intravenous (IV) fluids.

C. Solute depletion hyponatremia ($\downarrow$ Solutes + $\uparrow$ TBW; requires water intake).

  1. Renal solute loss.

    a. Diuretic.

    b. Solute diuresis: Bicarbonaturia, ketonuria, glucose, mannitol, or urea diuresis.

    c. Salt wasting nephropathy (i.e., cystic renal diseases, interstitial disease, chronic glomerular disease, partial obstruction).

    d. Mineralocorticoid deficiency.

  2. Nonrenal solute loss.

    a. Gastrointestinal loss (diarrhea, vomiting, pancreatitis, bowel obstruction).

    b. Cutaneous (sweating, burns).

    c. Blood loss.

    d. Excessive intake of water and sports drinks in athletes, combined with excessive body fluid losses.

Evaluation and Management Plan

A. Step 1—Choose therapy goal and timing of sodium correction based on the following (obtained from history).

  1. Acute hyponatremia with severe symptoms: Emergency treatment (more aggressive treatment).

    a. Sodium 129 mEq/L or less that fell within the past 48 hours, causing severe patient symptoms.

  2. Acute hyponatremia with moderately severe symptoms: Emergency treatment.

    a. Sodium 129 mEq/L or less that fell within the past 48 hours. causing moderate patient symptoms.

  3. Acute hyponatremia with mild symptoms: Nonemergency treatment (most cases).

    a. Sodium 129 mEq/L or less that fell within the past 48 hours, causing mild patient symptoms.

  4. Acute hyponatremia asymptomatic: Nonemergency treatment (most cases).

    a. Sodium 129 mEq/L or less that fell within the past 48 hours, without causing symptoms.

  5. Chronic hyponatremia with any symptoms: Nonemergency treatment.

    a. Sodium 129 mEq/L or less for greater than 48 hours or an unknown period of time, causing any related patient symptoms.

  6. Chronic hyponatremia asymptomatic: Outpatient treatment.

    a. Sodium 129 mEq/L or less for greater than 48 hours, without causing symptoms.

B. Step 2—Set up appropriate monitoring to provide safe care and prevent overcompensation of sodium levels.

  1. Emergency treatment.

    a. Monitor closely in an intensive care setting.

    b. Monitor complete fluid intake and output hourly.

      i. Do not allow water intake to exceed output as this will exacerbate hyponatremia.

    c. Perform neurological and symptom assessment frequently.

    d. Measure sodium levels every 2 to 4 hours; then take them once daily until stable and sodium greater than 130 mEq/L.

  2. Nonemergency treatment.

    a. Monitor in an ED, ICU, or other nursing floor with trained staff.

    b. Monitor complete fluid intake and output hourly.

      i. Do not allow water intake to exceed output as this will exacerbate hyponatremia.

    c. Perform neurological and symptom assessment frequently.

    d. Measure sodium levels every 4 to 6 hours; then take them once daily until stable and sodium greater than 130 mEq/L.

  3. Outpatient treatment.

    a. Only for chronic patients with stable but low sodium.

    b. Monitoring and follow-up vary according to cause of hyponatremia.

C. Step 3—Initiate volume correction if hypovolemic.

D. Step 4—Initiate sodium correction therapy according to severity of symptoms.

  1. Acute or severe symptomatic hyponatremia.

    a. Initial treatment: 3% sodium chloride 100 mL bolus over 10 to 20 minutes.

      i. Repeat as needed: Up to 3 times.

      ii. Goal: To raise sodium 5% or 4 to 6 mEq/L and resolve symptoms.

      iii. Once goal is met, change to 3% sodium chloride infusion initiated at 0.5 to 2 mL/kg/hr and titrated based on sodium levels until sodium reaches 130 mEq/L.

        1) Raise the sodium: 1 mEq/hour.

        2) Maximum rise in sodium: 10 mEq/L above baseline per 24 hours.

    b. Day 1 (first 24 hours): Maximum rise in sodium: 10 mEq/L or 10%.

    c. Following days: Raise the sodium 8 mEq/L or 10%.

  2. Acute or moderate symptomatic hyponatremia.

    a. Initial treatment: 3% sodium chloride infusion given at 0.5 to 2 mL/kg/hour and titrated based on sodium levels until sodium reaches 130 mEq/L.

    b. Day 1 (first 24 hours).

      i. Goal for day 1: To raise sodium 5% or 4 to 6 mEq/L and resolve symptoms.

      ii. Maximum rise in sodium: 10 mEq/L or 10%.

    c. Following days.

      i. Raise the sodium 8 mEq/L or 10%.

  3. Asymptomatic hyponatremia.

    a. Water diuresis (unless hypovolemic): Loop diuretics.

    b. If not resolved: 3% sodium chloride infusion initiated at 0.5 to 2 mL/kg/hour and titrated based on sodium levels until sodium reaches 130 mEq/L.

    c. Day 1 (first 24 hours).

      i. Maximum rise in sodium: 10 mEq/L or 10%.

    d. Following days.

      i. Raise the sodium 8 mEq/L or 10%.

E. Step 5—Other related interventions.

  1. Treatment of other electrolyte and acid–base disorders; correct hypokalemia to a potassium of 3.5 to 4.5 mEq/L.

  2. Strict fluid intake and output; restrict or supplement intake as needed.

3. Head trauma or hemodynamic instability: Consider consulting nephrology for continuous renal replacement therapy (CRRT) hyponatremia protocols.
   a. Slower sodium titration.
   b. Controlled management of sodium levels using CRRT.
4. Chronic hyponatremia.
   a. Initial therapy.
      i. Restrict all water intake (enteral and parenteral) to 1,000 to 2,000 mL/day.
      ii. Correct hypokalemia to a potassium of 3.5 to 4.5 mEq/L.
      iii. Euvolemic and hypovolemic patients.
         1) Administer isotonic saline or balanced crystalloid solution.
         2) Discontinue existing/chronic diuretics (assess as possible cause).
      iv. Hypervolemic patients.
         1) Further restrict all water intake (enteral and parenteral) to 800 to 1,500 mL/day.
         2) Give loop diuretics.
      v. Replace sodium deficit only if necessary.
         1) 3% sodium chloride infusion initiated at 0.5 to 2 mL/kg/hour and titrated based on sodium levels until sodium reaches 130 mEq/L.
         2) +/– desmopressin (dDAVP) 1 to 2 mcg IV or SC every 8 hours for 24 to 48 hours. Only use dDAVP to support a therapy plan that includes sodium replacement and water restriction; dDAVP alone will not correct hyponatremia. Do not use dDAVP in psychogenic polydipsia, or edematous hyponatremia (i.e., congestive heart failure [CHF], cirrhosis).
         3) Day 1 (first 24 hours): Maximum rise in sodium: 10 mEq/L or 10%.
         4) Following days: Raise the sodium 8 mEq/L or 10%.
   b. Patients with high urine cation concentrations.
      i. Give loop diuretics.
      ii. Give vasopressin type 2 (V_2) receptor antagonists, also called vaptans.
      iii. Give salt tablets.
      iv. If resistant to the previously noted therapies, consider demeclocycline, or urea in conjunction with nephrology (demeclocycline likely to damage kidney function).
5. Overcorrecting hyponatremia.
   a. Risks: Seizures, cerebral edema, osmotic demyelinating syndrome (ODS), and death.
   b. If baseline serum sodium is 120 mEq/L or more, no intervention necessary.
   c. If baseline serum sodium is less than 120 mEq/L or if correction exceeds 6 to 8 mEq/L or 10% per day.
      i. Give electrolyte free water (D_5W) 10 mL/kg and repeat as needed.
      ii. Consider also dDAVP 2 mcg IV.
      iii. Correct sodium level back to the most recent sodium that was within guidelines for correcting at 6 to 8 mEq/L or 10% per day.
      iv. Correct sodium quickly, within a few hours of overcorrecting.

Follow-Up
A. Follow-up depends on underlying cause of hyponatremia.
B. Follow-up should be managed by the primary service who is managing the underlying cause.

Consultation/Referral
A. Consult nephrology if hyponatremia is due to renal disorders.
B. Consult neurology for CNS disorders causing hyponatremia.

Special/Geriatric Considerations
A. A spectrum of diseases and disorders is associated with the geriatric population that predisposes them to hyponatremia, including pulmonary, endocrine, and CNS diseases, as well as cancers.
B. A careful assessment of overall fluid status in elderly patients should be ascertained.
C. Bone stress and fractures.
   1. Sodium is stored in bone. Hyponatremia induces osteoclasts and thus bone loss.
   2. Chronic hyponatremia is associated with a fourfold increase in osteoporosis (dose and time dependent), gait instability, falls in the elderly, and increased risk of fractures.
D. Cerebral edema.
   1. Sodium enters the brain only in plasma. Acute changes to plasma tonicity/osmolality cause water to shift in and out of astrocytes. Acute rises in osmolality cause astrocytes to shrink.
   2. Within 48 hours, astrocytes adapt to hyponatremia and intracellular osmolality becomes equal to plasma osmolality without changing cell volume due to adaptive solutes and osmolytes.
   3. However, this adaptation has consequences such as increased astrocyte susceptibility to injury and poor long-term outcomes.
E. ODS.
   1. Sudden rises in extracellular tonicity/osmolality caused by the treatment/overcorrection of hyponatremia can cause osmotic stress on astrocytes, resulting in demyelination.
   2. ODS initially seems to improve with improvement of hyponatremia.
   3. There is a delayed onset of additional symptoms: Seizures, behavior changes, delusions, swallowing and speech dysfunction, movement disorders, paralysis, and potentially death. Symptoms can be temporary or permanent.
F. Mortality: Mild hyponatremia is associated with increased mortality, but deaths from cerebral edema and ODS are rare.
G. Monitor sodium closely in high risk populations.
   1. Geriatrics.
   2. Liver disease.
   3. CHF.
   4. CKD.
H. Before treating hyponatremia, rule out and/or treat hypothyroidism, adrenal insufficiency, hyperglycemia, hypertriglyceridemia, and hyperproteinemia.
I. For refractory hyponatremia in patients with CHF, consider adding a low dose angiotensin-converting enzyme (ACE) inhibitor to the diuretic regimen. Consult nephrology and cardiology experts.
J. For patients with cirrhosis, primary therapy for hyponatremia is water restriction and a low salt diet. If diuretics are required, use loop diuretics in combination with potassium-sparing diuretics and monitor potassium carefully.

K. Thiazide diuretics impair urine-diluting capacity, thus exacerbating hyponatremia.

Bibliography

Hoorn, E. J., & Zietse, R. (2017). Diagnosis and treatment of hyponatremia: Compilation of the guidelines. *Journal of American Society Nephrology, 28*, 1–10. doi:10.1681/ASN.2016101139

Kraft, M. D., Btaiche, I. F., Sacks, G. S., & Kudsk, K. A. (2005, August). Treatment of electrolyte disorders in adult patients in the intensive care unit. *American Journal of Health System Pharmacy, 62*(16), 1663–1682. doi: 10.2146/ajhp040300

Spasovski, G., Vanholder, R., Allolio, B., Annane, D., Ball, S., Bichet, D., . . . Nagler, E. (2014, April). Clinical practice guideline on diagnosis and treatment of hyponatremia. *Nephrology, Dialysis, Transplantation, 29*(Suppl. 2), i1–i39. doi:10.1093/ndt/gfu040

Sterns, R. H. (2015). Disorders of plasma sodium. *The New England Journal of Medicine, 372*(1), 55–65. doi:10.1056/NEJMra1404489

Sterns, R. H., & Silver, M. S. (2016). Complications and management of hyponatremia. *Current Opinion Nephrology Hypertension, 25*(2), 114–119. doi:10.1097/MNH.0000000000000200

Sterns, R. H. (2018, September 18). Causes of hypotonic hyponatremia in adults. In J. P. Forman (Ed.), *UpToDate*. Retrieved from https://www.uptodate.com/contents/causes-of-hypotonic-hyponatremia-in-adults

Sterns, R. H. (2018, December 6). Overview of the treatment of hyponatremia in adults. In J. P. Forman (Ed.), *UpToDate*. Retrieved from https://www.uptodate.com/contents/overview-of-the-treatment-ofhyponatremia-in-adults;Sterns

Verbalis, J. G. (2014). Hyponatremia and hypoosmolar disorders. In D. S., Gipson, M. A. Perazella, & M. Tonelli (Eds.), *National Kidney Foundation's primer on kidney diseases* (6th ed., pp. 62–69). Philadelphia, PA: Elsevier Saunders.

Hypophosphatemia

Jessica S. Everitt, Divya Monga, and Catherine Wells

Definition
A. See Box 5.6.
B. Serum phosphorus less than 3.5 mg/dL.
C. Moderate hypophosphatemia less than 2.5 mg/dL.
D. Severe hypophosphatemia less than 1 mg/dL.

Incidence
A. Incidence in general population is typically asymptomatic and estimated to be around 1% to 5%.

The incidence rises sharply in patients with diabetic ketoacidosis, sepsis, or history of alcoholism.

Pathogenesis
A. Homeostasis of phosphate is maintained through gastrointestinal (GI) absorption and renal excretion.
B. Imbalances in either of these mechanisms can result in hypophosphatemia.

Predisposing Factors
A. Eating disorders.
B. Alcoholism.
C. Tumors.
D. Vitamin D deficiency.
E. Refeeding syndrome.
F. Malabsorption.

Subjective Data
A. Common complaints/symptoms.
  1. Depend on magnitude of hypophosphatemia: Moderate and severe before symptomatic.
  2. Muscle weakness.
    a. Diaphragmatic weakness and difficulty with ventilation or weaning mechanical ventilation.
    b. Impaired myocardial contractility.
  3. Neurological dysfunction.
    a. Irritability ranging to seizures or coma.
    b. Paresthesias.
  4. Hematologic dysfunction, including hemolysis and platelet dysfunction.

Physical Examination
A. Respiratory examination.
B. Musculoskeletal examination.
C. Neurological examination.
D. Gastrointestinal examination.

Diagnostic Tests
A. Serum phosphorus.
B. Total calcium and ionized calcium.

Differential Diagnosis
A. Decreased intestinal absorption.
  1. Malabsorption and chronic diarrhea.
  2. Antacid abuse, excessive calcium supplement use, or overdose of phosphate binders.
  3. Vitamin D deficiency.
  4. Alcoholism.
  5. Malnutrition, starvation, or anorexia.
B. Increased urinary losses.
  1. Primary hyperparathyroidism.
  2. Fanconi syndrome.
  3. Osmotic diuresis.
    a. Post-obstructive or resolving acute tubular necrosis (ATN) diuresis.
    b. Glucosuria.
  4. Acetazolamide.
  5. Rickets (X-linked or vitamin D dependent).
  6. Oncogenic osteomalacia.
  7. Enuresis/polyuria.
    a. Postoperative, especially immediately after kidney transplant.
    b. Extracellular volume expansion.
C. Redistribution (shift to intracellular space).
  1. Respiratory alkalosis.
  2. Diabetic ketoacidosis/treatment of hyperglycemia.
  3. Refeeding syndrome (shift of phosphorus intracellularly in response to carbohydrate load).
    a. Malnourished patients are at high risk with total parenteral nutrition.
  4. Alcohol withdrawal.
  5. Severe burns.
  6. Leukemic blast crisis.

Evaluation and Management Plan
A. Step 1—If acute, severe, or symptomatic, replace phosphate intravenously.
  1. Give intravenous repletion for symptomatic patients with moderate or severe hypophosphatemia or those who cannot tolerate or receive oral supplementation.
    a. Potassium phosphate or sodium phosphate may be given. Sodium phosphate is recommended unless the patient also has hypokalemia.
    b. The initial dose is 0.16 to 0.25 mmol/kg, not to exceed 0.5 mmol/kg.
      i. Give dose over a minimum of 4 to 6 hours.

ii. Reduce dose by 50% in patients with renal dysfunction.

B. Step 2—Assess for ongoing losses or further phosphorus replacement needs.

    1. Give intravenous replacement to patients who cannot take or absorb oral phosphorus or patients with ongoing symptoms.

    2. Use oral supplements in patients with asymptomatic mild hypophosphatemia.

        a. May cause or worsen diarrhea.

        b. Gastrointestinal absorption is variable.

        c. Oral formulations contain various amounts of phosphorus, sodium, and potassium.

        d. Common regimen is 250 mg of elemental phosphorus four times daily.

    3. If oral supplements fail to maintain phosphorous levels, supplement with intravenous phosphorus.

C. Step 3—Identify and treat cause.

D. Step 4—Treat other electrolyte and acid–base disorders.

Follow-Up

A. Follow-up should occur with the provider who treats the underlying condition causing the electrolyte imbalance.

Consultation/Referral

A. Depends on underlying condition causing hypophosphatemia.

B. Endocrinology should be consulted if the diagnosis is related to hyperparathyroidism.

C. Gastroenterology should be consulted if there is a malabsorption condition.

D. Nephrology should be consulted in renal phosphate wasting.

E. Psychiatry should be consulted for eating disorders.

Special/Geriatric Considerations

A. Elderly patients can develop osteomalacia and be prone to bone pain and fractures.

Bibliography

Kraft, M. D., Btaiche, I. F., Sacks, G. S., & Kudsk, K. A. (2005, August). Treatment of electrolyte disorders in adult patients in the intensive care unit. *American Journal of Health System Pharmacy, 62*(16), 1663–1682. doi:10.2146/ajhp040300

Moe, S. M., & Daoud, J. R. (2014). Disorders of mineral metabolism: calcium, phosphorous, and magnesium. In D. S. Gipson, M. A. Perazella, & M. Tonelli (Eds.), *National Kidney Foundation's primer on kidney diseases* (6th ed., pp. 100–112). Philadelphia, PA: Elsevier Saunders.

Yu, A. S. L., & Stubbs, J. R. (2019, February 12). Evaluation and treatment of hypophosphatemia. In A. Q. Lam (Ed.), *UpToDate*. Retrieved from https://www.uptodate.com/contents/evaluation-and-treatment-of-hypophosphatemia

Metabolic Acidosis

Mary Rogers Sorey

Definition

A. Low arterial pH and low HCO_3.

B. Low pCO_2 after respiratory compensation.

Incidence

A. Metabolic acidosis occurs frequently in acute and chronic renal disease and in patients with any type of poisoning from drugs or chemicals. It is a common finding in the hospital setting for a variety of reasons.

B. It is typically classified as having a normal anion gap (non-AG) or a high anion gap (AG).

Pathogenesis

A. Metabolic acidosis can be determined by calculating the AG, the first step in distinguishing the type of metabolic acidosis.

    1. The equation to calculate the AG: $AG = Na^+ - (Cl^- + HCO_3)$.

    2. The normal AG is 12 mEq/L.

B. The causes of metabolic acidosis can be a loss of bicarbonate or the addition of acid.

C. In metabolic acidosis caused by loss of bicarbonate, there is a non-AG.

    1. Gastrointestinal (GI) losses.

        a. Diarrhea.

        b. Ileostomy.

        c. Surgical drains.

    2. Renal losses.

        a. Proximal and distal renal tubular acidosis.

        b. Hypoaldosteronism.

D. In metabolic acidosis caused by addition of acid, the AG is elevated above 12.

    1. Renal failure or uremia.

    2. Lactic acidosis.

    3. Ketoacidosis.

        a. Diabetes.

        b. Ethanol.

        c. Starvation.

    4. Ingestion.

        a. Ethylene glycol.

        b. Methanol.

        c. Paraldehyde.

        d. Salicylate intoxication.

E. In metabolic acidosis, the PCO_2 falls predictably depending on HCO_3 concentration.

    1. To calculate expected change, $PCO_2 = (1.5\ HCO_3^-) + 8 \pm 2$.

    2. If the PCO_2 is not as expected, there is a respiratory acid–base disturbance, too.

F. In AG metabolic acidosis, - can be used to discover a second metabolic acid–base disorder.

    1. $Gap/HCO_3^- = $ (measured AG – ideal AG)/(ideal HCO_3 – measured HCO_3^-).

        a. If less than 1 then there is a non-AG metabolic acidosis present.

        b. If greater than 2 then there is a metabolic alkalosis present.

Predisposing Factors

A. There are none. Metabolic acidosis is dependent on cause, which determines the predisposing factors.

Subjective Data

A. Common complaints/symptoms.

    1. Increased respiratory rate.

    2. Drowsiness.

    3. Nonspecific.

B. Family and social history.

    1. Alcohol use or drug abuse.

    2. Occupational history and potential exposure to metals or chemicals.

    3. Genetic disorder associated with a family history of acidosis, typically discovered in childhood.

C. Review of systems.

1. Neurological: Blurred vision, vertigo, headache, confusion, generalized weakness.

2. Head, ear, eyes, nose, throat: Ringing in the ears, light bothering eyes, seeing floaters.

3. Respiratory—increased breathing.

4. Cardiovascular—chest pain, palpitations.

5. GI—diarrhea, vomiting, pain in the chest that feels like heartburn.

6. Renal—increased urination, increased thirst, urination at night.

7. Psychiatric: Any history of drug use or depression.

Physical Examination

A. Nonspecific physical examination that depends on the underlying cause.

1. Renal failure: Pallor, drowsiness, asterixis, pericardial rub.

2. Diabetic ketoacidosis: Reduced skin turgor, dry mucous membranes, fruity breath.

3. Sepsis—fever, confusion or coma, hypotension, Kussmaul respirations.

Diagnostic Tests

A. Serum electrolytes: Check serum bicarbonate.

B. Arterial blood gas (ABG): pH less than 7.40.

C. AG determination.

D. Base excess/deficit determination to determine the degree of acidosis.

E. CBC: Look for severe anemia which can affect oxygen delivery.

F. Urinalysis: Urine pH greater than 5.5 may be associated with certain renal diseases.

1. Calcium oxalate crystals seen in ethylene glycol toxicity.

G. Beta-hydroxybutyrate.

H. Lactate level.

I. Necessary in certain situations.

1. Salicylate levels.

2. Iron levels.

3. Aldosterone levels.

4. Ammonium levels.

Differential Diagnosis

A. For normal AG metabolic acidosis.

1. Abdomen.

a. Diarrhea.

b. Fistulas.

2. Renal.

a. Renal tubular acidosis: Addison's disease.

b. Carbonic anhydrase inhibitors.

c. Post hypocapnia.

d. Excessive chloride (large volumes of saline).

B. For a high AG metabolic acidosis, use the mnemonic MUDPILES to remember the differential diagnosis.

1. **M**ethanol.

2. **U**remia.

3. **D**iabetic ketoacidosis.

4. **P**araldehyde.

5. **I**nfection, iron, isoniazid, ibuprofen.

6. **L**actic acidosis.

7. **E**thylene glycol.

8. **S**alicylates.

Evaluation and Management Plan

A. General plan.

1. Treat with an alkali therapy to raise plasma pH greater than 7.20.

2. Calculate the sodium bicarbonate deficit to determine how much must be administered intravenously to raise the serum bicarbonate level to increase the pH greater than 7.20.

3. Determine the underlying cause of the metabolic acidosis and treat appropriately.

B. Pharmacotherapy.

1. Metabolic acidosis of any type. Sodium bicarbonate can be used, but treating the underlying issue is critical.

a. Be cautious of volume overload; loop diuretics can be used to reduce volume as needed.

2. Methanol or ethylene glycol poisoning. Fomepizole can be used to treat ethylene glycol poisoning.

3. Uremia. Sodium bicarbonate can be used to keep serum bicarbonate levels above 20 mEq/L.

4. Diabetic ketoacidosis. Insulin can be used to treat ketoacidosis.

5. Paraldehyde poisoning. Alkali therapy can be used to correct metabolic acidosis during supportive care; no specific antidote exists.

6. Infection, iron, isoniazid, or ibuprofen. Antibiotics can be used to treat sepsis and activated charcoal can be used for the treatment of poisoning caused by drugs and chemicals.

7. Lactic acidosis. Alkali therapy such as sodium bicarbonate or tromethamine can be used.

a. The role of alkali therapy can be controversial.

8. Ethylene glycol—Fomepizole or ethanol can be used to treat cases of poisoning.

9. Salicylates—Acetazolamide can treat salicylate poisoning by inducing alkaline diuresis.

Follow-Up

A. The patient needs to follow-up with the primary care provider and any appropriate service providers involved in regulating the underlying disease process that causes the metabolic acidosis.

Consultation/Referral

A. Refer to the appropriate service provider related to the cause of the metabolic acidosis.

B. Consult nephrology as quickly as possible in cases that may require hemodialysis.

C. Consult endocrine for patients who present with diabetic ketoacidosis.

Special/Geriatric Considerations

A. Metabolic complications are common in the elderly and can be exacerbated in chronic kidney disease.

B. Special care to monitor and detect metabolic disturbances should be instituted.

Bibliography

Kraut, J. A., & Madias, N. E. (2015, October 15). Metabolic acidosis of CKD: An update. *American Journal of Kidney Diseases, 67*(2), 307–317. doi:10.1053/j.ajkd.2015.08.028

Kraut, J. A., & Madias, N. E. (2016, September). Lactic acidosis: Current treatments and future directions. *American Journal of Kidney Diseases, 68*(3), 473–482. doi:10.1053/j.ajkd.2016.04.020

Rastegar, M., & G. T. Nagami (2017, February). Non-anion gap metabolic acidosis: A clinical approach to evaluation. *American Journal of Kidney Diseases, 69*(2), 296–301. doi:10.1053/j.ajkd.2016.09.013

Reddy, P., & Mooradian, A. D. (2009, October). Clinical utility of anion gap in deciphering acid-base disorders. *International Journal of Clinical Practice, 63*(10), 1516–1525. doi:10.1111/j.1742-1241.2009.02000.x

Thomas, C. P. (2018, October 10). Metabolic acidosis. In V. Batuman (Ed.), *Medscape*. Retrieved from https://emedicine.medscape.com/article/242975-overview

Nephrolithiasis

Juan A. Medaura

Definition

A. Formation of a kidney stone, an organized mass of crystals that grows on the surface of a renal papilla.

Incidence

A. Renal and ureteral stones are a common problem. In the United States, almost 2 million outpatient visits with urolithiasis as primary diagnosis were recorded in the year 2000.

B. The prevalence is increasing from 3.8% (1976–1980) to 8.4% (2007–2010). It coincidentally has increased in concordance with the rising incidence in obesity, insulin resistance, and metabolic syndrome.

C. The condition is more common in males than females. However, the ratio has gone from 1:4 to 1:1.4, as a result of a significant spike in the incidence of the condition in women in the past decades.

D. The average age of onset is 20s to 30s with a second peak in the mid-50s. Up to 16% of men and 8% of women will have at least one symptomatic stone by the age of 70 years.

E. It is more common in whites compared with blacks, Asians, and Hispanics.

F. It is more common in the south-eastern United States and more common in summer because of heat, sunlight exposure, and dehydration, leading to low urine volumes.

G. In stone formers, the rate of recurrence is 30% at 5 years, 50% at 10 years, and 80% at 20 years.

H. In the United States ~80% of kidney stones are calcium-containing stones, of which 80% are mainly calcium oxalate stones. Less often they are calcium phosphate stones.

Pathogenesis

A. Kidney stones occur as the result of an increased burden of a poorly soluble salt excreted into a volume of urine that is insufficient to dissolve it (supersaturation).

    1. In addition to an individual predisposition and/or other factors, there is, especially, lack of inhibitors of crystallization.

    2. Supersaturation of poorly soluble salts (i.e., calcium oxalate) in urine is one factor.

B. However, the main factor, especially in calcium-containing stones, is the accumulation of apatite (calcium phosphate) in the medullary interstitium; this may develop in idiopathic hypercalciuria.

    1. A stone starts to accumulate in the basement membrane of the thin loop of Henle and grows into the medullary interstitium, to finally form the "Randall's plaque" that will erupt breaking the urothelium of the papilla.

    2. This favors the deposition and aggregation of crystals, resulting in the organized stone.

Predisposing Factors

A. Idiopathic hypercalciuria.

B. Obesity, diabetes, and metabolic syndrome: Uric acid stones and calcium oxalate stones.

C. Dehydration, low fluid intake, and low urine volume (summer months, hot and/or dry weather, athletic, or occupational activities).

D. High dietary salt.

E. High oxalate food intake (e.g., spinach, nuts, chocolate, berries, tea, rhubarb, star fruit).

F. High animal protein diet.

G. Protein supplements.

H. Excessive vitamin C supplementation (metabolized to oxalate).

I. Low calcium diet with main meals of the day.

J. Bariatric surgery (gastric bypass).

K. Rapid weight loss/starvation.

L. Hypocitraturia, metabolic acidosis, hypokalemia, or hypomagnesemia.

M. Intestinal malabsorption.

N. Antibiotics (leading to loss of *Oxalobacter formigenes,* a protecting bacteria of the gut microbiota against excess oxalate absorption).

O. Chronic or recurrent urinary tract infection (UTIs) with urea-splitting organisms such as *Proteus, Providencia,* or *Ureaplasma* (struvite stones).

P. Medications: Topiramate, acetazolamide, atazanavir, indinavir, triamterene, sulfadiazine, sulfasalazine, or felbamate.

Q. Systemic diseases: Primary hyperparathyroidism, distal renal tubular acidosis (type 1), sarcoidosis/tuberculosis, medullary sponge kidney, malignancy, intestinal malabsorption (i.e., Crohn's disease), hyperthyroidism, and so forth.

Subjective Data

A. Common complaints/symptoms.

    1. Flank pain (radiates downward and anteriorly to the abdomen, pelvis, and groin/genitals).

    2. Nausea and vomiting.

    3. Hematuria (gross or microscopic).

    4. Stone passage.

B. Common/typical scenario.

    1. Fever.

    2. Dysuria.

    3. Calculous anuria.

    4. Interruption of urinary stream.

C. Review of systems.

    1. Establish onset and characteristics of the pain.

    2. Ask about witnessed stone passage.

    3. Ask about stone history.

        a. Age when first stone developed.

        b. Number of stones.

        c. Frequency of stone episodes.

        d. Size of stone (passed or still retained).

        e. Type of stone (if known).

        f. Kidney involved (left, right, or both).

        g. Need of urologic intervention (if yes, response to the intervention).

        h. UTI associated (yes or no).

    4. Inquire about diet, at-risk occupations (e.g., pilots, taxi drivers, teachers, athletes), family history, medications, dietary supplements, medical conditions, previous episodes of urolithiasis, and frequency of UTIs.

Physical Examination

A. The physical examination is most important for ruling out other conditions. Kidney and ureteral stones have no specific manifestations on physical examination.

B. Cerebrovascular accident (CVA) tenderness can be positive in some cases.

Diagnostic Tests

A. Noncontrast CT scan (stone protocol) is the gold standard.

B. Renal ultrasound (inexpensive, safe) is a good diagnostic tool to diagnose urolithiasis and rule out hydronephrosis, especially for frequent stone formers or patient with contraindication for radiation (i.e., pregnancy).

C. Plain radiography of the abdomen shot at 60 kV (kidney–ureter–bladder [KUB]) is useful for the frequent calcium stone former to reduce the amount of radiation and is more economic.

    1. Does not detect non-calcium stones (i.e., uric acid stones).

D. Laboratory analysis should be performed after the first kidney stone episode.

    1. Serum electrolytes, including calcium and phosphorus.

    2. Blood urea nitrogen (BUN) and creatinine.

    3. Uric acid level.

    4. In patients with hypercalcemia.

        a. Parathyroid hormone (PTH) level.

        b. 25-OH vitamin D.

        c. 1,25 dihydroxyvitamin D.

    5. A low-serum bicarbonate concentration.

        a. Urine pH.

            i. 6.0 or more: Suggests renal tubular acidosis.

            ii. Greater than 8 urine pH or pyuria: Should lead to urine cultures and consideration of struvite stones.

    6. Ancillary 24-hour urine collection for stone-risk profile is recommended in these situations.

        a. All children with kidney stones.

        b. Metabolically active stones (growing in size or in number within 1 year).

        c. Frequent stone formers (more than two to three episodes).

        d. Non-calcium (e.g., cystine, uric acid) stone formers.

        e. Patient in demographic group not typically prone to stone formation (e.g., African Americans).

Differential Diagnosis

A. Pyelonephritis (although in many situations coexist with nephrolithiasis).

B. Peritonitis.

C. In women: Ovarian torsion, ovarian cyst, or ectopic pregnancy.

Evaluation and Management Plan

A. General plan.

    1. Pain relief.

        a. Patients can be managed at home if they are able to take oral medications and fluids.

        b. Combination of nonsteroidal anti-inflammatory drugs (NSAIDs) and opioids is superior than each agent alone (i.e., morphine 5 mg + ketorolac 15 mg).

    2. Fluid intake.

        a. The mainstay of therapy is to increase the urine volume to more than 2 L per day.

        b. Therefore, the patient has to be encouraged to drink around 3 L of fluid per day. Because the risk of stone formation is highest during the night time, patients should be encouraged to drink plenty of fluids in the evening.

    3. Sodium intake.

        a. Urine sodium excretion augments urine calcium excretion.

        b. Hence, the patient should be instructed to limit dietary sodium to 2 g per day.

    4. Dietary calcium.

        a. It has been demonstrated that an adequate calcium intake in the diet decreases kidney stone incidence. This is likely due to intestinal binding of calcium to oxalate, preventing its absorption.

        b. An age- and gender-appropriate calcium diet is therefore recommended. Calcium supplementation outside of meals should be avoided.

B. Specific treatment (for each stone type).

    1. Calcium stones.

        a. Potassium citrate 30 to 60 mEq/day PO.

            i. Would start with 60 mEq/day if 24-hour urinary citrate is less than 150 mg/day.

            ii. Titrate dose to a 24-hour urinary citrate 320 to 640 mg/day and a urinary pH 6.0 to 7.0, to inhibit stone formation.

        b. Thiazide diuretic: Patients with hypercalciuria (24-hour urinary calcium >250 mg/day).

            i. Chlorthalidone 12.5 mg PO daily, or hydrochlorothiazide 12.5 mg PO daily, or indapamide 1.25 mg PO daily.

            ii. If the calcium excretion remains elevated in follow-up 24-hour urinary calcium several months after, the thiazide dose should be increased.

        c. Dietary oxalate restriction: Patients with hyperoxaluria (24-hour urinary oxalate >25–30 mg/day). Supplement each meal with calcium carbonate 1 to 1.5 g and snack to bind dietary oxalate in the intestine and prevent absorption.

        d. Specific therapy for malabsorptive disorder: First-line treatment for enteric hyperoxaluria.

    2. Uric acid stones.

        a. Potassium citrate: 30 to 60 mEq/day or twice daily orally to dissolve retained uric acid stones.

            i. For prevention of new stones: 30 to 60 mEq/day or three times a week titrating urinary pH to greater than 7.0.

            ii. Patient use of colorimetric pH-sensitive urine strips: Check the urinary pH 3 to 4 hours after taking potassium citrate.

        b. Low purine and low animal protein diet, if in follow-up the 24-hour urine uric acid is still high (>700 mg/day).

            i. May need to add allopurinol 100 mg/day PO, increasing weekly to 200 to 300 mg/day.

    3. Struvite stones (staghorn calculi).

        a. Aggressive medical and surgical treatment, since this can lead to renal failure.

            i. Early urologic intervention is advised.

        b. Antibiotic therapy, to prevent further stone formation due to urease splitting organisms.

    4. Cystine stones.

        a. Treatment to decrease cysteine concentration: Water intake as mainstay of therapy.

            i. Trying to achieve 3 to 4 L of urine a day.

ii. Goal urine cystine concentration less than 243 mg/L.

b. Low sodium diet 2 g/day.

c. Low animal protein diet.

d. Potassium citrate: Goal urine pH greater than 7.0 (maintained), which is a difficult task.

    i. Start 20 mEq TID and titrate up to a pH greater than 7.0.

e. Tiopronin 400 to 1,200 mg/day in three divided doses (comes in 100 mg tablets).

    i. Fewer side effects than D-penicillamine, but still can cause the same side effects (i.e., proteinuria, fever, rash, abnormal taste, arthritis, leukopenia, aplastic anemia, and hepatotoxicity).

C. Hospitalization.

  1. Stone greater than 5 mm (98% of stones <5 mm will pass spontaneously).

  2. Nausea and vomiting; unable to take oral medicine or fluids.

  3. Requiring parenteral therapy for pain.

  4. Pyelonephritis/UTI.

Follow-Up

A. For adult patients with history of only one calcium-containing kidney stone that passed spontaneously, no special follow-up is required.

B. For frequent stone formers (two to three or more episodes), children, or individuals who form non-calcium stones or rare stone types, they need a follow-up in 4 to 6 months with a 24-hour stone risk analysis to monitor the effect of therapy.

Consultation/Referral

A. Urology consultation is recommended for stones greater than 5 mm as the likelihood of spontaneous passage of stones of this magnitude is low, or consult when complications occur. UTI with obstruction is the most urgent indication for urologic consultation.

B. Nephrology consultation is recommended for frequent stone formers, patients who form non-calcium stones, those who form rare stone types, and those with nephrolithiasis and chronic kidney disease (CKD). Children should be referred to pediatric nephrology.

Special/Geriatric Considerations

A. Common in the **elderly** and is associated with multiple comorbidities, including hypertension, coronary artery disease, diabetes mellitus, and CKD.

Bibliography

Assimos, D. G., Krambeck, A., Miller, N. L., Monga, M., Murad, M. H., Nelson, C. P., & Matlaga, B. R. (2016). *Surgical management of stones: American Urological Association/Endourological Society Guideline.* Linthicum, MD: American Urological Association. Retrieved from https://www.auanet.org/education/guidelines/surgical-management-of-stones.cfm

Jindal, G., & Ramchandani, P. (2007, May). Acute flank pain secondary to urolithiasis: Radiologic evaluation and alternate diagnoses. *Radiologic Clinics of North America, 45*(3), 395–410, vii. doi:10.1016/j.rcl.2007.04.001

Singh, A., Alter, H. J., & Littlepage, A. (2007, November). A systematic review of medical therapy to facilitate passage of ureteral calculi. *Annals of Emergency Medicine, 50*(5), 552–563. doi:10.1016/j.annemergmed.2007.05.015

Wen, C. C., & Nakada, S. Y. (2007, August). Treatment selection and outcomes: Renal calculi. *The Urologic Clinics of North America, 34*(3), 409–419. doi:10.1016/j.ucl.2007.04.005

Worcester, E. M., & Coe, F. L. (2008, June). Nephrolithiasis. *Primary Care, 35*(2), 369–391. doi:10.1016/j.pop.2008.01.005

Ziemba, J. B., & Matlaga, B. R. (2017, September). Epidemiology and economics of nephrolithiasis. *Investigative and Clinical Urology, 58*(5), 299–306. doi:10.4111/icu.2017.58.5.299

Nephrotic Syndrome

Debra Hain

Definition

A. Nephrotic syndrome (NS) is a clinical syndrome with specific features of proteinuria and hypoalbuminemia or hypoproteinemia.

B. The National Kidney Foundation defines NS as total urine protein excretion in excess of 3,500 mg/d (equivalent to a total protein-creatinine ratio of >3,000 mg/g), with a decreased serum albumin concentration and edema with or without a decrease in glomerular filtration rate (GFR).

C. The term *nephritic syndrome* is an outdated term characterized by hematuria with red blood cell casts, hypertension, and edema with or without decreased GFR.

Incidence

A. Annual incidence in adults is three per 100,000 individuals.

B. About 80% to 90% of the NS cases are primary (idiopathic).

  1. Membranous nephropathy (MN) is the leading cause of idiopathic NS.

    a. MN NS is common in white individuals and focal segmental glomerulosclerosis (FSGS) is more common in black individuals.

    b. FSGS NS accounts for about 30% to 35% of NS cases.

  2. Minimal change disease (MCD) and immunoglobulin A nephropathy (about 15% of cases) are less frequent.

C. About 10% of NS cases are secondary (due to underlying medical conditions).

  1. Systemic lupus erythematosus (SLE).

  2. Malignancy.

  3. Infections (hepatitis B and C, HIV, and malaria).

  4. Diabetic nephropathy.

Pathogenesis

A. Pathogenesis of NS is related to increased glomerular permeability to albumin and other plasma protein as a consequence of a damaged basement membrane.

B. MN is characterized by immune deposits that form at the base of the foot processes of the glomerular visceral epithelial cell or podocyte.

C. FSGS is multifactorial, but the injury to the foot process on the podocytes seem to be the main cause. Mechanisms include a T-cell mediated circulating permeability factor, transforming growth factor (TGF), *B*-cell mediated matrix synthesis, and genetic podocyte abnormalities.

Predisposing Factors

A. Amyloidosis.

B. Diabetes mellitus.

C. Cryoglobulinemia.

D. Sjögren syndrome.

E. SLE.

F. Carcinoma.

G. Leukemia, lymphoma.

H. Melanoma.

I. Multiple myeloma.

J. Infection (bacterial, protozoan, viral).

K. Allergic reaction to insect stings or bites, antitoxins, position ivy, or oak.

L. Malignant hypertension.

M. Sarcoidosis.

N. Genetic syndromes (e.g., familial FSGS, hereditary nephritis [Alport syndrome]).

Subjective Data

A. Common complaints/symptoms.

  1. Progressive lower extremity edema.

  2. Significant fluid weight gain.

  3. Fatigue.

  4. Exertional dyspnea.

B. Common/typical scenario.

  1. Periorbital, genital edema.

  2. Ascites.

  3. Pleural or pericardial effusion.

  4. Adults who present with new onset of edema or ascites and do not have the typical dyspnea seen with heart failure or present with cirrhosis.

C. Review of systems.

  1. Determine onset and duration of symptoms.

  2. Determine if weight change has occurred (normal weight).

    a. If weight gain: How much and over what period of time?

  3. Ask if any changes in urine output; foamy urine?

  4. Identify medication or toxin exposure: Risk factors for HIV or hepatitis and symptoms that could be indicative of other causes for edema (e.g., heart failure).

  5. Underlying health conditions such as diabetes, SLE, or other systemic disease.

  6. Previous history of NS; if yes, when and, if known, what was the cause and treatment?

Physical Examination

A. Check vital signs, blood pressure, temperature, heart rate, and respirations; obtain body weight.

  1. Possible hypertension.

B. Inspect periorbital area, abdomen, and lower extremities assessing for edema or ascites.

C. Auscultate heart, lungs, and abdomen.

D. Palpate abdomen assessing for ascites and lower extremities for edema.

Diagnostic Tests

A. The goal of diagnostic testing is to (a) assess for complications; (b) identify underlying disease; and (c) possibly determine the histological type of idiopathic NS.

B. Serum and urine tests.

  1. Serum chemistry panel to evaluate kidney function (blood urea nitrogen [BUN], creatinine, estimated GFR), electrolytes.

  2. Assess for acute kidney injury (AKI; see section "Acute Kidney Injury" for specific information).

  3. Glucose for diabetes mellitus.

  4. Blood count and coagulation panel (abnormal suggestive of bleeding disorder).

  5. Serum albumin.

  6. Lipid panel to assess for hyperlipidemia.

  7. Urine dipstick to confirm proteinuria; protein-to-creatinine ratio from a random (spot) urine sample to evaluate for nephrotic-range proteinuria (24-hour urine collection is cumbersome for patients and the collection is done incorrectly).

    a. Early morning specimen is best.

    b. Protein-to-creatinine ratio greater than 3.0 to 3.5 mg protein/mg creatinine (300–350 mg/mmol).

    c. Spot urine may be inaccurate in person who exercises heavily or someone who is gaining or losing muscle mass.

    d. Hematuria or casts are suggestive of nephritis.

C. Additional tests depending on patient presentation.

  1. HIV screening.

  2. Liver panel; elevated transaminase may indicate viral hepatitis (if abnormal, obtain viral hepatitis panel).

  3. Serum or urine protein electrophoresis (amyloidosis or multiple myeloma).

  4. Rapid plasma regain to determine if syphilis present.

  5. Antinuclear antibodies, anti-double-stranded DNA antibody, and complement values (C3 and C4) if suspect connective tissue disorder.

D. Imaging studies.

  1. Chest x-ray: To evaluate for pleural effusion.

  2. CT or MRI: Possible to evaluate for neoplastic diseases as secondary cause.

  3. Ultrasound.

    a. Renal: For reduced GFR.

    b. Abdominal to evaluate for ascites.

    c. Lower extremity Doppler ultrasound, CT, MRI, or lung ventilation/perfusion scan if suspect thrombosis or pleural effusion.

  4. Echocardiography: For suspected heart failure.

E. Renal biopsy.

  1. The role of renal biopsy is controversial and there is a lack of evidence-based guidelines. In those with NS from a known secondary cause who are responding to treatment, the renal biopsy will not likely add to the treatment.

  2. It may prove beneficial when trying to determine best treatment and prognosis in adults with idiopathic NS of unknown histologic disease type and in those in which the provider is considering underlying SLE as the cause.

Differential Diagnosis

A. Liver disease (e.g., cirrhosis).

B. Heart failure.

C. Differential for AKI in NS.

  1. Allergic interstitial nephritis.

  2. AKI.

    a. Acute tubular necrosis.

    b. Prerenal azotemia.

  3. Adverse effects from drug therapy.

  4. Nonsteroidal anti-inflammatory drug (NSAID) nephropathy.

  5. Renal venous thrombosis.

Evaluation and Management Plan

A. General plan.

  1. Confirm NS (evidence of proteinuria and hypoalbuminemia); once confirmed, consult nephrology expert (e.g., physician, nurse practitioner).

  2. Assess for common causes (see section "Incidence").

  3. Assess for complications.

    a. Venous thrombosis.

      i. Renal veins affected; possible cause of pulmonary embolism.

ii. No evidence for prophylactic anticoagulation: Decision to treat should be considered individually.

  b. Infection, especially cellulitis.

    i. Maintenance of standard infection control practices.

    ii. No strong evidence supporting any specific intervention to prevent infection in adults with NS.

  c. AKI.

  d. Markedly elevated lipid levels.

B. Patient/family teaching points.

  1. Restrict sodium intake to less than 3 g per day.

  2. Restrict fluid to less than 1,500 mL per day.

C. Pharmacotherapy.

  1. Diuretic therapy to treat edema.

    a. Loop diuretics (act in renal tubule and must be protein-bound to be effective).

      i. Oral loop diuretics twice a day are more effective than once daily.

        1) Furosemide 40 mg PO twice daily or bumetanide 1 mg PO twice daily is used to start.

        2) The dose may be doubled every 1 to 3 days if edema not improved or patient experiencing hypervolemia.

        3) Maximum dose of furosemide is 240 mg per dose or 600 mg total per day. If no response to oral drug, consider intravenous form.

        4) Serum protein is decreased so higher dose may be necessary.

        5) Intravenous bolus of 20% human albumin prior to intravenous diuretic may be considered.

      ii. When edema is severe, it may be necessary to start with intravenous diuretics.

    b. Diuresis should be gradual and guided by daily weights (1–2 kg per day).

  2. Angiotensin-converting enzyme (ACE) inhibitors or angiotensin receptor blockers (ARBs) are used to reduce proteinuria.

  3. Immunosuppressive therapy: Should be prescribed in collaboration with nephrology expert.

    a. Corticosteroids: Used frequently (despite lack of supportive data).

    b. Azathioprine (Imuran).

    c. Biologics (rituximab, eculizumab).

    d. Cyclophosphamide.

    e. High dose immune globulin.

    f. Mycophenolate mofetil (CellCept).

Follow-Up

A. The prognosis is variable depending on the underlying cause, disease histology, and patient clinical factors.

  1. Many patients will improve and some will require dialysis.

  2. Patients with volume overload and cardiopulmonary decompensation for intravenous diuresis versus ultrafiltration for fluid removal require admission.

  3. Follow-up is on an individual basis, but patients should continue with nephrology expert and primary care provider.

Consultation/Referral

A. Nephrology expert.

B. Other specialist depending on underlying cause (e.g., infectious disease, endocrinology, liver specialist).

Special/Geriatric Considerations

A. Consider underlying kidney function when treating with medications.

B. In NS due to AKI requiring dialysis, avoid hypovolemia and hypotension to preserve residual kidney function. Resolution of AKI to baseline kidney function (without requiring dialysis) is possible.

C. Older adults may seem to have a creatinine within normal range due to loss of muscle mass. Use estimated GFR to determine kidney function.

Bibliography

Beck, L. H., & Salant, D. J. (2010). Membranous nephropathy: Recent travels and new roads ahead. *Kidney International, 77*(9), 765–770. doi:10.1038/ki.2010.34

Cattran, D. C., & Brenchley, P. E. (2017). Membranous nephropathy: Integrating basic science into improved clinical management. *Kidney International, 91*(3), 566–574. doi:10.1016/j.kint.2016.09.048

Floege, I. (2015). Introduction to glomerular disease: Clinical presentations. In R. J. Johnson, J. Feehally, & J. Floege(Eds.), *Comprehensive clinical nephrology* (5th ed., pp. 184–197). Philadelphia, PA: Elsevier Saunders.

Kerlin, B. A., Ayoob, R., & Smoyer, W. E. (2012). Epidemiology and pathophysiology of nephrotic syndrome—Associated thromboembolic disease. *Clinical Journal of the American Society of Nephrology, 7*(3), 513–520. doi: 10.2215/CJN.10131011

Kodner, C. (2009). Nephrotic syndrome in adults: Diagnosis and management. *American Family Physicians, 80*(10), 1129–1134.

Kodner, C. (2016). Diagnosis and management of nephrotic syndrome in adults. *American Family Physician, 93*(6), 479–485.

Korbet, S. M. (2012). Treatment of primary FSGS in adults. *Journal of the American Society of Nephrology, 23*(11), 1769–1776. doi:10.1681/ASN.2012040389

National Kidney Foundation. (2019). Retrieved from https://www.kidney.org/atoz/content/nephrotic

Nishi, S., Ubara, Y., Utsunomiya, Y., Okada, K., Obata, Y., Kai, H., & Sato, Y. (2016). Evidence-based clinical practice guidelines for nephrotic syndrome 2014. *Clinical and Experimental Nephrology, 20*(3), 342–370. doi:10.1007/s10157-015-1216-x

Radhakrishnan, J., & Cattran, D. C. (2012). The KDIGO practice guideline on glomerulonephritis: Reading between the (guide) lines—application to the individual patient. *Kidney International, 82*(8), 840–856. doi:10.1038/ki.2012.280

Segal, P. E., & Choi, M. J. (2012). Recent advances and prognosis in idiopathic membranous nephropathy. *Advances in Chronic Kidney Disease, 19*(2), 114–119. doi:10.1053/j.ackd.2012.01.007

Prostatitis

Catherine Harris

Definition

A. Inflammation of the prostate gland, which can be caused by infection or persistent irritation of the gland.

B. Can be acute or chronic, lasting for more than 3 months.

Incidence

A. Almost 10% of males will have prostatitis over their lifetime.

B. About 90% of these conditions will be related to chronic nonbacterial prostatitis.

Pathogenesis

A. Any bacteria can cause prostatitis, although 80% of pathogens are gram negative. Sexual transmission is very common.

B. Chronic nonbacterial prostatitis is inflammation of the prostate gland from persistent irritation that is nonbacterial.

Predisposing Factors

A. Blockage of urine out of the bladder.
B. Phimosis.
C. Injury to the perineum.
D. Foley catheters.
E. Procedures such as cystoscopy or biopsy of the prostate.
F. Benign prostatic hypertrophy (BPH).

Subjective Data

A. Common complaints/symptoms.
  1. Acute bacterial prostatitis: Fever, chills, malaise, dysuria, low abdominal pain, or urethral discharge.
  2. Chronic bacterial prostatitis: Intermittent dysuria or recurrent urinary tract infections (UTIs).
B. Common/typical scenario.
  1. Possible fever, chills, and malaise.
  2. Possible pain with intercourse or defecation.
  3. Arthralgias.
  4. Nocturia.
C. Family and social history.
  1. Ask about number of sexual partners or history of sexually transmitted infections (STIs).
D. Review of systems.
  1. Assess patient for discharge, pain, hematuria, back pain, and weight loss.

Physical Examination

A. Check for urethral discharge and inspect the foreskin and penis for any lesions or fluid.
B. Palpate testes and epididymides for inflammation and tenderness.
C. Check for costovertebral angle (CVA) tenderness.
D. Perform rectal examination to evaluate prostate for symmetry, swelling, and tenderness and to determine if the prostate gland is boggy.
E. Avoid massage if acute prostatitis is suspected.

Diagnostic Tests

A. Check for infection.
  1. Complete blood count (CBC) with differential.
  2. Urinalysis with urine culture.
  3. Gram stain and culture-expressed prostatic secretions (EPS).
  4. Presence of STI.
B. For chronic prostatitis, check:
  1. CBC, serum creatinine, and blood urea nitrogen (BUN).
  2. Ultrasound, MRI, or biopsy if necessary to rule out other possibilities.

Differential Diagnosis

A. Anal fistulas.
B. UTI.
C. Epididymitis.
D. Urethritis.
E. Urinary obstruction.
F. Pyelonephritis.

Evaluation and Management Plan

A. General plan.
  1. Acute prostatitis may need intravenous (IV) therapy for severe infection or if patient looks toxic.

  2. Increase fluid intake.
  3. Decrease caffeine and alcohol intake.
B. Patient/family teaching points.
  1. Teach patients how the infection is transmitted.
  2. Suggest that sexual partners may need treatment.
  3. Tell patients to use condoms.
  4. Tell patients to urinate when the urge comes.
C. Pharmacotherapy.
  1. Acute bacterial prostatitis.
    a. Broad-spectrum penicillin, third generation cephalosporins, or fluoroquinolones.
    b. Nonsteroidal anti-inflammatory drugs (NSAIDs) for treating discomfort may be considered.
  2. Chronic bacterial prostatitis.
    a. Fluoroquinolones for 4 to 6 weeks.
    b. NSAIDs.
    c. Alpha blockers, which reduce bladder outlet syndrome, may be beneficial.
D. Discharge instructions.
  1. Prevent infection with good hygiene.
  2. Complete the antibiotic treatment as prescribed, which may take up to 1 month.

Follow-Up

A. Evaluate the effectiveness of the treatment plan and resolution of symptoms.
B. Admit patients who appear toxic to the hospital for IV antibiotics.

Consultation/Referral

A. Consult urology for acute recurrent bacterial infections or persistent infections. Cystoscopy may be required.

Special/Geriatric Considerations

A. Prostatitis may lead to sepsis, particularly in patients with diabetes or chronic renal failure, patients on dialysis, immunocompromised patients, and postsurgical patients with urethral instrumentation. There should be a low threshold to hospitalize these patients if there is a concern.
B. Urinary retention association with acute prostatitis may also require hospitalization.

Bibliography

Center for Urology, Rochester, N. Y. (n.d.). Discharge instructions for prostatitis. Retrieved from http://www.cfurochester.com/pdf/discharge-prostatitis.pdf

5 Foods that can cause prostatitis. (n.d.). Retrieved from http://prostate.net/articles/foods-that-cause-prostatitis

Gupta, N., Mandal, A., & Singh, S. (2008). Tuberculosis of the prostate and urethra. *Indian Journal of Urology, 24*(3), 388–391. doi:10.4103/0970-1591.42623

Luzzi, G. (2007). Editorial letter. Chronic prostatitis. *New England Journal of Medicine, 356,* 423–424. doi:10.1056/NEJMc063135

Stevermer, J., & Easley, S. (2000, May). Treatment of prostatitis. *American Family Physician, 61*(10), 3015–3022.

Strauss, A., & Dimitrakov, J. (2010, March). New treatments for chronic prostatitis/chronic pelvic pain syndrome. *Nature Reviews Urology, 7*(3), 127–135.

Turek, P. J. (2019, December 6). In J. P. Taylor 3rd (Ed.), *Medscape.* Retrieved from http://emedicine.medscape.com/article/785418-overviewProstatitis

Yavasscaoglu, I., Oktay, B., Simpseck, U., & Ozyurt, M. (1999, March). Role of ejaculation in the treatment of chronic non-bacterial prostatitis. *International Journal of Urology, 6*(3), 130–134.

Pyelonephritis

Suzanne Barron

Definition

A. An infection (usually from bacteria but also from viruses, fungi, or parasites) that results in swelling of the kidney. It may affect one or both kidneys.
   1. Uncomplicated.
   2. Complicated—associated with obstruction, anatomic anomaly, or kidney stones.

Incidence

A. Population-based study of acute pyelonephritis in the United States found overall annual rates of 15 to 17 cases per 10,000 females and 3 to 4 cases per 10,000 males.
B. At least 250,000 cases of pyelonephritis are diagnosed annually in the United States.

Pathogenesis

A. Usually results from bacterial invasion by ascending from the lower urinary tract (urethra and bladder).
B. Can result from colonization of the vagina with fecal flora.
C. Hematogenous source—from bloodstream infection that reaches renal parenchyma (uncommon). Most likely gram-positive organisms from endocarditis.
D. Evidence suggests that bacteria attaches to the urothelium and causes an inflammatory response. Hemolysins allow for bacterial invasion by damaging cells. Infection is most commonly associated with gram-negative bacteria such as *Escherichia coli* and *Klebsiella pneumoniae*.

Predisposing Factors

A. Female sex: Shorter urethra, allowing organisms to ascend to bladder and kidneys.
B. Functional abnormalities: High post void residuals or incomplete bladder emptying, neurogenic bladder.
C. Anatomic conditions: Bladder outlet obstruction/BPH or vesicoureteral reflux.
D. Chronic indwelling catheters.
E. Nephrolithiasis.
F. Diabetes mellitus.
G. Immunosuppression.
H. Alcohol or drug abuse.
I. Previous history of pyelonephritis.
J. Pregnancy.
K. New or multiple sexual partners.
L. History of recent cystitis.

Subjective Data

A. Common complaints/symptoms.
   1. Flank pain.
   2. Fever.
   3. Nausea and vomiting.
   4. Weakness.
   5. Dysuria.
   6. Foul-smelling urine.
   7. Hematuria.
B. Common/typical scenario.
   1. Onset: Abrupt, usually 1 to 2 days of symptoms.
   2. Location/character.
      a. Sharp and persistent flank pain in one or both kidneys.

   b. Abdominal pain, suprapubic tenderness.
   c. Possible groin pain.
   d. Strong urge to urinate.
   e. Burning on urination.
3. Fevers/chills: Generally feeling unwell.
4. Possible past medical history of kidney stones, pyelonephritis, or neurogenic bladder with chronic indwelling catheter.
C. Family and social history.
   1. Family history.
      a. Congenital anomalies of genitourinary (GU) tract.
      b. Nephrolithiasis.
      c. Diabetes mellitus.
      d. History of frequent urinary tract infections (UTIs).
   2. Social history.
      a. Alcohol use.
      b. Drug use (intravenous [IV] drug abuse may be associated with hematogenous spread of staphylococcal infection to kidney).
      c. Multiple sexual partners.
      d. New sexual partners.
      e. Use of spermicide.
      f. Poor perineal hygiene (fecal incontinence, soiling).
D. Review of systems.
   1. Constitutional: Fevers, chills, or malaise.
   2. Cardiovascular: Palpitations or fast heart rate.
   3. Gastrointestinal—nausea and vomiting, abdominal pain, fecal incontinence.
   4. Genitourinary—flank pain, dysuria, foul-smelling urine, hematuria, urgency/frequency, incontinence.
   5. Neurological—confusion and dizziness, especially in elderly.
   6. Gynecologic—vaginal discharge.
   7. Endocrine—polyuria, polydipsia, polyphagia (symptoms of diabetes), night sweats.

Physical Examination

A. Vital signs: Evaluate for systemic inflammatory response/sepsis.
   1. Fever.
   2. Tachycardia.
   3. Hypotension.
B. Generalized: Check to see if the patient appears ill; he or she may have rigors.
C. Genitourinary—evaluate for cerebrovascular accident (CVA) tenderness (positive in most cases on side of infected kidney).
D. Abdominal—evaluate for suprapubic tenderness (without guarding) and rigidity to rule out other causes of abdominal pain (e.g., acute abdomen, appendicitis).
E. Respiratory—assess for crackles, decreased breath sounds (signs of pneumonia).
F. Gynecological examination—perform if necessary in females to rule out gynecological disorder or pelvic inflammatory disease.

Diagnostic Tests

A. Blood work.
   1. Complete blood count (CBC) with differential: Leukocytosis with neutrophil predominance.
   2. Basic metabolic panel: Renal failure. Uncommon unless obstruction or sepsis is present.
   3. Blood culture: Possible bacteremia.

B. Urinalysis.

1. Pyuria greater than 5 to 10 white blood cells (WBCs)/high power field (HPF).

2. Leukocytes positive.

3. WBC casts: Often indicative of pyelonephritis.

4. Nitrites: Positive in most cases if infection caused by gram-negative bacteria.

5. Red blood cells (RBCs): May be positive.

C. Urine culture.

1. Positive with greater than 100,000 bacteria/mL; 10,000 bacteria/mL in patients with catheterized urine samples.

2. Possibly negative if the patient was on antimicrobials prior to presentation.

D. Imaging: Not necessary in uncomplicated pyelonephritis but failure to respond to appropriate therapy requires imaging to rule out ureteral obstruction or abscess.

1. Abdominal x-ray (kidney–ureter–bladder [KUB]): Stones, intraparenchymal gas; may be emphysematous pyelonephritis.

2. CT scan (non contrast): Enlarged kidney with perinephric fat stranding.

3. Renal ultrasound: Imaging modality of choice for pregnant females (no radiation).

a. Shows renal enlargement with hypoechoic parenchyma and loss.

Differential Diagnosis

A. Abdominal disorders.

1. Appendicitis.

2. Cholecystitis.

3. Pancreatitis.

4. Diverticulitis.

5. Peptic ulcer disease.

B. Gynecologic disorders.

1. Ectopic pregnancy.

2. Pelvic inflammatory disease.

3. Ruptured ovarian cyst.

C. Urologic disorders.

1. Nephrolithiasis.

2. Epididymitis.

3. Renal or perinephric abscess.

4. Urethritis.

5. Cystitis.

Evaluation and Management Plan

A. General plan.

1. See Figure 5.2.

2. Obtain urinalysis and urine culture.

3. Obtain blood work: CBC, blood cultures, and basic metabolic panel.

4. Start broad-spectrum antibiotics.

a. Can tolerate oral agents (e.g., ciprofloxacin, trimethoprim, and sulfamethoxazole). Nitrofurantoin should be avoided (does not penetrate kidney well).

b. Unable to tolerate oral agents (e.g., ampicillin 2 g IV every 6 hours and gentamicin 1.5 mg/kg every 8 hours).

5. Use imaging studies for high suspicion of ureteral obstruction and abscess.

6. Hospitalize patients who have systemic inflammatory response syndrome (SIRS), sepsis, dehydration, or uncontrollable pain.

7. Consult urology if ureteral obstruction is found for stent placement or possible percutaneous nephrostomy drain.

B. Patient/family teaching points.

1. Increase fluids to promote hydration and flushing of the bacteria.

2. Encourage good hygiene and wiping from front to back after urinating to prevent bacteria from colonizing the urethra.

3. Urinate after sexual intercourse to help wash away bacteria.

4. Counsel patient and family that the patient may continue to have fever and flank pain for 2 to 3 days after appropriate treatment has been given.

5. Reinforce the importance of completing antibiotics for the recommended 14- to 21-day course.

C. Pharmacotherapy.

1. Once urine culture has finalized, switch to an appropriate antimicrobial for 14 to 21 days. Oral antibiotics can be used depending on susceptibilities.

2. Supportive care.

a. Phenazopyridine as possible help for dysuria.

b. Antipyretics such as acetaminophen to control fever.

c. Analgesics for appropriate pain management.

d. IV fluid hydration to prevent and treat dehydration and sepsis.

D. Discharge instructions.

1. Advise patients to seek medical care for any recurrent symptoms such as fevers, flank pain, nausea, and vomiting.

2. Advise patients to call if they are unable to tolerate oral antibiotic or develop adverse effects such as rash or diarrhea.

3. Advise patients to drink plenty of fluids.

Follow-Up

A. Instruct patients to follow-up within 4 to 6 weeks after completion of antibiotics with a repeat urine culture to verify that infection has cleared.

B. Advise patients to follow-up with recurrent symptoms because relapse can occur requiring a second 14-day course of antibiotics.

Consultation/Referral

A. Urology consult.

1. Obstructive ureteral stones.

2. Nephrolithiasis as a chronic nidus of infection.

3. Recurrent episodes of pyelonephritis, which warrant evaluation for anatomic anomalies.

B. Infectious disease consult: Complicated infections and recommendations of duration of treatment.

C. Home infusion consult/home health nursing: If IV antibiotics recommended.

D. Interventional radiology consult: If percutaneous nephrostomy tube is indicated due to ureteral obstruction or for percutaneous drain placement for an abscess.

Special/Geriatric Considerations

A. Diabetic patients; increased risk of developing emphysematous pyelonephritis.

B. Long-term/recurrent pyelonephritis patients: Development of significant renal scarring.

C. Geriatric individuals: Dosing of antibiotics based on renal function/creatinine clearance.

D. Pregnant patients: Increased risk of preterm delivery, sepsis, and adult respiratory distress syndrome.

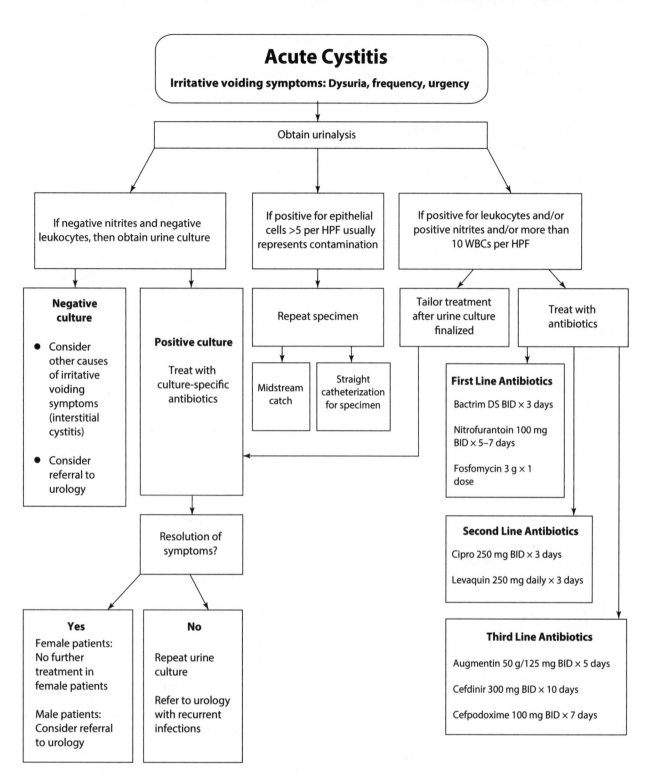

FIGURE 5.2 Acute cystitis algorithm.
HPF, high power field; WBC, white blood cells.

Bibliography

Czaga, C., Scholes, D., Hooton, T., & Stamm, W. (2007, August). Population-based epidemiologic analysis of acute pyelonephritis. *Clinical Infectious Diseases, 45*(3), 273–280. doi:10.1086/519268

Fulop, T. (2018, December 12). Acute pyelonephritis. In V. Batuman (Ed.), *Medscape*. Retrieved from http://emedicine.medscape.com/article/245559-overview

Naderi, A., & Reilly, R. (2008, December). Primary care approach to proteinuria. *The Journal of the American Board of Family Medicine, 21*(6), 569–574. doi:10.3122/jabfm.2008.06.070080

Urinary Incontinence

Suzanne Barron

Definition

A. Unintentional loss of urine.

B. Types.

1. Stress urinary incontinence (SUI): Occurs during physical exertion (sneezing, coughing, exercise).
2. Urgency incontinence (UI): Involuntary loss of urine associated with urgency (bladder spasms).
3. Mixed urinary incontinence: Combination of SUI and UI.
4. Overflow incontinence (OI): Occurs with urinary retention or high post void residuals. The overdistended bladder leads to leakage.
5. Functional incontinence: Loss of urine due to deficits of cognition and mobility.

Incidence

A. Urinary incontinence has been reported to affect 12% to 43% of women and 3% to 11% of men.
B. Prevalence rapidly increases in both genders after the age of 70, but severe incontinence in men is reported at about half that in women.

Pathogenesis

A. SUI: Hypermobility of the urethra and/or intrinsic sphincter deficiencies.
  1. Women: Related to the number of vaginal deliveries.
  2. Men: Rare, unless history of prostatectomy, trauma, or neurological disorder.
B. UI: Detrusor muscle over-activity.
  1. Detrusor myopathy.
  2. Detrusor neuropathy.
C. OI: Overdistention of the bladder with subsequent leakage from either impaired detrusor contractility or bladder outlet obstruction.
  1. Diabetes mellitus.
  2. Lumbosacral nerve disease.
  3. Multiple sclerosis.
  4. Spinal cord injuries.
  5. Prolapsed intervertebral discs.
  6. Severe cases of bladder outflow obstruction.

Predisposing Factors

A. Sex (female > male).
B. Advanced age.
C. Vaginal childbirth.
D. Cognitive impairment.
E. Chronic obstructive pulmonary disease (COPD).
F. Obesity.
G. Pelvic organ prolapse.
H. Smoking.
I. Pregnancy.
J. Previous history of pelvic surgery (hysterectomy, prostatectomy) or pelvic radiation.
K. Poor mobility.
L. Neurological disorders.
M. Anatomical disorders (e.g., vesicovaginal fistula).
N. Certain medications (diuretics, narcotic pain medication).
O. History of pelvic trauma.

Subjective Data

A. Common complaints/symptoms.
  1. SUI: Leakage of urine involuntarily when laughing, coughing, or sneezing.
  2. UI: Uncontrollable urge to urinate with associated leakage; occurs frequently.
  3. OI: Dribbling of urine, weak stream, and incomplete bladder emptying.

B. Common/typical scenario.
  1. Onset of symptoms: Gradual versus sudden.
  2. Associated pain with incontinence.
  3. Severity: Minimal amount of leakage versus large amount of leakage and soaking through clothes.
  4. Timing and frequency of the incontinence (after sneezing, only occurs at night).
  5. Aggravating factors (e.g., caffeine, citrus).
  6. Alleviating factors (pessary).
  7. Risk factors (vaginal prolapse, recent urinary tract infection [UTI], benign prostatic hypertrophy [BPH], neurological disorders, trauma).
C. Family and social history.
  1. Smoking.
    a. Tobacco: Irritant to the bladder, causing UI.
    b. Tobacco addiction: Possibly leading to a chronic cough and increased intra-abdominal pressure, damaging the muscles of the pelvic floor and resulting in SUI.
  2. Alcohol: Diuretic affect/central nervous system (CNS) depressant causing OI and UI.
  3. Illicit drugs: Abuse of prescription drugs such as opioids/sedatives causing OI or functional incontinence.
D. Review of systems.
  1. Constitutional: Fevers, chills, and weight gain.
  2. Neurological: Confusion, altered speech, altered mental status, lower extremity weakness, dizziness, tremors, decreased mobility, and paresthesia (saddle anesthesia).
  3. Respiratory: Chronic cough and chronic bronchitis.
  4. Cardiovascular: Shortness of breath or edema associated with congestive heart failure (CHF).
  5. Abdominal: Constipation, obstipation, or reflux that causes cough.
  6. Genitourinary: Frequency, urgency, hematuria, retention, incomplete bladder emptying, or suprapubic pain.
  7. Gynecologic: Pelvic organ prolapse or leakage of urine from vagina.
  8. Musculoskeletal: Lower back pain.

Physical Examination

A. Neurological.
  1. Assess mental status, motor strength, and sensory status, as well as deep tendon reflexes.
  2. Observe gait.
B. Respiratory: Assess for rhonchi and barrel chest.
C. Cardiovascular: Assess for JVD and edema.
D. Abdomen: Assess for suprapubic tenderness, palpable bladder, and abdominal/pelvic masses.
E. Genitourinary.
  1. Perform digital rectal examination (DRE) to evaluate for BPH, prostatitis, and prostate nodules.
  2. Evaluate for rectal fissures and/or fecal impaction.
F. Gynecologic.
  1. Perform Q-tip test: Used to demonstrate urethral hypermobility, which may indicate SUI.
    a. A sterile, well-lubricated Q-tip is placed into the urethra, and the patient is then told to cough or strain.
    b. The degree of Q-tip movement is measured. The test is considered positive if the Q-tip moves more than 30°.
  2. Evaluate for vaginal atrophy.
  3. Evaluate for pelvic organ prolapse.
G. Dermatological: Assess for excoriated skin due to incontinence or presence of fungal infection.

Diagnostic Tests

A. Urinalysis and urine culture: Evaluate for infectious source.

B. Blood work: Basic metabolic panel to evaluate renal function, which may indicate obstructive source.

C. Imaging: Generally not indicated.

D. Urodynamic studies/video-urodynamic studies.

   1. Filling study: Detrusor overactivity, leak point pressure.

   2. Voiding study: Urinary flow rate, post void residual, detrusor sphincter synergy.

E. Cystoscopy: If there is concern for fistula or malignancy.

Differential Diagnosis

A. UTI (Cystitis, prostatitis).

B. Interstitial cystitis.

C. Nocturnal enuresis.

D. Urethral diverticulum.

E. Vesicovaginal fistula.

F. Cauda equina syndrome.

G. Constipation/obstipation.

H. Bladder cancer.

I. Bladder outlet obstruction.

Evaluation and Management Plan

A. General plan.

   1. Obtain thorough history to determine type of urinary incontinence to target treatment.

   2. Obtain laboratory studies such as urinalysis, urine culture, and basic metabolic panel.

   3. If possible, obtain post void residual with bladder scan.

B. Patient/family teaching points.

   1. Encourage smoking cessation and avoidance of alcohol/caffeine.

   2. Encourage keeping a 24-hour voiding diary to help patients understand voiding patterns.

   3. Educate patient about timed voiding, which will help avoid significant bladder distention.

   4. Educate patients with SUI about how to perform Kegel exercises to strengthen pelvic floor muscles. Discuss the role of biofeedback in helping control these muscles.

   5. Educate patients with UI about bladder training (delay voiding for increasing periods of time by inhibiting the desire to void).

   6. Encourage weight loss in obese patients.

   7. Teach patients with overflow incontinence about how to perform clean intermittent catheterization if necessary.

C. Pharmacotherapy.

   1. SUI.

     a. Currently, no Food and Drug Administration (FDA) approved medication for SUI.

     b. Topical estrogen in post menopausal women: Mild benefit.

   2. UI.

     a. Anticholinergic medications: Act to inhibit bladder contractions and increase capacity.

       i. Most common: Oxybutynin and tolterodine.

       ii. Others: Trospium chloride, solifenacin, darifenacin, and fesoterodine.

     b. Tricyclic antidepressants.

       i. Direct relaxant effect on bladder muscle.

       ii. Not commonly used due to side effects.

     c. Beta 3-adrenergic receptor agonist (mirabegron): Associated with much less dry mouth and constipation (side effects of anticholinergic medications) but may cause hypertension.

D. Discharge instructions.

   1. Discuss with the patient to call with side effects of medication such as dry mouth, constipation, confusion, or vision changes.

   2. Instruct the patient to seek medical attention with any fevers, chills, flank pain, or hematuria, which may indicate UTI.

   3. Advise the patient about appropriate care of the skin due to incontinence. Keep the skin clean and dry. Wearing pads may help to protect the skin.

   4. Mention that stool softeners or mild laxatives may be needed to prevent constipation.

Follow-Up

A. Follow-up in 3 to 4 weeks for symptom assessment/response to therapy.

B. Biofeedback often requires multiple visits.

C. Instruct the patient to bring his or her voiding diary to follow-up appointment.

D. For patients on an anticholinergic, check post void residual to monitor for urinary retention.

Consultation/Referral

A. Refer to urologist/urogynecologist for persistent symptoms or concern for malignancy or anatomic abnormality.

   1. SUI.

     a. Periurethral bulking agents such as calcium hydroxylapatite.

     b. Pubovaginal sling placement.

     c. Surgical repair of pelvic organ prolapse.

     d. Surgery for BPH (transurethral resection of the prostate [TURP]).

     e. Artificial urinary sphincter for men.

     f. Fit for pessary.

   2. UI.

     a. Percutaneous tibial nerve stimulation.

     b. Intravesical botulinum toxin: High efficacy in patients who have failed other medical treatment.

   3. Cystoscopy to rule out malignancy or anatomic abnormality.

B. Refer to neurology/neurosurgery with any concern for spinal cord injury, compression (Cauda equine), or neurological disorder.

Special/Geriatric Considerations

A. Avoid anticholinergic medication in patients who have a history of acute angle glaucoma.

B. Anticholinergic medication may cause confusion in geriatric individuals.

C. Assess geriatric patients for polypharmacy. Various medications that are commonly given may cause overflow incontinence (antidepressants, calcium channel blockers, opioid pain medication, sedatives, antihistamines) or UI due to the high volume of urine (diuretics).

D. Consider the cost of pads in geriatric individuals who are on a fixed income. It is estimated that women with severe incontinence pay up to $900 per year for incontinence pads.

Bibliography

Albala, D., Morey, A., Gomella, L., & Stein, J. (2011). *Oxford American handbook of urology*, New York, NY: Oxford University Press.

Cameron, A., Jimbo, M., & Heidelbaugh, J. (2013). Diagnosis and office-based treatment of urinary incontinence in adults. Part two:

Treatment. *Therapeutic Advances in Urology, 5*(4), 189–200. doi:10.1177/1756287213495100

Cohn, J. A., Brown, E. T., Reynolds, W. S., Kaufman, M. R., Milam, D. F., & Dmochowski, R. R. (2016). An update on the use of transdermal oxybutynin in the management of overactive bladder disorder. *Therapeutic Advances in Urology, 8*(2), 83–90. doi:10.1177/1756287215626312

Gomella, L., Andriole, G., Burnett, A., Flanigan, R., Keane, T., Koo, H., & Thomas, R. (2015). *The 5-minute urology consult* 3rd ed. Philadelphia, PA: Lippincott Williams & Wilkins.

Herbruck, L. (2008). Stress urinary incontinence: An overview of diagnosis and treatment options. *Urology Nursing, 28*(3), 186–198. Retrieved from www.Medscape.com/viewarticle/57833_4

Hesch, K. (2007, July). Agents for treatment of overactive bladder: A therapeutic class review. *Proceedings (Baylor University Medical Center), 20*(3), 307–314.

Khandelwal, C., & Kistler, C. (2013, April). Diagnosis of urinary incontinence. *American Family Physician, 87*(8), 543–550.

MacDiarmid, S. (2008, Winter). Maximizing the treatment of overactive bladder in the elderly. *Reviews in Urology, 10*(1), 6–13.

Salzman, B., & Hersch, L. (2013, May). Clinical management of urinary incontinence in women. *American Family Physician, 87*(9), 634–640.

Subak, L., Brown, J., Kraus, S., Brubaker, L., Lin, F., Richter, H., . . . Grady, D. (2006). The "costs" of urinary incontinence for women. *Obstetric Gynecology, 107*(4), 908–916. doi: 10.1097/01.AOG.0000206213.48334.09

Thomas, B. (2015). *The pathophysiology of urinary incontinence: Part 2.* Retrieved from https://www.gmjournal.co.uk/the_pathophysiology_of_urinary_incontinence_part_2_25769830611.aspx

Urinary Tract Infection

Swetha Rani Kanduri & Karthik Kovvuru

Definition

A. Infection of the urinary tract in the absence of comorbidities such as diabetes, pregnancy, or physiologic and structural anomalies.

Incidence

A. Urinary tract infections (UTIs) account for about 7 million office visits annually, affecting men and women.
B. These infections are more common in young, sexually active women than men.
C. 30% to 40% of women will experience one episode/year.

Pathogenesis

A. UTIs are more common in women because the female urethra:
  1. Is shorter and in closer proximity to the rectum.
  2. Allows bacteria to colonize more easily.
B. UTIs peak in two different age groups in women.
  1. 20 to 40 age group: Predisposed by intercourse.
  2. 55 to 60 age group: Related to declining estrogen levels.

Predisposing Factors

A. Conditions that reduce urine flow.
  1. Outflow obstruction: Prostatic hyperplasia, prostatic carcinoma, urethral stricture, or foreign body (calculus).
  2. Neurogenic bladder.
  3. Inadequate fluid uptake.
B. Conditions that promote colonization.
  1. Sexual activity: Increased inoculation.
  2. Spermicide: Increased binding.
  3. Estrogen depletion: Increased binding.
  4. Antimicrobial agents: Decreased indigenous flora.
C. Conditions that facilitate ascent.
  1. Catheterization.

  2. Urinary incontinence.
  3. Fecal incontinence.
D. Conditions in older women, who may be at higher risk for UTIs due to a combination of factors.
  1. Atrophic changes.
  2. Impaired urethral function.
  3. Insufficient fluid intake.
  4. Constipation.
  5. Increased residual urine volume.

Subjective Data

A. Common complaints/symptoms.
  1. Foul-smelling urine.
  2. Dysuria, increased frequency, or urgency.
  3. Suprapubic pain and discomfort.
  4. Occasional hematuria.
B. Atypical symptoms in older patients.
  1. Confusion.
  2. Delirium.
  3. Falls or adverse behaviors.

Physical Examination

A. Possible suprapubic tenderness on palpation.
B. Increasing discharge from vagina.
C. Urinary meatus that may be erythematous or edematous.
D. Negative costovertebral angle (CVA) tenderness.
E. Negative pelvic or prostate examination.
F. Urological evaluation is required for men with UTI.

Diagnostic Tests

A. Urinalysis.
  1. Urine dipstick with clean catch urine necessary.
  2. Positive for blood, leukocyte esterase, or nitrate.
  3. Sensitivity of 75% to 96% and a specificity of 94% to 98%.
B. Urine gram stain.
  1. 10 white blood cells (WBC)/high power field (HPF; may not be present).
  2. Bacteria greater than 15 bacteria/HPF.
C. Urine culture.
  1. More than 10,000 bacteria/mL in fresh, midstream specimen.

Differential Diagnosis

A. Genital herpes (herpes simplex virus [HSV]).
B. Urethritis.
C. *Chlamydia.*
D. *Trichomonas.*
E. Vaginitis.
F. Prostatitis.
G. Nephrolithiasis.
H. Trauma.
I. Urinary tract tuberculosis.
J. Urinary tract neoplasm.
K. Intra-abdominal abscess.

Evaluation and Management Plan

A. General plan.
  1. See Figure 5.3.
  2. Advise patients on condition, timeline of treatment, and expected course of disease process.
  3. Collect urine culture before starting antibiotics.
  4. Complete all antibiotic regimens.

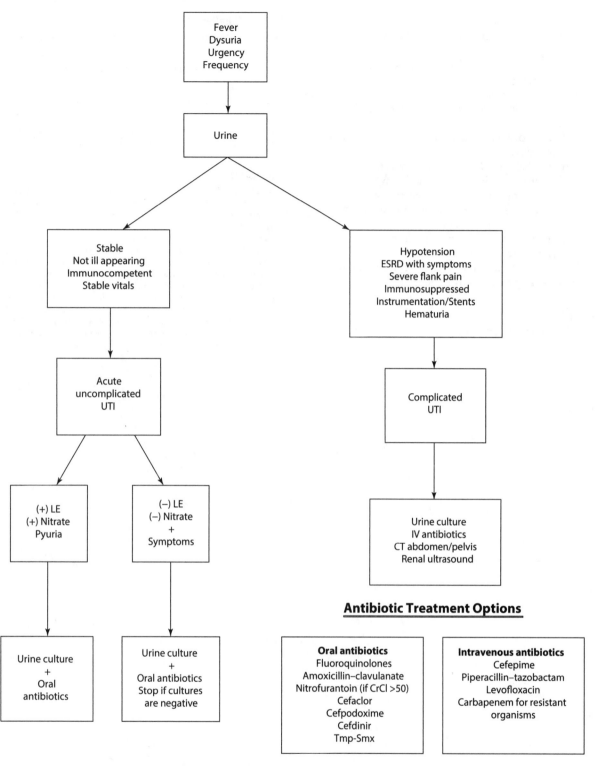

FIGURE 5.3 Urinary tract infection flipped in chronic kidney disease.
ESRD, end-stage renal disease; IV, intravenous; LE, leukocyte esterase; UTI, urinary tract infection.

B. Patient/family teaching points.

1. Counsel patients about appropriate use of medications (dose, frequency, side effects, need to complete entire course of medications).

2. Recommend increasing fluid intake to 8 to 10 glasses per day.

3. Suggest that sitting in a warm tub may relieve symptoms of dysuria.

4. For women, advise that they wipe front to back after a bowel movement.

5. For women, advise against using douches.

6. Tell patients to avoid bubble baths.

7. Advise that voiding after intercourse may be beneficial.

8. Use appropriate cleaning for sex toys and advise against sharing sex toys.

C. Pharmacotherapy.

1. First-line antibiotics.

    a. Bactrim, double strength orally twice a day for 3 days.

    b. Nitrofurantoin, 100 mg twice a day for 5 days.

    c. Fosfomycin 3 g single dose.

2. Second-line antibiotics.

    a. Ciprofloxacin 250 mg orally twice a day for 3 days.

    b. Amoxicillin/clavulanate 500/125 mg orally twice a day for 5 days.

3. Treatment during pregnancy.

    a. Ampicillin 500 mg orally every 8 hours for 3 to 7 days.

    b. Amoxicillin/clavulanate 500 mg every 8 hours for 3 to 7 days.

    c. Cephalexin 500 mg every 6 hours for 3 to 7 days.

    d. Nitrofurantoin 100 mg twice a day for 5 to 7 days (avoid during first trimester and at term).

    e. Bactrim DS twice a day for 5 days (avoid during first trimester and at term).

    f. Fosfomycin 3 g orally as single dose.

D. Discharge instructions.

1. Return to clinic for fever or if symptoms do not improve/progress in 48 to 72 hours.

Follow-Up

A. Follow-up with primary care provider.

Consultation/Referral

A. Consult or refer to urology only if complications occur.

Special/Geriatric Considerations

A. Geriatric patients may present with atypical symptoms and require close monitoring of intake versus output during UTI.

B. Patients with chronic kidney disease or end-stage renal disease (ESRD) may require antibiotic dose adjustments.

Bibliography

Lane, D. R., & Takhar, S. S. (2011, August). Diagnosis and management of urinary tract infection and pyelonephritis. *Emergency Medicine Clinics of North America, 29*(3), 539–552. doi:10.1016/j.emc.2011.04.001

Wagenlehner, F. M., Schmiemann, G., Hoyme, U., Fünfstück, R., Hummers-Pradier, E., Kaase, M., & Naber, K. G. (2011, February). National S3 guideline on uncomplicated urinary tract infection: Recommendations for treatment and management of uncomplicated community-acquired bacterial urinary tract infections in adult patients. *Urologe A, 50*(2), 153–169. doi:10.1007/s00120-011-2512-z

Workowski, K. A., & Bolan, G. A. (2015, June 5). Sexually transmitted diseases treatment guidelines, 2015. *Morbidity and Mortality Weekly Report. Recommendations and Reports. 64*(RR-03), 1–137. Retrieved from https://www.cdc.gov/mmwr/preview/mmwrhtml/rr6403a1.htm

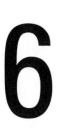

6 Neurology Guidelines

Nicole Thomer

Nicole Thomer and Syed Omar Shah

Definition

A. Deprivation of oxygen to the brain often due to cardiac arrest, but can occur from any cause including carbon monoxide poisoning, severe asthma attacks, suffocation, drowning, and strokes.

B. Can be classified into four categories.
  1. Diffuse cerebral hypoxia.
  2. Focal cerebral ischemia.
  3. Global cerebral ischemia.
  4. Cerebral infarction.

Incidence

A. No specific numbers are available to document the incidence or prevalence of anoxic brain injury.

B. Main cause of anoxic brain injury is cardiac arrest (82.4%).

C. Other main causes include: Poisoning, drug overdose, head trauma, stroke, seizures, and severe asthma attacks.

Pathogenesis

A. The delivery of oxygen to the brain is highly dependent on its metabolic demand. Overall, this drive is usually higher compared to the rest of the body.

B. Thus, any interruption of blood supply to its rich vasculature, even in short amounts of time such as a cardiac arrest, can cause significant brain injury.
  1. Primary brain injury.
    a. Decreased perfusion to the brain, leading to deprivation of oxygen, glucose, and other nutrients required for brain metabolism.
    b. Glutamate, an excitatory neurotransmitter, release. This, along with the release of other excitatory amino acid neurotransmitters, leads to the formation of free radicals and lipid peroxidation.
    c. Large amounts of sodium and calcium entering the cells. This leads to cytotoxic edema.
    d. Lost regulatory mechanisms of the cell. This results in cell death.
  2. Secondary brain injury.
    a. Microvascular dysfunction: Occurs from poor perfusion. Small capillaries and arterioles can continue to have low perfusion despite restoration of blood flow. This can result in cerebral edema.
    b. Cerebral edema: Can occur from microvascular dysfunction as well as cytotoxic edema from cell death.

  c. Impaired autoregulation: Pressure passive cerebral hemodynamics with a right shift in autoregulation.
  d. Hyperoxia: Occurs from increased free radicals.
  e. Hyperthermia: Occurs from increased metabolic demand and induction of apoptosis.

Predisposing Factors

A. In cardiac arrest, patients have risk factors associated with cardiac disease.

B. In other causes, patients tend to be younger, especially in respiratory-related anoxic brain injury cases.

Subjective Data

A. Patients with anoxic brain injury will not be able to provide any subjective information, so subjective data is not relevant in this situation.

B. However, the interviewer should obtain as much history from others as possible.
  1. Obtain a thorough patient social history through family, friends, or witnesses.
  2. Obtain any information about time, place, and onset.
    a. How long was the person in cardiac arrest or deprived of oxygen? Studies have shown that prolonged CPR (typically >15 minutes) has not led to a good prognosis. These people generally die from this injury within 6 weeks.
  3. Obtain the patient's medical history, medication use, any history of drug or alcohol abuse, or any recent complaints.

Physical Examination

A. Thorough neurological exam: Required.

B. Levels of consciousness.
  1. Coma: State of unresponsiveness. Patients are unaware of their surroundings and are unarousable.
  2. Vegetative state: State of wakefulness without awareness or return of sleep–wake cycles. This results from a severe anoxic injury.
    a. Persistent vegetative state: Vegetative state 1 month after injury.
    b. Permanent vegetative state (PVS): Irreversible. This may occur 3 months after a nontraumatic injury and 1 year following a traumatic brain injury.
  3. Minimal consciousness: State that does not fit the definition for PVS. Patients show limited evidence of awareness of themselves or environment that is reproducible. They may have brief periods of meaningful interaction (e.g., simple commands or tracking).

4. Locked-in syndrome: Sustained eye opening, awareness of environment with quadriplegia. Cognition is intact. Vertical eye movements and/or blinking of eyes to communicate.

5. Brain death: Death by irreversible cessation of cerebral blood flow. Absence of all brainstem functions is characteristic (see section "Brain Death" for additional information).

Diagnostic Tests

A. Diagnostic tests can be performed but these can be affected by timing and patient temperature. Overall, time is essential to the prognostication process. The longer a clinician waits to prognosticate, the better. In most cases, it is necessary to wait at least 72 hours after rewarming or postarrest without hypothermia to give a prognosis.

B. However, timing should be on a case-to-case basis. Some patients with hypothermia that requires heavy sedation should be given longer than 72 hours because hypothermia can delay drug metabolism.

C. Clinical examination: Traditionally the strongest predictor of outcome. Predictors of poor outcome include:

    1. Absent pupillary reflexes.

    2. Absent corneal reflexes.

    3. Motor response of extensor posturing or no movement.

D. Biochemical markers.

E. Neuroimaging.

    1. MRI of the brain: Loss of gray/white matter. This indicates significant brain injury and is a sign of poor prognosis.

    2. CT of the head: Initially, this can be normal but after about 3 days it shows brain edema and loss of gray/white differential.

F. Electrophysiology.

    1. Somatosensory evoked potential (SSEP).

    2. EEG: Used to determine the presence of underlying brain activity as well as seizures (commonly seen after an anoxic injury).

Differential Diagnosis

A. Seizure.

B. Hypoglycemia.

Evaluation and Management Plan

A. Hypothermia (see Chapter 7).

B. Supportive care.

    1. Ventilatory support.

    2. Seizure management: Continuous EEG monitoring during entire duration of hypothermia as well as post rewarming.

        a. This should be considered. It allows monitoring of not only seizures but the patient's background rhythms.

    3. Monitoring of basic labs and evidence of nosocomial infection.

    4. Monitoring for evidence of end organ damage.

C. Family counseling.

    1. Inform families of the studies that are performed, including the timeline of these studies; this helps set expectations.

    2. Review the results and provide the likelihood of a meaningful recovery versus the possibility of long-term placement.

Follow-Up

A. Case management consultation: Necessary for placement options (long-term facility vs. hospice care).

Consultation/Referral

A. Prompt consultation with a neurologist.

B. Potential consultation with palliative care.

Special/Geriatric Considerations

A. Poor neuroprognostication increases with age of patient and time sustained in a coma.

Bibliography

Heinz, U., & Rollnik, J. (2015). Outcome and prognosis of hypoxic brain damage patients undergoing neurological early rehabilitation. *BMC Research Notes, 8*, 243. doi:10.1186/s13104-015-1175-z

Romergyrko, G., Koenig, M., Jia, X., Stevens, R., & Peberdy, M. (2008). Management of brain injury after resuscitation from cardiac arrest. *Neurologic Clinics, 26*(2), 487–506. doi:10.1016/j.ncl.2008.03.015

Weinhouse, G., & Young, B. (2015). Hypoxic-ischemic brain injury in adults: Evaluation and prognosis. In J. L. Wilterdink (Ed.), *UptoDate*. Retrieved from https://www.uptodate.com/contents/hypoxic-ischemic-brain-injury-in-adults-evaluation-and-prognosis

Brain Death

Nicole Thomer and Syed Omar Shah

Definition

A. Often defined as the irreversible loss of all function of the brain, including the loss of brainstem functions.

    1. U.S. law associates brain death with cardiopulmonary death, but specific criteria are not mandatory.

    2. Some states, such as New Jersey, have very specific diagnostic mandates.

    3. Most clinicians rely on guidelines to help guide their decision making.

B. Three key findings suggest brain death and must be examined.

    1. Coma.

    2. Absence of brainstem reflexes.

    3. Apnea.

C. Once brain death criteria have been established and irreversible loss of brain function is proven, patients can be declared brain dead and therefore legally deceased.

Incidence

A. Brain death is declared in approximately 2.3% to 7.5% of all deaths annually.

Pathogenesis

A. Causes: Devastating, identifiable, and irreversible neurological injuries, such as subarachnoid hemorrhages.

B. Main processes resulting in brain death: Mass cerebral edema and downward herniation.

Physical Examination (Neurological Assessment)

A. Prerequisites for clinical examination. (Note that these could vary by institution; it is important to be familiar with institution guidelines.)

    1. Clear clinical or radiographic evidence of widespread brain injury that is compatible with a diagnosis of brain death.

2. Core body temperature greater than or equal to 36°C or 96.8°F.

3. Ruling out of the use of any drug or intoxication that could cause central nervous system (CNS) depression. This must be done through history taking through family and friends, clinical and laboratory testing, and drug screening.

4. Absence of severe metabolic disturbances as identified by clinical and laboratory data (i.e., severe electrolyte, endocrine, or acid–base abnormalities).

5. Systolic blood pressure greater than 100 mmHg.

6. Identification of an examiner. This can vary according to state and national laws. The examiner should be confident in his or her understanding of the criteria and comfortable performing all aspects of the examination.

B. Clinical examination: All of the following factors must be checked and confirmed to be absent to determine brain death.

  1. Level of consciousness/mental status.

    a. The patient must be in a nonmedically induced coma.

  2. Motor examination.

    a. The patient must have an absence of brain-originating responses to noxious stimuli.

    b. It is not uncommon to witness spinal mediated reflexive movements, which are not to be confused with purposeful movements. Examples of spinal-mediated movements include rhythmic facial nerve-innervated muscles, finger flexor movements, "Lazarus sign," triple flexion, positive Babinski sign, or fasciculations of trunk and extremities.

  3. Cranial nerve assessment.

    a. Pupillary response: Absent. Pupils are dilated and fixed in a neutral position.

    b. Ocular movement: Absence of oculovestibular reflexes.

      i. Cold calorics: Testing that injects ice cold water into the ear canal. The provider then watches the eyes for 2 minutes to ensure there are no findings of eye movements.

      ii. This is done on both ears.

    c. Brainstem reflexes.

      i. Absence of corneal reflexes.

      ii. Absence of a gag/sucking/rooting reflex.

      iii. Absence of a cough with tracheal suctioning.

    d. Respiratory function: Confirmation of apnea.

Diagnostic Tests

A. Apnea test.

  1. Prerequisites.

    a. Clinical examination has been performed as described earlier and the findings are consistent with brain death.

    b. Patient has been preoxygenated for 10 minutes and then an arterial blood gas is performed.

      i. A PaO_2 greater than 200 mmHg and a $PaCO_2$ greater than 35 to 45 mmHg must be present.

    c. Any prior evidence of CO_2 retention must be ruled out (e.g., patient with chronic obstructive pulmonary disease [COPD] or severe obesity).

      i. If a patient does have retention, an apnea test cannot be safely and accurately performed and thus a confirmatory ancillary test must be considered.

  2. Actual testing.

    a. Ensure that a physician, respiratory therapist, and nurse are present for the entirety of this test. Testing can range from 8 minutes up to 12 minutes, depending on the stability of the patient during testing. Disconnect the patient from the ventilator and provide oxygen via a nasal cannula at 6 L/min into the endotracheal tube at the level of the carina.

      i. Alternatively, use a T-piece system with oxygen flow at 12 L/min and use continuous positive airway pressure (CPAP) 10 to 20 cm H_2O, with oxygen flow at 12 L/min.

      ii. Observe for respiratory movements.

      iii. Ensure that all clothing is removed and the patient's chest is completely exposed.

      iv. If any respiratory movements are present, then place the patient back on the ventilator and abort the test.

    b. After the 8 to 12 minute test is performed, draw another arterial blood gas sample and result immediately, then place the patient back on the ventilator. Be sure not to place the patient on the ventilator before drawing the arterial blood gas.

      i. If the $PaCO_2$ is greater than or equal to 60 mmHg or greater than or equal to 20 mmHg above the baseline, then the test is confirmatory. Therefore, apnea is present.

  3. Complications during apnea testing.

    a. If respiratory instability defined as SaO_2 <90% or hemodynamic instability defined as systolic blood pressure less than 90 mmHg occurs, it is necessary to draw an arterial blood gas and place the patient back on the ventilator. If the earlier criteria are met prior to the 8-minute minimum, the test remains confirmatory.

    b. If the patient remains hemodynamically stable and maintains adequate saturations but the test is inconclusive, the test may be repeated for a longer period (10–15 minutes).

    c. If the patient does not meet criteria for confirmatory apnea, ancillary testing may be required.

  4. Observation period.

    a. Observing for adults is considered optional.

    b. Six hours is often recommended with longer periods, up to 24 hours, recommended in cases of hypoxic ischemic encephalopathy.

    c. The 2010 American Academy of Neurology guidelines found insufficient evidence to determine a minimally acceptable observation period.

B. Ancillary testing.

  1. Indications: Limitations to performing the clinical examination or apnea testing.

Reasons for considering ancillary testing include:

    a. Presence of factors that may affect accurate testing of cranial nerve functions (e.g., preexisting pupillary abnormalities complicating assessment of function and facial trauma).

    b. Inability to perform clinical examination or apnea testing.

    c. Inability to perform apnea testing because of preexisting CO_2 retention diagnosis.

    d. Presence of heavy sedation or neuromuscular paralysis.

  2. Specific tests.

    a. Angiography: "Gold Standard" for ancillary testing. A positive study reflects the absence of cerebral perfusion at or beyond the carotid bifurcation or circle of Willis and demonstrates that the external carotid system has blood flow. However, this is invasive, high risk, and requires transportation to the radiology department with an unstable patient. It also carries the risk of false positives when the cranial vault is breached by trauma, surgery, or ventricular drains.

b. Cerebral scintigraphy or nuclear testing. This method closely resembles the cerebral angiography. A positive finding consistent with no cerebral perfusion is the "hollow skull" appearance.

c. Transcranial ultrasound or transcranial Doppler. This method is safe, noninvasive, and inexpensive. However, this method is reliable only if there is a good quality signal and requires expertise in testing both anterior and posterior circulations. Abnormal findings include reverberating flow or small early systolic peaks without diastolic flow.

d. EEG. Testing should be performed for at least 30 minutes. This testing must demonstrate no electrical activity and no reactivity to visual, auditory, or sensory stimuli. Testing results can be skewed, especially in an ICU setting; outside activity can be mistaken for cortical activity. Also, the EEG may be flat or isoelectric but cannot evaluate a brainstem that may have viable neurons.

e. Somatosensory evoked potentials (SSEPS). In SSEPS, when the median nerve is stimulated and the response is bilateral absence of the parietal sensory cortex, brain death is indicated.

Differential Diagnosis

A. Various scenarios have been studied and closely resemble brain death. Conditions that therefore must be ruled out include:

1. Metabolic encephalopathy.
2. Drug intoxications.
3. Neuromuscular paralysis.
4. Guillain-Barre syndrome.
5. Locked-in syndrome.
6. Hypothermia.

Evaluation and Management Plan

A. Prognosis and pronouncement of death.

1. There are no published reports of neurological recovery after a diagnosis of brain death.

2. Once brain death criteria are met and determination of brain death is made, that person is legally dead, and a time of death is given. An attending physician must pronounce a person deceased.

3. Often, there are family objections and delays in discontinuation of life support. This can often be mitigated by good education as well as guidance for the family from the medical team. As the provider, it is important to include the family early in the process.

a. Be concise and clear in your communication to them. Be sensitive and ensure that an understanding of the process is being met. By doing so, when it comes time to remove life sustaining measures, the family has a better understanding as to why.

b. Once an understanding is reached, this would be an appropriate time to introduce the organ procurement team.

B. Organ procurement.

1. Each state has an organization that offers its services to hospitals and patients' families to discuss the opportunity for organ donation. This is most often an outlet for families to help cope in a devastating situation.

2. If a family does decide to donate organs, it may be necessary to treat certain medical problems to preserve

the patient's organs. Diabetes insipidus and pulmonary hypertension are two complications that develop early in patients who are diagnosed with brain death and are important to consider.

3. There are two types of organ donations after death.

a. Donation after cardiac death. If the person does not satisfy brain death criteria but does not have a meaningful recovery of life and the family decides to withdraw care but wants to proceed with donation, it can do so. The patient is extubated in the operating room and prepped for surgery, with transplant teams standing by. If the patient dies by cardiac death, he or she is reintubated and surgery is performed immediately for organ procurement. If the patient does not die within 60 minutes, surgery for donation legally cannot proceed and therefore the patient is made comfortable and allowed to die in a private room.

b. Donation after brain death. The patient has already been determined to be brain dead and given a time of death. He or she can then be taken to the operating room for organ procurement, once all arrangements have been made.

Bibliography

Baker, A., Beed, S., Fenwick, J., Kjerulf, M., Bell, H., Logier, S., & Shepherd, J. (2006). Number of deaths by neurological criteria, and organ and tissue donation rates at three critical care centres in Canada. *Canadian Journal of Anesthesia, 53*(7), 722–726. doi:10.1007/BF03021632

Burkle, C. M., Schipper, A. M., & Wijdicks, E. F. (2011). Brain death and the courts. *Neurology, 76*, 837–841. doi:10.1212/WNL.0b013e31820e7bbe

Gardiner, D., Shemie, S., Manara, A., & Opdam, H. (2012). International perspective on the diagnosis of death. *British Journal of Anaesthesia, 108*(Suppl. 1), i14–i28. doi:10.1093/bja/aer397

Hocker, S., Whalen, F., & Wijdicks, E. F. (2014). Apnea testing for brain death in severe acute respiratory distress syndrome: A possible solution. *Neurocritical Care, 20*, 298–300. doi:10.1007/s12028-013-9932-0

The Quality Standards Subcommittee of the American Academy of Neurology. (1995). Practice parameters for determining brain death in adults (summary statement). *Neurology, 45*, 1012–1014.

Wijdicks, E. F., Varelas, P. N., Gronseth, G. S., & Greer, D. M. (2010). Evidence-based guideline update: Determining brain death in adults. Report of the Quality Standards Subcommittee of the American Academy of Neurology. *Neurology, 74*, 1911–1918. doi:10.1212/WNL.0b013e3181e242a8

Headaches

Asha Avirachen and Muhammed Athar

Definition

A. Diffuse pain in some part of the head or pain located above the orbitomeatal line of the head.

B. The International Headache Society divides headaches into primary and secondary headaches.

1. Primary: Benign headaches without any abnormal pathology. More than 90% of headaches are primary. Three types are recognized.

a. Migraine: Characterized by attacks of moderate to severe throbbing headaches that are often unilateral in location, worsened by physical activity, and associated with nausea and/or vomiting, photophobia, and phonophobia. Migraine headaches may last from 4 to 72 hours.

i. Classic migraine: Migraine with aura—the aura usually only lasts up to 60 minutes.

ii. Common migraine: Migraine without aura.

iii. Status migrainosus: Migraine lasting more than 3 days.

b. Tension-type headache: Most common form of headache that can last from 30 minutes to 7 days. Characterized by bilateral mild to moderate non-throbbing pressure such as pain, without associated symptoms. Mostly described as tight band around the head.

c. Cluster headache: Less common. Brief episodes of severe unilateral throbbing pain, mostly in the retro-orbital area that usually last from 15 minutes to 3 hours. Ipsilateral autonomic symptoms such as eyelid edema, nasal congestion, and lacrimation may be present.

2. Secondary: Malignant headaches caused by structural lesion or organic pathology. Less than 10% of headaches are secondary.

a. Examples include headaches due to brain tumor, meningitis, substance withdrawal, and intracerebral hemorrhage.

Incidence

A. Many headache sufferers do not seek medical attention.
B. An estimated 23 million Americans and 240 million people worldwide have migraine headaches each year.
C. Migraine headaches occur in a 3:1 female-to-male ratio.
D. Episodic tension-type headaches are present in about 46% of the U.S. population.
E. Chronic tension-type headaches are present in approximately 2% of the U.S. population.

Pathogenesis

A. The exact mechanism involved in the development of primary headaches is unknown.
B. Headaches usually result from vasodilation/constriction of blood vessels.
C. Migraine headaches are thought to result from activation of meningeal and blood vessel nociceptors, combined with a change in central pain modulation.
D. Activation of trigeminal system results in release of neuropeptides, which, in turn, causes neurogenic inflammation and increase in vascular permeability and local dilation of blood vessels, causing pain and associated symptoms via the trigeminal pathway.
E. Decrease in levels of serotonin (5-hydroxytryptamine [5–HT]) have shown to induce migraine.

Predisposing Factors

A. Foods containing tyramine (aged cheeses, pickled foods), nitrites (cured meats), monosodium glutamate, or sulfites.
B. Alcoholic beverages, especially red wine and beer.
C. Emotional factors such as stress, anxiety, and depression.
D. Hormonal fluctuations.
E. Decreased sleep or sleep deprivation.
F. Medications: Estrogen, nitroglycerine, or ranitidine.
G. Physical fatigue.
H. Environmental: Weather, odors, sound, bright lights, and barometric changes.

Subjective Data

A. Common complaints/symptoms (red flag symptoms).
1. Every headache evaluation should begin with a search for certain signs and symptoms. The presence of any of these "red flag" symptoms warrants an urgent extensive workup.
2. Systemic symptoms (fever, weight loss) or secondary risk factors (HIV, systemic cancer).
3. Neurologic symptoms or abnormal signs (impaired alertness or consciousness, confusion, weakness, visual loss).
4. Onset: Sudden, abrupt, or split-second.
5. Increased age: New-onset and progressive headache, especially in middle age (>50 years [giant cell arteritis]).
6. Previous headache history: First headache or different headache (marked change in attack, frequency, severity, or clinical features).
B. Diagnostic criteria.
1. The gold standard for diagnosis of headache is a detailed interview and clinical examination.
2. Headache onset (age, sudden or gradual onset, factors associated with onset such as exercise, sexual activity, Valsalva maneuver, febrile illness).
3. Location of pain: Unilateral, bilateral, global.
4. Duration (see section "Definition" for details).
5. Frequency.
6. Quality: Throbbing, squeezing, band like, stabbing.
7. Severity (at onset, at peak, and duration from onset to peak).
8. Associated symptoms such as nausea, vomiting, blurred vision, nasal congestion, mood swings, and so forth.
9. Presence or absence of an aura: Visual scotomas, flashing lights, or facial numbness.
10. Aggravating and relieving factors: Body position or darkness.
C. History.
1. Medication history: Contraceptives, hormonal therapy, vitamins, herbals, and painkillers.
2. General medical history.
3. Family history of headaches.

Physical Examination

A. Perform a complete general examination with focus on the head and neck and a full neurological examination. Generally, these are normal, with no neurological deficits in primary headaches. A focal neurological deficit with acute headache predicts central nervous system (CNS) pathology.
B. Observe the body habitus. Patients with pseudo tumor cerebri tend to be obese.
C. Perform a funduscopic examination to rule out papilledema as in pseudo tumor cerebri or diseases with increased intracranial pressure (ICP).
D. Auscultate the skull and orbits for bruits as heard in arteriovenous malformation and fistulas.
E. Palpate and tap the sinus for tenderness in sinus inflammation.
F. Arteries may be tender and harder to palpate in temporal arteritis.
G. Palpate both temporomandibular joints for tenderness and crepitus while the patient opens and closes the jaw.

Diagnostic Tests

A. The diagnosis of primary headache is usually made on the basis of headache history, physical examination, and neurological examination. No specific diagnostic tests are available.
B. The diagnosis of secondary headache involves the following.

1. Complete blood count (CBC), chemistry panel, urinalysis, liver function test, and thyroid profile.
2. Sedimentation rate and C-reactive protein: Elevated in temporal arteritis.
3. Neurological imaging, which should be considered in patients with any of the following findings.
   a. Thunderclap headache/worst headache of life.
   b. Altered mental status.
   c. Meningismus.
   d. Papilledema.
   e. Acute neurological deficit.
   f. New onset headache after age 50.
   g. History of cancer or HIV or immunocompromised state.
4. CT of head: Best to rule out acute injury and bleed.
5. CT of paranasal sinuses: To rule out sinusitis.
6. MRI of brain (more sensitive than CT): Useful to rule out space occupying lesions, demyelinating lesions, ischemia, and abscess.
7. Magnetic resonance angiography (MRA): Helpful in identifying vascular abnormalities such as aneurysms and arteriovenous malformation.
8. Lumbar puncture: Useful in diagnosing infections, malignancy and subarachnoid hemorrhage, and idiopathic intracranial hypertension.
9. Tonometry: If symptoms suggest acute narrow angle glaucoma (visual halos, corneal edema, shallow anterior chamber).

Differential Diagnosis

A. Differential diagnosis.
B. Brain tumor.
C. Brain hemorrhage.
D. Seizure.
E. Meningitis.
F. Dissection.
G. Cerebral aneurysm.

Evaluation and Management Plan

A. Migraine headache.
   1. General interventions.
      a. Lifestyle modifications and trigger prevention should be emphasized.
      b. Analgesics such as aspirin, acetaminophen, ibuprofen, and naproxen can be used in mild headache. Opioids are generally avoided in primary headaches.
   2. Acute migraine: Abortive treatment in inpatient or ED setting.
      a. Nonsteroidal anti-inflammatory drugs (NSAIDs) and corticosteroids: Caution necessary in patients with hepatic or renal impairment, diabetes, or gastritis. One of the following drugs can be used.
         i. Ketorolac 30 mg IV.
         ii. Methylprednisolone 100 to 200 mg.
         iii. Dexamethasone 10 to 40 mg.
      b. Neuroleptics: Can be used alone and as pretreatment to ergot derivatives to offset nausea.
         i. Diphenhydramine 25 to 50 mg, lorazepam 0.5 to 1 mg, and/or benztropine 1 mg is often given before neuroleptic to prevent akathisia.
         ii. ECG: Check and avoid neuroleptics if QTc is prolonged.
      c. Anti-nausea medications can be used to alleviate the sense of nausea, but are also effective in controlling migraines in select patients.

         i. Metoclopramide 10 to 20 mg IV.
         ii. Prochlorperazine 10 to 20 mg IV, IM.
         iii. Droperidol 0.625 to 2.5 mg IV or IM.
         iv. Chlorpromazine 12.5 to 100 mg PO, IV (up to 50 mg only).
      d. Dihydroergotamine 0.5 to 1 mg IV push: Migraine-specific but also helpful in cluster headache. This drug must not be administered if a triptan has been taken in the preceding 24 hours, and it is contraindicated in patients with a history of, or at high risk for, myocardial infarction (MI), or stroke.
      e. Anticonvulsants: Can be useful; given as rapid infusions (over 10–20 minutes).
         i. Valproic acid: 500 to 1,000 mg; can also be useful for cluster headache.
         ii. Levetiracetam: 1,000 to 2,000 mg, maximum recommended dose is 3,000 mg/d.
      f. Magnesium sulfate: 1 to 2 g IV piggyback.
      g. Serotonin (5-HT) receptor agonists: Sumatriptan 6 mg SC or 10 mg intranasal.
   3. Migraine prophylaxis: Used when attacks exceed two per month or when acute attacks are refractory. One of the following drugs can be used.
      a. Beta adrenergic blockers: Propranolol—drug of choice.
      b. Tricyclic antidepressants: Amitriptyline 25 to 125 mg PO hs.
      c. Serotonin antagonists: Methysergide 1 to 2 mg PO TID.
      d. Calcium channel antagonist: Verapamil 40 to 80 mg TID.
      e. Anticonvulsant: Valproic acid total 250 mg BID or TID.
B. Tension-type headache.
   1. Usual abortive treatment can be any simple analgesic.
   2. Drug of choice for prophylaxis is amitriptyline 50 to 150 mg/d.
   3. Concurrent depression or anxiety disorder needs to be addressed if present.
C. Cluster headache.
   1. Abortive treatment.
      a. Inhalation of 100% of oxygen for 10 to 15 minutes.
      b. Sumatriptan 6 mg SC.
      c. Dihydroergotamine IV.
   2. Preventive therapy with one of the following.
      a. Verapamil—drug of choice—80 mg TID; max dose is 360 mg/d.
      b. Lithium 600 to 1,200 mg/d; monitor lithium levels.
      c. Topiramate 100 to 400 mg/d.
      d. Gabapentin 1,200 to 3,600 mg/d.
      e. Melatonin 9 to 12 mg/d.
D. Nonpharmacologic treatment for all types of headaches.
   1. Interventions such as acupuncture, biofeedback, nerve block, neurotoxin injections, neurostimulators, and behavioral and psychological therapies are found to be effective in managing headaches.

Follow-Up

A. Patients can follow-up with primary providers if headaches are infrequent.
B. Follow-up with a headache specialist for more complicated or refractory cases or treatment of persistent headaches.

Consultation/Referral

A. Refer to a headache specialist if there is concern for an underlying pathology for the headaches or if there are any unusual features or symptoms associated with the headaches.

B. Also consider referring patients who are refractory to conventional treatment.

Special/Geriatric Considerations

A. New onset of severe headache in pregnancy or postpartum period should be investigated to rule out cortical sinus thrombosis. MRI is considered safe during pregnancy.

B. Treatment of headache in pregnancy should be coordinated with obstetrician.

C. Metoclopramide and prochlorperazine are generally considered safe in pregnancy.

D. Ergotamines are absolutely contraindicated in pregnancy.

Bibliography

American Association of Neuroscience Nurses. (2004). Headaches. In M. Bader, & L. Littlejohns (Eds.), *AANN core curriculum for neuroscience nursing* (4th ed., Vol. 1, pp. 836–849). Maryland Heights, MO: Saunders.

Hainer, B., & Matheson, E. (2013). Approach to acute headache in adults. *American Family Physician, 87*(10), 682–687. Retrieved from https://www.aafp.org/afp/2013/0515/p682.html

Hickey, J. (2003). Headaches. In J. HIckey (Ed.), *The clinical practice of neurological and neurosurgical nursing* (5th ed., pp. 603–615). Philadelphia, PA: Lippincott Williams.

International Headache Society. (n. d.) Retrieved from http://www.ihs-headache.org

Singh, G., Gupta, P., Gupta, A., & Khanal, M. (2011). Clinical approach to a patient with headache. In *Neurology* (Vol. 1, pp. 514–517). Elsevier.

Young, W., Silberstein, S., Nahas, S., & Marmura, M. (2011). *Jefferson headache manual.* New York, NY: Demos Medical.

Intracerebral Hemorrhage

Bridget Gibson and Syed Omar Shah

Definition

A. A pathologic accumulation of blood within the parenchyma of the brain.

B. Often confused with intracranial hemorrhage, an umbrella term that encompasses subdural hematoma, epidural hematoma, and subarachnoid hemorrhage, as well as intracerebral hemorrhage (ICH).

Incidence

A. ICH affects 12 to 15 per 100,000 people. It increases with age, doubling every 10 years after age 35.

B. The incidence is higher in populations with higher frequencies of hypertension such as African Americans. The prevalence is increased in Asian populations compared with Caucasian populations because of environmental and genetic factors.

Pathogenesis

A. Hypertensive damage to intracranial blood vessels causing small vessel vasculopathy resulting from chronic or acute hypertension or drug abuse.

B. Autoregulatory dysfunction with excessive cerebral blood flow resulting from reperfusion or the hemorrhagic transformation of ischemic strokes.

C. Vascular malformations resulting from aneurysm rupture or hemorrhage of an arteriovenous malformation.

D. Coagulopathy resulting from anticoagulation, thrombolysis, or a bleeding disorder.

E. Hemorrhagic necrosis resulting from tumor or infection.

F. Venous outflow obstruction resulting from cerebral venous thrombosis.

G. Trauma.

Predisposing Factors

A. Modifiable risk factors: Hypertension, cocaine/stimulant use, low cholesterol levels, oral anticoagulants, and excessive alcohol intake.

B. Nonmodifiable risk factors: Age, male gender, African American/Japanese ethnicity, and cerebral amyloid angiopathy (CAA).

Subjective Data

A. Common complaints/symptoms.

    1. Headache, seizures, vomiting, or worsening score on the Glasgow Coma Scale (GCS).

    2. Focal neurological signs (such as unilateral limb weakness, facial weakness, or cranial nerve palsies) can present to varying degrees of severity depending on the location and size of hemorrhage.

    3. Frequency of clinical seizures within 1 week of ICH is 16% with majority occurring at onset.

B. Common/typical scenario.

    1. Severe headache with or without vomiting prompts patient to go to the hospital or the patient has a change in mental status and emergency personnel are called to the scene. Typically bystanders will report nothing unusual occurred until the moment of the intracranial injury.

C. Family and social history.

    1. Ask about smoking and alcohol use.

    2. Drug use is often associated with ICH in younger patients.

    3. Family history of stroke.

D. Review of systems.

    1. Neurological—ask about headache, any weakness, or difficulty speaking.

    2. Cardiac—ask about history of high blood pressure, if the patient is taking any blood thinning medications for irregular heart rate.

Physical Examination

A. Neurological—perform full neurological examination.

    1. Motor assessment—note any weakness of limbs.

    2. Sensory assessment—note any decrease in or lack of sensation on a limb.

    3. Assess cranial nerves for deficits, in particular the extraocular movements and facial nerves.

    4. Assess speech for difficulty speaking or finding words.

    5. Assess language for difficulty understanding.

    6. Determine level of consciousness.

    7. Check for symptoms that may provide a clue to a location of the hemorrhage.

        a. Basal ganglia/thalamus location: Hemisensory loss, hemiplegia, aphasia, homonymous hemianopsia, eye deviation away from lesion, upgaze palsy.

        b. Lobar location: Seizures, homonymous hemianopsia, plegia, or paresis of leg greater than arm.

        c. Cerebellar location: Ataxia, nystagmus, intractable vomiting, and/or symptoms related to obstructive hydrocephalus (drowsiness, leg weakness, impaired upgaze, blurred, or double vision).

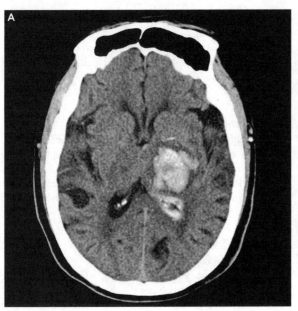 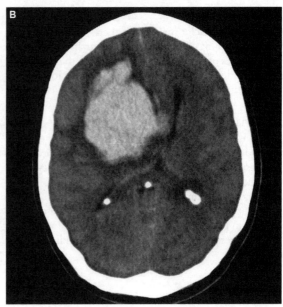

FIGURE 6.1 Head CT scans showing (A) basal ganglia hemorrhage due to hypertension, (B) right frontal hemorrhage due to amyloid angiopathy.

d. Pons location: Pinpoint pupils, quadriparesis, coma, locked-in syndrome.

Diagnostic Tests

A. Noncontrast head CT: Should be obtained as soon as possible and then 24 hours after admission (see Figure 6.1). Repeat imaging may be warranted if the patient bleeds on anticoagulation while reversal of coagulopathy is in process. Also, obtain a STAT noncontrast head CT with any neurological examination change.

    1. Fluid levels seen within hemorrhage on CT scan indicate a coagulopathy (slow oozing of blood over time as seen by different intensities of blood on CT scan).

    2. Hemorrhage volume calculation: ABC/2 (or ABC/3 for hemorrhages secondary to warfarin).

    3. A (diameter in cm on CT slice where hemorrhage is largest) ×

    4. B (largest diameter in cm 90° to A) ×

    5. C (number of 10 cm CT slices)/2

B. CT angiogram of head and neck: May be helpful to rule out subarachnoid hemorrhage, arteriovenous/cavernous malformation, and brain tumor.

C. MRI brain with and without contrast: Should be obtained 4 to 6 weeks posthemorrhage to evaluate for underlying mass if etiology remains unclear.

Differential Diagnosis

A. Clinical suspicion is warranted when there is a rapid alteration in neurological status often in conjunction with signs of an elevation in intracranial pressure. Increased intracranial pressure may be evidenced by change in level of consciousness, nausea, vomiting, or headache.

B. The type of neurological dysfunction brought about by ICH may indicate the location, etiology, and severity of the hemorrhage.

C. Conditions to rule out include arteriovenous malformations, severe hemiplegic migranes, seizures, cerebral aneurysms, and tumors.

Evaluation and Management Plan

A. General plan.

1. Determine the location of the hemorrhage, which will assist in secondary prevention.

    a. Hypertensive hemorrhages tend to occur in basal ganglia/thalamus greater than lobar more than cerebellum greater than pons.

    b. Amyloid hemorrhages are mostly in lobar locations.

    c. Hemorrhages secondary to vascular malformations, tumors, and coagulopathies can occur anywhere.

2. Medical management.

    a. Blood pressure.

      i. Hypertension is associated with hematoma expansion, neurological deterioration, dependency, and death. Early control is essential.

      1) Antihypertensive treatment of acute cerebral hemorrhage (ATACH) and intensive blood pressure reduction in acute cerebral hemorrhage (INTERACT) found reduction of systolic blood pressure less than 140 mmHg to be safe and beneficial in improving functional outcomes.

      2) Arterial line and peripheral intravenous lines should be placed for close monitoring and tight control of blood pressure.

      3) Continuous infusions should be used to maintain blood pressure parameters.

        a) Clevidipine, start 1 to 2 mg/hr (max 21 mg/hr).

        b) Labetalol, 1 to 2 mg/min (max 2 mg/min).

        c) Nicardipine, start 5 mg/hr (max 15 mg/hr).

    b. Coagulopathies.

      i. Any coagulopathies should be addressed and reversed if possible.

    c. Seizures.

      i. Clinical seizures should be treated with intravenous anti-epileptics.

      ii. Continuous EEG monitoring is necessary for patients with depressed mental status out of proportion to injury.

iii. Prophylactic anti-epileptic medication is not recommended.

d. Intracranial pressure.

i. Monitor intracranial pressure with an external ventricular device if patient has a Glasgow Coma Score of 8 or less.

e. Other medical issues.

i. Hypoglycemia and hyperglycemia should be avoided.

ii. Normothermia should be maintained.

iii. Deep venous thrombosis (DVT) prophylaxis: After radiographic evidence of hematoma stability, subcutaneous heparin should be considered for patients with lack of mobility after 1 to 4 days from onset.

3. Surgical management: Surgical management is not warranted in all cases of ICH and is limited in hypertensive hemorrhages to the acutely deteriorating patient as a lifesaving measure. Surgical management is the standard of care in subdural or epidural hematomas or in patients who have an ICH secondary to a tumor.

a. Craniotomy.

i. This procedure should be considered in patients with a subdural hematoma that is causing midline shift and increased intracranial pressure, epidural hematomas, and for removal of tumors associated with ICH.

ii. Patients with cerebellar ICH who deteriorate neurologically or have brainstem compression and/or hydrocephalus should undergo emergent surgical hematoma evacuation.

b. Decompressive hemicraniectomy.

i. This procedure may reduce mortality for comatose patients, those who have large hematomas with significant midline shift, or those with elevated ICP refractory to medical management.

ii. Decompressive hemicraniectomy is controversial because although it reduces mortality in comatose patients, morbidity is very profound and outcomes are generally poor, leading to significant impairments of motor, speech, language, and quality of life.

4. Determine prognosis.

a. Prognosis can be determined by using the ICH score.

i. This simple clinical grading scale (see Table 6.1) aids in prognostication at presentation.

ii. The total score (see Table 6.2) represents 30-day mortality risk based on a combination of criteria.

B. Patient/family teaching points.

1. Depends on the extent of the injury.

a. If patients are able to participate in their own care, they should be instructed on diet and lifestyle changes, blood pressure control, avoidance of alcohol, and smoking cessation.

b. If patients are unable to participate in their own care, families need to be given options to care for the patient at home or in a nursing home.

C. Pharmacotherapy.

1. There are no specific medications for the treatment of spontaneous ICH.

a. Antihypertensive medications to maintain normotension.

b. Antilipid medications for the treatment of atherosclerotic disease.

c. Patients who need to take antiplatelet medications or need anticoagulation should consult with the neurologist prior to starting.

D. Discharge instructions.

1. If the ICH is small, patients may return home with instructions to slowly return to daily activities.

2. If the patient requires rehabilitation, families should be given instructions to follow-up with the neurologist afterward.

3. If the patient requires a nursing home, follow-up can be on an as needed basis.

4. All patients should receive clearance from the neurologist prior to starting antiplatelet or anticoagulation therapy.

TABLE 6.1   ICH Score

	Points
Score on GCS	
3–4	2
5–12	1
13–15	0
Intracerebral Volume	
≥30 cm^3	1
<30 cm^3	0
Intraventricular Hemorrhage	
Yes	1
No	0
Location	
Infratentorial	1
Supratentorial	0
Age	
Age ≥80 y	1
Age <80 y	0

GCS, Glasgow Coma Scale; ICH, intracerebral hemorrhage.
Source: Hemphill, J. C., 3rd, Bonovich, D. C., Besmertis, L., Manley, G. T., & Johnston, S. C. (2001). The ICH score: A simple, reliable grading scale for intracerebral hemorrhage. *Stroke, A Journal of Cerebral Circulation, 32,* 891–897. doi:10.1161/STR.0000000000000069

TABLE 6.2   30-Day Mortality Risk for Spontaneous Intracranial Hemorrhage

ICH Score	Mortality (%)
0	0
1	13
2	26
3	72
4	97
5	100
6	100

ICH, intracerebral hemorrhage.

Follow-Up

A. Patients should follow-up with the neurologist in 6 to 8 weeks from discharge from the hospital or rehabilitation center.

B. Patients who require a nursing home can follow-up with specific issues on an as needed basis.

Consultation/Referral

A. Consult neurology on every ICH patient who comes into the hospital. All patients will require secondary prevention.

B. Consult neurosurgery if there is a concern for increased intracranial pressure or in patients with a GCS of less than 13. Patients who have large ICHs should be evaluated for possible surgery.

Special/Geriatric Considerations

A. Elderly patients who present with spontaneous ICH frequently have the condition amyloid angiopathy. There is no treatment for amyloid and recurrence is high, up to 30%.

B. Elderly patients with significant volume loss associated with aging or certain disease states, such as dementia or alcoholism, may tolerate larger ICHs with fewer deficits. However, recovery from any lost function in the elderly is generally poor.

Bibliography

Anderson, C. S., Heeley, E., Huang, Y., Wang, J., Stapf, C., Delcourt, C., . . . Chalmers, J. (2013). Rapid blood-pressure lowering in patients with acute intracerebral hemorrhage. *The New England Journal of Medicine, 368*, 2355–2365. doi:10.1056/NEJMoa1214609

Ariesen, M. J., Claus, S. P., Rinkel, G. J., & Algra, A. (2003). Risk factors for intracerebral hemorrhage in the general population: A systematic review. *Stroke, 34*, 2060–2065. doi:10.1161/01.STR.0000080678.09344.8D

Arima, H., Huang, Y., Wang, J. G., Heeley, E., Delcourt, C., Parsons, M., & Anderson, C. (2012). Earlier blood pressure-lowering and greater attenuation of hematoma growth in acute intracerebral hemorrhage: INTERACT pilot phase. *Stroke, 43*, 2236–2238. doi:10.1161/STROKEAHA.112.651422

De Herdt, V., Dumont, F., Hénon, H., Derambure, P., Vonck, K., Leys, D., & Cordonnier, C. (2011). Early seizures in intracerebral hemorrhage: Incidence, associated factors, and outcome. *Neurology, 77*, 1794–1800. doi:10.1212/WNL.0b013e31823648a6

Hemphill, J. C., Bonovich, C. D., 3rd, Besmertis, L., Manley, G. T., & Johnston, S. C. (2001). The ICH score: A simple, reliable grading scale for intracerebral hemorrhage. *Stroke, 32*, 891–897. doi:10.1161/01.STR.32.4.891

Hemphill, J. C., Greenberg, M. S., 3rd, Anderson, C. S., Becker, K., Bendok, B. R., Cushman, M., & Woo, D. (2015). Guidelines for the management of spontaneous intracerebral hemorrhage: A guideline for healthcare professionals from the American Heart Association/American Stroke Association. *Stroke, 46*, 2032–2060. doi:10.1161/STR.0000000000000069

Labovitz, D. L., Halim, A., Boden-Albala, B., Hauser, W. A., & Sacco, R. L. (2005). The incidence of deep and lobar intracerebral hemorrhage in Whites, Blacks, and Hispanics. *Neurology, 65*, 518–522. doi:10.1212/01.wnl.0000172915.71933.00

Mendelow, A. D., Gregson, B. A., Fernandes, H. M., Murray, G. D., Teasdale, G. M., Hope, D. T., & Barer, D. H. (2005). Early surgery versus initial conservative treatment in patients with spontaneous supratentorial intracerebral haematomas in the International Surgical Trial in Intracerebral Haemorrhage (STICH): A randomised trial. *Lancet, 365*, 387–397. doi:10.1016/S0140-6736(05)17826-X

Mendelow, A. D., Gregson, B. A., Rowan, E. N., Murray, G. D., Gholkar, A., & Mitchell, P. M. (2013). Early surgery versus initial conservative treatment in patients with spontaneous supratentorial lobar intracerebral haematomas (STICH II): A randomised trial. *Lancet, 382*, 397–408. doi:10.1016/S0140-6736(13)60986-1

Mould, W. A., Carhuapoma, J. R., Muschelli, J., Lane, K., Morgan, T. C., McBee, N. A., & Hanley, D. F. (2013). Minimally invasive surgery plus recombinant tissue-type plasminogen activator for intracerebral hemorrhage evacuation decreases perihematomal edema. *Stroke, 44*, 627–634. doi:10.1161/STROKEAHA.111.000411

Naff, N., Williams, M. A., Keyl, P. M., Tuhrim, S., Bullock, M. R., Mayer, S. A., & Hanley, F. D., Jr. (2011). Low-dose recombinant tissue-type plasminogen activator enhances clot resolution in brain hemorrhage: The intraventricular hemorrhage thrombolysis trial. *Stroke, 42*, 3009–3016. doi:10.1161/STROKEAHA.110.610949

Qureshi, A. I., Palesch, Y. Y., Martin, R., Novitzke, J., Cruz-Flores, S., Ehtisham, A., . . . Tariq, N. (2010). Effect of systolic blood pressure reduction on hematoma expansion, perihematomal edema, and 3-month outcome among patients with intracerebral hemorrhage: Results from the antihypertensive treatment of acute cerebral hemorrhage study. *Archives of Neurology, 67*, 570–576. doi:10.1001/archneurol.2010.61

Rincon, F., & Mayer, S. A. (2013). The epidemiology of intracerebral hemorrhage in the United States from 1979 to 2008. *Neurocritical Care, 19*, 95–102. doi:10.1007/s12028-012-9793-y

Stein, M., Misselwitz, B., Hamann, G. F., Scharbrodt, W., Schummer, D. I., & Oertel, M. F. (2012). Intracerebral hemorrhage in the very old: Future demographic trends of an aging population. *Stroke, 43*, 1126–1128. doi:10.1161/STROKEAHA.111.644716

van Asch, C. J., Luitse, M. J., Rinkel, G. J., van der Tweel, I., Algra, A., & Klijn, C. J. (2010). Incidence, case fatality, and functional outcome of intracerebral haemorrhage over time, according to age, sex, and ethnic origin: A systematic review and meta-analysis. *The Lancet Neurology, 9*(2), 167–176. doi:10.1016/S1474-4422(09)70340-0

Ischemic Stroke/Cerebrovascular Accident

Catherine Harris

Definition

A. A sudden interruption of blood flow to the brain.

B. Classification.
   1. Thrombotic strokes—55+%.
   2. Embolic strokes—10% to 30%.
   3. Lacunar strokes—10%.
   4. Cryptogenic strokes—10%.

Incidence

A. Approximately 800,000 strokes occur each year.
   1. 610,000 are first-time strokes.
   2. 185,000 are recurring strokes.

B. Stroke is the fifth leading cause of death.

C. Stroke is the leading cause of disability. There are approximately 7 million stroke survivors in the United States.

Pathogenesis

A. Stroke results from decreased cerebral blood flow that can be the result of an obstruction (e.g., thrombus or embolus), vasoconstriction, low blood flow states (shock), or anything that deprives oxygen or glucose to the brain.

B. Anaerobic metabolism and lactic acid production compromise surrounding brain tissue (penumbra), causing ischemia followed by infarction if blood flow is now restored.

Predisposing Factors

A. Nonmodifiable.
   1. Age greater than 55 years.
   2. Gender: Women greater than men.
   3. Race: African Americans have a 2 to 3x increased risk compared to Caucasians.
   4. Prior stroke or transient ischemic attack (TIA).
   5. Family history.

B. Modifiable.
   1. Hypertension.
   2. Hypercholesterolemia.
   3. Diabetes.
   4. Atrial fibrillation.
   5. Hypercoagulable states.
   6. Coronary artery disease.

7. Sleep apnea.
8. Smoking.
9. Alcohol consumption.
10. Use of oral contraceptives.
11. Obesity.
12. Drug use.

Subjective Data

A. Common complaints/symptoms.
  1. Depend on the location of the stroke (see section "TIA" discussion).
B. Common/typical scenario.
  1. Sudden, abrupt onset.
  2. Typical report of family members: Patient is perfectly fine one moment and then instantly changes.
  3. Relationship between typical symptoms and location of stroke (see section "TIA" discussion).
C. Review of systems.
  1. Ask patient about following (see Table 6.3).
    a. Headaches.
    b. Speech difficulties.
    c. Falls.
    d. Dropping objects.
    e. Weakness of arms/legs/face.
    f. Numbness/tingling.
    g. Loss of urine/bowel control.
    h. Visual changes—blurriness, double vision, loss of vision.

Physical Examination

A. Objective data.
  1. Level of consciousness.
  2. Visual examination.
  3. Motor and sensory examination.
  4. Speech assessment.
  5. Cognitive test.
  6. Cranial nerve examination.
B. Use the National Institute of Health Stroke Scale (NIHSS) to objectively score stroke severity. The tool uses a point range from 0 to 42, with severity increasing with score and can be accessed through the National Institutes of Health: www.ninds.nih.gov/sites/default/files/NIH_Stroke_Scale.pdf.
  1. Use dynamically to assess and then reassess the patient's condition.

TABLE 6.3	Typical Findings of Stroke Symptoms Based on Hemisphere
Left hemisphere	Right-sided weakness (face, arm, leg) Left gaze preference Speech slurred Aphasia
Right hemisphere	Left-sided weakness (face, arm, leg) Right gaze preference Speech slurred Flat affect May neglect the left side of the body
Brainstem or cerebellum	May have multiple cranial nerve palsies Ataxia Dysmetria Visual disturbances especially diplopia May have hemiparesis or quadriparesis Locked-in syndrome Vertigo

2. Scores greater than 13 indicate very severe stroke that may warrant surgical intervention and carry a very high probability of severe disability or death.

Diagnostic Tests

A. Initial tests to be done immediately.
  1. CT head.
    a. Should be done immediately if stroke is in the differential diagnosis. From the moment a stroke is suspected, a CT head should be completed within 25 minutes.
    b. Do NOT delay a CT head.
  2. Lab tests: Should be done simultaneously as preparing to go to CT head.
    a. Minimum: Obtain a glucose done prior to CT, but if the patient is a difficult stick, obtain the rest of the lab tests after CT of the head.
    b. Complete blood count (CBC), basic metabolic panel, prothrombin time (PT)/partial thromboplastin time (PTT)/international normalized ratio (INR).
  3. Electrocardiogram.
B. Other tests to be considered in select patients.
  1. CT angiogram (CTA)/CT perfusion (CTP): Shows blood vessels, area of occlusion, and if there is collateral circulation. It can quantify cerebral blood flow, blood volume, and the presence or absence of penumbra.
  2. MRI/magnetic resonance angiography: To evaluate extent of stroke.
  3. Arterial blood gas (ABG).
  4. Cerebral angiography: If a candidate for thrombectomy.
  5. Ultrasound of carotids: To evaluate for carotid plaque as the source of stroke.
  6. EEG: If seizure suspected.

Differential Diagnosis

A. Ischemic stroke.
B. Hemorrhagic stroke.
C. Migraine.
D. Bell's palsy.
E. Seizure.
F. Hypoglycemic/hyperglycemia episode.
G. Sepsis.
H. Vertigo.
I. Neuromuscular or neurodegenerative disease.
J. Brain tumor.
K. Meningitis.
L. Syncope.
M. Multiple sclerosis.

Evaluation and Management Plan

A. The treatment of stroke should be broken up into three main phases. In the first phase, after the stroke has been identified, the goal of treatment is to minimize the damage as quickly as possible. In the second phase of the treatment of stroke, the goal is to prevent further strokes from occurring. In the third phase of treatment, the goal is to return the patient to his or her functional baseline prior to the stroke occurring.
B. Phase I plan.
  1. Medical management.
    a. Blood pressure (BP) control—the goal of BP management is to avoid complications. BP that is lowered too rapidly can cause increased ischemia and BP that is too high may cause a hemorrhagic conversion.

i. If no thrombolytics are given, treat the following BP.

    1) Diastolic BP >140 mmHg: Intravenous infusion.

    2) Systolic BP >220 mmHg, diastolic BP 121 to 40 mmHg: Intravenous push medications.

    3) Systolic BP <220 mmHg or diastolic BP <120 mmHg: Monitor in the absence of other compelling indications.

ii. If thrombolytics are to be given or have been given, treat the following BP.

    1) Systolic BP >180 mmHg.

    2) Diastolic BP >105 mmHg.

  b. Glucose monitoring.

    i. The brain requires glucose for energy. Persistent hyperglycemia is associated with poor neurological outcomes. Hypoglycemia can cause worsening of ischemia.

    ii. Goal of glucose monitoring: Maintain euglycemia less than 180 mg/dL.

  c. Intravenous tissue plasminogen activator (tPA) administration.

    i. Given to patients with the diagnosis of ischemic stroke where intracranial hemorrhage has been ruled out who present within a 3-hour time frame for treatment from symptom onset.

    ii. Some patients may qualify for treatment with intravenous tPA up to 4.5 hours. However, this is not Food and Drug Administration (FDA) approved.

2. Surgical management.

  a. Endovascular intervention.

  b. Intra-arterial tPA administration.

    i. Intra-arterial delivery directly into the clot via endovascular intervention.

    ii. Given within 6 hours of symptom onset.

    iii. Delivered directly into the clot.

    iv. Often used with mechanical clot extraction in large vessel strokes.

  c. Carotid endarterectomy: Rarely done as an emergency.

  d. Hemicraniectomy used for large hemispheric strokes with significant edema.

C. Phase II plan: Medical management begins 48 to 72 hours after stroke presentation.

  1. Antiplatelet—low dose aspirin or clopidogrel should be initiated as soon as intracranial hemorrhage has been ruled out.

    a. Aspirin 81 to 325 mg.

    b. Clopidogrel.

  2. Anticoagulants—prescribe only if there is an increased cardioembolic risk as determined by the CHA$_2$DS$_2$-VAS$_c$ Score (see Table 6.4 and section "TIA" discussion).

  3. DVT prophylaxis.

  4. BP management (see Chapter 3).

D. Phase III plan: Rehabilitation.

  1. Speech.

  2. Physical therapy.

  3. Occupational therapy.

E. Patient/family teaching.

  1. Note that depression is very common after stroke.

  2. Provide education about the cognitive limitations of the patient.

  3. Emphasize that rehabilitation may last as long as 1 year.

4. Encourage lifestyle changes, including smoking cessation, physical activity, and changes in dietary intake.

Follow-Up

A. Patients need to follow-up with neurology.
If there has been any intervention, the patient should follow-up with the neurosurgeon.

Consultation/Referral

A. Provide referrals to rehabilitation, physical and occupational therapy, nutrition, and speech.

Special/Geriatric Considerations

A. Stroke in adults under 40 is rare.

  1. If it does occur in younger adults, a hypercoagulable workup should be initiated in the hospital.

  2. Also consider mechanical causes such as carotid dissection, arteriovenous malformations, or fistulas.

B. Older adults should not be denied treatment due to age alone.

  1. Make sure the patient is assessed for the degree of frailty to help the family make decisions on treatment.

  2. The goal of treatment is to return the patient to baseline. If the baseline for the patient is extremely poor at any age, this should play a stronger role in the decision-making process.

Bibliography

Adams, H. P., Jr., del Zoppo, G., Alberts, J. M., Bhatt, D. L., Brass, L., Furlan, A., , . . . Wijdicks, E. F. (2007, May). Guidelines for the early management of adults with ischemic stroke: A guideline from the American Heart Association/American Stroke Association Stroke Council, Clinical Cardiology Council, Cardiovascular Radiology and Intervention Council, and the Atherosclerotic Peripheral Vascular Disease and Quality of Care Outcomes in Research Interdisciplinary Working Groups: The American Academy of Neurology affirms the value of this guideline as an educational tool for neurologists. *Stroke, 38*(5), 1655–1711. doi:10.1161/STROKEAHA.107.181486

Goldstein, L. B., Bushnell, C. D., Adams, R. J., Appel, L. J., Braun, L. T., Chaturvedi, S., . . . Pearson, T. A. (2011, February). Guidelines for the primary prevention of stroke: A guideline for healthcare professionals from the American Heart Association/American Stroke Association. *Stroke, 42*(2), 517–584. doi:10.1161/STR.0b013e3181fcb238

Hughes, S. (2014, May 2). New AHA/ASA stroke secondary prevention guidelines. *Medscape Medical News*, (pp. 870–947). doi: 10.1161/STR.0b013e318284056a

Jauch, E. C., Saver, J. L., Adams, Jr., H. P., Bruno, A., Connors, J. J., Demaerschalk, B. M., Khatri, P., McMullan, P. W., . . . Howard Yonas, H. (2015, June 29). AHA/ASA focused update of the 2013 guidelines for the early management of patients with acute ischemic stroke regarding endovascular treatment: A guideline for healthcare professionals from the American Heart Association/American Stroke Association. *Stroke, 38*(5), 1655–1711.

Mozaffarian, D., Benjamin, E. J., Go, A. S., Arnett, D. K., Blaha, M. J., Cushman, M., . . . Turner, M. B. (2015, January 27). Heart disease and stroke statistics—2015 update: A report from the American Heart Association. *Circulation, 131*(4), e29–e322. 10.1161/CIR.0000000000000152

National Institutes of Health. (2003). NIH stroke scale. Retrieved from https://www.ninds.nih.gov/sites/default/files/NIH_Stroke_Scale.pdf

Status Epilepticus

Asha Avirachen and M. Kamran Athar

Definition

A. Five minutes or more of continuous clinical and /or electrographic seizure activity or recurrent seizure activity without return to baseline between seizures.

B. Classification of the type of status epilepticus (SE) based on semiology, duration, and underlying etiology.

    1. Convulsive SE: Associated with generalized tonic-clonic movements of extremities and mental status impairment; a life-threatening medical emergency.

    2. Nonconvulsive status epilepticus (NCSE): Seizure activity only seen on EEG without any correlating clinical findings; requires emergent treatment to prevent cortical neuronal damage.

    3. Refractory SE: Clinical or electrographic seizures that do not respond to adequate doses of initial benzodiazepines, followed by a second antiepileptic drug (AED) agent.

Incidence

A. Annual incidence of SE is 100,000 to 200,000 cases in the United States.

B. Refractory SE occurs in up to 43% of patients with SE.

C. Up to a third of neuro ICU patients have NCSE.

D. 10% of medical ICU patients develop NCSE.

Pathogenesis

A. SE results from a neuronal imbalance between excitatory and inhibitory neurotransmitters (gamma-aminobutyric acid [GABA], N-methyl-D-aspartate [NMDA], glutamate) within the central nervous system (CNS).

B. Prolonged epileptic seizures result in lack of oxygen and glucose in brain cells, stimulating the release of excessive amounts of glutamate. Glutamate alters membrane channels, leading to an influx of calcium, which in turn triggers oxygen free radicals. These make brain cells electrically stable and cause cell injury.

Predisposing Factors

A. Acute processes.

    1. Traumatic brain injury.

    2. Metabolic disturbances: Electrolyte abnormalities, hypoglycemia, and renal failure.

    3. CNS infections.

    4. Cerebrovascular pathology: Ischemic stroke, hemorrhage, cerebral sinus thrombosis, and hypertensive encephalopathy.

    5. Autoimmune encephalitis, paraneoplastic syndromes.

    6. Sepsis.

    7. Drugs: Toxicity; noncompliance with AEDs; and withdrawal from opioids, benzodiazepine, barbiturates, or alcohol.

    8. Anoxic brain injury.

B. Chronic processes.

    1. Preexisting epilepsy.

    2. CNS tumors.

    3. History of CNS pathology (traumatic brain injury, abscess, stroke).

    4. Chronic ethanol abuse.

Subjective Data

A. Common complaints/symptoms.

    1. Generalized convulsive status epilepticus (GCSE): Tonic extension of trunk and extremities, followed by clonic extension. Consciousness is usually lost.

    2. Myoclonic SE: Bursts of brief myoclonic jerks, which increase in intensity until a convulsion occurs. This condition is seen mostly in anoxic encephalopathy or metabolic disturbances, particularly renal failure.

    3. NCSE: Absence of awakening or returning to baseline even after 20 minutes of successful termination of clinical seizures. Symptoms may include coma, confusion, aphasia, staring, automatisms, facial twitching, eye deviation, and agitation.

B. Common/typical scenario.

    1. GCSE usually presents with the classic full body convulsions and the patient is not aware of the occurrence.

    2. Myoclonic SE typically is seen in what people describe as limb shaking or twitching. Patients are awake and are able to describe the sensation.

    3. In NCSE, patients do not have any signs of twitching or abnormal movements. The only clue to lead to NCSE is the absence of the patient waking up or returning to baseline after an event such as cardiac arrest, intracranial hemorrhage, or any surgery.

C. Family and social history.

    1. Most common cause of SE is a prior history of epilepsy.

    2. Ask about changes in antiepileptic medications.

    3. Alcohol and drug use can lower the seizure threshold in patients with a history of epilepsy.

D. Review of systems.

    1. In patients with GCSE or NCSE, a review of systems is generally not possible to the altered level of consciousness.

Physical Examination

A. Neurological examination.

    1. Assess for any sensory or motor deficits in all limbs.

    2. Assess for any speech, memory, or language impairment.

    3. Assess for cranial nerve palsies.

    4. Assess level of consciousness and response to stimuli.

Diagnostic Tests

A. Workup should occur simultaneously and in parallel with treatment.

    1. Finger stick glucose.

    2. Complete blood count (CBC), comprehensive metabolic panel (CMP), drug screen, AED levels, alcohol levels, arterial blood gas (ABG), serum magnesium, and calcium (total and ionized).

    3. CT of brain to rule out intracranial pathology.

    4. Continuous EEG monitoring: 24-hour EEG is the gold standard. Most typical pattern in SE is rhythmic high frequency (>12 hz) activity that increases in amplitude and decreases in frequency, finally terminating abruptly and leaving postictal low amplitude slowing.

    5. Brain MRI: Seizure focus may show up as a bright signal on diffusion weighted imaging (DWI) and dark signal on apparent diffusion coefficient (ADC) imaging in a nonvascular territory possibly with leptomeningeal enhancement.

    6. Lumbar puncture and cerebrospinal fluid (CSF) studies.

    7. Toxicology panel: Check for toxins that frequently cause seizures (i.e., isoniazid, tricyclic antidepressants (TCAs), antidepressants, theophylline, cocaine, sympathomimetic, organophosphates, and cyclosporine).

Differential Diagnosis

A. Movement disorders.

B. Herniation syndromes (decerebrate /decorticate posturing).

C. Psychiatric disorders: Psychogenic nonepileptic seizures, conversion disorder, acute psychosis, or catatonia.

Evaluation and Management Plan

A. General plan.

1. Treatment of SE should occur rapidly and continue sequentially until clinical and electrographic seizures are stopped.

2. Simultaneous assessment and management of airway, breathing, and circulation should be performed.

3. Do not withhold seizure medications because of fear of respiratory compromise.

4. Definitive control of SE should be established within 60 minutes of onset.

5. Emergent treatment.

    a. Stabilize patient (airway, breathing, circulation).

    b. Perform cardiac monitoring.

    c. Consider intubation as needed.

    d. Use nutritional resuscitation with 100 mg of thiamine IV followed by 50 mL of 50% dextrose IV push.

    e. Lorazepam (drug of choice for intravenous administration): 0.1 mg/kg IV at the rate of 2 mg/min (max 4 mg per dose); max total dose 8 mg.

    f. Midazolam is preferred for IM. 0.2 mg/kg IM; max dose 10 mg.

    g. Diazepam (preferred for rectal administration): One time dose of 10 mg per rectum.

6. Urgent treatment.

    a. Recommended AEDs include intravenous fosphenytoin or phenytoin (PHT), valproic acid, levetiracetam, and lacosamide. Initial total levels should be drawn after 2 hours of intravenous loading dose to determine maintenance dose and need to reload.

        i. Load with fosphenytoin 20 mg phenytoin sodium equivalent (PE)/kg at the rate of 150 mg/min. If using phenytoin, the rate should not be more than 50 mg/min. Cardiac monitoring should occur during infusion due to increased risk of QT prolongation and cardiac arrhythmia. An additional 10 mg/kg IV can be given if seizures persist. The maintenance dose is phenytoin 100 mg q8h. The target free phenytoin level is 2 to 3 mcg/mL. Check serum levels daily.

        ii. Valproic acid: Load with 20 mg/kg (max 2,000 mg) at a rate of 3 to 6 mg/kg/min. If seizure persists, additional 20 mg/kg can be given. Maintenance dose is 30 to 60 mg/kg/d in divided doses. Serum valproic goal is 70 to 100 mcg/mL. Check levels daily.

        iii. Levetiracetam is usually loaded with 1,000 mg. Maintenance dosing is 1,000 to 1,500 mg q12. Blood levels are not monitored.

        iv. Lacosamide: Load with 400 mg. Maintenance dosing is 100 to 200 mg twice daily. Max dose is 400 mg daily. Blood levels are not monitored.

7. Refractory therapy.

    a. If seizures persist, consider continuous infusion of AEDs. The most recommended are midazolam, propofol, and pentobarbital. Dosing of continuous infusion of AEDs should be titrated to cessation of electrographic seizures or burst suppression.

    b. A period of 24 to 48 hours of electrographic seizure control is recommended prior to slow withdrawal of continuous infusion of AEDs. It is recommended that EEG findings, not serum drug levels, guide therapy.

        i. Midazolam infusion: Load with 0.2 mg/kg, at an infusion rate of 2 mg/min. Begin continuous infusion: 0.05 to 2 mg/kg/hr. For breakthrough seizures: Give 0.1 to 0.2 mg/kg bolus and increase infusion by 0.05 to 0.1 mg/kg/hr every 3 to 4 hours.

        ii. Propofol infusion: Load with 1 to 2 mg/kg, infused over 1 minute. Begin continuous infusion at 20 to 200 mcg/kg/min. Use caution when administering high doses (>80 mcg/kg/min) for extended periods of time (>48 hours) to avert risk of propofol infusion syndrome. For breakthrough seizures: Increase infusion rate by 5 to 10 mcg/kg/min every 5 minutes until seizure cessation.

        iii. Pentobarbital infusion: Load with 3 to 5 mg/kg IVPB over 10 to 30 minutes. Begin continuous infusion at 0.5 to 5 mg/kg/hr. For breakthrough seizures: Titrate 1 mg/kg/hr every 10 minutes to continuous EEG of 4 to 6 bursts/minute.

Follow-Up

A. Patients will need to follow-up with an epileptologist to monitor and control the antiepileptic medications that will be required.

Consultation/Referral

A. A neurologist must be consulted on cases of SE. A neurologist with continuous EEG training and specialty training in epileptology is preferred.

B. Centers without the ability to perform or interpret continuous EEG in patients with SE or NCSE should consider rapid transfer to a higher level of care.

Special/Geriatric Considerations

A. Pregnancy: Lorazepam and fosphenytoin are recommended as initial and urgent therapy. Levetiracetam has shown to be safe in recent studies.

1. Eclampsia must be considered in patients with SE in pregnancy; delivering the fetus is the best therapy in this situation.

2. Also, magnesium sulfate is proved to be superior to AEDs in pregnant women with seizures and eclampsia.

B. Anoxic brain injury: Prognosis of SE after hypoxic or anoxic brain injury is really poor.

C. Ketamine, an NMDA receptor antagonist, has emerged as a potential treatment for refractory SE associated with autoimmune encephalitis.

Bibliography

Bleck, T. (2008). Seizures in the critically ill. In J. E. Parrillo & R. P. Dellinger (Eds.), *Critical care medicine: Principles of diagnosis and management in the adult* (3rd ed., pp. 1367–1383). Maryland Heights, MO: Mosby. doi:10.1016/b978-032304841-5.50068-6

Brophy, G. M., Bell, R., Classen, J., Alldredge, B., Bleck, T., Glauser, T., & Vespa, P. (2012). Guidelines for the evaluation and management of status epilepticus. *Neurocritical Care, 17,* 3–23. doi:10.1007/s12028-012-9695-z

Claassen, J., & Hirsch, L. J. (2009). Status epilepticus. In J. Frontera (Ed.), *Decision making in neurocritical care* (1st ed., Vol. 1, pp. 63–75). New York, NY: Thieme Medical.

Gilmore, R. L., Cibula, J. E., Eisenschenk, S., & Roper, S. N. (2013). Seizures. In J. Layon, A. Gabrielli, & W. Friedman (Eds.), *Textbook of neurointensive care* (2nd ed., Vol. 1, pp. 799–811). New York, NY: Springer Publishing Company.

Transient Ischemia Attack

Catherine Harris

Definition

A. Temporary blockage of blood flow to the brain (<24 hours) that does not result in permanent damage; often referred to as a "mini-stroke."
B. Majority of transient ischemia attacks (TIAs): Complete resolution in less than 10 minutes.

Incidence

A. It is estimated that up to 500,000 people a year have a TIA in the United States.
B. Up to 30% of people who report a TIA have a stroke within 5 years.
C. The incidence of a cerebrovascular accident (CVA) has been reported as high as 11% within 7 days.

Pathogenesis

A. A TIA occurs when there is blockage of blood to the brain from atherosclerosis, any type of emboli, decreased blood flow/volume to the brain, or constriction of the arteries in the brain.
B. The exact symptoms of a TIA correlate with the particular artery that is affected. The hallmark of a TIA is resolution of symptoms within 24 hours from onset.

Predisposing Factors

A. Medical factors.
　1. Hypertension.
　2. Diabetes.
　3. Hyperlipidemia.
　4. Coronary artery disease: Arrhythmias, heart defects, heart infections, or valvular disease.
　5. Peripheral artery disease.
　6. Obesity.
　7. Elevated homocysteine levels.
　8. Sickle cell disease.
B. Nonmodifiable risk factors.
　1. Family history.
　2. Age greater than 55 years.
　3. Gender (men more likely than women).
　4. Prior TIA.
　5. Race, with Hispanics and African Americans at higher risk.

C. Lifestyle factors.
　1. Cigarette smoking.
　2. Physical inactivity.
　3. Poor diet.
　4. Excessive alcohol intake.
　5. Illicit drug use.
　6. Oral contraceptive use.

Subjective Data

A. Common complaints/symptoms—the types of complaints a person would have depends on the area of the brain that is affected. In general, there are three main classifications of TIA/CVA based on circulation patterns.
　1. Anterior circulation symptoms.
　　a. Carotid artery: Contralateral motor and sensory loss to arm/leg.
　　b. Anterior cerebral artery: Confusion, personality changes, motor, or sensory loss in leg.
　　c. Middle cerebral artery (majority of TIAs/CVAs): Face asymmetry, motor or sensory loss in arm, slurred speech, or aphasia.
　2. Posterior circulation symptoms.
　　a. Contralateral motor or sensory loss.
　　b. Ipsilateral visual field loss.
　　c. Cortical blindness.
　　d. Dysarthria.
　　e. Dysphagia.
　　f. Diplopia.
　　g. Quadriparesis.
　3. Vertebrobasilar circulation symptoms.
　　a. Confusion.
　　b. Slurred speech.
　　c. Blurry vision or blindness.
　　d. Weakness of both arms or legs.
　　e. Difficulty walking, ataxia.
　　f. Paresthesias.
B. Common/typical scenario—a typical event is described as happening all of the sudden. One moment the person is fine, the next moment the symptoms occur. In the majority of the cases, the symptoms resolve within 10 minutes and the person is back to his or her previous self.
C. Family and social history.
　1. A family history of stroke can raise the risk of stroke, especially if before the age of 65.
　2. Smoking, physical inactivity, alcoholism, illicit drug use, and poor diet are all important factors to document.
D. Review of systems—typically all symptoms will have resolved by the time of the interview, but it is important to document which systems were affected.
　1. Visual fields—blurry vision, double vision, loss of vision, and/or sense of a curtain being pulled down over one eye (amaurosis fugax).
　2. Language—slurred speech, difficulty speaking, inability to find words, and/or inability to understand others.
　3. Extremities—weakness, numbness, tingling, and/or strange sensations.

Physical Examination

A. Cranial nerve testing—smile, stick out tongue, raise eyebrows, extraocular movements, and/or visual fields.
B. Motor strength.
C. Sensory testing.
D. Gait and posture—walking heel to toe and/or finger to nose test.

Diagnostic Tests

A. CT head.
B. MRI brain within 24 hours.
C. Carotid Doppler—to assess for carotid disease.
D. ECG—to assess for atrial fibrillation.
E. Transthoracic echocardiogram (TTE) to rule out any cardioembolic source.
F. Lab tests—glucose, chemistry profile, lipid panel.
　1. Consider hypercoagulable workup if younger than 40 years of age or based on history.
　2. Consider alcohol levels based on history.

Differential Diagnosis

A. Ischemic stroke.
B. Hemorrhagic stroke.
C. Migraine.
D. Bell's palsy.
E. Seizure.

F. Hypoglycemic/hyperglycemia episode.
G. Sepsis.
H. Vertigo.
I. Neuromuscular or neurodegenerative disease.
J. Brain tumor.
K. Meningitis.
L. Syncope.

Evaluation and Management Plan

A. General plan.
   1. Obtain results from diagnostic tests.
   2. Prevent further stroke from modification of risk factors.
   3. Manage blood pressure.
   4. Initiate lipid control.
   5. Maximize blood glucose control.
B. Patient/family teaching points.
   1. Assess family baseline understanding of TIAs/CVAs.
   2. Educate on risk factor modification.
   3. Educate on the role of diet/exercise in preventing future TIAs/CVAs.
   4. Educate on role of pharmacotherapy and adverse effects.
   5. Provide pamphlets and educational materials.
   6. Introduce smoking cessation plan if indicated.
   7. Introduce weight loss program if indicated.
C. Pharmacotherapy.
   1. Antiplatelet drugs—low dose aspirin or clopidogrel should be initiated as soon as intracranial hemorrhage has been ruled out.
      a. Aspirin 81 to 325 mg.
      b. Clopidogrel.
   2. Anticoagulants—prescribed only if there is an increased cardioembolic risk as determined by the CHA$_2$DS$_2$-VAS$_c$ Score (see Table 6.4).
   3. Thrombolytics—not indicated if there is resolution of symptoms.
D. Surgical intervention.
   1. Carotid endarterectomy if person is symptomatic with severe carotid stenosis (70%–99% blockage).
E. Discharge instructions.
   1. Warning signs of stroke.
   2. What to do if person suspects a stroke: Call 911.
   3. Possible Medic Alert bracelet if taking a blood thinner.

Follow-Up

A. Follow-up with primary care provider within 2 weeks.

Consultation/Referral

A. Refer all patients to neurology team.

TABLE 6.4 CHA$_2$DS$_2$-VAS$_c$ Score Criteria

Condition	No. of Points
Congestive heart failure	1
Hypertension	1
Age ≥75 y	2
Diabetes mellitus	1
CVA/TIA/Thromboembolic event	2
Vascular disease (prior MI, peripheral artery disease, aortic plaque)	1
Age 65–74	1
Female	1

Note: 0 points: No need for antiplatelet or anticoagulants; 1 point: None OR aspirin OR anticoagulant, depending on situation; ≥2 points: Start anticoagulant.

CVA, cerebrovascular accident; MI, myocardial infarction; TIA, transient ischemic attack.

Source: Lip, G. Y., & Halperin, J. L. (2010, June). Improving stroke risk stratification in atrial fibrillation. *American Journal of Medicine, 123*(6), 484–488. doi:10.1016/j.amjmed.2009.12.013

Special/Geriatric Considerations

A. Hypercoagulopathy can occur secondary to cancer, pregnancy, and in sickle cell disease. Patients under the age of 40 who present with TIA should undergo a hypercoagulable workup.

Bibliography

Easton, J. D., Saver, J. L., Albers, G. W., Alberts, M. J., Chaturvedi, S., Feldmann, E., . . . Sacco, R. L. (2009). Definition and evaluation of transient ischemic attack: A scientific statement for healthcare professionals from the American Heart Association/American Stroke Association Stroke Council, Council on Cardiovascular Surgery and Anesthesia: Council on Cardiovascular Radiology and Intervention; Council on Cardiovascular Nursing; and the Interdisciplinary Council on Peripheral Vascular Disease, The American Academy of Neurology affirms the value of this statement as an educational tool for neurologist. *Stroke, 40,* 2276–2293. doi:10.1161/STROKEAHA.108.192218

Giles, M. F., & Rothwell, P. M. (2007). Risk of stroke early after transient ischemic attack: A systematic review and meta-analysis. *Lancet Neurology, 6*(12), 1063–1072. doi:10.1016/S1474-4422(07)70274-0

Johnston, S. C. (2002). Transient ischemic attack. *New England Journal of Medicine, 347,* 1687–1692. doi:10.1056/NEJMcp020891

Kernan, W. N., Ovbiagele, B., Black, H. R., Bravata, D. M., Chimowitz, M. I., Ezekowitz, M. D., . . . Wilson, J. A. (2014). Guidelines for the prevention of stroke in patients with stroke and transient ischemic attack: A guideline for healthcare professionals from the American Heart Association/American Stroke Association. *Stroke, 45,* 2160. doi:10.1161/STR.0000000000000024

Lip, G. Y., & Halperin, J. L. (2010, June). Improving stroke risk stratification in atrial fibrillation. *American Journal of Medicine, 123*(6), 484–488. doi:10.1016/j.amjmed.2009.12.013

7 Targeted Temperature Management Guidelines

Sarah L. Livesay, Kiffon M. Keigher, Monique Lambert, Christina Shin, and Danielle Zielinski

Fever Management

Sarah L. Livesay, Kiffon M. Keigher, Monique Lambert, Christina Shin, and Danielle Zielinski

Definition

A. Therapeutic hypothermia, also called targeted temperature management (TTM), consists of intervention(s) for the management of fever and includes the use of antipyretic medications, surface cooling, and intravascular devices to reduce temperature.

B. Fever is defined by at least one core temperature measurement of ≥38.3°C on two consecutive days.

C. High fever is defined by one or more measurement of core temperature of ≥39.5°C.

D. Fevers of acute brain injury (either traumatic or vascular in nature) are independently associated with worse outcomes, which are associated with temperatures greater than 37.3°C in a number of studies.

   1. Fever control is important because it contributes to cerebral ischemia and possible worsening of cerebral edema, leads to increased intracranial pressures, and results in decreased levels of consciousness.

Incidence

A. The incidence of fever with traumatic brain injury (TBI) is difficult to quantify because targeted therapies are often initiated within hours of onset. However, it is estimated that there are approximately 1.4 million cases of TBI in the United States annually.

B. Patients with subarachnoid hemorrhage (SAH) have been shown to have a high incidence of fever development; SAH occurs in as many as 72% of patients diagnosed with SAH.

C. Patients with intracranial hemorrhage (ICH) have up to a 53% risk of fever development in some studies, and this risk increases to as much as 83% with patients who also have intraventricular hemorrhage (IVH).

Pathogenesis

A. Noninfectious, or central, fever is the physiological loss of ability to autoregulate body temperature. In ICUs, fever with a noninfectious source has been shown to have an earlier onset (within 72 hours of admission) than fever with an infectious source.

B. Infectious fevers occur in response to infection. Fever is associated with sepsis in up to 74% of hospitalized patients and as many as 90% of those with severe sepsis.

C. Heat shock proteins are induced by fever. These are critical for anti-inflammatory effects and cellular survival during stress.

D. Patients with neurological injury are at risk for both infectious and noninfectious fevers.

Predisposing Factors

A. Infectious processes.
   1. Bacterial.
      a. Urinary tract infection.
      b. Upper respiratory infection.
         i. Pneumonia.
         ii. Bronchitis.
         iii. Sinusitis.
      c. Central line infection.
      d. Bloodstream infection.
      e. Cerebrospinal fluid (CSF) infection.
         i. Ventriculitis.
         ii. Meningitis.
      f. Cellulitis.
      g. *Clostridium difficile* enteritis.
   2. Fungal.
   3. Viral.
      a. Influenza.
      b. Meningitis.
      c. Shingles.
      d. HIV/AIDS.
      e. Mumps/measles/rubella.
      f. Infectious mononucleosis.
      g. Herpes.

B. Surgical incisions, which should be monitored for signs and symptoms of infection.

C. Invasive lines and devices, which may predispose patients to infection.
   1. Foley catheters.
   2. Endotracheal tubes/tracheostomies.
   3. External ventricular drains/ventriculoperitoneal shunts/lumbar drains.
   4. Gastrostomy tubes.
   5. Central lines, arterial lines, pulmonary artery catheters, peripherally inserted central catheters, intravenous lines.

D. Some medications.
   1. Steroids.
   2. Antibiotics.
   3. Serotonergic drugs, which may lead to serotonin syndromes.
   4. Anesthetics, specifically volatile anesthetic agents, which are associated with malignant hyperthermia.
   5. Anticholinergic agents.
   6. Sympathomimetic agents.

E. Deep vein thrombosis (DVT).

F. Blood transfusion reactions.

G. Mechanical ventilation, which puts patients at increased risk for developing ventilator-associated infections.
H. Chronic medical illnesses, which may result in compromised immune systems and/or autoimmune disorders.

Subjective Data

A. Common complaints/symptoms.

> Patients with brain injuries may not be alert enough to reliably provide subjective complaints. Spinal cord injured patients may not be able to describe pain in detail due to sensory or thermoregulatory loss.

    1. Warm or overheated feeling.
    2. Chills.
    3. Generalized body aches.
    4. Sweating.
    5. Palpitations or fluttering of heart.
    6. Headache.
B. Other signs and symptoms.
    1. Decreased level of consciousness or altered mental status.
    2. Tachycardia.
    3. Tachypnea.
    4. Hypotension or hypertension.
    5. Increased intracranial pressure.
    6. Vasospasm in patients with SAH as evidenced by trending transcranial Doppler velocities and/or digital subtraction angiography (DSA), computed tomography angiogram (CTA), or magnetic resonance angiography (MRA) imaging.
    7. Positive cultures: Blood, CSF, pleural fluid, urine.
    8. Abnormal lab results: Elevated white blood cell (WBC) count, erythrocyte sedimentation rate (ESR), C-reactive protein (CRP).
C. Review of systems.
    1. Assess patient for fever or symptoms suggesting fever prior to hospital admission.
    2. Inquire about any recent or current known infections, cold/influenza symptoms, or abnormal rashes/skin lesions.
    3. Evaluate for any chills, shivering, or other symptoms suggestive of fever.
    4. Assess for loss of appetite, weight loss, dehydration, or nausea or vomiting or other gastrointestinal (GI) upset.

Physical Examination

A. Check blood pressure, pulse, respirations, and temperature.
    1. Temperature monitoring methods are essential in order to obtain accurate and reliable measurements. Continuous monitoring is ideal, but if this is not possible, patients' temperatures should be checked on an hourly basis using core methods.
        a. The most accurate source of core temperature monitoring is using a pulmonary artery catheter.
        b. Other core methods of temperature monitoring include intravesicular (bladder), esophageal, and rectal.
        c. Peripheral methods of temperature monitoring include tympanic membrane, axillary, and oral.
B. Look for any lines or drains that may be a nidus for infection.
    1. Urinary Foley catheter.
    2. Central venous catheters, arterial lines.
    3. Lumbar drain, ventricular drain.

    4. Any other surgical lines or drains.
    5. Lines for mechanical ventilation.
C. Examine skin thoroughly.
    1. Check for cellulitis.
    2. Recent surgical wounds.
    3. Any skin breakdown.
D. Auscultate heart and lungs.
    1. Listen for murmurs or consolidation.
E. Perform a neurological exam as appropriate for the patient's diagnosis.

Diagnostic Tests

A. All tests and imaging should be directed at ruling out infectious causes of fever as well as venous thromboembolism, transfusion reaction, drug fever, adrenal insufficiency, thyroid storm, and any other noninfectious, noncentral etiologies. Tests should be ordered with discretion and with the individual patient in mind.
B. Laboratory tests.
    1. Complete blood count with differential.
        a. Acute neurological injury can cause a rise in inflammatory markers, similar to an infectious response. The percentage of neutrophils, however, is likely higher in patients with infectious fever.
    2. Basic metabolic panel.
    3. Liver function tests and bilirubin.
    4. Amylase and lipase.
    5. ESR/CRP.
    6. Cortisol.
    7. Thyroid-stimulating hormone (TSH), triiodothyronine (T3), and thyroxine (T4).
    8. Procalcitonin.
C. Microbiology.
    1. HIV antibody.
    2. Heterophile antibody.
    3. Hepatitis serologies.
    4. Urine culture.
    5. Blood culture.
    6. CSF culture.
    7. Tuberculin skin test.
D. Imaging.
    1. Chest radiograph.
    2. CT of chest and abdomen.
    3. Ultrasonography.

Evaluation and Management Plan

A. If the fever is caused by an infectious source, source control is the priority, which involves removing any related lines or drains as well as choosing an effective antimicrobial agent.
B. If the fever is caused by a noninfectious, noncentral condition, it will need to be addressed accordingly. Possible causes are:
    1. Venous thromboembolism.
    2. Transfusion reaction.
    3. Drug fever.
    4. Adrenal insufficiency.
    5. Thyroid storm.
C. If other etiologies of fever have been ruled out and the most likely cause of a patient's fever is central and due to neurological injury, the following treatments can be used.
    1. Pharmacologic methods.
        a. Antipyretic agents: Acetaminophen, aspirin, or nonsteroidal anti-inflammatory drugs (NSAIDs).
            i. These agents are likely to be ineffective in brain-injured patients with impaired temperature regulatory mechanisms.

ii. Acetaminophen is the preferred agent because aspirin and NSAIDs have undesirable side effects such as platelet dysfunction and GI upset.
  b. Steroids: Not used because of multiple side effects.
2. External cooling.
  a. Evaporation.
    i. Water or alcohol sponge baths.
  b. Conduction.
    i. Ice packs.
    ii. Immersion in cold water.
    iii. Water-circulating cooling blankets or pads. Improved accuracy with newer technology provides constant monitoring of temperature and adjustment of circulating water to maintain desired body temperature.
  c. Convection.
    i. Fans.
    ii. Ambient air temperature control.
    iii. Air-circulating cooling blankets.
  d. Radiation.
    i. Skin exposure.
3. Invasive cooling.
  a. Cold saline boluses.
  b. Intravascular catheters.
D. Complications.

Many serious complications arise from induction of hypothermia as opposed to normothermia in a patient. Most of these adverse effects are not problematic until core body temperatures are 35°C or lower. However, a number of complications may occur when attempting maintenance of normal temperatures.

1. Hepatic and renal toxicity.
2. Catheter-related thrombosis and infection.
3. Skin breakdown.
  a. Surface cooling may predispose to skin lesions due to its intrinsic mechanism of action via contact with skin.
  b. This risk may be low depending on the type of material used, the temperature of the material, and the length of time of intense cooling.
  c. Skin should be monitored for blistering, bruising, or sign of breakdown from prolonged cold exposure.
  d. Circulating water temperature should be monitored continuously, and prolonged periods of cold circulating water should be avoided.
4. Subsequent infections.
5. Shivering.
  a. The metabolic effects of shivering can be considerable, resulting from increased energy expenditure.
  b. Shivering can produce heat, which is counterproductive.
  c. The implications and management of shivering are extensive (see the following section "Shivering During Targeted Temperature Management").

Follow-Up

A. There are no special follow-up needs for central fevers, because they are generally related to the initial neurological insult.
B. Follow-up and postdischarge monitoring is related to the patient's admission diagnosis as well as new issues that may have occurred during hospitalization.

Consultation/Referral

A. Inpatient consults are relevant to the diagnosis of each patient.
B. Examples of consults for noncentral fevers.
1. Infectious disease.
2. Wound/ostomy.
3. Hematology.
4. Endocrinology.
5. Pharmacy.
6. Others related to fever etiology.
C. Pastoral care.

Special/Geriatric Considerations

A. Geriatric individuals often have unique presentations and require special considerations when gathering a history and physical.
B. Treatment methods may also vary slightly due to multiple comorbidities and less reserve.
1. The elderly are more prone to ICU delirium and mental status changes while hospitalized, making history and physical examination challenging at times.
2. Skin breakdown is a regular concern in geriatric patients, because mobility and skin caliber are lower in these individuals, particularly with external cooling methods.
3. Geriatric patients may not always mount a febrile response to infection. They can become hypothermic in an infected state.
4. The effectiveness of different cooling methods increase with advanced age secondary to slower counterregulatory response to small temperature changes, decreased metabolism, decreased vascular response (and as a result, vasoconstriction), and often a lower body mass index (BMI).
5. Medications may need to be adjusted more frequently in the elderly, whether because of hepatic/renal function or low BMI.

Bibliography

Aiyagari, V., & Diringer, M. N. (2007). Fever control and its impact on outcomes: What is the evidence? *Journal of the Neurological Sciences, 261*(1), 39–46. doi:10.1016/j.jns.2007.04.030

Badjatia, N. (2009). Hyperthermia and fever control in brain injury. *Critical Care Medicine, 37*(37), S250–S257. doi:10.1097/ccm.0b013e3181aa5e8d

Bor, D. H. (2018). Approach to the adult with fever of unknown origin. In A. Bloom (Ed.), *UpToDate*. Retrieved from https://www.uptodate.com/contents/approach-to-the-adult-with-fever-of-unknown-origin

Commichau, C., Scarmeas, N., & Mayer, S. A. (2003). Risk factors for fever in the neurologic intensive care unit. *Neurology, 60*(5), 837–841. doi:10.1212/01.WNL.0000047344.28843.EB

Fernandez, A., Schmidt, J. M., Claassen, J., Pavlicova, M., Huddleston, D., Kreiter, K. T., & Mayer, S. A. (2007). Fever after subarachnoid hemorrhage: Risk factors and impact on outcome. *Neurology, 68*(13), 1013–1019. doi:10.1212/01.wnl.0000258543.45879.f5

Geri, G., Champigneulle, B., Bougouin, W., Arnaout, M., & Cariou, A. (2015). Common physiological response during TTM. *BMC Emergency Medicine, 15*(Suppl. 1), A14. doi:10.1186/1471-227X-15-S1-A14

Hocker, S. E., Tian, L., Li, G., Steckelberg, J. M., Mandrekar, J. N., & Rabinstein, A. A. (2013). Indicators of central fever in the neurologic intensive care unit. *JAMA Neurology, 70*(12), 1499–1504. doi:10.1001/jamaneurol.2013.4354

Hossmann, K.-A. (2012). The two pathophysiologies of focal brain ischemia: Implications for translational stroke research. *Journal of Cerebral Blood Flow & Metabolism, 32*(7), 1310–1316. doi:10.1038/jcbfm.2011.186

Laupland, K. B. (2009). Fever in the critically ill medical patient. *Critical Care Medicine, 37*(7), S273–S278. doi:10.1097/CCM.0b013e3181aa6117

Laupland, K. B., Shahpori, R., Kirkpatrick, A. W., Ross, T., Gregson, D. B., & Stelfox, H. T. (2008). Occurrence and outcome of fever in critically ill adults. *Critical Care Medicine, 36*(5), 1531–1535. doi:10.1097/CCM. 0b013e318170efd3

Lopez, G. A. (2016). Temperature management in the neurointensive care unit. *Current Treatment Options in Neurology, 18*(3), 12. doi:10.1007/s11940-016-0393-6

Luscombe, M., & Andrzejowski, J. C. (2006). Clinical applications of induced hyperthermia. *Continuing Education in Anesthesia, Critical Care & Pain, 6,* 23–27. Retrieved from https://academic.oup.com/bjaed/article/6/1/23/347011/Clinical-applications-of-induced-hypothermia

MacLaren, G., & Spelman, D. (2018). Fever in the intensive care unit. In G. Finlay (Ed.), *UpToDate.* Retrieved from https://www.uptodate.com/contents/fever-in-the-intensive-care-unit

McIntyre, L. A., Fergusson, D. A., Hébert, P. C., Moher, D., & Hutchison, J. S. (2003). Prolonged therapeutic hypothermia after traumatic brain injury in adults: A systematic review. *Journal of the American Medical Association, 289*(22), 2992–2999. doi:10.1001/jama.289.22.2992

McKinley, W., McNamee, S., Meade, M., Kandra, K., & Abdul, N. (2006). Incidence, etiology, and risk factors for fever following acute spinal cord injury. *The Journal of Spinal Cord Medicine, 29*(5), 501–506. doi:10. 1080/10790268.2006.11753899

Mrozek, S., Vardon, F., & Geeraerts, T. (2012). Brain temperature: Physiology and pathophysiology after brain injury. *Anesthesiology Research and Practice, 2012,* 13. doi:10.1155/2012/989487

O'Grady, N. P., Barie, P. S., Bartlett, J. G., Bleck, T., Carroll, K., Kalil, A. C., & Masur, H. (2008). Guidelines for evaluation of new fever in critically ill adult patients: 2008 update from the American College of Critical Care Medicine and the Infectious Diseases Society of America. *Critical Care Medicine, 36*(4), 1330–1349. doi:10.1097/CCM. 0b013e318169eda9

Porat, R., & Dinarello, C. A. (2018). Pathophysiology and treatment of fever in adults. In A. Bloom (Ed.), *UpToDate.* Retrieved from https://www.uptodate.com/contents/pathophysiology-and-treatment-of-fever-in-adults

Rabinstein, A. A., & Sandhu, K. (2007). Non-infectious fever in the neurological intensive care unit: Incidence, causes and predictors. *Journal of Neurology, Neurosurgery & Psychiatry, 78*(11), 1278–1280. doi:10.1136/jnnp.2006.112730

Ryan, M., & Levy, M. M. (2003). Clinical review: Fever in intensive care unit patients. *Critical Care, 7*(3), 221. doi:10.1186/cc1879

Scaravilli, V., Tinchero, G., & Citerio, G. (2011). Fever management in SAH. *Neurocritical Care, 15,* 287. doi:10.1007/s12028-011-9588-6

Schwarz, S., Häfner, K., Aschoff, A., & Schwab, S. (2000). Incidence and prognostic significance of fever following intracerebral hemorrhage. *Neurology, 54*(2), 354–361. doi:10.1212/WNL.54.2.354

Walter, E. J., Hanna-Jumma, S., Carraretto, M., & Forni, L. (2016). The pathophysiological basis and consequences of fever. *Critical Care, 20*(1), 200. doi:10.1186/s13054-016-1375-5

Yenari, M. A., & Hemmen, T. M. (2010). Therapeutic hypothermia for brain ischemia. *Stroke, 41*(10 Suppl. 1), S72–S74. doi:10.1161/STROKEAHA.110.595371

Hypothermia or Targeted Temperature Management After Cardiac Arrest

Definition

A. Hypothermia after cardiac arrest is the application of therapeutic cooling of the body for a prescribed period of time after cardiac arrest.

Incidence

A. Approximately 326,000 people in the United States experienced an out-of-hospital cardiac arrest in 2011, and approximately 11% of those who experienced a cardiac arrest survived to hospital discharge.

B. Approximately 209,000 people experienced an in-hospital cardiac arrest.

C. Survival statistics after in-hospital cardiac arrest are generally lower than out-of-hospital cardiac arrest.

Pathogenesis

A. Neuronal injury occurs as a consequence of the hypoxia-ischemia and reperfusion that occurs with cardiac arrest and return of circulation. When this cascade of injury results in altered consciousness or coma, it's often referred to as hypoxic-ischemic encephalopathy (HIE). However, there are multiple causes of HIE in addition to cardiac arrest.

B. Hypothermia or targeted temperature management (TTM) starts in the hours after return of spontaneous circulation (ROSC) decreases cerebral metabolism, interrupting multiple inflammatory pathways, and suppressing nitric oxide formation and suppressing programmed cell death.

Predisposing Factors

A. Coronary artery disease and other comorbid illnesses (such as diabetes, chronic kidney disease).

Subjective Data

A. The patient's history, functional status, and symptoms at the time of arrest may help determine the arrest etiology and assess if the patient or decision maker would want TTM as a postarrest intervention.

B. Criteria for TTM.

  1. Initial cardiac rhythm at time of arrest.

    a. TTM is indicated for patients who do not awaken after successful resuscitation with ROSC after an arrest with an initial rhythm of ventricular fibrillation (VF) or pulseless ventricular tachycardia (VT).

    b. While the strongest evidence supports TTM in patients with VT or VF initial rhythm, the therapy may be considered for patients with asystole or pulseless electrical activity (PEA) initial rhythms.

C. Common complaints/symptoms.

  1. Patients with HIE demonstrate impaired neurological function and should receive a complete neurological examination, including assessment of level of consciousness, brainstem function, motor function, respiratory pattern, and the presence of cranial nerve deficits. Impaired neurological function includes decreased level of arousal, inappropriate response to stimuli such as withdrawing from pain or decorticate or decerebrate posturing, and abnormal cranial nerve responses.

D. Other signs and symptoms.

  1. Other signs and symptoms depend on the cause of cardiac arrest and the timing from the arrest to ROSC, in addition to the comorbidities of individual patients.

Physical Examination

A. Check vital signs and perform telemetry monitoring.

B. Monitor for hypotension with possible compensatory tachycardia and signs of heart failure, including adventitious lung sounds, peripheral edema, or jugular venous distension.

C. Temperature.

D. Perfusion.

  1. Peripheral pulses may be weak, and there may be poor capillary refill.

E. Oxygenation status on ventilator, O_2 saturation.

F. Cardiac examination: Murmurs, rubs, or gallops, S4.

  1. New murmur may suggest papillary muscle dysfunction or septal rupture.

G. Neurological examination: Assessment of level of consciousness, brainstem function, motor function, respiratory pattern, and the presence of cranial nerve deficits.

Diagnostic Tests

A. Routine diagnostic tests include:

  1. EKG.

2. Full range of blood tests, including complete metabolic panel, complete blood count, cardiac enzymes, arterial blood gas, coagulation studies, and liver function tests.

    a. Evaluate for infection, bleeding risk, oxygenation status, and cardiac enzyme elevation.

3. Chest x-ray.

    a. Evaluate for pulmonary edema.

4. Transthoracic echocardiogram.

    a. May help identify the etiology of cardiac arrest or determine if urgent surgical repair is needed (e.g., aortic dissection, papillary muscle rupture, septal rupture, cardiac tamponade, wall rupture).

B. Patients must be assessed to determine if the benefit of TTM outweighs the risk. Generally speaking, patients are the best candidates for TTM if they meet the following criteria.

    1. Patient is unconscious, generally defined as a Glasgow Coma Score less than 8.

    2. Cardiac arrest is cardiac in origin.

        a. Patient must achieve ROSC after basic or advanced life support interventions.

        b. Cardiac arrest and resuscitation efforts were not prolonged (generally <30–50 minutes in clinical trials).

        c. As mentioned, the best evidence supports TTM in patients with an initial cardiac rhythm of VT or VF, which is usually cardiac in origin. TTM may be considered in other arrest etiologies as well. However, the outcome improvement is not as robust.

    3. Patients with any of the following conditions were not included in clinical trials and the risk of TTM may outweigh the benefit.

        a. Pregnancy.

        b. Intracranial hemorrhage or stroke.

        c. Bleeding diathesis.

        d. Active infection: Greater than 6 hours since ROSC.

        e. Systolic blood pressure (SBP) less than 80 mmHg despite fluid resuscitation, vasopressor agents, or advanced cardiac interventions (e.g., intra-aortic balloon pump).

Evaluation and Management Plan

A. General goal: To evaluate patient for TTM and initiate as quickly as possible after ROSC.

    1. Target temperature.

        a. Initial trials in hypothermia after cardiac arrest established a target temperature of 33°C for 24 hours. A recent trial compared 33°C to 36°C and found there was no difference in outcomes between the two temperatures. Therefore, either temperature may be used as the target for TTM (Nielsen et al., 2013).

        b. Certain patient criteria may cause the clinician to choose one temperature over another. For example, a higher temperature may be preferred in patients with bleeding or infection risk whereas a lower temperature may be helpful for patients with seizures or cerebral edema.

B. Hemodynamic goals.

    1. Avoid hypotension (SBP <90 mmHg, mean arterial pressure [MAP] <65 mmHg). Most published protocols titrate vasopressors to a MAP greater than 65 mmHg.

    2. Monitor arterial oxygen saturation, venous oxygen saturation, and urine output to determine end organ perfusion and titrate therapies accordingly.

C. Stages of TTM.

    1. Generally divided into three stages: Induction, maintenance, and rewarming.

        a. Induction.

            i. Induction of TTM should begin as quickly as possible after the patient is determined to be a candidate for therapy.

            ii. A smooth and well-coordinated induction includes coordination of medication administration, diagnostic tests, and application of the cooling device aimed at rapid reduction of temperature to goal.

        b. Maintenance at target temperature for 24 hours.

        c. Rewarming.

            i. After 24 hours at the target temperature, rewarming is started. Rewarming should occur slowly, particularly for patients who are cooled to 33°C, at a rate no faster than 0.1°C to 0.3°C.

            ii. Quick rewarming may precipitate rebound cerebral edema and elevated intracranial pressure, as well as other systemic complications.

    2. Post-rewarming, a fourth stage: Often discussed related to ongoing fever prevention and prognostication.

        a. After the patient returns to normal body temperature, interventions to prevent fever should be continued.

        b. Prognostication post-TTM may take additional time compared to patients after cardiac arrest who do not receive TTM.

    3. Cooling techniques.

        a. TTM is best implemented with advanced temperature technology.

        b. Cooling blankets and intravascular devices are available. There are benefits and drawbacks to each type of technology. Technology should be reviewed for accuracy and degree of temperature control.

            i. Surface cooling is easily applied by the nursing staff, leading to quick induction. Complications may include skin burns if the water temperature is allowed to be very cold for prolonged periods.

            ii. Intravascular cooling may decrease the occurrence of shivering. The intravascular line must be placed by a qualified practitioner, and this must be considered in the induction workflow. Intravascular catheters are associated with higher rates of deep venous thrombosis (DVT).

D. Complications.

    1. Cardiac.

        a. Bradycardia is often seen in hypothermia, usually at colder temperatures compared to warmer ones. Cardiac intervals (PR, QRS, QTc) can lengthen. This is generally well tolerated by the patient and resolves once rewarming has occurred.

        b. Central venous pressure (CVP) may increase due to vasoconstriction from cold temperatures.

    2. Pulmonary.

        a. Patients are at high risk for pulmonary edema following cardiac arrest, particularly if they received fluid for resuscitation or to induce TTM. Treatment should be individualized and commonly involves diuretics and oxygen support. Patients undergoing TTM at a lower temperature often experience a cold diuresis and will mobilize the excess fluid.

        b. During TTM, there is an increased solubility of O_2 and CO_2, which leads to a decrease in PaO_2 and

$PaCO_2$ and a left shift of the oxygen–hemoglobin dissociation curve. Ventilators may require frequent setting changes during induction of cooling. Arterial blood gas values should be corrected for temperature.

c. Normocarbia (end-tidal CO_2 of 30–40 mmHg or $PaCO_2$ of 35–45 mmHg) is a reasonable goal during TTM.

3. Endocrine.

a. In critically ill patients, tight control of low normal serum glucose levels is associated with increased frequency of hypoglycemic episodes. No one range is recommended for postcardiac arrest patients in guidelines. It is reasonable to avoid wide fluctuations in serum glucose.

b. At lower body temperature, there is a decreased production of insulin by the pancreas and decreased insulin sensitivity, resulting in higher exogenous insulin needs during hypothermia at lower target temperatures.

c. Hyperglycemia during HIE is associated with worse outcomes and should be avoided.

d. Increased lactate and ketone levels may be noted in blood or urine samples drawn during TTM to lower target temperatures.

4. Hypokalemia, hyperkalemia, and electrolyte imbalances.

a. As body temperature drops, serum potassium moves intracellularly, resulting in a serum hypokalemia that must be monitored with frequent lab checks and potassium supplementation. However, when the body rewarms, intracellular potassium then shifts extracellularly. Potassium replacement should be less aggressive toward the end of the maintenance period and during rewarming. Rewarming should be slow and controlled to minimize excessive potassium shifts.

b. Fluctuations in additional electrolytes such as calcium and magnesium may be seen and should be frequently monitored during TTM.

5. Neurological.

a. Seizures are estimated to occur in 12% to 22% of patients who are comatose after cardiac arrest. Clinical signs of seizures may be obscured by coma or sedatives and paralytics administered during TTM. Therefore, seizure activity may be subclinical and the only evidence on EEG monitoring.

b. The available evidence does not support prophylactic treatment and no specific antiseizure medication is identified as superior in this setting. It is reasonable to undergo frequent or continuous EEG monitoring in patients during TTM to identify subclinical seizures or status epilepticus.

6. Renal.

a. During TTM, particularly targeting a lower temperature, patients often experience a *cold diuresis*, or increased urine output during the induction period. This results as hypothermia increases venous return secondary to venous constriction. This, combined with an increase in atrial natriuretic peptide (ANP), decreased antidiuretic hormone (ADH), and tubular dysfunction from the cardiac arrest, may lead to large volume diuresis.

b. If uncorrected, this may lead to hypovolemia and hemoconcentration.

7. Hepatic and gastrointestinal.

a. The cardiac arrest and reperfusion of ROSC often results in decreased hepatic clearance, decreased hepatic blood flow, and decreased speed of enzymatic reactions. This may result in an increased amount of plasma drug levels and effects. This must be considered because many patients are on continuous vasopressors and receiving sedatives and analgesics during TTM.

b. During TTM, the gastrointestinal system demonstrates decreased motility and delayed gastric emptying. Patients may be at risk for developing gastric stress ulcers and should receive prophylaxis as indicated.

c. Postcardiac arrest, liver function testing should be monitored, and increased levels of amylase may occur even without acute pancreatitis. Patients may have elevated liver enzymes, and these should be monitored during TTM and therapy adjusted as necessary.

8. Hematological.

a. TTM results in platelet and neutrophil inhibition, particularly at lower target temperatures and longer duration. Patients are at risk for bleeding and infection.

b. In addition to neutrophil dysfunction, patients are at risk for infection as vasoconstriction may lead to decreased white blood cell (WBC) migration to the site of infection and a decreased inflammatory response.

E. Shivering during TTM.

1. Definition.

a. Shivering is an involuntary, rhythmic tremor that consists of oscillatory movements of various skeletal muscle groups. The act of shivering is both an anticipated consequence as well as an adverse effect of therapeutic hypothermia.

b. Shivering is usually greatest at temperatures between 34°C and 36°C.

2. Pathogenesis.

a. Core temperature is tightly regulated within the range of 36°C to 37°C. In healthy humans, peripheral vasoconstriction is triggered at 36.5°C and shivering typically starts at 35.5°C.

b. In patients with brain injury, peripheral vasoconstriction and shivering thresholds are often higher; thus, thermoregulatory defenses vigorously respond to drops in core temperature. Elderly patients also experience shivering at higher temperatures than those who are younger. Additional risk factors include male sex, and electrolyte derangement such as hypomagnesemia.

3. Consequence of shivering.

a. Increase in systemic and cerebral energy consumption.

b. Increase in metabolic demand.

c. Increase in oxygen and carbon dioxide production.

d. Increases in intraocular and in intracranial pressure.

e. Precipitation of hemodynamic changes including heart rate, respiratory rate, and blood pressure.

f. Hindering the process of cooling as heat is transferred from the core to the periphery.

g. Possible increased pain or bodily discomfort.

| TABLE 7.1 | The Bedside Shivering Assessment Scale |

Score	Definition
0	None: No shivering noted on palpation of the masseter, neck, or chest wall.
1	Mild: Shivering is localized to the neck and/or thorax only.
2	Moderate: Shivering involves gross movement of the upper extremities (in addition to the neck and thorax).
3	Severe: Shivering involves gross movements of the trunk and upper and lower extremities.

Source: Badjatia, N., Strongilis, E., Gordon, E., Prescutti, M., Fernandez, L., Fernandez, A., . . . Mayer, S. A. (2012). Metabolic impact of shivering during therapeutic temperature modulation: The Bedside Shivering Assessment Scale. *Stroke, 39*, 3242–3247. doi:10.1161/STROKEAHA.108.523654

4. Assessment.
    a. The most common and only validated tool for the assessment of shivering is the Bedside Shivering Assessment Scale (see Table 7.1).
        i. This scale measures the degree of shivering during induced hypothermia.
        ii. It assists in determining the efficacy of non-pharmacological and pharmacological interventions.
5. Management.
    a. Goals of therapy.
        i. Stopping or suppressing the vigorous central thermoregulatory reflex versus treating skeletal muscle contractions.
        ii. Using a multimodal approach to counter the effects of shivering, which includes both nonpharmacological and pharmacological therapy.
    b. Nonpharmacological agents.
        i. Skin counter-warming aims to reduce vasoconstriction by decreasing the shivering threshold by 1°C for every 4°C increase in mean skin temperature.
        ii. An air circulating blanket is an example of a device poised to counter the metabolic impact of shivering.
        iii. Focal hand warming has been proven successful in the reduction of shivering, while facial rewarming has conflicting data to support use in the treatment of shivering.
    c. Pharmacological agents.
        i. Sedatives and hypnotics.
            1) Propofol, dexmedetomidine, midazolam, and diazepam are agents utilized to reduce the shivering threshold.
            2) Propofol is also recommended as a continuous infusion for induced hypothermia. However, the risks associated with use include hypotension. Several pharmacokinetic studies have identified increased plasma concentrations during hypothermia. The practitioner must take caution in the titration of this potent sedative to avoid untoward effects.
            3) Dexmedetomidine has proven to be effective in countering shivering. The limiting factor may be related to the high cost of medication delivery.
            4) Diazepam IV at high doses (20 mg) has proven to successfully reduce core body temperature, and avoid unnecessary increases in oxygen consumption caused by discomfort.
        ii. Analgesics and opioids.
            1) Meperidine has proven to be most beneficial in the reduction of the shiver threshold.
            2) Precautions include respiratory depression, nausea and vomiting, and increased seizure potential with prolonged drug administration.
            3) Combination therapies tend to have a synergistic effect as in the case of meperidine and buspirone improving the effect of lowering the shivering threshold.
            4) Fentanyl and morphine are frequently used analgesics post cardiac arrest and induced hypothermia. Both effectively reduce the shiver threshold. However, caution must be used with morphine as it has a higher probability for hypotension.
        iii. Alpha-agonists.
            1) Clonidine is the most widely used alpha-agonist during induced hypothermia, as well as the most researched.
            2) A single dose has demonstrated to be as effective as meperidine in lowering the shivering threshold. Caution must be taken because clonidine can induce bradycardia and exacerbate bradycardia from induced hypothermia.
        iv. N-methyl-D-aspartate (NMDA) antagonists.
        v. Magnesium.
            1) Use of magnesium sulfate to control shivering has both neuroprotective qualities for brain-injured patients and acts to guard against hypomagnesemia, which is a common finding during induced hypothermic states.
            2) Often used in combination with meperidine for its thermoregulatory effect to reduce shivering, shorten time to target temperature, and improve overall patient comfort.
        vi. Neuromuscular blocking agents (NMBAs).
            1) Agents such as dantrolene, methylphenidate, and doxapram control the skeletal muscle contractions associated with shivering. However, they are often left as the last therapeutic option.
            2) Caution must be taken with NMBAs because induced hypothermia reduces clearance of NMBAs and may prolong paralysis well after normothermia has been reached.
6. Conclusions.
    a. Shivering left untreated adversely affects the patient, and it may negate the benefit of induced hypothermia and create unintended hemodynamic instability and life-threatening metabolic derangements.
    b. Shivering management can be successfully implemented with a multimodal approach utilizing both nonpharmacological and pharmacological interventions with no adverse events.

Consultation/Referral

A. Consult with cardiology to determine the etiology of cardiac arrest, perform acute interventions, and manage any dysrhythmias.

B. Consult with neurology and/or neurocritical care for the critical management of the patient during TTM and prognostication post-TTM.

C. Consult with critical care (or neurocritical care) as needed for critical management.

Special/Geriatric Considerations

A. Because liver and kidney impairment may be present following cardiac arrest, older patients are at further risk for adverse events and impaired drug metabolism. The medications identified as high risk in elderly patients (Beers criteria) should be avoided when possible.

B. Older patients may cool more quickly due to thinner skin and less body fat, which may also precipitate vasoconstriction and shivering. For these same reasons, these patients are at higher risk for skin breakdown.

Bibliography

American Geriatrics Society 2015 Beers Criteria Update Expert Panel. (2015). American Geriatrics Society 2015 updated Beers Criteria for potentially inappropriate medication use in older adults. *Journal of the American Geriatrics Society, 63,* 2227–2246.

Andresen, M., Gazmuri, J. T., Marín, A., Regueira, T., & Rovegno, M. (2015). Therapeutic hypothermia for acute brain injuries. *Scandinavian Journal of Trauma, Resuscitation and Emergency Medicine, 23*(1), 42. doi:10.1186/s13049-015-0121-3

Badjatia, N. (2012). Shivering: Scores and protocols. *Critical Care, 16*(Suppl. 2), A9. Retrieved from https://www.ncbi.nlm.nih.gov/pmc/articles/PMC3389469

Badjatia, N., Strongilis, E., Gordon, E., Prescutti, M., Fernandez, L., Fernandez, A., . . . Mayer, S. A. (2012). Metabolic impact of shivering during therapeutic temperature modulation: The Bedside Shivering Assessment Scale. *Stroke, 39,* 3242–3247. doi:10.1161/STROKEAHA.108.523654

Boddicker, K. A., Zhang, Y., Zimmerman, M. B., Davies, L. R., & Kerber, R. E. (2005). Hypothermia improves defibrillation success and resuscitation outcomes from ventricular fibrillation. *Circulation, 111*(24), 3195–3201. doi:10.1161/CIRCULATIONAHA.104.492108

Callaway, C. W., Donnino, M. W., Fink, E. L., Geocadin, R. G., Golan, E., Kern, K. B., . . . Zimmerman, J. Z. (2015). Part 8: Post–cardiac arrest care: 2015 American Heart Association guidelines update for cardiopulmonary resuscitation and emergency cardiovascular care. *Circulation, 132*(18 Suppl. 2), S456–S482. doi:10.1161/CIR.0000000000000262

Choi, H. A., Ko, S.-B., Presciutti, M., Fernandez, L., Carpenter, A. M., Lesch, C., & Badjatia, N. (2011). Prevention of shivering during therapeutic temperature modulation: The Columbia anti-shivering protocol. *Neurocritical Care, 14,* 389–394. doi:10.1007/s12028-010-9474-7

Geri, G., Champigneulle, B., Bougouin, W., Arnaout, M., & Cariou, A. (2015). Common physiological response during TTM. *BMC Emergency Medicine, 15,* A14. doi:10.1186/1471-227X-15-S1-A14. Retrieved from https://www.ncbi.nlm.nih.gov/pmc/articles/PMC4480975/

Liu-DeRyke, X., & Rhoney, D. H. (2008, April 4). *Pharmacological management of therapeutic hypothermia-induced shivering.* Retrieved from http://www.sccm.org/Communications/Critical-Connections/Archives/Pages/Pharmacological-Management-of-Therapeutic-Hypothermia-Induced-Shivering.aspx

Logan, A. S., Sangkachand, P., & Funk, M. (2011). Optimal management of shivering during therapeutic hypothermia after cardiac arrest. *Critical Care Nurse, 31*(6), e18–e30. doi:10.4037/ccn2011618

Lopez, G. A. (2016). Temperature management in the neurointensive care unit. *Current Treatment Options in Neurology, 18,* 12. doi:10.1007/s11940-016-0393-6

Luscombe, M., & Andrzejowski, J. C. (2006). Clinical applications of induced hyperthermia. *Continuing Education in Anesthesia, Critical Care & Pain, 6,* 23–27. Retrieved from https://academic.oup.com/bjaed/article/6/1/23/347011/Clinical-applications-of-induced-hypothermia

Mozaffarian, D., Benjamin, E. J., Go, A. S., Arnett, D. K., Blaha, M. J., Cushman, M., & Turner, M. B. (2015). Heart disease and stroke statistics—2015 update. *Circulation, 131,* e29–e322. doi:10.1161/CIR.0000000000000152

Nielsen, N., Wetterslev, J., Cronberg, T., Erlinge, D., Gasche, Y., Hassager, C., & Friberg, H. (2013). Targeted temperature management at 33°C versus 36°C after cardiac arrest. *New England Journal of Medicine, 369*(23), 2197–2206. doi:10.1056/NEJMoa1310519

Polderman, K. H., & Herold, I. (2009). Therapeutic hypothermia and controlled normothermia in the intensive care unit: Practical considerations, side effects, and cooling methods. *Critical Care Medicine, 37*(3), 1101–1120. doi:10.1097/ccm.0b013e3181962ad5

Povlishock, J. T., Buki, A., Koiziumi, H., Stone, J., & Okonkwo, D. O. (1999). Initiating mechanisms involved in the pathobiology of traumatically induced axonal injury and interventions targeted at blunting their progression. In A. Baethmann, N. Plesnila, F. Ringel, & J. Eriskat (Eds.), *Current progress in the understanding of secondary brain damage from trauma* (vol. 73, pp. 15–20). Vienna, Austria: Springer. doi:10.1007/978-3-7091-6391-7_3

Sandroni, C., & Geocadin, C. S. (2015). Neurological prognostication after cardiac arrest. *Current Opinion Critical Care, 21,* 209–214. doi:10.1097/MCC.0000000000000202

Scirica, B. M. (2013). Therapeutic hypothermia after cardiac arrest. *Circulation, 127,* 244–250. doi:10.1161/CIRCULATIONAHA.111.076851

Taccone, F. S., Cronberg, T., Friberg, H., Greer, D., Horn, J., Oddo, M., & Vincent, J.-L. (2014). How to assess prognosis after cardiac arrest and therapeutic hypothermia. *Critical Care, 18,* 202. doi:10.1186/cc13696

Van Poucke, S., Stevens, K., Marcus, A. E., & Lancé, M. (2014). Hypothermia: Effects on platelet functioning hemostasis. *Thrombosis Journal, 12,* 31. doi:10.1186/s12959-014-0031-z

Weant, K. A., Martin, J. E., Humphries, R. L., & Cook, A. M. (2010). Pharmacologic options for reducing the shivering response to therapeutic hypothermia. *Pharmacotherapy, 30,* 830–841. doi:10.1592/phco.30.8.830

Wijdicks, E. F., Hijdra, A., Young, G. B., Bassetti, C. L., & Wiebe, S. A. (2006). Practice parameter: Prediction of outcome in comatose survivors after cardiopulmonary resuscitation (an evidence-based review). *Neurology, 67,* 203–210. doi:10.1212/01.wnl.0000227183.21314.cd

Endocrine Guidelines

Catherine Harris

Adrenal Insufficiency

Kathryn Evans Kreider

Definition

A. Insufficient production of glucocorticoids and/or mineralocorticoids and adrenal androgens as a result of primary adrenal failure or failure of the pituitary or hypothalamus. Cortisol and mineralocorticoids are essential to life because of their role in energy and fluid homeostasis.

B. Primary adrenal insufficiency (PAI).

   1. Also known as Addison's disease.

   2. Deficiency in adrenal hormones as a result of direct injury to the adrenal glands.

C. Secondary adrenal insufficiency (SAI).

   1. Insufficient adrenal hormones due to lack of pituitary stimulation.

D. Tertiary adrenal insufficiency (TAI).

   1. Insufficient adrenal hormones due to lack of hypothalamic stimulation on the pituitary.

E. Adrenal crisis (AC).

   1. Potentially fatal condition that occurs when there is heightened need for cortisol in response to stress in the presence of adrenal insufficiency (AI).

   2. May be the initial presentation of AI.

Incidence

A. The prevalence of primary AI is 100 to 140 cases per million.

   1. Women more often affected.

   2. Peak age 30 to 50 years.

B. The prevalence of secondary AI is 150 to 280 cases per million.

   1. Women more often affected.

   2. Peak age around 60 years.

C. The risk of AC in patients with existing AI is 6.3% per patient year.

Pathogenesis

A. PAI is caused by destruction of the adrenal cortex, most often by antiadrenal antibodies.

   1. Hormone deficiency occurs when 90% of the cortex is lost.

   2. All adrenal hormones may be affected, including mineralocorticoids (aldosterone) and adrenal androgens.

B. Central AI includes SAI and TAI.

   1. SAI is a result of deficient ACTH from the pituitary gland leading to decreased adrenal stimulation.

2. TAI involves disruption of corticotropin-releasing hormone (CRH), vasopressin, or both, from the hypothalamus, resulting in decreased stimulation of the pituitary gland and reduced ACTH.

3. The hypothalamic–pituitary axis (HPA) is impaired.

4. Production of aldosterone and adrenal androgens is unaffected.

Predisposing Factors

A. Primary AI.

   1. Presence of other autoimmune conditions (e.g., autoimmune thyroid disease, type 1 diabetes mellitus, autoimmune polyendocrinopathy syndromes).

   2. Disseminated infection (e.g., tuberculosis, HIV, cytomegalovirus, fungal infections).

   3. Adrenal hemorrhage, metastases, or infiltration.

   4. Various genetic disorders (e.g., congenital adrenal hyperplasia, adrenoleukodystrophy).

   5. Use of medications associated with drug-induced AI (e.g., fluconazole, etomidate, phenobarbital, rifampin).

B. Secondary AI.

   1. Pituitary tumor or trauma.

   2. Infections or infiltrative processes (e.g., tuberculosis, meningitis, sarcoidosis).

   3. Pituitary surgery.

C. Tertiary AI.

   1. Most common cause: Long-term use of exogenous glucocorticoids.

   2. Hypothalamic dysfunction secondary to tumors or infiltrative processes.

D. AC.

   1. Abrupt cessation of glucocorticoid use.

   2. Acute physiologic stress in the presence of AI.

   3. Previous AC.

   4. Risk increased if significant comorbidity present.

Subjective Data

A. Common complaints/symptoms.

   1. Tends to be nonspecific with an insidious onset, including:

      a. Weakness and fatigue.

      b. Anorexia and weight loss.

B. Common/typical scenario.

   1. History of the present illness.

      a. Elicit information about onset, duration, and severity of symptoms.

      b. Obtain a detailed medical history.

      c. Inquire about recent illness, injury, trauma, surgery, and procedures.

      d. Evaluate for history of glucocorticoid use.

2. Other signs and symptoms.

   a. AI.

      i. Abdominal pain.

      ii. Myalgia or arthralgia.

      iii. Depression or anxiety.

      iv. Dizziness or postural hypotension.

      v. Salt craving.

      vi. Skin hyperpigmentation.

      vii. Decreased libido in women (if androgen deficient).

      viii. Loss of pubic and axillary hair in females (if androgen deficient).

      ix. Electrolyte imbalances including hyponatremia and hyperkalemia.

      x. Hypoglycemia.

   b. AC.

      i. Severe weakness.

      ii. Syncope.

      iii. Abdominal pain, nausea, and vomiting.

      iv. Back pain.

      v. Confusion.

Physical Examination

A. Vital signs.

   1. Orthostatic hypotension in AI.

   2. Hypotension in AC.

B. Skin.

   1. Hyperpigmentation, particularly sun-exposed areas, skin creases, mucous membranes, scars, and breast areolas.

   2. In females, pubic and/or axillary hair loss.

C. Signs of dehydration.

D. Cardiovascular examination.

E. Mental status examination.

   1. Altered consciousness and delirium in AC.

Diagnostic Tests

A. Diagnostic testing for AI should be performed in any hospitalized patient with symptoms suggestive of AI that are otherwise unexplained.

B. AI is usually diagnosed by a low morning (8 a.m.) serum cortisol level and a low stimulated cortisol level.

   1. Cortisol levels are usually at their highest levels in the morning; low levels should raise suspicion of AI.

   2. The diagnosis of AI is likely if the morning cortisol level is less than 5 mcg/dL, and less than 3 mcg/dL is highly suggestive.

   3. A low serum cortisol level (<5 mcg/dL) in addition to a high ACTH level (>66 pmol/L) is highly predictive of AI.

      a. ACTH twice the upper limit of normal of the reference range is consistent with PAI.

   4. A high ACTH with a normal cortisol level may be an early indicator of AI.

C. The most common stimulation test is the corticotropin stimulation test ("cort-stim"), also known as the ACTH test or cosyntropin test.

   1. This test is the gold standard for diagnosing primary (not secondary) AI.

   2. Cosyntropin is synthetic ACTH given to patients intramuscularly (IM) to stimulate the adrenal glands to produce cortisol.

   3. Cosyntropin testing can be done at any time of day.

      a. Testing is often done early morning (8 a.m.) so morning cortisol levels can be drawn simultaneously.

   4. Steps for performing the cort-stim test include:

      a. Draw baseline lab tests, including serum cortisol and ACTH.

      b. Administer 250 mcg of cosyntropin IM or intravenous (IV).

      c. After 30 or 60 minutes, draw peak serum cortisol level.

5. Peak serum cortisol levels less than 18 mcg/dL indicate AI.

   a. Certain conditions can alter cortisol measurements (alter cortisol-binding globulin [CBG]).

      i. Estrogen-containing contraceptives can falsely increase cortisol.

      ii. Patients with nephrotic syndrome, liver disease, or those with critical illness may have low CBG values and falsely low cortisol levels.

6. High ACTH levels (often >300 ng/L) are characteristic of PAI.

7. Renin and aldosterone should be measured to assess mineralocorticoid deficiency if there is a concern for PAI.

   a. PAI is associated with loss of the part of the adrenal gland that produces mineralocorticoid hormones.

      i. Elevated plasma renin and low or inappropriately normal aldosterone is typical.

8. If SAI or TAI is suspected (pituitary or hypothalamus dysfunction), it is recommended that an endocrinologist be consulted to assist with biochemical testing and confirmatory testing.

Differential Diagnosis

A. Malnutrition.

B. Gastrointestinal (GI) dysfunction.

C. Malignancy.

D. Failure to thrive.

E. Hyperthyroidism.

Evaluation and Management Plan

A. General plan: Replacement of glucocorticoid with physiologic dosing; hemodynamic stability.

B. Pharmacotherapy.

   1. If AI is diagnosed in the hospital and the patient is acutely ill/decompensating, stress-dose steroids should be used immediately and continued until the patient show signs of recovery.

   2. If AI or adrenal crisis is suspected in a hospitalized patient who is acutely ill, start stress-dose steroids prior to receiving results of diagnostic testing.

      a. Example: Hydrocortisone 50 mg IV q6h.

      b. Alternative: Hydrocortisone 100 mg IV given immediately, followed by 200 mg hydrocortisone given over 24 hours (continuous IV or intermittent injections).

   3. Stress dosing of steroids should be used for patients with previously diagnosed AI who present to the hospital with acute illness or injury.

   4. Patients should also be given a bolus of IV fluids for acute adrenal crisis.

      a. 1,000 mL saline or 5% dextrose in saline given within the first hour.

   5. If AI is diagnosed in the hospital and the patient is not acutely ill or demonstrating signs of AC, physiologic dosing may be started with careful consideration to other comorbid conditions and patient acuity.

   6. All patients with confirmed PAI require lifelong glucocorticoid therapy.

      a. Options—may be dosed based on body mass index or weight.

i. Hydrocortisone 15 to 20 mg in the morning and 5 to 10 mg in the afternoon (12–4 p.m.).
ii. Prednisolone 3 to 5 mg/d total in 1 to 2 daily doses.
b. Patients may occasionally be given glucocorticoid divided into three daily doses.
c. Dexamethasone should generally be avoided due to potential for Cushing-like features and overreplacement.
7. Mineralocorticoid replacement should be initiated in all patients who exhibit aldosterone deficiency.
a. Fludrocortisone should be initiated at doses of 50 to 100 mg/d.
b. Salt intake should not be restricted.
8. Response should be measured clinically for both glucocorticoid and mineralocorticoid replacement (blood pressure [BP], weight, energy levels, and signs of glucocorticoid excess; salt craving, postural hypotension, edema).
a. Electrolytes should be measured to confirm correct mineralocorticoid replacement.
b. Other biochemical tests are not recommended.
C. Discharge instructions.
1. Patient should be counseled on signs and symptoms of under- and overreplacement of cortisol.
2. Patients require a steroid emergency card and a medical alert bracelet.
3. Patient should be counseled extensively on "sick day rules."
a. Home management of illness with fever: Patients should double or triple home steroid dose for 2 to 3 days or until recovery; increase electrolyte-containing fluids.
b. Management of GI-related illness: Patient should inject 100 mg hydrocortisone IM if unable to tolerate oral administration.
c. Minor to moderate surgical stress: Double or triple home dosing until event is over.
4. Patients should have a prescription for IM hydrocortisone in case they are unable to take PO steroids.
5. Patients with mineralocorticoid deficiency should be counseled to increase salt intake on days of excess heat, sweating, or physical activity.

Follow-Up

A. Patients should follow-up with an outpatient provider every 3 to 6 months until clinically stable, with appointments every 6 to 12 months reasonable thereafter.
B. Patients should be evaluated at each clinical visit for signs and symptoms of over- and underreplacement.
1. Signs of overreplacement may include insomnia, weight gain, peripheral edema, or hypertension.
2. Signs of underreplacement are similar to the signs and symptoms of AI.
C. Patients should receive periodic clinical and biochemical evaluation to screen for other autoimmune conditions.
1. Type 1 diabetes.
2. Autoimmune thyroid disease.
3. Pernicious anemia.
4. Celiac disease.
5. Premature ovarian failure.

Consultation/Referral

A. Referral to an endocrinologist is recommended to assist with long-term steroid management.

Special/Geriatric Considerations

A. Pregnant patients should be evaluated at least once per trimester.
1. A glucocorticoid dose increase may be required in the third trimester.
2. Stress-dose steroids are required during labor.

Bibliography

Bornstein, S. R., Allolio, B., Arlt, W., Barthel, A., Don-Wauchope, A., Hammer, G. D., . . . Torpy, D. J. (2016). Diagnosis and treatment of primary adrenal insufficiency: An endocrine society clinical practice guideline. *Journal of Clinical Endocrinology and Metabolism, 101*(2), 364–389. doi:10.1210/jc.2015-1710

Charmandari, E., Nicolaides, N. C., & Chrousos, G. P. (2014). Adrenal insufficiency. *The Lancet, 383*(9935), 2152–2167. doi:10.1016/S0140-6736(13)61684-0

Husebye, E. S., Allolio, B., Arlt, W., Badenhopp, K., Bensing, S., Betterle, C., . . . Pearce, S. H. (2014). Consensus statement on the diagnosis, treatment and follow-up of patients with primary adrenal insufficiency. *Journal of Internal Medicine, 275*(2), 104–115. doi:10.1111/joim.12162

Smans, L. C., Van derValk, E. S., Hermus, A. R., & Zelissen, P. M. (2016). Incidence of adrenal crisis in patients with adrenal insufficiency. *Clinical Endocrinology, 84*, 17–22. doi:10.1111/cen.12865

Diabetes Mellitus—Type 1

Julie Stone

Definition

A. Due to autoimmune destruction of the pancreatic beta cells.
B. Previously referred to as insulin-dependent diabetes or juvenile-onset diabetes.
C. Further divided into two subgroups based on pathogenesis.
1. Immune-mediated diabetes.
a. Autoimmune-mediated destruction of pancreatic beta cells.
b. Often have other autoimmune disorders such as Hashimoto's thyroiditis, Graves' disease, Addison's disease, celiac disease, vitiligo, autoimmune hepatitis, myasthenia gravis, and pernicious anemia.
2. Idiopathic type 1 diabetes.
a. No known etiologies.
b. Permanent insulinopenia and prone to ketosis.
c. No evidence of autoimmunity.
d. African or Asian ancestry.
e. Strongly inherited; no human leukocyte antigen association.

Incidence

A. In 2012, approximately 1.25 million American children and adults had type 1 diabetes.
B. Worldwide incidence is increasing by approximately 3% per year.

Pathogenesis

A. Autoimmune destruction of pancreatic beta cells; 85% of type 1 diabetes patients have detectable circulating antibodies.
B. Rate of beta cell destruction can vary.
1. Rapid in infants and children.
2. Slow in adults.

Predisposing Factors

A. Presence of other autoimmune diseases.
B. Family history of diabetes.

C. Viruses.
D. Environmental toxins.

Subjective Data
A. Common complaints/symptoms.
   1. Polyuria (96%).
   2. Polydipsia.
   3. Weight loss.
   4. Fatigue.
B. Common/typical scenario.
   1. Patients frequently complain of fatigue and weakness. They may have muscle cramps, blurred vision, and significant polyuria, polydipsia, and polyphagia.
   2. Weight loss occurs over time despite normal or increased appetite.
C. Family and social history.
   1. Ask about family history since there is a strong link to family history.
   2. Ask about type of occupation, if the person is a shift worker, use of alcohol, smoking, or recreational drug use.
   3. Review how much exercise the person gets.
D. Review of symptoms.
   1. HEENT.
      a. Dental issues. Periodontal disease is associated with diabetes.
   2. Psychologic.
      a. Depression.
      b. Anxiety.
      c. Disordered eating.
      d. Psychosocial barriers/support.
      e. Barriers to self-management.
   3. Microvascular complications.
      a. Neuropathy.
      b. Nephropathy.
      c. Retinopathy.
   4. Macrovascular complications.
      a. Coronary artery disease.
      b. Cerebrovascular disease.
      c. Peripheral arterial disease.

Physical Examination
A. Height, weight, body mass index (BMI), waist circumference.
B. Vital signs.
C. Funduscopic examination.
D. Thyroid palpation.
E. Skin examination.
   1. Acanthosis nigricans (see Figure 8.1).
   2. Lipohypertrophy.
   3. Diabetic dermopathy.
   4. Skin tags.
F. Foot examination.
   1. Inspection, noting mycotic changes to nail or skin.
   2. Vascular examination.
      a. Hair patterns or lack of hair growth.
      b. Pulses (dorsalis pedis and posterior tibial).
      c. Temperature/color.
   3. Reflexes.
      a. Patellar.
      b. Achilles.
   4. Proprioception, vibration, and monofilament sensation.

Diagnostic Tests
A. Glycosylated hemoglobin (HgbA1C), fasting glucose, random glucose, or 2-hour glucose tolerance test to diagnose.
   1. HgbA1C greater than 6.5%.
   2. Fasting glucose greater than 126 mg/dL.
   3. Random glucose greater than 200 mg/dL with classic symptoms of hyperglycemia.
   4. 2-hour glucose tolerance test greater than 200 mg/dL.
B. Antibodies to check at time of diagnosis.
   1. Glutamic acid decarboxylase (GAD).
   2. Islet cell antibodies.
   3. Zinc antibodies.
C. HgbA1C on admission to hospital if no result available for past 3 months.
D. Yearly lab work.
   1. Fasting lipid panel.
   2. Liver function tests.
   3. Urine albumin-to-creatinine ratio.
   4. Serum creatinine and estimated glomerular filtration rate (GFR).
   5. Thyroid-stimulating hormone.
E. C-peptide and random glucose to determine insulin production by beta cells.

Differential Diagnosis
A. Steroid-induced diabetes.
B. Pancreatitis.
C. Cushing's disease.
D. Pancreatic endocrine tumor.
E. Gestational diabetes.
F. MODY type diabetes.
G. Latent autoimmune diabetes in adults (LADA).
H. Type 2 diabetes.
I. Cystic fibrosis-related diabetes.
J. Posttransplant diabetes.
K. Postpancreatectomy diabetes.

Evaluation and Management Plan
A. General plan. The recommended outpatient comprehensive treatment plan for type 1 diabetes according to the American Association of Diabetes Educators consists of the following seven self-care behaviors.
   1. Healthy eating: The patient should see a registered dietician for medical nutrition therapy counseling.
   2. Being active: At least 150 minutes of moderate to vigorous intensity physical activity spread out over a week is required. This can include resistance exercises and flexibility exercises.
   3. Monitoring: It is recommended to test glucose before meals and bedtime (more if needed).
   4. Medications (insulin).
      a. Delivery method options: Pens, vial and syringe, pump.
      b. Regimen choices (premixed insulin vs. basal and prandial).
      c. Proper storage of insulin.
      d. Preparation, administration, and site rotation of insulin injection.
      e. Disposal of sharps.
      f. Hypoglycemia symptoms.
   5. Problem solving.
   6. Healthy coping.
   7. Reducing risks.
B. Patient/family teaching points.
   1. Inpatient education focuses on survival skills only.
      a. Checking glucose.
      b. Taking medications.
      c. Diet.
      d. Hypoglycemia treatment.

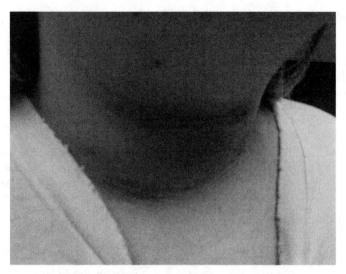

FIGURE 8.1 Acanthosis nigricans is a dark, velvety, hyperpigmentation of the skin, often found at the skin folds.
Source: Lyons, F., & Ousley, L. (2015). *Dermatology for the advanced practice nurse* (p. 55). New York, NY: Springer Publishing Company.

2. Outpatient education is more comprehensive and uses guidelines by the American Association of Diabetes Educators to direct the education. The patient should be referred to outpatient diabetes education at the time of diagnosis, yearly thereafter, and as needed or if therapy changes.

C. Pharmacotherapy.

1. Insulin: Mainstay of therapy.

   a. Initiate therapy using a 0.3 units/kg/d total daily dose.

   b. Follow 50/50 rule.

      i. Give one-half of the total daily dose as basal insulin (long-acting insulin).

      ii. Give one-half of the total daily dose as prandial insulin divided evenly between three meals (usually rapid-acting or short-acting insulin).

      iii. Add a gentle correction scale using the same rapid or short-acting insulin in number 2. Use 1 unit for every 50 points glucose is above 150 mg/dL.

   c. In the outpatient setting, the patient should learn carbohydrate counting, and then prandial insulin can be dosed as a ratio of 1 unit insulin to number of grams of carbohydrates.

   d. Consider insulin pump therapy at some point in the future.

2. Pramlintide.

   a. Delays gastric emptying, blunts secretion of glucagon, and enhances satiety.

   b. Food and Drug Administration (FDA) approved for use in adults with type 1 diabetes; most helpful in treating these patients.

   c. Helps with weight loss and reduces insulin dose.

D. Discharge instructions.

1. Verify the patient's understanding of how to take medications as prescribed.

   a. Dose.

   b. Route.

   c. Frequency.

   d. Relationship to meals.

   e. Proper disposal of sharps.

   f. Rotation of sites for subcutaneous insulin injections.

   g. Need for refrigeration.

2. Make sure the patient is familiar with dietary restrictions.

   a. The patient should aim for consistent amounts of carbohydrates per meal at first. Then the goal will be to learn to dose insulin to the amount of carbohydrates using carbohydrate counting.

3. Be sure the patient knows when glucose monitoring is important.

   a. Before meals and bedtime.

   b. Before and after exercise.

   c. Before driving.

   d. More often as needed.

Follow-Up

A. Recommend annual eye examination and podiatry examination.

B. Recommend outpatient education if appropriate.

C. Follow-up with endocrinologist or primary care provider. Specify how soon patient should be seen. Specify when to call provider.

D. Outline hypoglycemia treatment.

1. Rule of 15: 15 g of simple carbohydrates every 15 minutes until glucose is above 70 mg/dL (e.g., ½ cup juice, ½ cup pop, glucose gel, glucose tablets).

2. Carry glucose tablets or gel at all times.

3. Instruct the patient to carry a glucagon kit that can be administered by a friend or family member if the patient is unresponsive.

Consultation/Referral

A. Refer the patient to endocrinology for new diagnosis, uncontrolled HgbA1C, multiple complications of diabetes, or comorbid conditions affecting the diabetes control.

B. Refer the patient to nephrology for nephropathy.

C. Refer the patient to ophthalmology for yearly eye examination.

D. Refer the patient to podiatry for issues and/or yearly examination.

E. Refer the patient to a dentist (periodontal check, dental cleaning twice a year).

F. Refer the patient to psychology for coping with chronic disease.

Special/Geriatric Considerations

A. Pregnancy.

1. Retinopathy risk: Counsel patient on the risk of development or progression of retinopathy. Dilated eye examination should ideally occur preconception, each trimester, and 1 year postpartum.

2. Potentially teratogenic medications should be stopped.

3. Measurements of fasting and postprandial glucose are recommended.

4. HgbA1C is lower during pregnancy. Target in pregnancy is 6% to 6.5%.

5. Glycemic targets.

    a. Fasting 95 mg/dL or lower.

    b. 1-hour postprandial 140 mg/dL or lower.

    c. 2-hour postprandial 120 mg/dL or lower.

6. Changes in insulin requirements (see Table 8.1).

    a. First trimester.

    b. Second trimester.

    c. Third trimester.

7. Labor and delivery: Use regular insulin intravenous infusion and immediate postpartum until glucose is stable.

8. Postpartum care.

    a. Insulin sensitivity increases with delivery and returns to prepregnancy levels over 1 to 2 weeks.

    b. Prevent hypoglycemia with breastfeeding, erratic sleep, and eating that occurs postpartum.

B. Geriatric.

1. Determine glycemic goals based on expected life span, comorbid conditions, and ability of patient to self-manage disease.

2. Use hypoglycemia prevention.

Bibliography

Cefalu, W. T. (2017). Standards of medical care in diabetes–2017. *Diabetes Care, 40*(Suppl. 1), s1–s135. doi:10.2337/dc17-S003

Lyons, F., & Ousley, L. (2015). *Dermatology for the advanced practice nurse* (p. 55). New York, NY: Springer Publishing Company.

Menke, A., Orchard, T., Imperatore, G., Bullard, K., Mayer-Davis, E., & Cowie, C. (2013). The prevalence of type 1 diabetes in the United States. *Epidemiology, 24*, 773–774. doi:10.1097/EDE.0b013e31829ef01a

Mensing, C. (2011). *The art and science of diabetes self-management education desk reference* (2nd ed.). Chicago, IL: American Association of Diabetes Educators.

Statistics About Diabetes. (n. d.). Retrieved from http://www.diabetes.org/diabetes-basics/statistics/

Diabetes Mellitus—Type 2

Julie Stone

Definition

A. Relative (rather than absolute) insulin deficiency and peripheral insulin resistance.

B. Previously referred to as non-insulin-dependent diabetes or adult-onset diabetes.

Incidence

A. Accounts for 90% to 95% of all cases of diabetes.

B. According to the 2017 Centers for Disease Control and Prevention's National Diabetes Statistics Report, an estimated 30.3 million Americans or 9.4% of the population had diabetes in 2015 (see Table 8.2).

C. In 2015, an estimated 1.5 million new cases of diabetes was diagnosed among U.S. adults older than 18 years.

D. Diabetes was the seventh leading cause of death in 2015.

E. Prevalence varies among different ethnicities (see Table 8.3).

Pathogenesis

A. Specific etiologies are not known. There is no autoimmune destruction of beta cells.

B. Excess weight causes insulin resistance. Most patients with type 2 diabetes are overweight or obese.

C. Abdominal obesity contributes to increased risk.

D. Ketoacidosis seldom occurs.

E. Hyperglycemia develops gradually; it is often undiagnosed for years before the official diagnosis is made.

F. Insulin secretion is defective and unable to compensate for increased insulin resistance.

Predisposing Factors

A. Age; risk is higher as age increases.

B. Obesity, with body mass index (BMI) greater than or equal to 25 kg/m^2.

C. Lack of physical activity.

D. Women with prior gestational diabetes.

E. History of prediabetes.

F. History of metabolic syndrome.

G. Comorbidities of hypertension and dyslipidemia.

H. Higher rates in certain ethnic populations.

    1. African Americans.

    2. American Indian.

    3. Hispanic/Latino.

    4. Asian American.

I. Strong genetic predisposition.

J. Medications.

    1. Glucocorticoids.

    2. Thiazide diuretics.

    3. Atypical antipsychotics.

Subjective Data

A. Common complaints/symptoms.

    1. Polyuria.

    2. Blurred vision.

    3. Polydipsia.

    4. Malaise/fatigue.

TABLE 8.1 **Changing Insulin Requirements During Pregnancy**

Trimester	First	Second	Third
Insulin requirements	• Woman often has decrease in total daily insulin requirements. • May experience increased hypoglycemia.	• Woman often has rapidly increasing insulin resistance with need for weekly insulin dose adjustments.	• Woman often has a leveling off of insulin requirements or a small decrease.

TABLE 8.2 **Estimated Number and Percentage of Diagnosed and Undiagnosed Diabetes Among Adults Aged 18 Years and Older, United States, 2015**

Characteristic	Diagnosed Diabetes No. in Millions (95% CI)[a]	Undiagnosed Diabetes No. in Millions (95% CI)[a]	Total Diabetes No. in Millions (95% CI)[a]
Total	23.0 (21.1–25.1)	7.2 (6.0–8.6)	30.2 (27.9–32.7)
Age in years			
18–44	3.0 (2.6–3.6)	1.6 (1.1–2.3)	4.6 (3.8–5.5)
45–64	10.7 (9.3–12.2)	3.6 (2.8–4.6)	14.3 (12.7–16.1)
=65	9.9 (9.0–11.0)	2.1 (1.4–3.0)	12.0 (10.7–13.4)
Sex			
Women	11.7 (10.5–13.1)	3.1 (2.4–4.1)	14.9 (13.5–16.4)
Men	11.3 (10.2–12.4)	4.0 (3.0–5.5)	15.3 (13.8–17.0)
	Percentage (95% CI)[b]	**Percentage (95% CI)[b]**	**Percentage (95% CI)[b]**
Total	9.3 (8.5–10.1)	2.9 (2.4–3.5)	12.2 (11.3–13.2)
Age in years			
18–44	2.6 (2.2–3.1)	1.3 (0.9–2.0)	4.0 (3.3–4.8)
45–64	12.7 (11.1–14.5)	4.3 (3.3–5.5)	17.0 (15.1–19.1)
=65	20.8 (18.8–23.0)	4.4 (3.1–6.3)	25.2 (22.5–28.1)
Sex			
Women	9.2 (8.2–10.3)	2.5 (1.9–3.2)	11.7 (10.6–12.9)
Men	9.4 (8.5–10.3)	3.4 (2.5–4.6)	12.7 (11.5–14.1)

Note: [a]Numbers for subgroups may not add up to the total because of rounding.

[b]Data are crude, not age adjusted.

CI, confidence interval.

Data source: 2011–2014 National Health and Nutrition Examination Survey and 2015 U.S. Census Bureau data.

Source: National Center for Chronic Disease Prevention and Health Promotion. (2017). *National diabetes statistics report, 2017: Estimates of diabetes and its burden in the United States.* Retrieved from
https://www.cdc.gov/diabetes/pdfs/data/statistics/national-diabetes-statistics-report.pdf

TABLE 8.3 **Prevalence of Diagnosed and Undiagnosed Diabetes Among Adults Aged 18 Years and Older, United States, 2011–2014**

Characteristic	Diagnosed Diabetes Percentage (95% CI)	Undiagnosed Diabetes Percentage (95% CI)	Total Percentage (95% CI)
Total	8.7 (8.1–9.4)	2.7 (2.3–3.3)	11.5 (10.7–12.4)
Race/Ethnicity			
Asian, non-Hispanic	10.3 (8.6–12.4)	5.7 (4.0–8.2)	16.0 (13.6–18.9)
Black, non-Hispanic	13.4 (12.2–14.6)	4.4 (3.0–6.2)	17.7 (15.8–19.9)
Hispanic	11.9 (10.3–13.7)	4.5 (3.2–6.2)	16.4 (14.1–18.9)
White, non-Hispanic	7.3 (6.6–8.1)	2.0 (1.5–2.6)	9.3 (8.4–10.2)

Note: CI, confidence interval.

Data source: 2011–2014 National Health and Nutrition Examination Survey.

Source: National Center for Chronic Disease Prevention and Health Promotion. (2017). *National diabetes statistics report, 2017: Estimates of diabetes and its burden in the United States.* Retrieved from https://www.cdc.gov/diabetes/pdfs/data/statistics/national-diabetes-statistics-report.pdf

5. Frequent urinary tract infections (UTIs) or vaginal candidiasis.
6. Poor wound healing.
B. Common/typical scenario.
1. Patients frequently complain of fatigue and weakness. They may have muscle cramps, blurred vision, and significant polyuria, polydipsia, and polyphagia.
2. Weight loss occurs over time despite normal or increased appetite.
C. Family and social history.

1. Ask about family history since there is a strong link to family history.
2. Ask about type of occupation, if the person is a shift worker, use of alcohol, smoking, or recreational drug use.
3. Review how much exercise the person gets.
D. Review of symptoms.
1. HEENT.
a. Dental issues. Periodontal disease is associated with diabetes.

2. Psychologic.
   a. Depression.
   b. Anxiety.
   c. Disordered eating.
   d. Psychosocial barriers/support.
   e. Barriers to self-management.
3. Microvascular complications.
   a. Neuropathy.
   b. Nephropathy.
   c. Retinopathy.
4. Macrovascular complications.
   a. Coronary artery disease.
   b. Cerebrovascular disease.
   c. Peripheral arterial disease.

Physical Examination

A. Height, weight, BMI, waist circumference.
B. Vital signs.
C. Funduscopic examination.
D. Thyroid palpation.
E. Skin examination.
   1. Acanthosis nigricans (see Figure 8.1).
   2. Lipohypertrophy.
   3. Diabetic dermopathy.
   4. Skin tags.
F. Foot examination.
   1. Inspection, noting mycotic changes to nail or skin.
   2. Vascular examination.
      a. Hair patterns or lack of hair growth.
      b. Pulses (dorsalis pedis and posterior tibial).
      c. Temperature/color.
   3. Reflexes.
      a. Patellar.
      b. Achilles.
   4. Proprioception, vibration, and monofilament sensation.

Diagnostic Tests

A. Hemoglobin A1C (HgbA1C), fasting glucose, random glucose, or 2-hour glucose tolerance test to diagnose.
   1. HgbA1C greater than 6.5%.
   2. Fasting glucose greater than 126 mg/dL.
   3. Random glucose greater than 200 mg/dL with classic symptoms of hyperglycemia.
   4. 2-hour glucose tolerance test greater than 200 mg/dL.
B. HgbA1C on admission to hospital if no result available for past 3 months.
C. Yearly lab work for patients with diabetes.
   1. Fasting lipid panel.
   2. Liver function tests.
   3. Urine albumin-to-creatinine ratio.
   4. Serum creatinine and glomerular filtration rate (GFR).

Differential Diagnosis

A. Prediabetes.
B. Metabolic syndrome.
C. Stress hyperglycemia.
D. Medication-induced hyperglycemia.
E. Posttransplant diabetes.
F. MODY type diabetes.
G. Latent autoimmune diabetes.
H. Type 1 diabetes.
I. Ketosis-prone diabetes.
J. Pancreatitis.
K. Pancreatic insufficiency.

Evaluation and Management Plan

A. General plan. The recommended outpatient comprehensive treatment plan most helpful in treating type 2 diabetes according to the American Association of Diabetes Educators consists of the following seven self-care behaviors.
   1. Healthy eating: The patient should see a registered dietician for medical nutrition therapy counseling.
   2. Being active: At least 150 minutes of moderate to vigorous intensity physical activity spread out over a week. This can include resistance exercises and flexibility exercises.
   3. Glucose monitoring.
      a. Oral agents recommended one to two times a day before meals; can vary which meals.
      b. Insulin recommended before meals and bedtime.
   4. Medications: Oral agents, insulin, non-insulin (injectable).
      a. Delivery method options: Pens, vial and syringe, pump.
      b. Proper storage.
      c. Preparation, administration, and site rotation.
      d. Disposal of sharps.
      e. Hypoglycemia symptoms.
   5. Problem solving.
   6. Healthy coping.
   7. Reducing risks.
B. Patient/family teaching points.
   1. Inpatient education focuses on survival skills only.
      a. Checking glucose.
      b. Taking medications.
      c. Diet.
      d. Hypoglycemia treatment.
   2. Outpatient education is more comprehensive and uses guidelines by the American Association of Diabetes Educators to direct the education. The patient should be referred to outpatient diabetes education at the time of diagnosis, yearly thereafter, and as needed or if therapy changes.
C. Pharmacotherapy.
   1. Oral agents (see Table 8.4).
      a. Metformin: First-line agent.
      b. Sulfonylureas such as glimepiride.
      c. Meglitinides such as repaglinide.
      d. Thiazolidinediones such as pioglitazone.
      e. Alpha glucosidase inhibitors such as acarbose.
      f. Dipeptidyl peptidase-4 (DPP-4) inhibitors such as sitagliptin.
      g. Sodium glucose cotransporter-2 (SGLT2) inhibitors such as canagliflozin.
      h. Glucagon-like peptide-1 (GLP-1) receptor agonists such as exenatide.
   2. Insulin.
      a. Mainstay of therapy in hospital.
      b. Initiate therapy using one of three different calculations.
         i. For renal patients or those new to insulin: Start with 0.3 units/kg/day total daily dose.
         ii. For most patients: Start with 0.5 units/kg/day total daily dose.
         iii. For obese patients, insulin resistant patients, or those on steroids: Start with 0.7 units/kg/day total daily dose.
      c. 50/50 rule.
         i. Give one-half of the total daily dose as basal insulin (glargine, detemir, degludec).

TABLE 8.4 **Oral Agents Used to Treat Diabetes**

Oral Agent	Side Effects	Benefits and Considerations

Metformin (first-line agent)	• GI side effects; start low and go slow in titrating up dose
	• Extended-release form used to prevent GI side effects
		• Benefits
		  ° Inexpensive
		  ° Does not lead to hypoglycemia
		
		• Considerations
		  ° Renally cleared
		  ° Generally stop when hospitalized
		  ° Possible vitamin B_{12} deficiency when used long term
		  ° Lactic acidosis risk (rare: 1/30,000 patients)
		  ° Contraindications: Estimated GFR <30 mL/min/1.73 m^2, use with caution if estimated GFR <30 mL/min/1.73 m^2, acidosis, hypoxemia, and alcohol abuse

Sulfonylureas such as glimepiride	• Can cause hypoglycemia
	• Can cause weight gain
		• Benefits
		  ° Inexpensive
		
		• Considerations
		  ° Hepatically metabolized
		  ° Renally cleared
		  ° Caution required in renal and cardiac patients; have active metabolites
		  ° Generally stopped while in hospital

Meglitinides such as repaglinide	• Short action reduction in postprandial glucose
	• May cause hypoglycemia
		• Benefits
		  ° Moderate cost
		  ° Can use in hospital
		  ° Effective treatment for steroid-induced hyperglycemia such as once a day prednisone
		
		• Considerations
		  ° Hepatically metabolized
		  ° Renally cleared
		  ° Frequent dosing

Thiazolidinediones such as pioglitazone	• Edema/weight gain/CHF exacerbation
	  ° Contraindicated in New York Heart Association classes III and IV heart failure
	  ° Increased risk of MI in rosiglitazone; risk has not been shown in pioglitazone
		• Benefits
		  ° Does not cause hypoglycemia
		  ° Inexpensive
		• Considerations
		  ° Not used in hospital
		  ° Delayed onset: Can take up to 12 weeks to achieve peak effect

Alpha glucosidase inhibitors such as acarbose	• GI side effects: Gradual dose titration helps prevent	• Benefits
		  ° Minimal systemic absorption
		  ° Marked reduction in MI rates
		  ° Moderate cost
		
		• Considerations
		  ° Not used in hospital
		  ° Frequent dosing

DPP-4 inhibitors such as sitagliptin	• Minimal side effects
	• Rarely causes hypoglycemia
		• Benefits
		  ° Good oral agent for hospital use
		
		• Considerations
		  ° Renal dose adjustment (except for linagliptin)
		  ° Contraindicated in patients with history of pancreatitis
		  ° High cost

(continued)

TABLE 8.4	Oral Agents Used to Treat Diabetes	
Oral Agent	**Side Effects**	**Benefits and Considerations**

SGLT2 inhibitors such as canagliflozin	• Causes glucosuria
	• Increased risk of genitourinary infections
	• Polyuria, especially when also on diuretics
	• Can cause volume depletion, dehydration, dizziness, and hypotension
	• Cases of DKA
		• Benefits
		  ° Shown to improve cardiovascular disease outcomes
		  ° Empagliflozin (Jardiance) considered best at reducing cardiovascular events
		• Considerations
		  ° Not for use in hospital
		  ° High cost

GLP-1 receptor agonists such as exenatide	• Once-a-week preparations. Prolonged decreased appetite may occur in patients taking these preparations who are admitted to the hospital because medication is likely still having an effect	• Benefits
		  ° Can aid in weight loss
		  ° Can improve cardiovascular risk factors
		  ° Victoza (liraglutide) considered best at reducing cardiovascular events
		• Considerations
		  ° Should not be used in patients with history of medullary thyroid cancer or history of pancreatitis
		  ° Use in the hospital is being studied, but not currently recommended
		  ° Use with narcotic pain medications: Ileus has occurred with GLP-1 receptor agonist use postoperatively in conjunction with narcotic pain medications. Patients should wait until off narcotic pain medications and having no issues with constipation

CHF, congestive heart failure; DKA, diabetic ketoacidosis; DPP-4, dipeptidyl peptidase-4; GFR, glomerular filtration rate; GI, gastrointestinal; GLP-1, glucagon-like peptide-1; MI, myocardial infarction; SGLT2, sodium glucose co-transporter-2.

    ii. Give one-half of the total daily dose as prandial insulin divided evenly between three meals (lispro, aspart, glulisine).

    iii. Add a correction scale using the same rapid-acting insulin used previously.

D. Discharge instructions.

  1. Verify the patient understands how to take the medication as prescribed.

    a. Dose.

    b. Route.

    c. Frequency.

    d. Relationship to meals.

    e. Proper disposal of sharps (for injectables).

    f. Rotation of sites for subcutaneous injections.

    g. Storage.

  2. Make sure the patient is familiar with dietary restrictions.

    a. The patient should aim for consistent amounts of carbohydrates per meal at first. Then the goal will be to learn to dose insulin to the amount of carbohydrates using carbohydrate counting.

  3. Verify the patient is familiar with how to monitor glucose on an ongoing basis.

    a. For oral agents that do not typically cause hypoglycemia.

      i. One to two times a day before meals; can vary which meal.

      ii. Also acceptable: Have HgbA1C checked every 3 to 6 months with provider as an alternative to checking daily.

    b. For oral agents that can cause hypoglycemia.

      i. Consider initially checking glucose before each meal.

      ii. After a period of time, the patient may go to one to two times a day.

    c. For non-insulin injectable agents such as exenatide, one to two times a day (hypoglycemia is rare).

    d. For insulin.

      i. Before meals and bedtime.

      ii. Before and after exercise.

      iii. Before driving.

      iv. More often as needed.

Follow-Up

A. Recommend annual eye examination and podiatry examination.

B. Recommend outpatient education if appropriate.

C. Follow-up with endocrinologist or primary care provider. Specify how soon patient should be seen. Specify when to call provider.

D. Outline hypoglycemia treatment.

  1. Rule of 15: 15 grams of carbohydrates every 15 minutes until glucose above 70 mg/dL (e.g., ½ cup pop, ½ cup juice, glucose gel, glucose tablets).

  2. Carry glucose tablets or gel at all times.

  3. Instruct the patient (if on insulin) to carry a glucagon kit that can be administered by a friend or family member if the patient is unresponsive.

Consultation/Referral

A. Refer the patient to endocrinology for new diagnosis, uncontrolled HgbA1C, multiple complications of diabetes, and comorbid conditions affecting diabetes control.
B. Refer the patient to nephrology for nephropathy.
C. Refer the patient to ophthalmology every 2 years if negative examinations.
D. Refer the patient to podiatry for issues and/or yearly examination.
E. Refer the patient to a dentist for evaluation of gums and oral health problems associated with diabetes such as xerostomia, gingivitis, or signs of infection.
F. Refer the patient to psychology for coping with chronic disease.

Special/Geriatric Considerations

A. More than 25% of U.S. population older than 65 years has diabetes.
B. Diabetes in older adults is associated with higher mortality and reduced functional status.
C. Older adults with diabetes have a higher risk of microvascular and cardiovascular complications of the disease.

Bibliography

Cefalu, W. T. (2017). Standards of medical care in diabetes–2017. *Diabetes Care, 40*(Suppl. 1), s1–s135. doi:10.2337/dc17-S003
Garber, A. J., Abrahamson, M. J., Barzilay, J. I., Blonde, L., Bloomgarden, Z. T., Bush, M. A., . . . Umpierrez, G. E. (2017). Consensus statement by the American Association of Clinical Endocrinologists and American College of Endocrinology on the comprehensive type 2 diabetes management algorithm—2017 executive summary. *Endocrine Practice, 23*(2), 207–238. doi:10.4158/EP161682.CS
Menke, A., Orchard, T., Imperatore, G., Bullard, K., Mayer-Davis, E., & Cowie, C. (2013). The prevalence of type 1 diabetes in the United States. *Epidemiology, 24*, 773–774. doi:10.1097/EDE.0b013e31829ef01a
Mensing, C. (2011). *The art and science of diabetes self-management education desk reference* (2nd ed.). Chicago, IL: Publisher American Association of Diabetes Educators.
National Center for Chronic Disease Prevention and Health Promotion. (2017). *National diabetes statistics report, 2017: Estimates of diabetes and its burden in the United States.* Retrieved from https://www.cdc.gov/diabetes/pdfs/data/statistics/national-diabetes-statistics-report.pdf
Statistics About Diabetes. (n. d.). Retrieved from http://www.diabetes.org/diabetes-basics/statistics/

Diabetic Ketoacidosis

Julie Stone

Definition

A. Life-threatening emergency.
B. Absolute insulin deficiency.
C. Severe hyperglycemia.
D. Ketone body production.
E. Systemic acidosis.
F. Develops over 1 to 2 days.

Incidence

A. 18% of cases of diabetic ketoacidosis (DKA) in hospitals are children with type 1 diabetes.
B. 48% of cases of DKA in hospitals are adults with type 1 diabetes.
C. 34% of cases of DKA in hospitals are adults with type 2 diabetes.
D. Higher rate of DKA for persons age less than 45.
E. One to five episodes per 100 people per year.
F. Average mortality 5% to 10%.

Pathogenesis

A. Unchecked gluconeogenesis leads to hyperglycemia.
  1. Increased glucose production.
  2. Decreased glucose uptake.
B. Osmotic diuresis leads to dehydration.
C. Unchecked ketogenesis leads to ketosis.
D. Dissociation of ketone bodies into hydrogen ions and anions leads to anion gap metabolic acidosis; electrolyte abnormalities.

Predisposing Factors

A. Illness/Infection.
B. Myocardial infarction (MI)/cerebrovascular accident (CVA).
C. Omission of insulin.
D. Minority populations.
E. Newly diagnosed with type 1 diabetes.
F. Poor social support.
G. Mental illness.

Subjective Data

A. Common complaints/symptoms.
  1. Thirst.
  2. Polyuria.
  3. Abdominal pain.
  4. Nausea and vomiting.
  5. Profound weakness.
  6. Fatigue.
  7. Dyspnea.
B. Common/typical scenario. Patients with any form of diabetes who present with certain symptoms should be evaluated for DKA. These symptoms are abdominal pain, nausea, fatigue, and/or dyspnea.

Physical Examination

A. Fruity breath.
B. Vital sign assessment.
  1. Kussmaul respirations.
  2. Supine or orthostatic hypotension.
  3. Diminished peripheral pulses.
  4. Tachycardia.
  5. Hypothermia.
C. Skin examination.
  1. Dry mucous membranes.
  2. Poor skin turgor.

Diagnostic Tests

A. Glucose usually greater than 250 mg/dL.
B. Positive blood and urine ketones.
C. Elevated beta hydroxybutyrate.
D. High anion gap (>12 mEq/L).
E. Low arterial pH (<7.3).
F. Low bicarbonate (<15 mEq/L).
G. Serum hyperosmolality greater than 280 mOsm/L.

Differential Diagnosis

A. Lactic acidosis.
B. Other metabolic acidosis.
C. Starvation ketosis, ketogenic diet.
D. Euglycemic acidosis.
  1. Normal glucose.
  2. Clinical presentation of DKA.
  3. Seen with sodium-glucose cotransporter 2 (SGLT2) inhibitors.

E. Hyperglycemia without ketosis.

F. Hyperosmolar hyperglycemic syndrome.

Evaluation and Management Plan

A. Fluid replacement.

  1. Normal saline (NS) 1 to 2 L over 1 to 2 hours.

  2. Calculation of corrected serum sodium.

    a. High or normal serum sodium: ½ NS at 250 to 500 mL/hr.

    b. Low serum sodium: NS at 250 to 500 mL/hr.

  3. When glucose less than 250 mg/dL: D5%NS or ½ NS.

  4. Suggested rate for fluid replacement.

    a. First hour: 1 to 2 L.

    b. Second hour: 1 L.

    c. Third to fifth hours: 500 to 1,000 mL/hr.

    d. Sixth to 12th hours: 250 to 500 mL/hr.

B. Correction of hyperglycemia/metabolic acidosis.

  1. Intravenous regular insulin infusion.

    a. Bolus: 0.1 to 0.15 units/kg.

    b. Drip rate: 0.1 units/kg/hr.

    c. Check glucose every hour.

      i. If glucose does not decrease by 10% in the first hour, a second loading dose is indicted.

      ii. When glucose less than 250 mg/dL, slow rate to 0.05 to 1 units/kg/hr until resolution of ketoacidosis.

    d. Continue insulin infusion until anion gap closes (<14 mEq/L).

    e. Initiate subcutaneous basal insulin 2 hours prior to stopping drip.

    f. Refer to hospital DKA protocol.

  2. Acceptable to use subcutaneous insulin to treat DKA as well.

    a. Use insulin analogs: Lispro, aspart, or glulisine.

    b. Check glucose every 2 hours and give bolus of analog.

      i. Initial dose 0.2 to 0.3 units/kg.

      ii. Then 0.1 to 0.2 units/kg every 2 hours until glucose less than 250 mg/dL.

      iii. When glucose less than 250 mg/dL add dextrose to intravenous fluids as earlier.

      iv. Continue to give 0.05 to 0.1 unit/kg every 2 hours until anion gap closes.

C. Replacement of electrolyte losses.

  1. Watch for life-threatening hypokalemia, which can occur as insulin is infused.

  2. Monitor potassium closely and treat potassium losses aggressively. Anticipatory potassium replacement during treatment of DKA is usually required.

    a. If potassium is greater than 5.5 mEq/L, then no supplementation is immediately required. Reassess within 2 to 4 hours.

    b. If potassium is 4 to 5.4 mEq/L, give 20 mEq of replacement potassium.

    c. If potassium is 3.3 to 4 mEq/L, give 40 mEq of replacement potassium.

    d. If potassium is less than 3.3 mEq/L, hold starting insulin until potassium is replaced. Give potassium 20 to 30 mEq/hr until potassium is greater than 3.3 mEq/L.

  3. A sharp drop in serum phosphorus can also occur with insulin infusion. Treatment is usually not required.

  4. Bicarbonate is not usually given unless pH less than 7.0 mol/L.

D. Identification and treatment of precipitating causes.

  1. Nonadherence to insulin regimen or psychiatric issues.

  2. Insulin administration error or insulin pump malfunction.

  3. Poor sick day management.

    a. Patients often omit insulin when not eating or having nausea or vomiting.

    b. Patients often forget to check their glucose levels when feeling ill.

  4. Infections.

    a. Intra-abdominal.

    b. Pyelonephritis.

    c. Urinary tract infections (UTIs).

    d. Pneumonia.

    e. Influenza.

  5. MI.

  6. Pancreatitis.

  7. Steroid therapy prescribed with no instructions about adjusting insulin.

  8. CVA.

E. Conversion to a maintenance diabetes regimen; transition to subcutaneous insulin when glucose is less than 200 mg/dL and the anion gap is less than 14 mEq/L.

F. Patient/family teaching points.

  1. Sick day management.

  2. Survival skills.

  3. Glucose monitoring.

  4. Insulin administration.

  5. Use of ketone strips.

  6. Medical alert bracelet.

  7. Preventing DKA.

    a. Recognizing signs and symptoms.

    b. Frequency of glucose testing.

    c. Urine ketone testing.

    d. When to call for help.

G. Discharge instructions.

  1. Ensure the patient has prescriptions for insulin pen, insulin vial, and needles or syringes.

  2. Ensure the patient has prescriptions for glucometer, test strips, and lancets.

  3. Ensure the patient has ketone strips.

  4. Confirm that a follow-up appointment has been made.

  5. Give the patient physician contact phone numbers.

Follow-Up

A. Follow-up should occur with the endocrinologist for a management plan to regulate diabetes.

B. Patients may need to follow-up with social services for assistance with medications.

Consultation/Referral

A. Refer the patient to psychology/social work for assistance with purchasing medications and equipment and for emotional support.

B. Refer the patient to endocrinology for optimized management of diabetes.

Special/Geriatric Considerations

A. End-stage renal disease patients on dialysis.

  1. Absence of osmotic diuresis.

  2. Less volume depleted.

3. High serum potassium.

4. Insulin infusion: Only treatment required in a majority of patients.

5. Emergency hemodialysis: Possible treatment in cases where there is pulmonary edema, profound metabolic acidosis, or severe hyperkalemia with ECG changes.

B. DKA in pregnancy.

    1. DKA can occur rapidly and at a much lower glucose level in pregnant women with diabetes compared to non-pregnant women with diabetes.

    2. The effects of DKA on the fetus are not known. Ketoacids and glucose cross the placenta.

    3. There is a direct relationship between plasma ketone levels in pregnant diabetic women and lower IQ levels in the child.

    4. Presenting symptoms and treatment are the same as in women who are not pregnant.

    5. Certain metabolic changes predispose to ketosis.

        a. Increased insulin resistance.

        b. Insulin requirements that rise during pregnancy.

        c. More cases of DKA in second and third trimesters.

    6. Accelerated starvation.

        a. Use of large amounts of glucose for energy by fetus/placenta.

        b. Lower maternal glucose, leading to relative insulin deficiency.

        c. Increase in free fatty acids, which undergo conversion to ketones in liver.

    7. Emesis.

    8. Stress and fasting state: Can increase insulin antagonistic hormones, which along with dehydration can promote development of ketosis.

    9. Lowered buffering capacity.

    10. Increased minute alveolar ventilation in pregnancy leading to respiratory alkalosis, which is compensated by increased renal excretion of bicarbonate.

Bibliography

Cefalu, W. T. (2017). Standards of medical care in diabetes–2017. *Diabetes Care, 40*(Suppl. 1), s1–s135. doi:10.2337/dc17-S003

Menke, A., Orchard, T., Imperatore, G., Bullard, K., Mayer-Davis, E., & Cowie, C. (2013). The prevalence of type 1 diabetes in the United States. *Epidemiology, 24*, 773–774. doi:10.1097/EDE.0b013e31829ef01a

Mensing, C. (2011). *The art and science of diabetes self-management education desk reference* (2nd ed.). Chicago, IL: Publisher American Association of Diabetes Educators.

Statistics About Diabetes. (n. d.). Retrieved from http://www.diabetes.org/diabetes-basics/statistics/

Hyperglycemic Hyperosmolar State

Julie Stone

Definition

A. Severe relative insulin deficiency, resulting in profound hyperglycemia and hyperosmolality.

B. Absence of acidosis.

C. Develops over days to weeks.

D. Typically presents in type 2 diabetes or in patients with no prior diagnosis of diabetes.

Incidence

A. Hyperglycemic hyperosmolar state (HHS) represents less than 1% of hospital admissions of patient with diabetes.

B. Mortality is between 10% and 20%, which is 10 times higher than mortality for diabetic ketoacidosis (DKA).

C. Condition has been reported in children and young adults.

Pathogenesis

A. Extreme elevations in glucose.

B. Insulin deficiency.

C. Increased levels of counterregulatory hormones.

    1. Glucagon.

    2. Catecholamines.

    3. Cortisol.

    4. Growth hormone.

D. Increased gluconeogenesis.

E. Decreased use of glucose by peripheral tissues.

F. Higher hepatic and circulating insulin concentrations as well as lower glucagon in HHS compared to DKA.

G. Prevention of ketogenesis.

H. Severe hyperglycemia associated with a severe inflammatory state.

Predisposing Factors

A. Elderly patients with type 2 diabetes.

B. Patients with more comorbidities.

C. Infection.

    1. Pneumonia.

    2. Urinary tract infection (UTI).

D. No prior diagnosis of diabetes.

E. Stroke.

F. Myocardial infarction (MI).

G. Trauma.

H. Medications.

    1. Glucocorticoids.

    2. Thiazide diuretics.

    3. Phenytoin (inhibits endogenous insulin secretion).

    4. Beta-blockers.

    5. Atypical antipsychotics.

Subjective Data

A. Common complaints/symptoms.

    1. Dehydration presenting as a shock-like state.

    2. Mental confusion.

    3. Thirst.

    4. Polyuria.

    5. Nausea and vomiting.

    6. Weakness and fatigue.

Physical Examination

A. Ill appearing, likely with decreased level of consciousness.

B. Vital sign assessment.

    1. Tachycardia.

    2. Hypotension.

    3. Tachypnea.

    4. Decreased core temperature.

C. Neurologic findings. When HHS causes neurologic dysfunction, treatment of the HHS results in resolution of neurologic findings. When neurologic events cause HHS the neurologic findings remain after the resolution of the HHS.

    1. Seizures.

    2. Drowsiness and lethargy.

    3. Delirium to coma.

    4. Hemianopsia.

    5. Aphasia.

    6. Paresis.

    7. Positive Babinski sign.

    8. Myoclonic jerks.

    9. Nystagmus.

D. Dermatological findings.
1. Acanthosis nigricans (see Figure 8.1).
2. Diabetic dermopathy.
3. Dry mucous membranes.
4. Decreased skin turgor.
5. Necrobiosis on pretibial surfaces.

E. Funduscopic examination: Retinopathy, premature cataracts, xanthelasma.

F. Decreased urine output.

Diagnostic Tests

A. Plasma glucose: Greater than 600 mg/dL.
B. Arterial pH: Greater than 7.30 mol/L.
C. Serum bicarbonate greater than 18 mEq/L.
D. Urine or serum ketones: Absent or small.
E. Serum beta hydroxybutyrate less than 3 mmol/L.
F. Effective serum osmolality greater than 320 mOsm/L.
G. Anion gap variable.
H. Hemoglobin and hematocrit elevated due to volume contraction.
I. Leukocytosis usually present.
J. Hemoglobin A1C (HgbA1C).
K. Look for underlying cause using the following.
1. Chest x-ray.
2. Urine analysis.
3. Blood and urine cultures.
4. ECG.

Differential Diagnosis

A. DKA.
B. Hyperglycemia without DKA or HHS.
C. Dehydration.
D. Mental status changes or even coma.
E. Intoxication.
F. Sepsis.
G. Postictal state.
H. Diabetes insipidus.

Evaluation and Management Plan

A. Replacement of fluids.
1. Treatment of HHS requires more free water and greater volume replacement than in DKA: Can be as much as 10 L fluid deficit.
2. Rapid and aggressive intravascular volume replacement is necessary.
   a. Use isotonic sodium chloride initially.
   b. Replace one-half of volume in first 12 hours and then remainder over next 12-hour period.
   c. When glucose reaches 250 to 300 mg/dL, switch to D5%NS or ½NS.
3. Use caution in patients with heart failure and kidney disease as well as in those who are elderly.
B. Correction of hyperglycemia.
1. Use intravenous insulin or subcutaneous insulin in doses similar to DKA.
2. Understand that the use of insulin without concomitant vigorous fluid replacement increases the risk of shock.
3. Recheck glucose every 1 to 2 hours.
C. Replacement of electrolytes.
1. Potassium is not usually significantly elevated on admission.
2. Replacement of potassium is required as insulin drops are used. Add potassium to intravenous fluids starting at 5 mEq/L or less.

3. Recheck electrolytes every 2 to 4 hours as clinically indicated.
4. Phosphate, magnesium, and calcium are not routinely replaced.
D. Hospitalization.
1. All patients diagnosed with HHS require hospitalization and virtually all require ICU admission.
2. Neurological monitoring, with "neuro" checks every 2 hours, is important.
E. Detection and treatment of underlying pathology.
1. Some sources advocate prophylactic heparin treatment and broad-spectrum antibiotics until the underlying cause can be established.
F. Conversion to maintenance diabetes regimen prior to discharge.
1. The patient's extreme hyperglycemia usually indicates extensive beta cell dysfunction.
2. Initially patients require discharge on full insulin therapy.
3. Use HgbA1C to help determine glucose control prior to admission.
4. Make transition to subcutaneous insulin when glucose less than 200 mg/dL and the anion gap is less than 14 mEq/L.
G. Patient/family teaching points.
1. Sick day management.
2. Survival skills.
3. Glucose monitoring.
4. Insulin administration.
5. Medical alert bracelet.
H. Discharge instructions.
1. Ensure that the patient has prescriptions for insulin pen, insulin vial, and needles or syringes.
2. Ensure that the patient has prescriptions for glucometer, test strips, and lancets.
3. Confirm that a follow-up appointment has been made.
4. Give the patient physician contact phone numbers.

Follow-Up

A. Follow-up should occur with the endocrinologist for a management plan to regulate diabetes.
B. Patients may need to follow-up with social services for assistance with medications.

Consultation/Referral

A. Refer the patient to psychology for improving adherence to the diabetes regimen.
B. Refer the patient to social work and case management to assist with obtaining medications and resources as needed.

Special/Geriatric Considerations

A. Diabetes in older adults is associated with higher mortality and reduced functional status.
B. Older adults with diabetes have a higher risk of microvascular and cardiovascular complications of the disease.

Bibliography

Azoulay, E., Chevret, S., Didier, J., Neuville, S., Barboteu, M., Bornstain, C., . . . Schlemmer, B. (2001). Infection as a trigger of diabetic ketoacidosis in intensive care unit patients. *Clinical Infectious Disease, 32*, 30–35. doi:10.1086/317554

Joint British Diabetes Societies Inpatient Care Group. (2010, March). *The management of diabetic ketoacidosis in adults.* Retrieved from http://www .diabetes.nhs.uk/document.php?o=1336

Kamalakannan, D., Baskar, V., & Barton, D. M. (2003). Diabetic ketoacidosis in pregnancy. *Postgraduate Medical Journal, 79*, 454–457. doi:10.1136/pmj.79.934.454

Kitabchi, A. E., Umpierrez, G. E., Murphy, M. B., Barrett, E. J., Kreisberg, R. A., Malone, J. I., & Wall, B. M. (2004, January). Hyperglycemic crises in diabetes. *Diabetes Care, 27*(Suppl. 1), S94–S102. doi:10.2337/diacare.27.2007.S94

Pasuel, F. J., & Umpierrez, G. E. (2014). Hyperosmolar hyperglycemic state: A historic review of the clinical presentation, diagnosis, and treatment. *Diabetes Care, 37*, 3124–3131. doi:10.2337/dc14-0984

Wordsworth, G., Robinson, A., Ward, A., & Atkin, M. (2014). HHS—Full or prophylactic anticoagulation? *British Journal of Diabetes and Vascular Disease, 14*, 64–66. doi:10.15277/bjdvd.2014.011

Metabolic Syndrome

Julie Stone

Definition

A. Also called insulin resistance syndrome.

B. A group of traits linked to obesity that puts people at risk for both cardiovascular disease (CVD) and type 2 diabetes.

C. Must have three of the following.

    1. Waist circumference greater than 40 inches in men; greater than 35 inches in women (varies somewhat by ethnicity depending on which guidelines are used).

    2. Triglyceride level of 150 mg/dL or higher or taking medication for elevated triglyceride levels.

    3. High-density lipoprotein (HDL) below 40 mg/dL for men and below 50 mg/dL for women or taking medication for low HDL.

    4. Blood pressure above 130/85 mmHg or taking antihypertensives.

    5. Fasting glucose greater than 100 mg/dL or taking medication for elevated blood glucose.

D. Linked to type 2 diabetes, obesity, CVD, polycystic ovarian syndrome, nonalcoholic fatty liver disease, and chronic kidney disease.

E. Patients with metabolic syndrome are at twice the risk of developing CVD over the next 5 to 10 years as individuals without the syndrome. The risk of developing diabetes is five times higher for individuals with metabolic syndrome.

Incidence

A. About 34% of American adults are thought to have metabolic syndrome.

B. Risk increases as people age.

C. Prevalence is higher in non-Hispanic white men than Mexican American and non-Hispanic black men.

D. The condition is more common in Mexican American women than non-Hispanic black or non-Hispanic white women.

E. Prevalence is increasing globally due to increased obesity and sedentary lifestyles.

Pathogenesis

A. Contributing factors include increased free fatty acid levels, inflammatory cytokines from fat, and oxidative factors.

B. Patients with the characteristics of metabolic syndrome demonstrate a prothrombotic state and a proinflammatory state.

C. Elevated triglycerides and low HDL cholesterol is an atherogenic dyslipidemia condition.

D. The mechanism of how this constellation of risk factors contributes to development of type 2 diabetes and CVD is not completely understood.

Predisposing Factors

A. Sedentary lifestyle.

B. Western diet high in carbohydrates and fats, including saturated fats.

C. Obesity.

D. Family history of diabetes, heart disease, and hyperlipidemia.

Subjective Data

A. Typically, asymptomatic.

B. Patient presentation for a routine physical or a preoperative examination.

Physical Examination

A. Look for abdominal obesity: Record height, weight, body mass index (BMI), waist circumference, and waist to hip ratio.

B. Perform thorough cardiovascular examination.

C. Note skin findings consistent with obesity and insulin resistance.

    1. Skin tags.

    2. Acanthosis nigricans (see Figure 8.1).

D. Note presence of xanthelasma on medial aspect of eyelids, which is suggestive of hyperlipidemia.

Diagnostic Tests

A. Fasting lipid panel.

B. Fasting glucose.

Differential Diagnosis

A. Type 2 diabetes.

B. Prediabetes.

C. Hyperlipidemia.

D. Hypertension.

E. Obesity.

Evaluation and Management Plan

A. General plan. Treatment centers on two principles.

    1. Identify individuals with metabolic syndrome.

    2. Use risk factor modification to prevent CVD and type 2 diabetes.

B. Weight loss.

    1. Routinely measure weight and anthropometric measurements.

C. Healthy diet.

    1. Recommend saturated fat less than 7% of total calories.

    2. Reduce trans fats.

    3. Limit dietary cholesterol to less than 2,000 mg/d.

    4. Restrict total fat to 25% to 35% of total calories.

    5. Choose unsaturated fats.

    6. Limit simple sugars.

D. Increased physical activity.

    1. Encourage 30 to 60 minutes of moderate intensity aerobic activity, preferably daily, supplemented by increase in daily lifestyle activities.

E. Monitoring of blood glucose, lipoproteins, and blood pressure.

F. Treatment of individual risk factors following guidelines for hypertension, hyperlipidemia, and hyperglycemia.

G. Smoking cessation.

Follow-Up

A. Follow-up with primary care providers to monitor underlying problems and to treat cardiovascular risk factors.

Consultation/Referral

A. Endocrinology to manage any underlying problems with diabetes.

B. Cardiology to manage cardiovascular risk factors.

Special/Geriatric Considerations

A. The risk of metabolic syndrome increases with age.

B. People with metabolic syndrome are at increased risk of CVDs.

Bibliography

Aguilar, M., Bhuket, T., & Torres, S. (2015). Prevalence of the metabolic syndrome in the United States, 2003–2012. *Journal of the American Medical Association, 313*, 1973–1974. doi:10.1001/jama.2015.4260

Alberti, K. G., Eckel, R. H., Grundy, S. M., Zimmet, P. Z., Cleeman, J. I., Donato, K. A., . . . Smith, S. C., Jr. (2009). Harmonizing the metabolic syndrome: A joint interim statement of the International Diabetes Federation Task Force on Epidemiology and Prevention; National Heart, Lung, and Blood Institute; American Heart Association; World Heart Federation; International Atherosclerosis Society; and International Association for the Study of Obesity. *Circulation, 120*, 1640–1645. doi:10.1161/CIRCULATIONAHA.109.192644

American Association of Diabetes Educators. (2008). AADE7 self-care behaviors. *Diabetes Educator, 24*, 445–449.

American Diabetes Association. (2010, January). Diagnosis and classification of diabetes mellitus. *Diabetes Care, 33*(Suppl. 1), S62–S69. doi:10.2337/dc10-S062

American Diabetes Association. (2012, January). Standards of medical care in diabetes—2012. *Diabetes Care, 35*(Suppl. 1), S11–S63. doi:10.2337/dc12-s011

American Diabetes Association Professional Practice Committee. (2013, January). American Diabetes Association clinical practice recommendations: 2013. *Diabetes Care, 36*(Suppl. 1), S1–S110.

Pheochromocytoma

Kathryn Evans

Definition

A. A catecholamine-secreting tumor that typically produces one or more of the following hormones: Epinephrine, norepinephrine, or dopamine.

B. Cardiovascular morbidity and mortality may be high for undiagnosed pheochromocytomas (PCCs) due to catecholamine secretion.

C. PCCs enlarge over time and may cause mass effect if undiagnosed.

Incidence

A. 0.2% to 0.6% of patients in an outpatient setting with hypertension have a PCC.

B. Autopsy studies suggest that 0.05% to 1% of patients have undiagnosed PCCs.

C. Peak incidence is between the fourth and fifth decades of life.

D. Approximately 5% of adrenal incidentalomas are PCCs and 10% to 17% of PCCs may be malignant.

E. PCC should be considered in the workup for malignant hypertension, particularly when the patient reports paroxysmal symptoms, has an adrenal incidentaloma, or has a hereditary predisposition to PCC.

Pathogenesis

A. Catecholamine-producing neuroendocrine tumors arising from the adrenomedullary chromaffin cells.

B. Germline mutations: Present in at least one-third of patients presenting with PCC.

C. PCCs may be related to a hereditary condition.

Predisposing Factors

A. 30% of patients have a PCC as part of a genetic disorder.

B. Several genetic conditions predispose patients to PCC, including:

   1. Multiple endocrine neoplasia (MEN) type 2A.

   2. MEN type 2B.

   3. Von Hippel–Lindau syndrome.

   4. Neurofibromatosis type 1.

Subjective Data

A. Common complaints/symptoms.

   1. Signs and symptoms are present in about 50% of patients.

   2. Symptoms are typically paroxysmal.

   3. Classic triad of symptoms includes:

     a. Headache.

     b. Sweating.

     c. Tachycardia.

B. Other signs and symptoms.

   1. Cardiovascular (palpitations).

   2. Anxiety/panic attacks.

   3. Nausea.

   4. Abdominal/chest pain.

   5. Flushing.

   6. Weight loss.

   7. Weakness.

   8. Tremor.

   9. Pallor.

   10. Shortness of breath.

Physical Examination

A. Vital signs.

   1. Tachycardia.

   2. Hypertension.

   3. Weight loss.

B. Complete cardiovascular examination.

C. Skin examination.

   1. Pallor.

   2. Flushing.

Diagnostic Tests

A. Testing for PCC is necessary if there is:

   1. Previous history of PCC.

   2. Symptoms of PCC, especially if they occur in a paroxysmal manner.

   3. Adrenal incidentaloma.

   4. Hereditary predisposition to PCC.

B. Initial testing involves two types of metanephrine tests.

   1. Urinary fractionated metanephrines should be a 24-hour urine collection and include a creatinine level.

   2. Plasma-free metanephrines should be drawn with the patient in the supine position.

     a. Sympathetic activation occurs in the upright position and can falsely elevate catecholamine levels.

     b. Ideally, patients should be in the supine position for 30 minutes prior to blood draw.

C. False positive results are common.

   1. Physiologic stress such as hospitalization may elevate hormones and should be considered contributing factors to elevations.

   2. Multiple drugs can cause false positive results, including:

     a. Acetaminophen.

     b. Beta-blockers: Labetalol, sotalol.

c. Tricyclic antidepressants.
d. Sympathomimetics.
e. Buspirone.
f. Monoamine oxidase (MAO) inhibitors.
g. Cocaine.

3. Confirmatory testing is needed if positive results are believed to be influenced by any of these factors.
D. When biochemical results suggest a PCC, imaging is necessary. A CT scan should be ordered to locate the mass (CT preferred over MRI).
E. An MRI should be used in patients when a CT scan cannot be performed (e.g., allergy to CT contrast, or when attempting to limit radiation, such as in pregnant women).
F. All patients with PCCs should consider genetic testing to assess for other related conditions such as the MEN syndromes.

Differential Diagnosis

A. Labile essential hypertension.
B. Malignant hypertension.
C. Illegal drug use such as phencyclidine or cocaine.
D. Combining multiple pharmacologic agents such as MAO inhibitors, decongestants, or sympathomimetics.
E. Stroke.
F. Myocardial infarction.
G. Anxiety disorder.
H. Hyperthyroidism.
I. Hypoglycemia (including insulinoma).
J. Alcohol withdrawal.

Evaluation and Management Plan

A. General plan. Treatment involves surgery.
 1. Preoperative management.
  a. Preoperative medical treatment should occur for 7 to 14 days if possible to stabilize blood pressure (BP) and heart rate.
  b. Patients with hormonally active PCCs should undergo preoperative blockage with an *a*-adrenergic receptor blocker such as phenoxybenzamine or doxazosin. Calcium channel blockers can be used as secondary agents for further BP control.
  c. Beta-blockers can be added after initiation of an *a*-adrenergic receptor blocker to control heart rate. They should not be added before *a*-adrenergic receptor blockers due to the potential for hypertensive crisis if the *a*-adrenergic receptors are unopposed.
  d. *a*-Methyl-paratyrosine (metyrosine) can be used for a short time preoperatively in combination with an *a*-adrenergic receptor blocker to further stabilize BP and reduce blood loss and volume depletion during surgery.
  e. Initiating a continuous saline infusion the evening before surgery is another helpful approach to minimize volume depletion.
  f. Preoperative diet should include high sodium and high fluid intake to prevent hypotension after the tumor removal.
  g. Monitor heart rate, BP, and blood glucose in the pre- and postoperative periods.
 2. Operative procedure.
  a. Most PCCs can be removed via minimally invasive adrenalectomy.
  b. Open resection is recommended for large tumors greater than 6 cm or for invasive tumors.
 3. Postoperative management.

  a. The most common postoperative complications include hypertension, hypotension, and rebound hypoglycemia.
  b. Heart rate, BP, and glucose should be monitored for 24 to 48 hours.
  c. For patients who are at risk for adrenal insufficiency (AI) after surgery, particular attention should be paid to signs and symptoms of AI.
B. Patient/family teaching points.
 1. Consider genetic testing, if not already completed, for other potential family members at risk.
C. Discharge instructions (if standard accepted guidelines exist please use discharge template).
 1. Monitor BP at home, counseling particularly on the potential for low or labile BP.
 2. Monitor postoperative incision for any signs of infection.
 3. Discuss the symptoms of PCC and the recommendation for annual biochemical monitoring to ensure long-term disease remission.

Follow-Up

A. Biochemical testing should be repeated 2 to 4 weeks after surgery to ensure complete tumor resection.
B. Annual biochemical monitoring is recommended to assess for recurrent disease.

Consultation/Referral

A. Consultation with an endocrinologist and an endocrine surgeon is preferred for optimal patient outcomes.
B. It is recommended that patients with PCCs be treated by multidisciplinary teams at centers with expertise in this condition. Some studies suggest that there is lower postoperative mortality and shorter hospital stays in high-volume centers, but these data are not conclusive.

Special/Geriatric Considerations

A. Patients with metastatic disease or general complexity should always be referred to high-volume centers with expertise in the management of PCCs.

Bibliography

Lenders, J. W., Duh, Q.-Y., Eisenhofer, G., Gimenez-Roqueplo, A.-P., Grebe, S. K., Murad, M. H., . . . Young, W. F., Jr. (2014). Pheochromocytoma and paraganglioma: An endocrine society clinical practice guideline. *Journal of Clinical Endocrinology & Metabolism, 99*(6), 1915–1942. doi:10.1210/jc.2014-1498
Young, W. F., Jr. (2018, December 11). Clinical presentation and diagnosis of pheochromocytoma. In K. A. Martin (Ed.), *UpToDate*. Retrieved from https://www.uptodate.com/contents/clinical-presentation-and-diagnosis-of-pheochromocytoma

Prediabetes

Julie Stone

Definition

A. Failing pancreatic islet beta cells.
B. State of insulin resistance.
C. Caused by excess body weight, usually abdominal/visceral obesity.
D. Dyslipidemia.
E. Elevated triglycerides.
F. Low high-density lipoprotein (HDL) cholesterol.
G. Hypertension.

Incidence

A. In 2012, 86 million Americans age 20 and older had pre-diabetes; this is up from 79 million in 2010.

Pathogenesis

A. Insulin resistance. There is a marked decrease in insulin sensitivity 5 years prior to diagnosis of type 2 diabetes.
B. Relative insulin deficiency; beta cell dysfunction. Beta cell function is increased 3 to 4 years prior to the diagnosis of diabetes and then decreased immediately prior to the diabetes diagnosis.

Predisposing Factors

A. Obesity.
  1. Body mass index (BMI) greater than 25 in all but Asians.
  2. BMI greater than 23 in Asian Americans.
B. First-degree relative with diabetes.
C. Higher risk in certain ethnic populations.
  1. African Americans.
  2. Latino.
  3. Native Americans.
  4. Asian Americans.
  5. Pacific Islanders.
D. Women with history of gestational diabetes.
E. History of cardiovascular disease.
F. Hypertension greater than 140/90 mmHg.
G. HDL less than 35 mg/dL.
H. Triglycerides greater than 250 mg/dL.
I. Women with history of polycystic ovary syndrome.
J. Women who have given birth to a baby weighing over 9 lbs.
K. Physically inactive.
L. Physical findings of insulin resistance.
  1. Skin tags.
  2. Acanthosis nigricans (see Figure 8.1).
M. Obstructive sleep apnea.
N. Can have patient take American Diabetes Association risk test at www.diabetes.org.

Subjective Data

A. Common complaints/symptoms.
B. Usually asymptomatic.
C. Patient may present for routine physical or preoperative assessment.

Physical Examination

A. Record height, weight, BMI, waist circumference, waist to hip ratio.
B. Monitor for abdominal obesity.
C. Assess for signs of cardiovascular disease and peripheral vascular disease.
D. Check for the following signs/symptoms.
  1. Premature arcus cornealis.
  2. Xanthelasma.
  3. Polycystic ovarian syndrome symptoms.
    a. Acne.
    b. Hair loss.
    c. Hirsutism.
  4. Acanthosis nigricans (see Figure 8.1).
  5. Presence of skin tags.

Diagnostic Tests

A. Hemoglobin A1C (HgbA1C): 5.7% to 6.4%.
B. Fasting glucose: 100 to 125 mg/dL.
C. Random glucose: 140 to 199 mg/dL.

Differential Diagnosis

A. Metabolic syndrome.
B. Type 2 diabetes.
C. Obesity.
D. Hypertension.
E. Hyperlipidemia.

Evaluation and Management Plan

A. General plan: Lifestyle therapy.
  1. Treat cardiovascular risk factors.
    a. Dyslipidemia.
    b. Hypertension.
  2. Weight loss/management.
    a. This can be achieved through lifestyle, pharmacotherapy, surgery, or a combination of treatments.
    b. Bariatric surgery can be very effective in preventing progression of prediabetes to type 2 diabetes.
  3. Nutrition therapy.
  4. Physical activity.
  5. Sleep.
  6. Community engagement.
  7. Alcohol moderation.
  8. Smoking cessation.
B. Pharmacotherapy.
  1. No medications are approved by the Food and Drug Administration solely for the management of prediabetes and the prevention of type 2 diabetes.
  2. Medications should not be considered the only therapy. All medications should be combined with lifestyle modifications.
  3. Metformin reduces risk of type 2 diabetes mellitus (T2DM) in prediabetes patients by 25% to 30%.
  4. Acarbose reduces risk of T2DM in prediabetes patients by 25% to 30%.
  5. Consider with caution use of thiazolidinediones (prevent development of type 2 diabetes by 60%–75%) or glucagon-like peptide-1 (GLP-1) receptor agonists.

Follow-Up

A. Follow-up with primary provider as needed to manage risk factors.

Consultation/Referral

A. Refer the patient to a registered dietician for diet education/counseling.
B. Refer the patient to a psychologist/counselor for stress reduction and life coaching.
C. An exercise physiologist may help with planning a realistic exercise program.
D. Refer the patient to a lipid clinic for management of hyperlipidemia.

Special/Geriatric Considerations

A. The risk of diabetes increases with age.
B. Microvascular and cardiovascular complications are more common in the elderly and should be monitored closely.

Bibliography

Bock, G., Dalla Man, C., Campioni, M., Chittilapilly, E., Basu, R., Toffolo, G., . . . Rizza, R. (2006). Pathogenesis of pre-diabetes: Mechanisms of fasting and postprandial hyperglycemia in people with impaired fasting glucose and/or impaired glucose tolerance. *Diabetes, 55*, 3536–3549. doi:10.2337/db06-0319

Grundy, S. M. (2012). Pre-diabetes, metabolic syndrome, and cardiovascular risk. *Journal of the American College of Cardiology, 59*(7), 635–643. doi:10.1016/j.jacc.2011.08.080

Thyroid Disorder—Euthyroid Sick Syndrome

Lisa Coco

Definition
A. Term designated for those patients with nonthyroid illnesses who have abnormal thyroid tests and can be classified into the following categories.
   1. Low T3 syndrome (most common).
   2. Low T3 and low T4 syndrome.
   3. High T4 syndrome.
   4. Mixed form in which a combination of abnormalities may be found.

Incidence
A. Euthyroid sick syndrome can affect people of all races.
B. It affects both sexes equally.
C. It occurs in people of any age.

Pathogenesis
A. Almost 90% of the hormones secreted by the thyroid gland are T4 and approximately 10% are T3. Most of T4 is converted into T3 in the peripheral tissues, accounting for 90% of the production of T3. The more physiologically active hormone is T3, which is four times more potent than T4.
B. The most common factor in these conditions is reduced extrathyroidal conversion of T4 to T3.
C. With low T3 syndrome, the FT3 is low and the FT4 is normal.
D. The patient is clinically euthyroid and the leading cause in many circumstances is from systemic illness.
E. The low T3 resolves when the underlying illness clears.
F. The low T3 and low T4 syndrome is usually identified in severely ill patients.
G. The TSH early in the illness may be low or normal.
   1. As the illness progresses and recovery ensues, the thyroid-stimulating hormone (TSH) is often above normal.
   2. Patients who have severely low T3 and T4 levels generally do not do well; mortality approaches 84%.
   3. High T4 syndrome is caused by increased concentrations of thyroid-binding globulin produced in certain liver diseases causing high T4 levels. T4 usually returns to normal within 6 to 8 weeks as the disease stabilizes.

Predisposing Factors
A. Acute or chronic illness.
B. Medications.
C. Other endocrine disorders.
D. Burns.
E. Extreme heat or cold.
F. Starvation.

Subjective Data
A. Common complaints/symptoms.
   1. Most often, there are no associated symptoms. Careful history and physical examination will not reveal the typical features of hypothyroidism. Lab values will be abnormal.
   2. If there are symptoms, they are specific to each case.
B. Common/typical scenario.
   1. Patients are usually symptomatic. The condition is found typically during routine screening for thyroid disease.

C. Family and social history.
   1. No relevant family or social history.
D. Review of systems.
   1. Negative review of systems.

Physical Examination
A. There are no particular findings for patients with nonthyroidal illness.
B. The examination findings in each patient reflect the characteristics of the nonthyroidal disease.

Diagnostic Tests
A. Total T4.
B. Total T3.
C. TSH.
D. Free T4.
E. Reverse T3.
F. Free T3.

Differential Diagnosis
A. Hashimoto's thyroiditis.
B. Hyperthyroidism.
C. Hypopituitarism.
D. Hypothyroidism.
E. Thyroid dysfunction induced by amiodarone.

Evaluation and Management Plan
A. General plan.
   1. Monitor thyroid levels as needed if patient becomes symptomatic. Refer to healthcare provider.
B. Patient and family teaching.
   1. If symptoms of hypothyroidism or hyperthyroidism occur, call your healthcare provider.
C. Pharmacology.
   1. There is no evidence to date demonstrating the benefit of thyroid replacement in nonthyroidal illness.
D. Discharge instructions.
   1. No clear agreement on treatment exists. Hormone replacement with levothyroxine may not help these patients. Allowing for recovery time of the illness and checking thyroid function weeks after the illness resolves are the best treatment for euthyroid sick patients.

Follow-Up
A. Follow-up with primary care provider after release from the hospital.
B. Refer to endocrinology.

Consultation/Referral
A. Referral to an endocrinologist is recommended for monitoring of thyroid function tests both during and after recovery from nonthyroidal illness.

Bibliography
American Association of Clinical Endocrinologists. (2016). *Hyperthyroidism: Information for patients*. Retrieved from http://thyroidawareness.com/sites/all/files/hyperthyroidism.pdf
Brenner, Z., & Porsche, R. (2006). Amiodarone-induced thyroid dysfunction. *Critical Care Nurse, 26*(3), 34–41.
Burch, W. (1994). *Endocrinology* (3rd ed.). Baltimore, MD: Williams & Wilkins.
Burman, K., Ellahham, S., Fadel, B., Lindsay, J., Ringel, M., & Wartofsky, L. (2000). Hyperthyroid heart disease. *Clinical Cardiology, 23*(26), 402–408. doi:10.1002/clc.4960230605
Carroll, R., & Matfin, G. (2010). Endocrine and metabolic emergencies: Thyroid storm. *Therapeutic Advances in Endocrinology and Metabolism, 1*(3), 139–145. doi:10.1177/2042018810382481

Chowdhury, S., Ghosh, S., Mathew, V., Misgar, R., Mukhopadhyay, P., Mukhopadhyay, S., . . . Roychowdhury, P. (2011). Myxedema coma: A new look into an old crisis. *Journal of Thyroid Research, 2011,* 1–7. doi:10.4061/2011/493462

Dahlen, R., & Kumrow, D. (2002). Thyroidectomy: Understanding the potential for complications. *MEDSURG Nursing, 11*(5), 228–235.

Francis, J., & Jayaprasad, N. (2005). Atrial fibrillation and hyperthyroidism. *Indian Pacing and Electrophysiology Journal, 5*(4), 305–311.

Holcomb, S. (2002). Thyroid diseases: A primer for the critical care nurse. *Dimensions of Critical Care Nursing, 21*(4), 127–133. doi:10.1097/00003465-200207000-00003

Lee, S. (2018, March 15). Hyperthyroidism and thyrotoxicosis. In R. Khardori (Ed.), *Medscape.* Retrieved from http://emedicine.medscape.com/article/121865-overview

Manzullo, E. F., & Ross, D. S. (2019, February 26). Nonthyroid surgery in the patient with thyroid disease. In J. E. Mulder (Ed.), *UpToDate.* Retrieved from https://www.uptodate.com/contents/nonthyroid-surgery-in-the-patient-with-thyroid-disease

Merrill, E. (2013). A devastating storm. *The Medicine Forum, 14*(12), 24–25. doi:10.29046/TMF.014.1.012

The Nurse Practitioner: The American Journal of Primary Healthcare. (2005). *Thyroid Disorders, 30*(6), 51–52.

Roman, S. (2017). Current best practices in the management of thyroid nodules and cancer. (PowerPoint slides). Retrieved from https://reachmd.com/programs/cme/current-best-practices-in-the-management-of-thyroid-nodules-and-cancer/8470/transcript/16717/

Ross, D. (2018, September 27). Thyroid function in nonthyroidal illness. In J. E. Mulder (Ed.), *UpToDate.* Retrieved from https://www.uptodate.com/contents/thyroid-function-in-nonthyroidal-illness

Ross, D., & Sugg, S. (2018, September 25). Surgical management of hyperthyroidism. In J. E. Mulder (Ed.), *UpToDate.* Retrieved from https://www.uptodate.com/contents/surgical-management-of-hyperthyroidism

Tuttle, R. (2018, January 17). Differentiated thyroid cancer: Clinicopathologic staging. In J. E. Mulder (Ed.), *UpToDate.* Retrieved from https://www.uptodate.com/contents/differentiated-thyroid-cancer-clinicopathologic-staging/print

Umpierrez, G. (2002). Euthyroid sick syndrome. *Southern Medical Journal, 95*(5), 506–513. doi:10.1097/00007611-200295050-00007

Thyroid Disorder—Hyperthyroidism

Lisa Coco

Definition

A. If the thyroid-stimulating hormone (TSH) level is too low, the thyroid is producing too much hormone, specifically T3 and possibly T4. This is called hyperthyroidism.

B. Set of disorders that involve excess synthesis and secretion of thyroid hormones by the thyroid gland, which leads to the hypermetabolic state of thyrotoxicosis.

C. The main autoimmune cause of hyperthyroidism is Graves' disease.

D. Three main causes.

1. Diffuse toxic goiter (Graves' disease).
2. Toxic multinodular goiter.
3. Toxic adenoma.

Incidence

A. Hyperthyroidism affects approximately 3 million people.

B. Graves' disease.

1. This is the most common form of hyperthyroidism in the United States, causing approximately 60% to 80% of cases of thyrotoxicosis.
2. Its peak occurrence is at age 20 to 40 years.

C. Toxic multinodular goiter causes approximately 15% to 20% of thyrotoxicosis, occurring more frequently in regions of iodine deficiency. Toxic adenoma is the cause of approximately 3% to 5% of cases {9}.

Pathogenesis

A. Hyperthyroidism results from excess production of thyroid hormone from the thyroid gland.

B. Untreated toxicosis can increase the incidence of cardiovascular and pulmonary complications, skin and bone conditions, and eye disease.

Predisposing Factors

A. Genetic factors: Graves' disease often occurs in multiple members of a family.

B. Autoimmune thyroid disorders.

C. Hashimoto's disease.

Subjective Data

A. Common complaints/symptoms.

1. Palpitations, sweating, extreme fatigue, may have presence of goiter, and weight loss.

B. Common/typical scenario.

1. Patient presents with extreme fatigue or anxiety and/or significant weight loss over a short period of time and often complains of palpitations.

C. Family and social history.

1. May have a genetic or familial history.

D. Review of systems.

1. Cardiovascular: Ask about palpitations or recent increases in blood pressure medications.
2. Head, eyes, ears, nose, and throat (HEENT: Hair loss.
3. Psych: Insomnia, anxiety, irritability, nervousness, increased perspiration.
4. Endocrine: Menstrual irregularities, weight loss, heat intolerance, thinning skin.
5. Musculoskeletal—muscle weakness, myalgias, arthralgias.

Physical Examination

A. Constitutional—appears toxic.

B. Cardiovascular—systolic hypertension with a wide pulse pressure, tachycardia, atrial fibrillation.

C. HEENT: Palpable diffuse goiter, thyroid bruit, exophthalmos, periorbital edema, proptosis, lid lag.

D. Neurological/musculoskeletal—tremors, hyperreflexia.

E. Dermatological—warm moist skin, pretibial myxedema.

F. Psychological—anorexia, difficulty focusing.

Diagnostic Tests

A. TSH level: Most reliable screening measure. It is usually suppressed to an immeasurable level (<0.05 mIU/L) in thyrotoxicosis.

B. Free T4—may or may not be elevated.

C. Free T3—will be elevated.

D. Thyroid-stimulating immunoglobulin (TSI) or thyrotropin receptor antibodies (G1) to establish Graves' disease. Thyroid peroxidase (TPO) level or antimicrosomal antibodies are usually elevated with Graves' disease but are usually low or absent in toxic multinodular goiter and toxic adenoma.

E. Thyroid uptake scan to determine the pattern of uptake, which varies with the underlying disorder. Normal radioactive iodine uptake after 6 hours is 2% to 16%; after 24 hours, it is about 8% to 25%. In hyperthyroidism there will be markedly increased uptake.

Differential Diagnosis

A. Euthyroid sick syndrome.

B. Thyroiditis.

C. Goiter.

D. Struma ovarii.

E. Graves' disease.

Evaluation and Management Plan

A. General plan.

1. Symptom management—help the patient to establish symptom control with medications.

2. Further laboratory studies.

a. Repeat TSH every 6 weeks or as needed until symptoms controlled.

b. Check TSI and TPO to rule out Graves' disease or Hashimoto's thyroiditis, respectively.

3. Nuclear thyroid scanning to differentiate hyperthyroidism from thyroiditis.

B. Patient and family teaching.

1. Definitive treatment plan must be established and coordinated with endocrinology.

2. Reinforce need to see endocrinology on a regular basis.

3. If you develop flu-like symptoms while on antithyroid medications, call your provider immediately and stop your medications completely.

C. Pharmacotherapy.

1. Treatment consists of symptom relief with the following drugs.

a. Beta-blockers—titrate to heart rate less than 90 beats per minute and to reduce the sympathetic response associated with peripheral conversion of T4 to T3. Effects of beta-blockers are dramatic and rapid (within 10 minutes).

i. Propranolol best studied in this class of medications.

ii. Other beta-blockers have similar effects and can be used.

b. Antithyroid medications—prevents thyroid hormone synthesis.

i. Methimazole (Tapazole) is considered the first-line drug therapy.

ii. Propylthiouracil (PTU) is preferred in thyroid storm and first trimester of pregnancy.

c. Corticosteroids.

i. Dexamethasone contributes to blocking T4 to T3 conversion, which will control symptoms. Useful in emergencies, but has long-term complications to consider.

2. Radioactive iodine-131 therapy ablates thyroid tissue.

a. Thyroid cancer.

b. Hyperthyroidism not controlled with medical therapy.

3. Thyroidectomy: May be preferable to radioactive iodine-131 therapy.

a. May be required for large goiters causing airway constriction and severe dysphagia.

b. Thyroid cancers not responsive to radioactive iodine 131 therapy.

D. Imaging studies: Ultrasound, CT scan, and chest x-ray are routine. Fine needle aspiration for biopsy, vocal cord evaluation, or esophageal evaluation may be needed depending on the patient's presentation.

1. Monitor for thyroid storm, particularly in the first 18 hours postsurgery.

a. Treat with antithyroid medications until euthyroid.

b. Beta-blockers: Atenolol should be taken 1 hour before surgery to maintain blockade.

E. Discharge instructions.

1. Before discharge, refer the patient to outpatient endocrinology and to ophthalmology, if needed, for eye disease.

Follow-Up

A. Continue to monitor symptoms and thyroid levels.

B. Check TSH 6 weeks after discharge.

Consultation/Referral

A. Refer to endocrinology to manage symptoms and disease progression.

Special/Geriatric Considerations

A. In the acute care setting, the focus should be on the adverse effects of antithyroid medications.

1. Rash.

2. Urticaria.

3. Arthralgia.

B. Monitoring of results of lab studies is also important.

1. Complete blood count (CBC) for agranulocytosis if patient develops a fever or sore throat. Routine monitoring not recommended.

2. Hepatic profile for hepatitis.

C. In addition, monitor the development of fever (>100.5°F) or a sore throat; the medication will need to be stopped.

Bibliography

American Association of Clinical Endocrinologists. (2016). *Hyperthyroidism: Information for patients.* Retrieved from http://thyroidawareness.com/sites/all/files/hyperthyroidism.pdf

Brenner, Z., & Porsche, R. (2006). Amiodarone-induced thyroid dysfunction. *Critical Care Nurse, 26*(3), 34–41.

Burch, W. (1994). *Endocrinology* (3rd ed.). Baltimore, MD: Williams & Wilkins.

Burman, K., Ellahham, S., Fadel, B., Lindsay, J., Ringel, M., & Wartofsky, L. (2000). Hyperthyroid heart disease. *Clinical Cardiology, 23*(26), 402–408. doi:10.1002/clc.4960230605

Carroll, R., & Matfin, G. (2010). Endocrine and metabolic emergencies: Thyroid storm. *Therapeutic Advances in Endocrinology and Metabolism, 1*(3), 139–145. doi:10.1177/2042018810382481

Dahlen, R., & Kumrow, D. (2002). Thyroidectomy: Understanding the potential for complications. *MEDSURG Nursing, 11*(5), 228–235.

Francis, J., & Jayaprasad, N. (2005). Atrial fibrillation and hyperthyroidism. *Indian Pacing and Electrophysiology Journal, 5*(4), 305–311.

Holcomb, S. (2002). Thyroid diseases: A primer for the critical care nurse. *Dimensions of Critical Care Nursing, 21*(4), 127–133. doi:10.1097/00003465-200207000-00003

Lee, S. (2018, March 15). Hyperthyroidism and thyrotoxicosis. In R. Khardori (Ed.), *Medscape.* Retrieved from http://emedicine.medscape.com/article/121865-overview

Manzullo, E. F., & Ross, D. S. (2019, February 26). Nonthyroid surgery in the patient with thyroid disease. In J. E. Mulder (Ed.), *UpToDate.* Retrieved from https://www.uptodate.com/contents/nonthyroid-surgery-in-the-patient-with-thyroid-disease

Mathew, V., Misgar, R. A., Ghosh, S., Mukhopadhyay, P., Roychowdhury, P., Pandit, K., . . . Chowdhury, S. (2011). Myxedema coma: A new look into an old crisis. *Journal of Thyroid Research,* 1–7. doi: 10.4061/2011/493462

Merrill, E. (2013). A devastating storm. *The Medicine Forum, 14*(12), 24–25. doi:10.29046/TMF.014.1.012

The Nurse Practitioner: The American Journal of Primary Healthcare. (2005). *Thyroid Disorders, 30*(6), 51–52.

Roman, S. (2017). Current best practices in the management of thyroid nodules and cancer. (PowerPoint slides). Retrieved from https://reachmd.com/programs/cme/current-best-practices-in-the-management-of-thyroid-nodules-and-cancer/8470/transcript/16717/

Ross, D. (2018, September 27). Thyroid function in nonthyroidal illness. In J. E. Mulder (Ed.), *UpToDate.* Retrieved from Retrieved from https://www.uptodate.com/contents/thyroid-function-in-nonthyroidal-illness

Ross, D., & Sugg, S. (2018, September 25). Surgical management of hyperthyroidism. In J. E. Mulder (Ed.), *UpToDate.* Retrieved from https://www.uptodate.com/contents/surgical-management-of-hyperthyroidism

Tuttle, R. (2018, January 17). Differentiated thyroid cancer: Clinicopathologic staging. In J. E. Mulder (Ed.), *UpToDate.* Retrieved from https://www.uptodate.com/contents/differentiated-thyroid-cancer-clinicopathologic-staging/print

Umpierrez, G. (2002). Euthyroid sick syndrome. *Southern Medical Journal*, *95*(5), 506–513. doi:10.1097/00007611-200295050-00007

Thyroid Disorder—Hypothyroidism

Lisa Coco

Definition

A. If the thyroid-stimulating hormone (TSH) level is too high, the thyroid gland is not producing enough thyroid hormone, specifically T4 and possibly T3. This is called hypothyroidism.
B. Develops when the thyroid gland produces less than the normal amount of thyroid hormones. This leads to low serum levels of T4.
C. Results in the slowing of several bodily functions.
D. The main autoimmune cause of hypothyroidism is Hashimoto's disease.

Incidence

A. Hypothyroidism affects approximately 10 million people.
B. It affects approximately 10% of women and 3% of men in the outpatient setting.
C. Inhibits natural mechanism of metabolism in the body affecting many organ systems. Also associated with increased serum cholesterol levels, which may increase the risk for atherosclerosis and heart disease.

Pathogenesis

A. Insufficient production of thyroid hormone from thyroid gland.
B. Three causes.
  1. Primary: Occurs at the thyroid.
  2. Secondary: Results from problems with the pituitary.
  3. Tertiary: Results from problems at the level of the hypothalamus.

Predisposing Factors

A. Age and sex.
B. Family history.
C. Any autoimmune disorder: Autoimmune thyroiditis.
D. Subacute thyroiditis.
E. Radioactive iodine treatment.
F. Spontaneous onset.
G. Thyroid surgery or medications.
H. Postpartum thyroiditis.
I. Congenital condition.

Subjective Data

A. Common complaints/symptoms.
  1. Weight gain, fatigue, forgetfulness, dry hair/nail changes, cold intolerance, menstrual irregularities.
B. Common/typical scenario.
  1. Patient presents with persistent fatigue and inability to lose weight. The patient will complain that he or she just does not feel right.
C. Family and social history.
  1. May have a familial link.
D. Review of systems.
  1. Constitution—ask about recent viral infections, pervasive fatigue, drowsiness, forgetfulness, learning difficulties.
  2. Dermatological—dry brittle hair and nails, itchy skin.
  3. Psychological—recent depression, feeling sadness, decreased libido, irritability.
  4. Endocrine—cold intolerance, menstrual irregularities, miscarriages.
  5. Musculoskeletal—muscle cramps, soreness.

Physical Examination

A. Cardiovascular—low blood pressure, bradycardia, fluid retention.
B. HEENT—periorbital edema, assess for presence of goiter, dysphagia, eyebrow hair loss, possible scalp hair loss.
C. Neuro/musculoskeletal—lower extremity fluid retention, myalgia, arthralgia, hyporeflexia.
D. Dermatological—dry skin, coarse.

Diagnostic Tests

A. TSH (0.4–5 uIU/mL).
B. Free T4 (0.8–1.8 ug/dL).
C. Thyroid antibodies.
  1. Thyroid peroxidase (TPO) level (<35 IU/mL).

Differential Diagnosis

A. Anemia.
B. Addison's disease.
C. Anovulation.
D. Dysmenorrhea.
E. Cardiac tamponade.
F. Pericardial effusion.
G. Chronic fatigue syndrome.
H. Depression.
I. Thyroiditis.
J. Euthyroid sick syndrome.
K. Goiter.
L. Hypothermia.
M. Constipation.
N. Infertility.
O. Iodine deficiency.
P. Menopause.
Q. Hyperlipidemia.
R. Pituitary disorders.

Evaluation and Management Plan

A. General plan.
  1. Normalize thyroid levels by starting thyroid hormone replacement therapy.
  2. Routine laboratory testing every 6 weeks to adjust dose accordingly until stabilized.
B. Patient and family teaching.
  1. Teach patient signs and symptoms of hypothyroidism and when to call provider, including increase in fatigue, unexplained weight gain and fluid retention, increase in hair loss, arthralgias, and myalgias.
  2. Labs must be checked every 6 weeks for a period of time until the medications can be normalized to patient tolerance and TSH goal is reached.
C. Pharmacology.
  1. Treatment consists of administering the synthetic thyroid hormone levothyroxine.
    a. Dose is based on weight in kilograms multiplied by 1.6 and can be administered orally or intravenously in the hospital setting at 50% to 80% of the PO dose. It should be taken on an empty stomach with no food, no other medications or caffeine for 1 hour, and no supplements for 4 hours.

Follow-Up

A. Ensure patient adherence to treatment regimen.
B. Stress the importance of taking medication daily at approximately the same time.

C. Stress the importance of laboratory checks of TSH level every 6 to 8 weeks.

Consultation/Referral

A. Once discharged, referral to an outpatient endocrinologist is recommended.

Special/Geriatric Considerations

A. Keep TSH levels for geriatric patients in the midrange to avoid the incidence of cardiac side effects such as atrial fibrillation or tachycardia.

Bibliography

American Association of Clinical Endocrinologists. (2016). *Hyperthyroidism: Information for patients.* Retrieved from http://thyroidawareness.com/sites/all/files/hyperthyroidism.pdf

Brenner, Z., & Porsche, R. (2006). Amiodarone-induced thyroid dysfunction. *Critical Care Nurse, 26*(3), 34–41.

Burch, W. (1994). *Endocrinology* (3rd ed.). Baltimore, MD: Williams & Wilkins.

Burman, K., Ellahham, S., Fadel, B., Lindsay, J., Ringel, M., & Wartofsky, L. (2000). Hyperthyroid heart disease. *Clinical Cardiology, 23*(26), 402–408.

Carroll, R., & Matfin, G. (2010). Endocrine and metabolic emergencies: Thyroid storm. *Therapeutic Advances in Endocrinology and Metabolism, 1*(3), 139–145. doi:10.1177/2042018810382481

Chowdhury, S., Ghosh, S., Mathew, V., Misgar, R., Mukhopadhyay, P., Mukhopadhyay, S., . . . Roychowdhury, P. (2011). Myxedema coma: A new look into an old crisis. *Journal of Thyroid Research, 2011*, 1–7. doi:10.4061/2011/493462

Dahlen, R., & Kumrow, D. (2002). Thyroidectomy: Understanding the potential for complications. *MEDSURG Nursing, 11*(5), 228–235.

Francis, J., & Jayaprasad, N. (2005). Atrial fibrillation and hyperthyroidism. *Indian Pacing and Electrophysiology Journal, 5*(4), 305–311.

Holcomb, S. (2002). Thyroid diseases: A primer for the critical care nurse. *Dimensions of Critical Care Nursing, 21*(4), 127–133. doi:10.1097/00003465-200207000-00003

Lee, S. (2018, March 15). Hyperthyroidism and thyrotoxicosis. In R. Khardori (Ed.), *Medscape.* Retrieved from http://emedicine.medscape.com/article/121865-overview

Manzullo, E. F., & Ross, D. S. (2019, February 26). Nonthyroid surgery in the patient with thyroid disease. In J. E. Mulder (Ed.), *UpToDate.* Retrieved from https://www.uptodate.com/contents/nonthyroid-surgery-in-the-patient-with-thyroid-disease

Merrill, E. (2013). A devastating storm. *The Medicine Forum, 14*(12), 24–25. doi:10.29046/TMF.014.1.012

The Nurse Practitioner: The American Journal of Primary Healthcare. (2005). *Thyroid Disorders, 30*(6), 51–52.

Roman, S. (2017). Current best practices in the management of thyroid nodules and cancer. (PowerPoint slides). Retrieved from https://reachmd.com/programs/cme/current-best-practices-in-the-management-of-thyroid-nodules-and-cancer/8470/transcript/16717/

Ross, D. (2018, September 27). Thyroid function in nonthyroidal illness. In J. E. Mulder (Ed.), *UpToDate.* Retrieved from https://www.uptodate.com/contents/thyroid-function-in-nonthyroidal-illness

Ross, D., & Sugg, S. (2018, September 25). Surgical management of hyperthyroidism. In J. E. Mulder (Ed.), *UpToDate.* Retrieved from https://www.uptodate.com/contents/surgical-management-of-hyperthyroidism

Tuttle, R. (2016). Differentiated thyroid cancer: Clinicopathologic staging. In J. E. Mulder (Ed.), *UpToDate.* Retrieved from https://www.uptodate.com/contents/differentiated-thyroid-cancer-clinicopathologic-staging/print

Umpierrez, G. (2002). Euthyroid sick syndrome. *Southern Medical Journal, 95*(5), 506–513. doi:10.1097/00007611-200295050-00007

Thyroid Disorder—Myxedema Coma

Lisa Coco

Definition

A. A rare (0.22/one million annually) but severe life-threatening form of decompensated hypothyroidism associated with a high mortality rate.

B. Major precipitating factors: Infection and discontinuation of thyroid supplements.

Incidence

A. At present, there are over 300 cases reported in the literature. Myxedema coma is rare and generally unrecognized, with 80% of patients older than 60 years of age.

B. Myxedema coma can occur in younger women with 36 known cases occurring with pregnant females.

C. A commonly ignored background factor in myxedema coma/crisis is the discontinuation of thyroid supplements in critically ill patients.

Pathogenesis

A. Low intracellular T3 secondary to hypothyroidism is the basic underlying pathology.

Predisposing Factors

A. Certain medications.

B. Infection and septicemia.

C. Trauma.

D. Withdrawal of thyroid supplements.

E. Underlying cardiovascular disease.

Subjective Data

A. Complaints/symptoms.

    1. Decreased mentation and extreme lethargy.

B. Common/typical scenario.

    1. Very few cases have occurred in the United States, but usually related to having underlying hypothyroidism. Most likely to be seen in the ICU after hypothyroid medication is discontinued for an extended period of time and a precipitating event occurs, such as sepsis.

C. Family and social history.

    1. Ask about discontinuation of thyroid medications.

D. Review of systems.

    1. Unable to assess due to mental status.

Physical Examination

A. Cardiovascular—hypotension, bradycardia, ECG changes.

B. Respiratory—decreased breath sounds, respiratory depression.

C. Neurological—poor cognitive function, generalized weakness.

Diagnostic Tests

A. Thyroid-stimulating hormone (TSH).

B. Free T4.

C. Nonspecific labs to rule out other disorders including complete blood count, urinalysis, blood and urine culture, and serum electrolytes.

Differential Diagnosis

A. Cerebrovascular accident.

B. Acute psychosis.

C. Hypoglycemia.

D. Hypoxia.

E. Sepsis.

F. Hypothermia.

G. Acute myocardial infarction (MI).

H. Intracranial hemorrhage.

I. Panhypopituitarism.

J. Adrenal insufficiency.

K. Hyponatremia.
L. Gastrointestinal (GI) bleeding.
M. Conversion disorder.

Evaluation and Management Plan

A. General plan.
    1. Consult with endocrinologist. This is a medical emergency with a high (25% to 60%) risk of mortality. If an endocrinologist is not available, confer with a critical care specialist. The advanced practice provider (APP) should not manage this type of patient alone.
    2. Be aware that cardiovascular morbidity occurs, including cardiogenic shock, respiratory depression, hypothermia, and coma.
    3. Achieve normothermia. Warming occurs with administration of thyroid hormone, in most cases both T3 and T4, with gradual slow rewarming via a warming blanket.
    4. Focus on stabilization of cardiac status. Cardiac support is given through the administration of thyroid hormone and intravenous fluids with the stabilization of electrolytes and blood glucose.
    5. Achieve optimum ventilation. Ventilation is given through administration of oxygen and, if needed, central or bilevel positive airway pressure or mechanical ventilation.
B. Patient and family teaching.
    1. Explain to the patient and family the severity of myxedema crisis and the course of treatment in the intensive care setting.
C. Pharmacology.
    1. Give intravenous triiodothyronine and thyroxine replacement with gradual slow rewarming.
    2. Resuscitation and ICU management should be a multidisciplinary team approach.
D. Discharge instructions.
    1. Poor outcomes are associated with myxedema coma; may need nursing home placement, long-term acute care hospital, or even palliative care/hospice if clinical course is complicated.

Follow-Up

A. Follow-up is dependent on individual outcome.

Consultation/Referral

A. Consultation with an endocrinologist.
B. May need to consider a palliative care consult due to high mortality rate.
C. Social work consult for placement or family support may be needed.

Special/Geriatric Considerations

A. Poor outcomes are associated with myxedema coma in all age groups.
B. Myxedema coma is rare, with fewer than 40 cases reported and presentation of advanced hypothyroidism in pregnancy is very unusual.

Bibliography

American Association of Clinical Endocrinologists. (2016). *Hyperthyroidism: Information for patients.* Retrieved from http://thyroidawareness.com/sites/all/files/hyperthyroidism.pdf

Brenner, Z., & Porsche, R. (2006). Amiodarone-induced thyroid dysfunction. *Critical Care Nurse, 26*(3), 34–41.

Burch, W. (1994). *Endocrinology* (3rd ed.). Baltimore, MD: Williams & Wilkins.

Burman, K., Ellahham, S., Fadel, B., Lindsay, J., Ringel, M., & Wartofsky, L. (2000). Hyperthyroid heart disease. *Clinical Cardiology, 23*(26), 402–408.

Carroll, R., & Matfin, G. (2010). Endocrine and metabolic emergencies: Thyroid storm. *Therapeutic Advances in Endocrinology and Metabolism, 1*(3), 139–145.

Chowdhury, S., Ghosh, S., Mathew, V., Misgar, R., Mukhopadhyay, P., Mukhopadhyay, S., . . . Roychowdhury, P. (2011). Myxedema coma: A new look into an old crisis. *Journal of Thyroid Research, 2011*, 1–7. doi:10.4061/2011/493462

Dahlen, R., & Kumrow, D. (2002). Thyroidectomy: Understanding the potential for complications. *MEDSURG Nursing, 11*(5), 228–235.

Francis, J., & Jayaprasad, N. (2005). Atrial fibrillation and hyperthyroidism. *Indian Pacing and Electrophysiology Journal, 5*(4), 305–311.

Holcomb, S. (2002). Thyroid diseases: A primer for the critical care nurse. *Dimensions of Critical Care Nursing, 21*(4), 127–133. doi:10.1097/00003465-200207000-00003

Lee, S. (2018, March 15). Hyperthyroidism and thyrotoxicosis. In R. Khardori (Ed.), *Medscape.* Retrieved from http://emedicine.medscape.com/article/121865-overview

Manzullo, E. F., & Ross, D. S. (2019, February 26). Nonthyroid surgery in the patient with thyroid disease. In J. E. Mulder (Ed.), *UpToDate.* Retrieved from https://www.uptodate.com/contents/nonthyroid-surgery-in-the-patient-with-thyroid-disease

The Nurse Practitioner: The American Journal of Primary Healthcare. (2005). *Thyroid Disorders, 30*(6), 51–52.

Roman, S. (2017). Current best practices in the management of thyroid nodules and cancer. (PowerPoint slides). Retrieved from https://reachmd.com/programs/cme/current-best-practices-in-the-management-of-thyroid-nodules-and-cancer/8470/transcript/16717/

Ross, D. (2018, September 27). Thyroid function in nonthyroidal illness. In J. E. Mulder (Ed.), *UpToDate.* Retrieved from https://www.uptodate.com/contents/thyroid-function-in-nonthyroidal-illness

Ross, D., & Sugg, S. (2018, September 25). Surgical management of hyperthyroidism. In J. E. Mulder (Ed.), *UpToDate.* Retrieved from https://www.uptodate.com/contents/surgical-management-of-hyperthyroidism

Tuttle, R. (2018, January 17). Differentiated thyroid cancer: Clinicopathologic staging. In J. E. Mulder (Ed.), *UpToDate.* Retrieved from https://www.uptodate.com/contents/differentiated-thyroid-cancer-clinicopathologic-staging/print

Umpierrez, G. (2002). Euthyroid sick syndrome. *Southern Medical Journal, 95*(5), 506–513. doi:10.1097/00007611-200295050-00007

Thyroid Disorder—Thyroid Storm

Lisa Coco

Definition

A. State of severe hyperthyroid crisis that causes organ dysfunction.
B. An acute, life-threatening, hypermetabolic state induced by excessive release of thyroid hormones.
C. The severe end of the spectrum of thyrotoxicosis.

Incidence

A. Thyroid storm is most often seen in the context of underlying Graves' hyperthyroidism.
B. Although quite rare, it can complicate thyrotoxicosis of any etiology and has a high mortality rate that may approach 10% to 20%.
C. Thyroid marker levels do not adequately address the differences between thyroid storm and hyperthyroidism. To differentiate the severity and potential morbidity of the disease, the Burch-Wartofsky Point Scale (BWPS) can predict the risk of thyroid storms independently from thyroid levels.
D. Thyrotoxicosis is three to five times more common in females, predisposing them to this condition.

Pathogenesis

A. Patients with thyroid storm have relatively higher levels of free thyroid hormones.

Predisposing Factors

A. Regardless of the underlying etiology, the transition to a state of thyroid storm usually requires a second superimposed insult. Most often, this is infection.

B. Other associated causes are:

1. Trauma.

2. Surgery.

3. Thyroid surgery.

4. Myocardial infarction (MI).

5. Diabetic ketoacidosis (DKA).

6. Pregnancy.

7. Parturition.

8. Abrupt cessation of antithyroid medications.

9. Excessive ingestion of thyroid hormone.

Subjective Data

A. Common complaints/symptoms.

1. Irritability, emotional lability, and anxiety.

2. Increased appetite with poor weight gain.

3. Heat intolerance and excessive sweating.

4. Fatigue.

5. Respiratory distress.

6. Nausea and vomiting, diarrhea, and abdominal pain.

B. Common scenario.

1. Severe florid hyperthyroidism evidenced by extreme irritability, high heart rate, cardiac arrhythmia, nausea, and/or vomiting; in addition, the patient may present with a possible psychosis.

C. Family and social history.

1. None.

D. Review of systems.

1. May be difficult to speak to during the acute phase.

2. Ask about extreme irritability, fatigue, anxiety.

3. Ask about palpitations.

Physical Examination

A. General: Appears toxic.

B. Cardiovascular—hypertension with pulse pressure, cardiac arrhythmias, fever.

C. HEENT—goiter, exophthalmos.

D. Neurological—tremors, seizure activity, hyperflexia.

Diagnostic Tests

A. Thyroid-stimulating hormone (TSH).

B. Free T4.

C. Free T3.

D. Liver function tests.

E. Complete blood count (CBC).

F. Comprehensive metabolic panel.

G. Imaging studies, which may include:

1. Chest x-ray (CHF).

2. Head CT (exclude other neurological conditions).

3. ECG (cardiac arrhythmias).

Differential Diagnosis

A. Anticholinergic or adrenergic drug intoxication.

B. Anxiety disorders.

C. Central nervous system infections.

D. Heart failure.

E. Hypertension.

F. Hypertensive encephalopathy.

G. Hyperthyroidism.

H. Malignant hyperthermia.

I. Panic disorder.

J. Pheochromocytoma.

K. Septic shock.

Evaluation and Management Plan

A. General plan.

1. Medical treatment of thyroid storm aims to stop thyroid hormone production within the gland, inhibit the release of thyroid hormone, and inhibit conversion of T4 to T3.

2. An acute care or ICU is most appropriate for management.

3. Antithyroid treatment should be continued until euthyroidism is achieved, at which point a final decision regarding oral medications, surgery, or radioactive iodine therapy can be made.

a. Occasionally, patients may be severely agitated, limiting further intervention.

b. Sedatives such as haloperidol or benzodiazepine can be given.

4. Management of airway, breathing, circulation, disability, and examination (ABCDE) is crucial.

5. With high fever, acetaminophen is preferable to aspirin, which can increase serum T4 and T3 concentrations by interfering with protein binding.

6. Cooling blankets can also be used with close attention to slow cooling to decrease metabolic demand.

7. Other elements of supportive care: Intravenous fluids, electrolyte replacement, and nutritional support.

8. Intubation or noninvasive positive pressure ventilation may also be needed with arterial blood gas (ABG) analysis.

B. Patient and family teaching.

1. Explanation of what thyroid storm is and the importance of management should be discussed with the patient and family. The need for the ICU is the most appropriate for management to provide careful monitoring.

C. Pharmacotherapy.

1. Beta-blockers. Propranolol is the first-line choice for beta-blockers providing antiadrenergic effects and inhibits peripheral conversion of T4 to T3.

2. Propylthiouracil (PTU) is the thionamide of choice in severe, life-threatening thyroid storm because it blocks conversion of T4 to T3.

a. PTU should be administered orally or via nasogastric tube in the awake or unresponsive patient with a loading dose of 600 mg followed by a dose of 200 to 250 mg every 4 to 6 hours.

b. PTU is preferred in the first trimester because it causes less severe birth defects.

3. Methimazole.

a. Methimazole is recommended for severe non-threatening thyroid storm because it has a longer half-life than PTU, normalizes T3 more rapidly, and has less hepatotoxicity.

b. Methimazole is administered in a loading dose of 40 mg po with a dose of 20 to 30 mg every 4 to 6 hours (max 120 mg/d).

4. Potassium iodine (SSKI): 5 ggts po q6h.

5. Steroids: 100 mg hydrocortisone IV; then 100 mg q8h.

D. Definitive therapy: Thyroidectomy.

Consultation/Referral

A. Endocrinology should be consulted on all cases.

Follow-Up

A. Follow-up care with an endocrinologist posthospitalization is recommended.

Special/Geriatric Considerations

A. With pregnancy, lithium carbonate at a dose of 300 mg every 8 hours can be used when there is a contraindication to thionamide therapy. Lithium inhibits thyroid hormone release from the thyroid gland.

Bibliography

American Association of Clinical Endocrinologists. (2016). *Hyperthyroidism: Information for patients.* Retrieved from http://thyroidawareness.com/sites/all/files/hyperthyroidism.pdf

Brenner, Z., & Porsche, R. (2006). Amiodarone-induced thyroid dysfunction. *Critical Care Nurse, 26*(3), 34–41.

Burch, W. (1994). *Endocrinology* (3rd ed.). Baltimore, MD: Williams & Wilkins.

Burman, K., Ellahham, S., Fadel, B., Lindsay, J., Ringel, M., & Wartofsky, L. (2000). Hyperthyroid heart disease. *Clinical Cardiology, 23*(26), 402–408.

Carroll, R., & Matfin, G. (2010). Endocrine and metabolic emergencies: Thyroid storm. *Therapeutic Advances in Endocrinology and Metabolism, 1*(3), 139–145. doi:10.1177/2042018810382481

Chowdhury, S., Ghosh, S., Mathew, V., Misgar, R., Mukhopadhyay, P., Mukhopadhyay, S., . . . Roychowdhury, P. (2011). Myxedema coma: A new look into an old crisis. *Journal of Thyroid Research, 2011*, 1–7. doi:10.4061/2011/493462

Dahlen, R., & Kumrow, D. (2002). Thyroidectomy: Understanding the potential for complications. *MEDSURG Nursing, 11*(5), 228–235.

Francis, J., & Jayaprasad, N. (2005). Atrial fibrillation and hyperthyroidism. *Indian Pacing and Electrophysiology Journal, 5*(4), 305–311.

Holcomb, S. (2002). Thyroid diseases: A primer for the critical care nurse. *Dimensions of Critical Care Nursing, 21*(4), 127–133. doi:10.1097/00003465-200207000-00003

Idrose, A. M. (2015). Acute and emergency care for thyrotoxicosis and thyroid storm. *Acute Medicine and Surgery, 2*(3), 147–157. Published online 2015 May 12. doi:10.1002/ams2.104

Lee, S. (2018, March 15). Hyperthyroidism and thyrotoxicosis. In R. Khardori (Ed.), *Medscape.* Retrieved from http://emedicine.medscape.com/article/121865-overview

Manzullo, E. F., & Ross, D. S. (2019, February 26). Nonthyroid surgery in the patient with thyroid disease. In J. E. Mulder (Ed.), *UpToDate.* Retrieved from https://www.uptodate.com/contents/nonthyroid-surgery-in-the-patient-with-thyroid-disease

Merrill, E. (2013). A devastating storm. *The Medicine Forum, 14*(12), 24–25. doi:10.29046/TMF.014.1.012

The Nurse Practitioner: The American Journal of Primary Healthcare. (2005). *Thyroid Disorders, 30*(6), 51–52.

Roman, S. (2017). Current best practices in the management of thyroid nodules and cancer. (PowerPoint slides). Retrieved from https://reachmd.com/programs/cme/current-best-practices-in-the-management-of-thyroid-nodules-and-cancer/8470/transcript/16717/

Ross, D. (2018, September 27). Thyroid function in nonthyroidal illness. In J. E. Mulder (Ed.), *UpToDate.* Retrieved from https://www.uptodate.com/contents/thyroid-function-in-nonthyroidal-illness

Ross, D., & Sugg, S. (2018, September 25). Surgical management of hyperthyroidism. In J. E. Mulder (Ed.), *UpToDate.* Retrieved from https://www.uptodate.com/contents/surgical-management-of-hyperthyroidism

Tuttle, R. (2018, January 17). Differentiated thyroid cancer: Clinicopathologic staging. In J. E. Mulder (Ed.), *UpToDate.* Retrieved from https://www.uptodate.com/contents/differentiated-thyroid-cancer-clinicopathologic-staging/print

Umpierrez, G. (2002). Euthyroid sick syndrome. *Southern Medical Journal, 95*(5), 506–513. doi:10.1097/00007611-200295050-00007

9 Psychiatric Guidelines

Dawn Vanderhoef

Bipolar Disorder

Dawn Vanderhoef

Definition

A. Manic episode (see Table 9.1).

1. Distinct period of abnormal and persistent elevated, expansive, or irritable mood and abnormally and persistent increase in goal-directed activity or energy, lasting at least a week and nearly all day.

2. During the period of mood disturbance and increased energy or activity, three of the following symptoms (four if mood is irritable) are present to a significant degree and represent a noticeable change from usual behavior.

a. Inflated self-esteem or grandiosity.

b. Decreased need for sleep.

c. More talkative.

d. Flight of ideas.

e. Distractibility.

f. Increase in goal-directed activities.

g. Excessive involvement in activities that have a high risk for painful consequences.

3. The mood disturbance is sufficiently severe to cause marked impairment in social, occupational functioning, or to necessitate hospitalization to prevent harm to self or others.

4. The episode is not attributable to the physiological effects of a substance or to another medical condition.

5. NOTE: A full manic episode that emerges during antidepressant treatment but persists at a fully syndromal level beyond the physiological effect of treatment is sufficient evidence for a manic episode.

B. Hypomanic episode (see Table 9.1).

1. Distinct period of elevated expansive or irritable mood, lasting at least 4 days, that is clearly different from non-depressed mood.

2. Three or more (four if mood is irritable): Grandiosity, decreased sleep, pressured speech, racing thoughts, hyperverbal, distractible, increase in goal-directed activity, and excessive involvement in pleasurable activities that may have negative consequences.

3. Change in behavior is uncharacteristic for the person.

4. Other people notice the change in mood and functioning.

5. Episode does not cause marked impairment in social or occupational functioning, it does not require hospitalization, and there is no psychosis.

6. Symptoms are not due to substance use or a general medical condition.

C. Bipolar depression.

1. Prolonged sadness.

2. Pessimism.

3. Changes in appetite.

4. Indifference.

5. Loss of energy.

6. Persistent lethargy.

7. Inability to concentrate.

8. Recurring thoughts of death or suicide.

D. Bipolar I or bipolar II disorder.

1. Bipolar I: Has one or more manic episodes or mixed episodes: A distinct period of abnormally and persistently increased goal-directed activity or energy lasting at least 1 week and present nearly every day, for most of the day, with three or more of the following: Grandiosity/inflated self-esteem, decreased need for sleep, more talkative/pressured speech, flight of ideas/racing thoughts, distractibility, increase in goal-directed behavior, or excessive engagement in high-risk activities. *The Diagnostic and Statistical Manual of Mental Disorders*(5th ed.; *DSM-5*) has six separate criteria sets.

a. bipolar disease (BPD) I single manic episode.

b. Most recent episode hypomanic.

c. Most recent episode manic.

d. Most recent episode mixed.

e. Most recent episode depressed.

f. Most recent episode unspecified.

2. Bipolar II: Has one or more major depressive episodes and at least one hypomanic episode.

a. Specifiers are used to indicate the nature of the current episode: hypomanic or depressed.

b. If depressed, specifiers are mild, moderate, severe without psychotic features or severe with psychotic features, chronic, with catatonic features, with melancholic features, with atypical features, or with postpartum onset.

Incidence

A. 12-month prevalence for bipolar I disorder is 0.6% with lifetime male-to-female ratio of 1:1.

Age of onset is about 18 years of age, earlier than in major depressive disorder.

B. 90% of individuals with a single manic episode have a recurrent mood episode.

C. 60% of manic episodes occur immediately before a major depressive episode.

D. 12-month prevalence for bipolar II disorder is 0.3%.

TABLE 9.1	Mania and Hypomania Comparisons

	Manic Episode	Hypomanic Episode
Duration	1 week or more	4 days or more
Mood	Abnormally and persistently high, irritable, or expansive	
Activity/energy	Persistently increased	
Symptoms that are changes from usual behavior	Three or more of grandiosity, ↓ need for sleep, ↑ talkativeness, flight of ideas or racing thoughts, distractibility (self-report or that of others), agitation, ↑ goal-directed activity, poor judgment	
Severity	Results in psychotic features, hospitalization, or impairment at work, social, and personal levels	Clear change from usual functioning and others notice this change and NO psychosis, hospitalizations, or impairment
Other	Rule out substance/medication-induced symptoms with mixed features, if appropriate	

Source: Adapted with permission from Morrison, J. (2014). DSM-5 *made easy: The clinician's guide to diagnosis.* New York, NY: Guilford Press.

Pathogenesis

A. Up to 70% to 80% heritability.
B. Brain changes.
  1. Decreased size and activity in the prefrontal cortex with limbic hyperactivity and decreased hippocampal volume.
  2. The amygdala is larger and more active in bipolar disorder.
  3. Disrupted glutamate and gamma-aminobutyric acid (GABA) regulation with greater norepinephrine and dopamine activity in mania.

Predisposing Factors

A. Environmental: Separated, widowed individuals have higher rates.
B. Genetics: Family history is one of the strongest and most consistent predictors for bipolar disorder. Individuals with psychiatric features likely have subsequent episodes with psychotic features.
C. Gender: Females are more likely to have rapid cycling and mixed states and are more likely to have depressive episodes along with a greater likelihood of alcohol use disorders.
D. Suicide: Lifetime risk is 15 times greater than that in the general population.

Subjective Data

A. Common complaints/symptoms.
  1. Mania.
    a. Racing thoughts.
    b. Flight of ideas.
    c. Increased focused activity.
    d. Thoughts of grandiosity.
    e. Excessive talking or pressured speech.
  2. Depressive episodes.
    a. Depressed mood.
    b. Loss of energy or fatigue.
    c. Diminished interest in anything.
    d. Weight loss.
    e. Feelings of worthlessness.
B. Common/typical scenario.
  1. A typical scenario starts with an unusual shift in mood and energy. The person may have excessively elevated mood for about a week and then become depressed.
C. Family and social history.
  1. Inquire about family history of mental illness.
  2. Inquire about periods of depression or manic episodes.

3. Inquire about patterns of prolonged sleep alternating with excessively elevated mood.
  4. Inquire about lifestyle and stressful life events.
D. Review of systems.
  1. Noncontributory.

Mental State Examination

A. Conduct a Mental State Examination.
B. General description: Manic patients are excited, talkative, and sometimes amusing. Hyperactivity is common and at times is psychotic and disorganized.
C. Mood and affect: Mood is euphoric but also can be irritable. A low frustration tolerance is common as is labile mood with shifts from laughing to crying to irritability.
D. Perceptual disturbances.
  1. Delusions are common in manic patients.
  2. Mood-congruent manic delusions have themes of wealth, extraordinary abilities, or power.
  3. Hallucinations may also be present.
E. Thought: Distractibility and flight of ideas are common.
F. Impulse control: 75% of manic patients are assaultive and threating.
G. Judgment and insight: Impairment is a hallmark.
H. Reliability: Commonly unreliable historians.

Diagnostic Tests

A. Used to rule out a medical cause of the psychiatric symptoms.
B. Endocrine disorders.
  1. Hyperthyroid.
  2. Diabetes.
  3. Cushing's syndrome.
  4. Addison disease.
C. Neurological disorders.
  1. Epilepsy.
  2. Cerebrovascular disease.
  3. Tumors.
  4. Head trauma.
  5. Lupus.
  6. Multiple sclerosis.
D. Infectious disease.
  1. HIV/AIDS.
  2. Lyme disease.
  3. Syphilis.
E. Medications/substances associated with mania.
  1. Amphetamines.
  2. Cocaine.

3. Corticosteroids.
4. Hallucinogens.
5. Levodopa.
6. Opiates.
7. Phencyclidine (PCP).

F. Screening instruments: Positive screen DOES NOT indicate a disorder; REQUIRES validation with comprehensive interview/assessment.
1. Mood Disorder Questionnaire (MDQ).
2. Young Mania Rating Scale.
3. Bipolar Depression Rating Scale (BDRS).
4. Hypomania Checklist (HCL-32): Self-report.

Differential Diagnosis

A. Major depressive disorder.
B. Schizophrenia.
C. Generalized anxiety disorder.
D. Posttraumatic stress disorder.
E. Substance-induced mood disorder.
F. Attention deficit hyperactivity disorder.
G. Personality disorders.

Evaluation and Management Plan

A. General plan.
1. Treatment of bipolar disorders is complex—antidepressants should be avoided unless an individual has refractory depression unresponsive to an atypical antipsychotic (AA) and mood stabilizer. Antidepressant treatment can make an individual cycle or become refractory to treatment.
2. If an antidepressant is used to treat the depressive episode it should be discontinued after 6 to 9 months of sustained remission of the episode.
3. Refer to AAs in the Posttraumatic Stress Disorder section.
B. Patient/family teaching points.
1. Compliance with treatment plan can be challenging.
2. Teach patient and family warning signs and symptoms.
3. Teach patient coping skills to deal with life stressors.
4. Encourage patient to learn more about biology behind the disease to increase compliance.
5. Provide information on local support groups and other national resources.
C. Pharmacotherapy.
1. *Gold standard* is Lithium, which has an indication for acute mania, prophylaxis of depression and suicide, and is adjunct to antidepressant treatment in unipolar depression.
   a. *Elimination* is almost entirely by the kidneys; therefore, once a day dosing is recommended. Lithium 300 mg = 0.3 mEq/L plasma concentration.
   b. *Therapeutic range* 0.5 to 1.0 mEq/L.
   c. *Drug–drug interactions:* Diuretics, angiotensin-converting enzyme (ACE) inhibitors, digoxin, nonsteroidal anti-inflammatory drugs (NSAIDs), Flagyl.
   d. *Pregnancy:* Avoid use due to risk of Ebstein's anomaly.
   e. *Laboratory tests:* Prior to treatment, check pregnancy test in females, creatinine, thyroid profile, and complete blood count (CBC; can cause leukocytosis) and repeat every 6 months. Patients over 40 years of age should have an EKG.
   f. Side effects of lithium at different levels can be seen in Table 9.2.

TABLE 9.2   Lithium Toxicity and Side Effects

Lithium Level (mEq/L)	Side Effects
1.0–1.5	Tremor
1.5–2.0	Cog-wheeling, tremor, nausea, drowsiness
2.0–3.0	Ataxia, confusion
>3.0	Delirium, coma, seizures, death

2. Valproate (Depakote) is indicated for acute mania and rapid cycling. Also used in prophylaxis. It is highly protein bound and metabolized by the liver. Extended release has about 8% to 20% lower bioavailability than intervention radiology (IR).
   a. *Drug–drug interactions:* ASA, CYP2D6 and 3A4, avoid with heavy alcohol consumption.
   b. *Box warning:* Pancreatitis.
   c. *Laboratory tests:* Liver function tests, CBC, and pregnancy test in females. Recheck liver function tests, CBC, and valproic acid (VPA) level every 6 months. Response is based on evaluation of patient; laboratory ranges were developed in persons with seizure disorders.
3. Carbamazepine (Tegretol) is indicated for acute mania and prophylaxis.
   a. Highly protein bound, interaction with CYP3A4, and is a strong autoinducer.
   b. Lowers the effectiveness of oral birth control pills.
   c. *Laboratory tests:* Liver function tests, CBC, pregnancy test in females, and follow-up testing every 6 months with carbamazepine level. 2007 Food and Drug Administration (FDA) Alert: Genetic testing required in persons with human leukocyte antigen (HLA) allele, which occurs in individuals from Asia, including South Asian Indians.
4. Lamotrigine (Lamictal) is indicated for bipolar maintenance; it has been found effective in bipolar II disorder as well.
   a. Follow recommended dosing and guidelines if a patient is on valproate.
   b. Risk of Stevens-Johnson syndrome if a patient missed more than 5 days; need to be retitrated.
   c. Oral contraceptives lower lamotrigine levels.

Follow-Up

Patients with bipolar disorder should be followed by a psychiatric specialist.

Consultation/Referral

A. Consultation and referral to a primary care provider is warranted if there are comorbid physical health conditions.

Special/Geriatric Considerations

A. Support group.
1. Depression and Bipolar Support Alliance.
2. National Alliance on Mental Illness (NAMI).

Bibliography

American Psychiatric Association. (2013). *Diagnostic and statistical manual of mental disorders* (5th ed.). Arlington, VA: American Psychiatric Publishing.

Morrison, J. (2014). *DSM-5 made easy: The clinician's guide to diagnosis.* New York, NY: Guilford Press.

Pliszka, S. R. (2016). *Neuroscience for the mental health clinician* (2nd ed.). New York, NY: Guilford Press.

Sadock, B. J., Sadock, V. A., & Ruiz, P. (2015). *Kaplan & Sadock's synopsis of psychiatry: Behavioral sciences/clinical psychiatry* (11th ed.). Philadelphia, PA: Wolters Kluwer.

Stahl, S. M. (2013). *Stahl's essential psychopharmacology: Neuroscientific basis and practical applications* (4th ed.). New York, NY: Cambridge University Press.

Stahl, S. M. (2014). *Stahl's essential psychopharmacology: Prescriber's guide* (5th ed.). New York, NY: Cambridge University Press.

Major Depressive Disorder

Dawn Vanderhoef

Definition

A. Five (or more) of the following symptoms present during the same 2-week period and represent a change from previous functioning. At least one of the symptoms must be either (a) depressed mood or (b) loss of interest or pleasure.

  1. Depressed mood most of the day, nearly every day, by subjective report (sad, empty, hopeless) or observed by others (appears tearful).

  2. Markedly diminished pleasure in all or most activities.

  3. Significant weight loss (more than 5% in a month) or decrease or increase in appetite nearly every day.

  4. Insomnia or hypersomnia nearly every day.

  5. Psychomotor agitation or retardation nearly every day (observable by others, not merely subjective feelings of restlessness or being slowed down).

  6. Fatigue or loss of energy nearly every day.

  7. Feelings of worthlessness or excessive or inappropriate guilt (which may be delusional) nearly every day.

  8. Diminished ability to think or concentrate, indecisiveness, nearly every day (subjective or observed).

  9. Recurrent thoughts of death (not just dying), recurrent suicidal ideation without a specific plan, or a suicide attempt or a specific plan.

B. Symptoms cause clinically significant distress or impairment in social, occupational, or other areas of functioning.

C. The episode is not attributable to the physiological effects of a substance or to another medical condition.

D. With postpartum onset: If symptoms are within 4 weeks postpartum. Commonly includes psychosis.

E. Mnemonic: **SIGE CAPS**.

  1. **S**leep disturbance.

  2. **I**nterest and pleasure decrease.

  3. **G**uilt.

  4. **E**nergy lower.

  5. **C**oncentration decrease.

  6. **A**ppetite increase or decrease.

  7. **P**sychomotor agitation or retardation.

  8. **S**uicidal/hopeless.

Incidence

A. 12-month prevalence is approximately 7% with increase in 18- to 29-year-olds.

B. Females have 1.5- to 3-fold higher rates than males beginning in early adolescence.

C. Mean age of onset is 40 years of age with 50% of persons having an onset between the ages of 20 and 50 years.

Pathogenesis

A. Heritability: 50%.

B. 8% to 17% risk if first degree relative has diagnosis.

  1. Neurochemical imbalance: Most basic level is the monoamine hypothesis, an imbalance in the following neurotransmitters.

  a. Norepinephrine.

  b. Dopamine.

  c. Serotonin.

Predisposing Factors

A. No close interpersonal relationships.

B. Divorced or separated.

C. More common in rural than urban areas.

D. Stressful life events precede first episode.

E. Depression in older persons is common. Individuals with the following are at higher risk of developing depression: Lower socioeconomic status, loss of spouse, current physical illness, and social isolation.

Subjective Data

A. Common complaints/symptoms.

  1. Agitation or restlessness.

  2. Psychomotor retardation.

  3. Flat affect.

  4. Loss of energy.

  5. Feeling of worthlessness.

  6. Diminished ability to concentrate.

  7. Loss of pleasure in activities.

  8. Recurrent thoughts of death.

B. Common/typical scenario.

  1. Patients may not seek attention for depression but typically complain of other symptoms, such as insomnia, headaches, abdominal upset, and difficulty concentrating.

C. Family and social history.

  1. Depression can be familial.

  2. Social history is noncontributory.

D. Review of systems.

  1. Noncontributory.

Mental State Examination

A. General description: Psychomotor retardation, hand wringing, stooped posture, downcast gaze.

B. Mood and affect: 50% persons deny depressed feelings/constricted affect.

C. Speech: Decreased rate and volume with limited response to questions.

D. Perceptual disturbances: Assess for hallucinations (auditory are most common), delusions, paranoia.

E. Thought content: Negative worldviews, rumination, and guilt. Assess for suicidal (10%–15% commit suicide) and homicidal ideation.

F. Cognition: Cognitive impairment seen in 50% to 70% of depressed patients.

G. Impulse control: If the patient has psychotic symptoms, may consider harming others. HIGH RISK for self-harm exists when energy is improving; the individual can carry out the plan.

H. Suicide assessment.

  1. Ask about ideation: Onset, duration, frequency, active thoughts, lethality, stressors, use of substances.

  2. Ask about plan: Wish to die, means, and understands consequences.

  3. Ask about means: Access to carry out plan, taken steps to prepare to end life, lethality.

  4. Ask about intent: Protective or risk factors.

  5. Screening instrument: Columbia Suicide Severity Rating Scale.

I. High risk populations for suicide.

  1. Older single white males.

  2. Divorced/widowed.

3. Unemployed.
4. Psychosis.
5. Homeless.
6. LGBT.
7. Veterans.
8. Comorbid physical and/or substance use disorder.
9. Previous attempt and/or family history.
10. Access to lethal means.

J. Homicidal assessment.
   1. Ideation, means, plan, and intent.
   2. Assess for anger, rage, and interpersonal conflict.
   3. If actively homicidal: Inpatient psychiatric hospitalization, notify law enforcement and Duty to Warn: Tarasoff v. Regents of the University of California (1976)—must notify victim.

Diagnostic Tests

A. Thyroid profile.
B. Complete blood count.
C. Comprehensive metabolic panel.
D. And based on history: Vitamin D level, folate level, B_{12}, or thiamine level.
E. Medical rule outs.
   1. Endocrine disorders: Hypothyroidism, diabetes, adrenal dysfunction.
   2. Neurological disorders: Dementia, seizures, tumors, Parkinson's disease, sleep apnea, cerebrovascular accident (CVA), neoplasms.
   3. Cardiac disease: Congestive heart failure, hypertension.
   4. Infection: Mononucleosis, HIV/AIDS, pneumonia, TD.
   5. Nutrition deficits: Anemia, low vitamin D/folate/B_{12}/thiamine.
   6. Other: Side effects of medications such as cardiac medications, hypnotics, antibacterial medications, antineoplastic medications, analgesics, antiepileptics, or antiparkinsonian drugs.
F. Screening instruments (in public domain): Positive screen DOES NOT indicate a disorder; REQUIRES validation with comprehensive interview/assessment.
   1. Patient Health Questionnaire (PHQ)—2.
   2. Patient Health Questionnaire (PHQ)—9.
   3. Mood Disorders Questionnaire (MDQ).
   4. Edinburgh Postnatal Depression Scale (EPSD).
   5. Geriatric Depression Scale.

Differential Diagnosis

A. Bipolar disorder, depressed phase.
B. Mood disorder due to general medical condition.
C. Eating disorder.
D. Substance-induced mood disorder.
E. Adjustment disorder.

Evaluation and Management Plan

A. General plan.
   1. Meets criteria for major depressive disorder, single episode or recurrent, and, if postpartum onset, psychosis or suicide/homicidal ideation.
   2. If patient is not actively suicidal, homicidal, or psychotic, discuss treatment options.
   3. Psychotherapy for mild symptoms or if patient refuses medication.
   4. Prior to starting antidepressant treatment, bipolar disorder has been ruled out.

B. Patient/family teaching points.
   1. Teach patients about early signs of relapse and rationale of treatment choices made.
   2. Family members need to be taught about depression and how to be supportive.
   3. Encourage patient to learn more about biology behind the disease to increase compliance.
   4. Provide information on local support groups and other national resources.
C. Pharmacotherapy.
   1. Medication treatment options.
      a. *Selective serotonin reuptake inhibitors.*
         i. Boxed warning for increase in suicidal thinking up to age 24 (for all antidepressants in all classes).
         ii. Risk of serotonin syndrome.
         iii. Discontinuation syndrome—abrupt discontinuation of medication that is more common in medications with short half-lives.
            1) Mnemonic **FINISH**.
               a) **F**lu-like symptoms.
               b) **I**nsomnia.
               c) **N**ausea.
               d) **I**mbalance.
               e) **S**ensory disturbance.
               f) **H**yperarousal.
            2) Treatment: Place back on medication.
         iv. Serotonin syndrome (risk with any medication that increases serotonin levels).
            1) Mnemonic **HARMED** (medical emergency).
               a) **H**yperthermia.
               b) **A**utonomic instability.
               c) **R**igidity.
               d) **M**yoclonus.
               e) **E**ncephalopathy.
               f) **D**iaphoresis.
            2) Treatment.
               a) Stop medication.
               b) Supportive measures and cyproheptadine (Periactin) can be helpful.
      b. *Serotonin norepinephrine reuptake inhibitors (SNRIs).*
      c. Other antidepressants.
         i. Noradrenergic and specific serotonergic antidepressant (NaSSA) more sedating at lower doses; increased appetite; can lower white blood cell (WBC); Sol Tab.
         ii. Norepinephrine dopamine reuptake inhibitor (NDRI).
            1) Avoid with history of seizure disorder or eating disorder; weight neutral and little to no sexual dysfunction.
            2) Attention deficit/hyperactivity disorder (ADHD) off label; less likely to switch into mania/DOSE BASED ON FORMULATION.
            3) Zyban—smoking cessation.
            4) Serotonin antagonist reuptake inhibitor (SARI): Sleep agent; risk of priapism; orthostasis; QTc prolongation.
            5) Multimodal antidepressant.
               a) SSRI—5HT1a agonist (low sexual dysfunction).
               b) 5HT1a partial agonist.
               c) 5HTc, 1D (improved cognition).

d) 7 antagonist—vortioxetine (Trintellix): Little/no sexual dysfunction, improved cognition, gastrointestinal (GI) upset, hyponatremia, bleeding.
   6) Serotonin partial agonist reuptake inhibitor (SPARI).
   d. *Tricyclic Antidepressants (TCAs).*
   i. Side effects: Sedation, weight gain, hypotension, anticholinergic toxicity (treatment with physostigmin), and QTc prolongation (EKG over 40 or with history of cardiovascular disease).
   ii. Lethal in overdose.
   iii. Use caution when given with anticoagulants, which increases risk for bleeding.
   iv. Need to check blood levels (therapeutic ranges).
   e. *Monoamine oxidase inhibitors (MAOIs).*
   i. Not used as first- or second-line treatment due to need for dietary changes and drug–drug interactions.
   ii. Risk for hypertensive crisis with tyramine (treatment with phentolamine).
   iii. Need education on tyramine free diet, such as to avoid dairy, fish, and processed meats.
   iv. Many drug–drug interactions: Demerol, OTC flu/cold medications, lithium, serotonergic agents, stimulants.
   v. Even with MAOI patches, dietary changes should be made.

Follow-Up
A. Weekly follow-up for the first month.
B. High risk of suicide as energy improves and mood stays low.

Consultation/Referral
A. Consultation with or referral to a psychiatric specialist if patient fails two full (adequate trial both time and dose) antidepressant trials.
B. Referral for psychotherapy as appropriate.

Special/Geriatric Considerations
A. Women of childbearing age: Assess Food and Drug Administration (FDA) pregnancy risk (with all psychotropic medications).
B. Postpartum depression: Important to assess for postpartum depression (PPD) with psychosis.
C. Older adults: Assessment of depression in older adults with cognitive problems, as pseudodementia may be present. White, widower, older males are at high risk of suicide. Considerations related to aging and drug–drug interactions.

Bibliography
American Psychiatric Association. (2013). *Diagnostic and statistical manual of mental disorders* (5th ed.). Arlington, VA: American Psychiatric Publishing.
Caplan, J. P., & Stern, T. A. (2008). Mnemonics in a nutshell: 32 aids to psychiatric diagnosis. *Current Psychiatry, 7*(10), 27–33.
Pliszka, S. R. (2016). *Neuroscience for the mental health clinician* (2nd ed.). New York, NY: Guilford Press.
Sadock, B. J., Sadock, V. A., & Ruiz, P. (2015). *Kaplan & Sadock's synopsis of psychiatry: Behavioral sciences/clinical psychiatry* (11th ed.). Philadelphia, PA: Wolters Kluwer.
Stahl, S. M. (2013). *Stahl's essential psychopharmacology: Neuroscientific basis and practical applications* (4th ed.). New York, NY: Cambridge University Press.
Stahl, S. M. (2014). *Stahl's essential psychopharmacology: Prescriber's guide* (5th ed.). New York, NY: Cambridge University Press.

Posttraumatic Stress Disorder

Dawn Vanderhoef

Definition
A. Exposure to actual or threatened death, serious injury, or sexual violation in one (or more) of the following ways.
   1. Directly experiencing the traumatic event(s).
   2. Witnessing, in person, the event(s) that occurred to a close family member or close friend, resulting in actual or threatened death.
   3. Learning that the traumatic event(s) occurred to a close family member or close friend. In cases of actual or threatened death of a family member or friend, the event(s) must have been violent or accidental.
   4. Experiencing repeated or extreme exposure to aversive details of the traumatic event(s) (e.g., first responders collecting human remains; police officers repeatedly exposed to details of child abuse).
B. Presence of one (or more) of the following intrusive symptoms associated with the traumatic event(s), beginning after the traumatic event(s) occurred.
   1. Recurrent, involuntary, and intrusive distressing stories or memories of the traumatic event(s).
   2. Recurrent distressing dreams in which the content and/or affect of the dream related to the traumatic event(s) are expressed.
   3. Dissociative reactions (flashbacks) in which the individual feels or acts as if the traumatic event(s) were recurring.
   4. Intense or prolonged psychological distress at exposure to internal or external cues that symbolize or resemble an aspect of the traumatic event(s).
   5. Marked physiological reactions to internal or external cues that symbolize or resemble an aspect of the traumatic event(s).
C. Persistent avoidance of stimuli associated with the traumatic event(s), beginning after the traumatic event(s) occurred, as evidenced by one or both of the following.
   1. Avoidance of or efforts to avoid distressing memories, thoughts, or feelings about or closely associated with the traumatic event(s).
   2. Avoidance of or efforts to avoid external reminders (people, places, conversations, activities, objects, situations) that trigger distressing memories, thoughts, or feelings about or closely associated with the traumatic event(s).
D. Negative alterations in cognition and mood associated with the traumatic event(s) beginning or worsening after the traumatic event(s) occurred, as evidenced by two (or more) of the following.
   1. Inability to remember an important aspect of the traumatic event(s) (typically due to dissociative amnesia and not the other factors such as head injury, alcohol, or drugs).
   2. Persistent and exaggerated negative beliefs or expectations about oneself, others, or the world.
   3. Persistent, distorted cognitions about the cause or consequences of the traumatic event(s) that lead the individual to blame himself/herself or others.
   4. Persistent negative emotional state (horror, fear, anger, guilt, shame).
   5. Markedly diminished interest or participation in significant activities.
   6. Feelings of detachment or estrangement from others.
   7. Persistent inability to experience positive emotions.

E. Marked alterations in arousal and reactivity associated with the traumatic event(s) beginning or worsening after the traumatic event(s) occurred, as evidenced by two (or more) of the following.

    1. Irritable behavior and angry outbursts typically expressed as verbal or physical aggression toward others/objects.

    2. Reckless or self-destructive behavior.

    3. Hypervigilance.

    4. Exaggerated startle response.

    5. Problems with concentration.

    6. Sleep disturbances (falling/staying asleep or restless sleep).

F. Duration of the disturbance is more than 1 month.

G. The disturbance causes clinically significant distress or impairment in social, occupational, or other important areas of functioning.

H. The disturbance is not attributed to the physiological effects of a substance or another medical condition.

Incidence

A. 9% to 15% lifetime incidence, and lifetime prevalence is about 8% of the general population.

B. Lifetime prevalence is 10% in women and 4% in men and is more common in young adults.

C. More common in single, divorced, widowed, and socially withdrawn individuals.

D. Risk factor is severity, duration, and proximity of the person's exposure to the trauma.

E. Symptoms usually develop within the first 3 months of the trauma, but a delay can exist.

Pathogenesis

A. Activation of the amygdala, increase in epinephrine and norepinephrine, and changes in cortisol production.

B. Activation of the hypothalamus–pituitary–adrenal axis (HPA) and reduction of the hippocampus/frontal cortex.

Predisposing Factors

A. Childhood trauma.

B. Intimate partner violence.

C. Personality disorder.

D. Female.

E. Genetic vulnerability.

F. Recent life change.

G. Perception of external locus of control.

H. Alcohol and substance use.

I. Rape, military combat, and ethnically motivated genocide.

J. Medical rule out: Posttraumatic stress disorder (PTSD) commonly exists with chronic pain syndromes and irritable bowel syndrome.

K. Other psychiatric disorders commonly coexist with PTSD and all other disorders.

Subjective Data

A. Common symptoms.

    1. Patients who have PTSD have considerable stress that interferes with their ability to interact in society.

B. Common or typical scenario.

    1. May involve the patient withdrawing from society, job loss, divorce, or even substance abuse.

C. Family/social history.

    1. Ask about family situation, support system, or use of any drugs or alcohol.

D. Review of systems.

    1. Psychiatric: Ask about depression, anxiety, constant fear, suicidal thoughts, or complaints of chronic pain.

Mental State Examination

A. General.

    1. Agitated.

    2. Anxious.

    3. Irritable.

B. Attitude.

    1. Describe if patient is friendly, cooperative, hostile, or defensive.

C. Mood.

    1. General mood of patient.

D. Affect.

    1. Can be described as expansive, euthymic, constricted, or blunted.

E. Speech.

    1. Quantity, rate, and volume.

F. Thought process and content.

    1. How is the patient thinking?

Diagnostic Tests

A. Screening instruments.

    1. Posttraumatic Stress Disorder Checklist for *Diagnostic and Statistical Manual of Mental Disorders* (5th ed.; *DSM-5*) (PCL-S).

    2. Clinician-Administered PTSD Scale for PTSD (CAPS-5).

    3. Trauma Screening Questionnaire (TSQ).

    4. Short Screening Scale for PTSD.

    5. Short Form of the PTSD Checklist.

Differential Diagnosis

A. Adjustment disorder.

B. Acute stress disorder—Distinguished from PTSD based on time frame: Duration is restricted to 3 days to 1 month.

C. Anxiety/obsessive-compulsive disorder.

D. Major depression.

E. Personality disorders.

F. Conversion disorder.

G. Psychotic disorders.

H. Traumatic brain injury.

Evaluation and Management Plan

A. General plan.

    1. Psychotherapy.

        a. Trauma-focused therapy.

        b. Cognitive behavioral therapy (CBT).

        c. Exposure therapy.

        d. Eye movement desensitization and reprocessing (EMDR).

B. Pharmacotherapy.

    1. Selective serotonin reuptake inhibitors (SSRIs) are the only Food and Drug Administration (FDA) approved treatment for PTSD and have the strongest evidence: Paroxetine (Paxil) and sertraline (Zoloft) are the only medications with FDA approval.

    2. Benzodiazepines are not indicated in the treatment of PTSD.

    3. Serotonin norepinephrine reuptake inhibitors (SNRIs) like venlafaxine XR (Effexor SR) and mirtazapine (Remeron) have been shown to be helpful.

    4. Prazosin has been studied to treat nightmares: Starting dose 1 mg with range up to 40 mg.

Follow-Up

A. Coordination with a psychiatric specialist for ongoing treatment and follow-up.

B. Trauma-informed care and interventions have the best outcomes.

Consultation/Referral

A. Consider referral for integrative treatments (Confusion Assessment Method [CAM]): Mindfulness, yoga, acupuncture, and massage.

Special/Geriatric Considerations

A. Adaptive coping in elderly patients may be impaired and lead them to engage in substance abuse to manage PTSD symptoms.

B. Older adults may not identify symptoms in the context of a psychological framework, making them less likely to seek treatment.

C. There may be a stigma in older adults about seeking psychological assistance.

Bibliography

American Psychiatric Association. (2013). *Diagnostic and statistical manual of mental disorders* (5th ed.). Arlington, VA: American Psychiatric Publishing.

Pliszka, S. R. (2016). *Neuroscience for the mental health clinician* (5th ed.). New York, NY: Guilford Press.

Sadock, B. J., Sadock, V. A., & Ruiz, P. (2015). *Kaplan & Sadock's synopsis of psychiatry: Behavioral sciences/clinical psychiatry* (11th ed.). Philadelphia, PA: Wolters Kluwer.

Stahl, S. M. (2013). *Stahl's essential psychopharmacology: Neuroscientific basis and practical applications* (4th ed.). New York, NY: Cambridge University Press.

Stahl, S. M. (2014). *Stahl's essential psychopharmacology: Prescriber's guide* (5th ed.). New York, NY: Cambridge University Press.

Schizophrenia

Dawn Vanderhoef

Definition

A. Psychiatric disorder that affects behavior.

B. People with varying degrees of schizophrenia can have chronic and severe alterations in the way they think, feel, and behave.

Incidence

A. 1% with a lifetime prevalence of 0.6% to 1.9%.

B. Equally prevalent in men and women, but onset differs with more men having onset before age 25 with a peak age of 10 to 25 years of age and a peak in females age 25 to 35 with up to 10% of women having onset after age 40.

Pathogenesis

A. The pathogenesis of schizophrenia is unknown.

B. It is a uniquely human condition that appears to be caused by a complex interaction of genes and environment.

C. Genetic studies have shown a strong hereditary association, but the understanding of why or how schizophrenia occurs is unknown.

Predisposing Factors

A. Decreased cortical volume in temporal cortex and increased ventral size with decrease in gamma-aminobutyric acid (GABA) interneurons. Genetic estimates of up to 46% in monozygotic twins.

B. Born in winter or spring.

C. Raised in urban areas.

D. Early or prenatal infections.

E. Birth complications.

F. Substance use disorders.

Subjective Data

A. Common complaints/symptoms.
   1. One of the top three + one for 1 month.
      a. Delusions.
      b. Hallucinations (auditory and visual are most common; gustatory, olfactory, and tactile are more common due to an organic etiology).
      c. Disorganized speech.
      d. Grossly disorganized or catatonic behavior.
      e. Negative symptoms (restricted affect, poverty of speech, decreased interests, decrease dsense of purpose, decreased social drive).
   2. Impairment in function such as work, interpersonal relations, self-care, academic, or occupational issues.
   3. Continuous symptoms that last for 6 months or longer.

B. Common/typical scenario.
   1. Patients commonly present with hallucinations or disorganized speech.
   2. Symptoms may be vague in the beginning stages.
   3. The first psychotic episode may start in the teen years up to the mid-30s.

C. Family and social history.
   1. Family and close friends may describe a noticeable change in personality.
   2. Family history of schizophrenia may be pertinent, but the link is not very strong.

D. Review of systems.
   1. Rule out schizoaffective disorder, major depressive disorder, and bipolar disorder.
   2. Rule out due to substance use or general medical condition.
   3. Positive and negative symptoms.
      a. Positive symptoms: Hallucinations, delusions, disorganized behavior, paranoia.
      b. Negative symptoms: Affect flattening, alogia, avolition, apathy, anhedonia, abstract thinking loss.

Mental State Examination

A. General description: Disheveled, agitated, obsessively groomed, silent, or immobile.

B. Mood and affect: Reduced emotional responsiveness and/or overly active and inappropriate emotions (extremes of rage, happiness, and anxiety).

C. Perceptual disturbances.
   1. Auditory hallucinations are most common (voices threating, accusatory, or insulting).
   2. Command hallucinations put the patient and others at risk of harm.
   3. Visual hallucinations are also common.
   4. Tactile, olfactory, and gustatory disturbances are unusual and often associated with an underlying medical/neurological cause.

D. Thought.
   1. Content: Delusions (persecutory, grandiose, religious, somatic).
   2. Belief that outside sources control thoughts or behavior.
   3. Process: Way ideas form, including flight of ideas, thought blocking, impaired attention, poverty of thought, poor abstraction, clang associations, thought

broadcasting (others can hear their thoughts), or thought insertion (people place thoughts into their minds).

E. Violence.

1. Delusions may lead to violent behavior.

2. In an acute setting, intramuscular medication may be needed (benzodiazepine such as lorazepam or antipsychotic medication).

3. Suicide is common; 20% to 50% of persons with schizophrenia attempt suicide.

4. Homicide is no more likely than in the general population: Associated with bizarre hallucinations or delusions with predictors of previous violence, dangerous behavior, or hallucinations/delusions with violent content.

F. Orientation/memory/cognitive impairment: Usually oriented to person, place, and time. Memory and cognition are likely to be impaired.

G. Judgment and insight: Poor insight may lead to poor adherence along with poor judgment in the acute phase of illness.

H. Reliability: Dependent on the phase of illness.

I. Medication protective in suicidal ideation clozapine (Clozaril).

Diagnostic Tests

A. Broad screening: Complete blood count (CBC), blood glucose, comprehensive metabolic panel, urine drug screen, liver function tests.

B. Exclude specific disorders: Thyroid panel, vitamin B_{12}, folate, HIV, RPR (with prevalence of syphilis , this should be part of screening).

C. Other tests: EEG, chest x-ray, CT scan/MRI (first episode scan is part of the work up).

D. Screening instruments.

1. Brief Psychiatric Rating Scale (BPRS).

2. Scale for Assessment of Negative/Positive Symptoms (SANS / SAPS).

3. Positive and Negative Symptoms Syndrome Scale (PANSS).

Differential Diagnosis

A. Schizophreniform (less than 6 months of symptoms).

B. Schizoaffective disorder.

C. Brief psychotic disorder.

D. Delusional disorder.

E. Bipolar disorder.

F. Major depressive disorder.

G. Substance-induced disorder.

H. Psychotic disorder due to general medical condition (as with all psychiatric disorders, onset of symptoms is more commonly insidious: An abrupt change in mental status is likely related to an organic cause).

I. Medical rule outs.

1. Epilepsy.

2. Neoplasm.

3. AIDS.

4. Vitamin B_{12} deficiency.

5. Heavy metal poisoning.

6. Diabetes mellitus.

7. Cardiovascular disease.

8. Lung disease and cancer (due to high rates of nicotine use in up to 90% of patients—due in part to impairment of nicotine receptors in the brain).

Evaluation and Management Plan

A. General plan.

1. Risk of neuroleptic malignant syndrome (NMS) on antipsychotic medication.

2. Mnemonic **FEVER**.

a. Fever.

b. Encephalopathy.

c. Vital sign instability.

d. Enzyme elevation and creatinine phosphokinase (CPK).

e. Rigidity.

3. Cardinal signs/symptoms of NMS: Acute mental status changes with fluctuating consciousness, lead pipe rigidity, autonomic instability.

4. Labs: Leukocytosis and increased CPK, aspartate aminotransferase (AST), alanine aminotransferase (ALT), and myoglobinuria.

5. Treatment: Stop offending agent. Supportive care often in ICU setting.

B. Pharmacotherapy treatment of NMS.

1. Bromocriptine: Dopamine agonist used to restore lost dopaminergic tone.

2. Dantrolene: Direct acting skeletal muscle relaxant.

3. Antipsychotic medications.

a. *Medication class box warning*: Increase mortality in elderly patients with dementia-related psychosis. *Warning* for increased risk of hyperglycemia and diabetes mellitus.

b. *Expert guidelines on screening for all persons treated on AA medications:* At baseline, assess family and personal history of cardiovascular disease, weight (body mass index [BMI]), blood pressure, waist circumference, and fasting lipid/glucose; weight is done every 4 weeks; and blood pressure and fasting labs are completed again in 12 weeks. Glucose and lipid changes can occur in the absence of weight gain.

c. *Risk of tardive dyskinesia* on both atypical and typical antipsychotics exists and assessment of abnormal movements using the Abnormal Involuntary Movement Scale (AIMS) is recommended every 6 months.

d. *Risk of dystonic reactions:* Cervical, torticollis, oculogyric crisis, blepharospasms, larynogospasm. Acute treatment: Intermuscular benzotropine (Cogentin), diphenhydramine (Benadryl), or IV benzodiazepine.

Follow-Up

A. Follow-up with a psychiatric specialist: Should not be treated in primary care setting.

B. Smoking cessation programs.

Consultation/Referral

A. Consultation with primary care providers and referral for ongoing medical follow-up given the high prevalence of medical comorbidities.

B. Referral to psychosocial intervention/training programs and National Alliance on Mental Illness (NAMI).

C. Referral for cooccuring disorders treatment may be necessary given the high rates of comorbid substance use disorders.

Special/Geriatric Considerations

A. More than two-fifths of older adults with schizophrenia show clinical signs of depression and rates of suicide may be higher.

Bibliography

American Psychiatric Association. (2013). *Diagnostic and statistical manual of mental disorders* (5th ed.). Arlington, VA: American Psychiatric Publishing.

Pliszka, S. R. (2016). *Neuroscience for the mental health clinician* (2nd ed.). New York, NY: Guilford Press.

Sadock, B. J., Sadock, V. A., & Ruiz, P. (2015). *Kaplan & Sadock's synopsis of psychiatry: Behavioral sciences/clinical psychiatry* (11th ed.). Philadelphia, PA: Wolters Kluwer.

Stahl, S. M. (2013). *Stahl's essential psychopharmacology: Neuroscientific basis and practical applications* (4th ed.). New York, NY: Cambridge University Press.

Stahl, S. M. (2014). *Stahl's essential psychopharmacology: Prescriber's guide* (5th ed.). New York, NY: Cambridge University Press.

Tasman, A., & Mohr, W. (2011). *Fundamentals of psychiatry.* Hoboken, NJ: Wiley-Blackwell.

Substance Use Disorders

Dawn Vanderhoef

Definition

A. Abuse: Maladaptive pattern of use as evidenced by one or more of the following occurring within a 12-month period.
   1. Recurrent substance use with failure to fulfill major role obligations.
   2. Recurrent use in physically hazardous situations.
   3. Recurrent substance-related legal problems.
   4. Continued use despite persistent or recurrent social or interpersonal problems.
B. Dependence: Maladaptive pattern of use as evidenced by three or more of the following occurring at any time within the same 12-month period.
   1. Tolerance.
   2. Withdrawal.
   3. Substance taken in larger amounts over a longer period of time.
   4. Persistent desire/effort to cut down or control use.
   5. Increasing time spent obtaining, using, and recovering from use.
   6. Important social, occupational, or recreational activities given up.
   7. Continued use despite knowledge of adverse effects.
   8. With physiological dependence: Evidence of tolerance or withdrawal.
   9. Without physiological dependence: No evidence of tolerance or withdrawal.
C. Substances of addiction: Alcohol; caffeine; cannabis; hallucinogens; inhalants: opioids; sedatives/hypnotics/anxiolytics; stimulants; tobacco; other/unknown substances.

Incidence

A. Alcohol abuse 9.4% versus dependence 14%.
B. Cannabis 8.5%.
C. Opioids 1.4%.
D. Sedatives 1%.
E. Amphetamines 2%.
F. Cocaine 2.8%.
G. Hallucinogens 1.7%.

Pathogenesis

A. Has both a genetic and environmental risk with complex neurobiology.

Predisposing Factors

A. Age of first use matters: Odds of alcoholism as an adult go down by 14% for each year a youth does not drink after age 14.
B. Access.
C. Peer groups.

Subjective Data

A. Common complaints/symptoms.
   1. Craving, irrepressible urge to seek and consume drug substance.
B. Common/typical scenario.
   1. Patients commonly present for either another medical condition or a complication associated with use of the substance.
C. Family and social history.
   1. Behaviors may be learned or there may be a genetic predisposition to addictive substances.
D. Review of systems.
   1. Psychological—irritable, anxious, restless.
   2. Cardiac—racing heart rate, feeling of palpitations.

Mental State Examination

A. General.
   1. Agitated.
   2. Anxious.
   3. Irritable.
B. Attitude.
   1. Describe if patient is friendly, cooperative, hostile, or defensive.
C. Mood.
   1. General mood of patient.
D. Affect.
   1. Can be described as expansive, euthymic, constricted, or blunted.
E. Speech.
   1. Quantity.
   2. Rate.
   3. Volume.
F. Thought process and content.
   1. How is the patient thinking?

Diagnostic Tests

A. Comprehensive metabolic panel (CMP).
B. Liver function tests.
C. Blood alcohol level.
D. Serum drug screen.
E. Pregnancy test.
F. HIV.
G. EKG.
H. Screening.
   1. Screening, brief intervention, and referral to treatment (SBIRT).
     a. Screening: A healthcare professional assesses for risky substance use behaviors using standardized screening tools such as CAGE.
     b. Brief intervention: A healthcare professional engages a patient showing risky substance use behaviors in a short conversation.
   2. A standard drink.
     a. 2 oz of beer/ale/malt liquor.
     b. 1.5 oz of spirits such as vodka, tequila, gin, whiskey, or rum.
     c. 5 oz of wine.
   3. Positive screen for at-risk drinking.
     a. Men: Greater than 14 drinks a week or greater than 4 on occasion.
     b. Women: Greater than 7 drinks a week or greater than 3 drinks on occasion.
     c. Elders: Greater than 7 drinks a week or greater than 1 drink on occasion.

4. CAGE assessment: One yes is a positive screen and needs further assessment.

    a. Have you ever felt the need to CUT down on your substance use?

    b. Have people ANNOYED you by criticizing your substance use?

    c. Have you ever felt GUILTY about your substance use?

    d. Have you ever felt the need to drink/use first thing in the morning as an EYE opener?

Differential Diagnosis

A. Attention deficit hyperactivity disorder (ADHD).
B. Bipolar disorder.
C. Trauma-related disorders.
D. Major depression.
E. Anxiety disorders.
F. Other substance use disorders.

Evaluation and Management Plan

A. Motivational interviewing to assess readiness and increase ambivalence.
B. Treatment is based on severity, individual motivation taking into account abstinence, or harm reduction.
C. Withdrawal.
D. Hierarchy of detoxification: Sedative/hypnotics, alcohol, then opioids.
E. Assessment of alcohol withdrawal and providing intervention: Risk of seizures after 48 hours of last drink and risk of DTs after 72 hours of last drink.
F. Alcohol withdrawal assessment: Clinical Institute for Withdrawal Assessment for Alcohol (CIWA-AR) and detox is most commonly attempted with a benzodiazepine.
G. Opioid withdrawal assessment: Clinical Opiate Withdrawal Scale (COWS) and detox commonly with opiates such as buprenorphine or phenobarbital.
H. Alcohol cravings: Naltrexone/Vivitrol, acamprosate, ondansetron, or disulfiram (Antabuse)—need to provide education about products to avoid adverse reactions.
I. Opioid replacement: Methadone, buprenorphine (can be prescribed by nurse practitioners [NPs] with additional training), Suboxone.
J. Nicotine replacement: NRT options (patch, gum, inhaler), bupropion (Zyban) same as Wellbutrin, varenicline (Chantix)

Follow-Up

A. Follow-up with a substance use disorder specialist for medications and therapy.

Consultation/Referral

A. Consultation for medical comorbidities.
B. Referral to outpatient support groups such as Alcoholics Anonymous (AA), Narcotics Anonymous (NA), Cocaine Anonymous (CA), Opioids Anonymous (OA).
C. Referral to treatment: A healthcare professional provides a referral to brief therapy or for additional services.

Special/Geriatric Considerations

A. Substance abuse in the elderly is a rapidly growing problem and may be triggered by retirement; death of a close family member, friend, or even pet; financial strains; or mental or physical decline.
B. Elderly patients may have a decreased ability to metabolize drugs or alcohol.

Bibliography

American Psychiatric Association. (2013). *Diagnostic and statistical manual of mental disorders* (5th ed.). Arlington, VA: American Psychiatric Publishing.

Morrison, J. (2014). *DSM-5 made easy: The clinician's guide to diagnosis.* New York, NY: Guilford Press.

Sadock, B. J., Sadock, V. A., & Ruiz, P. (2015). *Kaplan & Sadock's synopsis of psychiatry: Behavioral sciences/clinical psychiatry* (11th ed.). Philadelphia, PA: Wolters Kluwer.

Substance Abuse and Mental Health Services Administration. (2019). Recovery and recovery support. Retrieved from https://www.samhsa.gov/find-help/recovery

Psychiatric Patient Medical Clearance

Dawn Vanderhoef

Definition

A. Guidelines exist, but no clear definition of what "medical clearance" should include.
B. Review local institutional guidelines.

    1. Purpose: Clearance of a psychiatric patient to transfer to a setting with fewer medical resources.

    2. Guideline: Within reasonable medical certainty, there is no contributing medical condition causing the psychiatric complaints.

C. Assessment for risk of violence STAMP—Staring and eye contact, Tone and volume of voice, Anxiety, Mumbling, and Pacing.
D. Training in nonviolent crisis intervention and de-escalation.

Subjective Data

A. Common complaints/symptoms.

    1. Delirium.

    2. Confusion.

    3. Agitated behavior.

B. Common/typical scenario.

    1. Patients come to the ED or are brought by family or medical services because of an alteration in disposition.

C. Family and social history.

    1. Inquire about drug use, or any medications.

    2. Inquire about falls.

    3. Inquire about family history of mental illness.

    4. Biopsychosocial history.

        a. What led to ED presentation?

        b. Risk to self/others or inability to care for self due to mental status changes.

        c. Rule out organic or substance-induced causes.

        d. Identify needed medical treatments.

    5. History.

        a. History taking will provide guidance as to what medical testing should occur. Collateral data from a family member, caseworker, group home staff, or someone who knows the patient is critical.

        b. Is this an existing or new psychiatric illness?

        c. Assessment of mental status for acute (more commonly organic in nature) or insidious (more commonly psychiatric in nature) onset, drug interaction, or toxicity (new medication/medication change/overtaking medication).

        d. Relapse of a psychiatric disorder due to nonadherence.

D. Review of systems.

    1. Dermatologic—ask about bruising or breaks in skin.

    2. Neurological—ask about dizziness, confusion, or weakness.

Mental State Examination

A. Mental State Examination: Assessment of risk to self, risk to others, or risk of violence (see suicide/homicide risk assessment noted previously).

B. Quick confusion scale.

    1. Five items: What year is it? What month is it? About what time is it? Count backward from 20 to 1. Repeat a phrase.

    2. Correlation with Mental State Examination.

Diagnostic Tests

A. No high yield laboratory tests.

B. Consider.

    1. Drug screen and blood ethanol level.

    2. Anything triggered by return of spontaneous circulation (ROSC) to include American Society of Anesthesiologists (ASA) or acetaminophen level.

    3. Human chorionic gonadotropin (HCG).

    4. Basic metabolic panel (BMP).

    5. Complete blood count (CBC).

    6. Liver function test (LFT).

    7. HIV.

    8. Rapid plasma reagin (RPR).

    9. Unstable angina (UA).

Differential Diagnosis

A. Fasting glucose/metabolic disorders.

B. Meningitis (drop coin to see if patient can look down).

C. Substance use (look up nose for substance use).

D. Seizure—postictal (assess tongue for lacerations)

E. Traumatic brain injury.

F. Delirium.

G. Drug overdose.

H. Syphilis.

Evaluation and Management Plan

A. Assess capacity: Consent to treatment and competency: Does this patient have a legal guardian (incompetence can only be determined by the court)?

B. Involuntary commitment: Know your state laws about the process AND transportation.

C. Duty to protect (see earlier) and duty to report (children, older adults, and those without capacity).

D. Inpatient/outpatient or referral to community resource.

Consultation/Referral

A. Psychiatry if available in the hospital or one can use telemedicine. ED protocols for evaluation of psychiatric cases have been developed by the American College of Emergency Physicians.

B. Consult case management to help the patient find needed resources for outpatient management.

C. Consult social work if drugs are involved or the patient is homeless.

Special/Geriatric Considerations

A. Geriatric patients are more likely to present with delirium to the ED related to medical conditions.

B. Elderly patients with psychiatric disorders are more likely to have multiple psychotic disorders, mood disorders, and dementia and less likely to have schizophrenia or substance disorders.

Bibliography

American College of Emergency Physicians. (2009). *Massachusetts medical clearance guidelines.* Retrieved from https://www.acep.org/global assets/uploads/uploaded-files/acep/advocacy/state-issues/psychiatric-hold-issues/ma-medical-clearance-guidelines-toxic-screen-ma.pdf

American Psychiatric Association. (2013). *Diagnostic and statistical manual of mental disorders* (5th ed.). Arlington, VA: American Psychiatric Publishing.

Boudreaux, E. D., Niro, K., Sullivan, A., Rosenbaum, C. D., Allen, M., & Camargo, C. A. (2011). Current practices for mental health follow-up after psychiatric emergency department/psychiatric emergency service visits: A national survey of academic emergency departments. *General Hospital Psychiatry, 33*(6), 631–633. doi:10.1016/j.genhosppsych.2011.05.020

New Jersey Hospital Association. (2011). *Consensus statement: Medical clearance protocols for acute psychiatric patients referred for inpatient admission.* Retrieved from http://www.njha.com/media/33107/ClearanceProtocolsforAcutePsyPatients.pdf

Nordstrom, K., Zun, L. S., Wilson, M. P., Stiebel, V., Ng, A. T., Bregman, B., . . . Nouri, T. (2012). Medical evaluation and triage of the agitated patient: Consensus statement of the American Association for Emergency Psychiatry project BETA medical evaluation workgroup. *Western Journal of Emergency Medicine, 13*(1), 3–10. doi:10.5811/westjem.2011.9.6863

Tang, S., Patel, P., Khubchandani, J., & Grossberg, G. (2014). The psychogeriatric patient in the emergency room: Focus on management and disposition. *ISRN Psychiatry, 2014,* 5. doi:10.1155/2014/413572

Infection Guidelines

Rose Milano

Colitis: Infective

Jennifer W. Parker

Definition

A. Inflammation of the colon caused by an infectious agent (i.e., bacteria, virus, or parasites). Colitis is diagnosed when the patient has diarrhea (passage of three or more unformed stools per day and has evidence of inflammation in the colon based on at least one of the following.

  1. Positive fecal markers: Elevated leukocytes, positive lactoferrin, or positive calprotectin.

  2. Dysentery: Many small volume stools containing obvious blood or mucus (often associated with fever and abdominal pain).

  3. Mucosal inflammation as identified by colonoscopy or sigmoidoscopy.

B. Duration of symptoms.

  1. Acute: 14 days or fewer (most are infectious and self-limiting).

  2. Persistent: 14 to 30 days.

  3. Chronic: 30 or more days (most are noninfectious).

C. Pseudomembranous colitis caused by the bacteria *Clostridioides difficile* in the acute care setting: Of special concern; to be highlighted in this chapter.

Incidence

A. The vast majority of colitis is viral; only 1.5% to 5.6% of stool cultures produce positive results.

B. Severe diarrhea (four or more liquid stools/day for more than 3 days) is generally bacterial.

C. In the past 10 years, *C. difficile* infection (CDI) has been increasing in the United States—not only in the healthcare setting but also in community. Here are the 2011 estimated incidence rates in the United States for CDI, which can no longer be considered just a healthcare-acquired disease.

  1. Community-acquired CDI: 51.9 cases per 100,000. The rate of first recurrence was 13.5%, and the death rate within 30 days was 1.3%.

  2. Healthcare-acquired CDI: 95.3 cases per 100,000. The rate of first recurrence was 20.9%, and a death rate within 30 days was 9.3%.

Pathogenesis

A. Diarrhea represents altered changes in the flow of water and electrolytes within an osmotic gradient. Normally the gastrointestinal (GI) tract absorbs about 8 to 9 L of fluid a day, excreting about 200 mL of water in stool.

B. Enteric pathogens, acting primarily on transporter cells or the lateral spaces between cells (which are regulated by tight junctions), alter the balance toward significantly greater excretion and less absorption.

C. Pathogens can alter absorption by either direct or indirect modulation.

  1. Direct modulation involving.

   a. Epithelial ion transport processes.

    i. Evidence from the literature proposes that the rapid onset of diarrhea induced via enteropathogenic *Escherichia coli* (EPEC) may result from direct effects on intestinal epithelial ion transport processes.

   b. Barrier function.

  2. Indirect modulation involving.

   a. Inflammation.

    i. *Shigella* and *Salmonella* species cause an inflammatory diarrhea characterized by fever and polymorphonucleocytes (PMNs) in the stool.

    ii. PMNs regulate absorption through cytokine secretion but also have a more direct role through the secretion of a precursor to adenosine, activating certain transmembrane conductance regulators.

   b. Neuropeptides.

    i. *C. difficile* and rotavirus infection also work indirectly through modulation of ion transport subsequent to cytokine secretion and activation of enteric nerves via neuropeptides.

   c. Loss of absorptive surface.

    i. *Giardia* lead to the loss of brush border absorptive surface and diffuse shortening of villi.

    ii. Similarly, EPEC cause effacement of microvilli, which decreases the surface area for nutrient absorption and causes increased osmolarity of the intestinal contents and malabsorption.

    iii. Major causes in the United States.

     1) Viruses: Norovirus, rotavirus, adenoviruses, and astrovirus.

     2) Bacteria: *Salmonella, Campylobacter, Shigella,* enterotoxigenic *E. coli,* and *C. difficile.*

     3) Protozoa: *Cryptosporidium, Giardia, Cyclospora,* and *Entamoeba.*

D. CDI (nosocomial and community acquired) account for almost all cases of pseudomembranous colitis (acute colitis characterized by the formation of an adherent inflammatory membrane that overlays injury site).

  1. There is multifactorial activation with enterotoxin A and cytotoxin B. In addition, there is a new strain with increased productions of enterotoxin A and cytotoxin B, as well as binary toxin, with fluoroquinolone resistance.

2. Besides the direct effect of the toxins on tight junctions, and in contrast to other pathogens, *C. difficile* leads to activation of neuropeptides, resulting in inflammation via a necroinflammatory reaction, which activates mast cells, nerves, vascular endothelium, and immune cells.

Predisposing Factors

A. Hospitalization, previous CDI, greater than 65 years of age, recent abdominal surgery, use of proton pump inhibitors (PPI), and living conditions (long-term care facilities).
B. International travel: *Shigella, Campylobacter, Salmonella,* enteroinvasive *E. coli* (EIEC), enteroaggregative *E. coli* (EAEC), and others.
C. Foodborne: *Staphylococcus aureus, Bacillus cereus, Clostridioides perfringens,* or *E. coli.*
D. Other risk factors.
  1. Antibiotic exposure, healthcare exposure.
  2. Exposure to *C. difficile.*
  3. HIV or other immune deficiency.
  4. Chemotherapy.
  5. Enteric tube feeding or other GI tract manipulation.
  6. Inflammatory bowel disease (IBD) or other chronic GI disease.

Subjective Data

A. Common complaints/symptoms.
  1. Mild: Watery diarrhea three or more times a day, abdominal cramping.
  2. Severe: Watery diarrhea 10 or more times a day with abdominal cramping and pain.
    May also be associated with fever, dehydration, and rapid heart rate.
B. Common/typical scenario.
  1. Careful, detailed history of present illness: Important because it can suggest likely cause of the diarrhea.
    a. Duration—acute, persistent, chronic, or change in periodicity.
    b. Frequency and characteristics of stool.
      i. Small bowel origin—watery, large volume, abdominal cramping, bloating, or gas.
      ii. Large bowel origin—frequent, regular small volume stools, often tenesmus with bowel movements, and inflammatory signs (i.e., fever and bloody or mucoid stools) are common.
      iii. Inflammatory signs suggest enteric viruses (e.g., cytomegalovirus [CMV], adenovirus), invasive bacteria (e.g., *Salmonella, Shigella, Campylobacter*), or cytotoxic pathogen such as *C. difficile.*
C. Family and social history.
  1. Food exposure—raw or undercooked meat, seafood, unpasteurized dairy products. Timing is important.
    a. Less than 6 hours with nausea and vomiting, likely *S. aureus* or *B. cereus.*
    b. 8–16 hours—likely *C. perfringens.*
    c. Greater than 16 hours—viral or possibly *E. coli* enterotoxigenic pathogen.
  2. Other exposures.
    a. Animals (e.g., poultry, petting zoos): *Salmonella.*
    b. Travel to resource limited areas (increased risk of pathogens and certain bacteria).
    c. Occupation—Day-care centers likely for *Giardia, Shigella,* or *Cryptosporidium.*
    d. Recent hospitalizations—increased likelihood of CDI.
    e. Antibiotic use—increased likelihood of CDI.

f. Use of PPI—can increase risk of infectious diarrhea.
D. Review of systems.
  1. Neurologic—lightheadedness, dizziness.
  2. Dermatologic—dry skin.
  3. Genitourinary—frequency of urination and color.
  4. Abdominal—diarrhea, nausea, pain anywhere in the abdomen, bloody stools, loss of appetite, bloating, or distension.

Physical Examination

A. Volume status: Hypovolemia.
  1. Dry mucous membranes.
  2. Tenting of skin or diminished skin turgor.
  3. Change in mental status.
  4. Dizziness, lightheadedness, and orthostatic blood pressure.
  5. Hypotension.
B. Complications: Ileus or peritonitis.
  1. Abdominal distention.
  2. Abdominal tenderness with percussion or gentle palpitation.
  3. Rebound tenderness.
  4. Abdominal rigidity.

Diagnostic Tests

A. Blood studies: Often not needed for patients with infectious diarrhea but helps determine status of the acutely ill patient.
  1. Serum electrolytes if volume depletion is a concern: Screening for hypokalemia and acute kidney injury (AKI).
  2. Complete blood count (CBC)—may be of limited help.
    a. Platelet count—concern for hemolytic uremic syndrome.
    b. Leukocytosis—consistent with CDI.
  3. Blood cultures—if high fever is present, or sepsis is a concern.
  4. Lactate, CPR, procalcitonin (PCT) level if patient has signs and symptoms of sepsis.
B. Stool studies: Often unnecessary if patients have no comorbidities: Infectious colitis generally resolves on its own. However, these tests should be completed for those with severe illness, high-risk comorbidities, or suggestive history.
  1. Fecal leukocytes—findings of white blood cell (WBC) count on a test result does *not* differentiate between IBD and infectious colitis.
  2. Acute bloody diarrhea: Bacterial colitis.
    a. Cultures for enterohemorrhagic *E. coli* (EHEC) and *Entamoeba.*
    b. Shiga toxin direct testing: For many strains of Shiga toxin-producing *E. coli* (STEC).
  3. Stool culture.
    a. *Shigella, Salmonella,* and *Campylobacter* are routinely sought.
    b. If STEC, noncholera *Vibrio,* or *Yersinia* is suspected, alert the lab to look for these, because specialized techniques are required.
  4. Ova and parasites (O&P): For patients with persistent diarrhea or who are immunocompromised. Unlike bacterial pathogens, which are shed continuously, O&P are shed intermittently.
  5. *C. difficile* toxin: For patients who currently take or have recently taken antibiotics *or* have been hospitalized or recently been in a healthcare facility.

C. Imaging (CT): Not usually warranted unless patient is presenting with acute abdomen.

D. CDI.

    1. Leukocytosis: Can be marked in severe disease (>15,000 cells/μL).

    2. Volume depletion—elevated creatinine (Cr), blood urea nitrogen (BUN), reduced estimated glomerular filtration rate (GFR).

    3. Elevated lactate.

    4. Predictors of mortality.

        a. WBC greater than 35,000 cells/μL or less than 4,000 cells/μL.

        b. Significant banding (>10%).

        c. Immunosuppression.

        d. Cardiorespiratory failure.

    5. Need to differentiate *C. difficile* colonization from infection.

        a. Only perform CDI testing on loose stools (unless concern for ileus) when there is a reasonable likelihood of CDI.

        b. Stool studies.

            i. Culture: Gold standard for identification of *C. difficile*.

                1) Sow times; requires follow-up with toxigenic testing, because not all strains produce toxins.

                2) Usually reserved for epidemiologic studies.

            ii. Enzyme immunoassay—rapid.

                1) Sensitivity of 75% to 94% and specificity of 83% to 98% for identification of toxins A and B.

                2) Low sensitivity may require further diagnostic testing in face of high clinical suspicion and negative test results.

            iii. Polymerase chain reaction—superior to enzyme immunoassay.

                1) Used by most U.S. hospitals.

                2) High sensitivity and specificity—single sample is sufficient.

                3) Generally 24 to 48 hours turnaround.

                4) *Does not* differentiate colonization from infection.

Differential Diagnosis

A. IBD (i.e., ulcerative colitis, Crohn's disease).

B. Ischemic colitis—vasculitis common in Henoch–Schönlein purpura.

C. Immunodeficiency syndromes (e.g., common variable immunodeficiency, chronic granulomatous disease, Wiskott–Aldrich syndrome, and immunodysregulation polyendocrinopathy enteropathy X-linked [IPEX] syndrome).

D. Irritable bowel syndrome.

E. Celiac disease.

Evaluation and Management Plan

A. General plan.

    1. Supportive care.

        a. Fluid and electrolyte administration to keep up with losses.

            i. Oral is preferred hydration. Severe disease may require oral rehydration solution.

            ii. Monitor electrolytes and repletion as necessary.

    2. Low fat, low dairy (except yogurt or other fermented dairy items) diets: Preferred; banana, rice, applesauce, and toast (BRAT) diet.

    3. Holding of anti-motility therapy (e.g., loperamide, bismuth subsalicylate): Can be harmful with some pathogens; generally all right with inflammatory diarrhea.

B. Pharmacotherapy.

    1. Antibiotics.

    2. Empiric therapy.

        a. Not widely recommended (despite reducing length of illness) because of promotion of antibiotic resistance, likely changes in gut flora, and increased risk of CDI.

        b. However, recommended for certain conditions:

            i. Severe disease: Greater than six stools per day, fever, hypovolemia requiring hospitalization.

            ii. Bloody or mucoid stools (likely invasive bacterial infection) unless fever is low or absent.

            iii. Comorbidities (especially immunocompromising and cardiac diseases), including age greater than 70.

        c. *Oral* fluoroquinolones for 3 to 5 days: Preferred treatment for empiric therapy for acute diarrhea of unknown source.

            i. Ciprofloxacin: 500 mg BID.

            ii. Levofloxacin: 500 mg daily.

            iii. Fluoroquinolone intolerant patients: Oral azithromycin 500 mg PO daily for 3 days or erythromycin 500 mg PO BID for 5 days.

    3. History of antibiotic therapy or recent hospitalizations: Treatment for CDI.

        a. Discontinuation of offending antibiotic (if possible).

        b. *Avoidance* of anti-motility medications.

        c. Enhanced contact precautions: Handwashing before and after patient contact.

        d. Antibiotic therapy: Best to wait for diagnostic confirmation if possible; no treatment if positive toxin assay but asymptomatic.

            i. Mild-moderate.

                1) Vancomycin 125 mg PO QID × 10 to 14 days.

                2) Fidaxomicin 200 mg BID × 10 days.

                3) Metronidazole 500 mg PO TID × 10 to 14 days (not first-line treatment; use only if other options not available.) Not for use in recurrent CDI infections.

            ii. Severe (WBC >15,000 cells/μL × serum albumin <3 g/dL, and /or Cr ≥1.5 baseline).

                1) Vancomycin 125 mg PO QID × 10 to 14 days.

            iii. Fulminant or complicated.

                1) Vancomycin 125 mg PO QID × 10 to 14 days, *plus.*

                2) Metronidazole 500 mg IV q 6 to 8 hours, *plus.*

                3) Vancomycin via nasogastric tube or rectally.

            iv. Recurrent, antibiotic resistant (but recurrent is not equivalent to resistant); after initial treatment, recurrence in 15% to 20% of cases generally 5 to 8 days after treatment. It is important to distinguish a spontaneous recurrence versus antibiotic triggered resistance.

                1) Repeat same or alternate antibiotic. Recurrences beyond the second infection should not be treated with metronidazole due to possible neurotoxic effects with prolonged use and decreased effectiveness.

2) Vancomycin pulses and/or tapers for extended duration.

3) Vancomycin for 2 weeks, then rifaximin for 2 weeks (generally not used now that fecal microbiota treatment is available).

4) High dose vancomycin in combination with *Saccharomyces boulardii* (*not* in immuno-suppressed patients).

5) Fecal microbiota treatment: Used in cases of multiple recurrent CDI, moderate CDI with no response to standard antibiotic therapy for 1 week, or severe or fulminate CDI with no response to treatment in 48 hours; relatively high success rate (nearly 90% for recurrent CDI). It involves fecal enemas, colonoscopy with delivery of fecal material, and nasogastric tube delivery of fecal material.

6) Colectomy.

v. Probiotics: Generally, *not* appropriate for patients being treated for CDI.

4. Probiotics: Should be started within 48 hours of initiation of antibiotic treatment on **any patient receiving antibiotics other than for CDI** to lower risk of *C. difficile*.

C. Patient/family teaching points.

1. Prevent the spread of *C. difficile* with aggressive handwashing. Do not rely on hand sanitizers because they are ineffective in destroying *C. difficile* spores.

2. Patients need to have a private room.

3. All staff and visitors must wear isolation gowns and gloves while in the room.

D. Discharge.

1. Avoid unnecessary antibiotics.

2. Report new or worsening symptoms.

3. Clean surfaces at home with chlorine-based disinfectants.

4. Drink fluids to prevent dehydration.

Follow-Up

A. There is generally no role for repeat laboratory testing/testing for a cure with *C. difficile*.

B. Assays may remain positive during recovery.

Consultation/Referral

A. In severe, unresponsive cases, gastroenterology and/or surgery may need to be consulted.

Special/Geriatric Considerations

A. Elderly patients are generally characterized as having decreased immune function.

B. Short- and long-term hospitalizations have become a critical risk factor in the development of colitis in this population.

C. Mortality rates are also significantly higher in elderly patients.

Bibliography

Barkley, T. W., Jr., Myers, C. M. (2014). *Practice considerations for adult-gerontology acute care nurse practitioners.* West Hollywood, CA: Barkley and Associates.

DuPont, H. L. (2012). Approach to the patient with infectious colitis. *Current Opinion in Gastroenterology, 28*, 39–46. doi:10.1097/MOG.0b013e32834d3208

Hodges, K., & Ravinder, G. (2010). Infectious diarrhea: Cellular and molecular mechanisms. *Gut Microbes, 1*(1), 4–21. doi:10.4161/gmic.1.1.11036

Kelly, C. P. Lamont, J. T., & Bakken, J. S. (2019, March 1). Clostridioides (formerly clostridium) difficile infection in adults: Treatment and prevention. In E. L. Baron (Ed.), *UpToDate.* Retrieved from https://www.uptodate.com/contents/clostridioides-formerly-clostridium-difficile-infection-in-adults-treatment-and-prevention

Lamont, J. T. (2018, October 25). Clostridioides (formerly clostridium) difficile infection in adults: Clinical manifestations and diagnosis. In E. L. Baron (Ed.), *UpToDate.* Retrieved from https://www.uptodate.com/contents/clostridioides-formerly-clostridium-difficile-infection-in-adults-clinical-manifestations-and-diagnosis

Liubakka, A., & Vaughn, B. P. (2016). *Clostridioides difficile* infection and fecal microbiota transplant. *Advanced Critical Care, 27*(3), 324–337. doi:10.4037/aacnacc2016703

McDonald, L. C., Gerding, D. N., Johnson, S., Bakken, J. S., Carroll, K. C., Coffin, S. E., ... Wilcox, M. H. (2018). Clinical practice guidelines for *Clostridioides difficile* in adults and children: 2017 update by the Infectious Disease Society for Healthcare Epidemiology of America (SHEA). *Clinical Infectious Disease, 66*, 987. doi:10.1093/cid/ciy149

Piccoli, D. A. (2019, January 4). Colitis. In C. Cuffari (Ed.), *Medscape.* Retrieved from http://emedicine.medscape.com/article/927845-overview

Shen, N. T. (2017). Timely use of probiotics in hospitalized adults prevents *Clostridioides difficile* infection: A systematic review with meta-regression analysis. *Gastroenterology, 152*, 1889–1900. doi: 10.1053/j.gastro.2017.02.003

Wedro, B. (2016, June 20). *Colitis.* Retrieved from http://www.emedicinehealth.com/colitis/article_em.htm

Encephalitis

Dominick Osipowicz

Definition

A. Inflammation of the brain parenchyma.

B. Viral encephalitis: An acute viral infection of the brain parenchyma, characterized by a moderate elevation of white blood cells in the cerebrospinal fluid (CSF) and focal neurological deficits. These include but are not limited to altered mental status, cognitive impairments, aphasia, hemiparesis, paresthesias, and behavioral changes.

C. Bacterial or fungal encephalitis: Rare.

D. Paraneoplastic and autoimmune encephalitis: Beyond the scope of this text but should be considered in the setting of known history of or concern for cancer and a sterile CSF analysis. Etiology of disease is related to an inflammation of the brain parenchyma secondary to an antibody attack of the neuronal surface cells and/or synaptic proteins.

Incidence

A. Despite its rarity in contrast to bacterial meningitis, encephalitis remains a significant health concern associated with a high rate of morbidity and mortality.

B. Incidence is related to global distribution patterns of viral infections with the herpes virus and arthropod-borne viruses.

Pathogenesis

A. Encephalitis is characterized as an inflammation of the brain parenchyma due to infectious, postinfectious, or non-infectious etiology with symptoms of altered mental status, focal neurological deficits, and seizures.

B. Viral infection is the most common cause of encephalitis in adults. Herpes simplex virus (HSV) is the leading cause of encephalitis worldwide.

C. In addition to HSV, common causes of infectious encephalitis are varicella herpes zoster virus (VZV), cytomegalovirus (CMV), West Nile Virus, influenza, HIV, mumps, rabies, and measles. Also, more than a dozen species of arthropod-borne viruses are known to cause encephalitis.

Predisposing Factors
A. Recent viral illness.
B. Mosquito bites.
C. Tick bites.
D. Exposure to pig, bat, duck, and rodent feces.
E. Rabid animal bites.
F. Travel to areas with known infective vectors.
G. Immunocompromised state.
H. Immunosuppressive therapy.
I. Organ transplantation.

Subjective Data
A. Common complaints/symptoms.
  1. Presentation varies from mild confusion and inappropriate behavior to comatose state.
  2. Affected patients present with cortical findings as viruses gravitate toward the brain parenchyma.
  3. Cortical symptoms include but are not limited to altered mental status, cognitive impairment, aphasias, hemiparesis, paresthesias, and behavioral changes.
  4. Meningeal irritation should not be a symptom. However, it may be seen in patients with meningoencephalitis.
B. Family and social history.
  1. Familial history is often noncontributory.
  2. Social history may reveal recent viral illness and travel abroad, particularly to sub-Saharan Africa and exposure to rodents, ticks, and mosquitoes.
  3. History of cancer or concern for cancer diagnosis may be a factor.
C. Review of systems.
  1. General: Fatigue, weakness, fever, or chills.
  2. Head, ear, eyes, nose, and throat (HEENT): Headaches.
  3. Neurological: Lethargy, syncope, seizures, muscle weakness, altered sensation, altered speech, or disorientation.

Physical Examination
A. Altered mental status: Presence or absence of normal brain function. This is the important distinguishing feature between encephalopathy and meningitis.
B. Focal neurological deficits: Including, but not limited to, cognitive impairments, aphasia, hemiparesis, paresthesias, and behavioral changes.
C. Seizure activity.
D. Nuchal rigidity (unlikely): Including tenderness to palpation and pain with flexion and extension.

Diagnostic Tests
A. A noncontrast CT of the head: Required.
  1. Patients will likely have altered mental status, focal neurological deficits, and new onset seizures, which raise concern for elevated intracranial pressure; this allows for ruling out a space occupying lesion.
  2. CT scan of the head with temporal lobe edema that does not follow a vascular pattern is the classic presentation of HSV encephalitis.
B. MRI: Shows demyelination, which may be present in other clinical states with similar presentation.
C. Lumbar puncture: Gold standard for a diagnosis of viral encephalitis.
  1. CSF analysis.

  a. Cell count/differential, glucose, protein and gram stain, and bacterial culture.
  b. Abnormal CSF suggestive of viral encephalitis.
    i. Elevated opening pressure.
    ii. CSF white blood cell (WBC) count elevated but less than $250/\mu L$ and lymphocyte dominant.
    iii. CSF red blood cells (RBC) count may be present in HSV encephalitis.
    iv. CSF glucose greater than 60 mg/dL and CSF/serum ratio of greater than 0.6.
    v. CSF protein elevated but less than 150mg/dL.
    vi. Culture and polymerase chain reaction (PCR) test for virus.
      1) If culture is negative but strong clinical and radiological suspicion for HSV/VZV encephalitis remains, repeat lumbar puncture in 3 to 5 days and continue treatment.
  2. Contraindications to lumbar puncture.
    a. Systemic anticoagulation.
    b. Thrombocytopenia.
    c. Coagulopathy.
    d. Open sacral wound at level L3 to L5.
    e. CT head with evidence of increased intracranial pressure and/or mass lesion.
D. EEG: Often abnormal in acute encephalitis.
E. Relevant blood work: CBC, basal metabolic profile (BMP), partial thromboplastin time (PTT)/prothrombin time (PT)/international normalized ratio (INR), lactate, and arterial blood gas.
F. Blood cultures.

Differential Diagnosis
A. Viral encephalitis.
B. Bacterial meningitis.
C. Epidural abscess.
D. Nonconvulsive status epilepticus.
E. Subarachnoid hemorrhage.

Evaluation and Management Plan
A. General plan: Viral encephalitis.
  1. Rule out bacterial meningitis due to high risk of morbidity and mortality.
  2. Patient presentation suggestive of central nervous system (CNS) infection.
  3. Follow SEPSIS 3.0 guidelines for fluid resuscitation management of septic shock.
  4. Begin broad-spectrum antibiotics as well as antiviral therapy and glucocorticoids if appropriate.
  5. Obtain a "Stat" CT head without contrast to rule out alternative diagnoses.
  6. Use lumbar puncture with CSF analysis for definitive treatment, and if available meningitis/encephalitis PCR for rapid identification of causative pathogen.
  7. Arrange for hemodynamic management and supportive care.
  8. Admit to ICU for appropriate level of care.
  9. Consider MRI of the brain in patients who fail to improve despite treatment to evaluate alternative diagnoses.
  10. Consider EEG brain for patients with fluctuating neurological examination or a suppressed level of consciousness.
B. Patient/family teaching points.
  1. Worsening neurological examination may lead to acute respiratory failure requiring intubation and mechanical ventilation.

2. Seizures may require treatment with anti-epileptics and in severe cases intubation and mechanical ventilation for treatment with potent sedatives.

3. Evidence of cerebral edema on head CT may prompt aggressive medical management with mannitol and hypertonic saline, including surgical decompression.

4. Evidence of hydrocephalus on head CT may prompt neurosurgical evaluation and intervention.

5. Long-term neurological sequelae are likely with encephalitis.

C. Pharmacotherapy.

1. Definitive diagnosis of encephalitis: Based on CSF analysis and culture data.

2. HSV/VZV encephalitis: Acyclovir 10 mg/kg IV q8 hours for a duration of 21 days.

    a. Kidney function should be assessed because acyclovir is nephrotoxic.

3. CMV encephalitis: Ganciclovir 5 mg/kg IV q12 hours + Foscarnet 60 mg/kg q8 hours until symptoms improve.

4. HIV encephalitis.

    a. Highly Active Antiretroviral Therapy (HAART): Resume or initiate.

    b. Patient-specific treatment plan: Refer to infectious disease guidelines for treatment of HIV/AIDS.

5. De-escalation of antimicrobial therapy based on negative cultures or preferably definitive meningitis/encephalitis PCR test.

6. Patients presenting with seizure activity: Prompt initiation of antiepileptics and discontinuation of medications known to reduce seizure potential.

D. Discharge instructions.

1. Patients should be instructed to seek emergency care if they experience signs and symptoms of fever, headache, neck pain, confusion, and muscle weakness.

Follow-Up

A. Patients with neurological sequelae on discharge are to obtain follow-up with a neurologist.

Consultation/Referral

A. Consider infectious disease consult for atypical pathogens or patients who do not respond to traditional therapy.

B. Consult neurology for patients with neurological sequelae.

Special/Geriatric Considerations

A. Viral encephalitis in elderly patients may often present with mild confusion, lethargy, and nonspecific neurological findings. The provider must be vigilant to recognize patients at high risk for CNS infection and promptly initiate treatment.

Bibliography

Dalmau, J., & Rosenfeld, M. R. (2018, December 10). Paraneoplastic and autoimmune encephalitis. In A. F. Eichler (Ed.), *UpToDate*. Retrieved from https://www.uptodate.com/contents/paraneoplastic-and-autoimmune-encephalitis

Gaieski, D. F., Nathan, B. R., & O'Brien, N. F. (2015). *Emergency neurological life support: Meningitis and encephalitis*. New York, NY: Springer Science+Business Media.

Gluckman, S. J. (2017, October 15). Viral encephalitis in adults. In J. Mitty (Ed.), *UpToDate*. Retrieved from https://www.uptodate.com/contents/viral-encephalitis-in-adults

Wijdicks, E. F. M., & Rabinstein, A. A. (2012). *Neurocritical care*. (pp. 27–43). New York, NY: Oxford University Press.

Endocarditis: Infective

Robin Miller

Definition

A. An infection involving the cardiac valves (native or prosthetic), mural endocardium, or intracardiac devices.

B. Termed a vegetation.

C. Acute endocarditis.

1. Rapid damage to cardiac structures with extracardiac seeding; fulminant illness can develop in days to 2 weeks.

2. If untreated, can lead to death within weeks.

D. Subacute endocarditis.

1. Indolent course.

2. Slow and progressive damage to cardiac structures.

3. Gradually progressive unless associated with embolic event or ruptured mycotic aneurysm.

E. Short incubation period (<6 weeks) and long incubation period (>6 weeks) are preferred classifications.

F. Heart side used for classification.

1. Right sided—generally from intravenous (IV) drug use.

2. Left sided—more common in IV drug use and non-drug users.

Incidence

A. Uncommon; 3 to 7 per 100,000 person-years.

B. Life-threatening infection; third to fourth most common after fatal infective (IE) process after sepsis, pneumonia, and intra-abdominal abscess.

C. 5% to 15% of affected patients have negative blood cultures.

Pathogenesis

A. Endothelial injury allows either direct infection or the development of a platelet and fibrin thrombus that serves as a site of bacterial attachment.

B. Primary portals of entry include:

1. Oral cavity.

2. Skin.

3. Upper respiratory tract.

4. Sites of focal infection.

C. Microorganisms adhere to endothelium, which is often abnormal or damaged. Platelets aggregate at the site.

D. If the organism is resistant to normal bactericidal activity of serum and microbicidal peptides released by platelets, proliferation will occur with formation of microcolonies. Platelet deposition is induced.

E. Tissue factor is elicited from the endothelium and causes a localized procoagulant state.

F. Fibrin deposition occurs. This together with platelet aggregation and microorganism proliferation all generate a vegetation.

1. Organisms deep within vegetation are metabolically inactive and resistant to antimicrobials.

2. Surface microorganisms are shed into the bloodstream continuously.

G. Clinical manifestations of IE are a result of cytokine release.

H. Microorganisms associated with IE are dependent on classification (see Table 10.1).

Predisposing Factors

A. IV drug use predominantly.

B. Advanced age.

TABLE 10.1   **Classification of Microorganisms Associated With Infective Endocarditis**

| | Native Valve Endocarditis | | Prosthetic Valve Endocarditis. Time of Onset Related to Salve surgery in Months | | | Implantable Cardiac Device | Intravenous Drug Use |
	Hospital-acquired	Community-acquired	<2	2–12	>12		
Organism	*Staphylococcus aureus.* Enterococci. Streptococci	Streptococci. *S. aureus.* Entero-cocci	Coagulase-negative Staphylo-cocci. *Staphylo-coccus aureus.*	Coagulase-negative *Staphylo-cocci. Staphylo-coccus aureus.* Enterococci	Streptococci. *Staphylo-coccus aureus.* Enterococci. Coagulase-negative Staphylococci	*Staphylococcus aureus.* Coagulase-negative *staphylo-cocci*	*Staphylococcus aureus.* Strepto-cocci.

Source: Brusch, J. L. (2007). Infective endocarditis and its mimics in the critical care unit. In B. A. Cunha (Ed.), *Infectious diseases in critical care* (2nd ed., pp. 261–262). New York, NY: Informa Healthcare; Thuny, F., Grisoli, D., Collart, F., Habib, G., & Raoult, D. (2012). Management of infective endocarditis: Challenges and perspectives. *Lancet, 379*(9819), 965–975 doi:10.1016/S0140-6736(11)60755-1

C. Degenerative valve disease.

D. Prosthetic valves or other cardiac devices.

E. Chronic rheumatic heart disease (especially in developing countries).

F. Impaired immune system.

G. Hemodialysis.

H. Unrepaired cyanotic congenital heart defect.

Subjective Data

A. Common complaints/symptoms.

   1. Flu-like symptoms, including fever and chills.

   2. Night sweats.

   3. Anorexia and weight loss.

   4. Chest pain with breathing.

   5. Shortness of breath.

B. Common/typical scenario.

   1. Depends on the type of IE, location, and patient risk factors.

   2. Fever: Common in most types of IE.

   3. Physical examination findings: Can vary based on location of lesion.

   4. Need to identify if there has been a recent surgery or illness.

C. Family and social history.

   1. IV drug use.

D. Review of systems.

   1. General: Malaise, chills, or sweats.

   2. Cardiovascular: Recent surgery, dyspnea, or chest pain or pressure.

   3. Respiratory: Dyspnea or cough.

   4. Skin: Discoloration of fingers and toes, pain in fingers and toes, or cutaneous lesions.

   5. Musculoskeletal: Generalized musculoskeletal pain.

   6. Neurological: Vision changes or headache.

   7. With arterial emboli, review of systems (ROS) can include:

      a. Flank pain.

      b. Hematuria.

      c. Abdominal pain.

Physical Examination

A. Cardiac manifestations.

   1. New regurgitant cardiac murmurs (85% of cases): Indicates valve involvement.

   2. S3 heart sound (with heart failure).

B. Noncardiac manifestations.

   1. Janeway lesions: Red spots on palms of hands or soles of feet.

   2. Osler's nodes: Red tender spots under the skin of fingers or toes.

   3. Subungual hemorrhage.

   4. Discoloration of skin, distal phalanges, or extremities (especially with arterial occlusion from emboli).

   5. Conjunctival hemorrhage.

   6. Petechiae.

Diagnostic Tests

A. Blood cultures.

   1. Three sets of blood cultures.

   2. Peripheral venipuncture, different sites.

   3. First and third sets drawn at least 1 hour apart.

B. Other cultures.

   1. Serologic testing for organisms difficult to identify by blood culture alone (i.e., *Bartonella, Legionella*).

   2. At time of surgery, detection of pathogens from valve tissue by polymerase chain reaction (PCR) is validated.

C. Other tests.

   1. Complete blood count (CBC) with differential.

   2. Complete metabolic panel.

   3. Erythrocyte sedimentation rate (ESR), C-reactive protein (CRP), procalcitonin (PCT).

   4. Chest radiograph.

   5. EKG.

      a. With abscess formation, progressive heart block can occur.

D. Echocardiogram.

   1. Transthoracic echocardiogram (TTE) in all suspected cases less than 12 hours after initial evaluation.

   2. Transesophageal echocardiogram (TEE) in the following circumstances.

      a. Inability to assess valve adequately in TTE.

      b. Suspected IE but negative TTE.

      c. High likelihood for IE: TEE first.

      d. For recurrent IE.

      e. If vegetation is noted.

      f. Clinical suspicion for 3 to 5 days after initial TEE.

E. Other imaging modalities.

   1. Coronary CT angiography (chest CT angiography [CTA] coronary).

      a. In those undergoing surgery for IE.

      b. Preoperative screening: Evaluation for central nervous system (CNS) and intra-abdominal lesions.

c. Limitations.
    i. Radiation exposure.
    ii. Nephrotoxicity associated with contrast dye.
    iii. Lack of sensitivity to evaluate valve lesions.
2. MRI.
    a. Tool to detect cerebral embolic events (typically silent) and evaluate for mycotic aneurysms.
    b. Not routinely used.
F. Modified Duke criteria for diagnosis.
    1. Based on clinical, laboratory, and echocardiographic findings.
        a. Definite IE.
            i. Two major criteria or
            ii. One major criterion and three minor criteria or
            iii. Five minor criteria.
        b. Possible IE.
            i. One major criterion and one minor criterion or.
            ii. Three minor criteria.
        c. Rejected.
            i. Firm alterative diagnosis.
            ii. Resolution of IE syndrome with antibiotic therapy less than 4 days.
            iii. No pathological evidence of IE at surgery/autopsy with antibiotics less than 4 days.
            iv. Does not meet the previous criteria.
    2. Major criteria.
        a. Positive blood culture.
            i. Typical microorganisms identified on two separate blood cultures.
                1) *Viridans streptococci, Streptococcus bovis,* HACEK group (fastidious gram-negative coccobacillary organisms. HACEK stands for *Haemophilus* species, *Aggregatibacter* species, *Cardiobacterium hominis, Eikenella corrodens,* and *Kingella* species), *Staphylococcus aureus.*
                2) Community-acquired enterococci in the absence of a primary focus.
            ii. Persistently positive blood culture, consistent with IE.
                1) At least two positive cultures of blood samples drawn greater than 12 hours apart or all of three cultures or,
                2) A majority of four or more separate cultures of blood (with first and last sample drawn at least 1 hour apart).
            iii. Single positive blood culture for *Coxiella burnetii* or anti-phase 1 IgG antibody titer of 1:800 or more.
            iv. Evidence of endocardial involvement: Echocardiogram positive for IE.
                1) Oscillating intracardiac mass on valve or supporting structures, in the path of regurgitant jets, or on implanted material in the absence of an alternative anatomic explanation.
                2) Abscess.
                3) New partial dehiscence of prosthetic valve or new valvular regurgitation (worsening or changing or preexisting murmur not sufficient).
    3. Minor criteria.
        a. Predisposing factors, or IV drug use.
        b. Fever: Temperature greater than 38°C.
        c. Vascular phenomena: Major arterial emboli, septic pulmonary infarcts, mycotic aneurysm, intracranial

hemorrhage, conjunctival hemorrhages, and Janeway lesions.
        d. Immunological phenomena: Glomerulonephritis, Osler nodes, Roth spots, and rheumatoid factor.
        e. Microbiological evidence: Positive blood culture but does not meet a major criterion as previously noted or serological evidence of active infection with organism consistent with IE.

Differential Diagnosis

A. Bacteremia from other focal infection.
B. Heart failure.
C. Valve dysfunction not associated with IE (e.g., cord rupture).
D. Peripheral arterial disease.
E. Pulmonary embolism.
F. Heart block related to conduction disease.
G. Mesenteric ischemia.
H. Chronic obstructive pulmonary disease (COPD).
I. Leukemia.

Evaluation and Management Plan

A. General plan.
    1. Empiric antimicrobial coverage (see Pharmacotherapy) is warranted if acute IE is suspected.
    2. Blood cultures need to be repeated every 24 to 48 hours until negative.
    3. Surgical intervention needs to be considered, especially in the patients indicated here. Definitive treatment may not be possible without valve replacement and/or removal of implantable cardiac devices.
        a. Indications for surgical intervention.
            i. Moderate to severe refractory heart failure due to valve regurgitation.
            ii. Partially dehisced and unstable prosthetic valve.
            iii. Persistent bacteremia despite optimal antimicrobial therapy.
            iv. *S. aureus* prosthetic valve IE with intracardiac complications.
            v. Prosthetic valve endocarditis relapse despite optimal antimicrobial therapy.
            vi. Ruptured abscess.
            vii. Valve obstruction by vegetation.
        b. Considerations for surgical intervention.
            i. Perivalvular abscess with or without progressive conduction delays.
            ii. Large (>10 mm) hypermobile vegetation noted on TTE (known increased risk of embolic events); recommendation increases strength with associated prior embolic events or valvular regurgitation.
            iii. Persistent unexplained fever (>10 days) in culture-negative valve endocarditis.
            iv. Poorly responsive or relapsed endocarditis associated with highly resistant microorganisms, such as enterococci or *S. aureus.*
B. Patient/family teaching points.
    1. Discussion about potential complications and progression of disease.
    2. Early therapy warranted; will need adherence to antimicrobial therapy to prevent resistant organisms.
    3. Surgical options need to be discussed, especially as they relate to possible removal of implantable cardiac devices.
    4. Education regarding need for central line and long-term IV antibiotics, likely at home; or skilled nursing facility (SNF) if IV drug use is a concern.

5. Education around abstinence from IV drugs, if indicated.

C. Pharmacotherapy.

   1. Primary goal: To eradicate infection by sterilizing vegetations.

   2. Prolonged IV antimicrobial therapy: Required.

   3. Empiric antimicrobial therapy: To be initiated when IE is suspected, after initial blood cultures have been drawn.

   4. Typical length of parenteral therapy: 4 to 6 weeks.

   5. For patients who undergo surgery, intraoperative tissue cultures should be obtained, with antimicrobial coverage narrowed to identified organisms.

   6. For IE associated with implantable cardiac device, antimicrobial therapy is instituted but considered adjunct to device removal (if possible).

   7. For common antimicrobial coverage based on the identified microorganism (see Table 10.2).

D. Discharge instructions.

   1. Instructions about IV antibiotics and central line care, if indicated, should be provided.

Follow-Up

A. Follow-up depends on what therapy is initiated and needed interventions.

   1. A visit with the patient's primary care physician should occur within 3 weeks of discharge.

   2. If surgical intervention was required, a visit with the surgical team should occur within 1 to 2 weeks of discharge.

   3. Depending on the length of antimicrobial therapy and patient factors, a visit with an infectious disease provider should occur within 1 week of planned antimicrobial discontinuation.

Consultation/Referral

A. An infectious disease consult should be obtained to determine appropriate antimicrobial therapy as well as needed duration and follow-up.

B. A cardiac surgery consult may be warranted when surgical indications are present.

C. If indicated, a substance abuse/addiction team consult may be needed.

TABLE 10.2	Antimicrobial Coverage in Infectious Endocarditis Based on Causal Microorganism

Organism	Antibiotic	Duration	Notes
Streptococcus			
	Penicillin G 12–24 million U/24 hr (continuously or in 4–6 divided doses) IV *or* ceftriaxone 2 g/24 hr IV *or* vancomycin 30 mg/kg per 24 hr IV in 2 divided doses *plus* gentamicin 3 mg/kg per 24 hr IV (if prosthetic valve) for first 2 weeks	4–6 weeks	For relative penicillin resistance, use higher dose of penicillin G. Vancomycin should be used in patients who cannot tolerate penicillin. If microorganism is susceptible to ceftriaxone, use as first-line agent.
Staphylococcus (most common is *Staphylococcus aureus*)			
Methicillin-susceptible *S. aureus* (MSSA) of native valve (no foreign devices)	Nafcillin, oxacillin 12 g/24 hr IV in 4–6 equally divided doses OR cefazolin 6 g/24 hr IV in 3 divided doses OR vancomycin 30 mg/kg per 24 hr IV in 2 divided doses OR daptomycin >8 mg/kg/dose IV	6 weeks	Use penicillin if organism is sensitive; dosing based on sensitivity and renal function; check creatinine kinase
Methicillin-resistant <u>S. aureus</u> (MRSA) of native valve (no foreign devices)	Vancomycin 30 mg/kg per 24 hr IV in 2 divided doses	6 weeks	
MSSA of prosthetic valve	Nafcillin, oxacillin 12 g/24 hr IV in 6 equally divided doses *PLUS* gentamicin 3 mg/kg per 24/h IV in 2–3 divided doses (2 weeks) *PLUS* rifampin 900 mg/24hr PO in 3 divided doses	6–8 weeks	Use gentamicin for 2-week period to determine susceptibility prior to adding rifampin
MRSA of prosthetic valve	Vancomycin 30 mg/kg per 24 hr IV in 2 divided doses *PLUS* gentamicin 3 mg/kg per 24/hr IV in 2–3 divided doses (2 weeks) *PLUS* rifampin 900 mg/24 hr PO in 3 divided doses	6–8 weeks	Use gentamicin for 2-week period to determine susceptibility prior to adding rifampin
Enterococcus			
	Penicillin G 18–30 million U/24 hr IV continuously or in 6 divided doses *PLUS* gentamicin 3 mg/kg (ideal body weight) per 24/hr IV in 2–3 divided doses	4–6 weeks	
	Ampicillin 2 g IV every 4 hr *PLUS* gentamicin 3 mg/kg (IBW) per 24/hr IV in 2–3 divided doses	4–6 weeks	

(continued)

(*continued*)

TABLE 10.2 **Antimicrobial Coverage in Infectious Endocarditis Based on Causal Microorganism**

Organism	Antibiotic	Duration	Notes
	Vancomycin 30 mg/kg per 24 hr IV in 2 divided doses. *PLUS* gentamicin 3 mg/kg (IBW) per 24/hr IV in 2–3 divided doses	4–6 weeks	For penicillin allergic patients
	Ampicillin 2 g IV every 4 hr *PLUS* ceftriaxone 2 g IV every 12 h	6 weeks	For *Enterococcus faecalis* strains with high level of resistance (ampicillin + gentamicin preferable)

IV, intravenous; MRSA, Methicillin-resistant *S. aureus*; MSSA, Methicillin-susceptible *S. aureus*.

D. For those with persistent bacteremia without surgical options, it is appropriate to consider a palliative care consultation.

Special/Geriatric Considerations

A. Prophylaxis should be targeted at the viridans group of streptococci.
B. Antibiotic prophylaxis should be considered for patients with the following conditions.
   1. Prosthetic cardiac valve or prosthetic material used for cardiac valve repair.
   2. Previous IE.
   3. Congenital heart disease (CHD).
   4. Unrepaired cyanotic CHD including palliative shunts and conduits.
   5. Repaired congenital heart defect with prosthetic material or device within past 6 months.
   6. Repaired CHD with residual defects at site or adjacent to site of a prosthetic patch or device.
   7. Cardiac transplantation recipients with cardiac valvulopathy.
C. Prophylactic antimicrobials should be considered when patients with the conditions listed in B undergo the following procedures.
   1. Dental procedures that involve manipulation of gingival tissue or the periapical region of the teeth or perforation of the oral mucosa.
   2. Invasive procedures of the respiratory tract that involve incision or biopsy of the respiratory mucosa, such as tonsillectomy and adenoidectomy.
   3. Elective cystoscopy or other urinary tract manipulation in those with an enterococcal urinary tract infection or colonization.
D. General treatment principle: Single dose administered prior to procedure (if not administered before, must be given within 2 hours of procedure).
E. Pharmacotherapy.
   1. Standard oral regimen: Amoxicillin 2 g PO, 30 to 60 minutes prior to procedure.
   2. If unable to take oral therapy: Ampicillin 2 g IV, 30 to 60 minutes prior to procedure.
   3. Penicillin allergy: Cephalexin 2 g PO OR clindamycin 600 mg PO OR azithromycin 500 mg PO, 30–60 minutes prior to procedure.

Bibliography

Brusch, J. L. (2007). Infective endocarditis and its mimics in the critical care unit. In B. A. Cunha (Ed.), *Infectious diseases in critical care* (2nd ed., pp. 261–262). New York, NY: Informa Healthcare.
Cahill, T. J., Baddour, L. M., Habib, G., Hoen, B., Salaun, E., Pettersson, G. B., . . . Prendergast, B. D. (2017, January). Challenges in infective endocarditis. *Journal of the American College of Cardiology, 69*(3), 325–344. doi:10.1016/j.jacc.2016.10.066
Karchmer, A. W. (2005). Infective endocarditis. In R. O. Bonow, D. L. Mann, D. P. Zipes, & P. Libby (Eds.), *Braunwald's heart disease: A textbook of cardiovascular medicine* (7th ed., pp.1633–1658). Philadelphia, PA: WB Saunders.
Slipczuk, L., Codolosa, J. N., Davila, C. D., Romero-Corral, A., Yun, J., Pressman, G. S., & Figueredo, V. M. (2013). Infective endocarditis epidemiology over five decades: A systematic review. *PLOS ONE, 8*(12), e82665. doi:10.1371/journal.pone.0082665
Thuny, F., Grisoli, D., Collart, F., Habib, G., & Raoult, D. (2012, March 10). Management of infective endocarditis: Challenges and perspectives. *Lancet, 379*(9819), 965–975. doi:10.1016/S0140-6736(11)60755-1

Influenza

David Bergamo

Definition

A. An acute respiratory illness caused by the influenza virus, an orthomyxovirus.

Incidence

A. 3 to 5 million severe cases and 250,000 to 500,000 deaths annually worldwide.
B. Annually, since 2010, in the United States.
   1. Between 9.2 and 35.6 million related illnesses.
   2. Hospitalization rate between 140,000 and 710,000.
   3. Death rates range between 12,000 and 56,000.

Pathogenesis

A. A single-stranded RNA virus attaches to the epithelial cells in the respiratory tract and replicates inside of them. Ongoing destruction and eradications of these cells occurs.
B. Infectious particles are released through "budding," causing rapid invasion of neighboring cells and a cyclical process.

Predisposing Factors

A. All individuals are at risk. Influenza vaccination can decrease risk. However, this decrease changes annually, pending vaccination efficacy.
B. Those at higher risk for complications include children younger than 5 years of age, adults older than 65 years old, pregnant women, long-term care facility residents, Alaskan Natives, and American Indians.
C. Other high risk groups include patients with underlying neurological, cardiac, or pulmonary conditions; immunosuppressed individuals (with conditions such as hypogammaglobulinemia, HIV, or cancer); obese patients; and those with other significant comorbid conditions.

Subjective Data

A. Common complaints/symptoms.
1. Fever.
2. Diffuse myalgias.
3. Fatigue.
4. Cough and respiratory symptoms, including rhinorrhea and sore throat.
5. Headache.
B. Common/typical scenario.
1. Symptoms: Abrupt in onset; some patients may remember exact time.
2. Abrupt onset of fever with myalgia and respiratory symptoms during influenza season (late fall to early spring): High likelihood for influenza.
C. Family and social history.
1. Positive comorbid conditions or hereditary immunodeficiencies.
2. Recent exposure to individuals with symptoms of influenza: Symptoms generally appear 2 days after exposure (airborne, touching contaminated surfaces).
3. Crowded environments.
D. Review of systems.
1. Neuro: Anorexia, dizziness, or weakness.
2. Gastrointestinal (GI) symptoms: Uncommon in adults.
3. Respiratory: Nonproductive cough (productive cough is more common in pneumonia).
4. HEENT: Runny nose, sore throat.

Physical Examination

A. Relatively benign, with nonspecific findings.
B. Constitutional: Ill appearing, fatigued appearing.
C. Fever: Usually 100°F–104°F; rarely much higher other than in complicated cases.
D. Possible hyperemia or cervical lymphadenopathy (more common in younger patients).
E. Mild tachycardia from hypoxia, dehydration, and fever.
F. Pharyngitis.
G. Conjunctivitis.
H. Pulmonary findings: Possibly dry cough, focal wheezing, or rhonchi.
I. Skin: May appear flushed, warm to hot, with diaphoresis depending on the core body temperature.

Diagnostic Tests

A. Clinical diagnosis in patients with influenza symptoms during influenza season or during outbreaks. The combination of fever with cough, sore throat, and myalgia can improve diagnostic accuracy. In periods of outbreak, patients with combinations of any of these symptoms may be reasonably treated with neuraminidase inhibitors without testing.
B. Rapid influenza tests.
1. Polymerase chain reaction (PCR): Most sensitive and specific and can differentiate subtypes.
2. Rapid antigen tests: Result obtained in 15 minutes; less sensitive.
3. Gold standard: Viral culture; may take 72 hours to obtain results.

Differential Diagnosis

A. HIV.
B. Pneumonia.
C. Cytomegalovirus (CMV).
D. Legionnaires' disease.
E. Hantavirus pulmonary disease.
F. Acute respiratory distress syndrome (ARDS).
G. Other viral upper respiratory infections (URIs).
H. Tick- and mosquito-borne illnesses.
1. However, these tend to present in different seasons or patients have exposure history or travel history.

Evaluation and Management Plan

A. General plan.
1. Usually self-limited; duration can be shortened with the use of neuraminidase inhibitors.
2. Airborne isolation.
3. Supportive care.
B. Patient/family teaching points.
1. Handwashing is key to help prevent spread.
2. Annual influenza vaccines for all those who can receive them (most individuals).
C. Pharmacotherapy.
1. Neuraminidase inhibitors.
   a. Oseltamivir (Tamiflu).
      i. Most commonly used agent; can cause nausea and vomiting.
      ii. Treatment: 75 mg BID for 5 days, starting within 48 hours of symptom onset.
      iii. Prophylaxis: 75 mg daily for 10 days within 48 hours of contact with infected person.
   b. Zanamivir (Relenza).
      i. Inhaled agent that should not be used in patients with pulmonary disease.
      ii. Should be avoided in lactose intolerant patients (powder mixture contains lactose/milk proteins).
   c. Peramivir (Rapivab).
      i. Intravenous formulation for those who cannot use oral route.
      ii. Treatment: 600 mg IV 1 dose.
   d. Laninamivir.
      i. Still under development: Nasal spray.
   e. All neuraminidase inhibitors: Can cause neuropsychiatric effects based on their mechanism of action. Less commonly, they may cause skin reactions, including erythema multiforme or Stevens–Johnson syndrome.
   f. Adamantane antivirals (amantadine and rimantadine).
      i. Target M2 protein of influenza A and therefore not active against influenza B; little to no activity against current influenza A strains.
      ii. Amantadine and rimantadine not currently recommended for treatment of influenza A, due to high levels of resistance among many circulating strains of influenza.
      iii. Amantadine and rimantadine are safe in children older than 1 year of age.
   g. Ribavirin.
      i. Nucleoside analog active against influenza A and B.
      ii. Not Food and Drug Administration (FDA) approved; rarely used except with consultation of infectious disease specialists via inhaled route.
   h. Baloxavir marboxil.
      i. FDA approved.
      ii. Influenza treatment 40 to less than 80 kg: 40 mg as a single dose within 48 hours of onset of influenza symptoms.
      iii. 80 kg: 80 mg as a single dose within 48 hours of onset of influenza.

Follow-Up

A. Follow-up other than regular visits with primary care physician is usually not required.

Consultation/Referral

A. If hospitalized, consider consultation with infectious disease and pulmonary specialists.
B. If illness is significant, a critical care specialist may be required.
C. In general, influenza tends to be an outpatient illness cared for by primary care and urgent care providers.

Special/Geriatric Considerations

A. Annual influenza vaccination is indicated in all patients who are at least 6 months of age *except*:
    1. Patients who have had a severe allergic reaction to prior influenza vaccine (this does not include minor flu-like symptoms).
    2. Those with a severe allergic reaction to egg proteins if receiving the live attenuated vaccine (nasal).
B. Immunocompromised patients, pregnant women, and patients 50 years of age or older should *not* receive live attenuated vaccine.
C. Adults under the age of 65 with no significant comorbidities generally have self-limiting disease.
D. Children younger than 5 years of age, but especially under 2 years, are at higher risk of influenza complications.
E. Patients older than 65 years have an increased risk of developing complications.

Bibliography

Centers for Disease Control and Prevention. (2016). *National and state healthcare associated infections progress report.* Retrieved from http://www.cdc.gov/HAI/pdfs/progress-report/hai-progress-report.pdf

Centers for Disease Contro and Prevention. (2019, February 19). Disease burden of influenza. Retrieved from https://www.cdc.gov/flu/about/disease/burden.htm

Longo, D., Fauci, A., Kasper, D., Hauser, S., Jameson, J., & Loscalzo, J.(Eds.). (2015). *Harrison's principles of internal medicine* (19th ed.). New York, NY: McGraw Hill.

Meningitis

Dominick Osipowicz

Definition

A. Inflammation of the meninges, the three membranes surrounding the brain and spinal cord.
B. Types of meningitis.
    1. Bacterial meningitis: Acute infection of the meninges and cerebrospinal fluid (CSF), characterized by an elevated number of white blood cells and positive bacterial cultures in the CSF. This type of meningitis has the highest rate of morbidity and mortality of all forms of disease.
    2. Viral meningitis: Acute viral infection of the meninges and CSF, characterized by a moderate elevation of white blood cells in the CSF with negative bacterial cultures. Often referred to as aseptic meningitis due to lack of growth in CSF cultures, it is often self-limiting without treatment.
    3. Fungal meningitis: Acute fungal infection of the meninges and CSF, characterized by a moderate elevation of white blood cells in the CSF, generally with negative bacterial cultures but positive for antibodies of fungal organisms. Like bacterial meningitis, it is associated with significant morbidity and mortality.
    4. Drug-induced meningitis (rare): Acute inflammation of the meninges, characterized by a moderate elevation of white blood cells in the CSF with negative blood cultures and history of using nonsteroidal anti-inflammatory drugs (NSAIDs), certain antibiotics, intravenous immune globulin, and antiepileptic drugs.

Incidence

A. In 2015, there were 8.7 million cases of meningitis worldwide.
B. More than one million cases of *bacterial* meningitis occur every year, worldwide.
C. Meningitis is one of the top 10 causes of death from infection. Fatalities from meningitis are in excess of 100,000 every year.
D. Like bacterial meningitis, fungal meningitis is associated with a significant morbidity and mortality.

Pathogenesis

A. Many pathogens responsible for meningitis, including bacteria, possess surface components that enhance mucosal colonization.
    1. After bacterial colonization, invasion across the epithelium occurs by intra- or inter-cellular pathways, often mediated by specific adhesions of the bacterial surface.
    2. Following invasion, bacteria survive normal immunological forces via evasion of the complement system, often due to polysaccharide capsules, and then cross the blood–brain barrier. Complement activation may occur in the CSF, often causing meningeal tissue damage. In the CSF, bacteria can multiply to high concentrations due to the low humoral immunity activity in CSF. The clinical disease process is due to the interaction of the host inflammatory response and bacterial components once the bacteria enter the CSF.
    3. Once inflammation is present, a series of injuries to the blood–brain barrier epithelium lead to vasogenic brain edema, loss of cerebrovascular regulation, and increased intracranial pressure (ICP), ultimately leading to motor, sensory, or cognitive deficits.
B. Bacterial meningitis: Characterized as a rapidly progressing systemic bacterial illness presenting with fever, headache, and neck stiffness.
C. Cortical brain function: Generally remains intact as brain parenchyma is spared.
D. Types of meningitis and associated causal pathogens.
    1. Bacterial meningitis.
        a. Misdiagnosed, undiagnosed, or untreated bacterial meningitis: Associated with a high rate of morbidity and nearly 100% mortality.
        b. Most common bacterial pathogens: *Streptococcus pneumoniae, Listeria monocytogenes, Neisseria meningitis, Haemophilus influenzae,* and *Staphylococcus aureus.*
            i. Adults: Most common pathogen is *S. pneumoniae.*
            ii. Elderly (age >60): Highly susceptible to *L. monocytogenes.*
    2. Viral meningitis.
        a. Diagnosis of exclusion given the limited diagnostic tools for isolating individual pathogens.
        b. Most common viral pathogens: Human simplex virus (HSV), varicella-zoster virus (VZV), HIV, West Nile Virus (WNV), and enteroviruses.

3. Fungal meningitis.

    a. Most common fungal pathogens: *Cryptococcus neoformans* and *Coccidioides immitis*.

4. Drug-induced meningitis.

    a. Proposed mechanism of action: Combination of delayed hypersensitivity reaction and direct meningeal irritation.

    b. Common causative agents: NSAIDs, certain antibiotics, intravenous immune globulin, and antiepileptic drugs.

Predisposing Factors

A. Immunocompromised state.

B. Use of immunosuppressive therapy.

C. Organ transplantation.

D. Environmental exposure.

E. Use of intravenous drugs.

F. Lack of immunizations for meningococcus (*Neisseria meningitides*), pneumococcus (*S. pneumoniae*), and *H. influenzae*.

G. Recent brain surgery or trauma (concern for *S. aureus*).

H. Bacterial meningitis is more likely to affect the elderly and individuals who are immunocompromised.

Subjective Data

A. Common complaints/symptoms.

1. Severe headache.

2. Nuchal rigidity: Inability to flex neck forward passively due to increased muscle tone and stiffness; present in 70% of cases of bacterial meningitis.

3. Hyperthermia/hypothermia.

4. Altered mental status.

B. Common/typical scenario.

1. Classic triad of meningitis: Fever, neck stiffness, and headaches.

    a. Found in less than 50% of patients.

    b. However, two out of three symptoms should raise suspicion for meningitis.

2. Nonspecific symptoms: Altered mental status, lethargy, malaise, nausea, vomiting, diarrhea, photophobia, muscle aches, cough, and sore throat.

C. Family and social history.

1. Family history: Generally noncontributory.

2. Social history: Recent illness; travel abroad, particularly sub-Saharan Africa; exposure to rodents, ticks, mosquitos; or individuals residing in close quarters (e.g., students in dormitory housing).

3. Medication history positive for NSAIDs, certain antibiotics, intravenous immune globulin, or antiepileptic drugs.

D. Review of systems.

1. General: Fatigue, weakness, fever, or chills.

2. Head, ear, eyes, nose, and throat (HEENT): Headaches, neck pain, or neck stiffness.

3. Neurological: Lethargy.

4. Skin: Rash.

Physical Examination

A. Nuchal rigidity, including tenderness to palpation and pain with flexion or extension.

B. Kernig test: Pain induced by attempting full extension of the knee while the hip is flexed at 90°. Specificity is high, but sensitivity is limited.

C. Brudzinski test: Passive flexion of the neck induces flexion of the hips. Specificity is high, but sensitivity is limited.

D. Lethargy and suppressed level of consciousness.

E. Focal neurological deficits, including cranial nerve palsies.

F. Papilledema.

G. Petechial or ecchymotic rash. Petechial rash is relatively specific for meningococcal meningitis, which is caused by *N. meningitides*.

Diagnostic Tests

A. Lumbar puncture: Gold standard for diagnosis of bacterial meningitis (ideally performed prior to or simultaneously with antibiotic administration) with CSF analysis.

1. CSF analysis.

    a. Assessment of cell count/differential, glucose, protein gram stain, and bacterial culture.

    b. Normal CSF.

        i. Normal opening pressure less than 20 mmHg.

        ii. CSF WBC less than $5/\mu L$.

        iii. CSF RBC (absent).

            1) CSF Glucose greater than 60 mg/dL and CSF/serum ratio of greater than 0.6.

        iv. CSF Protein less than 50 mg/dL.

        v. Sterile culture.

    c. Abnormal CSF suggestive of bacterial meningitis.

        i. Elevated opening pressure.

        ii. CSF WBC greater than $1,000/\mu L$ and neutrophil dominant.

        iii. CSF RBC (absent).

        iv. CSF Glucose less than 40 mg/dL and CSF/serum ratio of less than 0.4.

        v. CSF Protein greater than 200 mg/dL.

        vi. Culture results in a positive growth for bacterial organism.

    d. Abnormal CSF suggestive of viral/aseptic meningitis.

        i. Elevated opening pressure.

        ii. CSF WBC less than $250/\mu L$ and lymphocyte dominant.

        iii. CSF RBC (absent).

        iv. CSF Glucose greater than 60 mg/dL.

        v. CSF Protein less than 150 mg/dL.

        vi. Sterile culture.

    e. Abnormal CSF suggestive of fungal meningitis (results may be nonspecific).

        i. Elevated opening pressure.

        ii. CSF WBC less than $500/\mu L$ and lymphocyte dominant.

        iii. CSF RBC (absent).

        iv. CSF Glucose less than 40 mg/dL and CSF/serum ratio of less than 0.4.

            1) Bacteria ingest glucose, causing a decreased level associated with bacterial meningitis.

        v. CSF Protein greater than 250 mg/dL.

        vi. Sterile culture.

            1) Proceed with fungal cultures and fungal antibody testing.

    f. WBC/RBC adjustment.

        i. A false positive WBC elevation: Often noted in a traumatic lumbar puncture or a patient with subarachnoid bleed.

        ii. Acceptable ratio of WBC/RBC should be approximately 1:700.

2. Relative contraindications to lumbar puncture.

    a. Systemic anticoagulation.

    b. Thrombocytopenia.

    c. Coagulopathy.

    d. Open sacral wound at level L3 to L5.

e. CT of the head with evidence of increased ICP and/or mass lesion.

B. Laboratory tests.

1. Relevant blood work including complete blood count (CBC), basal metabolic profile (BMP), partial thromboplastin time (PTT)/prothrombin time (PT)/international normalized ratio (INR), lactate, and arterial blood gas.

2. Blood cultures.

C. A noncontrast CT of the head: Required for certain patients.

1. Those who present with signs and symptoms concerning for elevated ICP, altered level of consciousness, new-onset seizures, or focal neurological deficits.

2. Those with immunocompromised status.

3. Those with a history of prior central nervous system (CNS) infection, trauma, stroke, cancer, and surgery.

Differential Diagnosis

A. Viral encephalitis.

B. Epidural abscess.

C. Nonconvulsive status epilepticus.

D. Subarachnoid hemorrhage.

E. Meningeal tear or CSF leak.

Evaluation and Management Plan

A. General plan.

1. Bacterial meningitis.

a. Blood cultures.

b. Broad spectrum antibiotic therapy and glucocorticoids if appropriate.

c. Administration of antivirals if there is concern for encephalitis.

d. Obtain "Stat" CT of the head if altered mental status, focal neurological deficit, immunocompromised status, or new onset seizures.

e. Lumbar puncture (ideally performed prior to or simultaneously with antibiotic administration) with CSF fluid analysis for definitive treatment, including meningitis/encephalitis polymerase chain reaction (PCR) for rapid identification of causative pathogen if available.

f. Continued hemodynamic management and supportive care.

g. MRI of the brain should be considered if the patient fails to improve despite appropriate therapy.

2. Viral meningitis.

a. Spinal fluid suggestive of viral meningitis.

b. De-escalation of antibiotic therapy.

c. Supportive treatment, including but not limited to:

i. Rest.

ii. Fluid resuscitation.

iii. Antipyretics and analgesics as needed.

3. Fungal meningitis.

a. Spinal fluid analysis is likely to be abnormal but may be nonspecific, sending CSF for fungal cultures and fungal antibody testing.

b. Addition of antifungal medication to antibiotic therapy for bacterial meningitis.

c. Supportive treatment as previously noted.

4. Drug-induced meningitis.

a. Treatment as previously noted pending results of lumbar puncture.

b. De-escalation of antibiotic and antiviral therapy.

c. Immediate cessation of causative agent.

d. Supportive treatment.

B. Patient/family teaching points.

1. Worsening neurological examination may lead to acute respiratory failure requiring intubation and mechanical ventilation.

2. Seizures may require treatment with antiepileptics and, in severe cases, intubation and mechanical ventilation for treatment with potent sedatives.

3. Evidence of cerebral edema on head CT may prompt aggressive medical management with mannitol and hypertonic saline, as well as surgical decompression.

4. Evidence of hydrocephalus on head CT may prompt neurosurgical evaluation and intervention.

5. Neurological sequelae including hearing loss and visual symptoms are very likely post recovery in bacterial meningitis.

C. Pharmacotherapy.

1. Dexamethasone 10 mg IV q6 hours (prior to initiation of antibiotics if able).

a. Evidence is inconclusive, but certain studies suggest that dexamethasone correlates with a decrease in mortality and mitigates incidence of hearing loss in patients with *S. pneumoniae* meningitis.

2. Ceftriaxone 2 g IV q12 hours (*N. meningitidis, H. influenzae*).

a. Lactam allergy: Substitute with chloramphenicol 50 to 100 mg/kg/day IV divided q6 hours.

b. Has good meningeal coverage.

3. Vancomycin 20 mg/kg IV q12 hours (*S. pneumoniae*).

4. Ampicillin 2 g IV q6 hours (if suspicious for Listeria monocytogenes).

a. B-lactam allergy: Substitute with trimethoprim-sulfamethoxazole 5 mg/kg IV q6 hours.

5. Acyclovir 10 mg/kg IV q8 hours (if suspicious for HSV encephalitis).

6. Imipenem 1 gram IV q6 hours (if trauma or neurosurgical manipulation).

7. Fluconazole 400 mg IV daily (if suspicious for *C. neoformans* and *C. immitis*). Dosing can be increased to 800 to 1,200 mg daily for critically ill patients.

D. Discharge instructions.

E. Instruct patient to seek emergency care if presenting with fever, headache, and stiff neck because this may indicate a worsening infection.

Follow-Up

A. Patients with neurological sequelae on discharge are encouraged to follow-up with a neurologist.

Consultation/Referral

A. Consider an infectious disease consult for patients with atypical pathogens or patients who do not respond to traditional therapy.

Special/Geriatric Considerations

A. Gerontology patients with a fulminant bacterial meningitis may present with atypical symptoms and deny neck pain or headache. Confusion and lethargy may be the only presenting symptoms.

B. Provider must be vigilant to recognize high-risk patient for CNS infection so that treatment is not delayed.

Bibliography

Gaieski, D. F., Nathan, B. R., & O'Brien, N. F. (2015). *Emergency neurological life support: Meningitis and encephalitis*. New York, NY: Springer Science+Business Media.

Tunkle, A. R. (2018, August 30). Clinical features and diagnosis of acute bacterial meningitis in adults. In J. Mitty (Ed.), *UpToDate*. Retrieved from https://www.uptodate.com/contents/clinical-features-and-diagnosis-of-acute-bacterial-meningitis-in-adults

Wijdicks, E. F. M., & Rabinstein, A. A. (2012). *Neurocritical care*. New York, NY: Oxford University Press .

Necrotizing Fasciitis

Dana A. Albinson

Definition

A. Severe bacterial infection of the fascia (connective tissue that covers and separates the muscles and other internal organs) and overlying subcutaneous fat that causes extensive tissue death.

Incidence

A. Necrotizing fasciitis can occur at any age; however, the mean age is around 50 years.
B. Hospitalizations due to necrotizing fasciitis are gender neutral.
C. Necrotizing fasciitis occurs randomly and is not linked to similar infections in others.

Pathogenesis

A. The most common way of getting necrotizing fasciitis is when the bacteria enter the body through a break in the skin, such as a cut, scrape, burn, insect bite, or puncture wound.
B. The infection spreads along the muscle fascia as a result of its relatively poor blood supply, and muscle tissue may be spared. In addition, overlying tissue can appear unaffected.
C. Necrotizing fasciitis is typically classified based on the microbial source of infection.
  1. Type I—polymicrobial with aerobic and anaerobic bacteria, such as *Clostridioides, Peptostreptococcus*, and *Bacteroides* species.
  2. Type II—monomicrobial and generally caused by group A streptococcus (GAS; also known as hemolytic streptococcal gangrene).

Predisposing Factors

A. Type I: Certain comorbid conditions.
  1. Diabetes.
  2. Obesity.
  3. Cardiovascular disease.
  4. Peripheral vascular disease.
  5. Liver disease.
  6. Kidney disease.
  7. Cancer.
  8. Other chronic health conditions that weaken the body's immune system.
B. Type II: Risk factors in healthy individuals (no past medical history).
  1. Skin injury—laceration or burn.
  2. Blunt trauma.
  3. Surgery.
  4. Childbirth.
  5. Varicella.
  6. Intravenous drug use.

Subjective Data

A. Common complaints/symptoms.
  1. Pain—usually out of proportion to how the area looks; followed by anesthesia (due to thrombosis of small vessels).
  2. Swelling.
  3. Redness.
  4. Fever.
  5. Chills.
  6. Fatigue.
B. Family and social history.
  1. A detailed history is important, as it can suggest the likely cause of the infection.
  2. A careful history, including several factors, should be taken.
    a. Indicate if any trauma occurred at the site.
    b. Onset and duration of symptoms.
    c. Speed at which erythema is spreading.
    d. Existence of any comorbid conditions (past medical history).
    e. Any recent swimming in lakes, ponds, or areas of concern.

Physical Examination

A. Early on, healthy appearance, but possible rapid progression to ill/septic appearance.
B. Acute tenderness at site of infection.
C. Skin with area of rapidly increasing erythema, bullae, skin necrosis, and/or crepitus; sometimes with dusky or purplish discoloration.
  1. Skin color can change in a few days from red/purple to patchy blue/gray, followed in 3 to 5 days with skin breakdown with bullae with thick pink/purple fluid and frank cutaneous gangrene.
D. Increased warmth and induration at site.
E. Possible crepitus at site.
F. Difficult to palpate muscle groups due to induration, with edema of subcutaneous tissue.
G. If the skin is open, gloved fingers can pass easily between the two layers and may reveal yellowish-green necrotic fascia.
H. If the skin is not open, a scalpel may be needed to open the site.

Diagnostic Tests

A. Lab work.
  1. Complete blood count (CBC), basal metabolic profile (BMP), and blood and tissue cultures are necessary.
  2. Lab findings are often nonspecific but may include leukocytosis with a marked left shift; coagulopathy; and elevated creatine kinase (CK), lactate, and creatinine.
B. Imaging: Noncontrast CT and MRI scans (especially in abdominal wall infections).
  1. These can be helpful if gas is identified in the soft tissue and/or fascial planes.
  2. MRI can be overly sensitive.
C. Surgical exploration.
  1. Do *not* delay surgical exploration for results from blood, skin, or wound cultures.
  2. Surgical exploration is the only way to confirm diagnosis. Histopathology of tissue will show extensive tissue damage, including:
    a. Thrombosis of blood vessels.
    b. Abundant bacteria along fascial planes.
    c. Infiltration of acute inflammatory cells.

Differential Diagnosis

A. Acute epididymitis.

B. Cellulitis.

C. Orchitis.

D. Toxic shock syndrome.

E. Deep vein thrombosis (DVT).

F. Brown recluse spider bite.

Evaluation and Management Plan

A. Surgical emergency. Debridement needs to be done early to minimize tissue loss and possible amputation, and debridement will require review in the operating room every 24 hours.

B. Empiric antibiotics. These should be started immediately. Agents should be broad based to cover gram-negative and gram-positive organisms and anaerobes. More target-specific antibiotics may be started once tissue cultures and sensitivities are available.

  1. Clindamycin is the antibiotic of choice to cover necrotizing fasciitis for its antitoxin effects.

  2. In addition, the patient requires carbapenems (e.g., imipenem, meropenem, or ertapenem—please note that ertapenem does not cover pseudomonas) or beta lactamase inhibitor (e.g., piperacillin/tazobactam, ampicillin sodium/sulbactam sodium, or Ticarcillin/clavulanic acid), as well as an agent active against methicillin-resistant *Staphylococcus aureus* (MRSA; e.g., vancomycin, daptomycin, or linezolid).

C. Intravenous fluids. Massive fluids may be necessary due to diffuse capillary leak and hypotension. Also, nutritional support needs to be implemented to help support wound healing.

Follow-Up

A. Repeat imaging of area to make sure there is no lingering infection.

B. Follow-up with infectious disease after completion of antibiotics.

C. Follow-up with surgery as needed.

Consultation/Referral

A. Consult surgery emergently for surgical intervention.

B. Infectious disease for antibiotic duration.

C. Depending on extent of injury, may need plastics consult for flap.

D. Wound care.

Special/Geriatric Considerations

A. Necrotizing fasciitis is the most frequently overlooked infectious process of the skin in the elderly.

B. Skin and soft tissue represent a common site of infection, and it is a recognized focus of sepsis in the elderly.

Bibliography

Centers for Disease Control and Prevention. (n.d.). *Necrotizing fasciitis: A rare disease, especially for the healthy*. Retrieved from https://www.cdc.gov/features/necrotizingfasciitis

Edlich, R. (2018, October 17). Necrotizing fasciitis workup. In M. S. Bronze (Ed.), *Medscape*. Retrieved from http://emedicine.medscape.com/article/2051157-workup

Ghosh, A., & Johnstone, J. (2013). Necrotizing fasciitis in an immuno-compromised elderly woman. *Canadian Journal of Infectious Diseases and Medical Microbiology, 24*(1), 38–39. doi:10.1155/2013/489587

Goh, T., Goh, L. G., Ang, C. H., & Wong, C. H. (2013). Early diagnosis of necrotizing fasciitis. *British Journal of Surgery, 101*(1), e119–e125. doi:10.1002/bjs.9371

Misiakos, E. P., Bagias, G., Patapis, P., Sotiropoulos, D., Kanavidis, P., & Machairas, A. (2014). Current concepts in the management of necrotizing fasciitis. *Frontiers in Surgery, 1,* 36. doi:10.3389/fsurg.2014.00036

Oud, L., & Watkins, P. (2015). Contemporary trends of the epidemiology, clinical characteristics, and resource utilization of necrotizing fasciitis in Texas: A population-based cohort study. *Critical Care Research and Practice, 2015,* 1–9. doi:10.1155/2015/618067

Southwick, F. S. (2008). *Infectious diseases: A clinical short course* (2nd ed, pp. 268–271). New York, NY: McGraw-Hill Professional Publishing.

Osteomyelitis

Rose Milano

Definition

A. Represents a wide spectrum of inflammatory bone disorders due to bacteria, mycobacteria, or fungi.

B. Multifaceted presentations of bone infection; no universally accepted system of classification.

C. Classification is most commonly based on the pathogenesis, chronicity, or location.

D. Known as a disease of the very young and the very old.

Incidence

A. The incidence of osteomyelitis in the United States is largely unknown. It may be as high as 16% after foot puncture (30%–40% in patients with diabetes). The rate of occurrence of vertebral osteomyelitis is estimated at 2.4 cases per 100,000. The prevalence of osteomyelitis is estimated as 1 case per 5,000 in children.

B. The prevalence of bone and joint infections in adults is increasing because of (1) longer life expectancy, (2) increasing use of bone fixation and prosthetic implants, and (3) higher rate of diabetes.

Pathogenesis

A. Hematogenous source: Spread by seeding from bacteria in blood.

  1. Primary sources of initial infection: Urinary tract, skin and soft tissue, and intravascular catheters, as well as endocarditis.

  2. Usually monomicrobial.

  3. Most common in children due to seeding in the metaphysis of long bones, particularly the femur and tibia. Such osteomyelitis is rare in adults, but when it does occur it is most frequent in the vertebrae of the spine.

B. Contiguous source: Spread from adjacent soft tissues and joints.

  1. Exogenous: Often spread following surgery or trauma with direct inoculation.

  2. Generally polymicrobial, but can be monomicrobial.

  3. Accounts for 80% of chronic osteomyelitis infection.

  4. Bimodal age distribution with differing sources.

    a. Older individuals: Decubitus ulcers, chronic soft tissue injuries, dental infections, and joint arthroplasties.

    b. Younger individuals: Open fracture or bone surgery.

C. Secondary disease: From vascular insufficiency or peripheral neuropathy.

  1. Most often related to diabetes.

  2. Results from chronic, progressive deep skin/soft tissue infection, generally in the foot from diabetic foot syndrome.

D. Infectious causes: Multifactorial mechanisms in hosts at high risk.

  1. Most commonly due to hematogenous seeding.

2. Intravenous drug abuse.

3. HIV infection.

4. Sickle cell disease: Accounts for about one third of cases.

E. Histological changes.

1. Infection: Results in bone edema and vascular congestion, leading to small vessel thrombosis.

2. Medullary and periosteal blood supplies: Compromised; bone becomes necrotic.

3. Sequestra: Fragments of dead bone that detach from living bone.

4. Dead bone: Becomes colonized by a biofilm of bacteria that is often resistant to antibiotics, so debridement in addition to antibiotics is necessary for chronic, well-established osteomyelitis.

F. Microorganisms: Often a function of the location of the osteomyelitis infection.

1. *Staphylococcus aureus:* Most frequent cause of all types of osteomyelitis.

2. Coagulase-negative staphylococci: Most common cause of prosthetic-associated infection.

3. Streptococci and other anaerobic bacteria: Associated with diabetic foot lesions and decubitus ulcers.

4. *Aspergillus* spp., *Candida albicans,* and *Mycobacteria* spp. most common in immunocompromised hosts.

Predisposing Factors

A. Compromised host.

B. Immunocompromise (HIV: High correlation secondary to unsterilized needles. The very young experience mostly in the long bones while the very old have more occurrences in the vertebrae).

C. Intravenous drug abuse or alcohol abuse.

D. Diabetes.

E. Malignancies.

F. Impaired circulation.

G. Liver cirrhosis.

H. Sickle cell disease.

I. Chronic steroid use.

J. Bone or joint surgery.

K. Traumatic injury involving the bone.

Subjective Data

A. Common complaints/symptoms.

1. Gradual onset of symptoms over several days.

2. Spinal osteomyelitis.

a. Pain: Determined by the location of the infection in the spine; generally dull pain with and without movement.

b. Fever (only in 64% of cases, due to degree of immunocompromise and age).

c. Local tenderness, warmth, erythema, and swelling.

d. Motor weakness or radicular pain.

e. Spinal deformity in patients with prolonged course of treatment.

3. Long bone and pelvis.

a. Acute osteomyelitis: Can present as septic arthritis because it affects the metaphysis to the joint.

b. Tenderness, warmth, erythema, and swelling.

4. Chronic osteomyelitis.

a. Pain, erythema, and swelling.

b. Occasional draining sinus tract.

c. More likely with presence of prosthetic material, extensive tissue ulceration, or vascular insufficiency.

B. Common/typical scenario.

1. Complaints of pain, swelling, and possibly low-grade fever.

2. Symptoms develop over days to weeks.

C. Family and social history.

1. Past medical history: Comorbidities leading to increased risk.

2. Recent surgeries, implants, and so on.

3. History of diabetes with ulcers.

4. Decubitus ulcers.

5. Peripheral vascular disease.

6. Intravenous (IV) drug abuse.

7. Sickle cell disease.

8. Recent trauma.

9. Urinary tract infection (UTI) or pyelonephritis.

D. Review of systems.

1. Constitutional: Possible night sweats, fatigue, malaise, or lethargy.

2. Genitourinary: Signs and symptoms of UTI; loss of bowel or bladder control.

3. Musculoskeletal: Pain, swelling, or redness at site.

4. Skin: Purulent drainage from open wound.

5. Musculoskeletal: Weakness in lower extremities.

Physical Examination

A. Location of any skin lesions (in case of diabetic foot ulcers [> 2 × 2 cm] or exposed bone, osteomyelitis is likely).

B. Positive neurological examination with areas of weakness or sensory loss (particularly in suspected spinal osteomyelitis).

C. Presence of vascular and arterial insufficiency.

D. Probe to the bone in pedal ulcers using sterile, blunt metal tool.

1. Positive result: Hard, gritty surface of bone.

Diagnostic Tests

A. Laboratory studies: Generally nonspecific initially.

1. CBC.

a. Leukocytosis: Common in acute osteomyelitis but less common in chronic cases.

2. ESR greater than 70 mm/h: Indicative of osteomyelitis.

3. CRP elevated.

4. Blood cultures: Most useful when patient is febrile.

B. Imaging studies.

1. Accuracy dependent on intensity of the inflammation, chronicity of the infection, site, vascularity, and associated pathology.

2. Simply support or refute clinical suspicion.

3. Plain films generally used for the initial study.

a. Most sensitive but least specific of all the diagnostic modalities.

b. Cortical abnormality with periosteal new bone formation: Suggestive of osteomyelitis.

c. Most useful when symptoms have persisted for more than 2 weeks.

4. MRI: High negative predictive value and highly sensitive.

a. First choice for suspected spinal osteomyelitis.

5. Radionuclide bone skeletal scintigraphy (i.e., three-phase bone scan) combined with CT: May be used if MRI is not possible due to indwelling hardware.

C. Bone biopsy: Combined with histologic findings of inflammation and bone necrosis.

1. May be done using open or percutaneous approach, with open being preferable because the sensitivity of percutaneous biopsy is poor.

Differential Diagnosis

A. Spinal osteomyelitis with symptoms of backache.
   1. Influenza, or virus with flu-like symptoms.
   2. Pyelonephritis.
   3. Pancreatitis.
   4. Osteoporotic fracture.
   5. Disc herniation.
B. Long bone osteomyelitis.
   1. Septic arthritis.
   2. Bone tumor.
   3. Occult or pathological fracture.
   4. Soft tissue infection.
   5. Charcot arthropathy.
   6. Bursitis.
   7. SAPHO syndrome (synovitis, acne, pustulosis, hyperostosis, and osteitis).
   8. Gout.

Evaluation and Management Plan

A. General plan.
   1. Bone probing for foot ulcerations suspected of being osteomyelitis.
   2. Prolonged duration of antibiotic treatment is necessary.
   3. Bone biopsy: Open approach preferable to needle biopsy.
      a. Identification of causative organism with gram stain and culture, including aerobic, mycobacterial, and fungal culture.
   4. Surgical debridement: May be required for chronic osteomyelitis.
   5. Removal of hardware: May be required.
   6. Adjunctive therapies: Hyperbaric oxygen therapy.
B. Patient/family teaching points.
   1. Prolonged duration of antibiotic treatment is necessary.
   2. Recurrence is common.
C. Pharmacotherapy.
   1. Antibiotic selection based on cultures identifying causative agent and susceptibilities. Empiric treatment against methicillin-resistant *Staphylococcus aureus* (MRSA) should be completed when culture data are available (piperacillin-tazobactam, ampicillin-sulbactam, ticarcillin-clavulanate; penicillin allergic: clindamycin, metronidazole, ciprofloxacin, levofloxacin; if MRSA is suspected, vancomycin).
   2. Prolonged duration of treatment; generally outpatient parenteral antibiotic therapy.
      a. Measurement of C-reactive protein (CRP) weekly: To determine serial trends.
D. Discharge instructions.
   1. Complete the course of antibiotics as prescribed.
   2. Follow wound care instructions as prescribed.
   3. Avoid injury to the area where the infection is located.
   4. Report new or worsening symptoms, especially pain, redness, swelling, or drainage in the affected area.

Follow-Up

A. Based on the location of disease and duration of treatment.
   1. Long-term oral antibiotic therapy (3–6 months) may be required if orthopedic hardware must remain in place.

Consultation/Referral

A. Orthopedic consult.
B. Radiology consult to assist with determining the best mode of diagnostics.

C. Infectious disease consult to determine type and duration of antibiotics.

Special/Geriatric Considerations

A. Incidence peaks in geriatric patients because of prosthetic implants and chronic health diseases such as peripheral vascular disease and diabetes.
B. The most common sites of infection in the elderly are in joint replacements and the spine.

Bibliography

Calhoun, J. H., & Manring, M. M. (2005, December). Adult osteomyelitis. *Infectious Disease Clinics of North America, 19*(4), 765–786. doi:10.1016/j.idc.2005.07.009

Paluska, S. A. (2004). Osteomyelitis. *Clinics in Family Practice, 6,* 127–156. doi:10.1016/S1522-5720(03)00130-2

Peritonitis

Jennifer W. Parker

Definition

A. Inflammation of the peritoneum: The thin layers (visceral and parietal) of tissue that line the inner wall of the abdomen, covering most of the organs.
B. Considered an **acute abdomen**.
C. Types.
   1. Primary peritonitis: Most often seen as spontaneous bacterial peritonitis (SBP).
      a. Considered to be infection of peritoneum/ascitic fluid without a surgically treatable source.
   2. Secondary peritonitis: Most common form.
      a. Considered to be inflammation of the peritoneum secondary to a surgically treatable source.
   3. Tertiary peritonitis: Recurring or chronic peritonitis after adequate treatment of the original disease.

Incidence

A. May be difficult to establish and varies with disease process and type of peritonitis.
   1. Patients with an all cause diagnosis of cirrhosis were reported.
   2. Patients with ascites have an incidence rate as high as 18%.
   3. Patients with peritoneal dialysis may have rates as high as 12%.

Pathogenesis

A. Peritonitis may be generalized or localized (i.e., abscesses, the leading cause of persistent infection/tertiary peritonitis), and infectious or sterile (i.e., chemical or mechanical).
B. Primary peritonitis (generally SBP) is an acute infection of ascitic fluid, resulting from translocation of bacteria across the gut wall and/or mesenteric lymphatics or, less frequently, due to hematogenous seeding in the presence of bacteremia.
   1. SBP is a complication of any disease that causes ascites, including cirrhosis, heart failure, and Budd–Chiari syndrome. From 10% to 30% of patients with liver cirrhosis develop SBP.
   2. Majority (>90%) of SBP is monomicrobial, with most commonly gram-negative organisms including *Escherichia coli* (40%) and *Klebsiella pneumoniae* (7%); or gram-positive organisms such as *Streptococcus pneumoniae*

(15%), other *Streptococcus* strains (15%), and *Staphylococcus* species (3%).

C. Secondary peritonitis is intra-abdominal sepsis generally from a perforated viscus resulting from direct spillage of the luminal organ into the peritoneum.

    1. Causes include perforated peptic ulcer, diverticulitis, appendicitis, necrotizing pancreatitis, or iatrogenic perforation.

    2. Pathogens differ from the proximal to distal end of the gastrointestinal (GI) tract (gram-positive is predominant in the upper GI tract, unless the patient is on long-term proton pump inhibitor (PPI) treatment, when gram-negative may become more populous). Contamination from distal small bowel or colon is generally polymicrobial and may include fungi.

    3. Women can experience localized peritonitis from an infected fallopian tube or a ruptured ovarian cyst, as well as pelvic inflammatory disease.

D. Peritoneal-dialysis-associated peritonitis.

    1. Causes include and are almost always due to catheter-related infection and are related to touch contamination with pathogenic skin bacteria.

    2. Abdominal pain, cloudy peritoneal effluent due to white cell counts greater than 100 cells/mm^3, purulent drainage at catheter site, or a swollen, tender tunnel site may appear.

E. Secondary peritonitis: Acute or chronic.

    1. Onset can be sudden as when secondary to appendicitis or cholecystitis, or it can be associated with chronic diseases (especially GI) such as Crohn's disease or peptic ulcer disease (PUD); trauma; or recent surgery.

Predisposing Factors

A. Primary peritonitis (SBP): Cirrhosis of the liver with ascites.

    1. Any diagnosis of cirrhosis.

    2. Contaminated dialysate.

B. Secondary peritonitis: Peritonitis with surgically treatable source.

    1. Perforation of intestinal tract, abdominal organs.

    2. Trauma.

    3. Peritoneal dialysis.

    4. Previous history of peritonitis.

Subjective Data

A. Common complaints/symptoms.

    1. Primary peritonitis (SBP): Fever and abdominal pain, often accompanied by change in mental status from hepatic encephalopathy and/or sepsis.

    2. Secondary peritonitis: Acute abdominal pain, worse with movement, variable location of pain, high fever, and nausea and vomiting.

        a. Pain can be generalized and dull initially (visceral peritoneum involvement) and then become more localized and severe (parietal layer involvement).

B. Common/typical scenario.

    1. Diagnosis of peritonitis is primarily clinical; thus, history is important.

    2. Specific historical factors include knowledge of previous peritonitis, causes of immunosuppression including the use of immunosuppressive agents, recent abdominal surgery or trauma, presence of diseases (e.g., inflammatory bowel disease, diverticulitis, PUD) that may predispose to intra-abdominal perforations/infections, and travel history.

        a. Primary peritonitis (SBP): Cirrhosis of the liver; hepatitis C, now with ascites.

C. Social history.

    1. Alcohol dependency.

    2. Intravenous (IV) drug use.

    3. Blood transfusion.

D. Review of systems.

    1. Primary peritonitis (SBP).

        a. Constitutional: Feeling poorly, fever, loss of appetite, or generalized weakness.

        b. Neurological: Change in mental status or dizziness/lightheadedness (secondary to hypotension).

        c. Respiratory shortness of breath, dyspnea on exertion, and inability to take a deep breath.

        d. GI: Diffuse abdominal pain, abdominal tenderness, fever, and often ascites.

    2. Secondary peritonitis.

        a. Constitutional: Fever, chills, diaphoresis, or loss of appetite.

        b. Neurological: Lightheadedness/dizziness (secondary to hypotension).

        c. Cardiac: Tachycardia secondary to pain.

        d. Respiratory: Shortness of breath, dyspnea (secondary to pain).

        e. GI: Acute abdominal pain (worse with movement), nausea and vomiting, and constipation or diarrhea.

Physical Examination

A. General appearance: Ill and in severe discomfort.

    1. Peritonitis can often proceed quickly to septic shock and multiple organ dysfunction syndrome (MODS).

B. Vital signs.

    1. Temperature: Often greater than 38°C, but if patient is in shock, may become hypothermic.

    2. Tachycardia from presence of inflammatory mediators; fever and hypovolemia from vomiting/shock/third spacing.

    3. Hypotension: Primarily as patients progress with dehydration and shock.

C. Abdominal (patient should be supine, with a pillow underneath knees; this may allow for improved relaxation of abdominal wall).

    1. Tenderness to palpitation.

        a. The region of greatest tenderness overlies the site of maximal irritation/pathologic process, even with generalized pain.

    2. Rigidity: Voluntary in anticipation to or response to palpitation or involuntary from peritoneal irritation.

        a. Involuntary rigidity makes peritonitis highly likely.

    3. Increased pain with movement: Possible severe pain caused by coughing or flexing of the hips.

    4. Rebound tenderness (i.e., positive Bloomberg sign): As peritoneum snaps back into place with sudden removal of pressure.

    5. Distension.

    6. Hypoactive to absent bowel sounds: Reflecting generalized ileus (less likely with highly localized infection).

    7. Masses or hernias (occasionally).

    8. Ascites: Especially in SBP.

D. Genitourinary: Oliguria or anuria as patient becomes hypotensive.

E. Integumentary: Presence of signs of liver failure such as jaundice or angiomata if SBP results from cirrhosis.

Diagnostic Tests

A. For all patients.

1. Paracentesis: For all patients with new ascites and/or hospitalization of cirrhotic patients *prior to* receiving antibiotics.

   a. A cell count of 250 or more polymorphonuclear leukocytes (PMN) suggests infection. Patients should be started on broad-spectrum antibiotics immediately, with narrowing of antibiotic treatment following results of culture of ascitic fluid.

   b. Analysis of ascitic fluid should also include Gram's stain; fluid chemistries; serum-ascites albumin gradient; ascitic fluid total protein concentration; and ascitic fluid glucose, lactate dehydrogenase, amylase, and bilirubin concentrations. All of these can help the diagnosis of SBP and/or differentiate SBP from secondary peritonitis.

2. Plain and upright abdominal films: Evaluation for free air or dilation of large or small bowel.

   a. Free air is present in most cases of anterior gastric and duodenal perforation, less frequent with small bowel and colonic perforations, and rarely present with perforations of the appendix.

   b. Upright films are useful for identifying free air under the diaphragm (usually on the right), which is indicative of viscus perforation.

3. Chest x-ray: Elevated diaphragm.

4. CT of abdomen with enteral and IV contrast: Evidence of surgically treatable source, ascites, or mass. CT is the optimal diagnostic study for peritoneal abscess and related visceral pathology.

5. Blood cultures: Often positive.

B. For patients on peritoneal dialysis.

1. Peritoneal fluid analysis: With WBC greater than 100 cells/mm^3; more than 50% of those are polymorphonuclear leukocytes.

   a. Low WBC is found even in cases of peritonitis, usually due to the short length of dialysate dwell time, or a poor host immune response.

   b. Gram's stain of fluid should be completed.

2. Peritoneal fluid culture: Most commonly gram-positive organisms, such as coagulase-negative *Staphylococcus*.

3. Peripheral WBC and blood cultures.

4. Culture of purulent drainage from exit site.

Differential Diagnosis

A. Primary peritonitis (SBP).

1. Important to differentiate from secondary peritonitis because of high mortality associated with unnecessary versus postponed surgery.

2. Other conditions to be considered with ascitic patients: Peritoneal carcinomatosis, tuberculous peritonitis, and alcoholic hepatitis.

B. Secondary peritonitis: Associated with many thoracic and abdominal conditions.

1. Thoracic conditions leading to diaphragmatic irritation (e.g., empyema).

2. Retroperitoneal processes: Renal abscess, pyelonephritis, cystitis, and urinary retention.

3. External hernia with intestinal incarceration.

4. Familial Mediterranean fever.

5. Gynecological disorders: Salpingitis, endometriosis, teratoma, and dermoid cysts.

6. Neoplasms.

7. Vascular conditions: Mesenteric embolus or nonocclusive ischemia, ischemic colitis, and portal or mesenteric vein thrombosis.

8. Splenosis.

9. Vasculitis: Systemic lupus erythematosus and allergic vasculitis.

Evaluation and Management Plan

A. All types of peritonitis: Essential to provide aggressive fluid management to maintain hemodynamic stability.

1. If at all possible: Avoid vasopressors.

B. Primary peritonitis (SBP).

1. Empiric antibiotic therapy should be given as soon as possible (but preferably after paracentesis for culture).

   a. Cefotaxime 2 g every 8 hours is recognized to produce good results in ascitic fluid.

   b. Other third generation cephalosporins and fluoroquinolones may also be appropriate, although resistance to fluoroquinolones is an increasing concern.

2. Any nonselective beta blocker should be discontinued.

3. IV albumin (1.5 g/kg body weight within 6 hours of diagnosis and 1.0 g/kg on day 3) is beneficial with renal dysfunction (Cr >1.0 mg/dL, BUN >30 mg/dL or total bilirubin is >4 mg/dL).

4. Diuretic therapy concentrates ascitic fluid, thereby raising opsonic activity, which limits recurrence of SBP.

5. Use of PPIs, which are associated with increased risk of SBP, should be limited.

C. Secondary peritonitis.

1. Prompt initiation of empiric antibiotic treatment after all cultures have been drawn is necessary to cover gram-negative aerobes, enteric streptococci, and anaerobes (e.g., Cefotaxime 2 g IV every 8 hours with metronidazole 500 mg IV every 8 hours).

2. Emergent operative management to eliminate the contamination source is important.

3. Frequently, patients must be *nil per os* (NPO) with possible nasogastric tube placement—depending on the source of infection.

4. Nutritional demands need to be met; many patients develop an ileus after surgery. Consideration of enteral versus parenteral feeding should take place early in the course of treatment. Sepsis will increase nutritional demands.

Follow-Up

A. Primary peritonitis (SBP).

1. Repeat paracentesis is generally not necessary if patient has cirrhosis and monomicrobial infection.

   a. With an atypical course of SBP, repeat paracentesis in 48 hours.

2. Prophylaxis is recommended for the many ascitic patients to prevent repeat SBP, including:

   a. Patients with ascites with GI bleed.

   b. Patients with low protein levels in ascitic fluid (<1 g/dL).

   c. Patients with history of SBP.

3. Prophylactic regimens include:

   a. Ciprofloxacin—750 mg weekly.

   b. Trimethoprim-sulfamethoxazole five doses (Monday to Friday) of double strength tablets weekly.

   c. Norfloxacin—400 mg daily (Note: Long-term prophylaxis with fluoroquinolones is recognized to lead to high level fluoroquinolone resistance).

Consultation/Referral

A. Peritonitis, with the associated high mortality rates, often requires multiple consults, including:

1. Surgery (secondary peritonitis).

2. Infectious disease.

3. GI.

4. Nutrition.

5. Critical care.

6. Renal (for peritoneal-dialysis-associated peritonitis).

Special/Geriatric Considerations

A. Elderly patients may not present with profound guarding and/or abdominal rigidity, which are classic findings of peritonitis.

B. Fever and tachycardia are more common, although these signs are much less specific to peritonitis.

C. Careful history should be taken, and peritonitis cannot be ruled out with just a physical examination in elderly patients.

Bibliography

Barkley, T. W., Jr., & Myers, C. M. (2014). *Practice considerations for adult-gerontology acute care nurse practitioners.* West Hollywood, CA: Barkley and Associates.

Burkart, J. M. (2018, June 1). Clinical manifestations and diagnosis of peritonitis in peritoneal dialysis. In S. Motwani (Ed.), *UpToDate.* Retrieved from www.uptodate.com/contents/clinical-manifestatiosn-and-diagnsosis-of-peritonitis-in-peritoneal-dialysis

Daley, B. J. (2017, January 11). Peritonitis and abdominal sepsis. In P. K. Roy (Ed.), *Medscape.* Retrieved from http://emedicine.medscape.com/article/180234-overview

Runyon, B. A. (2018, April 11). Spontaneous bacterial peritonitis in adults: Diagnosis. In K. M. Robson (Ed.), *UpToDate.* Retrieved from www.uptodate.com/contents/spontaneous-bacterial-peritontis-in-adults-diagnosis

Runyon, B. A. (2018, September 21). Spontaneous bacterial peritonitis in adults: Treatment and prophylaxis. In K. M. Robson (Ed.), *UpToDate.* Retrieved from www.uptodate.com/contents/spontaneous-bacterial-peritontis-in-adults-treatments-and-prophylaxis

Sabatine, M. S. (Ed.). (2017). *Pocket medicine: The Massachusetts General Hospital handbook of internal medicine* (6th ed.). Philadelphia, PA: Wolters Kluwer.

Systemic Inflammatory Response Syndrome (SIRS)/Bacteremia/Sepsis

Rose Milano

Definition

A. Systemic Inflammatory Response Syndrome (SIRS): Clinical syndrome that is a form of dysregulated inflammation; can be present with or without infection; considered the clinical expression of host response to inflammation resulting from nonspecific insult.

1. SIRS is considered to be present when two or more of the following signs are present:

a. Temperature greater than 38°C (100.4°F) or less than 36°C (96.8°F).

b. Heart rate more than 90 beats per minute.

c. Respiratory rate greater than 20 breaths per minute or arterial carbon dioxide ($PaCO_2$) of less than 32 mmHg.

d. Abnormal white blood cell count (>12,000/μL or <4,000/μL or >10% immature forms; i.e., bands).

B. Bacteremia: Traditionally, essentially synonymous with septicemia; today, defined as the presence of viable bacteria in the blood.

1. Signs and symptoms range from asymptomatic, noninfectious to full blown sepsis.

C. Sepsis (general): A continuum of severity ranging from infection and/or SIRS, to sepsis, severe sepsis, and septic shock.

D. Sepsis: Traditionally, clinical syndrome with a collection of signs (objective) and symptoms (subjective); patient meets SIRS criteria and has a source of infection (this definition has been changed). Severe sepsis: Usually defined as sepsis with persistently low blood pressure, despite fluid resuscitation.

1. According to the Surviving Sepsis 2016 Campaign, sepsis is a life-threatening dysfunction caused by a dysregulated host response to infection (and category of severe sepsis has been removed).

2. Organ dysfunction is defined by an increase over baseline in the sequential organ failure assessment (SOFA) score (see Table 10.3). In critically ill patients, SOFA has a higher predictive value of in-hospital mortality than the SIRS criteria. Patients who meet SOFA criteria have greater than 10% predicted mortality.

a. SOFA score.

i. Mortality prediction score based on evaluation of organ dysfunction.

ii. Based on six different criteria: Respiratory, cardiovascular, hepatic, coagulation, renal, and neurological.

iii. Calculated on day of admission to the ICU and daily thereafter, until discharged from the ICU.

iv. Recommended that one uses the worst value to calculate the patient's daily score.

b. Quick SOFA score (qSOFA).

i. System used as a prompt to recognize patients with infections who are likely to be septic, yet not in the ICU.

ii. Developed with the intention to be used in the prehospital, ED, non-ICU floors in a hospital.

iii. Bedside scoring system that assesses three components.

1) 1 point: Systolic blood pressure less than or equal to 100 mmHg,

2) 1 point: Respiratory rate greater than or equal to 22 breaths per minute.

3) Altered mental status: Glasgow Coma Score of less than 15.

iv. Per the Surviving Sepsis Guidelines: A patient with an infection and a qSOFA score of 2 or more has a higher risk of death or prolonged ICU stay.

E. Septic shock: Sepsis, a vasodilatory or distributive shock, defined by the 2016 Surviving Sepsis Campaign as including the criteria for sepsis, and even with adequate fluid resuscitation meets the following conditions:

1. Unresponsive to fluid resuscitation.

2. Serum lactate levels more than 2 mmol/L.

3. Need for vasopressors to maintain mean arterial pressure (MAP) of 65 mmHg or more.

Incidence

A. SIRS.

1. The incidence of SIRS increases as the level of care unit acuity increases.

2. Progression of SIRS was noted to be: 26% developed sepsis, 18% developed severe sepsis, and 4% developed septic shock within 28 days of admission.

TABLE 10.3   **Sequential Organ Failure Assessment**

SOFA Score	0	1	2	3	4
Respiratory PaO2/FiO2	≥400	<400	<300	<200 (+) respiratory support	<100 (+) respiratory support
Coagulation	≥150,000				
Platelets × 10³ /mm³		<150,000	<100,000	<50,000	<20,000
Hepatic					
Bilirubin mm/dL	<1.2	1.2–1.9	2.0–5.9	6.0–11.9	>12
Cardiovascular Catecholamine doses ug/kg/min for at least 1 hour.	MAP ≥70 mmHg	MAP <70 mmHg	Dopamine <5 OR dobutamine (any dose)	Dopamine 5.1–15 OR epinephrine OR norepinephrine.	Dopamine >15 OR. epinephrine OR norepinephrine >0.1
Neurological					
Glasgow Coma Score	15	13–14	10–12	6–9	< 6
Renal Creatinine mg/dL OR Urine Output mL/day	<1.2	1.2–1.9	2.0–3.4	3.5–4.9 <500 mL/day	>5.0 <200 mL/day

B. Bacteremia.

1. Often asymptomatic, transient, and without consequences.

2. 25% to 45% with significant bacterial counts develop sepsis.

C. Sepsis.

1. One of the leading causes of death in the United States; between 230,000 and 370,000 people die of sepsis annually in the United States.

2. Sepsis is diagnosed in more than 25% of all hospitalized patients. The incidence of sepsis diagnosis has increased over the past 10 years.

3. Septic shock is associated with higher mortality than sepsis alone (40% vs. 10%).

4. Sepsis develops in 80% of patients prior to being admitted to a hospital.

5. 7 out of 10 patients diagnosed with sepsis had recently seen a healthcare worker or had a chronic disease requiring frequent medical care.

Pathogenesis

A. SIRS.

1. An insult/injury occurs, followed by local cytokine production, a local inflammatory response.

  a. Inflammatory cascade is an important piece of pathophysiology.

  b. Local cytokines are released to the systemic circulation, further provoking local response.

2. This leads to growth factor stimulation, with the recruitment of platelets and macrophages.

3. The acute phase of the response is controlled by a decrease in proinflammatory mediators and release of endogenous antagonists. If homeostasis is not restored with cytokine release into the systemic circulation, significant reaction occurs.

4. Continued exposure to injury/illness results in continuation of this inflammatory cascade, leading to progressive illness.

B. Bacteremia.

1. Sources of gram-negative bacteremia: Gastrointestinal (GI) tract, genitourinary tract, or from the skin on patients with decubitus ulcers.

2. Staphylococcal bacteremia: Common in patients with intravenous (IV) catheters and IV drug abusers.

3. Infection above the diaphragm causing bacteremia: Most likely gram-positive organism.

4. Infection below the diaphragm causing bacteremia: Most likely gram-negative bacillus.

C. Sepsis.

1. Sources of infections most likely associated with sepsis: Infections of the respiratory tract, gastrointestinal tract, genitourinary tract, and the skin. If the nervous system becomes involved, the mortality is greatest.

2. Bacterial infections: Most common cause of sepsis.

  a. Common causal bacteria: *Staphylococcus aureus*, group A *Streptococcus, Escherichia coli, Klebsiella* species, *Enterobacter* species, and *Pseudomonas aeruginosa*.

  b. Fungal and viral sources: Also possible causes.

3. Immunocompromised patients: Susceptible to fungal bloodstream infections from *Candida* species.

4. Culture Negative Severe Sepsis (CNSS).

  a. Sepsis without a documented microbiological source.

  b. Affects 28% to 49% of hospitalized patients with sepsis.

5. Sepsis: A complex interaction between a host's response to an invading pathogen and the pathogen itself.

  a. Most of the time, the response to an invading pathogen is a normal reaction in order to maintain overall integrity of the host. The normal host response may include fever and leukocytosis.

  b. Any pathogen that violates at the tissue level is potentially able to evade the host's humeral and cellular immune system leading to widespread, systemic infection.

  c. Although the early phases of sepsis are proinflammatory in nature, if not controlled, these may progress to a significant immunosuppressed phase where the host is at an increased risk for secondary infections, along with reactivation of latent viruses.

   i. Initially, pro-inflammatory molecules enter the bloodstream in an effort to ward off the pathogen.

ii. With sepsis, an overactive immune response to an infection causes the natural checks and balances to fail. Rather than dissipating, the activated inflammatory forces spread beyond the infected area.

iii. As these pro-inflammatory molecules travel they cause dilation and endothelial damage, leading to leakage of fluid out of the intravascular system and interstitial edema accumulation.

iv. This vascular leakage causes disruption of oxygen, nutrients, waste products, and fluids through the capillary walls.

v. If left unchecked, eventually organs become hypoxic and begin to fail.

d. A patient's response to sepsis is highly dependent on a variety of both host variables (i.e., age, comorbidities, genetics) and pathogen factors (i.e., virulence, susceptibility to treatment).

Predisposing Factors

A. SIRS.
  1. Infection.
  2. Autoimmune disorders.
  3. Pancreatitis.
  4. Vasculitis.
  5. Thromboembolism.
  6. Burns.
  7. Surgery.
B. Bacteremia.
  1. IV drug user.
  2. Presence of indwelling catheter (i.e., urinary catheter, IV catheter).
  3. Presence of multiple abscesses.
  4. History of structural heart disease and/or prosthetic heart valve.
  5. History of recent dental procedure.
  6. History of recent surgical treatment of an abscess or infected wound.
C. Sepsis.
  1. Younger than 1 year or over 65 years of age.
  2. Weakened immune system.
  3. Comorbid diseases.
  4. Unrecognized, untreated, or undertreated infection.
  5. Any condition listed under bacteremia.

Subjective Data

A. Common complaints/symptoms.
  1. Condition specific.
    a. SIRS.
      i. Temperature greater than 100.4°F.
      ii. Heart rate greater than 90.
      iii. Respiratory rate greater than 20.
      iv. Abnormal WBC count (>12,000 or <400,000).
    b. Bacteremia.
      i. Possibly asymptomatic or only a mild fever.
      ii. Other symptoms: Tachypnea, shivering, chills, persistent fever, altered sensorium, hypotension, and GI symptoms. This suggests development of sepsis and should be treated as such.
      iii. Thus, the remainder of this section will be directed toward sepsis specifically.
    c. Sepsis.
      i. Acute fever with or without chills.
      ii. Altered mental status (related to fever or hypoxia).

iii. Hypotension.
      iv. Tachycardia (unless on beta-blockers, calcium channel blockers, or if presenting late with systemic organ failure).
      v. Tachypnea with hypoxia.
      vi. Cool, clammy skin (depending on status of end organ perfusion).
      vii. Abdominal pain if intra-abdominal source of infection.
B. Common/typical scenario.
  1. Possibly asymptomatic.
  2. qSOFA score: 2 or more.
  3. Nonspecific symptoms such as weakness, fatigue, malaise.
C. Family and social history.
  1. Use of IV drugs.
  2. Family history of diabetes, hepatic disease, cardiovascular disease, or immunosuppression.
  3. Medical history: Important because it can suggest a likely source of the infection as the cause of the inflammatory response. It helps to identify the following:
    a. Comorbidities.
    b. Recent infections.
    c. Recent procedures/medical treatments.
    d. Implanted devices.
D. Review of systems: Highly variable depending on source of infection.
  1. Constitutional—fever, chills, malaise, or fatigue.
  2. Respiratory—dyspnea, cough, or increased oxygen needs.
  3. Cardiovascular—chest pain or palpitations.
  4. Gastrointestinal—ocalized or diffuse abdominal pain.
  5. Genitourinary—dysuria or decreased urine output.
  6. Neurological—altered mental status.
  7. Integumentary—cool/cold clammy skin, rash at IV sites, purulent wound, erythema, or warmth.

Physical Examination

A. General: Asymptomatic or generally ill appearing, complaining of fever, chills, or shivering.
B. Neurological: Altered mental status from baseline, ranging from confusion, malaise, and fatigue to lethargic to obtunded to comatose.
C. Respiratory: Tachypnea, dyspnea, cough, respiratory distress, or sputum production.
D. Cardiovascular: Tachycardia with or without murmur; jugular vein distention.
E. Gastrointestinal: Diffuse severe abdominal pain with peritonitis; pain localized depending on source of infection.
  1. Right upper quadrant with gallbladder source.
  2. Right lower quadrant with appendix source.
  3. Left lower quadrant with diverticulitis.
F. Genitourinary: Costovertebral angle tenderness with acute pyelonephritis or tender prostate on examination, with possible prostatitis.
G. Musculoskeletal: Swelling, joint tenderness, or warmth from septic arthritis.
H. Dermatological.
  1. Cool, clammy, and diaphoretic—septic shock.
  2. Rash, erythema, and induration—cellulitis.

Diagnostic Tests

A. Laboratory.
  1. Complete blood count (CBC) to check for leukocytosis with left shift, anemia, and thrombocytopenia.

2. Blood cultures, at least two sets aerobic and anaerobic prior to antibiotic administration.

3. Urinalysis with culture if indicated.

4. Chemistry panel to check renal and hepatic function.

5. Cardiac enzymes to rule out cardiac cause.

6. Lactate level (marker of tissue perfusion).

7. Procalcitonin level to guide length of antimicrobial therapy.

    a. Low levels may indicate reduction of the likelihood of bacterial infection.

B. Imaging.

    1. Chest x-ray.

    2. Abdominal ultrasound if suspect biliary tract obstruction.

    3. Possible CT scan or MRI: Superior to ultrasound when looking for any potential sources of infection, except those related to the biliary tree.

        a. Consider specific CTs if suspect concomitant traumatic injury; useful in base workup on mechanism of injury.

C. Miscellaneous.

    1. EKG if suspect cardiac cause.

    2. Possible lumbar puncture if suspect infection of the neurological system.

Differential Diagnosis

A. Pulmonary embolism.

B. Acute myocardial infarction.

C. Acute pancreatitis.

D. Diabetic ketoacidosis.

E. Massive aspiration.

F. Upper or lower GI hemorrhage.

G. Diuretic-induced hypovolemia.

H. Systemic vasculitis.

I. Cholecystitis.

J. Renal calculi.

Evaluation and Management Plan

A. General plan.

    1. Based on recommendations from the 2016 Surviving Sepsis Campaign: International Guidelines for Management of Sepsis and Septic Shock.

    2. Sepsis and septic shock are medical emergencies, and it is recommended that treatment and resuscitation begin immediately.

    3. The source of insult should be identified to prevent progressive dysfunction (SIRS). Recommend source control for infection should occur as soon as medically and logistically possible.

    4. Surviving sepsis interventions, or "Bundles." "Time of presentation" is defined as the time of triage in the ED or, if presenting from another care venue, from the earliest chart annotation consistent with all elements of severe sepsis or septic shock ascertained through chart review.

        a. Tasks to be accomplished within 3 hours of presentation.

            i. Measure lactate level.

            ii. Obtain blood cultures prior to administering antimicrobials.

            iii. Administer broad spectrum antimicrobials.

            iv. Administer 30 mL/kg crystalloids for hypotension or lactate 4 mmol/L or more.

        b. Tasks to be accomplished within 6 hours of presentation.

            i. In the event of persistent hypotension after initial fluid administration (MAP <65 mmHg) or if initial lactate was 4 mmol/L or more, reassess volume status and tissue perfusion and document findings.

            ii. Give vasopressors (for hypotension that does not respond to initial fluid resuscitation) to maintain a MAP of 65 mmHg or more.

            iii. Remeasure lactate if initial lactate elevated.

    c. Assessment of volume status and tissue perfusion indicators.

        i. Perform a focused examination including vital signs, cardiopulmonary status, capillary refill, pulse, and skin findings _OR two of the following_.

        ii. Measure central venous pressure (CVP).

        iii. Measure central venous oxygen saturation (ScvO2).

        iv. Obtain a bedside cardiovascular ultrasound.

        v. Perform dynamic assessment of fluid responsiveness with passive leg raise or fluid challenge.

    d. Fluid therapy.

        i. Resuscitate patients with sepsis-induced hypotension using at least 30 mL/kg of IV crystalloid solution over 3 hours.

        ii. If additional fluids are required after initial resuscitation, base IV crystalloid infusion rates on frequent assessment of hemodynamic status.

    e. Antimicrobial therapy.

        i. Start administration of IV antimicrobials as soon as possible, within 1 hour, after diagnosis.

        ii. Administer empiric combination antimicrobial therapy using drugs from at least two different antimicrobial classes to target the most likely pathogens for initial management, pending culture results.

            1) Do not use combination therapy for routine treatment of neutropenic sepsis.

        iii. Narrow empiric antimicrobials as soon as pathogens have been identified by culture/sensitivity results and/or adequate clinical improvements are noted.

        iv. 7 to 10 days of antimicrobial therapy is adequate for most serious infections associated with sepsis.

        v. Perform daily assessment for de-escalation of antimicrobial therapy.

        vi. Understand that procalcitonin levels can be used to support shortening the duration of antimicrobial therapy.

    f. Vasoactive agent therapy (recommended).

        i. Aim for an initial target MAP of 65 mmHg.

        ii. Select norepinephrine as a first choice of vasopressor.

    g. Corticosteroids.

        i. Understand that these agents are not recommended if adequate fluid resuscitation and vasopressor therapy are able to restore hemodynamic stability.

        ii. Recognize that if fluids and vasopressors are not successful, then a daily dose of hydrocortisone 200 mg can be attempted.

    h. Mechanical ventilation.

        i. Strongly recommend prone over supine positioning of adult patients with sepsis-induced adult respiratory distress syndrome (ARDS).

        ii. Strongly recommend a PaO_2/FIO_2 ratio of less than 150.

        iii. Do not use high frequency oscillatory ventilation (HFOV) in adult sepsis-induced ARDS.

iv. Do not use beta-2 agonists to treat adult sepsis-induced ARDS without bronchospasms.

v. Suggest using lower over higher tidal volumes in adult sepsis-induced respiratory failure without ARDS.

i. Glucose control.

    i. Initiate an insulin infusion once blood glucose levels are more than 180 mg/dL for two consecutive readings.

    ii. Aim for an upper glucose limit that targets less than or equal to 180 mg/dL.

    iii. Monitor blood glucose levels every 1 to 2 hours until stable, then every 4 hours, while on insulin infusion in the ICU.

j. Nutrition.

    i. Start early enteral feeding as soon as patient can tolerate.

    ii. Use enteral feeding as opposed to parenteral feeding.

    iii. Within the first 7 days of caring for a critically ill adult septic patient, start IV glucose and advance enteral feedings as tolerated over administering parenteral feedings.

    iv. Give trophic/hypocaloric enteral feedings according to patient tolerance.

    v. Do not routinely monitor gastric residual volumes in adult septic patients, unless they are at a high risk for aspiration.

    vi. Suggest use of prokinetics for adult septic patients with feeding intolerance.

k. Renal replacement therapy.

    i. Do not recommend for adult sepsis with acute kidney injury, unless there are other definitive indications for dialysis.

B. Patient/family teaching points.

  1. To be completed within 72 hours of ICU admission.

  2. Goals of care.

  3. Prognosis.

  4. End-of-life care planning.

Follow-Up

A. Follow-up with the discharging provider and infectious disease provider.

Consultation/Referral

A. Consult critical care team to manage patients with sepsis.

B. Consult infectious disease provider to assist in managing antibiotic selection.

C. Consult appropriate surgical service for source control if sepsis is related to a structure in the body.

Special/Geriatric Considerations

A. Pregnancy.

  1. Most common cause of sepsis in pregnant patients is obstruction of the urinary tract.

    a. This may be caused by either hormonal effects of the pregnancy (hydroureters) or the mechanical obstruction of the uterus impinging on the ureters.

B. Geriatrics.

  1. Blunted responses: May have insult without meeting criteria.

  2. Medication effects: Blunt heart rate, respiratory rate, and temperature.

  3. Possible peritonitis without rebound tenderness.

Bibliography

Abraham, E. (2016). New definitions for sepsis and septic shock: Continuing evolution but with much still to be done. *Journal of American Medical Association, 315*(8), 757–758. doi:10.1001/jama.2016.0290

Centers for Disease Control and Prevention. (2016). *National and state healthcare associated infections progress report.* Retrieved from http://www.cdc.gov/HAI/pdfs/progress-report/hai-progress-report.pdf

Delinger, R. P., Schorr, C. A., & Levy, M. M. (2017). A user's guide to the 2016 Surviving Sepsis Campaign. *Intensive Care Medicine, 43*(3), 299–303. doi:10.1007/s00134-017-4681-8

Gaieski, D. F., Edwards, J. M., Kallen, M. J., & Carr, B. G. (2013). Benchmarking the incidence and mortality of severe sepsis in the United States. *Critical Care Medicine, 41*(5), 1167–1174. doi:10.1097/CCM.0b013e31827c09f8

Gupta, S., Sakjuja, A., Kumar, G., McGrath, E., Nanchal, R. S., & Kashani, K. B. (2016). Culture negative severe sepsis: Nationwide trends and outcomes. *Chest, 150*(6), 1251–1259. doi:10.1016/j.chest.2016.08.1460

Head, L. W., & Coopersmith, C. M. (2016). Evolution of sepsis management: From early goal directed therapy to personalized care. *Advances in Surgery, 50*(1), 221–234. doi:10.1016/j.yasu.2016.04.002

Longo, D., Fauci, A., Kasper, D., Hauser, S., Jameson, J., & Loscalzo, J. (Eds.). (2015). *Harrison's principles of internal medicine* (19th ed.) New York, NY: McGraw Hill.

MacClaren, A., & Spelman, G. (2018, July 6). Fever in the intensive care unit. In G. Finlay (Ed.), *UpToDate.* Retrieved from https://www.uptodate.com/contents/fever-in-the-intensive-care-unit

Marino, P. M. (2014). *The ICU book* (4th ed). Philadelphia, PA: Wolters Kluwer/Lippincott Williams & Wilkins.

O'Grady, N. M., Barie, P. S., Bartlett, J. G., Bleck, T., Carroll, K., Kalil, A. C., . . . Masur, H. (2008). Guidelines for evaluation of new fever in critically ill adult patients: 2008 update from the American Association of Critical Care Medicine and the Infectious Diseases Society of America. *Critical Care Medicine, 36*(4), 1330–1349. doi:10.1097/CCM.0b013e318169eda9

Rhodes, A., Evans, L. E., Alhazzani, L. E., Levy, M. M., Antoneilli, M., Ferrer, R., & Dellinger, P. (2017). Surviving sepsis campaign: International guidelines for management of sepsis and shock: 2016. *Intensive Care Medicine, 43*(3), 304–377. doi:10.1007/s00134-017-4683-6

Singer, M., Deutschman, C. S., Seymour, C. W., Shankar-Hari, M., Annane, D., Bauer, M., & Angus, D. A. (2016). The third international consensus definitions for sepsis and septic shock (Sepsis-3). *Journal of the American Medical Association, 315*(8), 801–810. doi:10.1001/jama.2016.0287

Septic Arthritis

Rose Milano

Definition

A. Infection of a joint, generally caused by bacteria, but can be caused by fungi or mycobacteria.

B. Devastating form of acute-onset arthritis; considered an orthopedic emergency.

C. Although all types of septic arthritis are infectious, not all types of infectious arthritis are classified as septic. Systemic diseases that can trigger an inflammatory response in joints include:

  1. Lyme disease.

  2. Chikungunya: Mosquito-borne illness (in the family of alphaviruses).

  3. Rubella.

  4. Parvovirus.

  5. Hepatitis B and C.

Incidence

A. Incidence is 2 to 10 per 100,000 in general population.

B. The incidence is increased in patients with rheumatoid arthritis or joint prostheses, 30 to 70 per 100,000.

C. The prevalence has been estimated to range from 8% to 27% in adults presenting with one or more acutely painful joints.

D. Mortality has been at the persistent rate of 5% to 15% over the past 25 years.

Pathogenesis

A. Hematogenous seeding from bacteremia. Bacteria cause acute synovitis after entering the closed joint space within hours. The synovium is very vascular with no membrane barriers, making it susceptible to seeding by bacteria.

1. Synovial reaction: Results in swift entry of acute and chronic inflammatory cells.

2. Release of cytokines and proteases, which causes cartilage degradation.

3. Bone loss: Evident within a few days.

4. Generally monomicrobial.

5. Most cases (75%): Involvement of only one joint (monoarticular).

    a. Polyarticular infection is commonly seen in rheumatoid arthritis.

B. Joint surgery, joint aspiration, or local steroid injections: Often polymicrobial infections.

C. Puncture wounds or bites: Also possibly inoculant into the joint.

D. Bacteria most often involved.

1. *Staphylococcus aureus:* Primary cause.

2. Beta hemolytic streptococci: Next most common.

3. *Neisseria gonorrhoeae:* Most common pathogen among younger, sexually active adults, causing more than 75% of septic arthritis cases.

E. In intravenous (IV) drug users, gram-negative bacilli implicated most often.

1. *Klebsiella pneumoniae.*

2. *Escherichia coli.*

3. *Pseudomonas aeruginosa.*

Predisposing Factors

A. Age greater than 80 years.

B. Immunocompromised status.

C. Preexisting joint disease (gout, systemic connective tissue disorders).

D. Diabetes mellitus.

E. Rheumatoid arthritis.

F. Disseminated gonococcal infections in young healthy adults. Develops in 1% to 3% of untreated cases of gonorrhea.

G. All substance abuse, particularly IV drug use.

H. Skin infections; cutaneous ulcers.

I. Previous intra-articular corticosteroid injections.

Subjective Data

A. Common complaints/symptoms.

1. Native joints: Acute joint pain, swelling, warmth, erythema, decreased range of motion, fever, or malaise.

2. Prosthetic joints: Possibly minimal symptoms.

B. Common/typical scenario.

1. History of joint swelling, pain, fever, general malaise, or chills of acute onset.

2. Other recent infection (e.g., urinary tract infection [UTI], cellulitis; cutaneous infections from IV drug use; sexually transmitted diseases, particularly gonorrhea; endocarditis).

3. Recent orthopedic surgery or joint replacement: Can be early onset, delayed onset (3–24 months), or late onset (24 months after surgery).

4. History of rheumatoid arthritis; receiving anti-tumor necrosis factor (TNF).

    a. Anti-TNF therapy associated with doubling of risk of septic arthritis.

    b. Can result in higher mortality because septic arthritis can be mistaken for an acute rheumatoid arthritis flare up and lead to delay in treatment.

5. History of immunosuppressive diseases, including:

    a. Liver disease.

    b. Diabetes.

    c. Solid tumors.

    d. Lymphomas.

    e. HIV.

C. Family and social history.

1. History of IV drug use.

2. Smoking history.

3. Sexually active with multiple partners (gonococcal bacterial arthritis).

D. Review of systems.

1. Constitutional: Fatigue, malaise, lethargy, decreased appetite, or recent trauma.

2. Gastrointestinal: Unintentional weight loss, or diarrhea.

3. Genitourinary (GU): Frequent infections.

4. Musculoskeletal: Pain in joint(s), joint swelling, decreased range of motion, or arthritis.

5. Skin: Lesions, erythema, cutaneous wounds, needle marks, or bites.

6. Hematologic/lymphatic: Swollen lymph nodes or exposure to Lyme disease.

Physical Examination

A. Low grade fever.

1. Chills and spiking fever atypical.

2. Fever less likely in older adults.

B. Possible joint swelling, warmth, erythema, and limited range of motion.

C. Generally monoarticular. Polyarticular disease is present in about 20% of cases, generally in patients with rheumatoid arthritis or other systemic connective tissue disease.

1. Knee most common (50%).

2. Hip (20%).

3. Ankle (7%).

4. Wrists (7%).

5. Sacroiliac joints (1%–4%).

6. Axial joint septic arthritis (sternoclavicular, sternomanubrial joints): Most common in IV drug abuse.

D. Joint effusion.

E. Limited active and passive range of motion.

F. Prosthetic joint infections: Later physical findings often minimal.

1. Slight to no swelling.

2. May have draining sinus.

Diagnostic Tests

A. Synovial fluid aspiration.

1. Synovial fluid leukocyte count and neutrophil percentage: Reliable measure before cultures available. Synovial fluid leukocyte count greater than $50,000/mm^3$ with polymorphonuclear leukocyte predominance is usually indicative of septic arthritis but can also be seen in gout.

2. Cytology: Used to exclude gout or other crystal arthritis types. Mycobacteria and fungi may also be identified by cytology.

3. Cultures.

    a. Complete blood count.

i. Leukocytosis present in most cases but has low sensitivity and specificity.

b. Inflammatory markers.

i. Erythrocyte sedimentation rate (ESR): Useful only in patients with native joint infections without underlying hematological or rheumatological conditions.

ii. C-reactive protein (CRP): Typically elevated, but also lacks specificity.

c. Radiologic studies.

i. Plain films not usually helpful except to rule out an injury that might produce similar symptoms.

ii. CT better than plain films in identifying joint effusion, soft tissue swelling, and abscesses.

iii. MRI sometimes useful in native joint infections. Newer machines may allow for assessment of prosthetics.

4. Bone scintigraphy: Sensitive in identifying joint infections but is not specific enough to distinguish infection from other pathologies.

B. Other diagnostics.

1. CT or ultrasound guided biopsy: Used in axial skeletal joints and sternoclavicular joints.

2. Open biopsy: Highest sensitivity and specificity but is rarely done.

3. Arthroscopy: Useful to evaluate for septic arthritis of the knee.

Differential Diagnosis

A. Traumatic effusion.

B. Hemarthrosis.

C. Bursitis.

D. Cellulitis.

E. Acute synovitis (inflammation of synovial membrane).

F. Gout or pseudo gout.

G. Viral arthritis (rubella, hepatitis B and C, HIV).

H. Lyme disease.

I. Reactive arthritis—seronegative spondyloarthropathies such as Reiter's syndrome, psoriatic arthritis, ankylosing spondylitis, inflammatory bowel disease-related arthritis.

J. Endocarditis—can present with sterile synovitis or joint pain similar to septic arthritis. Fifteen percent of patients with infective endocarditis have concomitant septic arthritis or osteomyelitis.

Evaluation and Management Plan

A. General plan.

1. Considered a medical emergency.

2. Early treatment (<7 days from onset): Improved outcome.

3. Antibiotics: First-line treatment.

a. Empiric treatment aimed at most common bacteria of staphylococci and streptococci.

b. Concomitant infections such as UTIs: Possible use of antibiotics for gram-negative bacteria.

c. Prosthetic joint infections: Vancomycin if methicillin-resistant coagulase-negative staphylococci.

4. Drainage.

a. Hip, shoulder, and sacroiliac joints: Not easily drained with needle aspiration; may require open arthrotomy.

b. Sternomanubrial and sternoclavicular joints: Generally managed with open irrigation and debridement.

5. Splinting.

a. Knees splinted in extension.

b. Elbows splinted at 90°.

c. Hips in balanced suspension with no rotation.

d. Joint range of motion to begin when infection improved.

6. Removal of prosthetic joint often necessary.

7. Dental prophylaxis: Should be considered in patients who have prosthetic joints and immunosuppression, diabetes, or rheumatoid arthritis.

B. Pharmacotherapy.

1. Antibiotic therapy: Initiated empirically, then tailored based on gram stain/cultures after joint aspiration.

a. Most common pathogens: *S. aureus*, *Staphylococcus epidermidis*, and methicillin-resistant *Staphylococcus aureus* (MRSA), so empiric coverage can be initiated for gram-positive organisms (vancomycin).

b. Ceftriaxone: Empiric coverage for gonococcal infection.

2. Symptom management with acetaminophen and ibuprofen if no contraindications.

C. Patient/family teaching.

1. Antibiotics are used to treat the infection in septic arthritis.

2. If source control is not achievable with antibiotics alone, the fluid in the joint may be drained.

3. If there is extensive fluid, reaccumulation of fluid, or treatment is ineffective, surgery may be an option.

D. Discharge.

1. Rest painful joints as needed.

2. Elevate joints to reduce swelling and pain.

3. Exercise may help keep joints flexible and reduce pain, but once joints become painful remember to rest them.

4. Nonsteroidal anti-inflammatory drugs (NSAIDs) help reduce swelling, pain, and fever.

Follow-Up

A. Follow-up with the orthopedics team.

B. Infectious disease.

C. Physical therapy may be helpful.

Consultation/Referral

A. Consult rheumatology for assistance with diagnosis.

B. Consult orthopedics for anticipated surgical intervention.

C. Infectious disease consult for duration, route, and type of antibiotics.

Special/Geriatric Considerations

A. Immunocompromised patients.

1. Fungal septic arthritis: More common with Candida species, Aspergillus, Histoplasma, Cryptococcus, and Sporothrix.

2. Fungal infections: Challenging to diagnose and treat.

B. Geriatric patients.

1. Inflammatory response: Possibly blunted due to age. Patients may not have overt symptoms such as fever and significant joint swelling, which could delay diagnosis.

2. Advanced age: Significant risk factor for poor outcome.

3. Female predominance after age 80.

4. Removal of prosthetics in patients with advanced age: May not be possible.

5. High index of suspicion: Warranted in geriatric patients in any recently symptomatic joint or worsening of preexisting joint disease.

Bibliography

Del Pozo, J. L., & Patel, R. (2009, August 20). Clinical practice. Infection associated with prosthetic joints. *New England Journal of Medicine, 361*(8), 787–794. doi:10.1056/NEJMcp0905029

Garcia-De La Torre, I. (2003, February). Advances in the management of septic arthritis. *Rheumatic Disease Clinics of North America, 29*(1), 61–75. doi:10.1016/S0889-857X(02)00080-7. Retrieved from https://www.sciencedirect.com/science/article/pii/S0889857X02000807

Osmon, D. R., Berbari, E. F., Berendt, A. R., Lew, D., Zimmerli, W., Steckelberg, J. M., . . . Wilson, W. R. (2013, January). Executive summary: Diagnosis and management of prosthetic joint infection: Clinical practice guidelines by the Infectious Diseases Society of America. *Clinical Infectious Diseases, 56*(1), 1–10. doi:10.1093/cid/cis966

Zimmerli, W., Trampuz, A., & Ochsner, P. E. (2004, October 14). Prosthetic-joint infections. *The New England Journal of Medicine, 351*(16), 1645–1654. doi:10.1056/NEJMra040181

Tuberculosis

Rose Milano

Definition

A. An infectious disease characterized by the growth of tubercles (nodules).

B. One of the oldest diseases known to affect humans, most frequently affecting the lungs, although up to 1one third of cases occur outside of the pulmonary system.

Incidence

A. One of the top 10 leading causes of death worldwide, tuberculosis (TB) ranks higher than malaria and HIV. TB is a leading killer of HIV-positive individuals; in 2015, 35% of deaths in those with HIV were due to TB.

Pathogenesis

A. General information.
  1. Cause: Bacterium *Mycobacterium tuberculosis*.
  2. Dispersion: Spread by *M. tuberculosis* bacilli-infected airborne droplets, through coughing, sneezing, speaking, and singing.

B. Primary tuberculosis.
  1. Active disease that develops in previously unexposed patients.
  2. Almost always starts in the alveoli of the lungs.

C. Latent tuberculosis infection (LTBI).
  1. Exposure to *M. tuberculosis* without development of active disease. *M. tuberculosis* can stay dormant in the exposed host for decades.
  2. Noncontagious: Can turn into active TB disease if left untreated. About 5% to 10% of persons who do not receive treatment for LTBI infection develop active TB disease at some time in their lives.

D. Extra-pulmonary TB: Can affect any organ/system in the body. It may occur in 10% to 40% of infected individuals; the most common sites are:
  1. Lymph nodes (tuberculous lymphadenitis).
  2. Pleura.
  3. Upper airways.
  4. Genitourinary tract.
  5. Skeletal.
  6. Central nervous system (CNS/meninges).
  7. Gastrointestinal (GI).
  8. Pericardium (tuberculous pericarditis).
  9. Miliary/disseminated TB.

E. Drug-resistant TB.
  1. Certain strains of *M. tuberculosis* bacillus are resistant to the drugs normally used to treat the disease.

F. Previous exposure.

  1. Individuals with positive tuberculosis skin test (TST) are less susceptible to a new *M. tuberculosis* infection than individuals with a negative TST.
  2. Previous latent or active TB infections may not confer protective immunity.

Predisposing Factors

A. Decreased immune status of the host.
  1. HIV.
  2. Posttransplant patient on immunosuppressive therapy.
  3. Cancer patient on chemotherapy.
  4. Intravenous (IV) drug abuse history.

B. Malnutrition.

C. History of smoking tobacco/alcohol abuse/intravenous drug use.

D. Chronic renal failure/hemodialysis.

E. Recent infection with pulmonary fibrotic changes.

F. Post jejunoileal bypass/gastrectomy.

G. Elderly individuals with comorbidities and inconsistent immune response.

H. Crowded living conditions.

I. Healthcare workers.

J. Migration from/travel to a country with a high volume of TB cases.

K. Extremes in age: Very young and very old.

Subjective Data

A. Common complaints/symptoms.
  1. Early active TB disease: May be asymptomatic.
  2. Fever.
  3. Unexplained productive cough for more than 2 weeks (cough is seldom a presenting symptom in HIV patients).
  4. Hemoptysis: Sign of advanced infection.
  5. Loss of appetite/weight loss.
  6. Malaise/fatigue.
  7. Night sweats.

B. Common/typical scenario.
  1. Generally, exposure from infected droplets by coughing, sneezing, speaking, or singing.
  2. Slow symptom progression (over months).
    a. Worsening productive cough.
    b. Low grade fever.
    c. Night sweats.
    d. Fatigue.
    e. Weight loss.
  3. Hemoptysis and/or pleuritic pain, which indicates severe disease.
  4. Detailed medical history: TB.
    a. Presence of TB symptoms: If so, for how long?.
    b. Known exposure to individuals with infectious TB disease: When?
    c. Residence in high-risk congregate settings, such as prisons, long-term care facilities, and homeless shelters.
    d. Past medical diagnosis of latent TB or previous known TB disease and previous treatment.
    e. Comorbid diseases, which may increase risk of TB progression, including:
      i. HIV.
      ii. Diabetes mellitus.

C. Family and social history.
  1. TB: An infectious disease with no known genetic predisposition.
  2. Social stigma/poor knowledge about TB: Possibly difficult to obtain accurate history.

3. Recent travel to areas of known high prevalence of TB, such as Central/South America, Russia, Africa, Eastern Europe, and Asia.
D. Review of systems.
  1. General: Fever, night sweats, weight loss, and fatigue.
  2. Vision: Icteric sclera.
  3. Head/neck: Headache, neck pain, swelling/soreness of lump in throat, and hoarseness.
  4. Respiratory: Shortness of breath, cough, coughing up blood, and pleuritic chest pain.
  5. Neurological: Change in level of consciousness/ mental status, generalized weakness.
  6. Endocrine: Fatigue, polyuria, polydipsia, polyphagia, and weight loss.
  7. Musculoskeletal: Bone/joint pain.
E. Mental health: Alcohol/drug abuse.
F. Skin/hair: Presence/change in lesions/lumps.

Physical Examination

A. General.
  1. Many individuals with primary TB are asymptomatic (about 90% early onset).
  2. Once symptoms present, constitutional symptoms include weakness, fatigue, fever, chills, night sweats, loss of appetite, and jaundice.
B. Head, ear, eyes, nose, throat (HEENT; TB of eyes, mouth, nose).
  1. Headache (meningeal TB).
  2. Nonhealing oral ulcers/dysphagia (GI tract TB).
  3. Icteric sclera.
  4. Bleeding gums.
  5. Epistaxis.
  6. Hoarseness.
C. Neck (lymphatic TB/pericardial TB).
  1. Lymphadenitis.
  2. Jugular venous distention (late sign of pericardial tamponade).
D. Neurological (meningeal TB).
  1. Altered mental status, confusion.
  2. Coma.
E. Respiratory (pulmonary TB).
  1. Decreased, absent, coarse breath sounds.
  2. Dyspnea, tachypnea, sputum production, cough, and hemoptysis (pulmonary TB).
F. Skin.
  1. Jaundice.
  2. Pruritic rash, which may lead to ulcers and abscesses.
  3. Various stages of bruising.

Diagnostic Tests

A. Mantoux TST.
  1. Small "wheel" of tuberculin fluid is injected under the skin.
  2. Positive skin test means the individual has been infected with the TB bacteria.
    a. Greater than 5 mm induration is positive for:
      i. HIV.
      ii. Recent exposure.
      iii. Fibrotic changes on chest x-ray.
      iv. Organ transplant.
      v. Patients on immunosuppression medications.
    b. Greater than 10 mm induration is positive for:
      i. IV drug users.
      ii. Recent immigrants from high-risk areas.
      iii. Residents/employees of high-risk congregate settings.
      iv. Microbial lab personnel.
    c. Greater than 15 mm or more induration is positive for:
      i. Any individual, even with no risk factors.
  3. A negative skin test does not exclude a diagnosis of latent TB or active TB disease.
  4. Targeted TST programs are recommended for use only in high-risk groups.
B. Approved TB blood tests in the United States: Interferon gamma release assays (IGRAs).
  1. QuantiFERON-TB test.
  2. T-SPOT TB test.
C. Acid-fast bacilli (AFB) testing: Smear and culture.
  1. Culture remains the gold standard for diagnosis and identifying drug susceptibility and genotyping.
  2. Sputum specimens should be obtained from all individuals suspected of having active TB disease, both pulmonary and extra-pulmonary, with or without respiratory symptoms.
    a. At least three sputum specimens should be collected at consecutive intervals, 8 to 12 hours apart.
    b. At least one of the specimens should be an early morning specimen.
D. Imaging: Cannot be used alone to distinguish active TB from latent TB.
  1. Chest x-ray with a posterior–anterior view is the standard approach.
    a. Although abnormalities may be seen anywhere on a chest x-ray, TB lesions are most often noted in the apical and posterior sections of the upper lobes or superior sections of the lower lobes.
    b. Chest x-rays can be used to rule out active pulmonary TB in an asymptomatic, immunocompetent individual with a positive TST or IGRA.
  2. Chest CT is recommended if any suspicions for TB are noted after chest x-ray.

Differential Diagnosis

A. Pulmonary TB.
  1. Nontuberculous mycobacterial (NTM) infection.
  2. Fungal infections.
  3. Sarcoidosis.
  4. Lung abscess.
  5. Septic emboli.
  6. Lung cancer.
  7. Lymphoma.
  8. Actinomycosis.
B. Extra-pulmonary TB.
  1. Fungal infections.
  2. Non-TB bacterial infections.
  3. Syphilis.
  4. Nodular vasculitis.
  5. Leprosy.
  6. Cat-scratch disease.
  7. Rheumatoid arthritis.
  8. Lupus vulgaris.
  9. Pott disease.
  10. Histoplasmosis.
  11. Constrictive pericarditis.
  12. Bronchiectasis.

Evaluation and Management Plan

A. General plan: If properly treated, TB caused by drug-susceptible strains is curable in the vast majority of cases. If untreated, the disease may be fatal within 5 years in 50% to 65% of cases.

1. Medical evaluation for TB disease.
   a. Medical history.
   b. Physical examination.
   c. Test for *M. tuberculosis* infection (IGRA or TST).
   d. Chest x-ray.
   e. Bacteriologic examination of clinical specimens.
2. Goals of treatment if active TB disease has been diagnosed.
   a. Curing the individual.
   b. Preventing morbidity and mortality.
   c. Preventing emergence of multidrug resistant (MDR)-TB.
   d. Interrupting transmission of disease by making patients with active TB disease become patients with latent noninfectious TB.
3. LTBI: Who should receive treatment?
   a. Individuals with positive IGRA or TST and greater than 5 mm induration.
      i. Those with HIV.
      ii. Those who have had recent contact with person who has active TB disease.
      iii. Those with fibrotic chest x-ray findings and history of prior TB disease.
      iv. Those with organ transplants or other known immunosuppressive conditions, including those who have been receiving the equivalent of 15 mg of prednisone daily for longer than 1 month.
   b. Individuals with positive IGRA or TST and greater than 10 mm induration.
      i. Those who have recently (less than 5 years) arrived in the United States from areas where prevalence of TB is high (Asia, Africa, Eastern Europe, Russia, and Latin America).
      ii. Those who are known IV drug users.
      iii. Those who are residents/employees of high-risk cluster/congregate settings (prisons, nursing homes, homeless shelters, hospitals).
      iv. Those who work in a mycobacteriology lab setting.
      v. Those individuals with comorbidities known to increase the risk of infection to active disease (leukemia, diabetes, cancer, renal failure, gastrectomy).
      vi. Those with an un-accounted weight loss of 10%.
   c. Direct observation therapy (DOT): For individuals who have active TB disease or are at high risk for TB disease *if* they are suspected to be noncompliant with prescribed medications.
B. Patient/family teaching points.
   1. Provide information about the disease process.
   2. Explain the prescribed medication regimen and the importance of completing the entire treatment, even if the patients are asymptomatic.
   3. Give information about possible side effects of the LTBI medications prescribed and when to call the medical provider. Possible side effects include:
      a. Fever.
      b. Unexplained anorexia.
      c. Coffee or cola-colored urine.
      d. Icterus.
      e. Skin rash.
      f. Paresthesias of upper/lower extremities.
      g. Fatigue/weakness.
      h. Abdominal tenderness, especially right upper quadrant.
      i. Easily bruisable.
      j. Joint pain.
      k. Nausea/vomiting.
C. Pharmacotherapy.
   1. Latent TB.
      a. It is imperative to rule out active TB disease prior to initiating LTBI therapies. If mono-therapy with Isoniazid is prescribed for active TB disease, drug resistance may develop.
      b. Mono-therapy with Isoniazid (INH): 6-month dosing regimen.
      c. Mono-therapy with INH: 9-month dosing regimen.
      d. INH and rifapentine (RPT) regimen: 12 doses.
      e. Rifampin (RIF) mono-therapy: 4 month regimen.
         i. Active TB disease.
         ii. Treatment must be for at least 6 months.
         iii. Most, but not all, of the *M. tuberculosis* bacilli are killed within the first 8 weeks of treatment.
         iv. Undertreatment of the bacilli surviving the initial 8 weeks of treatment can cause the individual to become ill again, potentially with MDR-TB.
         v. Although the Food and Drug Administration has approved 10 medications to treat active TB disease, four core medications are used as first-line drugs.
            1) INH.
            2) RIF.
            3) Ethambutol (EMB).
            4) Pyrazinamide (PZA).
         vi. Dosing regimens: Available at the Centers for Disease Control and Prevention website: www.cdc.gov/tb/topic/treatment/tbdisease.htm.
D. Discharge instructions.
   1. Provide documentation of the following.
      a. TST or IGRA results.
      b. Medications to be taken (dose and timing).
      c. Possible side effects of medications to watch for.
      d. Duration of drug treatment, with date of last dose.
   2. Give details of when individual is required to be tested for TB.
   3. Name signs and symptoms of active TB disease and stress the importance of seeking medical care if symptoms should arise.
   4. Give information about the consequences of noncompliance with the prescribed medication regimen.
   5. Describe TB infection control measures and the potential need for isolation.

Follow-Up

A. Assess the state of infection and the infection's response to therapy.
   1. Negative culture results are the most important objective measure of response to treatments.
   2. Individuals with previously reported positive culture are considered positive until two consecutive negative monthly specimens can be obtained.
B. Check individuals monthly during treatment.
   1. Monitor compliance with prescribed medication regimen.
   2. Monitor for signs and symptoms of active TB disease.
   3. Monitor for signs and symptoms of side effects of medications, especially hepatitis.
      a. Jaundice.
      b. Loss of appetite.
      c. Fatigue.
      d. Muscle and/or joint aches.

C. Recognize that active hepatitis and/or end-stage liver disease is a relative contraindication for use of INH or RIF.

    1. Individuals with baseline abnormal liver function tests (LFTs) need regular monitoring with physical examination and laboratory evaluation of LFTs.

D. Understand that follow-up recommendations after treatment for active TB disease has been completed include the following:

    1. Individuals with a positive response to a 6- to 9-month treatment regimen with both INH and RIF do not require routine follow-up but they should be educated to promptly report a prolonged cough, fever, or weight loss to their medical provider.

    2. Individuals with TB bacilli who were resistant to INH and RIF should be monitored for 2 years after completing the alternative treatment option.

Consultation/Referral

A. TB disease treatment regimens for specific situations require special management and should be administered in consultation with a TB expert.

B. Certain individuals with known or suspected TB should be evaluated by a TB specialist.

    1. Pregnant women.

    2. Breastfeeding women.

    3. Infants and children.

    4. HIV-infected individuals.

    5. Individuals with known hepatic disease.

    6. Individuals with extra-pulmonary TB disease.

    7. Individuals with drug-resistant TB disease.

    8. Individuals with culture-negative TB disease.

    9. Individuals with renal insufficiency or end-stage renal disease.

Special/Geriatric Considerations

A. Individuals are no longer considered contagious when they meet *all three* of the following criteria.

    1. Three consecutive negative AFB sputum smears collected at 8- to 24-hour intervals with at least one being an early morning specimen.

    2. Symptoms have improved clinically.

    3. Compliance with prescribed treatment regimen for at least 2 weeks or longer.

B. Special consideration for treatment interruption during initial phase.

    1. Interruption is equal to or greater than 14 days; restarting the treatment from the beginning is recommended.

    2. Interruption is less than 14 days; continuing treatment to complete the total number of doses as originally planned, as long as they are completed within 3 months, is recommended.

C. Special consideration for treatment interruption during the continuation phase.

    1. If greater than or equal to 80% of the doses have been given *and* sputum AFB is negative on initial testing, then further dosing may not be needed.

    2. If greater than or equal to 80% of the doses have been given *and* sputum AFB is positive on initial testing, then continue and complete therapy as initially prescribed.

    3. If less than 80% of the doses have been given *and* the interruption is less than 3 months duration, then continue and complete therapy as initially prescribed.

    4. If less than 80% of the doses have been given *and* the interruption is more than 3 months in duration, then restart therapy from the beginning of the **initial** phase.

D. The rate of TB increases in elderly individuals who live at home.

E. There is a two- to three-fold additional increased incidence rate of active TB among nursing home residents.

F. Atypical presentation is not uncommon in older individuals.

    1. Approximately 75% present with lung involvement.

    2. Miliary TB, meningitis TB, skeletal TB, and genitourinary TB increase with advanced age.

    3. Many do not present with cough, hemoptysis, fever, night sweats, or weight loss.

    4. Many present with a change in functional capacity, chronic fatigue, cognitive impairment, anorexia, or unexplained low grade fever.

    5. Nonspecific, unexplainable symptoms that persist for weeks to months should alert medical providers to consider the possibility of unrecognized TB.

Bibliography

Centers for Disease Control and Prevention. (2013). *Core curriculum on tuberculosis: What the clinician should know* (6th ed.). Atlanta, GA: Author. Retrieved from https://www.cdc.gov/tb/education/corecurr/pdf/corecurr_all.pdf

Centers for Disease Control and Prevention. (n.d.). Tuberculosis. Retrieved from https://www.cdc.gov/tb/default.htm

Ehlers, S., & Schaible, U. E. (2013). The granuloma in tuberculosis: Dynamics of a host-pathogen collusion. *Frontiers in Immunology, 3*(411), 1–9. doi:10.3389/fimmu.2012.00411

Ellner, H. J. (2016). Tuberculosis. In L. Goldman & A. L. Schafer (Eds.), *Goldman-Cecil medicine* (25th ed.). 2030–2039. Philadelphia, PA: Elsevier Saunders.

Lewinsohn, D. M., Leonard, M. K., LoBue, P. A., Cohn, D. L., Daley, C. L., Desmond, E., . . . Woods, G. L. (2016). Official American Thoracic Society/Infectious Diseases of America/Centers for Disease Control and Prevention clinical practice guidelines: Diagnosis of tuberculosis in adults and children. *Clinical Infectious Diseases, 64*(2), e1–e33. doi:10.1093/cid/ciw694

Marino, P. M. (2014). *The ICU book* (4th ed.). Philadelphia, PA: Wolters Kluwer/Lippincott, Williams & Wilkins.

Mason, P. H., Roy, A., Spillane, J., & Singh, P. (2016). Social, historical and cultural dimensions of tuberculosis. *Journal of Biosocial Science, 48*(2), 206–232. doi:10.1017/S0021932015000115

Mathew, A. S., & Takalkar, A. M. (2007). Living with tuberculosis: The myths and the stigma from the Indian perspective. *Clinical Infectious Diseases, 45*(9), 1247. doi:10.1086/522312

Mattu, A., Grossman, S. A., & Rosen, P. L., (Eds.). (2016). *Geriatric emergencies: A discussion-based approach.* Hoboken, NJ: John Wiley & Sons.

Rajagopalan, S. (2001). Tuberculosis and aging: A global health problem. *Clinical Infectious Disease, 33*, 1034–1039. doi:10.1086/322671

Raviglione, M. C. (2015). Mycobacterial diseases: Tuberculosis. In D. L. Kasper, S. L. Hauser, L. J. Jameson, A. S. Fauci, D. L. Longo, & J. Loscalzo (Eds.), *Harrison's principles of internal medicine.* (pp. 1102–1122). San Francisco, CA: McGraw-Hill.

Weber, C. G. (2014, July 11). *Clinical infectious disease-2017 (The clinical medicine series)* [Kindle] Pacific Primary Care Software PC.

World Health Organization. (2018). *Tuberculosis fact sheet.* Retrieved from http://www.who.int/mediacentre/factsheets/fs104/en

11 Peripheral Vascular Guidelines

Fiona Unac

Acute Limb Ischemia

Fiona Unac

Definition
A. Acute limb ischemia (ALI) is a sudden decrease in limb perfusion that causes a potential threat to limb viability.

Incidence
A. The incidence of ALI is approximately 1.5 cases per 10,000 persons per year.

Pathogenesis
A. Arterial emboli that travel to the extremities predominantly originate from the heart.
B. Paradoxical emboli occur when venous thrombus traverse a cardiac defect and lodge in the arterial circulation.
C. Arterial thrombosis can occur where there is an atherosclerotic plaque or arterial aneurysm at sites of prior revascularization or in patients with thrombophilic conditions.
D. Arterial trauma can occur with interventional catheterization procedures, as well as blunt or penetrating injuries.

Predisposing Factors
A. Atrial fibrillation.
B. Recent myocardial infarction.
C. Aortic atherosclerosis.
D. Large vessel aneurysmal disease (e.g., aortic aneurysm, popliteal aneurysm).
E. Prior lower extremity revascularization (angioplasty/stent, bypass graft).
F. Risk factors for aortic dissection.
G. Arterial trauma.
H. Deep vein thrombosis (paradoxical embolism).

Subjective Data
A. Common complaints/symptoms.
   1. The "Six P's" is the classic presentation of ALI in patients without underlying occlusive vascular disease.
      a. Paresthesia.
      b. Pain.
      c. Pallor.
      d. Pulselessness.
      e. Poikilothermia (cold).
      f. Paralysis.
   2. The sudden and dramatic development of ischemic symptoms in a previously asymptomatic patient is most consistent with an embolus.

B. Common/typical scenario.
   1. Other signs and symptoms.
      a. Patients with known peripheral artery disease or those who have undergone prior revascularization may develop symptoms slower (hours to days), depending if collateral channels provide flow around the occlusion.
      b. Upper limb ischemia is seldom limb threatening. Patients often present with a cold feeling and numbness, rather than pain in the arm. Duplex ultrasonography can confirm diagnosis. The arm often improves with anticoagulation. There should be a low threshold to undertake embolectomy if there is doubt about limb viability.
      c. Blue toe syndrome is typically due to embolic occlusion of digital arteries with atherothrombotic material from proximal arterial sources. There is often a strong pedal pulse and a warm foot. Identification and eradication of the embolic source should be undertaken.

C. Family and social history.
   1. Elicit onset, duration, and intensity of the "Six P's" of ALI (paresthesia, pain, pallor, pulselessness, poikilothermia, and paralysis).
   2. Question the patient about previous peripheral artery disease, prior lower extremity revascularization, and aortic or popliteal aneurysm.
   3. Question the patient about atrial fibrillation, coronary artery disease, recent myocardial infarction, valve disease, and deep vein thrombosis.
   4. Inquire into the patient's history of limb trauma.
   5. Ask the patient about any condition that is a contraindication for administering pharmacological thrombolytic agents.

D. Review of systems.
   1. Musculoskeletal: Ask about the following.
      a. Temperature and pain of extremity.
      b. Any numbness, tingling, or weakness.

Physical Examination
A. Check temperature, pulse, respirations, and oxygen saturation.
B. Take blood pressure on both arms.
C. Inspect: Observe affected limb and compare with contralateral limb for mottling, pale, rubra, or necrosis.
D. Auscultate.
   1. Heart and lungs.
   2. Carotid, abdominal aorta pulses.
   3. Pulse of affected limb with the contralateral limb.
      a. Arm: Brachial.
      b. Leg: Femoral, popliteal.

E. Palpate.

1. Palpate and compare the pulses of the affected limb with the contralateral limb.

a. Arm: Brachial, radial, ulnar pulses.

b. Leg: Femoral, popliteal, dorsalis pedis, post tibial pulses.

2. Check capillary refill of affected limb and compare with contralateral limb.

3. Check limb strength and movement of affected limb and compare with contralateral limb.

4. Check limb sensation of affected limb and compare with contralateral limb.

F. Handheld Doppler.

1. Assess pulses of affected limb with the contralateral limb and note if the pulse is monophasic, biphasic, or triphasic.

a. Arm: Brachial, radial, ulnar pulses.

Diagnostic Tests

A. 12-Lead ECG to assess for underlying atrial fibrillation or myocardial infarction.

B. If distal leg pulses detected on handheld Doppler, obtain an ankle–brachial index (ABI). An ABI of about 0.3 is diagnostic of subcritical acute ischemia (refer to lower extremity peripheral artery disease for measuring ABI).

C. Full serum chemistry panel, including urea, creatinine, complete blood count, and baseline coagulation studies.

D. Vascular imaging.

1. The availability of specific imaging modality and the time required to perform and interpret the study should be weighed against the urgency for revascularization.

2. Patients should be anticoagulated prior to and during imaging.

3. CT is the investigation of choice.

4. Percutaneous angiography is the best choice when an endovascular solution to the arterial occlusion is likely.

Differential Diagnosis

A. Chronic critical limb ischemia.

B. Acute extremity compartment syndrome.

C. Extensive deep vein thrombosis.

D. Raynaud phenomenon.

E. Nonischemic limb pain from acute gout, neuropathy, spontaneous hemorrhage, or traumatic soft tissue injury.

Evaluation and Management Plan

A. General plan.

1. Systemic anticoagulation with unfractionated heparin.

a. Anticoagulation minimizes the risk of further clot propagation and prevents microvascular thrombosis of underperfused distal vessels.

2. Supportive measures.

a. Keep NPO by mouth until a definitive treatment plan has been determined.

b. Intravenous hydration, supplemental oxygen, and analgesia.

c. Results of vital signs, EKG, and serum panel will guide further therapy.

3. Treatment selection.

a. ALI treatment depends on the extent of limb ischemia (refer to Table 11.1).

b. Class I: ALI may require medical therapy only. Revascularization if contemplated can be performed electively.

c. Class II: ALI may require revascularization to preserve the affected extremity.

i. Class IIa: Percutaneous endovascular options are more effective in patients with ischemia of less than 2 weeks duration. Surgical revascularization is more effective in patients with ischemia of more than 2 weeks.

ii. Class IIb: Requires emergency revascularization. Treatment options will depend on timeliness, personnel, and resource availability.

d. Class III ALI. Revascularization is usually futile, and primary amputation should be considered.

4. Endovascular treatment options.

a. Catheter-directed thrombolysis.

b. Pharmacomechanical thrombectomy.

c. Catheter-directed thrombus aspiration.

d. Percutaneous mechanical thrombectomy.

5. Surgical revascularization options.

a. Balloon catheter thrombectomy or embolectomy.

b. Bypass procedures.

c. Endarterectomy.

d. Hybrid procedures combining open and endovascular techniques.

B. Pharmacological.

1. There are no pharmacological treatment options for ALI.

2. This is a surgical emergency.

3. Systemic anticoagulation with a heparin drip may be started to minimize further clot propagation and to prevent microvascular thrombosis.

4. Administer an initial bolus of 100 mg/kg followed by an intravenous infusion of 1,000 U/hr.

5. If an urgent operation is not undertaken, the heparin should be titrated to maintain an activated partial thromboplastin (aPTT) between 60 and 100 seconds.

6. Postoperatively, patients will need to be started on long-term oral anticoagulation.

C. Discharge.

1. Patients will need to be maintained on anticoagulation after surgery and will need to follow-up with vascular surgery for the surgical wound. Patients need to be taught about side effects of anticoagulation therapy and signs and symptoms of effective wound healing.

Follow-Up

A. Outpatient vascular specialty after 4 to 6 weeks.

B. Outpatient cardiology (if emboli likely to have originated from the heart) after 4 to 6 weeks.

Consultation/Referral

A. ALI is an emergency.

B. Immediate transfer to hospital for urgent vascular consult.

Special/Geriatric Considerations

A. Patients with ALI are usually elderly.

Bibliography

Cronenwett, J. L., & Johnston, K. W. (2014). *Rutherford's vascular surgery* (8th ed). Philadelphia, PA: Elsevier Saunders.

Gerhard-Herman, M. D., Gornick, H. L., Barrett, C., Barshes, N. R., Corriere, M. A., Drachman, D. E., . . . Walsh, M. E. (2016). 2016 AHA/ACC guideline on the management of patients with lower extremity peripheral artery disease: A report of the American College of Cardiology/American Heart Association Task Force on Clinical Practice Guidelines. *Journal of the American College of Cardiology, 69*, 1465–1508. doi:10.1016/j.jacc.2016.11.008

TABLE 11.1	Factors Affecting Risk of AAA Rupture		
	Low Risk	**Average Risk**	**High Risk**
Diameter	<5 cm	5–6 cm	>6 cm
Expansion	<0.3 cm/y	0.3–0.6 cm/y	>0.6 cm/y
Smoking/COPD	None, mild	Moderate	Severe/steroids
Family history	No relatives	One relative	Numerous relatives
Hypertension	Normal blood pressure	Controlled	Poorly controlled
Shape	Fusiform	Saccular	Very eccentric
Wall stress	Low (35 N/cm$^{2)}$)	Medium (40 N/cm$^{2)}$)	High (45 N/cm^2)
Sex	...	Male	Female

AAA, abdominal aortic aneurysm; COPD, chronic obstructive pulmonary disease.
Source: Rahimi, S. A. (2019, January 8). Abdominal aortic aneurysm. In V. L. Rowe (Ed.), *Medscape*. Retrieved from https://emedicine.medscape.com/article/1979501-overview

Mitchell, M. E., & Carpenter, J. P. (2018, March 15). Clinical features and diagnosis of acute lower extremity ischemia. In K. A. Collins (Ed.), *UpToDate*. Retrieved from https://www.uptodate.com/contents/clinical-features-and-diagnosis-of-acute-lower-extremity-ischemia
Rasmussen, T. E., Clouse, W. D., & Tonnessen, B. H. (2011). *Handbook of patient care in vascular diseases* (5th ed.). Philadelphia, PA: Wolters Kluwer Health.

Aortic Vessel Diseases: Aneurysms of the Aorta

Ponrathi Athilingam

Definition

A. An aortic aneurysm is an abnormal enlargement or bulging of the wall of the aorta.
B. An aneurysm can occur anywhere in the vascular tree.
C. The bulge or ballooning may be defined as a:
  1. Fusiform: Uniform in shape, appearing equally along an extended section and edges of the aorta.
  2. Saccular aneurysm: Small, lopsided blister on one side of the aorta that forms in a weakened area of the aorta wall.
D. An aneurysm can develop anywhere along the aorta.
  1. Abdominal aortic aneurysms (AAAs): Occur in the section of the aorta that runs through the abdomen (abdominal aorta).
  2. Thoracic aortic aneurysms: Occur in the chest area and can involve the aortic root, ascending aorta, aortic arch, or descending aorta.
  3. Thoracoabdominal aortic aneurysms: Involve the aorta as it flows through both the abdomen and chest.

Incidence

A. Approximately three to four per 100,000 per year.
  1. Intraperitoneal rupture (20%).
  2. Retroperitoneal rupture (80%).
  3. Aortocaval fistula (3%–4%).
  4. Primary aortoduodenal fistula (less than 1%).

Pathogenesis

A. Once the aorta reaches a critical diameter (about 6 cm in the ascending aorta and 7 cm in the descending aorta), it loses all distensibility, so that a rise in blood pressure to around 200 mmHg (as can occur physiologically during stress or exertion) can exceed the arterial wall strength and may trigger dissection or rupture. This is an emergency that warrants immediate intervention; often surgical.
B. Often occurs as:
  1. Retroperitoneal leak or rupture: If blood leaks into the space around the aorta behind the gut cavity then the leak is "contained" by the tissues and the patient is more likely to survive long enough to get to the hospital.
  2. Free intraperitoneal rupture: If the rupture is into the gut cavity (the peritoneal cavity) then there are no tissues to "contain" the escape of blood from the aorta, and it is much less likely that the patient will survive long enough to be taken to the hospital. Virtually all the blood in the circulation can escape into the peritoneal cavity.

Predisposing Factors

A. Genetic: Familial thoracic aortic aneurysm and dissection (TAAD).
B. Connective tissue disorders (Marfan's syndrome, Ehlers–Danlos syndrome type IV, and Loeys–Dietz syndrome, which partly resembles Marfan's syndrome).
C. Aortitis from giant cell arteritis.
D. Rheumatoid arthritis.
E. Behçet's disease.
F. Takayasu's arteritis or retroperitoneal fibrosis.
G. Infection, such as syphilis and HIV.
H. Trauma.
I. Weightlifting.
J. Cocaine and amphetamine use.

Subjective Data

A. Common complaints/symptoms.
  1. Most people are unaware that they have an aneurysm because, in most cases, there are no symptoms. However, as aneurysms grow, symptoms may include:
    a. Pulsating enlargement or tender mass felt by a physician when performing a physical examination.
    b. Pain in the back, abdomen, or groin that may be prolonged and not relieved with position change or pain medication.
  2. A ruptured aneurysm usually produces sudden, severe pain and other symptoms, such as loss of consciousness or shock, depending on the location of the aneurysm and the amount of bleeding.

B. Common/typical scenario.
   1. Thoracic aneurysm dissection rupture.
      a. TAAs are easily missed or misdiagnosed for cardiac ischemia.
      b. Patients complain of sudden intense and persistent chest or back pain, pain that radiates to the back, trouble breathing, low blood pressure causing feelings of fainting, loss of consciousness, and trouble swallowing.
   2. Abdominal aneurysm dissection or rupture.
      a. With AAA rupture patients complain of a sudden onset of severe lower back pain that may radiate to the groin, hypotension, or transient lower limb paralysis.
      b. Classic triad of symptoms: Pain, hypotension, and a pulsatile mass.
      c. Most abdominal aneurysms rupture into the retroperitoneal cavity.
      d. Rarely, AAA may rupture into the abdominal veins or the bowel. This may or may not be associated with retroperitoneal rupture.
      e. Emergent surgery is warranted once diagnosis is confirmed with echocardiogram, CT scan, or MRI.
      f. Rupture of an aneurysm is one of the most fatal surgical emergencies, with an overall mortality rate of 90%.
C. Family/social history.
   1. Family history is an independent risk factor for more rapid growth of aortic aneurysms and should be assessed.
   2. First-degree family history of aortic aneurysm or bicuspid aortic valve also elevates risk.
   3. Ask about smoking, which also increases risk of aortic aneurysm.
D. Review of systems.
   1. HEENT: Ask about any hoarseness or difficulty swallowing.
   2. Respiratory: Ask if the patient is having any shortness of breath, coughing, difficulty breathing, or chest pain.
   3. Musculoskeletal: Ask about back pain.

Physical Examination

A. Transient lower limb paralysis.
B. Right hypochondrial pain.
C. Nephroureterolithiasis.
D. Groin pain.
E. Testicular pain.
F. Testicular ecchymosis (blue scrotum sign of Bryant).
G. Iliofemoral venous thrombosis.
H. Inguinoscrotal mass mimicking a hernia.
I. Patient may show decreased red blood cell (RBC) or hemoglobin due to internal blood loss and increased white blood cell (WBC).

Diagnostic Tests

A. An echocardiogram, MRI, or CT scan may help to differentiate the diagnosis.
   1. Echocardiogram.
   2. CT and MRI only if the aorta is calcified.
B. Aortic angiogram or arteriogram: An arteriogram or angiogram accurately and directly depicts the vasculature; therefore, it clearly delineates the vessels and any abnormalities.
   1. An abdominal aneurysm would only be visible on an x-ray if it were calcified.
   2. CT scan and ultrasound don't give a direct view of the vessels and don't yield as accurate a diagnosis as the arteriogram.

Differential Diagnosis

A. Acute gastritis.
B. Appendicitis.
C. Urinary tract infection (UTI).
D. Diverticulitis.
E. Pancreatitis.
F. Cholelithiasis.
G. Small bowel obstruction.
H. Myocardial infarction.

Evaluation and Management Plan

A. General plan.
   1. Uncomplicated aneurysm.
      a. The goals of treatment include:
         i. Preventing the aneurysm from growing.
         ii. Preventing or reversing damage to other body structures.
         iii. Preventing or treating a rupture or dissection.
         iv. Allowing the patient to continue doing normal daily activities.
         v. Follow-up and screening for risk to prevent occurrence, which is key.
         vi. Evaluation of risk factors.
      b. Primary management is rigorous blood pressure control.
      c. Smoking cessation.
      d. Antiplatelet therapy where appropriate.
B. Dissecting or ruptured aneurysm.
   1. Rupture of aneurysm is an emergency: Patient is often in shock and needs immediate intervention.
      a. Open repair when a rupture occurs as an emergency surgery.
      b. Emergency endovascular repair for ruptured AAA, thanks to new technology, is now feasible?
      c. Operative risk is based on patients' comorbidities and hospital factors (Table 11.1).
   2. Type of repair.
      a. Open repair of an AAA involves an incision of the abdomen to directly visualize the aortic aneurysm.
      b. Endovascular aneurysm repair (EVAR).
C. Patient/family teaching points.
   1. Patients should seek attention if they feel chest pain or they just suddenly "don't feel right."
   2. A strong pulse sensation near the navel or bulge from the abdomen is also a reason to contact a provider right away. Deep constant or severe back or flank pain may be the only symptom a patient has of an expanding aneurysm.
D. Pharmacotherapy.
   1. Uncomplicated aneurysm.
      a. Statins: The role of statin therapy in AAA is unproven, but statins are advised because AAA patients have increased cardiovascular disease (CVD) risk.
      b. Other medical treatment: There is some evidence that the following may reduce the rate of expansion of small aneurysms, but their role is not yet clear.
         i. Doxycycline or roxithromycin.
         ii. Angiotensin-converting enzyme (ACE) inhibitors or losartan.
         iii. Statins.
         iv. Low-dose aspirin.
         v. Evaluate annually for risk of rupture, and follow-up.

E. Discharge instructions.

  1. Patients with incidentally discovered AAA should be taught to recognize signs and symptoms of an emergency and be given instructions on what to do next.

  2. Patients who undergo surgery should be taught effective wound care and to assess for signs and symptoms of healing.

Follow-Up

A. Surgical intervention for aneurysm (abdominal or thoracic).

  1. Patients with an incidentally discovered AAA that is less than 3 cm in diameter require no further follow-up.

  2. With AAAs 4 to 5 cm in diameter, elective repair may be of benefit for patients who are young, have a low operative risk, and have a good life expectancy.

  3. If the AAA is 3 to 4 cm in diameter, annual ultrasound imaging should be used to monitor for further dilatation. AAAs 4 to 4.5 cm in diameter should be evaluated with ultrasonography every 6 months, and patients with AAAs greater than 4.5 cm in diameter should be referred to a vascular surgeon.

  4. The decision to treat an unruptured AAA is based on:

    a. Operative risk.

    b. Risk of rupture.

    c. Patient's estimated life expectancy.

Consultation/Referral

A. Consultation should be made immediately to vascular surgery or cardiothoracic surgery for evaluation and general management of patients.

Special/Geriatric Considerations

A. Age is an important predictor of mortality in patients with aortic dissection with or without surgical intervention.

B. Treatment with endovascular aortic aneurysm repair should be strongly considered, particularly in octogenarians.

Bibliography

Bown, M. J., Fishwick, G., Sayers, R. D., & Bell, P. R. (2007). Repair of ruptured abdominal aortic aneurysm by endovascular technique. *Advances in Surgery, 41*, 63–80. doi:10.1016/j.yasu.2007.05.005

Hiratzka, L. F., Bakris, G. L., Beckman, J. A., Bersin, R. M., Carr, V. F., Casey, D. E., Jr., . . . Williams, D. M. (2010). 2010 ACCF/AHA/AATS/ACR/ASA/SCA/SCAI/SIR/STS/SVM guidelines for the diagnosis and management of patients with thoracic aortic disease. *Circulation, 121*(13), e266–e369. doi:10.1161/CIR.0b013e3181d4739e

LeFevre, M. L. (2014, August 19). Screening for abdominal aortic aneurysm: U.S. Preventive Services Task Force recommendation statement. *Annals of Internal Medicine, 161*(4), 281–290. doi:10.7326/M14-1204

Moulakakis, K. G., Mylonas, S. N., Dalainas, I., Kakisis, J., Kotsis, T., & Liapis, C. D. (2014, May). Management of complicated and uncomplicated acute type B dissection: A systematic review and meta-analysis. *Annals of Cardiothoracic Surgery, 3*(3), 234–246. doi:10.3978/j.issn.2225-319X.2014.05.08

Mussa, F. F., Horton, J. D., Moridzadeh, R., Nicholson, J., Trimarchi, S., & Eagle, K. A. (2016). Acute aortic dissection and intramural hematoma: A systematic review. *Journal of the American Medical Association, 316*, 754–763. doi:10.1001/jama.2016.10026

Rahimi, S. A. (2019, January 8). Abdominal aortic aneurysm. In V. L. Rowe (Ed.), *Medscape*. Retrieved from https://emedicine.medscape.com/article/1979501-overview

Svensson, L. G., Kouchoukos, N. T., Miller, D. C., Bavaria, J. E., Coselli, J. S., Curi, M. A., & Sundt, T. M., 3rd. (2008). Expert consensus document on the treatment of descending thoracic aortic disease using endovascular stent-grafts. *The Annals of Thoracic Surgery, 85*(1), S1–S41. doi:10.1016/j.athoracsur.2007.10.099

Westaby, S., & Bertoni, G. B. (2007, February). Fifty years of thoracic aortic surgery: Lessons learned and future directions. *The Annals of Thoracic Surgery, 83*(2), S832–S834. doi:10.1016/j.athoracsur.2006.10.098

Carotid Artery Disease

Ponrathi Athilingam

Definition

A. Atherosclerosis (waxy substance) plaque builds up inside the carotid arteries and causes carotid artery disease.

B. There are two common carotid arteries, one on each side of the neck. They each divide into internal and external carotid arteries.

  1. The internal carotid arteries supply oxygen-rich blood to brain.

  2. The external carotid arteries supply oxygen-rich blood to face, scalp, and neck.

Incidence

A. Carotid artery stenosis is one of the risk factors for stroke. The overall prevalence of asymptomatic carotid artery stenosis $\geq$ 50% in the general population is estimated.

B. The prevalence is higher in patients who harbor additional atherosclerotic lesions such as coronary artery disease.

C. Patients with severe asymptomatic carotid stenosis have an annual risk of 2% to 5% for stroke.

D. Among those 70 years and older, prevalence is increased to 12.5%.

Pathogenesis

A. Atherosclerosis of the carotid arteries is a diffuse, degenerative disease of the arteries resulting in plaques that consist of necrotic cells, lipids, and cholesterol crystals in the intima of carotid arteries.

B. Arterial narrowing leads to locally increased velocities. A hemodynamic effect is reached when pressure and flow volume are diminished in the poststenotic segment.

C. These plaques can cause stenosis, can crack, or cause injury, allowing platelets to stick to the site to form thrombi and/or rupture, causing embolization, which can cause stroke.

Predisposing Factors

A. Smoking.

B. High cholesterol levels in the blood.

C. High blood pressure.

D. Family history of atherosclerosis.

E. Sedentary lifestyle.

F. Diabetes or metabolic syndrome.

Subjective Data

A. Common complaints and symptoms.

  1. Amaurosis fugax (fleeting or transient ipsilateral visual loss).

  2. Transient ischemic attacks (TIAs).

  3. Crescendo TIAs.

  4. Stroke-in-evolution.

  5. Cerebral infarction.

B. Common/typical scenario.

  1. Patients may be asymptomatic with carotid artery disease.

  2. Sometimes it is found on routine surveillance.

  3. Patients oftentimes present with stroke symptoms which depend on the location of the brain.

4. Typically the patient with a stroke from carotid artery disease presents with weakness of extremities and speech difficulties.

C. Family and social history (pertinent findings—positive/negative).

1. Ask about family history, which has a strong association.

2. Ask about smoking, dietary habits, and physical activity.

D. Review of systems (pertinent findings—positive/negative).

1. Neurology—ask about the following:

a. Numbness.

b. Tingling or weakness.

c. Speech difficulties.

d. Confusion.

e. Trouble swallowing.

f. Visual disturbances.

Physical Examination

A. Thorough history.

B. Carotid bruit heard on auscultation.

C. Fundoscopic examination, if patient presents with amaurosis fugax, hypertensive, or history of TIAs.

D. Cardiac auscultation for murmur.

Diagnostic Tests

A. Imaging of the carotid artery is recommended in all patients with symptoms of carotid territory ischemia. This recommendation is based on the significant incidence of clinically relevant carotid stenosis in this patient group and the efficacy of carotid endarterectomy (CEA) for clinically significant lesions in reducing overall stroke (Grade 1, level of evidence A).

B. Imaging should be strongly considered for patients who present with amaurosis fugax, evidence of retinal artery embolization on fundoscopic examination, or asymptomatic cerebral infarction and are candidates for CEA. This recommendation is based on the intermediate stroke risk in this group of patients and the efficacy of CEA in reducing the risk of subsequent stroke (Grade 1, level of evidence A).

C. Routine screening is *not* recommended to detect clinically asymptomatic carotid stenosis in the general population.

D. Diagnosis.

1. Carotid duplex ultrasonography, with or without color: Screening test of choice to evaluate for carotid stenosis.

2. Computed tomographic angiography (CTA) is preferable to MRI/magnetic resonance angiography (MRA) for delineating calcium.

3. Carotid angiography.

4. Carotid MRA: May be useful in collaborating the finding of an occluded carotid with duplex sonography; however, this modality tends to overstate the significance of the stenosis.

5. Aortic arch and carotid arteriography: To evaluate the percentage of stenosis.

Differential Diagnosis

A. Stroke.

B. Intracerebral hemorrhage.

C. Neck trauma.

D. Headache.

E. Vertebral dissection.

F. Vertigo.

Evaluation and Management Plan

A. General plan.

1. For neurologically symptomatic patients with 50% stenosis or asymptomatic patients with 60% stenosis diameter reduction, optimal medical therapy is indicated (Grade 1, level of evidence B).

a. Grading carotid artery stenosis by ultrasound.

i. Low degree stenosis 0% to 40%.

ii. Moderate stenosis 50% to 60%.

iii. Hemodynamically relevant stenosis greater than 70%.

iv. Other simplistic grade is mild stenosis (less than 50%), moderate stenosis (50%–70%), and severe stenosis (70% or greater).

2. Antiplatelet therapy in asymptomatic patients with carotid atherosclerosis is recommended to reduce overall cardiovascular morbidity although it has not been shown to be effective in the primary prevention of stroke.

3. Surgical management.

a. Carotid artery angioplasty and stenting.

i. Indication for carotid angioplasty and stenting (CAS).

1) Symptomatic patients with a high-grade stenosis (>70%) who are at high risk for CEA.

2) Patients who are at high risk for CEA and have asymptomatic carotid stenosis greater than 80%.

3) CAS is preferred over CEA in *symptomatic* patients with 50% stenosis and prior ipsilateral operation, tracheal stoma, or external beam irradiation resulting in fibrosis of the tissues of the ipsilateral neck.

b. CEA.

i. Indications for CEA.

1) Symptomatic patients with greater than 70% stenosis—clear benefit was found in the North American Symptomatic Carotid Endarterectomy Trial (NASCET).

2) Symptomatic patients with greater than 50% to 69% stenosis—benefit is marginal; appears to be greater for male patients.

3) Asymptomatic patients with greater than 60% stenosis—benefit is significantly less than for symptomatic patients with greater than 70% stenosis.

4) Generally, symptomatic patients with greater than 50% stenosis and healthy, asymptomatic patients with greater than 60% stenosis warrant consideration for CEA.

5) Patients who present with repetitive (crescendo) episodes of transient cerebral ischemia unresponsive to antiplatelet therapy should be considered for urgent CEA.

6) CEA is preferred over CAS in patients 70 years of age, with long (>15 mm) lesions, pre-occlusive stenosis, or lipid-rich plaques that can be completely removed safely by a cervical incision in patients who have a virgin, nonradiated neck.

7) Patients with symptomatic carotid stenosis will benefit from CEA prior to or concomitant with coronary artery bypass graft. The timing of the intervention depends on clinical presentation and institutional experience.

8) Patients with severe bilateral asymptomatic carotid stenosis (including stenosis and contralateral occlusion) should be considered for CEA prior to or concomitant with coronary artery bypass graft.

   ii. Contraindications for CEA.

     1) Patients with a severe neurological deficit following a cerebral infarction.

     2) Patients with an occluded carotid artery.

     3) Concurrent medical illness that would significantly limit the patient's life expectancy.

     4) Anatomic issues that would be unfavorable for CEA include the following:

       a) Lesions that extend above C2.

       b) Prior irradiation of the neck.

       c) Prior neck operation.

B. Patient/family teaching points.

  1. Review lifestyle changes.

    a. Smoking cessation.

    b. Weight loss.

    c. Increasing physical activity.

    d. Consuming a healthy diet low in fat and cholesterol.

  2. Remind patients to take medication daily.

  3. Blood pressure management.

  4. Optimum blood sugar control in diabetes.

  5. Manage comorbid conditions.

  6. Educate patient on warning for stroke and regular follow-up.

  7. Patients should be instructed to seek help immediately if they have any worsening symptoms or signs and symptoms of a stroke.

C. Pharmacotherapy.

  1. Perioperative medical management of patients undergoing carotid revascularization should include blood pressure control (<140/80) or beta-blockade (HR 60–80).

  2. Management of cholesterol with statin therapy (low-density lipoprotein [LDL] 100 mg/dL).

  3. Perioperative antithrombotic therapy for CEA should include aspirin (81–325 mg).

    a. Antiplatelet agents (e.g., aspirin, ticlopidine, clopidogrel).

    b. Anticoagulants (e.g., warfarin)—Note that use of warfarin in patients with noncardiac emboli is controversial. Anticoagulation is not recommended for the treatment of TIA or acute stroke unless there is evidence of a cardioembolic source.

D. Discharge instructions.

  1. Eat a healthy diet.

  2. Limit salt.

  3. Maintain a healthy weight.

  4. Exercise as directed.

  5. Limit alcohol.

  6. Smoking cessation.

Follow-Up

A. Medical therapy recommendation by guideline after intervention.

  1. Aspirin (30–325 mg/d) irreversibly acetylates the cyclooxygenase of platelets, thus inhibiting platelet synthesis of thromboxane.

2. Ticlopidine (250 mg q12h) is a thienopyridine that irreversibly alters the platelet membrane and inhibits platelet aggregation. It is approximately 10% more effective than aspirin. Toxicity includes neutropenia and diarrhea.

3. Clopidogrel (75 mg/d) is used if the risk of neutropenia is low.

4. Warfarin (titrated international normalized ratio [INR] 2–3) use in patients with noncardiac emboli is controversial.

5. Antiplatelet therapy with cilostazol may reduce the progression of carotid artery stenosis after stent implantation.

B. Other recommendations for follow-up.

  1. A postoperative duplex ultrasound, within 30 days, is recommended to assess the status of the endarterectomized vessel.

  2. Imaging after CAS or CEA is indicated to follow contralateral disease progression in patients with contralateral stenosis 50%.

  3. In patients with multiple risk factors for vascular disease, follow-up duplex may be indicated with lesser degrees of stenosis. The likelihood of disease progression is related to the initial severity of stenosis (Grade 2, level of evidence C).

  4. Risk factor modification: Lifestyle or medical interventions are implemented in order to address the following risk factors: Hypertension, hypercholesterolemia, and smoking.

Consultation/Referral

A. Referral to a cardiologist.

B. Vascular surgeon is recommended.

C. Intervention cardiologist.

Special/Geriatric Considerations

A. Benefits of CAS versus CEA should be strongly considered in the elderly.

B. While elderly patients who had CEA had fewer incidents of stroke than those who had CAS, mortality, they had an increased risk of mortality and an increased rate of AMI.

Bibliography

Brown, K., Itum, D. S., Preiss, J., Duwayri, Y., Veeraswamy, R. K., Salam, A., & Brewster, L. P. (2015). Carotid artery stenting has increased risk of external carotid artery occlusion compared with carotid endarterectomy. *Journal of Vascular Surgery, 61*(1), 119–124. doi:10.1016/j.jvs.2014.06.008

Mas, J. L., Trinquart, L., Leys, D., Albucher, J. F., Rousseau, H., Viguier, A., & Chatellier, G. (2008, October). Endarterectomy Versus Angioplasty in Patients with Symptomatic Severe Carotid Stenosis (EVA-3S) trial: Results up to 4 years from a randomised, multicentre trial. *Lancet Neurology, 7*(10), 885–892. doi:10.1016/S1474-4422(08)70195-9

Moore, W. S., Popma, J. J., Roubin, G. S., Voeks, J. H., Cutlip, D. E., Jones, M., & Brott, T. G. (2016, April). Carotid angiographic characteristics in the CREST trial were major contributors to periprocedural stroke and death differences between carotid artery stenting and carotid endarterectomy. *Journal of Vascular Surgery, 63*(4), 851–858.e1. doi:10.1016/j.jvs.2015.08.119

Ricotta, J. J., Aburahma, A., Ascher, E., Eskandari, M., Faries, P., Lal, B. K., & Moore, W. S. (2011, September). Updated Society for Vascular Surgery guidelines for management of extracranial carotid disease. *Journal of Vascular Surgery, 54*(3), e1–e31. doi:10.1016/j.jvs.2011.07.031

von Reutern, G. M., Goertler, M. W., Bornstein, N. M., Del Sette, M., Evans, D. H., Hetzel, A., , . . . Yasaka, M. (2012). Grading carotid stenosis using ultrasonic methods. *Stroke, 43*, 916–921. doi:10.1161/STROKEAHA.111.636084

Peripheral Artery Disease: Lower Extremity

Fiona Unac

Definition

A. Lower extremity peripheral artery disease (PAD) is the obstruction of blood flow in the lower extremity arteries.

Incidence

A. The incidence of lower extremity PAD increases with age.
   1. 5% of adults over 50 years of age.
   2. 14.5% of adults over 70 years of age.

Pathogenesis

A. Lower extremity PAD is frequently caused by atheroma in the walls of the arteries.
B. PAD, coronary artery disease, and cerebral artery disease are all manifestations of atherosclerosis and commonly occur together.

Predisposing Factors

A. Age 70 years and older.
B. Age 50 to 69 years with a history of smoking or diabetes.
C. Age 40 to 49 with diabetes and at least one other risk factor for atherosclerosis.
D. Known atherosclerosis at other sites (e.g., coronary, carotid, renal artery disease).
E. Hypertension.
F. Smoking.
G. Hyperlipidemia.
H. Homocysteinemia.
I. Diabetes.

Subjective Data

A. Common complaints/symptoms.
   1. The PAD Fontaine Classification score lists the common symptoms in accordance with disease progression.
B. Common/typical scenario.
   1. Patient will report painful cramping during walking or exercise.
   2. Elicit onset, duration, location, and intensity of pain. (Intermittent claudication pain is typically a muscle tightness in the buttock, thigh, or calf that comes on with exercise and is relieved at rest.)
   3. Inquire what aggravates and relieves the pain.
      a. Is the leg pain worse when legs are elevated or down?
      b. Is there resting pain or nocturnal cramping? (With critical limb ischemia, resting leg pain is aggravated when the legs are elevated.)
   4. Question the patient about cardiovascular-related conditions: Coronary artery disease, myocardial infarction, carotid artery disease, trans-ischemic attack, or strokes.
   5. Question the patient about other medical conditions such as diabetes, chronic kidney disease, heart failure, chronic obstructive pulmonary disease, and hematology conditions.
   6. Inquire about musculoskeletal conditions such as osteoarthritis and spinal degeneration.
C. Review of systems.
   1. Musculoskeletal.
      a. Inquire about aching, tightness, or squeezing pain in the calf, thigh, or buttocks.

b. Ask about pain before walking versus pain that starts during walking.

Physical Examination

A. Atherosclerotic disease is a diffuse process. Therefore, the examination, regardless of the complaint (intermittent claudication, angina, transient ischemic attack), should include the entire arterial system.
   1. Check blood pressure in both arms, heart rate, and rhythm.
   2. Inspect full length of upper and lower extremities: Dry, shiny hairless skin, muscle atrophy, color, necrotic and/or gangrenous ulcers, or evidence of distal embolization in the fingers and/or toes (blue toe syndrome).
   3. Auscultate.
      a. Heart to listen for arrhythmias, gallops, and murmurs.
      b. Carotid, brachial, abdominal aorta, femoral, and popliteal pulses to listen for bruits.
      c. Lung fields.
   4. Palpate.
      a. Abdomen to assess for a pulsatile mass (aortic aneurysm).
      b. Leg: Femoral, popliteal, dorsalis pedis, and post tibial pulses.
      c. Arm: Brachial, radial, ulnar pulses.
      d. Check capillary refill, strength, and sensation of upper and lower extremities.
   5. Beurger test to assess for positional rubra (with significant PAD, foot is paler with elevation and then rubrous or cyanotic in the dependent position).
   6. 10 g monofilament foot test to assess for peripheral neuropathy.

Diagnostic Tests

A. Ankle–brachial index has a high sensitivity and specificity for the identification of PAD. Inclusion of the toe–brachial index or continuous wave Doppler (if tissue is intact) assessment increases detection of serious PAD.
B. Radiological imaging of arterial leg circulation such as ultrasound, CT, or MRI is best reserved for vascular services as part of the treatment decision and workup.
C. Abdominal aorta screening is recommended due to the correlation between PAD and abdominal aortic aneurysm. Ultrasound is the modality of choice.
D. Hematologic evaluation: Complete blood count, fasting blood glucose, fasting lipids, serum creatinine, urinalysis.

Differential Diagnosis

A. Arterial aneurysm.
B. Arterial dissection.
C. Embolism.
D. Popliteal entrapment syndrome.
E. Adventitial cystic disease.
F. Thromboangitis obliterans (Buerger's disease).
G. Limb trauma.
H. Nonarterial etiologies for limb pain: Neurogenic, musculoskeletal causes, pathologic.

Evaluation and Management Plan

A. General plan.
   1. Peripheral arterial disease management is dependent on symptom severity, comorbid condition, and whether or not a patient will experience a meaningful benefit from a technically successful procedure.

2. Patients with PAD should have a cardiovascular risk reduction plan.

   a. Smoking cessation is critical.

   b. Treatment of diabetes if applicable to achieve an HbA1c less than 5.5 mmol/L.

   c. Healthy diet and exercise.

   d. Hematologic evaluation (see section "Diagnostics Tests"). Results will guide further therapy.

   e. Additional management plan for patients with intermittent claudication (Fontaine IIa and IIb) includes:

      i. Structured exercise program.

      ii. Referral to vascular service if intermittent claudication is lifestyle limiting and patient may benefit from revascularization treatment.

3. Critical limb ischemia (Fontaine III) and necrosis and gangrene (Fontaine IV) management plan will depend on progression of limb symptoms, comorbid conditions, and conduit availability.

   a. Supportive measures may include:

      i. Wound management.

      ii. Antibiotic therapy if underlying cellulitis or wound infection (consider Flucloxacillin).

      iii. Pain management.

   b. Vascular treatment may include:

      i. Endovascular revascularization.

      ii. Bypass surgery.

      iii. Digit or limb amputation.

B. Patient/family teaching points.

1. Patients should seek out a provider if they experience pain, numbness, tingling, weakness, or significant temperature change in their extremities.

2. Patients should also report open sores that do not heal.

C. Pharmacotherapy.

1. Antiplatelet therapy with long-term low-dose aspirin.

2. Treatment of hyperlipidemia with a statin to achieve a low-density lipoprotein level less than 100 mg/dL (<70 mg/dL if PAD and a history of coronary or cerebral artery disease).

3. Treatment of hypertension to achieve a blood pressure less than 140/90 mmHg (<130/80 mmHg for patients with diabetes or renal failure).

4. Consider pharmacology therapy. In the United States only pentoxifylline and cilostazol have achieved Food and Drug Administration (FDA) approval for the treatment of intermittent claudication.

D. Discharge.

1. Patients need to be taught to make healthy dietary changes, keep cholesterol levels down, maintain a healthy weight, and stop smoking.

Follow-Up

A. Three-month primary care review of cardiovascular risk management.

B. If treated percutaneously or surgically, outpatient vascular review after 4 to 6 weeks.

Consultation/Referral

A. Consultation and referral are dependent on symptom status. Patients with lower extremity PAD have a wide spectrum of symptoms.

1. Fontaine Classification I: Asymptomatic. Conservative management.

2. Fontaine Classification IIa: Intermittent claudication greater than 200 m (and nonlifestyle limiting). Conservative management.

3. Fontaine Classification IIb: Intermittent claudication less than 200 m (or lifestyle limiting). Refer to vascular service.

4. Fontaine Classification III: Nocturnal or resting pain. Referral to vascular service.

5. Fontaine Classification IV: Necrosis and gangrene. For hospital admission, vascular consult.

Special/Geriatric Considerations

A. Patients with PAD are usually elderly.

B. Younger patients are usually diabetic.

Bibliography

Cronenwett, J. L., & Johnston, K. W. (2014). *Rutherford's vascular surgery* (8th ed.). Philadelphia, PA: Elsevier Saunders.

Mitchell, M. E., & Carpenter, J. P. (2017). Overview of acute arterial occlusion of the extremities (acute limb ischaemia). Retrieved from www.uptodate.com

Neschis, D. G., & Golden, M. A. (2018, June 11). Clinical features and diagnosis of lower extremity peripheral artery disease. In K. A. Collins (Ed.), *UpToDate*. Retrieved from https://www.uptodate.com/contents/clinical-features-and-diagnosis-of-lower-extremity-peripheral-artery-disease

Rasmussen, T. E., Clouse, W. D., & Tonnessen, B. H. (2011). *Handbook of patient care in vascular diseases* (5th ed.). Philadelphia, PA: Wolters Kluwer Health.

Tehan, P. E., Bray, A., & Chuter, V. H. (2016). Non-invasive vascular assessment in the foot with diabetes: Sensitivity and specificity of the ankle brachial index, toe brachial index and continuous wave Doppler for detecting peripheral arterial disease. *Journal of Diabetes and Its Complications, 30*(1), 155–160. doi:10.1016/j.jdiacomp.2015.07.019

Peripheral Artery Disease: Upper Extremity

Fiona Unac

Definition

A. Upper extremity arterial disease is the obstruction of blood flow in the large and/or small arterial vessels of the upper extremity arteries.

Incidence

A. Upper extremity arterial disease is relatively rare. It accounts for less than 5% of patients presenting with limb ischemia.

Pathogenesis

A. Arterial vasospasm: Raynaud's phenomenon, ergotism, vinyl chloride exposure.

B. Arterial obstruction.

1. Atherosclerosis (main cause of upper extremity arterial disease).

2. Thoracic outlet compression.

3. Embolic (e.g., cardiac or thoracic outlet in origin), aneurysms.

4. Arteritis (e.g., Takayasu arteritis or giant cell arteritis).

5. Fibromuscular disease.

6. Hypersensitivity angiitis.

7. Iatrogenic, cold, or vibration injury.

8. Dialysis steal syndrome.

9. Connective tissue disease (e.g., scleroderma, rheumatoid arthritis, systemic lupus).

10. Myeloproliferative disorders and hypercoagulable states.

11. Infection from injection of drugs and arterial procedures.

C. Bilateral symptoms may be from a systemic cause such as a connective tissue disorder.

D. Unilateral symptoms may be from a discrete occlusive lesion.

Predisposing Factors

A. Dependent on pathogenesis.

B. Patients who present with upper extremity ischemia range from young adults with nonatherosclerotic causes to elderly patients with atherosclerosis.

C. Risk factors include smoking, hypercholesterolemia, hypertension, diabetes, and age.

Subjective Data

A. Common complaints/symptoms.
   1. Most patients with upper extremity arterial disease are asymptomatic; the condition is only detected by finding asymmetric arm blood pressures.

B. Common/typical scenario.
   1. Raynaud's phenomenon: Predictable sequence of color changes in finger and/or hand.
      a. Pallor (white), followed by cyanosis (blue) and then rubor (red).
      b. Often associated with finger numbness.
      c. Pain is generally not severe, unless ulceration is present.
      d. Symptoms are activated by exposure to cold and emotional stimuli.
   2. Arm intermittent claudication is an unusual presentation of arm ischemia due to excellent collateral blood flow around the shoulder. However, active adults, particularly manual laborers, may experience arm claudication from subclavian or brachial artery stenosis.
   3. Dizziness, or even syncope, during arm exertion may be from subclavian steal syndrome.
   4. Patients with chronic upper extremity ischemia may complain of change in sensation, hand temperature, and muscle pain with use.
   5. Tissue necrosis includes gangrene and poorly healing ulcerations of the fingers. (Patients may dismiss small ulcers caused by microemboli as inconsequential bruises or sores.)
   6. Acute limb ischemia is covered previously.

C. Family and social history.
   1. Elicit onset, duration, location, and intensity; aggravates and relieves pain.
   2. Inquire about signs and symptoms of connective tissue disease such as dry eyes, difficulty swallowing, dry mouth, and arthritis.
   3. Question the patient about any history of trauma, including upper extremity access for peripheral or coronary catheterization.
   4. Inquire about occupational and recreational history regarding exposure to vibrating tools or toxins, as well as repetitive trauma.
   5. Question the patient about cardiovascular-related conditions: Coronary artery disease, myocardial infarction, carotid artery disease, transient ischemic attack, or strokes.
   6. Question the patient about other medical conditions such as diabetes, chronic kidney disease, heart failure, chronic obstructive pulmonary disease, or hematology conditions.
   7. Inquire about musculoskeletal conditions such as osteoarthritis or rotator cuff injury.

D. Review of systems.
   1. Musculoskeletal: Ask about arm pain with movement and at rest; ask about any swelling.
   2. Dermatology: Ask about ulceration of fingers or discoloration.

Physical Examination

A. Take blood pressure in both arms.
   1. 10 mmHg or more difference suggests a hemodynamically significant innominate, subclavian, or axillary artery stenosis.
   2. In cases of suspected claudication, arm blood pressure, should be measured at rest and after 2 to 5 minutes of exercise.

B. Inspect.
   1. Hands and fingers and note temperature, color, capillary refill, ulcers, and any other lesions.
   2. Fingers for clubbing, which is associated with chronic pulmonary disease. (Patients with clubbing and cold fingers may have low arterial oxygen levels as the basis for their complaint).
   3. Fingers for telangiectasia and sclerodactyly, which is commonly seen with advanced scleroderma as well as other connective tissue diseases.
   4. Check for splinter hemorrhages in the nail beds, which is seen with emboli.

C. Auscultate.
   1. Heart to listen for arrhythmias, gallops, and murmurs.
   2. Supraclavicular and infraclavicular fossa to listen for bruits which may indicate a possible subclavian artery stenosis. A supraclavicular pulsatile mass is associated with a subclavian aneurysm or cervical rib.

D. Palpate.
   1. Upper extremity pulses.
      a. Axillary and proximal brachial artery: The upper medial arm in the groove between the biceps and triceps muscles.
      b. Brachial artery: The antecubital fossa just medial to the biceps tendon.
      c. Radial artery: The wrist over the distal radius.
      d. Ulnar artery: The wrist over the distal ulna.
   2. Carotid, abdominal aorta, femoral, popliteal, dorsalis pedis, post tibial pulses.

E. Handheld Doppler.
   1. Assess upper extremity pulses including digital pulses and note if the pulse is monophasic, biphasic, or triphasic.

F. Neurological examination, including muscle mass, muscle strength, and sensation to assess for compression of the neurovascular bundle (see section "Thoracic Outlet Syndrome").

G. Additional bedside examination.
   1. Allen's test is recommended if there is a difference in arm blood pressure or if there is a reduced radial or ulnar pulse.
      a. Allen's test should be conducted on both arms.
      b. A positive Allen's test suggests that there is adequate dual blood supply to the hand.
         i. Elevate the hand and ask the patient to clench his or her fist for 30 seconds.
         ii. Pressure is applied over the ulnar and radial arteries to occlude both of them.
         iii. The hand is then opened. It should appear blanched.
         iv. One artery is tested by releasing the pressure over that artery to see if the hand flushes (color should return within 5–15 seconds).

v. The other artery is then tested in a similar fashion.

2. Adson's test and Roos test can assist in assessing for thoracic outlet syndrome (see section "Thoracic Outlet Syndrome").

Diagnostic Tests

A. Vascular laboratory: Segmental pressure measurements of the upper extremity and finger pressure measurements and waveforms.

B. Radiological imaging of arterial arm circulation such as duplex ultrasound, CT, and MRI is best reserved for vascular services as part of the treatment decision and workup.

C. Hematologic evaluation.

1. Erythrocyte sedimentation rate, C-reactive protein, antiphospholipid antibodies, antinuclear antibody titer, and rheumatoid factor to screen for underlying autoimmune disease.

2. Platelet count, since thrombocytosis can mimic Raynaud's phenomenon.

3. Serum protein electrophoresis since serum protein abnormalities may be associated with vasospasms.

4. For patients at risk of or with suspected atherosclerotic disease, fasting lipids, fasting glucose, or serum creatinine.

Differential Diagnosis

A. Multiple etiologies; see "Pathogenesis" section.

B. Differential diagnosis includes neurogenic, musculoskeletal, and pathological causes.

Evaluation and Management Plan

A. General plan.

1. All patients with upper extremity arterial disease should have a cardiovascular risk reduction plan based on their 5-year cardiovascular risk assessment.

2. Treat underlying cause.

a. Primary Raynaud's phenomenon.

i. Conservative management; patients advised to minimize cold exposure and stress.

b. Emboli: Manage arrhythmia and anticoagulate.

c. Connective tissue diseases: Management of disease process.

d. Occupational and recreational factors: Advise patients to minimize exposure.

3. Supportive measures.

a. Wound management.

b. Antibiotic if underlying cellulitis or wound infection (consider Flucloxacillin).

c. Pain management.

4. Vascular treatment may include:

a. Endovascular revascularization.

b. Bypass surgery.

c. Digit or limb amputation.

B. Patient/family teaching points.

1. Patients should seek out a provider if they experience any pain, numbness, tingling, weakness, or significant temperature change in their extremities.

2. Patients should also report open sores that do not heal.

C. Pharmacotherapy.

1. Frequent or severe symptoms.

a. Nifidipine 30 to 180 mg/d or amiodipine 5 to 20 mg/d.

2. Start with lowest dose and gradually increase, if needed, depending upon the response.

D. Discharge instructions (if standard accepted guidelines exist, please use discharge template).

1. Make healthy dietary changes.

2. Keep cholesterol levels down.

3. Maintain a healthy weight.

4. Smoking cessation.

Follow-Up

A. Depend on pathogenesis: Outpatient follow-up with vascular, cardiology, or rheumatology service.

B. Three-month primary care review of cardiovascular risk management.

Consultation/Referral

A. Consultation and referral is dependent on pathogenesis and severity of symptoms.

1. If clinical presentation is suggestive of large vessel disease, refer to vascular service.

2. If hematological screening is positive for autoimmune disease, refer to rheumatology service.

3. Acute limb ischemia for urgent hospital admission (see "Acute Limb Ischemia" section).

4. Necrosis and gangrene. For hospital admission, seek a vascular consult.

Special/Geriatric Considerations

A. Elderly patients may not report or experience intermittent claudication.

B. Elderly patients may have decreased blood flow and other circulatory problems that put them at special risk of being unaware of any issues or problems.

Bibliography

Barshes, N. R. (2017, November 22). Overview of upper extremity peripheral artery disease. In K. A. Collins (Ed.), *UpToDate*. Retrieved from https://www.uptodate.com/contents/overview-of-upper-extremity-peripheral-artery-disease

Cronenwett, J. L., & Johnston, K. W. (2014). *Rutherford's vascular surgery* (8th ed.). Philadelphia, PA: Elsevier Saunders.

Mitchell, M. E., & Carpenter, J. P. (2017). Overview of acute arterial occlusion of the extremities (acute limb ischaemia). Retrieved from www.uptodate.com

Rasmussen, T. E., Clouse, W. D., & Tonnessen, B. H. (2011). *Handbook of patient care in vascular diseases* (5th ed.). Philadelphia, PA: Wolters Kluwer Health.

Peripheral Vascular Disease

Ponrathi Athilingam

Definition

A. Peripheral vascular disease (PVD) refers to diseases of the blood vessels located outside the heart and brain.

B. Peripheral arterial disease (PAD) develops only in the arteries. PAD is the most common form of PVD.

Incidence

A. The Centers for Disease Control and Prevention (CDC) reports approximately 12% to 20% of people over age 60 develop PAD; it affects 15% to 20% of persons older than 70 years of age.

B. PAD affects about 8.5 million Americans.

C. The prevalence of PAD, both symptomatic and asymptomatic, is greater in men than in women, especially in young persons. At very advanced ages almost no differences exist between the sexes. However, age remains the main marker of PAD risk.

D. The estimated prevalence of intermittent claudication in persons aged 60 to 65 years is 35%. However, the prevalence in persons 10 years older (70–75 years) rises to 70%.

Pathogenesis

A. PVD is a slow and progressive circulation disorder caused by narrowing, blockage, or spasms in a blood vessel. PAD is considered a set of chronic or acute syndromes, generally derived from the presence of occlusive arterial disease, which causes inadequate blood flow to the limbs.

B. On most occasions, the underlying disease process is arteriosclerotic disease, mainly affecting the vascularization to the lower limbs.

C. From the pathophysiologic point of view, ischemia of the lower limbs can be classified as functional or critical due to an imbalance between the needs of the peripheral tissues and the blood supply.

D. Functional ischemia occurs when the blood flow is normal at rest but insufficient during exercise, presenting clinically as intermittent claudication.

E. Critical ischemia is produced when the reduction in blood flow results in a perfusion deficit at rest and is defined by the presence of pain at rest or trophic lesions in the legs.

Predisposing Factors

A. Age over 50.
B. Postmenopausal women have a higher risk.
C. Overweight and obesity.
D. Dyslipidemia.
E. Hyperhomocysteinemia.
F. History of cerebrovascular disease or stroke.
G. History of heart disease.
H. History of diabetes.
I. High blood pressure.
J. Family history of high cholesterol, high blood pressure, or PVD.
K. Kidney disease on hemodialysis.
L. Lifestyle choices that can increase risk of developing PVD include:
    1. Sedentary lifestyle or not engaging in physical exercise.
    2. Unhealthy dietary habits.
    3. Smoking increases risk by seven times.
    4. Drug use.
    5. Excessive alcohol.

Subjective Data

A. Common complaints/symptoms.
    1. The first signs of PVD begin slowly and irregularly.
    2. Fatigue or cramping in legs and feet that gets worse with physical activity due to the lack of blood flow are the earliest signs the patients often report.
    3. Leg cramps when lying in bed may occur.
    4. Poor hair growth often below knees.
    5. Legs and arms may turn reddish blue or pale.
    6. Skin in the extremities may appear pale and thin.
    7. Pulses in the extremities may be weak.
    8. Ulcers and wounds in legs and toes that will not heal.
    9. Toes may appear blue in color and the toenails become thick and opaque.
    10. Patient often experiences severe burning in toes.
    11. In severe cases, pain may occur even at rest, particularly at night when the legs are raised in bed.

    12. In a small number of cases (often untreated), tissue death (gangrene) of a foot may result.
    13. If an artery higher upstream is narrowed, such as the iliac artery, pain may be experienced in the thighs or buttocks while walking.
B. Common/typical scenario.
    1. Patients will typically present with intermittent claudication, which is cramping with exercise that resolves with rest.
    2. If the patient has severe disease progression, he or she may present with pain in the legs that occurs at rest.
C. Family and social history.
    1. Ask about family history of any vascular disease or diabetes.
    2. Ask about smoking, if the patient has a sedentary lifestyle or poor eating habits.
D. Review of systems.
    1. Musculoskeletal: Ask about leg cramps, pain at rest, or if patients raise their legs at night.
    2. Neurology: Ask about numbness or severe burning in toes.
    3. Dermatology: Ask about discoloration of extremities, ulcers, or wounds that don't heal, and/or nails that have become thick and opaque.

Physical Examination

A. Basic examination of PVD includes assessment for the presence of pulses in the lower limbs including the femoral, popliteal, pedal, and posterior tibial arteries.

B. Auscultation of the abdomen will enable identification of the presence of murmurs, which are indicative of disease in the aorta or the iliac arteries. Auscultation of the inguinal region may reveal the presence of lesions in the external iliac or femoral bifurcation vessels.

C. Check the temperature, color, and capillary refill of the foot. Patients with claudication do not usually show a reduction in temperature or capillary filling.

D. Leg dangling test: A reduction in temperature and paleness, with or without cyanosis or dangling erythrosis, are common in patients with critical ischemia.

E. Patients with PAD have a higher risk for developing critical limb ischemia (CLI).
    1. The patients with CLI should undergo expedited evaluation and treatment of factors that are known to increase the risk of amputation.
    2. Patients with CLI in whom open surgical repair is anticipated should undergo assessment of cardiovascular risk.
    3. Patients with CLI and skin breakdown should be referred to healthcare providers with specialized expertise in wound care.
    4. Patients at risk for CLI (those with diabetes, neuropathy, chronic renal failure, or infection) who develop acute limb symptoms represent potential vascular emergencies and should be assessed immediately and treated by a specialist competent in treating vascular disease.
F. Chronic foot and leg ulcers (see Table 11.2).
G. Stages of PVD.
    1. Stage I is characterized by the absence of symptoms. It includes patients who have an extensive occlusive arterial lesion in the legs, or have high risk but present no symptoms of arterial failure. In these situations, the patients may present with critical ischemia straight from an asymptomatic stage.
    2. Stage II is characterized by the presence of intermittent claudication. The intermittent claudication that is

| TABLE 11.2 | How to Differentiate Foot Ulcer and Pain |

Neuropathic Ulcer	Ischemic Ulcer
Often painless	Extremely painful
Normal pulses	Absent pulses
Typically punched-out appearance	Irregular margins
Often located on sole or edge of foot or metatarsal head	Commonly located or starts on toes
Presence of calluses	Calluses absent or infrequent
Loss of sensation, reflexes, and vibration sense	Variable sensory findings present
Increase in blood flow (arteriovenous shunting)	Decrease in blood flow
Dilated veins	Collapsed veins
Dry, warm foot	Cold foot
Bone deformities	No bony deformities
Red appearance	Pale, cyanotic

Sources: Armstrong, D. G., & Lavery, L. A. (1998, March 15). Diabetic foot ulcers: Prevention, diagnosis and classification. *American Family Physician, 57*(6):1325–1332. Retrieved from https://www.aafp.org/afp/1998/0315/p1325.html; Cleveland Clinic. (n.d.). Leg and foot ulcers. Retrieved from http://my.clevelandclinic.org/heart/disorders/vascular/legfootulcer.aspx; Frykberg, R. G. (2002, November 1). Diabetic foot ulcers: Pathogenesis and management. *American Family Physician, 66*(9), 1655–1663. Retrieved from http://www.aafp.org/afp/2002/1101/p1655.html; Jeffcoate, W. J., & Harding, K. G. (2003). Diabetic foot ulcers. *The Lancet, 361*(9368), 1545–1551. doi:10.1016/S0140-6736(03)13169-8

typical in patients with PAD is defined as the appearance of pain in muscle masses caused by walking and which ceases immediately after stopping exercise. Of note: A great number of patients report pain in the legs associated with walking, but not with the presence of arterial disease. The stage II is itself divided into groups.

    a. Stage IIa includes patients with non-invalidating claudication that impedes walking long distances.

    b. Stage IIb refers to patients with short claudication or claudication that impedes activities of daily living.

3. Stage III constitutes a more advanced phase of ischemia and is characterized by the presence of symptoms at rest. The predominant symptom is usually pain, although the patient often reports paresthesia and hypoesthesia.

4. Stage IV is characterized by the presence of tropical lesions. It is due to the critical reduction of distal perfusion pressure, which is insufficient to maintain tissue tropism. These lesions are situated in the more distal areas of the limb, usually the toes, although on occasions they may present in the malleolus or the heel.

Diagnostic Tests

A. The diagnosis is usually made by the typical symptoms, history, and physical examination.

B. Homocysteine level to rule out hyperhomocysteinemia.

C. An ankle–brachial index (ABIs), toe–brachial index (TBI), and/or exercise ABI must be ordered.

D. Pulse volume recording or plethysmography: Recording the pulse wave volumes along the limb by plethysmography is particularly useful in patients in whom arterial calcification prevents a reliable recording of systolic pressures. Transmetatarsal or digital recording provides important information about the state of the vascularization in this zone.

E. Segmental pressure examination or Doppler recording of velocimetric wave can also provide very useful information by means of evaluating the changes in the different components of the arterial velocimetric wave.

F. Duplex ultrasound of the extremities is useful to diagnose anatomic location and degree of stenosis of PAD. May be used in select candidates for endovascular intervention, surgical bypass, and to select the sites of surgical anastomosis. This may also be used for surveillance following femoral-popliteal bypass using venous conduit (but not prosthetic grafts).

G. Imaging techniques are indicated if surgical or endovascular repair is contemplated after identification of a susceptible lesion.

    1. Computed tomography angiography (CTA) produces an excellent arterial picture; however, it requires iodinated contrast. CTA may be considered to diagnose anatomic location and presence of significant stenosis in patients with lower extremity PAD and as a substitute for magnetic resonance angiography (MRA) for those patients with contraindications to MRA.

    2. MRA has virtually replaced contrast arteriography for PAD diagnosis. The advantages of MRA include:

        a. Excellent arterial picture and no ionizing radiation; noniodine-based intravenous contrast medium rarely causes renal insufficiency or allergic reaction. However, about 10% of patients cannot utilize MRA because of claustrophobia, having a pacemaker/implantable cardioverter-defibrillator, or because they are obese.

        b. The major challenge with MRA is: Gadolinium use in individuals with an estimated glomerular filtration rate (eGFR) less than 60 mL/min has been associated with nephrogenic systemic fibrosis (NSF)/nephrogenic fibrosing dermopathy.

        c. The MRA is useful to diagnose anatomic location and degree of stenosis of PAD as well as in selecting patients with lower extremity PAD as candidates for endovascular intervention.

Differential Diagnosis

A. For leg pain or claudication with normal physiological testing, a provider needs to consider (not PAD related).

    1. Symptomatic Baker's cyst.

    2. Chronic compartment syndrome.

    3. Spinal stenosis.

    4. Nerve root compression: Arthritis—hip, ankle, or foot.

Evaluation and Management Plan

A. General plan.

    1. The two main goals of PVD treatment are to stop the disease from progressing and manage pain and symptoms so patients can remain active. The treatments are aimed to lower risk for serious complications.

    2. Antiplatelet therapy.

    3. Smoking cessation, as well as avoiding environmental smoking and secondhand smoking.

    4. Good glycemic control.

    5. Surgical management.

        a. Endovascular revascularization.

i. Endovascular procedures are effective as a revascularization option for patients with lifestyle-limiting claudication.

ii. Endovascular procedures are recommended to establish in-line blood flow to the foot in patients with nonhealing wounds or gangrene. A staged approach may be done in patients with ischemic rest pain.

b. Surgical revascularization: Bypass or graft to restore blood flow. Surgical revascularization is performed; bypass to the popliteal artery with autogenous vein is recommended in preference to prosthetic graft material.

c. Angioplasty of the blocked peripheral artery is a procedure to open narrowed or blocked blood vessels that supply blood to your legs. Fatty deposits can build up inside the arteries and block blood flow.

B. Patient/family teaching points.

1. Pain management to enhance activity.

2. Exercise and physical activity. Structured exercise program and home-based exercise program.

    a. Any exertional limitation of the lower extremity muscles or any history of walking impairment, described as fatigue, aching, numbness, or pain.

    b. The primary site(s) of discomfort in the buttock, thigh, calf, or foot, and relation of such discomfort to rest or exertion.

3. Look for any poorly healing or nonhealing wounds of the legs or feet.

4. Note any pain at rest localized to the lower leg or foot and its association with the upright or recumbent positions.

5. Watch for postprandial abdominal pain that reproducibly is provoked by eating and is associated with weight loss.

6. Family history of a first-degree relative with an abdominal aortic aneurysm.

7. Pulse intensity should be assessed and should be recorded numerically from 0 to 3 (0 = absent, 1 = diminished, 2 = normal, and 3 = bounding).

C. Pharmacotherapy.

1. Statin therapy.

2. Antihypertensive therapy: Angiotensin-converting enzyme (ACE) inhibitors.

3. Oral anticoagulation (warfarin) in improving lower extremity bypass patency demonstrated improved patency among the subgroup of patients with autogenous vein bypass grafts.

4. Cilostazol increases blood flow and relieves symptoms of claudication.

D. Discharge instructions.

1. Patients should be encouraged to maintain a healthy diet, stop smoking, control diabetes, and begin an exercise program.

Follow-Up

A. PVD is a lifelong chronic medical condition. Ongoing care focuses on cardiovascular risk reduction with medical therapy, optimizing functional status with structured exercise and, when indicated, revascularization.

B. Patients with PVD who have undergone lower extremity revascularization (surgical and/or endovascular) should be followed up with periodic clinical evaluation and ABI measurement.

C. Duplex ultrasound is recommended for routine surveillance after femoral-popliteal or femoral-tibial-pedal bypass with a venous conduit. Minimum surveillance intervals are approximately 3, 6, and 12 months, and then yearly after graft placement.

Consultation/Referral

A. Interdisciplinary care team members must be included.

B. Care team members may include:

1. Vascular medical and surgical specialists (i.e., vascular medicine, vascular surgery, interventional radiology, interventional cardiology).

2. Orthopedic surgeons and podiatrists.

3. Endocrinologists.

4. Infectious disease specialists.

5. Radiology and vascular imaging specialists.

6. Physical medicine and rehabilitation clinicians.

7. Orthotics and prosthetics specialists.

8. Social workers.

9. Exercise physiologists.

10. Physical and occupational therapists.

11. Nutritionists/dieticians.

Special/Geriatric Considerations

A. Elderly may not experience intermittent claudication because of comorbidities that limit walking such as arthritis, spinal stenosis, heart failure, and pulmonary disease. Hence, management of comorbidities is vital in management of PAD.

B. Elderly also need a more sensitive diagnostic test for PAD for the identification of patients with asymptomatic PVD.

C. They may also benefit from early diagnosis by screening for asymptomatic PAD.

D. It would be beneficial for the elderly to have an established structured or supervised exercise program rather than an unsupervised exercise program.

E. Cilostazol increases maximal walking distance, pain free walking distance, and quality of life for the elderly population.

Bibliography

Alonso-Coello, P., Bellmunt, S., McGorrian, C., Anand, S. S., Guzman, R., Criqui, M. H., . . . Spencer, F. A. (2012, February). Antithrombotic therapy in peripheral artery disease: Antithrombotic Therapy and Prevention of Thrombosis, 9th ed.: American College of Chest Physicians Evidence-Based Clinical Practice Guidelines. *Chest, 141*(2 Suppl.), e669S–e690S. doi:10.1378/chest.11-2307

Armstrong, D. G., & Lavery, L. A. (1998, March 15). Diabetic foot ulcers: Prevention, diagnosis and classification. *American Family Physician, 57*(6), 1325–1332. Retrieved from https://www.aafp.org/afp/1998/0315/p1325.html

Cleveland Clinic. (n.d.). Leg and foot ulcers. Retrieved from http://my.clevelandclinic.org/heart/disorders/vascular/legfootulcer.aspx

Frykberg, R. G. (2002, November 1). Diabetic foot ulcers: Pathogenesis and management. *American Family Physician, 66*(9), 1655–1663. Retrieved from http://www.aafp.org/afp/2002/1101/p1655.html

Gerhard-Herman, M. D., Gornick, H. L., Barrett, C., Barshes, N. R., Corriere, M. A., Drachman, D. E., . . . Walsh, M. E. (2016). 2016 AHA/ACC Guideline on the management of patients with lower extremity peripheral artery disease: A report of the American College of Cardiology/American Heart Association Task Force on Clinical Practice Guidelines. *Journal of the American College of Cardiology, 69*, 1465–1508. doi:10.1016/j.jacc.2016.11.008

Jackson, E. A., Munir, K., Schreiber, T., Rubin, J. R., Cuff, R., Gallagher, K. A., . . . Grossman, P. M. (2014, June 17). Impact of sex on morbidity and mortality rates after lower extremity interventions for peripheral arterial disease: Observations from the Blue Cross Blue Shield of Michigan Cardiovascular Consortium. *Journal of American College of Cardiology, 63*(23), 2525–2530. doi:10.1016/j.jacc.2014.03.036

Jeffcoate, W. J., & Harding, K. G. (2003). Diabetic foot ulcers. *The Lancet, 361*, 1545–1551. doi:10.1016/S0140-6736(03)13169-8

Suzuki, J., Shimamura, M., Suda, H., Wakayama, K., Kumagai, H., Ikeda, Y., . . . Morishita, R. (2016, April). Current therapies and investigational drugs for peripheral arterial disease. *Hypertension Research, 39*(4), 183–191. doi:10.1038/hr.2015.134

Thoracic Outlet Syndrome

Cara M. Staley

Definition

A. Thoracic outlet syndrome (TOS) is a constellation of signs and symptoms that arise from compression of the neurovascular bundle just above the first rib and behind the clavicle, within the confined space of the thoracic outlet.

Incidence

A. TOS is uncommon and its true incidence is unknown.
B. Most patients are 20 to 50 years old, less than 5% are teenagers, and 10% are older than 50.
C. 70% are female.

Pathogenesis

A. Neurogenic (nTOS) arises from brachial plexus compression.
  1. It accounts for more than 95% of TOS cases.
  2. Associated with developmental anomalies of the thoracic outlet and fibrosis of the scalene muscle.
  3. Most common causes are hyperextension neck trauma (motor vehicle accident whiplash) and repetitive stress injuries.
B. Venous (vTOS) arises from subclavian vein compression.
  1. It accounts for 3% of TOS cases.
  2. Often a result of developmental anomalies of the costoclavicular space and repetitive arm activities.
  3. In vTOS a focal area of scarred subclavian intima narrows the lumen. Thrombus is the final event that occludes the vein.
  4. Typically asymptomatic until a venous thrombolytic event occurs.
C. Arterial (aTOS) arises from subclavian artery compression.
  1. It accounts for 1% of TOS cases.
  2. Almost always associated with a cervical rib or anomalous rib.
  3. aTOS subclavian artery stenosis is accompanied by poststenotic dilatation that gives the appearance of an aneurysm. Thrombus forms in the dilatation.
  4. Usually asymptomatic until the arterial emboli dislodges.

Predisposing Factors

A. Cervical rib or anomalous rib.
B. Congenital cervical fibrocartilaginous band associated with an incomplete cervical rib.
C. Muscular anomalies.
D. Chronic inflammatory change due to trauma.
E. Fractured first rib or clavicle.
F. Neck mass, for example, goiter, apical lung cancers, thyroid cancers, lymphoma.
G. Repetitive occupational overhead arm movements (e.g., box stacking), or sporting movements (e.g., pitching, swimming).

Subjective Data

A. Common complaints/symptoms.
  1. Neurogenic TOS: Pain, dysesthesia, numbness, and weakness, which may not be localized in specific nerve distribution. Symptoms are reproducibly aggravated by elevation or sustained use of the arms or hands.
  2. Venous TOS: Pain, cyanosis, edema. Paresthesia in the fingers is typically from swelling in the hand rather than nerve compression. Collateral venous patterning over the ipsilateral shoulder, neck, and chest wall indicates compensatory superficial venous flow from subclavian vein stenosis or occlusion.
  3. Arterial TOS: Pain, pallor, paresthesia, coldness to hand. Symptoms develop spontaneously unrelated to work or trauma.
B. Common/typical.
  1. Common causes of TOS include physical trauma from car accidents, sports, or repetitive injuries.
  2. Sometimes having an anatomical defect such as an extra rib can cause this.
  3. Patients may complain of numbness or tingling in their arm or fingers and have a weak grip.
C. Family and social history.
  1. Elicit onset, duration, location, intensity, aggravators, and relievers of symptoms.
  2. Ask about occipital headaches and pain over the trapezius, neck, chest, and shoulder. (Patients with symptoms confined to the forearm and hand are more likely to have carpal or cubital tunnel syndrome, not nTOS).
  3. Enquire about any history of neck trauma (e.g., whiplash, clavicle fracture, fall on slippery surface, or tripping down stairs).
  4. Enquire about occupational and recreational history of repetitive stress injury (e.g., hours on keyboards, assembly lines).
  5. Rule out any secondary causes of upper extremity deep vein thrombosis or arterial thrombosis such as central venous catheters, pacemakers, or peripheral or coronary catheterization.
D. Review of systems.
  1. Musculoskeletal: Ask about arm pain or swelling.
  2. Cardiovascular: Ask about cold fingers.
  3. Dermatology: Ask about any changes in skin color such as lack of color or bluish discoloration.
  4. Neurology: Ask about numbness, tingling, or weakness of extremity.

Physical Examination

A. Perform a standard neurological test.
B. Take blood pressure in both arms. Lower systolic pressure in the affected arm may suggest aTOS.
C. Inspect.
  1. Neck and supraclavicular area for pulsatile and nonpulsatile mass.
  2. Hands and fingers: Swelling and cyanosis (vTOS), pale, cold, ischaemic changes (aTOS).
  3. Skin overlying the ipsilateral shoulder, neck and chest wall for collateral venous patterning (vTOS).
D. Auscultate.
  1. Heart to listen for arrhythmias, gallops, and murmurs.
  2. Supraclavicular and infraclavicular fossa to listen for bruits or a thrill (aTOS).

E. Palpate.

1. Carotid and upper extremity pulses. Reduced or absent (aTOS).

2. Palpate scalene muscle to assess for tenderness (nTOS).

F. Perform provocative maneuvers.

1. Adson test.

a. Palpate the radial pulse and then move the patient's upper extremity into an extended, abducted, and externally rotated position.

b. Patient then rotates and laterally flexes the neck to the ipsilateral side while inhaling deeply.

c. A positive test results in reduction or obliteration of the radial pulse.

2. Elevated arm stress test (EAST) or Roos test.

a. Patient seated with arms abducted at 90° in external rotation, elbows flexed to 90°, head in neutral position.

b. Patient opens and closes hands.

c. The test has a high negative predictive value for nTOS if the patient performs the maneuver for 3 minutes.

Diagnostic Tests

A. The predominant clinical signs and symptoms direct the nature of further evaluation depending on the type of TOS.

1. Cervical spine x-ray: Identify bony abnormalities such as cervical ribs, anomalous ribs, or rib/clavicular fracture calluses.

2. Ultrasound: The initial imaging test to evaluate aTOS or vTOS. Provocative shoulder/arm maneuvers are performed under ultrasound.

3. Cross sectional imaging (CT or MR) and/or electromyography is best reserved for TOS specialists.

4. Hematologic evaluation: There are no specific blood tests for TOS. However, hematologic tests are helpful in ruling out other causes. See the "Diagnostic Test" section "Upper Extremity Arterial Disease."

Differential Diagnosis

A. Neurogenic TOS.

1. Carpal tunnel syndrome.

2. Ulnar nerve compression.

3. Rotator cuff tendinitis.

4. Neck strain/sprain.

5. Fibromyositis.

6. Cervical disc disease.

7. Cervical arthritis.

8. Brachial plexus injury.

B. Arterial TOS.

1. Embolization from other sources.

2. Vasculitis.

3. Radiation arteritis.

4. Connective tissue disorders.

5. Arterial dissection.

6. Atherosclerotic upper extremity disease.

7. Thromboangiitis obliterans.

8. Traumatic.

C. Venous TOS.

1. Acute thrombosis.

2. Lymphedema.

3. Rheumatologic disorders.

4. Cellulitis and allergic reactions.

5. Metabolic or global causes of limb swelling such as heart failure or myxedema.

Evaluation and Management Plan

A. General plan.

1. Treatment is indicated only for symptomatic patients. Having a cervical rib or other rib anomaly does not indicate a need to intervene.

2. Prevention and rehabilitation: Minimizing work-related overuse syndromes. Input from physical therapists.

3. Thrombolysis.

4. Severe arterial ischemia usually requires surgical embolectomy (with or without intraoperative thrombolysis).

5. Thoracic outlet decompression.

B. Patient/family teaching points.

1. Patients need to avoid repetitive movements and heavy lifting.

2. Diet and exercise can improve symptoms as well.

3. Stretching daily can keep muscles strong and prevent increased pressure on the thoracic outlet.

C. Pharmacotherapy.

1. Medical therapy: Interscalene injection of anesthetic agents, steroids, or botulinum toxin type A.

2. Anticoagulation.

D. Discharge instructions.

1. Patients should follow-up with their primary care provider.

2. Surgery may be indicated if medical treatment and physical therapy are not effective.

3. Untreated symptoms can lead to permanent nerve damage, so patients should report any worsening symptoms.

Follow-Up

A. As guided by appropriate specialist services (neurology, vascular, or general surgery).

Consultation/Referral

A. Acute ischemia: For hospital admission, seek vascular consult.

B. Non-acute, progressive symptoms referral to TOS specialist.

1. Such as complaints of shoulder, neck, head, chest, and arm problems with activity, elevation, or dangling; with supraclavicular or intraclavicular tenderness, and the absence of obvious cervical disc, rotator cuff, or carpal tunnel pathology.

Special/Geriatric Considerations

A. TOS is a complex disease in terms of its etiologies, pathophysiology, diagnosis, and management.

B. TOS is associated with a high incidence of insurance claims and worker compensation issues.

C. Early identification that TOS potentially exists and referral to specialist services is important.

Bibliography

Goshima, K. G. (2019, January 31). Overview of thoracic outlet syndromes. In K. A. Collins (Ed.), *UpToDate*. . Retrieved from https://www.uptodate.com/contents/overview-of-thoracic-outlet-syndromes

Illig, K. A., Thompson, R. W., Freischlag, J. A., Donahue, D. M., Jordon, S. E., & Edgelow, P. I. (Eds.). (2013). *Thoracic outlet syndrome*. Philadelphia, PA: Springer Publishing Company.

12 Hematology Guidelines

Mary L. Wilby

Anemia

Mary L. Wilby

Definition
A. Anemia is characterized by a lower than normal number of red blood cells (RBCs) and/or level of hemoglobin causing decreased oxygen-carrying capacity.

Incidence
A. Iron deficiency is the most common cause of anemia worldwide with women and children most often affected.
B. Other causes of anemia vary based on age, gender, and geographical region. Anemias in high income North American countries, including the United States, are most frequently the result of gastrointestinal hemorrhage, hemoglobinopathy, and chronic kidney disease.
C. Approximately 240,000 ED visits in the United States result in anemia as the primary hospital discharge diagnosis.

Pathogenesis
A. Anemia can be a consequence of bleeding, hemolysis, or inadequate bone marrow function, or nutritional deficiency.
B. Blood loss anemia results in a loss of iron containing RBCs. Hemolysis results in destruction of RBCs but iron is retained in the body.
C. Microcytic anemia is characterized by RBCs of reduced size. While most commonly associated with iron deficiency, microcytic anemia can be associated with anemia of chronic disease (ACD), thalassemia, and sideroblastic anemia.
D. Macrocytic anemias are characterized by greater than normal mean corpuscular volume. Causes are most often associated with vitamin B_{12} and folate deficiency; antimetabolite drugs, including methotrexate; and other causes that interfere with cell metabolism.
E. Pernicious anemia is associated with vitamin B_{12} deficiency caused by the absence of intrinsic factor, a glycoprotein secreted by parietal cells needed for absorption of vitamin B_{12}. Absence of intrinsic factor may be congenital, but is most often caused by an autoimmune-mediated atrophic gastritis.
F. Normocytic anemia, characterized by normal size RBCs, may be associated with ACD, hemolysis, acute blood loss, and volume overload. In the acute care setting, hemolysis may be associated with hemolytic uremic syndrome (HUS), thrombotic thrombocytopenic purpura (TTP), disseminated intravascular coagulation (DIC), or heart valve abnormalities.

Predisposing Factors
A. Use of nonsteroidal anti-inflammatory drugs (NSAIDs).
B. Peptic ulcer disease.
C. Chronic kidney disease.
D. Uterine fibroids/menorrhagia.
E. Family history of thalassemia, sickle cell disease, or hereditary spherocytosis.
F. Recent blood transfusion.
G. Nutritional deficiency.
H. Alcohol abuse.
I. Cancer.
J. Connective tissue diseases.
K. Chronic infection such as HIV or tuberculosis (TB).
L. Pregnancy.
M. Intestinal disorders including diverticulosis, inflammatory bowel disease, or celiac disease.

Subjective Data
A. Common complaints/symptoms.
   1. Signs and symptoms of anemia may vary depending on the severity, speed of development, age, and comorbidities of the individual. Tissue hypoxia and the pathologic process contribute to complaints.
   2. Fatigue, weakness, headache, shortness of breath, palpitations, and angina may occur.
   3. Decreased oxygen to the brain often results in confusion, visual changes, and fainting.
   4. Chronic blood loss may not cause symptoms until hemoglobin drops below 8 g/dL.
B. Common/typical scenario.
   1. Other signs and symptoms.
      a. Pale skin, nail beds, conjunctiva, and mucous membranes result from shifting of blood away from cutaneous tissues.
      b. Flow-type systolic murmurs may be associated with altered blood viscosity. High output heart failure and ventricular hypertrophy may occur with severe anemia, especially individuals with established heart disease.
      c. Hemolytic anemia may be associated with increased bilirubin causing jaundice, splenomegaly, and dark-colored urine.
C. Family and social history.
   1. Onset and duration of symptoms.
   2. Family history of blood disorder.
   3. Associated abdominal pain.
   4. Changes in diet, bowel habits.
   5. Menstrual history including timing and amount of bleeding.
   6. Medication history.

D. Review of systems.

1. Head, ear, eyes, nose, and throat (HEENT): Ask about premature graying of hair or burning sensation of tongue.

2. Neurology: Ask about numbness or tingling sensations.

3. Genitourinary: Ask about urine color.

4. Gastrointestinal: Ask about stool color, any blood in stool, abdominal pain, or cramping.

5. Ask about dietary habits or unusual habits such as pagophagia.

6. Dermatology: Ask about any rashes or redness of skin.

7. Psychiatric: Ask about fatigue.

Physical Examination

A. Check vital signs including pulse, respirations, and blood pressure.

B. Oral mucosa may be cracked or dry; tongue may be thickened and smooth with vitamin deficiency.

C. Cardiac examination, noting rate, rhythm, and presence of murmurs.

D. Lung examination, noting rate and adventitious sounds.

E. Abdominal examination, noting evidence of bleeding, distension, peristalsis, abnormal bowel sounds, tenderness, and masses.

F. Rectal examination, noting presence of blood in stool.

G. Skin and mucous membrane examination, noting petechiae, bruising, or pallor of skin, nail beds, and mucous membranes including conjunctiva.

H. Neurological disturbances may be associated with long-standing vitamin B_{12} deficiency; peripheral neuropathy, alterations in deep tendon reflexes, impaired vibratory sensation, alterations in balance, and impaired mental status may be present.

Diagnostic Tests

A. Complete blood count (CBC) including RBC indices.

B. Reticulocyte count.

C. Hemoglobin electrophoresis.

D. Coombs test (antiglobulin test).

E. Serum ferritin.

F. Serum iron.

G. Vitamin B_{12} level.

H. Folate level.

I. Haptoglobin.

Differential Diagnosis

A. Acute blood loss.

B. Chronic blood loss.

C. Hemolysis.

D. Aplastic anemia.

E. Leukemia.

Evaluation and Management Plan

A. General plan.

1. See Figure 12.1 for overview of anemia evaluation.

2. Treatment of anemia is based on identifying and eliminating or ameliorating the cause.

3. The severity of the anemia and its accompanying symptoms determine treatment.

4. Transfusion is often indicated if/when hematocrit drops to 27% or less.

5. Risks associated with transfusion include fluid overload, transfusion reaction, and iron overload, which must be taken into consideration.

6. Iron deficiency may be treated with increased intake of dietary iron and supplemental iron. Dietary sources are frequently insufficient and oral and/or intravenous supplementation are often required.

7. ACD may require treatment when patients become symptomatic with use of medication to stimulate erythropoiesis such as erythropoietin alpha and darbepoietin alfa.

B. Patient/family teaching points.

1. Nutritional deficiencies of iron, vitamin B_{12}, and folic acid should be corrected with changes to diet.

2. If taking ferrous sulfate, patients should avoid tea and coffee, which can affect absorption of the drug.

C. Pharmacotherapy.

1. Treatment of anemia is to correct the underlying condition and supplement with ferrous sulfate until anemia is corrected and for several months after it is corrected.

2. Ferrous sulfate 325 mg three times a day is the standard pharmacological treatment.

3. Vitamin C 500 units per day can promote absorption of ferrous sulfate.

4. Patients with severe anemia from chronic kidney failure, chemotherapy, or HIV can benefit from epoetin injections.

a. Dose of epoetin will depend on the severity of anemia, but typically starts at 50 to 100 units per kilogram administered subcutaneously three times per week. Patient will require adequate iron stores prior to starting epoetin injections.

D. Discharge instructions (If standard accepted guidelines exist please use discharge template).

1. Patients are not routinely admitted for anemia unless they are hemodynamically unstable.

2. Discharge planning for a patient who is found to be anemic in the hospital would be to follow-up with the primary care provider for a further evaluation and workup of anemia in nonacute setting.

Follow-Up

A. Once iron stores have been replenished, there is no need to retest iron studies unless there is evidence of a change in the patient's symptoms or physical examination.

B. Follow-up to identify the cause of the anemia is discussed in the following.

C. Conditions that are unresolved warrant follow-up.

D. ACD often requires ongoing treatment and follow-up under specialist care depending on the cause of the underlying disease.

E. Patients with aggressive forms of thalassemia should be under care of a hematologist.

F. Patients with vitamin B_{12} deficiency require ongoing care for monitoring B_{12} levels and monitoring of liver function if taking parenteral therapy.

G. Follow-up for patients with folic acid deficiency should consist of periodic monitoring of CBC and serum folate levels.

Consultation/Referral

A. Iron deficiency associated with occult blood loss often requires referral to a gastroenterologist for upper endoscopy and/or colonoscopy as well as additional testing to identify the source of bleeding.

B. In the case of menorrhagia, referral for follow-up gynecologic care may be needed. Follow-up care of individuals with ACD is dependent on the underlying cause.

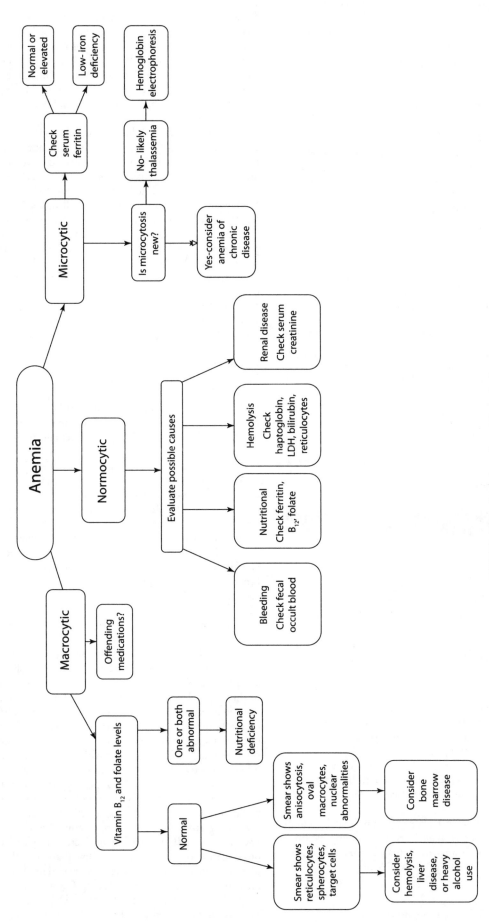

FIGURE 12.1 Overview of anemia evaluation. LDH, lactate dehydrogenase.

C. Referral for care by nephrology, rheumatology, hematology, oncology, gastroenterology, or other specialists may be required.

D. Use of erythrocyte stimulating factors should be directed by a hematologist or other qualified specialist.

E. Thalassemia may require consultation with hematology for ongoing monitoring.

F. Evidence of sideroblastic anemia should prompt consultation with hematology.

Special/Geriatric Considerations

A. Adults over 50 with occult blood in the stool or iron deficiency anemia should be referred for colonoscopy given the increased risk for gastrointestinal malignancy associated with aging.

B. In some cases the risk associated with the procedure, including perforation, may outweigh the benefits.

Bibliography

Centers for Disease Control and Prevention National Center for Disease Statistics. (2017). Anemia or iron deficiency. Retrieved from https://www.cdc.gov/nchs/fastats/anemia.htm

Grossman, S. (2014). Disorders of hemostasis. In S. C. Grossman & C. M. Porth (Eds.), *Porth's pathophysiology: Concepts of altered health states* (9th ed., pp. 648–664). Philadelphia, PA: Wolters Kluwer Health/Lippincott Williams & Wilkins.

Kassebaum, N., Jasrasaria, R., Naghavi, M., Wulf, S., Johns, N., Lozano, R., . . . Murray, C. (2014). A systematic analysis of global anemia burden from 1990 to 2010. *Blood, 123*, 615–624. doi:10.1182/blood-2013-06-508325

Porter, B. O., & Winland-Brown, J. E. (2015). Hematological and immune problems. In L. M. Dunphy, J. E. Winland-Brown, B. O. Porter, & D. J. Thomas (Eds.), *Primary care the art and science of advanced practice nursing* (4th ed., pp. 920–1025). Philadelphia, PA: F. A. Davis.

Rote, N., & McCance, K. (2014). Structure and function of the hematological systems. In K. McCance & S. Huether (Eds.), *Pathophysiology: The biologic basis for disease in adults and children* (7th ed., pp. 945–981). St. Louis, MO: Elsevier.

Bleeding Diatheses

Mary L. Wilby

Definition

A. Bleeding disorders may occur as a result of abnormalities in platelet number or function, coagulation factors, fibrinolysis, and blood vessel integrity.

B. Deficiencies or inhibitors of clotting factors, whether acquired or inherited, can result in bleeding disorders.

Incidence

A. Bleeding disorders occur frequently in seriously ill patients, and causes may vary from prolonged global clotting tests or isolated thrombocytopenia to composite defects, such as consumption coagulopathies.

B. A prolongation of global clotting times, such as the prothrombin time (PT) or the activated partial thromboplastin time (aPTT), may be apparent in 14% to 28% of critically ill patients.

C. The incidence of a low platelet count (platelet count <150,000 per microliter) in an intensive care population is 35% to 44%. Platelet counts of less than 100,000 per microliter may be seen in another 30% to 50% of patients.

Pathogenesis

A. Hemostasis is the process of clot formation at the site of blood vessel injury. Abnormal bleeding is often a result of the absence or dysfunction of one or more of the elements needed in clot formation.

B. Most clotting factors are synthesized by the liver. A final step dependent on vitamin K is required for Factors II, VII, IX, and X, and procoagulant proteins C and S. Factor VIII, von Willebrand factor (vWF), and tissue plasminogen activator are produced in the endothelium, including that of the liver. The liver reticuloendothelial system is responsible for metabolizing most clotting factors and fibrin degradation products (FDPs).

C. Coagulation factor inhibitors are antibodies that neutralize a specific clotting factor's function. Alloantibodies occur in patients with inherited factor deficiency. Autoantibodies arise in patients without an inherited factor deficiency. The most commonly inhibited factor is Factor VIII.

D. Low platelet counts in critically ill individuals are frequently the result of increased platelet turnover due to thrombin generation, platelet activation, and enhanced platelet-vessel wall interaction. Sepsis is a frequent cause for thrombocytopenia in seriously ill patients. The severity of sepsis may be correlated with the reduction in the platelet count.

E. Drug-induced thrombocytopenia has been associated with a variety of prescription and over-the-counter (OTC) medications including quinine and some sulfa-containing antibiotics. Antigen–antibody responses lead to the destruction of platelets.

F. Immune thrombocytopenic purpura (ITP) occurs as a result of antibody-induced destruction of platelets. Primary ITP can occur without any known risk factors while secondary ITP is a result of an acute or chronic underlying disorder, such as AIDS, systemic lupus erythematosus, lymphoma, or hepatitis C.

G. Thrombotic thrombocytopenic purpura (TTP) is a rare condition that manifests with a combination of low platelet count, hemolytic anemia, renal failure, neurological abnormalities, and fever. This rare disorder stems from introducing certain platelet aggregating substances into the circulation. In many cases this is triggered by a lack of an enzyme that breaks down vWF, causing platelet aggregation and adherence to vascular endothelium. While this condition may occur in otherwise healthy people, it is also found in individuals with autoimmune disorders, HIV infection, and pregnancy.

H. Disseminated intravascular coagulation (DIC) is a systemic process that can cause both thrombosis and hemorrhage. The processes associated with coagulation and fibrinolysis become abnormally activated within the vessels and promote ongoing coagulation and fibrinolysis. Consumption of platelets is associated with constant generation of thrombin. Microvascular thrombi, along with inflammation, may cause injury to the microvasculature, resulting in organ dysfunction. Consumption of platelets and low levels of other factors increase the risk for hemorrhagic complications, especially in perioperative patients or those undergoing other invasive procedures. Thrombin generation is triggered and promoted by a lack of thrombin-generating inhibitory mechanisms. Impaired fibrin degradation, due to elevated circulating levels of plasminogen activator inhibitor-type 1 (PAI-1), further promotes intravascular fibrin deposition. Patients with DIC have a low or decreasing platelet count, prolongation of coagulation tests, low plasma levels of coagulation factors and inhibitors, and increased markers of fibrin formation or degradation, including D-dimer or FDPs. No single diagnostic test is used to confirm DIC. The presence of a condition associated with DIC and a combination of laboratory tests are necessary to confirm the diagnosis.

I. Von Willebrand disease (VWD) is the most common form of inherited bleeding disorder, resulting from a deficiency or defect of vWF. Individuals with VWD have defects in both platelet function and the coagulation pathway.

J. Hemophilia A is the most common form of hemophilia, accounting for approximately 85% of hemophilia cases. Caused by an x-linked recessive gene, it affects males most often. Although it is a genetic disorder, a number of cases occur without a family history of bleeding. Deficiency or defects of Factor VIII are associated with excessive bleeding, most often occurring in soft tissue, joints, and the gastrointestinal (GI) tract. Bleeding may be spontaneous or associated with trauma.

Predisposing Factors
A. TTP.
B. Hemolytic-uremic syndrome.
C. Chemotherapy-induced microangiopathic.
D. Hemolytic anemia.
E. Severe malignant hypertension.
F. Hemolysis, elevated liver enzymes, low platelet count (HELLP) syndrome of pregnancy.
G. Preeclampsia.
H. Retained products of conception.
I. Malignancy, especially leukemia.
J. Blood transfusion reaction.
K. Systemic infection.
L. Connective tissue disease.
M. Pancreatitis.
N. Liver disease.
O. Surgery or trauma.
P. Burns.
Q. Snake venom.

Subjective Data
A. Common complaints/symptoms.
  1. Bruising.
  2. Nose bleeds.
  3. Bleeding gums.
  4. Menorrhagia.
  5. Weakness.
  6. Fatigue.
  7. Abdominal discomfort.
B. Common/typical scenario.
  1. Other signs and symptoms.
    a. Immediate bleeding after vessel injury is frequently associated with platelet disorders.
    b. Large ecchymoses and large, diffusely spreading deep tissue hematomas are common with coagulation disorders.
    c. Bleeding into synovial joints is characteristic of inherited coagulation disorders such as hemophilia.
    d. Petechiae.
    e. Oozing from venipuncture sites.
    f. Uncontrolled postpartum bleeding.
C. Family and social history.
  1. History of HIV infection and malignancy.
  2. History of liver or kidney disease, or malabsorption that is often associated with bleeding.
  3. Medication history including anticoagulants, nonsteroidal anti-inflammatory drugs (NSAIDs), oral contraceptives, antibiotics, alcohol, and dietary vitamins K and C.
  4. Response to previous hemostatic challenges, including trauma, tooth extraction, pregnancy, surgery, sports, and menstruation.
  5. Family history of bleeding disorders.
D. Review of systems.
  1. Hematological: Ask about past bleeding problems, any history of anemia, bleeding after any type of surgical procedure or dental procedure, or any transfusions.
  2. GI: Ask about dietary habits or antibiotic use which might contribute to vitamin K deficiency; ask about liver disease or black tarry stools.
  3. Genitourinary: Ask about any kidney diseases or hematuria.
  4. Endocrine.
    a. Ask women about menses.
    b. Ask about medications the patient is taking for other conditions.
  5. Dermatological: Ask about bruising or ecchymosis.

Physical Examination
A. Signs of bleeding (e.g., petechiae, mucosal bleeding, soft tissue bleeding, ecchymoses). In hospitalized patients, bleeding from multiple sites can indicate DIC or TTP. Acute extensive mucocutaneous bleeding in a patient previously without symptoms should suggest ITP.
B. Organ enlargement.
C. Joint abnormalities.
D. Signs of systemic disease including fever and lymphadenopathy.

Diagnostic Tests
A. Complete blood count (CBC).
B. Bleeding time.
C. PT.
D. aPTT.
E. Platelet function analysis.
F. Examination of a peripheral blood smear.
The following may be required in the presence of abnormalities in screening tests described earlier.
G. Factor deficiencies and inhibitors.
H. Fibrinogen.
I. Fibrin and FDPs.

Differential Diagnosis
A. Anticoagulant overdose.
B. Acquired Factor VIII inhibitors.
C. Local surgical complications.
D. Physical abuse.

Evaluation and Management Plan
A. General plan.
  1. Bleeding associated with deficiency of vitamin K can be treated with parenteral vitamin K. Normalization of clotting studies usually follows within several hours. Fresh frozen plasma may be needed in the event of hemorrhage or if emergency surgery is necessary.
  2. Individuals with acute or chronic liver disease may require treatment of alterations in clotting functions, fibrinolytic systems, or platelet function. When multiple coagulation factors are involved, infusion of fresh frozen plasma is a preferred treatment. Additional treatments may include exchange transfusion and platelet infusion.

3. DIC treatment should be directed at reducing the burden of the underlying disease, controlling thrombosis, and preserving organ function. Controlling the underlying condition is necessary to reduce the stimulus for abnormal clotting and restoring a normal balance of clotting factors. The role of heparin is limited but has been effective when DIC is associated with retained products of conception and when acute promyelocytic leukemia is present. It is contraindicated when there is evidence of central nervous system (CNS), GI, or postoperative bleeding. Interventions for restoring the balance of coagulation factors and platelets include infusion of fresh frozen plasma, cryoprecipitate, and platelets.

4. Individuals with hemophilia should avoid trauma whenever possible. Medications that interfere with platelet function, including NSAIDs, should be avoided.

5. VWD type 1 and some forms of type 2 can be treated with desmopressin to promote hemostasis, treat mucocutaneous bleeding, and prevent bleeding associated with minor procedures. Therapy with antifibrinolytic agents such as tranexamic acid is also beneficial in VWD. Treatment with oral contraceptives or a levonorgestrel-releasing intrauterine device can be very beneficial for women with VWD experiencing menorrhagia. Infusion of von Willebrand concentrate is also an option when desmopressin is not effective.

B. Patient/family teaching points.

1. Patients should contact their primary care provider prior to any dental procedures or surgical interventions.

2. Bruising may be spontaneous or recurrent and patients may experience prolonged bleeding after minor cuts or abrasions.

3. Women of childbearing age will need high risk obstetrics and should carefully plan pregnancies.

C. Pharmacotherapy.

1. Pharmacological treatment will be based on the underlying cause of bleeding diathesis and is fairly limited.

2. In the acute setting, blood products can be used to control bleeding disorders.

3. Avoidance of medications that interfere with platelet function should be evaluated.

4. Hypoprothrombinemia can be treated acutely with parenteral vitamin K.

5. Minor bleeding or elevated international normalized ratio (INR)—2.5 to 5 mg oral vitamin K one time may be sufficient, or can be repeated in 24 hours if needed.

6. Patients who have internal bleeding or who are at high risk for bleeding can be given intravenous vitamin K 5 to 10 mg diluted in IVF and infused over 20 minutes. These patients should also receive prothrombin complex concentrate (PCC).

D. Discharge instructions (If standard accepted guidelines exist please use discharge template).

1. Patient should be instructed on how to recognize signs and symptoms that warrant immediate attention.

2. Patients should also be given instructions on how to control a bleeding source.

Follow-Up

A. In general, medications such as aspirin and NSAIDs should be avoided in patients with abnormal bleeding.

B. Conditions that may pose special risks for individuals with bleeding disorders, including hypertension that may lead to intracranial bleeding, need close monitoring and treatment.

C. Procedures necessary for preventive care and screening should be planned in cooperation with the patient's hematologist.

D. Dental care and screening colonoscopy can usually be performed with decreased risk for bleeding when supervised carefully and given appropriate hemostatic coverage.

Consultation/Referral

A. Treatment of underlying conditions is important in controlling bleeding in individuals with bleeding diatheses.

B. Consultation with a gastroenterologist/hepatologist is important in management of advanced liver disease.

C. When thrombocytopenia is present, consultation with a hematologist is warranted.

D. If DIC or thrombocytopenia is associated with sepsis, consultation with an infectious disease specialist is indicated.

E. Bleeding associated with malignancy requires referral to hematology oncology.

F. Bleeding in the setting of pregnancy-related complications requires immediate referral to OB/GYN.

Special/Geriatric Considerations

A. Bleeding disorders in the elderly pose special challenges.

B. A number of acquired disorders can present in older adults as a result of alterations in coagulation factors, medications, and comorbid conditions more common with aging.

C. Older adults are more likely to be receiving medications to treat thrombotic disorders and evidence of bleeding may be dismissed as a side effect of anticoagulants and antiplatelet drugs.

D. Increased risk for bleeding associated with anticoagulants as well as NSAIDs accompanies many physiological changes of aging.

E. Thrombocytopenia in the elderly may be associated with ITP, leukemia, or DIC associated with malignancy or sepsis.

F. Though rare, there is risk for acquired hemophilia and acquired von Willebrand syndrome in older adults.

Bibliography

Baz, R., & Mekhail, T. (2013). *Bleeding disorders*. Cleveland Clinic Center for Continuing Education, Disease Management. Retrieved from http://www.clevelandclinicmeded.com/medicalpubs/diseasemanagement/hematology-oncology/bleeding-disorders/

Capriotti, T., & Frizzell, J. P. (2016). *Pathophysiology: Introductory concepts and clinical perspectives* (pp. 285–304). Philadelphia, PA: F. A. Davis.

Drews, R. E. (2017). Approach to the adult patient with bleeding diathesis. In L. Leung (Ed.), *UpToDate*. Retrieved from https://www.uptodate.com/contents/approach-to-the-adult-with-a-suspected-bleeding-disorder

Grossman, S. (2014). Disorders of hemostasis. In S. C. Grossman & C. M. Porth (Eds.), *Porth's pathophysiology: Concepts of altered health states* (9th ed., pp. 648–664). Philadelphia, PA: Wolters Kluwer Health/Lippincott Williams & Wilkins.

Kruse-Jarres, R. (2015). Acquired bleeding disorders in the elderly. *ASH Education Book, 2015*(1), 231–236.

Kruse-Jarres, R., Singleton, T. C., & Leissinger, C. A. (2014). Identification and basic management of bleeding disorders in adults. *Journal of the American Board of Family Medicine, 27*(4), 549–564. doi:10.3122/jabfm.2014.04.130227

Leung, L. (2018, November 12). Overview of hemostasis. In P. Mannucci (Ed.), *UpToDate*. Retrieved from https://www.uptodate.com/contents/overview-of-hemostasis

Levi, M., & Sivapalaratnam, S. (2015). Hemostatic abnormalities in critically ill patients. *Internal and Emergency Medicine, 10*, 287–296. doi:10.1007/s11739-014-1176-2

Lillicrap, D. (2013). Von Willebrand disease: Advances in pathogenetic understanding, diagnosis, and therapy. *Blood, 122*(23), 3735–3740. doi:10.1182/blood-2013-06-498303

Schwartz, A., & Rote, N. S. (2014). Alterations in leukocyte, lymphoid, and hemostatic function. In K. L. McCance, S. E. Huether, V. L. Brashers, & N. S. Rote (Eds.), *Pathophysiology: The biologic basis for disease in adults and children* (pp. 1008–1054). St. Louis, MO: Elsevier/Mosby.

Coagulopathies

Mary L. Wilby

Definition

A. Strictly speaking, coagulopathy describes a condition that disturbs the blood's ability to clot. For purposes of this text, coagulopathy will refer to hypercoagulability. Bleeding disorders are described elsewhere in this chapter.

B. Hypercoagulability, sometimes referred to as thrombophilia, is an enhanced state of hemostasis that increases the risk for thrombosis and blood vessel occlusion.

C. These conditions are typically created in the presence of increased platelet function or increased activity of the coagulation system. Arterial thrombi are most often associated with turbulent blood flow and are composed of platelets.

D. Hypercoagulability disorders have been characterized as primary (hereditary) or secondary (acquired).

Incidence

A. Approximately 30% of those who present with deep vein thrombosis or pulmonary emboli are found to have Factor V Leiden. Factor V Leiden is seen primarily in individuals of European descent and in approximately 5% of whites in the United States.

B. Antiphospholipid antibodies are present in 3% to 5% of the general population and are more prevalent in individuals with systemic lupus erythematosus.

C. Venous thromboembolism (VTE) is not uncommon in the presence of malignancy. Tumor type and stage, location of the tumor, treatment, and comorbid conditions influence risk. It is estimated that as many as 10% of cancer patients develop VTE.

Pathogenesis

A. Most hereditary thrombophilic disorders are associated with mutations in coagulation proteins, fibrinolytic proteins, platelet receptors, and various other factors. Factor V Leiden, a condition in which a Factor V mutation interacts with protein C, leading to increased clot formation, is the most common hereditary condition.

B. Other inherited hypercoagulable states are rarer and include prothrombin gene mutation, hyperhomocysteinemia, antithrombin deficiency, and protein C and protein S deficiency.

C. Antiphospholipid syndrome is the most common acquired hypercoagulable condition. When present, antiphospholipid antibodies are directed against phospholipid–protein complexes causing risk for both arterial and venous thrombus formation.

D. Protein C and protein S deficiency may also become acquired in some disease states.

E. Increased platelet function may manifest as enhanced platelet adhesion, with clot formation and decreased blood flow. Disturbances in blood flow, as with a therosclerotic plaques, cause endothelial tissue damage. Increased sensitivity of platelets to substances that influence platelet aggregation may increase platelet activity.

F. Elevation in platelet counts above 1,000,000/μL, referred to as thrombocytosis, is associated with both thrombosis and bleeding. Primary thrombocytosis is a myeloproliferative disorder associated with a disorder of hematopoietic cells in the bone marrow. Secondary thrombocytosis is often associated with disease states that trigger thrombopoietin production, increasing platelet production. These conditions include surgery, cancer, and chronic inflammatory disorders.

Predisposing Factors

A. Surgery.
B. Cancer.
C. Chronic inflammatory disorders.
D. Atherosclerosis.
E. Diabetes mellitus.
F. Smoking.
G. Pregnancy.
H. Oral contraceptive use.
I. Estrogen replacement therapy.
J. Obesity.
K. Heart failure.
L. Nephrotic syndrome.
M. Polycythemia.
N. Sickle cell disease.

Subjective Data

A. Common complaints/symptoms.
  1. Patients with thrombocytosis may experience painful burning and throbbing in digits associated with arteriole occlusion.
  2. Painful, swollen extremity (usually unilateral).
B. Common/typical scenario.
  1. Other signs and symptoms.
    a. Neurological impairment consistent with transient ischemic attack or stroke.
    b. Chest pain associated with cardiac ischemia.
    c. Dyspnea associated with pulmonary emboli.
    d. Visual disturbance with retinal ischemia.
C. Family and social history.
  1. History of fetal loss in women with antiphospholipid syndrome.
  2. History of unprovoked thrombosis in adults under 45 years of age.
  3. Family history of multiple individuals with VTE.
D. Review of systems.
  1. Hematologic: Ask about bruising or previous clotting episodes of the arterial or venous system, such as stroke, myocardial infarction, or small vessel thrombosis.
  2. Rheumatology: Ask about autoimmune disorders.
  3. Obstetrics: Ask about spontaneous abortions.
  4. Dermatology: Ask about skin discoloration.

Physical Examination

A. Physical examination may yield nonspecific findings.
B. Evidence of arterial thrombosis may manifest in signs of stroke, myocardial infarction, DVT, PE, or digital ischemia.
C. Skin necrosis is associated with warfarin therapy.

Diagnostic Tests

A. Complete blood count (CBC).
B. Prothrombin time.
C. Activated partial thromboplastin time.
D. Antiphospholipid antibodies.
E. Protein C—may be low in acute thrombosis.
F. Protein S—may be low in acute thrombosis.
G. Antithrombin III—may be low in acute thrombosis.

Differential Diagnosis

A. Paroxysmal nocturnal hematuria.
B. Homocysteinemia.
C. Heparin-induced thrombocytopenia.
D. Atherosclerosis.
E. Sickle cell disease.
F. Myeloproliferative diseases.

Evaluation and Management Plan

A. General plan.

  1. Not all thrombotic episodes are associated with hypercoagulable risk factors and not all individuals with risk factors develop thrombosis.

  2. Workup for coagulopathy is indicated with the presence of idiopathic or recurrent VTE, VTE before the age of 40, VTE with strong family history, VTE in an atypical site, or warfarin-induced skin necrosis.

  3. Treatment involves reducing or eliminating factors that lead to thrombosis.

B. Patient/family teaching points.

  1. Women need to avoid oral contraceptives or hormone replacement therapy.

  2. Patients may need to be treated with lifelong anticoagulation to prevent further clotting.

  3. Patients must be instructed on how to manage bleeding diathesis if on anticoagulation agents.

C. Pharmacotherapy.

  1. Acute events require treatment with anticoagulants including heparin, warfarin, and other agents.

  2. Immune suppression may be needed in some cases when the condition is refractory to anticoagulants.

D. Discharge instruction.

  1. Patients will need to follow-up with hematology.

  2. Any dental procedures or surgical interventions must be done in conjunction with the patient's primary care provider.

Follow-Up

A. Monitoring of anticoagulation therapy posthospitalization is critical to preventing recurrence.

B. Patients should be cautioned to avoid trauma while receiving anticoagulant therapy.

C. Patients with modifiable risk factors including tobacco use or use of estrogen-containing oral contraceptives should be counseled about their use.

Consultation/Referral

A. Consultation with a hematologist is critical in the diagnosis and management of patients with hypercoagulable disorders.

B. It is also important that laboratory testing is completed at a facility with experience in utilizing specialized tests.

Special/Geriatric Considerations

A. Aging is accompanied by increased risk of both arterial and venous thrombosis.

B. While mechanisms are not entirely clear, a number of coagulation factors, including Factors V, VII, VIII, IX, and von Willebrand factor (vWF), increase with aging. This coupled with other comorbid conditions such as malignancy and structural changes in vascular endothelium contribute to an increased risk for thrombosis in older adults.

C. Special consideration is given for the use of anticoagulation in older adults to minimize the risk for bleeding. Careful monitoring of vitamin K antagonists is necessary.

D. Use of direct oral anticoagulants (DOAs) may be an alternative in some cases.

E. Education and monitoring to decrease risk for falls and other forms of trauma are essential for older adults receiving anticoagulation therapy.

Bibliography

Bauer, K. A. (2019, February 27). Risk and prevention of venous thromboembolism in adults with cancer. In L. Leung (Ed.), *UpToDate*. Retrieved from https://www.uptodate.com/contents/risk-and-prevention-of-venous-thromboembolism-in-adults-with-cancer

Grossman, S. (2014). Disorders of hemostasis. In S. C. Grossman & C. M. Porth (Eds.), *Porth's pathophysiology: Concepts of altered health states* (9th ed., pp. 648–664). Philadelphia, PA: Wolters Kluwer Health/Lippincott Williams & Wilkins.

Hogan, C. (2015). Thrombophilia and hypercoagulable states. In F. J. Domino, R. A. Baldor, J. Golding, & M. B. Stephens (Eds.), *The 5 minute clinical consult premium, 2016* (24th ed., pp. 1092–1093). Philadelphia, PA: Wolters Kluwer Health.

Nakashima, M. O., & Rogers, H. J. (2014). Hypercoagulable states: An algorithmic approach to laboratory testing and update on monitoring of direct oral anticoagulants. *Blood Research, 49*(2), 85–94. doi:10.5045/br.2014.49.2.85

Previtali, E., Bucciarelli, S., Passamonti, S. M., & Martinelli, I. (2011). Risk factors for venous and arterial thrombosis. *Blood Transfusion, 9*, 120–138. doi:10.2450/2010.0066-10

Robert-Ebadi, H., & Righini, M. (2010). Anticoagulation in the elderly. *Pharmaceuticals, 3*(12), 3543–3569. doi:10.3390/ph3123543

Schick, P. (2018, January 5). Hereditary and acquired hypercoagulability. In S. Nagalla (Ed.), *Medscape*. Retrieved from https://emedicine.medscape.com/article/211039-overview

Schwartz, A., & Rote, N. S. (2014). Alterations in leukocyte, lymphoid, and hemostatic function. In K. L. McCance, S. E. Huether, V. L. Brashers, & N. S. Rote (Eds.), *Pathophysiology the biologic basis for disease in adults and children* (pp. 1008–1054). St. Louis, MO: Elsevier Mosby.

Deep Vein Thrombosis

Mary L. Wilby

Definition

A. Deep vein thrombosis (DVT) describes clot formation in the deep veins, most often in the lower extremities.

B. DVT increases the risk for venous thromboembolism (VTE) to the pulmonary circulation.

C. See Figure 12.2.

Incidence

A. More than 900,000 VTE events occur each year in the United States. Nearly one-third of these result in death.

B. Up to 50% of cases are believed to be idiopathic, with an additional 15% to 25% associated with cancer, and 20% associated with surgery.

C. Pulmonary embolism (PE) can occur in up to 50% of patients with untreated DVT.

D. The mortality rate associated with PE is 25% to 30%.

Pathogenesis

A. Three factors often referred to as Virchow's triad promote venous thrombosis. These three factors are (a) venous stasis, (b) damage to venous endothelium, and (c) hypercoagulable states. Buildup of clotting factors and platelets promotes thrombus formation in the vessel, often adjacent to a valve. Inflammation associated with the clot promotes additional platelet aggregation, causing the clot to grow proximally.

B. Bed rest and/or immobility are factors often associated with venous stasis.

C. Hypercoagulability may be associated with increased activity of clotting factors or inherited or acquired conditions in which factors that would normally inhibit clotting are deficient.

D. Venous injury can result from surgery, trauma, and venous catheters.

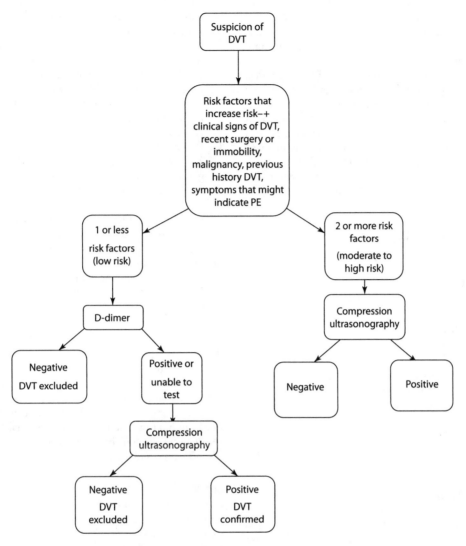

FIGURE 12.2 Diagnosis of DVT.
DVT, deep vein thrombosis; PE, pulmonary embolism.

E. Localized symptoms are the result of inflammation and venous obstruction, but symptoms may not be apparent if the vein is deep within the leg because of incomplete occlusion and collateral circulation.

Predisposing Factors

A. Immobility.
B. Obesity.
C. Prolonged dependency (including air travel).
D. Age.
E. Heart failure.
F. Trauma.
G. Medications.
H. Malignancy.
I. Central venous catheters.
J. Pregnancy.
K. Oral contraceptives.
L. Hormone replacement.
M. Nephrotic syndrome.
N. Antiphospholipid antibody syndrome.
O. Hospitalization (especially orthopedic surgery, trauma, spinal cord injury, gynecologic disorders).
P. Inherited clotting disorders including Factor V Leiden mutation, prothrombin mutations, antithrombin deficiency,

hyperhomocysteinemia, elevated Factor VIII activity, protein C deficiency, and protein S deficiency.

Subjective Data

A. Common complaints/symptoms.
  1. Pain.
  2. Swollen extremity.
  3. Muscle tenderness.
B. Common/typical scenario.
  1. Other signs and symptoms.
    a. Fever.
    b. Increased erythrocyte sedimentation rate.
    c. Increased white blood cell count.
C. Family and social history.
  1. History of recent surgery or trauma.
  2. History of cancer, liver disease, autoimmune disorder, or cardiovascular disease.
  3. Previous history of blood clotting or bleeding problems.
  4. Family history of stroke or other thrombosis.
  5. Immobility.
  6. Recent prolonged travel.
D. Review of systems.
  1. Musculoskeletal: Ask about extremity pain with or without movement, edema, and redness.

Physical Examination

A. Physical examination alone is less reliable than when coupled with thorough history.

B. Unexplained extremity swelling, pain, warmth, or erythema may be noted. Pain is frequently described as a cramp or ache in the calf or thigh.

C. The location of the thrombus may influence physical findings. Swelling in the foot and ankle and calf pain are associated with thrombi in the venous sinuses in the soleus muscle and posterior tibial and peroneal veins. Thrombi in the femoral vein are associated with pain in the popliteal area and distal thigh while those in the ileofemoral veins are manifested by pain and swelling involving the whole leg.

D. Upper extremity swelling along with pain and venous distention may indicate upper extremity DVT.

Diagnostic Tests

A. Serum D-dimer concentration.
B. Lower extremity ultrasonography.
C. CT.
D. MRI.
E. Venogram.

Differential Diagnosis

A. Trauma.
B. Infection.
C. Peripheral artery disease.
D. Chronic venous insufficiency.
E. Postthrombotic syndrome.
F. Lymphedema.
G. Erythema nodosum.
H. Insect bites.
I. Muscle strain.

Evaluation and Management Plan

A. General plan.

1. Prompt diagnosis of DVT is facilitated by combining medical history and physical examination, D-dimer testing, and appropriate use of imaging studies.

2. Hospitalized patients are typically treated with intravenous heparin and monitored for signs of bleeding.

3. Thrombolytic therapy should be reserved for massive PE or extensive DVT.

4. Contraindications to outpatient management of DVT include surgery within 7 days, cardiopulmonary instability, and severe symptomatic venous obstruction.

5. Additional contraindications for outpatient treatment include platelet count less than 50,000/lL, other medical or surgical conditions requiring inpatient management, medical nonadherence, geographical or telephone inaccessibility, impaired hepatic function, impaired renal function (e.g., rising serum creatinine), and inadequate home healthcare support.

6. The optimal duration of therapy is dictated by the presence of modifiable risk factors for thrombosis.

7. Long-term anticoagulation is an important consideration for individuals with unprovoked VTE or ongoing prothrombotic risk factors such as cancer and antiphospholipid antibody syndrome.

8. Short-term therapy is sufficient for most patients with VTE associated with transient triggers such as major surgery.

9. Inferior vena cava (IVC) filters should be considered for patients with acute VTE and contraindications to anticoagulation. Retrievable filters are preferable.

10. Warfarin is contraindicated in pregnancy while low molecular weight heparin (LMWH), dalteparin, and fondaparinux are pregnancy Category B.

B. Patient/family teaching points.

1. Patients must be taught to recognize concerning signs for bleeding diathesis while on anticoagulation.

2. Depending on the medication ordered, patients may need to have routine blood work completed.

3. Patients need to set reminders to take the medications the same time each day to optimize efficacy of the medication.

C. Pharmacotherapy.

1. Low dose fractionated or nonfractionated heparin given subcutaneously is the mainstay of treatment.

2. The availability of LMWH, fondaparinux, and direct oral anticoagulants (DOACs) has increased the options for acute outpatient treatment of DVT and PE.

a. DOACs can be as effective as LMWH and vitamin K antagonists such as warfarin.

D. Discharge instructions (If standard accepted guidelines exist please use discharge template).

1. Patients will need to follow-up with hematology as an outpatient.

Follow-Up

A. Patients with DVT should gradually resume activity and avoid immobility.

B. Monitoring of anticoagulation and bleeding risk can be done as an outpatient.

C. Individuals receiving warfarin need regular monitoring of prothrombin time and international normalized ratio (INR).

D. Platelets should be monitored in patients receiving LMWH and fondaparinux.

Consultation/Referral

A. Consultation with interventional radiology is necessary when considering use of thrombolytics, thrombectomy, stents, or placement of IVC filter.

B. Ongoing follow-up should be provided for patients requiring IVC filter to reduce risks for filter thrombosis.

Special/Geriatric Considerations

A. Increasing age and renal impairment increase risk for VTE in older adults while at the same time increasing risk for bleeding associated with anticoagulant therapy.

B. DOAs may offer an acceptable alternative to warfarin as monitoring is simpler.

C. Alteration in renal function may necessitate dose adjustments or serve as a contraindication for their use.

Bibliography

Behravesh, S., Hoang, P., Nanda, A., Wallace, A., Sheth, R. A., Deipolyi, A. R., & Oklu, R. (2017). Pathogenesis of thromboembolism and endovascular management. *Thrombosis, 2017*, 1–14. doi:10.1155/2017/3039713

Brashers, V. L. (2014). Alterations in cardiovascular functioning. In K. L. McCance, S. E. Huether, V. L. Brashers, & N. S. Rote (Eds.), *Pathophysiology the biologic basis for disease in adults and children* (pp. 1129–1193). St. Louis, MO: Elsevier Mosby.

Conelius, J. (2014). Disorders of blood flow in the systemic circulation. In S. C. Grossman & C. M. Porth (Eds.), *Porth's pathophysiology: Concepts of altered health states* (pp. 739–765). Philadelphia, PA: Wolters Kluwer Health/Lippincott Williams & Wilkins.

Geldhof, V., Vandenbrielem, C., Verhamme, P., & Vanassche, T. (2014). Venous thromboembolism in the elderly: Efficacy and safety of non-VKA oral anticoagulants. *Thrombosis Journal, 12*, 21. doi:10.1186/1477-9560-12-21

Keller, K., Prochaska, J. H., Coldewey, M., Gobel, S., Ullmann, A., Jünger, C., . . . Wild, P. S. (2015). History of deep vein thrombosis is a discriminator for concomitant atrial fibrillation in pulmonary embolism. *Thrombosis Research, 136*(5), 899–906. doi:10.1016/j.thromres.2015.08.024

Streiff, M. B., Agnelli, G., Connors, J. M., Crowther, M., Eichinger, S., Lopes, R., . . . Ansell, J. (2016). Guidance for the treatment of deep vein thrombosis and pulmonary embolism. *Journal of Thrombosis and Thrombolysis, 41*, 32–67. doi:10.1007/s11239-015-1317-0

Talfur, D. V., & Talfur, A. (2015). Deep vein thrombosis. In F. J. Domino, R. A. Baldor, J. Golding, & M. B. Stephens (Eds.), *The 5 minute clinical consult premium, 2016* (24th ed., pp. 1092–1093). Philadelphia, PA: Wolters Kluwer Health.

Weber, J. (2014). Venous thromboembolic disease. *Journal of the American Osteopathic College of Radiology, 3*(3), 2–7.

Wilbur, J., & Shian, B. (2012). Diagnosis of deep vein thrombosis and pulmonary embolism. *American Family Physician, 86*(10), 913–919. Retrieved from https://www.aafp.org/afp/2012/1115/p913.html

Sickle Cell Crisis

Mary L. Wilby

Definition

A. Vaso-occlusive crisis (VOC) involving the bones is the most consistent and characteristic feature of sickle cell disease (SCD).

B. VOCs and their accompanying pain present most frequently in the extremities, chest, and back, although multiple sites may be involved.

Incidence

A. Approximately 5% of the world's population carries an abnormal hemoglobin gene, with SCD being the most predominant form.

B. The greatest burden of the disease lies in sub-Saharan Africa. SCD affects nearly 100,000 individuals in the United States, the majority of whom are African American.

Pathogenesis

A. SCD occurs as a result of change in the amino acids of the beta globin chain of the hemoglobin molecule. Under circumstances where deoxygenation occurs, causing a reaction leading to "sickling" of the red blood cell, reoxygenation allows the cell to return to its normal shape; however, repeated sickling damages the cells, leaving them permanently sickled.

B. Chronic hemolysis and high viscosity and vascular occlusion are the two main pathologic processes leading to the symptom most often associated with SCD. Infarction occurs as a result of stasis of the rigid sickle cells in the vascular beds of organs as a result of decreased blood flow. Sickled cells lose their flexibility and are unable to pass through the capillaries. Additionally, sickle cells tend to exhibit more adhesiveness to vascular endothelium and other blood cells, contributing to the obstruction of blood flow.

C. Bone pain crisis is one of the most common manifestations of SCD. Pain occurs as a result of activating afferent nerves in bones experiencing ischemia. Long bones including the femur and humerus, as well as ribs, vertebrae, pelvis, and sternum, are common sites of pain, often with multiple sites affected at once. Painful crises may vary in intensity.

D. When arising in other sites, pain can be confused with, or can be an early indication of, another acute complication such as stroke, liver or splenic sequestration, or constipation associated with opioid use. The etiology of the pain must be identified in order to rule out potential causes of pain other than an uncomplicated VOC, such as cardiac ischemia, pneumonia, or other abdominal complications. VOC can occur in the presence of other complications, making diagnosis more challenging. No diagnostic test is able to rule in or to rule out a VOC. Diagnostic tests are most useful in ruling out other causes of pain.

E. Acute abdominal pain may result from vaso-occlusion of mesenteric vasculature, sequestration of blood in the spleen, biliary tract disease, or non-SCD related conditions. Sequestration most often occurs in the spleen, but the liver and lymph nodes may also be sites of sequestration. If not recognized and treated rapidly, acute sequestration may result in shock and death. Mesenteric syndrome is a rare complication. The patient may present with generalized abdominal pain, localized or rebound tenderness, and rigidity. Paralytic ileus with vomiting, distention, and absence of bowel sounds along with dilated bowel loops, and air-fluid levels on abdominal x-ray are hallmarks.

Predisposing Factors

A. Exposure to cold.
B. Dehydration.
C. Infection.
D. Physical exertion.
E. Tobacco smoke.
F. Alcohol use.
G. Drug abuse.
H. High altitude.
I. Hypoxic conditions.
J. Physical pain.
K. Pregnancy.
L. Hot weather.
M. Emotional stress.
N. Onset of menses.

Subjective Data

A. Common complaints/symptoms.
  1. Extremity pain.
  2. Chest pain.
  3. Back pain.
B. Common/typical scenario.
  1. Other signs and symptoms.
    a. Abdominal pain.
    b. Tachycardia.
    c. Tachypnea.
    d. Fever.
    e. Pallor.
    f. Jaundice.
C. Family and social history.
  1. Recent history of precipitating factors.
  2. Previous VOC.
  3. Comorbid conditions.
  4. Current treatment regimen, including analgesics and other medications, as well as transfusions.
D. Review of systems.
  1. Ask about pain and where it is located.
    a. Pain can affect any part of the body.
  2. Ask about any infections, cough, or fever.
  3. Cardiac.
    a. Chest pain.
    b. Palpitations.
  4. Neurology.
    a. Any weakness or shaking.

Physical Examination

A. Vital signs.
B. Oxygen saturation.

C. Skin and mucous membranes, noting pallor or jaundice.
D. Hydration status.
E. Cardiac examination.
F. Lung examination.
G. Abdominal examination.
H. Neurological examination.

Diagnostic Tests
A. Complete blood count (CBC).
B. Blood and urine cultures if febrile.
C. Chest x-ray if pulmonary symptoms.
D. EKG to rule out ischemia.
E. Chemistry panel.
F. Liver function testing.
G. Urinalysis.

Differential Diagnosis
A. Avascular necrosis.
B. Acute chest syndrome.
C. Gout.
D. Bone infarction.
E. Osteomyelitis.
F. Joint infection.
G. Cerebrovascular accident.
H. Pneumonia.
I. Asthma.

Evaluation and Management Plan
A. General plan.
  1. Treatment of bone pain crisis includes providing adequate analgesia, hydration, prophylactic or therapeutic antibiotics after collection of appropriate cultures, and oxygenation when hypoxia is evident.
  2. Oral hydration may be inadequate, making intravenous hydration necessary.
  3. Pain management is best directed by the patient's report of pain.
    a. Analgesia should be offered within 30 minutes of presentation with an acute painful event.
    b. Before prescribing analgesics for an acute painful sickle cell episode, the provider should inquire about and consider any analgesia taken by the patient for this painful episode prior to his or her arrival at the hospital.
      i. The effectiveness of pain relief should be assessed frequently. If the patient with severe pain has not had relief, a second dose of strong opioid should be offered. Patient-controlled analgesia should be considered if repeated boluses of strong opioid medications are needed within a 2-hour period.
      ii. Frequent monitoring for adverse events associated with strong opioids, including respiratory depression and excessive sedation, is advised.
      iii. An alternative diagnosis should be considered if the patient does not respond to standard treatment for an acute crisis.
      iv. Consideration of exchange blood transfusion should be given in situations where pain is unrelieved with conventional measures.
      v. Nonpharmacologic measures include:
        1) Physical therapy.
        2) Relaxation.
        3) Distraction techniques.
        4) Music therapy.
        5) Meditation, which may be beneficial.
        6) Prophylactic incentive spirometry, which is recommended to reduce the risk for acute chest syndrome.
B. Patient/family teaching points.
  1. Preventing sickle cell crises is the keystone management approach.
  2. Patients need to be taught how to recognize their own triggers and to have a self-assessment and treatment plan at home.
  3. Prevention of infection is also important.
    a. Reinforcing proper hygiene is key.
    b. Reinforcing universal precautions is essential.
  4. Remind patients that the use of live vaccines is contraindicated in sickle cell due to the immunosuppressive therapy they receive.
C. Pharmacotherapy.
  1. A dose of a strong opioid should be offered to all patients with severe pain (7 or greater on a 0–10 scale) and those with moderate pain (4–7 on a 0–10 scale) who have already received some analgesia before their arrival at the hospital.
  2. Severe VOC requires parenteral opioid analgesia and hydration in a hospital setting.
  3. The dose of the analgesia should be titrated with the severity of the pain until adequate control is achieved with a scheduled dose regimen, with short-acting agents for breakthrough pain.
  4. Meperidine should be avoided because of neurotoxicity associated with high doses.
  5. A weak opioid may be considered for those with moderate pain who have not yet received some form of analgesic. Except when contraindicated, acetaminophen, or nonsteroidal anti-inflammatory drugs (NSAIDs), should be offered to all patients via a suitable route in addition to opioids.
  6. All patients receiving opioids should receive laxatives on a regular basis as well as antiemetics and antipyretics as needed.
D. Discharge instructions (If standard accepted guidelines exist please use discharge template).
  1. Long-term follow-up is essential.
  2. Teach patients to recognize signs of infection and what to do when the signs manifest.

Follow-Up
A. Patients with SCD should have regular follow-up with their hematologist.
B. Those with frequent readmissions for painful crises should be considered for treatment, with hydroxyurea used to increase fetal hemoglobin.
C. Routine laboratory evaluation should include CBC, electrolytes, renal, and liver function tests.
D. Adults should receive all age-appropriate immunizations including pneumococcal vaccines, influenza, and meningococcal vaccines.

Consultation/Referral
A. Referral for pain management services may be warranted for individuals with chronic pain and when there is concern for opioid abuse.
B. Referral to ophthalmology for annual retinal examination should be considered for all patients.

Special/Geriatric Considerations
A. Improved treatment of patients with SCD has progressively increased their survival over the past 30 years.

B. While the average life expectancy of patients with SCD in the 1970s was less than 20 years, mean life expectancy in the 1990s among those with the most severe form of the disease increased to 42 years for men and 48 years for women.

C. Cases of individuals living into their 50s and 60s have been well documented, with additional recent cases indicating some individuals lived into their 80s.

D. Those who survive into later life are more likely to have long-term disease complications including renal insufficiency.

Bibliography

Adewoyin, A. S. (2015). Management of sickle cell disease: A review for physician education in Nigeria (sub-Saharan Africa). *Anemia, 2015,* 791498. doi:10.1155/2015/791498

Ballas, S. K., Pullte, D. E., Lobo, C., & Riddick-Burden, G. (2016). Case series of octogenarians with sickle cell disease. *Blood, 128,* 2367–2369. doi:10.1182/blood-2016-05-715946

Field, J. J., Vichinsky, E. P., & DeBraun, M. R. (2018, September 7). Overview of the management and prognosis of sickle cell disease. In S. L. Schrier & D. H. Mahoney, Jr. (Eds.), *UpToDate.* Retrieved from https://www.uptodate.com/contents/overview-of-the-management-and-prognosis-of-sickle-cell-disease

Lanzkron, S., Carroll, C. P., & Haywood, C., Jr. (2013). Mortality rates and age at death from sickle cell disease: U.S., 1979–2005. *Public Health Reports, 128,* 110–128. doi:10.1177/003335491312800206

National Heart, Lung, and Blood Institute. (2014). *Evidence-based management of sickle cell disease: Expert panel report, 2014.* Washington, DC: U.S. Department of Health and Human Services.

Porter, B. O., & Winland-Brown, J. E. (2015). Hematological and immune problems. In L. M. Dunphy, J. E. Winland-Brown, B. O. Porter, & D. J. Thomas (Eds.), *Primary care the art and science of advanced practice nursing* (4th ed., pp. 920–1025). Philadelphia, PA: F. A. Davis.

13 Oncology Guidelines

Jerrad M. Stoddard

Brain/Central Nervous System Malignancies

Jerrad M. Stoddard

Definition

A. Brain tumors most commonly arise from distant metastasis of other primary malignancies.
B. Subtypes and classification: Primary brain tumors are classified according to the histologic pattern of cell differentiation.
  1. Gliomas.
    a. Most commonly occurring primary brain tumors.
    b. Several types, including:
      i. Glioblastomas (most common).
      ii. Astrocytomas.
      iii. Oligodendrogliomas.
      iv. Ependymomas.
  2. Meningiomas.
  3. Nerve sheath tumors.
  4. Pituitary tumors.
  5. Primary central nervous system (CNS) lymphoma (associated with HIV/AIDS and immunosuppression).

Incidence

A. The U.S. incidence rate of primary brain and CNS tumors in patients 20 years of age and older is 28.6 per 100,000 persons.
B. The incidence rate for children (ages 0–19) is much lower, 5.6 per 100,000 persons.
C. The 5-year overall survival rate for all malignant brain tumors is ~34%.
D. Survival rates depend on histologic subtype. For example, the 5-year overall survival rates for anaplastic astrocytoma and glioblastoma are 28% and 5%, respectively.

Pathogenesis

A. Primary brain tumors proliferate from brain tissue most commonly from glial tissue.
  1. Tumors that arise from glial tissue include astrocytomas, oligodendrogliomas, and ependymomas.
  2. Nonglial primary type brain tumors are meningiomas, schwannomas, craniopharyngiomas, germ cell tumors, and pineal region tumors.
B. Typically primary brain tumors do not metastasize, although they can.
C. Secondary or metastatic brain tumors originate from another part of the body and spread to the brain.
  1. Several types of secondary brain tumors spread quickly to the brain, including lung, breast, melanoma, colon, and kidney cancer.

Predisposing Factors

A. Ionizing radiation.
B. Exposure to cured foods.
C. HIV/AIDS.
D. Immunosuppression.
E. Cytomegalovirus (CMV) infection.
F. Familial predisposition.
  1. Neurofibromatosis type 1 (NF1) and type 2 (NF2).
  2. Li–Fraumeni syndrome.
  3. Turcot syndrome.

Subjective Data

A. Common complaints/symptoms.
  1. Patients with low-grade tumors may initially be asymptomatic.
  2. Symptoms are related to compression of intracranial structures and/or increased intracranial pressure (ICP).
  3. Nausea and/or vomiting may occur due to increased ICP.
  4. Neurological symptoms.
    a. Seizures.
    b. Headaches.
    c. Focal neurological deficits.
    d. Syncope.
    e. Visual changes.
    f. Gait instability.
  5. Symptoms/signs associated with pituitary tumors (e.g., prolactinomas).
    a. Bitemporal hemianopsia due to compression of the optic chiasm.
    b. Spontaneous bilateral nipple discharge.
    c. Hypogonadism.

Physical Examination

A. Assess for evidence of primary tumors (most commonly lung followed by melanoma, renal cell, breast, and colorectal).
B. A full neurological exam must be performed in all patients with suspected brain tumors.
  1. Mini-Mental State Exam.
  2. Motor strength in all extremities.
  3. Sensory testing.
  4. Visual field testing.
  5. Reflexes.
  6. Cranial nerve testing.
  7. Gait and cerebellar assessment.
  8. Rectal tone.

Diagnostic Tests

A. Contrast enhanced MRI (diagnostic standard).

B. Single photon emission CT (SPECT) imaging may be used to detect defects in the blood-brain barrier and may be considered to distinguish benign from malignant brain lesions.
C. Consider lumbar puncture (contraindicated if evidence of elevated intracranial pressure).
D. Hormone evaluation for pituitary tumors.
E. Consider metastatic disease.
   1. If metastatic disease is suspected, search for primary tumor (most commonly lung primary).
   2. Biopsy of brain lesion is not necessary if metastatic disease is confirmed.

Differential Diagnosis

A. Gliomas.
B. Meningiomas.
C. Nerve sheath tumors.
D. Pituitary tumors.
E. Primary CNS lymphomas.

Evaluation and Management Plan

A. General plan.
   1. Management of brain tumors is dependent on definitive pathology for diagnosis.
   2. Biopsy or total resection (if possible) is recommended for all suspected brain malignancy.
   3. The blood–brain barrier limits CNS penetration of many chemotherapies.
   4. Treatment approach varies depending on grade.
      a. Low-grade glioma (grade I or II).
         i. Maximal safe resection is recommended for all patients.
         ii. Low-risk patients.
            1) Observation postoperatively is reasonable due to slow growth.
            2) MRI should be obtained every 3 to 6 months for the first 5 years, then annually.
         iii. High-risk patients.
            1) Age greater than 40, subtotal resection, or unfavorable molecular features.
            2) Consider radiation and adjuvant chemotherapy.
      b. High-grade glioma (grade III or IV).
         i. Maximal safe resection.
         ii. Combination therapy with adjuvant radiation therapy and chemotherapy following resection.
         iii. Chemotherapy.
         iv. Targeted therapy.
   5. Seizure prophylaxis.
      a. Patients with no prior history of seizures generally do not require prophylactic anticonvulsants.
      b. Patients undergoing surgical resection of supratentorial tumors should be placed on prophylactic anticonvulsants.
B. Acute care issues in brain/CNS cancers.
   1. Seizures.
   2. Cerebral edema.

Follow-Up

A. Follow-up with the team on a regular basis is important, including medical oncology, radiation oncology, and the neurosurgeon.

Consultation/Referral

A. Referral to a neurosurgeon for biopsy/resection.

1. Histologic review of the biopsy is the most crucial component of diagnosing brain tumors.
2. Histologic classification dictates therapeutic approach.
3. Pathologic review.

Special/Geriatric Considerations

A. Prognosis of the patient is highly dependent on tumor location, the ability to resect it, tumor type, and age of patient.
B. Patients may develop seizures related to the location or aggressiveness of the tumor.

Bibliography

Ostrom, Q. T., Gittleman, H., Fulop, J., Liu, M., Blanda, R., Kromer, C., . . . Barnholtz-Sloan, J. S. (2015). CBTRUS Statistical Report: Primary brain and central nervous system tumors diagnosed in the United States in 2008–2012. *Neuro Oncology, 17*(Suppl. 4), iv1–iv62.

Breast Cancer

Alicia John

Definition

A. Uncontrolled growth of breast cells, usually forming a tumor that can be felt as a lump or seen on a x-ray.
B. Malignant tumors invade the surrounding tissues or metastasize to distant body areas.
C. Breast cancer can be curable, and early detection yields a favorable prognosis.

Incidence

A. Breast cancer is the most commonly diagnosed cancer in American women, and approximately 12.4% of women in the United States will develop invasive breast cancer during their lifetime.
B. After increasing for more than 20 years, breast cancer incidence rates in women have stabilized since 2000, possibly related to fewer women using hormone replacement therapy after menopause.
C. Breast cancer is the second leading cause of cancer deaths in women, second only to lung cancer.
D. The chance that a woman will die from breast cancer is about 1 in 36 (~3%).
E. The median age of diagnosis of breast cancer for women in the United States is 68.
F. Fewer than 5% of women diagnosed with breast cancer in the United States are younger than 40.
G. Risk of breast cancer increases with age, and is highest for women over the age of 70.
H. Breast cancer is much less common in men than in women, with men in the United States experiencing a 1 in 1,000 lifetime risk of developing breast cancer.

Pathogenesis

A. Ductal carcinoma in situ (DCIS).
   1. DCIS is considered noninvasive or preinvasive breast cancer.
   2. The cells that line the ducts of the breast have become dysplastic but remain contained within the walls of the ducts and have not spread into the surrounding breast tissue.
   3. DCIS accounts for approximately 20% of new diagnoses of breast cancer.

B. Lobular carcinoma in situ (LCIS).

1. LCIS is a collection of abnormal cellular growth inside one or more of the milk-producing glands in the breast (called lobules).

2. As the abnormal cells have not grown outside of the lobules, it is considered "in situ."

3. Although it is not considered cancer, it is associated with a higher risk of developing invasive cancer in the future.

4. LCIS is not very common and usually occurs in premenopausal women.

5. LCIS is considered higher risk as it typically does not cause symptoms and can be difficult to see on imaging, making it difficult to detect.

6. It is usually found incidentally when the breast is biopsied for some other reason.

C. Invasive ductal carcinoma (IDC).

1. This is the most common type of breast cancer and accounts for approximately 80% to 85% of all new breast cancer diagnoses.

2. IDC (or infiltrating) starts within the duct and grows into the adipose tissue of the breast.

3. Breaking beyond the ductal wall means it now has the capability to spread to other areas of the body through lymphatic spread.

D. Invasive lobular carcinoma (ILC).

1. ILC starts in the milk-producing glands (lobules) and has invaded into the adipose tissue of the breast and therefore can metastasize to other parts of the body.

2. Accounts for about 10% of breast cancers.

3. It is considered higher risk as it can be difficult to see on imaging, making detection and monitoring for recurrence difficult.

E. Inflammatory breast cancer (IBC).

1. IBC is a rare but aggressive form of invasive breast cancer, and accounts for about 1% to 3% of all breast cancers.

2. There may not be a palpable mass or tumor, so it may not be seen on imaging. Sometimes skin thickening can be seen on mammogram.

3. Often mistaken as cellulitis of the breast, as it presents with redness, warmth, and edema to the skin of the breast, often causing an orange peel appearance.

a. This is caused not by infection but by cancer cells blocking lymph vessels in the skin, causing congestion.

b. If cellulitis is suspected and the patient fails to respond after a course of antibiotics, timely or prompt mammogram and biopsy should be considered.

4. Time is of the essence with IBC given the strong potential for rapid progression.

5. IBC is considered a more aggressive breast cancer and is associated with poorer prognosis when compared to IDC.

F. Other less common breast cancers and tumors: Angiosarcoma, medullary, mucinous, Paget's disease, papillary, phyllodes, tubular.

Predisposing Factors

A. Nonmodifiable.

1. Family history.

2. Genetic mutation or diagnosis (including *BRCA1/2* gene mutations, Cowden syndrome, and Li–Fraumeni syndrome).

3. Race (white women are more likely to develop breast cancer than other ethnicities).

4. Gender (women > men).

5. Personal history of breast cancer.

6. Breast cellular changes (such as hyperplasia).

B. Modifiable.

1. Smoking.

2. Obesity (fat cells produce estrogen).

3. Increased alcohol consumption (alcohol can limit your liver's ability to control blood levels of the hormone estrogen).

4. Sedentary lifestyle.

5. Exposure to estrogen (nulliparity, early onset of menorrhea, delayed onset of menopause, hormone replacement therapy, never breastfeeding).

6. Use of oral contraceptives (there is an immediate increased risk, but that risk resolves over time after discontinuation).

7. Prior radiation to the breast or chest wall.

Subjective Data

A. Common complaints/symptoms.

1. Localized disease.

a. Pain, swelling, or redness in the breast.

b. Nipple changes, inversion, or discharge.

c. Skin changes, thickening, dimpling, or scaling in the breast or nipple.

d. With lymphatic spread, patients may experience painful or enlarged lymph nodes in the axilla, chest, or neck.

2. Metastatic disease.

a. Weight loss and/or change in appetite.

b. Persistent, nagging, or worsening pain (visceral or bone/joint).

c. Shortness of breath or cough.

d. Headache.

e. Fatigue.

B. Common/typical scenario.

1. Due to increased awareness and screening, breast cancer can frequently be found on screening mammograms, by self-breast examination, or by providers performing breast surveillance examinations.

2. When patients present with symptoms outside of the breast, they likely have already developed metastatic disease.

Physical Examination

A. In addition to evaluating for disease in the primary site (breast), evaluate for possible metastatic disease.

B. The most common sites of breast cancer metastases are brain, bone, liver, and lung.

C. Check vital signs including pulse oximetry.

D. A thorough baseline cardiac examination is important, as some chemotherapies used to treat breast cancer are associated with risk for cardiotoxicity. Many chemotherapies used to treat breast cancer can cause neuropathies, so it is important to assess for any preexisting neuropathies at baseline that may not be related to cancer (such as diabetic neuropathy or prior nerve damage due to injury).

E. Breast examination.

1. Should be performed in the sitting position with arms at side and raised above head, and again while lying supine with the same arm positions. If a patient has a self-palpated mass, ask the patient in which position he or she was best able to feel the mass. Do not forget to also examine the nipple–areolar complex.

2. Once the mass is located, measure with a disposable measuring tape by isolating the mass between the thumb and forefinger and noting the distance between your digits. Note which quadrant of the breast the mass is in.

3. Assess the skin of the breast, including skin overlying the mass and the nipple for changes such as redness, peau d'orange appearance, edema, scaliness, or even an open lesion.

4. If the patient notes nipple discharge, the breast can be gently pressed to try and elicit the discharge so the output can be evaluated. If unable to easily express discharge, do not utilize increasing pressure. Sometimes the patient will have discharge that has collected in a bandage or her bra that can be evaluated. Note the color, amount, and consistency.

5. Lymph nodes should also be evaluated in the sitting and supine positions. Include bilateral evaluation of axilla, supraclavicular, infraclavicular, cervical, and mandibular regions. If lymph nodes are palpated, note size, consistency, if fixed or mobile, and if patient reports tenderness with palpation.

F. Evaluate for metastatic disease.

1. Pulmonary: Observe for signs of dyspnea, increased work of breathing, or retractions; evaluate for pleural effusions (auscultation, percussion, and cacophony).

2. Musculoskeletal: Bone tenderness, impaired range of motion.

3. Abdomen: Assess for hepatomegaly, ascites, mass, or tenderness.

4. Neurological: Incoordination, focal deficits, visual changes, hearing changes, decreased strength.

Diagnostic Tests

A. History and physical examination.

B. Diagnostic bilateral mammogram with tomosynthesis, which provides higher resolution when evaluating someone who has a known mass or breast abnormality; ultrasound of the breast as necessary (or as recommended by the radiologist).

C. Breast biopsy and clip placement. Ultrasound of nodal basin on the ipsilateral side.

D. Pathology review; determination of hormone receptor status (estrogen/progesterone receptor and human epidermal growth factor receptor 2 [HER2]).

E. Breast MRI when indicated. This is usually recommended by the radiologist if dense breast tissue obscures the mass, there is a question of the size of the mass, or concern is observed for involvement of the chest wall.

F. Breast cancer is predictable. It starts in the breast, moves to the regional lymph nodes, and then metastasizes to distant sites in the body. If nodal ultrasound is negative and there are no findings on physical examination to suggest metastasis, systemic staging is not indicated (per National Comprehensive Cancer Network [NCCN] guidelines). If a suspicious node is noted on imaging or examination, proceed with biopsy of lymph node. If positive, proceed with metastatic workup.

1. Complete blood count (CBC), comprehensive metabolic panel (CMP).

2. CT chest, abdomen, pelvis with contrast.

3. Bone scan.

4. PET scan, if indicated.

G. Diagnosis.

1. Tissue sample or biopsy is required for diagnosis. Pathology results will help guide the next step of workup, referral/provider evaluation, and recommended interventions.

2. It is imperative to send biopsy sample(s) for estrogen/progesterone (ER/PR) and HER-2/neu testing, as these results are required for prognostication and therapy recommendations.

H. Staging: Breast cancer is staged utilizing the American Joint Committee on Cancer (AJCC) tumor, node, metastasis (TNM) system.

Differential Diagnosis

A. DCIS.

B. LCIS.

C. IDC.

D. ILC.

E. IBC.

F. Paget's disease.

G. Abscess.

H. Fibroadenoma.

Evaluation and Management Plan

A. General plan.

1. Unless there is metastatic disease at the time of presentation, all patients that can tolerate surgery will be offered surgical intervention.

2. Depending on stage, some patients will also be offered chemo and/or radiation.

3. If the cancer is estrogen or progesterone positive, they may also be offered adjuvant hormone therapy.

4. Surgery.

5. Radiation therapy.

6. Chemotherapy.

7. Hormone therapy.

a. About two out of three breast cancers are hormone receptor-positive.

b. These cells have estrogen (ER-positive) and/or progesterone (PR-positive) receptors on the cell surface that stimulate cell proliferation in the presence of estrogen or progesterone, respectively.

B. Acute care issues in breast cancer.

1. Breast cancer patients are typically only admitted for surgical resection.

a. Some procedures, such as segmental mastectomy, are outpatient procedures.

b. More involved procedures, such as total mastectomy or those receiving immediate breast reconstruction, may require postoperative admission.

2. Neutropenic fever (also see sections on Leukemias).

a. Neutropenia may occur as a chemotherapy side effect, and neutropenic patients are highly susceptible to infection.

b. Neutropenic fever can be life-threatening and can rapidly lead to sepsis.

c. Diagnostics include CBC with differential, blood cultures, urinalysis with culture, chest x-ray, sputum culture (if appropriate), intravenous (IV) fluid support (if appropriate), antipyretics, and empiric broad-spectrum antibiotics.

d. Use of granulocyte stimulating colony factor (G-CSF) may be considered for neutropenia.

3. Metastatic symptoms.

a. The most common sites of metastatic spread from breast cancer are bone, brain, liver, and lung.

b. Patients with metastatic disease may be admitted for pain management or symptoms resulting from an organ system being affected by disease such as:

i. Fluid retention or transaminitis from hepatic metastasis.

ii. Confusion related to brain metastasis.

iii. Pain and/or fracture from metastasis to the bone.

TABLE 13.1   **Breast Cancer Follow-Up**

	NCCN	ACS/ASCO
History physical examination	Year 1, every 3–4 mo Year 2, every 4 mo Year 3–5, every 6 mo Year 6+, annually	Year 1–3, every 3–6 mo Year 4–5, every 6–12 mo Year 6+, annually
Signs of recurrence	No recommendation	Educated and counseled about signs and symptoms
Mammography	6 mo after post-BCS radiation therapy Annually thereafter	Annually
MRI	No recommendation	Not recommended for routine screening unless patient meets high-risk criteria for increased surveillance
Pelvic examination	Annually, for woman on tamoxifen Annual exam if uterus present	No recommendation
Routine blood tests	No recommendation	No recommendation
Imaging studies	No recommendation	No recommendation
Tumor marker testing	No recommendation	No recommendation

ACS, American Cancer Society; ASCO, American Society of Clinical Oncology; BCS, Breast Cancer Society; NCCN, National Comprehensive Cancer Network.

Follow-Up

A. See Table 13.1.

Consultation/Referral

A. Medical oncology.
B. Breast surgical oncology.
C. Radiation oncology (can be done prior to or after surgery and/or chemotherapy; or for palliation if metastatic).
D. Fertility specialist, if appropriate.
E. Cardiology referral may be indicated prior to chemotherapy or surgery as chemotherapeutic regimens (i.e., anthracyclines) can cause cardiotoxicity or lead to evaluate for anesthesia clearance.
F. Genetic counseling: If indicated according to NCCN guidelines.
G. Any patient with suspected breast cancer needs to be seen urgently by a specialist or breast clinic.
H. Consider referrals to support groups and psychiatry for assistance in coping.

Special/Geriatric Considerations

A. Treatment guidelines for elderly patients with breast cancer are limited.
B. Treatment recommendations should be decided in conjunction with the patient and based on life expectancy as well as the patient's functional status, comorbidities, and social support.

Bibliography

National Cancer Institute. (n.d.). Fast stats. Retrieved from https://seer.cancer.gov/faststats/selections.php?series=cancer
NCCN. (2017, November 10). Clinical practice guidelines in oncology. *Breast cancer* (Version 3. 3017). Fort Washington, PA: National Comprehensive Cancer Network.
Runowicz, C. D., Leach, C. R., Henry, N. L., Henry, K. S., Mackey, H. T., Cowens-Alvarado, R. L., & Ganz, P. A. (2016). American Cancer Society/American Society of Clinical Oncology breast cancer survivorship care guideline. *CA: A Cancer Journal for Clinicians, 66*, 43–73. doi:10.3322/caac.21319

Gastrointestinal Cancers: Colorectal Cancer

Cheryl Pfennig, Karen A. Beaty, Erin Michelle Dean, Rae Brana Reynolds, and Leigh A. Samp

Definition

A. Cancer that forms in the tissues of the colon.
B. Most colon cancers are adenocarcinomas and develop from polyps.

Incidence

A. Colorectal cancer is the third most common cancer in both men and women, and is also the third leading cause of cancer deaths.
B. In 2016, there were an estimated 134,490 cases diagnosed in the United States: 39,220 cases of rectal cancer and 95,270 cases of colon cancer.
C. The incidence of colon cancer has continued to decline over the past three decades, likely associated with improved screening and treatment of colorectal polyps. Despite this decline, there were still an estimated 49,140 deaths from colon and rectal cancer in 2016.
D. Greater than 90% of new cases of colorectal cancer occur in patients over the age of 50, with the median onset age at 73.
E. While the risk of colorectal cancer increases with age, in recent years there has been a significant increase in the incidence of colorectal cancer in younger patients.

Pathogenesis

A. Colorectal cancer is a complex process that derives from the epithelial cells lining the colon.
B. Genetic mutations, either inherited or acquired, are thought to occur that irritate the lining, causing inflammation and necrosis of the colon.
C. Over time, lesions can develop which can disrupt cellular DNA and cause dysplasia, which can lead to the development of cancer.

Predisposing Factors

A. Approximately 2% to 5% of colorectal cancers are hereditary, while the majority of cases are sporadic.

B. Risk factors associated with the development of colorectal cancer include:

    1. Dietary factors including the consumption of red meat, processed meat, and animal fat.

    2. Cigarette smoking.

    3. Inflammatory bowel disease (e.g., ulcerative colitis).

    4. History of a prior colorectal cancer or adenomatous polyps.

    5. Obesity.

    6. Familial syndromes: Familial adenomatous polyposis (FAP) or hereditary nonpolyposis colorectal cancer (HNPCC).

Subjective Data

A. Common complaints/symptoms.

    1. Colorectal cancer is often asymptomatic, with symptoms appearing once the disease has become more advanced. Screening colonoscopies often detect early, asymptomatic colorectal cancers.

    2. The most common presenting signs and symptoms include:

        a. Abdominal pain.

        b. Anorectal pain.

        c. Iron deficiency anemia.

        d. Weight loss.

        e. Fatigue.

        f. Hematochezia.

        g. Melena.

        h. Bowel changes.

            i. Constipation.

            ii. Diarrhea.

            iii. Urgency.

            iv. Frequency.

            v. Tenesmus.

            vi. Mucous discharge.

        i. Nausea/vomiting.

        j. Urinary dysfunction.

        k. Erectile dysfunction.

Physical Examination

A. Gastrointestinal.

    1. Percussion.

        a. Dull areas may be present over the tumor site.

        b. A protuberant, tympanic abdomen may be indicative of an obstruction.

    2. Auscultate for bowel sounds in all four quadrants.

        a. Absent or decreased bowel sounds are often indicative of obstruction.

    3. Palpate for tenderness and/or masses in all four quadrants.

        a. Larger tumors of the colon are often palpable on physical examination in nonobese patients.

        b. Liver is one of the two most common sites for colorectal metastasis, and patients with advanced liver metastasis may have tender hepatomegaly.

    4. Digital rectal examination to assess for tumor location, circumferential nature, and sphincter tone.

B. Gynecologic examination in females with rectal cancer is important secondary to the proximity of the rectum to the vagina. Vaginal examination should be performed to evaluate for posterior vaginal wall involvement and to rule out rectovaginal fistula.

C. Evaluate for metastatic disease: Primarily liver, lung, and/or lymph nodes.

Diagnostic Tests

A. The workup for colorectal cancers includes diagnostic studies to help determine the extent of disease, as well as the presence of metastatic disease.

B. Colon cancer workup.

    1. Colonoscopy, complete to the cecum with adequately prepped colon.

    2. Pathology review of biopsies.

    3. Laboratory studies: Complete blood count (CBC), comprehensive metabolic panel (CMP), carcinoembryonic antigen (CEA) level.

    4. CT scan of the chest, abdomen, and pelvis with intravenous (IV) and oral contrast.

C. Rectal cancer workup.

    1. Colonoscopy, complete to the cecum with adequately prepped colon.

    2. Pathology review of biopsies.

    3. Laboratory studies: CBC, CMP, CEA.

    4. CT scan of the chest, abdomen, and pelvis with IV and oral contrast.

    5. Pelvic MRI is the preferred staging study; however, if not available, perform endorectal ultrasound.

    6. Flexible sigmoidoscopy or rigid proctoscopy is often performed by a surgeon to verify the tumor location for radiation treatment planning and surgery planning.

    7. Enterostomal therapist referral is made for patient education and ostomy site marking.

D. Diagnosis and staging.

    1. Colorectal cancer diagnosis is established via tissue biopsy. Colonoscopy is the most common mode to obtain a tissue diagnosis, although an image-guided biopsy of a tumor may confirm the diagnosis.

    2. Adenocarcinomas are the most common histologic subtype, accounting for greater than 90% of all cases. Less common histologic subtypes include: Mucinous carcinoma, signet-ring cell carcinoma, squamous cell carcinoma, and undifferentiated carcinoma.

    3. Confirmed tissue diagnosis and a complete workup provide the necessary data to clinically stage colorectal cancer. Proper clinical staging is important, as it influences treatment planning and serves as an indicator for prognosis.

    4. Staging for colorectal cancer is similar to the staging of many cancers, and utilizes the tumor, node, metastasis (TNM) system.

Differential Diagnosis

A. Inflammatory bowel disease.

B. Ileus.

C. Ischemic bowel.

D. Diverticulosis.

Evaluation and Management Plan

A. General plan.

    1. The primary treatment for colorectal cancer is surgery; however, disease stage and presence of metastatic disease can alter the treatment modalities offered as well as their sequencing.

    2. Chemotherapy agents are commonly administered in the adjuvant setting; however, they may be administered in patients with locally advanced disease or with metastatic disease at presentation.

    3. Radiation therapy.

    4. Surgical management for colorectal cancers.

        a. Should include resection of the primary tumor, as well as the lymphatic, venous, and arterial supply.

b. Treatment side effects are a potential threat from all three treatment modalities with the most common including:

 i. Bowel dysfunction.

 ii. Sexual dysfunction.

 iii. Genitourinary dysfunction.

 iv. Neuropathies.

B. Acute care issues in colorectal cancer.

 1. Colorectal cancer patients will be admitted to the hospital following surgical resection or for urgent situations including bowel obstructions or perforations.

 2. Postoperative hospitalization varies by surgical approach. The average hospital stay is 2 to 7 days, with a shorter average stay for patients who have undergone a minimally invasive surgical approach.

  a. Postoperative management is focused on return of bowel function, ostomy care (if applicable), and pain control.

 3. Patients admitted for complications such as bowel obstruction or perforation are managed based on the severity of the complication.

  a. Bowel obstruction.

   i. Nothing by mouth (NPO) and bowel rest.

   ii. Nasogastric tube.

   iii. Surgery: Exploratory laparotomy with possible bowel resection.

  b. Perforation.

   i. NPO and bowel rest.

   ii. Surgery is indicated in the majority of cases to remove the area of perforation and to wash out the abdomen.

   iii. Antibiotics.

Follow-Up

A. Colon cancer recurrence typically occurs within 3 years of resection; therefore, patients should have routine follow-up for at least 5 years after resection.

B. Colonoscopy is necessary after resection for surveillance.

Consultation/Referral

A. Gastroenterology referral for screening is critical in patients who are high risk for colorectal cancer.

B. Any patient with suspected colon cancer should be referred to surgery immediately. Surgery is the only curative option for localized cancer and should not be delayed.

C. Medical oncology referral for treatment and surveillance.

D. Refer patients to support groups.

Special/Geriatric Considerations

A. Most patients with colorectal cancer are older than 70 years old.

B. Elderly patients may be undertreated and are underrepresented in clinical trials, making treatment guidelines difficult.

C. Life expectancy, quality of life, and patient's functional status should be taken into consideration when determining a plan of action.

Bibliography

Jasperson, K. W., Tuohy, T. M., Neklason, D. W., & Burt, R. W. (2010). Hereditary and familial colon cancer. *Gastroenterology, 138*(6), 2044–2058.

National Cancer Institute. (2016, September 12). Surveillance, epidemiology, and end results program. Retrieved from https://seer.cancer.gov/faststats/selections.php?series=cancer

Gastrointestinal Cancers: Gastric Cancer

Cheryl Pfennig, Karen Beaty, Erin Michelle Dean, Rae Brana Reynolds, and Leigh A. Samp

Definition

A. A malignant tumor of the stomach.

B. Most cancers of the stomach are adenocarcinomas: Malignant tumors that develop from the cells in the lining of the stomach.

Incidence

A. Gastric cancer is the third most common cause of cancer-related mortality worldwide.

B. In the United States, approximately 22,220 patients are diagnosed annually, 10,990 of whom are expected to die from gastric cancer.

C. The worldwide incidence of gastric cancer has declined over the past few decades, partly due to the recognition of risk factors such as *Helicobacter pylori* and dietary risks.

D. The overall 5-year relative survival rate of all people with stomach cancer in the United States is about 30%.

Pathogenesis

A. Gastric cancer is a malignant neoplasm that arises anywhere between the gastroesophageal junction and pylorus.

B. Most tumors are epithelial in origin and classified as adenocarcinomas.

C. *H. pylori* infection is strongly associated with the presence of precancerous lesions that manifest into cancer proliferation. Over 80% of gastric cancers are thought to be attributed to *H. pylori* infection.

Predisposing Factors

A. Chronic gastritis caused by:

 1. Chronic *H. pylori* infection.

 2. Pernicious anemia.

 3. Diet.

  a. Diet high in salt and salt-preserved foods, nitrates, nitrites, fried foods, processed meats, alcohol.

  b. Diets low in vegetables (diets high in fruits, vegetables, and fiber are protective against gastric cancer).

B. Obesity.

C. Smoking.

D. Prior gastric surgery.

E. Prior abdominal radiation.

F. Male gender.

G. African American race.

H. Inherited germline mutations in *TP53*, *BRCA2*, and *CDH1*.

Subjective Data

A. Common complaints/symptoms.

 1. Unintentional weight loss secondary to insufficient caloric intake caused by tumor related anorexia, nausea, abdominal pain, early satiet-, and/or dysphagia.

 2. Bowel changes: Melena or black tarry stools, constipation if treating pain, nausea, anemia, change in nature or pattern of bowel habits if an obstructing tumor.

 3. Persistent vague, epigastric abdominal pain.

 4. Dysphagia, especially for tumors in the proximal stomach or gastroesophageal junction.

 5. Fatigue secondary to anemia from bleeding tumors.

Physical Examination

A. Focused areas of the physical examination for suspected gastric cancer should include:

1. Vital signs.

a. Evaluate weight and recent trends for unintentional weight loss.

b. Heart rate: Tachycardia suggestive of dehydration secondary to poor oral intake.

2. Head, ear, eyes, nose, and throat (HEENT).

a. Evaluate oral mucosa for paleness suggestive of anemia.

b. Evaluate tongue for evidence of thrush.

c. Quality of dentition.

3. Palpate neck and cervical nodal chains for adenopathy suggestive of metastasis.

4. Abdominal examination.

a. Observe for contour of the abdomen and distention, evidence of cachexia.

b. Evaluate the skin, subcutaneous tissue, and umbilicus.

c. Auscultate abdomen noting the frequency and character of bowel sounds, normally 5 to 30 gurgling sounds per minute.

d. Palpation: Prior to palpation, ask about any tender areas and palpate this area last; commonly tender in the epigastric region secondary to reflux.

e. Evaluate for abdominal firmness suggesting carcinomatosis and ascites.

f. Evaluate for nodularity in the umbilical area suggestive of a Sister Mary Joseph nodule demonstrating umbilical metastasis.

g. Palpate for hepatosplenomegaly suggestive of metastasis.

Diagnostic Tests

A. Complete history and physical examination.

B. Laboratory tests including complete blood count (CBC) with differential and comprehensive metabolic panel (CMP).

C. Upper gastrointestinal (GI) series with barium swallow as initial screening for patients with dysphagia.

D. CT of the chest, abdomen, and pelvis.

E. Esophagogastroduodenoscopy (EGD) for tissue diagnosis and anatomic location.

F. Endoscopic ultrasound (EUS) if no evidence of distant metastatic disease.

G. Diagnostic laparoscopy with biopsy and peritoneal lavage to evaluate for radiographically occult metastatic disease and carcinomatosis.

H. Diagnosis: Tissue diagnosis and anatomic localization of the primary tumor are best obtained by upper GI endoscopy.

I. Staging.

1. Gastric cancers that are 5 cm or more from the gastroesophageal junction are staged using the tumor, node, metastasis (TNM) system as gastric cancers.

2. Gastric cancers that are less than 5 cm from the gastroesophageal junction are staged using the TNM system as esophageal cancers.

Differential Diagnosis

A. Gastritis.

B. Gastroenteritis.

C. Esophagitis.

D. Esophageal cancer.

E. Peptic ulcer disease.

F. Neoplasm.

Evaluation and Management Plan

A. General plan and treatment.

1. Tissue diagnosis and staging evaluation are required for treatment planning.

2. Surgical resection is required for cure of gastric cancer.

3. Surgery followed by chemotherapy +/− radiation is the mainstay of treatment.

4. Surgery.

5. Advanced metastatic disease (stage IV) is treated with palliative chemotherapy or on a clinical trial.

B. Acute care issues in gastric cancer.

1. Gastric cancer patients are often only admitted for surgical resection.

2. Postoperative gastric surgery patients without complications will spend 7 to 10 days in the hospital after surgery.

3. The primary focus in the postoperative inpatient setting is nutrition, pain control, monitoring lab work, wound care, and early ambulation.

a. Routine blood work including CBC with differential, electrolyte panel, blood urea nitrogen (BUN), and creatinine must be monitored for anemia, infection, electrolyte imbalance/need for replacement, and kidney function.

b. The incision site will be monitored daily for signs of infection and proper healing.

c. The postgastrectomy patient will have a nasogastric tube in place. Once there is no evidence of anastomotic leak, the nasogastric tube may be removed.

d. Supplemental jejunostomy tube feedings will be initiated on postoperative day one and will continue until oral intake is adequate.

e. Oral feeding is started 4 to 7 days postoperatively.

f. Upper GI studies are done as indicated (fever, tachycardia, tachypnea, leukocytosis).

g. Early ambulation reduces risk of postoperative pneumonia, ileus, and thrombosis. The goal is to have the patient out of bed the day after the procedure as tolerated.

h. Postoperative cancer patients have a hypercoagulable state; prophylactic enoxaparin is initiated postoperatively and continued for 28 days.

Follow-Up

A. Postgastrectomy complications.

1. Duodenal stump or anastomotic leak.

a. Anastomotic leak: Arises from any of the suture/staple lines of the anastomosis.

b. Duodenal stump leak: Most feared complication of gastrectomy.

c. Symptoms: Severe abdominal pain, fever, tachycardia, hypotension.

d. CT abdomen is indicated.

i. Findings: Pneumoperitoneum, extraluminal contrast, fluid collection, and/or abscess.

e. Upper GI series (with Gastrografin) may also be performed to assess leak.

f. Treatment.

i. Broad-spectrum antibiotics.

ii. Consider percutaneous drainage of fluid collection/abscess by interventional radiology.

iii. If leak persists or patient is hemodynamically unstable, patient should be taken to the operating room for exploration, drainage, and repair.

2. Dumping syndrome.

   a. Postgastrectomy patients commonly have rapid transit and report diarrhea.

   b. Dumping syndrome is characterized by diaphoresis, abdominal cramps, and watery diarrhea shortly after intake of concentrated sweets and hyperosmolar liquids.

   c. Diagnosis is based on clinical symptoms.

      i. Gastric emptying studies or upper GI series may be performed.

   d. Treatment.

      i. Primary goal includes dietary changes with frequent small meals that are high in fiber and low in carbohydrates. Avoid food triggers (e.g., simple sugar).

      ii. Octreotide may help but is not typically required.

Consultation/Referral

A. In patients with suspected gastric cancer, consults should be made to gastroenterology, radiation oncology, medical oncology, and surgery.

Special/Geriatric Considerations

A. Most cases of gastric cancer affect the elderly.

B. Aggressive treatment and surgery should not be withheld from patients solely due to chronological age.

C. Life expectancy, quality of life, and patient's functional status need to be taken into consideration in conjunction with patient wishes.

Bibliography

National Cancer Institute. (2016, September 12). Surveillance, epidemiology, and end results program. Retrieved from https://seer.cancer.gov/faststats/selections.php?series=cancer

Siegel, R., Ma, J., Zou, Z., & Jemal, A. (2014). Cancer statistics, 2014. *CA: A Cancer Journal for Clinicians, 64*(1), 9–29.

Zhu, A. L., & Sonnenberg, A. (2012). Is gastric cancer again rising? *Journal of Clinical Gastroenterology, 46*, 804–806.

Gastrointestinal Cancers: Hepatic Cancer

Cheryl Pfennig, Karen Beaty, Erin Michelle Dean, Rae Brana Reynolds, and Leigh A. Samp

Definition

A. Hepatocellular carcinoma (HCC) is the most common form of primary liver cancer in adults.

B. Other cancers that begin in the liver include intrahepatic cholangiocarcinoma (about 10%–20%) and less common tumors such as angiosarcomas, hemangiosarcomas, hepatoblastomas, and malignant epithelioid hemangioendotheliomas.

Incidence

A. Liver cancer occurs primarily in people ages 55 to 64, with a median age of 63 at diagnosis.

B. Liver and bile duct cancers are relatively rare when compared with other cancers.

C. In 2016, an estimated 39,230 cases were diagnosed in the United States, and about 27,170 people died of liver and intrahepatic cholangiocarcinoma.

D. The survival rate among individuals with liver cancer varies based on staging at the time of diagnosis.

E. Surveillance, epidemiology, and end results (SEER) data estimates that 43% of patients present with localized disease (confined to the primary site), 27% have disease that has spread to regional lymph nodes, and 18% present with distant metastases.

F. The 5-year relative survival rates for each are 30.9%, 10.9%, and 3.1%, respectively.

G. The incidence and mortality rates of HCC are on the rise in the United States.

Pathogenesis

A. There is a strong association with inflammation, necrosis, fibrosis, and cirrhosis in the development of HCC.

B. Some gene mutations have been identified as the cause of uncontrolled division of cells in the liver, leading to development of cancer.

C. HCC has several different subtypes, each with different growth patterns.

Predisposing Factors

A. Male sex.

B. Chronic hepatitis B and C virus infections.

C. Alcohol-related cirrhosis.

D. Nonalcoholic fatty liver disease (NAFLD).

E. Exposure to certain chemicals (e.g., nitrites, hydrocarbons, and polychlorinated biphenyls).

F. Dietary intake of aflatoxins (toxic metabolites produced by certain fungi in foods and feeds).

G. Metabolic disorders such as hemochromatosis, Wilson's disease, and Alpha-1 antitrypsin deficiency.

Presence of hepatocellular adenoma (unclear risk of malignant transformation to HCC).

Subjective Data

A. The presentation of liver cancer is dependent upon the stage of disease.

B. Common complaints/symptoms.

   1. Fatigue.

   2. Abdominal pain/bloating.

   3. Palpable mass in the right upper quadrant.

   4. Signs and symptoms of liver disease: Ascites, jaundice, splenomegaly, portal hypertension.

   5. Nausea.

   6. Decreased appetite and early satiety.

   7. Unexplained weight loss.

   8. Fever.

Physical Examination

A. Check vital signs.

B. Head and neck.

   1. Evaluate for scleral icterus.

   2. Palpate the neck and supraclavicular area for adenopathy. Look for jugular venous distinction.

C. Pulmonary system.

   1. Observe the patient for signs of dyspnea, increased work of breathing, or retractions.

   2. Auscultate all lung fields.

D. Cardiovascular system: Auscultate heart sounds.

E. Gastrointestinal system.

   1. Perform a thorough abdominal examination.

   2. Pay close attention to the right upper quadrant.

   3. Assess for a fluid wave/evidence of ascites, hepatomegaly, an umbilical hernia, and caput medusae.

F. Musculoskeletal system.

   1. Observe for signs of muscle wasting and cachexia.

2. Evaluate lower extremities for pitting edema.
G. Central nervous system: Assess cranial nerves II—XII.
H. Skin: Assess for jaundice, palmar erythema, and spider angiomata.

Diagnostic Tests

A. Laboratory evaluation should include complete blood count (CBC), comprehensive metabolic panel (CMP), prothrombin time/partial thromboplastin time/international normalized ratio (PT/PTT/INR), and prealbumin.
B. Tumor markers: Alpha fetoprotein (AFP) and cancer antigen 19–9 (CA 19–9).
C. CT of the chest, abdomen, and pelvis with contrast.
D. MRI of the abdomen and chest x-ray in patients with PO/IV contrast allergy.
E. EKG if considering surgery.
F. Liver tumor biopsy is *generally* not necessary when considering surgery in the setting of classic imaging findings, elevated tumor markers, and the presence of known risk factors. Patients with fatty liver disease may be referred for biopsy of their underlying (nontumoral) liver to evaluate for percent steatosis and fibrosis, as this impacts their candidacy for surgical resection.
G. Diagnosis.
  1. Diagnosis typically requires a combination of laboratory data, imaging, and biopsy results.
  2. Laboratory data.
    a. Tumor markers are often elevated in patients with liver cancer and can be followed to assess response to therapy or monitored for disease progression.
    b. AFP, while neither specific nor sensitive for HCC, is elevated in 50% to 90% of all patients with HCC.
    c. CA 19–9 is a useful tumor marker and often elevated in cholangiocarcinoma.
  3. Imaging.
    a. Ultrasonography may be used as the initial screening technique in patients being monitored for chronic hepatitis; however, surgical resectability and treatment planning is always based on dedicated, multiphasic imaging of the chest, abdomen, and pelvis.
    b. Triple phase CT assesses the blood flow to liver tissue during early arterial, late arterial, and portal venous phases.
    c. CT imaging typically shows arterial phase enhancement in HCC due to increased vascular supply of the tumor from the hepatic artery.
    d. Metastatic adenocarcinomas and cholangiocarcinomas typically enhance during the portal phase on CT.
  4. Biopsy.
    a. Tissue sampling/biopsy is recommended if the patient is not a candidate for surgery and targeted therapy or systemic chemotherapy is being considered.
    b. Tissue for pathologic confirmation can be obtained through a percutaneous image-guided biopsy of the liver nodule/mass.
H. Staging.
  1. The staging of HCC, like the majority of cancers, follows the American Joint Committee on Cancer (AJCC) tumor, node, metastasis (TNM) system.
  2. Higher numbers indicate more advanced disease.

Differential Diagnosis

1. Cirrhosis.
2. Hepatocellular adenoma.
3. Cholangiocarcinoma.

Evaluation and Management Plan

A. General plan.
  1. Patients with HCC may be offered surgery, targeted therapy/chemotherapy, radiation therapy, liver-directed therapy, or referral for transplantation depending upon multiple factors present at diagnosis including:
    a. Geographic distribution of disease.
    b. The presence of metastatic disease.
    c. Age and comorbidities.
    d. Cirrhosis.
    e. Liver reserve.
  2. Surgery.
  3. Targeted therapy/chemotherapy.
  4. Radiation therapy.
  5. Liver-directed therapy includes percutaneous treatments.
    a. Radiofrequency/laser/microwave ablation.
    b. Cryotherapy.
    c. Ethanol injection.
    d. Transarterial chemoembolization (TACE).
    e. Radioembolization.
  6. Liver transplantation.
B. Acute care issues in hepatic cancer.
  1. Liver cancer patients are often only admitted to the hospital after surgical resection or transplantation.
  2. Patients either undergo a partial hepatectomy (removal of a portion of the right or left liver, which may or may not require resection of an entire segment) or a complete right or left hepatectomy. These surgeries can be performed laparoscopically, open, or via a minimally invasive approach. The gallbladder is sometimes removed at the time of liver resection.
  3. Liver-directed therapies are generally performed in the outpatient setting but can occasionally require hospital admission.

Follow-Up

A. Postoperative liver surgery patients, without complications, will spend an average of 3 to 7 days in the hospital, depending upon the type of surgery performed (laparoscopic vs. open).
B. The primary focus in the postoperative inpatient setting is pain control, early ambulation, monitoring blood counts and liver function tests, wound/drain management, pulmonary toileting to avoid pneumonia, and prevention of blood clots.
C. Patients are evaluated by the inpatient dietician who stresses the importance of adequate protein and fluid intake in the perioperative period and after discharge.

Consultation/Referral

A. Most patients are treated by a multidisciplinary team including both surgical and medical oncologists who formulate a treatment plan based upon clinical staging.
B. Radiation oncologists may be consulted if radiation therapy is being considered.
C. Prior to surgery, patients are often referred to internal medicine to optimize and manage medical comorbidities in the perioperative period.
D. Patients with active hepatitis virus infections are managed by either infectious disease or hepatology specialists.

Special/Geriatric Considerations

A. Surgical resection is the only potentially curative treatment for most hepatic cancers.
B. Decisions to aggressively treat or not treat hepatic cancer in the geriatric population should not be based on age alone.

C. Factors such as life expectancy, quality of life, and patient functional status should be taken into consideration.

Bibliography

National Cancer Institute. (2016, September 12). Surveillance, epidemiology, and end results program. Retrieved from https://seer.cancer.gov/faststats/selections.php?series=cancer

Gastrointestinal Cancers: Pancreatic Cancer

Cheryl Pfennig, Karen Beaty, Erin Michelle Dean, Rae Brana Reynolds, and Leigh A. Samp

Definition

A. Adenocarcinoma of the pancreas (referred to as pancreatic cancer) originates from the exocrine cells of the pancreas.
B. Pancreatic cancer comprises more than 95% of pancreatic malignancies.

Incidence

A. Pancreatic cancer is the fourth leading cause of cancer deaths in the United States with an estimated 53,070 new cases and 41,780 deaths from pancreatic cancer in 2016.
B. The overall risk of developing pancreatic cancer increases after 50 years of age and the majority of patients with disease are between the ages of 60 and 80 years.
C. The only potentially curative therapy for pancreatic cancer is surgical resection of the involved portion of the pancreas in patients with localized disease. Unfortunately, 80% of patients have metastatic and locally advanced disease at initial diagnosis, which precludes curative resection for the majority of patients.
D. In patients who have undergone resection with curative intent, only 10% to 27% of patients survive at least 5 years after surgical resection. Meanwhile, the 5-year overall survival rate for all pancreatic cancer stages combined remains low at 8%.

Pathogenesis

A. Pancreatic cancer is caused by mutations to DNA.
B. Insults to DNA can be hereditary or environmental such as alcohol, smoking, drugs, and obesity.
C. Acute pancreatitis and recurrent acute pancreatitis can develop into chronic pancreatitis, which can convert to pancreatic cancer.
D. Most cases of pancreatic cancer are adenocarcinomas.

Predisposing Factors

A. Cigarette smoking.
B. Alcoholism.
C. Obesity.
D. Chronic pancreatitis.
E. Diabetes mellitus.
F. Family history.
G. Genetic mutations.

Subjective Data

A. Common complaints/symptoms.
   1. Pain.
   2. Jaundice.
   3. Weight loss.
   4. Steatorrhea.
   5. Nausea.
   6. Hyperglycemia.
   7. Diabetes mellitus.
B. Common/typical scenario.
   1. The pancreas is located proximal to the stomach, small intestine, and bile duct so clinical manifestations of pancreatic cancer usually affect the anatomy and function of these adjacent structures. For example:
      a. A pancreatic tumor obstructing the biliary system could cause jaundice.
      b. Nausea, digestive problems, and weight loss may result from obstruction of the upper digestive tract.
      c. Steatorrhea can result from an obstruction of the pancreatic duct that prevents the passage of digestive enzymes into the intestines.

Physical Examination

A. Head and neck: Inspect for scleral icterus and palpate for cervical and supraclavicular lymphadenopathy.
B. Integumentary: Inspect for jaundice.
C. Abdomen: Inspect and palpate for mass effect, ascites, hepatosplenomegaly, and pain.
D. Weight assessment: Measure weight at each visit especially when nutritionally compromised.
E. Complete a full examination including cardiopulmonary, musculoskeletal, and neurology assessment to evaluate the patient's overall fitness for oncology treatment.

Diagnostic Tests

A. Laboratory data.
   1. Complete blood count (CBC).
   2. Comprehensive metabolic panel (CMP).
   3. Prealbumin for nutrition status assessment.
   4. CA 19–9.
B. Diagnostic imaging.
   1. Multiphase helical CT scan.
      a. A CT scan with contrast can correctly predict resectability in pancreatic cancer with 80% to 90% accuracy.
   2. Endoscopic evaluation.
      a. Esophagogastroduodenoscopy (EGD).
      b. Endoscopic retrograde cholangiopancreatography (ERCP).
C. Staging: The American Joint Committee on Cancer (AJCC) has developed a staging system based on tumor, node, metastasis (TNM) status for pancreatic cancer.

Differential Diagnosis

A. Acute pancreatitis.
B. Cholangitis.
C. Cholecystitis.
D. Gastric cancer.
E. Peptic ulcer disease.

Evaluation and Management Plan

A. General plan.
   1. Chemotherapy, radiation, and surgery are utilized in the treatment of pancreatic cancer.
   2. The modalities employed and the sequence in which they are administered often depend on the clinical stage of disease.
   3. Neoadjuvant therapy for pancreatic cancer refers to chemotherapy and/or radiation administered prior to surgery.
   4. Surgery.

a. The majority of pancreatic cancers arise from the pancreatic head and these lesions, if resectable, are treated with a pancreaticoduodenectomy, commonly known as the Whipple procedure.

b. Resectable pancreatic tail cancers are treated with a distal pancreatectomy which can also involve a splenectomy depending on the splenic vessel involvement of the tumor.

5. Chemotherapy.

6. Radiation.

Follow-Up

A. Routine follow-up is essential.

B. Patients should have CT imaging at 3- to 6-month intervals for the first 2 years and then annually.

Consultation/Referral

A. Consults should be made to gastroenterology, medical oncology, radiation oncology, and general surgery.

Special/Geriatric Considerations

A. Prognosis for pancreatic cancer is very poor and largely incurable.

B. The 5-year relative survival rate is 7% for all stages of pancreatic cancer.

Bibliography

Bose, D., Katz, M. H., & Fleming, J. B. (2012). Pancreatic adenocarcinoma. In B. W. Feig & C. D. Ching (Eds.), *The MD Anderson cancer center surgical oncology handbook* (5th ed., pp.). Philadelphia, PA: Wolters Kluwer/Lippincott Williams & Wilkins.

Chatterjee, D., Katz, M. H., Rashid, A., Varadhachary, G. R., Wolff, R. A., Wang, H., . . . Wang, H. (2012). Histologic grading the extent of residual carcinoma following neoadjuvant chemoradiation in pancreatic ductal adenocarcinoma: A predictor for patient outcome. *Cancer, 118*(12), 3182–3190.

Fernandez-del Castillo, C. (2019, January 18). Clinical manifestations, diagnosis, and staging of exocrine pancreatic cancer. In D. M. F. Savarese & K. M. Robson (Eds.), *UpToDate*. Retrieved from https://www.uptodate.com/contents/clinical-manifestations-diagnosis-and-staging-of-exocrine-pancreatic-cancer

Karmazanovsky, G., Fedorov, V., Kubyshkin, V., & Kotchatkov, A. (2005). Pancreatic head cancer: Accuracy of CT in determination of resectability. *Abdominal Imaging, 30*(4), 488–500.

Katz, M. H., Wang, H., Fleming, J. B., Sun, C. C., Hwang, R. F., Wolff, R. A., . . . Evans, D. B. (2009). Long-term survival after multidisciplinary management of resected pancreatic adenocarcinoma. *Annals of Surgical Oncology, 16*(4), 836–847.

National Cancer Institute. (2016, September 12). Surveillance, epidemiology, and end results program. Retrieved from https://seer.cancer.gov/faststats/selections.php?series=cancer

Gynecologic Cancers: Cervical Cancer

Valerie F. Villanueva, Amelita B. Marzan, Annamma Sam, and Cynae Johnson

Definition

A. Types of cervical cancer.

1. The most common type of invasive cervical cancer is squamous cell carcinoma (about 70%–80%).

2. The second most common subtype is adenocarcinoma (10%–15%).

3. Other types include adenosquamous carcinoma, adenoid cystic carcinomas, neuroendocrine tumors of the cervix, undifferentiated cervical cancer, and mixed epithelial and mesenchymal tumors.

Incidence

A. Cervical cancer remains the fourth most common cancer of women worldwide with a mortality rate of ~52%.

B. Approximately 86% of deaths from cervical cancer are in the developing world.

C. Cervical cancer is the third most common gynecologic cancer (after uterine and ovarian cancer) and the 12th most common cancer of women in the United States.

D. An estimated 12,990 new cases of invasive cervical cancer were diagnosed in 2016 and approximately 4,120 deaths from cervical cancer occurred in the United States in 2016.

Pathogenesis

A. Caused by an abnormal growth of cells. Human papillomavirus (HPV) must be present for cervical cancer to develop.

Predisposing Factors

A. Early age of sexual activity: The relative risk of having cervical cancer is 2.5 if the age of first sexual exposure is less than 18 years of age.

B. Multiple sexual partners: Relative risk is 2.8 if the number of partners is five or more.

C. Lower socioeconomic status.

D. Promiscuous sexual partners.

E. Tobacco use.

F. Immunocompromised conditions.

G. In utero exposure to diethylstilbestrol (DES) increases the risk of clear cell carcinoma of the cervix.

H. HPV infection.

1. HPV is a double-stranded DNA virus that belongs to the Papillomaviridae family.

2. There are more than 100 different types of HPV identified, and they are divided into two groups.

a. Low-risk HPV.

b. High-risk HPV.

Subjective Data

A. Common complaints/symptoms.

1. At early stages, many patients are asymptomatic.

2. Postcoital bleeding (most common).

3. Thin, clear, or blood-tinged vaginal discharge.

4. Abnormally heavy or prolonged menses.

5. Vaginal bleeding becomes heavier, frequent, and may become continuous with progressive disease.

6. Pelvic pain, often seen with advanced disease.

B. Common/typical scenario.

1. The most common cervical lesions are exophytic and friable, arising from the ectocervix.

2. Endocervical lesions are more commonly adenocarcinomas arising from the mucus-producing glands.

3. Cervix may be firm with or without mass or ulceration.

4. May find an ulcerated tumor eroding through the cervix.

Physical Examination

A. When patients present with symptoms suggestive of cervical cancer, they should undergo complete physical examination including a pelvic examination.

B. It is important to determine if the disease has spread into the parametria or the pelvic sidewalls.

C. Rectovaginal examination is also important to assess the spread.

Diagnostic Tests

A. Pelvic examination, including Pap smear.

B. If no lesions are noted, perform a colposcopy to identify any abnormalities.

C. Histologic confirmation is important for accurate diagnosis. If a visible lesion is noted, obtain a biopsy. The best site to take the biopsy is from the edge of the tumor, where the transition from invasive to noninvasive can be clearly seen.

D. Once diagnosis is confirmed by biopsy, the following tests may be beneficial.

  1. Laboratory data: Complete blood count (CBC) and comprehensive metabolic panel (CMP).

  2. Chest x-ray.

  3. CT imaging to assess extrauterine spread and adenopathy.

  4. MRI (best imaging modality to assess extent of disease).

  5. PET scan to assess for lymphatic metastasis.

  6. Cystoscopy.

  7. Proctoscopy.

  8. Exam under anesthesia (EUA) may be needed for a thorough examination.

E. Staging.

  1. Cervical cancer is staged clinically.

  2. Staging is used to determine the treatment and prognosis.

Differential Diagnosis

A. Cervicitis.

B. Endometrial carcinoma.

C. Vaginitis.

D. Pelvic inflammatory disease.

Evaluation and Management Plan

A. General plan.

  1. Treatments for cervical cancer depend on the age of the patient, type of cervical cancer, stage, and desire for children.

  2. Prognostic factors.

    a. Pathologic types.

    b. Tumor size.

    c. Depth of invasion.

    d. Lymphovascular invasion.

    e. Nodal metastases.

  3. Surgery is the treatment of choice for stage I–IIA1 cervical cancer.

  4. Most patients with stage I disease do not require further treatment if they do not have adverse prognostic factors (see following).

  5. Surgical options depend on the stage of cancer and/or are based on the fertility needs.

    a. Simple hysterectomy.

    b. Radical hysterectomy.

    c. Fertility preserving surgeries.

    d. Pelvic exenteration surgery: Type of radical surgery that removes organs from urinary, gastrointestinal, and gynecological systems.

  6. Chemotherapy.

  7. Radiation therapy.

B. Acute care issues in cervical cancer.

  1. Cervical cancer patients are only admitted for certain types of surgeries.

    a. Radical hysterectomy.

    b. Pelvic exenteration.

    c. Other surgeries, including simple hysterectomy and fertility preserving surgical procedures, can be done as outpatient.

  2. Radiation therapy.

  3. Other situations where cervical cancer patients may need inpatient admission include postoperative complications or due to chemotherapy side effects including nausea, vomiting, and neutropenic fever.

Follow-Up

A. The goals of postoperative management include pain control, fluid and electrolyte balance, early ambulation, and return of bowel and bladder function.

B. Follow-up care should focus on identifying, preventing, and controlling long-term and late effects of cervical cancer.

C. Coordination of all the patient's providers should be navigated by the primary/leading care provider.

D. Follow-up standards for frequency of follow-up have not been established.

Consultation/Referral

A. Gynecologist, gynecologic oncology, radiation oncology, and surgery.

Special/Geriatric Considerations

A. Cervical cancer is common in elderly women, and treatment disparities are significantly associated with mortality in this population.

B. Despite evidence that elderly women tolerate treatment well, they are less likely to be offered surgery and adjuvant radiation.

Bibliography

Bruni, L., Barrionuevo-Rosas, L., Albero, G., Serrano, B., Mena, M., Gómez, D, . . . de Sanjosé, S. (2016, December 15). *ICO Information Centre on HPV and Cancer (HPV Information Centre)*. Human Papillomavirus and Related Diseases in the World.

Eskander, R. N., & Bristow, R. E. (Eds.). (2014). *Gynecologic oncology: A pocketbook*. New York, NY: Springer Science + Business Media.

National Cancer Institute. (2016, September 12). Surveillance, epidemiology, and end results program. Retrieved from https://seer.cancer.gov/faststats/selections.php?series=cancer

Noor, R., Tay, E. H., & Low, J. (2014). *Gynaecologic cancer: A handbook for students and practitioners*. Boca Raton, FL : Pan Stanford.

Siegel, R., Naishadham, D., & Jemal, A. (2013). Cancer statistics, 2013. *CA: A Cancer Journal for Clinicians, 63*(1), 11–30.

Gynecologic Cancers: Endometrial Cancer

Valerie F. Villanueva, Amelita B. Marzan, Annamma Sam, and Cynae Johnson

Definition

A. Endometrial cancer develops in the uterus and is the most common type of malignancy of the female reproductive system.

B. The majority of all uterine cancers arise from the endometrium (the inner layer) of the uterus. However, uterine leiomyosarcoma is a type of endometrial cancer that develops in the myometrium (the muscle layer) of the uterus.

Incidence

A. It is estimated that 60,050 new uterine cancer cases were diagnosed in 2016, with 10,470 deaths resulting from the disease.

B. Uterine sarcomas are rare, accounting for approximately 9% of all uterine malignancies.

C. A woman's lifetime risk of developing endometrial cancer is approximately 2.8%.

D. Endometrial cancer represents 3.6% of all new cancer cases in the United States.

E. The majority of women are diagnosed between ages 45 and 74, with a median age of 62.

Pathogenesis

A. Endometrial cancer is usually preceded by endometrial hyperplasia, which is an overgrowth of the uterine lining.

B. Adenocarcinomas comprise 80% of endometrial cancers.

Predisposing Factors

A. Major risk factors.
   1. Obesity.
   2. Diabetes.
   3. Hypertension.

B. Other risk factors.
   1. Increased levels of unopposed estrogen.
   2. Early age at menarche.
   3. Nulliparity.
   4. Late age at menopause.
   5. Older age of 55 or more.
   6. Tamoxifen use for greater than 5 years.
   7. Previous pelvic radiation therapy.
   8. A personal family history of breast or ovarian cancer.
   9. Family history of hereditary nonpolyposis colorectal cancer (HNPCC or Lynch syndrome).

Subjective Data

A. Common complaints/symptoms.
   1. About 90% of women diagnosed with endometrial cancer have abnormal uterine bleeding (i.e., postmenopausal bleeding, recurrent metrorrhagia, or menorrhagia).
   2. Asymptomatic women can present with an abnormal Pap smear showing atypical or malignant endometrial cells.

B. Common/typical scenario: Endometrial cancer can be discovered incidentally on ultrasonography, CT, or MRI with a thickened endometrial lining.

C. Family and social history: An accurate history of present illness as well as past medical conditions, family, and social history should be taken.

Physical Examination

A. The physical examination should involve a general inspection of the body for abnormalities, palpation of the inguinal and supraclavicular nodes, and inspection of the vulva, anus, vagina, and cervix to evaluate for metastatic lesions.

B. Bimanual and rectovaginal examination should be performed to evaluate the uterus, cervix, adnexa, parametria, and rectum.

C. The size, mobility, and axis of the uterus should be assessed.

D. A biopsy should be performed for any suspicious genital tract lesions detected on examination.

Diagnostic Tests

A. Histologic evaluation of endometrial tissue is required for diagnosis.

B. Once endometrial cancer is confirmed, additional studies are needed for treatment planning.
   1. Complete blood count (CBC) with differential.
   2. Serum electrolytes.
   3. Kidney and liver function tests.
   4. EKG.
   5. Transvaginal ultrasound.
   6. CT chest, abdomen, and pelvis with intravenous (IV) and oral contrast to rule out extrauterine spread in high-grade malignancies.
   7. MRI of the abdomen and pelvis.
   8. Chest x-ray (can be used as alternative to CT).
   9. CA-125—can be elevated in some uterine subtypes.
   10. Colonoscopy, sigmoidoscopy, or barium enema.
   11. Genetic testing.

C. Staging: Staging of endometrial cancer is defined by the International Federation of Gynecology and Obstetrics (FIGO) criteria.

Differential Diagnosis

A. Determine source of bleeding.
   1. Cervix.
   2. Vulva.
   3. Vagina.

B. Bleeding can be caused by:
   1. Polyps.
   2. Endometritis.
   3. Neoplasm.
   4. Atrophic changes.

Evaluation and Management Plan

A. General plan.
   1. Treatment is determined based on disease stage and histologic features.
      a. Stage I.
      b. Stage II or III.
      c. Stage IV.
   2. Treatment can continue as long as treatment response is favorable.
   3. There are four basic types of treatment for women with endometrial cancer.
      a. Surgery: The standard of care for treatment of endometrial cancer is hysterectomy.
      b. Radiation therapy.
      c. Hormone therapy.
      d. Chemotherapy.
   4. Fertility-sparing therapy—may be initiated in premenopausal patients with Grade 1 well-differentiated tumor; stage FIGO IA tumor without involvement of myometrium on MRI, absence of lymphovascular invasion, and without intraabdominal disease or adnexal mass.
      a. Hormone therapy with megestrol and medroxyprogesterone (most common).
      b. Levonorgestrel.

B. Acute care issues in endometrial cancer.
   1. Endometrial cancer patients are often admitted for surgical management. Surgery can be performed either open laparotomy or minimally invasive via laparoscopic or robotic approach.
   2. Postoperative laparotomy patients without complications will spend 3 to 5 days in the hospital after surgery, compared to 1 to 2 days recovery for patients undergoing minimally invasive surgery (MIS).

Follow-Up

A. Follow-up should occur every 3 to 4 months for the first 2 years and then every 6 months for 5 years.

B. PET/CT has been shown to be more sensitive or specific than CT alone for recurrence but further investigation is being evaluated.

C. Pap smears for detection of local recurrence has not been demonstrated.

Consultation/Referral

A. Gynecology oncology, medical oncology, radiation oncology, and surgery.

Special/Geriatric Considerations

A. Prognosis is favorable for endometrial cancer.

B. Diagnosis at an early stage of the disease process is a key factor for good prognosis.

C. Surgery is a safe option for elderly women, which significantly extends life with a low rate of complications.

Bibliography

National Cancer Institute. (2016, September 12). Surveillance, epidemiology, and end results program. Retrieved from https://seer.cancer.gov/faststats/selections.php?series=cancer

Nordal, R. R., & Thoresen, S. O. (1997). Uterine sarcomas in Norway 1956–1992: Incidence, survival, and mortality. *European Journal of Cancer, 33*(6), 907–911.

Pecorelli, S. (2009). Revised FIGO staging for carcinoma of the vulva, cervix and endometrium. *International Journal of Gynecology and Obstetrics, 105*(2), 103–104. doi:10.1016/j.ijgo.2009.02.012

Pecorelli, S. (2010). Corrigendum to "Revised FIGO staging for carcinoma of the vulva, cervix, and endometrium". *International Journal of Gynecology and Obstetrics, 108*(2), 176. doi:10.1016/j.ijgo.2009.08.009

Gynecologic Cancers: Ovarian Cancer

Valerie F. Villanueva, Amelita B. Marzan, Annamma Sam, and Cynae Johnson

Definition

A. Ovarian cancers are classified by cells they are derived from.

B. There are three main types of ovarian cancer: Epithelial tumors (accounting for 95%), germ cell tumors, and sex cord stromal tumors.

Incidence

A. It is the second most common cancer among women, with endometrial cancer being first, but it is the most lethal of all gynecologic malignancies.

B. In a woman's lifetime, there is a 1.3% risk of developing ovarian cancer and 1 in 100 risk of dying from ovarian cancer.

C. Approximately 22,280 new cases were reported in 2016.

Pathogenesis

A. The origin and pathogenesis of epithelial ovarian cancer are poorly understood though dedifferentiation of cells overlying the ovary is thought to be an important source.

B. Ovarian cancer typically spreads by local extension with significant dissemination within the peritoneal cavity.

C. Ovarian cancer often goes undetected as symptoms are vague and there is no approved screening test. Therefore, patients are typically diagnosed with advanced stages.

Predisposing Factors

A. Age.

B. Family history of ovarian, breast, or colon cancer.

C. Genetic predisposition.

D. Reproductive and endocrine abnormalities.
  1. Infertility.
  2. Endometriosis.
  3. Hormonal replacement therapy.

E. Obesity (body mass index of ≥30).

Subjective Data

A. Common complaints/symptoms.
  1. Abdominal bloating.
  2. Increase in abdominal girth.
  3. Pelvic/abdominal pain.
  4. Early satiety.
  5. Difficulty eating.
  6. Nausea and vomiting.
  7. Fatigue.

B. Common/typical scenario.
  1. Ovarian cancer was dubbed the "silent killer" due to women presenting with vague symptoms.
  2. Additionally, there are no approved screening methods for ovarian cancer.
  3. Because of the vague symptoms, the majority of women are not diagnosed until they have advanced stage disease.

Physical Examination

A. In patients with early disease, physical examination findings are uncommon.

B. Ovarian/pelvic mass, fluid in the abdomen (ascites), pleural effusion, and abdominal mass or a bowel obstruction may be present in advanced disease.

C. Physical examination includes, and is not limited to:
  1. General assessment.
  2. Survey of the lymphatic system.
  3. Abdomen: Assess for pain, palpable masses, fluid waves, bowel sounds.
  4. Pelvic examination: Assess for bleeding, masses, position of cervix if present, uterine size.
  5. Rectovaginal examination: Assess for bleeding, masses, uterosacral ligaments, and cul-de-sac.

Diagnostic Tests

A. Ultrasound, CT, or MRI of the abdomen/pelvis.

B. Tumor markers.

C. Complete blood count and comprehensive metabolic panel.

D. Urinalysis to rule out other causes of pain (urinary tract infection [UTI], kidney stones).

E. Diagnosis.
  1. Final diagnosis is based on the pathologic review of tissue specimen obtained through surgery or biopsy.
  2. Initial surgery (exploratory laparotomy vs. laparoscopic). If there is a strong clinical suggestion for ovarian cancer, laparotomy is preferred for diagnosis and staging.
  3. Fine needle aspiration (FNA) or diagnostic paracentesis should be performed in patients with diffuse carcinomatosis or ascites without an obvious ovarian mass.

F. Staging: Ovarian cancer is clinically staged based on the Federation International de Gynecologue et d'Obstetrique (FIGO) staging system.

Differential Diagnosis

1. Adnexal tumors.

2. Ectopic pregnancy.

3. Cysts.
4. Endometriosis.
5. Cervicitis.
6. Cancer of surrounding structures.
7. Pelvic inflammatory disease.
8. Uterine leiomyomas.

Evaluation and Management Plan

A. General plan.
   1. All women diagnosed with ovarian, fallopian tube, or peritoneal cancer should have genetic counseling and be considered for genetic testing.
   2. Surgery.
   3. Chemotherapy.
   4. Radiation therapy: Not used as first-line treatment; however, it may be used occasionally to treat small, localized recurrent tumors.
   5. Hormonal therapy.
   6. Targeted therapy.
   7. Biotherapy/immunotherapy.

Follow-Up

A. Follow-up for ovarian cancer is based on National Comprehensive Cancer Network (NCCN) guidelines for tumor type and stage.
B. Many providers recommend pelvic examination every 2 to 4 months for the first 4 years after resection and every 6 months for 3 years thereafter.

Consultation/Referral

A. Gynecological oncologist: Typically will involve surgery, medical oncology, and radiation oncology.
B. Gastroenterologist: Patients may present with primarily gastrointestinal complaints.
C. Palliative care: Due to the very poor prognosis, may be beneficial early on.

Special/Geriatric Considerations

A. Ovarian cancer increases with advancing age, peaking in the seventh decade of life.
B. Discuss aggressive treatment with the patient, based on life expectancy, quality of life goals, and functional status.

Bibliography

National Cancer Institute. (2016, September 12). Surveillance, epidemiology, and end results program. Retrieved from https://seer.cancer.gov/faststats/selections.php?series=cancer

Prat, J. (2014). Staging classification for cancer of the ovary, fallopian tube, and peritoneum. *International Journal of Gynaecology and Obstetrics, 124*(1), 1–5.

Head and Neck Cancers

Susan Varghese

Definition

A. Head and neck cancers can arise in the oral cavity, pharynx, larynx, nasal cavity, paranasal sinuses, and salivary glands and include a variety of histopathologic tumors.

Incidence

A. In the United States, head and neck cancer accounts for 3% of malignancies, with approximately 63,030 Americans developing head and neck cancer annually and 13,000 dying from the disease.
B. Head and neck squamous cell carcinoma (HNSCC) comprises more than 90% of head and neck cancers.

Pathogenesis

A. Pathophysiology of cancers of the head and neck usually begin in squamous cells of the mucosal lining of the aerodigestive tract.
B. Viral infection, smoking, and alcohol consumption can encourage differentiation of squamous cells.

Predisposing Factors

A. Tobacco products.
B. Alcohol.
C. Viral infections.
   1. Epstein–Barr virus (nasopharyngeal cancers).
   2. Human papilloma virus (HPV; oropharyngeal cancers).
      a. HPV is accepted as a risk factor in the development of squamous cell carcinomas of the oropharynx, especially cancers of the lingual and palatine tonsil and base of tongue.
      b. HPV vaccine reduces HPV oral infection, but the impact on HNSCC incidence is yet unknown.
D. Betel nut use: Combination of areca palm nuts, betel leaf, slaked lime, +/− tobacco commonly used in South Asia.
E. Radiation exposure.
F. Periodontal disease.
G. Immunodeficiency (immunosuppressant use, HIV/AIDS, bone marrow, or organ transplantation).
H. Occupational exposure.
I. Genetic factors (polymorphisms, Fanconi anemia, etc.).
J. Iron deficiency (Plummer-Vinson) associated with elevated risk of squamous cell carcinoma.
K. Gastroesophageal reflux or laryngopharyngeal reflux (laryngeal cancers).

Subjective Data

A. Common complaints/symptoms.
   1. Symptoms and signs vary depending on the subtype and location of the tumor.
   2. Patient may be asymptomatic, but common symptoms include:
      a. Oral mass.
      b. Dsyphagia.
      c. Pain: Odynophagia and/or otalgia.
      d. Dysarthria.
      e. Cervical adenopathy.
      f. Hoarseness.
      g. Hearing loss.
      h. Facial numbness, paresthesias, or paralysis.
      i. Trismus.
      j. Loose teeth.
   3. Patients may present with precursor lesions that transform into oral cancer.
      a. Can develop from area of leukoplakia or erythroplakia.
      b. Transformation of severe dysplasia or carcinoma in situ.

Physical Examination

A. Identify the key elements of the mass: The size, firmness, associated pain, and overlying skin changes.

B. Head and neck: Assess for dysarthria, tongue mobility; visual examination and palpation of mucous membranes, floor of the mouth, tongue, buccal and gingival mucosa, palates, and posterior pharyngeal wall.
C. Ears: Inspect ear canal for drainage and tympanic membrane; grossly assess hearing.
D. Lymphatics: Palpate the neck for cervical lymphadenopathy.
E. Neurological: Assess cranial nerves II through XII; assess for facial twitching.

Diagnostic Tests

A. History and physical examination.
B. Direct laryngoscopy and biopsy of the primary site.
C. CT or MRI of the head and neck.
D. PET/CT (optional, preferred in lymph node positive disease).
E. Chest imaging as clinically indicated.
F. Fine needle aspiration (FNA) and/or biopsies of primary tumor and/or nodal disease.
G. Videostroboscopy for patients with dysphonia.
H. Epstein–Barr virus (EBV) quantitative polymerase chain reaction (PCR; for nasopharyngeal cancers).
I. Dental, nutrition, speech/swallowing evaluation, and audiogram if indicated.
J. Staging.
  1. Staging for all oral cancers utilizes the tumor, node, metastasis (TNM) staging outlined by the American Joint Committee on Cancer (AJCC).
  2. TNM staging varies depending on the primary tumor site.

Differential Diagnosis

A. Inflammatory process.

Evaluation and Management Plan

A. General plan: Subtypes and treatment.
  1. Treatment for all head and neck cancers depends on TNM stage at diagnosis.
  2. Treatment recommendations vary depending on primary site of tumor. However, generalized guidelines are outlined here.
    a. Early stage (localized) disease (stage I or II): Definitive radiation therapy (RT) and/or localized resection may be all that is indicated.
    b. Advanced disease (stage III or IV) or resections without clear margins.
      i. Adjuvant or neoadjuvant chemotherapy or radiation may also be indicated in addition to surgery.
      ii. High risk of local recurrence and distant metastasis.
B. Acute care issues in head and neck cancers.
  1. Patients with HNSCC are rarely admitted except for postoperative management.
  2. RT sequelae.
    a. Sore throat.
    b. Dry mouth.
    c. Alteration in taste.
    d. Swelling in the neck.
    e. Soft tissue necrosis leading to chondritis (<1%).
    f. Sensation of lump in the throat.
  3. Xerostomia.
    a. Due to salivary gland destruction/injury.
    b. May be prevented by administering amifostine during RT.

    c. Management.
      i. Submandibular gland transfer.
      ii. Pilocarpine.
      iii. Hyperbaric oxygen.
  4. Mucositis.
    a. Frequent severe complication of RT and chemoradiotherapy.
    b. Management.
      i. Avoid acidic or spicy foods.
      ii. Monitor closely for infections (e.g., oral candidiasis or herpes simplex virus).
      iii. Topical anesthetics.
      iv. Doxepin rinse.
      v. Palifermin (keratinocyte growth factor).
  5. Weight loss and malnutrition.
    a. Due to difficulty eating, mucositis, trismus, and difficult mastication.
    b. Management.
      i. Consider parenteral, enteral, or oral nutritional support.
      ii. Refer to nutritionist.

Follow-Up

A. Follow-up should occur every 1 to 2 months for the first 6 months after the completion of treatment and every 2 to 3 months in the next 6 months, then every 3 to 4 months during the second year and then every 6 months from years 3 to 5.

Consultation/Referral

A. Otolaryngology, medical oncology, and radiation oncology.
B. Nutritionist for weight loss and malnutrition.

Special/Geriatric Considerations

A. Patients older than 70 years should not be denied chemotherapy based solely on age.
B. Discuss aggressive treatment with the patient.
C. Take life expectancy, quality of life, and patient's functional status into consideration.

Bibliography

National Cancer Institute. (2016, September 12). Surveillance, epidemiology, and end results program. Retrieved from https://seer.cancer.gov/faststats/selections.php?series=cancer
Poon, C. S., & Stenson, K. M. (2018, November 19). Overview of the diagnosis and staging of head and neck cancer. In R. F. Connor (Ed.), *UpToDate*. Retrieved from https://www.uptodate.com/contents/overview-of-the-diagnosis-and-staging-of-head-and-neck-cancer
Popescu, C. R., Bertesteanu, S. V., Mirea, D., Grigore, R., Ionescu, D., & Popescu, B. (2010). The epidemiology of hypopharynx and cervical esophagus cancer. *Journal of Medicine and Life, 3*, 396–401.

Leukemias: Acute Leukemias

Alexis C. Geppner

Definition

A. Acute leukemias are a group of rare clonal hematopoietic/stem cell neoplasms involving myeloid or lymphoid precursor cells.
B. These malignant clones replace the normal bone marrow causing ineffective hematopoiesis, resulting in granulocytopenia, anemia, and thrombocytopenia.

C. Acute leukemia is categorized broadly into acute myeloid/myelogenous leukemia (AML) and acute lymphoblastic leukemia (ALL).

Incidence

A. AML.

1. An estimated 19,950 people were diagnosed with AML in the United States in 2016.

2. The incidence of AML is similar to that of solid tumors with an exponential rise after age 40. The median age of patients is roughly 67 years.

3. Approximately 83% of patients with newly diagnosed AML are greater than 45 years old.

B. ALL.

1. An estimated 6,590 people were diagnosed with ALL in the United States in 2016.

2. Approximately 57% of new cases are diagnosed before age 20, indicating that ALL is primarily a disease of younger patients.

Pathogenesis

A. Leukemia develops as a series of genetic changes within a single hematopoietic precursor cell, resulting in alteration of normal hematopoietic growth and differentiation. Accumulation of large numbers of abnormal, immature cells incapable of differentiating into mature hematopoietic cells results.

B. AML.

1. Thought to be related to the transformation of a single hematopoietic stem cell into a malignant undifferentiated cell with endless proliferation; results in accumulation of abnormal, immature myeloid cells in the bone marrow, and peripheral blood.

2. Can occur de novo or secondary to previous cytotoxic therapy (therapy-related or secondary AML).

C. ALL.

1. Thought to be the result of genetic insults that block lymphoid differentiation and drive aberrant cell proliferation and survival.

2. Two subtypes depending on lymphocyte lineage affected: T-lymphocytes (T-ALL) or B-lymphocytes (B-ALL).

Predisposing Factors

A. Gender: Male to female ratio is 4.1 to 1.

B. Race and ethnicity: Slightly higher in European descent; acute promyelocytic leukemia (APL) more common in Hispanic population.

C. Chemical or pesticide exposure: Particularly benzene, petroleum products, and ionizing radiation.

D. Smoking: Most significant controllable risk factor.

E. Prior chemotherapy or high-dose radiation exposure: Alkylating agents, topoisomerase II inhibitors, anthracyclines, and taxanes.

F. Genetic disorders: Down syndrome, Bloom syndrome, Fanconi anemia, Diamond–Blackfan anemia, Shwachman–Diamond syndrome, Li–Fraumeni syndrome, Klinefelter syndrome, Neurofibromatosis type 1, Kostmann syndrome (severe congenital neutropenia), ataxia–telangiectasia, Wiskott–Aldrich syndrome.

G. Blood disorders: Myelodysplastic syndrome (MDS), polycythemia vera (PV), and myelofibrosis (MF).

H. Viruses: RNA retroviruses, parvovirus B19.

Subjective Data

A. Common complaints/symptoms.

1. Patients are often symptomatic due to the disease's impact on normal hematopoiesis, causing pancytopenia and/or leukocytosis; however, patients can be initially asymptomatic.

a. Thrombocytopenia: Easy bruising and bleeding (especially of the mucosal surfaces), epistaxis, petechiae/purpura.

b. Anemia: Dyspnea, orthopnea, headaches, pallor.

c. Fatigue often precedes diagnosis for a number of months.

d. Leukopenia/dysfunctional white blood cells: Fever, persistent infections not responsive to antibiotics.

2. Bone pain/joint pain (due to marrow proliferation).

3. Altered mental status, intermittent/persistent cranial nerve palsies, priapism (due to leukostasis or leukemia infiltrating the central nervous system [CNS]).

4. Ocular, cardiac, pulmonary, or cerebral dysfunction (due to hyperleukocytosis).

5. Palpable lymphadenopathy and/or abdominal distention/bloating.

6. Unexplained weight loss.

7. Loss of appetite.

8. Night sweats (possibly due to the release of cytokines).

Physical Examination

A. Check vital signs including pulse oximetry, height, and weight.

B. Head and neck.

1. Evaluate conjunctiva for pallor (anemia) and ocular fundus for hemorrhage or white plaques (related to nerve fiber ischemia).

2. Evaluate pupils for symmetry and reactivity to light and accommodation (acute brain bleed or CNS infiltration).

3. Carefully examine oropharynx for bleeding, herpetic lesions/aphthous ulcers, oral candidiasis, or gingival hypertrophy (leukemic involvement of the gums: Common in monocytic variants of AML).

4. Evaluate neck/cervical area for lymphadenopathy due to leukemic infiltration, often seen in ALL rather than AML.

C. Cardiovascular system.

1. Auscultate heart sounds in all four quadrants. Tachycardia may be present if the patient is profoundly anemic or septic.

2. Assess for signs of pericardial effusion or cardiac tamponade (hypotension, muffled heart sounds, pericardial friction rub, jugular venous distension [JVD]).

D. Pulmonary system.

1. Inspect and observe for signs of dyspnea, retractions, and work of breathing.

2. Auscultate and percuss all lung fields for signs of infection/leukostasis to include pneumonia, pleural effusion, pulmonary embolism, mediastinal mass, or pneumothorax.

3. Mediastinal adenopathy is found in 80% of cases of T-cell ALL.

E. Gastrointestinal system.

1. Inspect abdomen for distention.

2. Auscultate for bowel sounds in all four quadrants.

3. Palpate for hepatosplenomegaly (HSM) due to infiltration of the liver and spleen with leukemia cells. HSM is often found in ALL rather than AML. Massive HSM is rare in de novo acute leukemia and should raise the suspicion of leukemia evolving from a prior hematologic disorder (e.g., chronic myeloid leukemia [CML] or MDS) or ALL.

F. Integumentary system.

1. Inspect skin for pallor (anemia), petechiae and ecchymosis (thrombocytopenia or disseminated intravascular coagulopathy [DIC]), or infiltrative lesions (leukemia cutis/myeloid sarcoma).

a. Leukemic involvement of the skin occurs in 13% or more of patients and is often found in AML with a monocytic of myelomonocytic component.

b. Cutis lesions are often nodular and violaceous/blue-gray in color.

2. Erythematous to violaceous tender nodules and plaques suggest acute neutrophilic dermatosis (Sweet syndrome).

G. CNS.

1. Perform a full neurological examination to evaluate for focal neurological deficits secondary to leukemic involvement.

2. CNS involvement occurs in 3% to 5% of adult ALL and is rare in AML, but can be seen.

3. CNS involvement is usually restricted to the leptomeninges.

Diagnostic Tests

A. Complete history, including family history.

B. Physical examination.

C. Laboratory data: Complete blood count (CBC), comprehensive metabolic panel (CMP), lactate dehydrogenase (LDH), prothrombin time/international normalized ratio (PT/INR), partial thromboplastin time (PTT), thyroid-stimulating hormone and free T4 levels (TSH/T4), fibrinogen, vitamin B_{12}, reticulocyte count, ferritin, total iron-binding capacity (TIBC), D-Dimer, erythropoietin, B-type natriuretic peptide (BNP), type and screen, and infectious disease screening (hepatitis B/C and HIV).

D. Chest x-ray or CT imaging of the chest.

E. Bone marrow aspiration and biopsy: Morphology, immunohistochemistry, flow cytometry, molecular, and cytogenetic analysis.

F. PET/CT if staging for ALL or myeloid sarcoma or clinical suspicion for extramedullary disease.

G. Lymph node biopsy if necessary for staging of ALL.

H. CT chest with mediastinal biopsy for T-ALL.

I. Lumbar puncture in patients with neurological symptoms.

J. CT or MRI with contrast if neurological symptoms and/or suspicion of leukemic meningitis.

K. Human leukocyte antigen (HLA) typing if a potential allogeneic stem cell transplant candidate.

L. Echocardiogram for patients with a history or symptoms of cardiac disease, or prior exposure to cardiotoxic agents, such as anthracyclines.

M. Central venous access: Peripheral intravenous central catheter (PICC) or central venous catheter (CVC).

N. Diagnosis.

1. Bone marrow aspiration/biopsy required for diagnosis of all types of acute leukemia.

2. Lymph node biopsy may be necessary to aid in diagnosis of ALL.

3. Perform lumbar puncture at diagnosis in all pediatric patients with ALL and all patients with neurological symptoms.

O. Classification of acute leukemia.

1. Diagnosis of acute leukemia requires ≥20% blasts (myeloblasts or lymphoblasts) in the bone marrow or peripheral blood.

2. Two main classification systems.

a. French–American–British (FAB).

b. World Health Organization (WHO).

Differential Diagnosis

A. Acute myeloid leukemia.

B. Lymphomas.

C. Aplastic anemia.

D. Idiopathic thrombocytopenic purpura.

Evaluation and Management Plan

A. General plan.

1. The general approach is based on the subtype of leukemia, age, and performance status.

2. Treatment for all patients with acute leukemia (AML and ALL) can be subdivided into two or three phases.

a. Induction chemotherapy.

b. Consolidation chemotherapy.

c. Maintenance chemotherapy.

Follow-Up

A. Supportive care.

1. Myelosuppression is anticipated as a consequence of both leukemia and the treatment of leukemia with chemotherapy.

2. Blood work required two to three times weekly with transfusional support.

3. Broad-spectrum prophylactic antimicrobial therapy during myelosuppression, which increases susceptibility to opportunistic infections.

B. Disease monitoring.

1. Bone marrow aspirate/biopsy 14 to 21 days following start of therapy to document hypoplasia.

2. Repeat in 7 to 14 days if hypoplasia is indeterminate or not documented. If documented, repeat at the time of hematologic recovery.

Consultation/Referral

A. Hematology oncology once ALL is suspected.

Special/Geriatric Considerations

A. Elderly patients tend to have a poor overall prognosis compared to younger patients, which may be related to some intrinsic poorly understood aspects of the tumor or even host factors.

B. Despite poor prognosis, treatment options should not be based on chronological age alone and should be discussed in detail with the patient.

Bibliography

National Cancer Institute. (2016, September 12). Surveillance, epidemiology, and end results program. Retrieved from https://seer.cancer.gov/faststats/selections.php?series=cancer

Stock, W. S., & Thirman, M. J. (2017, August 4). Pathogenesis of acute myeloid leukemia. In A. G. Rosmarin (Ed.), *UpToDate*. Retrieved from https://www.uptodate.com/contents/pathogenesis-of-acute-myeloid-leukemia

Zuckerman, T., & Rowe, J. M. (2014). Pathogenesis and prognostication in acute lymphoblastic leukemia. *F1000Prime Reports, 6*, 59.

Leukemias: Chronic Leukemias

Allyson Price

Definition

A. Chronic leukemias are blood cancers that arise from hematopoietic stem cells in the bone marrow.
B. Two general subtypes.
   1. Chronic myeloid leukemia (CML): Myeloproliferative neoplasm (MPN) characterized by uncontrolled proliferation of mature and maturing granulocytes.
   2. Chronic lymphocytic leukemia (CLL): Monoclonal disease characterized by accumulation of mature B-cell lymphocytes.

Incidence

A. CML.
   1. Approximately 14% of newly diagnosed leukemia in the United States.
   2. Approximately 1 in every 555 persons will develop CML in a lifetime within the United States.
   3. Average age of diagnosis is approximately 64 years old; rarely seen in children.
   4. Approximately 1,070 people died of CML in 2016.
B. CLL.
   1. Most common type of adult leukemia in the United States with approximately 30% of adults diagnosed with leukemia.
   2. Mean age of diagnosis is approximately 70 years old.

Pathogenesis

A. CML.
   1. Caused by a reciprocal translocation of chromosome 22 (BCR) and chromosome 9 (ABL) resulting in fusion gene BCR-ABL1, also known as the Philadelphia chromosome.
     a. Results in expression of an oncoprotein leading to elevated and uncontrolled kinase activity, allowing unregulated cell division (i.e., proliferation of mature and maturing granulocytes).
     b. Overall promotes leukemogenesis.
   2. Three phases.
     a. Chronic.
     b. Accelerated.
     c. Blast.
   3. CLL.
     a. Heterogeneous disease.
     b. Incidental diagnosis often seen on imaging or routine complete blood count (CBC).
     c. Can remain indolent, not requiring treatment for years.
     d. Aggressive disease requires more upfront treatment; can have complications such as hemolytic anemia, hypogammaglobulinemia, or progression to Richter's transformation.

Predisposing Factors

A. Exposure to ionizing radiation.
B. Family history.
C. Exposures to certain chemicals: Agent orange, herbicides, pesticides.
D. Gender: More common in males.
E. Race/ethnicity: More common in North America and Europe in comparison to Asia.

Subjective Data

A. Common complaints/symptoms.
   1. Typically asymptomatic.
   2. Fatigue and malaise.
   3. Weight loss.
   4. Excessive sweating or night sweats.
   5. Abdominal fullness/discomfort with or without early satiety.
   6. Bleeding or bruising easily.
   7. Bone pain.
   8. B symptoms: Fevers, drenching night sweats, or unintentional weight loss.
   9. Lymphadenopathy.
   10. Organomegaly.
B. Common/typical scenario.
   1. Presentation varies.
   2. Most common symptom in majority of cases is presence of enlarged lymph nodes.
   3. Patients frequently complain of petechiae, tiredness, and fatigue.
   4. Staging.
     a. Prognostic factors for CLL: Advanced age, increased number of prolymphocytes, diffuse pattern of bone marrow infiltration, short time of lymphocyte doubling.
     b. Two staging systems.
       i. Rai (see Table 13.2).
       ii. Binet (see Table 13.3).

Physical Examination

A. Monitor vitals to ensure hemodynamic stability.
B. Routine physical examination.
C. Abdomen: Evaluation for organomegaly.
D. Skin: Assess for petechiae or bruising.
E. Lymphatics: Assess for cervical, axillary, and inguinal adenopathy.

Diagnostic Tests

A. CML.
   1. CBC.
     a. White count normal or elevated.

TABLE 13.2   **Rai Staging for CLL**

Rai Staging		
Stage	**Risk**	**Defining Characteristics**
0	Low risk	Lymphocytosis[a] in blood and marrow only.
I	Intermediate risk	Lymphocytosis[a] and presence of ymphadenopathy.
II	Intermediate risk	Lymphocytosis[a] and presence of splenomegaly and/or hepatomegaly.
III	High risk	Lymphocytosis[a] and presence of anemia.
IV	High risk	Lymphocytosis[a] and presence of thrombocytopenia.

Note: [a]Defined as greater than 15,000 lymphocytes/mm^3.
CLL, chronic lymphocytic leukemia.
Source: Adapted from Rai, K. R., Sawitsky, A., Cronkite, E. P., Chanana, A. D., Levy, R. N., & Pasternack, B. S. (1975). Clinical staging of chronic lymphocytic leukemia. *Blood, 46*(2), 219–234

TABLE 13.3   Binet Staging for CLL

Binet Staging		
Stage	**Risk/Survival**	**All Criteria Must Be Met**
A	Low risk	• Up to two areas of enlarged lymph nodes >1 cm in diameter • Platelets > 100 ×10⁹/L • Hemoglobin ≥ 10 g/dL
B	Intermediate risk	• Three or more areas of enlarged lymph nodes >1 cm in diameter • Platelets > 100 ×10⁹/L • Hemoglobin ≥ 10 g/dL
C	High risk	• Three or more areas of enlarged lymph nodes >1 cm in diameter • Platelets < 100 ×10⁹/L • Hemoglobin < 10 g/dL

CLL, chronic lymphocytic leukemia.
Source: Adapted from Desai, S., & Pinilla-Ibarz, J. (2012). Front-line therapy for chronic lymphocytic leukemia. *Cancer Control, 19*, 26–3.

b. Absolute basophilia and absolute eosinophilia on blood smear.

c. Leukemia hiatus—finding in peripheral blood from CBC showing greater percent of myelocytes versus more mature metamyelocytes.

d. Platelets normal or elevated.

e. Normocytic, normochromic anemia.

2. Peripheral blood quantitative polymerase chain reaction (qPCR) for BCR-ABL1.

3. Bone marrow aspiration and biopsy.

B. CLL.

1. CBC with differential: ≥5,000 monoclonal B lymphocytes/μL.

2. Comprehensive metabolic panel (CMP), immunoglobulins, direct antiglobulin test, infectious disease panel including HIV, hepatitis B, and hepatitis C; lactate dehydrogenase (LDH), beta-2 microglobulin.

3. Clonality of circulating B lymphocytes confirmed by flow cytometry on peripheral blood.

4. Fluorescent in situ hybridization (FISH) and conventional cytogenetics performed on peripheral blood or bone marrow aspiration.

5. Bone marrow aspiration/biopsy.

6. Chest x-ray or CT imaging to assess for lymphadenopathy.

7. PET/CT scan.

Differential Diagnosis

1. Acute leukemias.

Evaluation and Management Plan

A. General plan: Goal of treatment for CML is to prohibit the disease from progressing to accelerated or blast phase.

B. Therapy.

  1. CML.

    a. Tyrosine kinase inhibitors (TKIs): Gold standard treatment of CML.

    b. Stem cell transplant.

  2. CLL.

    a. Indications for initiating therapy include:

      i. Constitutional symptoms referable to relating to CLL; also known as tumor burden.

      ii. Progressive marrow failure; depicted through suppression of counts or progression of anemia and thrombocytopenia.

      iii. Autoimmune anemia +/− thrombocytopenia poorly responsive to steroids.

      iv. Splenomegaly (>6 cm) or progressing in size.

      v. Lymphadenopathy (>10 cm) or progressing in size.

      vi. Progressive lymphocytosis, greater than 50% increase in 2 months or lymphocyte doubling time (LDT) less than 6 months.

    b. Observation is acceptable if all of the following are met.

      i. Absolute monoclonal B lymphocyte count less than 5,000/mm³.

      ii. All lymph nodes less than 1.5 cm.

      iii. No anemia.

      iv. No thrombocytopenia.

    c. Frontline therapy: Monoclonal antibodies used in CLL.

  3. CML response to therapy.

    a. Typically patients are monitored for cytogenetic and molecular responses with repeat bone marrow aspirations every 3 to 6 months for the first year or once a complete cytogenetic remission has been achieved.

    b. Hematologic response.

      i. Normalization of CBC including white blood cell (WBC) less than 10k and platelets less than 450.

      ii. No immature cells in peripheral blood.

      iii. Goal to achieve hematologic response within 1 month of starting therapy.

    c. Cytogenetic response: Goal is to achieve complete cytogenetic remission within 1 year of starting therapy. If not obtained, change of therapy is indicated.

    d. Molecular response: No indication to switch therapy if molecular response is not obtained.

C. Acute care issues in leukemias.

  1. Neutropenic fever.

    a. Fever (temperature ≥ 100.5°F) in the setting of absolute neutrophil count (ANC) less than 500/mm³.

    b. Common in patients undergoing cytotoxic systemic chemotherapy causing profound neutropenia or patients receiving immunosuppressive agents like IV steroids.

    c. Assess vital signs for hemodynamic stability: Fever, tachycardia, and hypotensive or altered mental status.

    d. Need full assessment on physical examination.

    e. Diagnostic tests: Blood and urine cultures, chest x-ray, discontinue peripheral line (i.e., peripheral intravenous central catheter [PICC] line); stool culture for *Clostridium difficile* and vancomycin-resistant enterococci (VRE), respiratory panel via nasal or throat swab.

    f. Treatment: Tylenol PRN, initiate broad-spectrum antimicrobials while awaiting culture results, IV fluids, supplemental oxygen.

i. Most commonly isolated organisms are gram-positive organisms such as *Staphylococcus epidermidis* and gram-negative organisms such as *Pseudomonas aeruginosa, Escherichia coli,* and *Klebsiella.*

ii. Empiric antibiotic options include intravenous cefepime/ceftazidime, piperacillin-tazobactam, vancomycin, and/or imipenem/meropenem.

iii. Antibiotics should be continued until the patient is no longer neutropenic.

iv. If the infection persists despite antibiotic therapy, consider removal of an indwelling catheter.

v. If the neutropenic patient remains febrile for greater than 1 week while on broad-spectrum antibiotics, a fungal infection should be suspected.

2. Hyperleukocytosis.

a. Medical emergency seen in patients experiencing CML blast crisis or CLL in more aggressive settings.

b. It is defined by a WBC greater than 100,000k caused by rapid, uncontrolled leukemic cell proliferation; however, this value is an arbitrary threshold.

c. Three main complications: Disseminated intravascular coagulation (DIC), tumor lysis syndrome (TLS), leukostasis.

   i. DIC.

   ii. TLS.

     1) Most common disease-related emergency in adults with hematologic cancers.

     2) Classically: Hyperuricemia, hyperkalemia, hyperphosphatemia, and hypocalcemia.

       a) Hyperuricemia: Gout attacks, renal insufficiency.

       b) Hyperkalemia: Cardiac arrhythmias (peaked T waves on EKG), muscle cramps, paresthesia, nausea, vomiting, diarrhea.

       c) Hyperphosphatemia/hypocalcemia: Hypotension, arrhythmias, tetany/muscle cramps, confusion, seizures.

     3) Management.

       a) Goals are to prevent moderate to severe metabolic abnormalities and subsequent clinical complications.

       b) Monitor: Serum electrolytes, renal function, urine output, neurological status, EKG.

       c) Avoid: Nephrotoxic agents, exogenous electrolyte supplementation.

       d) Hydration is the most important factor for renal perfusion; rate is dependent on risk factors and subsequent comorbidities.

       e) Treating electrolyte imbalance.

         i) Hyperuricemia.

           – Allopurinol: Hypoxanthine analog.

           – Rasburicase: Guidelines for administration include high LDH, high WBC, large tumor mass, significantly elevated serum uric acid level.

         ii) Hyperkalemia.

           – Kayexalate or other sodium polystyrene sulfonate.

           – Calcium gluconate (if EKG changes).

           – Lasix, Regular insulin $+D_{50}W$, Albuterol via nebulizer.

         iii) Hyperphosphatemia.

           – Phosphate binders: Sevelamer, aluminum hydroxide.

           – Dialysis in severe cases.

         iv) Hypocalcemia.

           – Correct hyperphosphatemia first!

           – Caution with additional calcium supplementation.

         v) Hemodialysis in severe cases.

         vi) Cardiac monitoring for dysrhythmias.

3. Leukostasis.

a. "Symptomatic hyperleukocytosis"; medical emergency.

b. Characterized by extremely high WBC ($>100 \times 10^6$/L) resulting in decreased tissue perfusion secondary to increased blood viscosity and inflammation from cytokine release.

c. Pulmonary signs and symptoms: Dyspnea, shortness of breath, hypoxia demonstrated through pulse oximetry; imaging revealing diffuse or alveolar infiltrates; increased oxygen supplementation needs.

d. Neurological signs and symptoms: Headache, confusion, altered mental status, visual changes, gait instability; imaging demonstrating intracranial hemorrhage or areas of ischemia.

e. Approximately 80% of patients with leukostasis are febrile; typically treated with empiric antibiotics.

f. Diagnosis is made empirically when a patient presents with a high white count manifesting in respiratory or neurological distress.

g. Treatment.

   i. Hemodynamic stabilization with rapid cytoreduction in conjunction with prophylaxis for TLS due to rapid cessation of leukocytosis.

   ii. Cytoreduction.

     1) Achieved with hydroxyurea (Hydrea), induction chemotherapy, and leukapharesis.

     2) Prophylactic platelet transfusions and correction of coagulopathy dependent on clinical presentation.

     3) Adequate fluid restoration and prophylactic treatment of TLS with reduction in uric acid level and restoring electrolyte balance.

4. Autoimmune hemolytic anemia and autoimmune thrombocytopenia.

a. Autoimmune hemolytic anemia.

   i. Laboratory findings.

     1) Positive Coombs test.

     2) Decreased hemoglobin.

     3) Increased reticulocyte count.

     4) Elevated LDH.

     5) Elevated indirect bilirubin.

   ii. First-line treatment is steroids.

   iii. Consider intravenous immunoglobulin (IVIG), Rituxan, or splenectomy in steroid-refractory patients.

b. Immune thrombocytopenia (ITP).

   i. Characterized by rapid decrease in platelet count.

   ii. Laboratory findings.

     1) Decreased platelet count.

2) Hemoglobin and WBC within expected ranges (may be low due to disease or chemotherapy).

3) Normal coagulation studies (prothrombin time [PT]/partial thromboplastin time [PTT]).

4) Peripheral smear to rule out platelet clumping (pseudothrombocytopenia).

iii. Diagnosis of exclusion. Must rule out other causes of thrombocytopenia (e.g., medications, microangiopathy, infections).

iv. Treatment.

   1) Frontline treatment is IV steroids tapered to PO steroids.

   2) IVIG raises platelet count more rapidly than steroids.

   3) Rituxan and/or splenectomy can be considered in steroid-refractory patients.

5. Central nervous system (CNS) disease.

   a. Evaluation for CNS disease both in CML blast crisis and CLL.

      i. Signs/symptoms: Headaches, visual changes, unexplained neuropathy, altered mental status.

   b. Imaging including CT head/brain or MRI brain.

   c. Lumbar puncture to assess cell count and differential and flow cytometry; cerebrospinal fluid (CSF) cytology.

   d. Treatment: Intrathecal chemotherapy until CNS clears of malignant cells.

6. Differentiation syndrome.

   a. Often seen in patients with acute promyelocytic leukemia (APL).

   b. Fever often associated with increasing WBC, shortness of breath, hypoxemia, and pleural or pericardial effusions.

   c. Treatment.

      i. Initiate dexamethasone (10 mg twice daily x 3–5 days tapering over 2 weeks) at first sign of respiratory compromise.

      ii. Interrupt administration of all-trans-retinoic acid (ATRA) until hypoxia resolves.

      iii. For those at high risk for differentiation syndrome, begin prophylaxis with corticosteroids (prednisone 0.5 mg/kg on day 1 or dexamethasone 10 mg every 12 hours) tapered over several days.

      iv. With difficult to treat patients, may begin cytoreduction, hydroxyurea, or anthracycline.

Follow-Up

A. Routine follow-up for all patients should occur once every 6 to 12 months and include a physical examination and CBC.

B. Patients with CLL have a higher risk of developing other types of cancer. Follow-up should occur if patients notice any new or worsening symptoms.

Consultation/Referral

A. Hematology oncology.

B. Additional referrals to surgery for port access or infectious disease may be made at the discretion of the team.

Special/Geriatric Considerations

A. CLL primarily affects the elderly population.

B. A careful assessment of the elderly patient should be taken into consideration when determining a plan of action.

C. Chronological age should not be the sole determinant of treatment options. Life expectancy, quality of life, and patient functional status should be considered as well.

Bibliography

Baccarani, M., Pileri, S., Steegmann, J., Muller, M., Soverini, S., & Dreyling, M. (2012). Chronic myeloid leukemia: ESMO Clinical Practice Guidelines for diagnosis, treatment, and follow-up. *Annals of Oncology, 23*(Suppl. 7), vii72–vii77.

Desai, S., & Pinilla-Ibarz, J. (2012). Front-line therapy for chronic lymphocytic leukemia. *Cancer Control, 19*, 26–36.

Elinoff, J. M., Salit, R. B., & Ackerman, H. C. (2011). The tumor lysis syndrome. *The New England Journal of Medicine, 365*(6), 571–572.

Greenberg, E. M., & Probst, A. (2013). Chronic leukemia. *Critical Care Nursing Clinics, 25*, 459–470.

National Cancer Institute. (2016, September 12). Surveillance, epidemiology, and end results program. Retrieved from https://seer.cancer.gov/faststats/selections.php?series=cancer

Rai, K. R., Sawitsky, A., Cronkite, E. P., Chanana, A. D., Levy, R. N., & Pasternack, B. S. (1975). Clinical staging of chronic lymphocytic leukemia. *Blood, 46*(2), 219–234.

Schiffer, C. A. (2017, November 27). Hyperleukocytosis and leukostasis in hematologic malignancies. In A. G. Rosmarin (Ed.), *UpToDate*. Retrieved from https://www.uptodate.com/contents/hyperleukocytosis-and-leukostasis-in-hematologic-malignancies

Woessner, D., & Lim, C. (2013). Disrupting BCR-ABL in combination with secondary leukemia-specific pathways in CML cells lead to enhanced apoptosis and decreased proliferation. *Molecular Pharmaceutics, 10*, 270–277.

Leukemias: Myelodysplastic Syndromes

Madeleine Nguyen-Cao

Definition

A. Myelodysplastic syndromes (MDS) encompass an array of myeloid clonal hemopathies with a wide range of clinical presentations.

B. They are characterized by the morbidities of their cytopenias and the ominous potential to evolve into acute myeloid leukemia (AML).

Incidence

A. The incidence rate of MDS is approximately 4.9 per 100,000 people per year.

B. MDS is a disease of older individuals (median age at diagnosis: 70–75 years of age) with incidence peaking at 59.8 per 100,000 people among those who are 80 years of age and older.

Pathogenesis

A. MDS develops when a clonal population of dysplastic hematopoietic stem cells overtakes healthy bone marrow cells.

B. MDS can be characterized as primary (de novo) or secondary to a prior potent chemotherapy regimen for other cancers.

Predisposing Factors

A. More common in males.

B. Increases with age.

C. Exposure to chemotherapy or radiation therapy.

Subjective Data

A. Common complaints/symptoms: Patient presentation is typically related to cytopenias and may include:

1. Fever.
2. Cough.
3. Malaise.
4. Fatigue.
5. Bruising.
6. Gingival bleeding.
7. Epistaxis.
8. Recurrent infections.
B. Medical history.
   1. Timing, severity, and pace of abnormal cytopenias.
   2. Transfusion history.
   3. Pneumonias, urinary tract, and other frequent infections.

Physical Examination

A. Vital signs: Assess for tachycardia due to anemia or weight.
B. General: Assess for pallor or weakness.
C. Head, ear, eyes, nose, and throat (HEENT): Assess oral cavity for hemorrhagic bullae or gingival bleeding and eyes for hemorrhagic conjunctiva.
D. Cardiopulmonary: Assess for signs of heart failure and adventitious breath sounds consistent with infection.
E. Gastrointestinal: Assess for hepatosplenomegaly and hematochezia.
F. Skin: Assess for petechiae.

Diagnostic Tests

A. Laboratory.
   1. Complete blood count (CBC) with differential.
   2. Peripheral blood smear.
   3. Comprehensive metabolic panel (CMP) with serum uric acid and lactate dehydrogenase (LDH).
   4. Thyroid function tests.
   5. Serum erythropoietin, vitamin B_{12}, folate, and iron studies.
   6. Fluorescence in situ hybridization (FISH) to detect BCR-ABL fusion transcript to exclude chronic myeloid leukemia (CML) diagnosis.
   7. Human leukocyte antigen (HLA)—typing for high-risk patients being considered for allogeneic hematopoietic cell transplantation.
B. Bone marrow aspirate and biopsy.
C. Diagnostic criteria.
   1. MDS diagnostic criteria is primarily based on the following World Health Organization (WHO) guidelines correlated with the clinical presentation (see Table 13.4).
   2. Risk stratification and prognostic scoring system.

Differential Diagnosis

1. Anemias.
2. Neutropenia.

Evaluation and Management Plan

A. General plan.
   1. Treatment of MDS is based on the stage and mechanism of the disease that predominates the particular phase of the disease process.
   2. In the early phases, when increased bone marrow apoptosis results in ineffective hematopoiesis, retinoids and hematopoietic growth factors are indicated.
   3. Treatment is focused on supportive management of cytopenias (e.g., blood and platelet transfusions, growth factors) and prolonging the time to disease progression (i.e., transformation to AML).

   4. Supportive care pharmacotherapy.
     a. Thrombocytopenia: Romiplostim (Nplate), eltrombopag (Promacta).
     b. Anemia: Darbepoetin (Aranesp).
     c. Neutropenia: Neupogen (Filgastrim) and antimicrobial prophylaxis.
     d. Iron overload from repeated transfusions: Iron chelation therapy.
B. Pharmacotherapy.
   1. Hypomethylating agents.
   2. Biologic response modifiers.
   3. High-intensity idarubicin-, cytarabine-, fludarabine-, and topotecan-based regimens.
C. Other treatments: Allogeneic hematopoietic stem cell transplant.
D. Disease progression to AML is defined by the presence of 20% or more myeloid blasts in bone marrow or peripheral blood. This is associated with poor prognosis and response to standard treatment options.

Follow-Up

A. Focus on response to therapy and monitor for signs or symptoms of disease progression.
B. Frequency of visits determined by the oncologist; will include CBCs to monitor hematological response.
C. A bone marrow aspirate may be warranted if concern for disease progression.

Consultation/Referral

A. Patients with MDS need to be referred to hematology-oncology.

Special/Geriatric Considerations

A. Management of the disease in the elderly population presents a challenge due to concomitant morbidities, which preclude toleration of intensive chemotherapy regimens.
B. Patients with MDS have high utilization rates of EDs and require frequent transfusions. Comorbidities, including diabetes, liver disease, and infections, tend to be higher in elderly MDS patients.

Bibliography

Arber, D. A., Orazi, A., Hasserjian, R., Thiele, J., Borowitz, M., LeBeau, M., & Vardiman, J. W. (2016). The 2016 revision to the World Health Organization classification of myeloid neoplasms and acute leukemia. *Blood, 127*(20), 2391–2405.

Gerds, A. T., Gooley, T. A., Estey, E. H., Appelbaum, F. R., Deeg, H. J., & Scott, B. L. (2012). Pretransplantation therapy with azacitadine vs induction chemotherapy and posttransplantation outcome in patients with MDS. *Biology of Blood and Marrow Transplantation, 18,* 1211–1218.

Germing, U., Kobbe, G., Hass, R., & Gatterman, N. (2013). Myelodysplastic syndromes: Diagnosis, prognosis, and treatment. *Deutsches Ärzteblatt International, 110*(46), 783–790.

Greenberg, P. L. (1997). The role of hemopoietic growth factors in the treatment of myelodysplastic syndromes. *International Journal of Pediatric Hematology/ Oncology, 4,* 231–238.

Ma, X. (2012). Epidemiology of myelodysplastic syndromes. *American Journal of Medicine, 125*(7 Suppl), S2–S5. doi:10.1016/j.amjmed.2012.04.014

Ma, X., Does, M., Raza, A., & Mayne, S. T. (2007). Myelodysplastic syndromes: Incidence and survival in the United States. *Cancer, 109,* 1536–1542.

National Cancer Institute. (2016, September 12). Surveillance, epidemiology, and end results program. Retrieved from https://seer.cancer.gov/faststats/selections.php?series=cancer

Thiele, J., Kvasnicka, H. M., Facchetti, F., Franco, V., van der Walt, J., & Orazi, A. (2005). European consensus on grading bone marrow fibrosis and assessment of cellularity. *Haematologica, 90*(8), 1128–1132.

TABLE 13.4   2008 and 2016 WHO Classifications of MDS

2008 WHO Classification	2016 WHO Classification
Refractory cytopenia with unilineage dysplasia (RCUD) encompassing refractory anemia (RA), refractory neutropenia (RN), and refractory thrombocytopenia (RT)	MDS with single lineage dysplasia (MDS-SLD)
Refractory cytopenia with multilineage dysplasia (RCMD)	MDS with multilineage dysplasia (MDS-MLD)
Refractory anemia with ringed sideroblasts (RARS)	**MDS with ringed sideroblasts (MDS-RS)**
	MDS-RS with single lineage dysplasia (MDS-RS-SLD)
	MDS-RS with multilineage dysplasia (MDS-RS-MLD)
MDS associated with isolated del(5q)	MDS with isolated del(5q)
	MDS with excess blasts (MDS-EB)
Refractory anemia with excess blasts-1 (RAEB-1)	MDS-EB-1
Refractory anemia with excess blasts-2 (RAEB-2)	MDS-EB-2
MDS, unclassified (MDS-U)	**MDS, unclassifiable (MDS-U)**
	With 1% blood blasts
	With single lineage dysplasia and pancytopenia
	Based on defining cytogenetic abnormality
Refractory cytopenia of childhood	Refractory cytopenia of childhood

MDS, myelodysplastic syndrome; WHO, World Health Organization.

Leukemias: Myeloproliferative Neoplasms

Shannon B. Holloway

Definition

A. Myeloproliferative neoplasms (MPNs) are characterized by clonal myeloproliferation without dysplastic features.
B. Essential thrombocythemia (ET), polycythemia vera (PV), and primary myelofibrosis (PMF) result in clonal proliferation of hematopoietic stem cells.

Incidence

A. The reported worldwide annual incidence rate of MPNs ranges from 0.44 to 5.87 per 100,000 with the lowest incidence rates being reported in Japan and Israel.
B. PV is the most prevalent Philadelphia-negative MPN in the United States and is estimated to affect about 148,000 people.

Pathogenesis

A. MPNs are characterized by the overproduction of mature blood cells deriving from the three primary myeloid lineages.
B. Typically predominate in one lineage depending on the disease.

Predisposing Factors

A. Age greater than 65.
B. History of thrombosis.

Subjective Data

A. Common complaints/symptoms.

1. Most patients with MPNs are typically asymptomatic and abnormal blood counts (e.g., thrombocytosis or elevated hematocrit) often prompt further evaluation.
2. Common symptoms according to the myeloproliferative neoplasm symptom assessment form (MPN-SAF) include:
   a. Abdominal pain.
   b. Early satiety.
   c. Abdominal discomfort.
   d. Inactivity.
   e. Vasomotor symptoms: Headaches/lightheadedness.
   f. Difficulty concentrating/sleeping.
   g. Night sweats.
   h. Pruritus (particularly after warm showers).
   i. Bone pain.
   j. Fever.
   k. Unintentional weight loss that lasts greater than 6 months.
   l. Depressed mood.
B. Common/typical scenario.
   1. Some patients present with bleeding or thrombosis. If there are small vessel disturbances due to thrombosis, patients may experience headaches, migraines, dizziness, lightheadedness, coldness of the fingers and toes, and/or burning and erythema of the smaller extremities.
   2. There can be life-threatening presentations associated with thrombosis, such as transient ischemic attack, myocardial infarction, stroke, deep vein thrombosis (DVT), pulmonary embolism (PE), or clotting in usual areas such as abdominal veins.
   3. Patients with a platelet count of 1.5 million or more are at risk for spontaneous bleeding and may experience frequent epistaxis, easy bruising, menorrhagia, or gastrointestinal bleeding.

Physical Examination

A. Skin: Facial plethora (flushed face), excoriations from scratching secondary to pruritus, petechiae.
B. Abdomen: Splenomegaly, hepatomegaly, abdominal distention, tenderness to palpation typically in the left upper quadrant.
C. Head and neck: Epistaxis, hemorrhagic bullae, or gingival bleeding in oral cavity.

Diagnostic Tests

A. Complete blood count (CBC) with differential.
B. Comprehensive metabolic panel (CMP) with serum uric acid and lactate dehydrogenase (LDH).
C. Erythropoietin level and iron studies.
D. Vitamin B_{12} level.
E. Evaluate for acquired Von Willebrand disease.
  1. Prothrombin time/international normalized ratio (PT/INR) and partial thromboplastin time (PTT).
  2. Factor VIII.
  3. Gold standard: Ristocetin activity test.
F. Peripheral blood smear.
G. Bone marrow aspiration and biopsy.
H. Abdominal ultrasound to assess splenomegaly/hepatomegaly.
I. CT scan of abdomen and pelvis with contrast to assess splenomegaly/hepatomegaly and for obscure venous thrombosis.
J. Diagnosis: According to the World Health Organization (WHO) diagnostic criteria, laboratory findings and a bone marrow aspiration and biopsy are necessary to confirm a diagnosis of ET, PV, and PMF.

Differential Diagnosis

A. Acute lymphoblastic leukemia.
B. Acute myeloid leukemia (AML).
C. Chronic lymphocytic leukemia.
D. Chronic myelogenous leukemia.
E. Non-Hodgkin lymphoma.

Evaluation and Management Plan

A. General plan.
  1. The overall goal of treatment for patients with ET and PV is to prevent thrombosis and bleeding.
  2. The most frequent complication of ET/PV is thrombosis, which can include myocardial infarction, PE, DVT, or cerebrovascular accident.
  3. There is a risk stratification process that assesses a patient's risk for thrombohemorrhagic complications.
B. Treatment of ET.
  1. Low-risk patients.
    a. Managed with observation.
    b. Low-dose aspirin can be added to a low-risk patient's regimen on a case-by-case basis.
  2. High-risk patients.
    a. Treated with a cytoreductive agent.
    b. In addition, all high-risk patients must be on low-dose aspirin.
    c. Patients with a history of thrombosis should be treated with anticoagulant therapy.
C. Treatment of PV.
  1. Low-risk patients.
    a. Therapeutic phlebotomy and daily low-dose aspirin are indicated for low-risk patients.
  2. High-risk patients.
    a. Initially treated with phlebotomy to attain hematocrit goal of less than 45% and are then placed on a cytoreductive agent such as hydroxyurea or interferon alpha.
    b. The recommendation is for these patients to take a daily low-dose aspirin.
  3. Common complaints/symptoms: Pruritus is a common symptom of PV and can be treated with proper hematocrit control and the use of antihistamines or antipruritic agents such as hydroxyzine.
  4. Patients with preexisting thrombus must be treated with anticoagulation.
D. Staging of myelofibrosis (MF).
  1. Risk stratification.
    a. Three main prognostic scoring systems are used for MF risk stratification.
      i. International Prognostic Scoring System (IPSS) is used at initial diagnosis and scores are based on age, hemoglobin level, leukocyte count, and circulating peripheral blasts.
      ii. Diagnostic International Prognostic Scoring System (DIPSS) is used if karyotyping is not available during the course of treatment.
      iii. Diagnostic International Prognostic Scoring System-plus (DIPSS-plus) is used if karyotyping is available during the course of treatment and includes platelet count and transfusion needs, as well as unfavorable karyotype.
  2. MF grading based on bone marrow biopsy.
E. Treatment of MF.
  1. The treatment approach for PMF, post-PV, or post-ET MF is the same.
  2. Referral to specialized centers with experts in MF and stem cell transplantation is recommended.
  3. Watch and wait approach is appropriate for low-risk patients.
  4. Immunotherapy and targeted therapy.
  5. Allogeneic hematopoietic stem cell transplant is the only curative option.
  6. Disease progression to AML is defined by the presence of 20% or more myeloid blasts in bone marrow or peripheral blood. This is associated with poor prognosis and response to standard treatment options.

Follow-Up

A. Changes in symptom status should be reported immediately to providers; prompt evaluation should include a CBC at a minimum.
B. Follow-up to monitor response to treatment should occur every 3 to 6 months, or more frequently if there is a change in symptoms.

Consultation/Referral

A. Refer to an oncologist specializing in MPNs.
B. MPNs are relatively rare, and smaller community type oncologists may not have extensive experience in treatment options or access to major clinical trials that could benefit patients.

Special/Geriatric Considerations

A. Supportive care should be an integral part of treatment.
B. MPNs are more prevalent in the elderly, who are at increased risk for cardiovascular and other comorbidities, such as congestive heart failure, peripheral vascular disease, stroke, thromboembolism, renal disease, liver disease, and infections.

Bibliography

Barbui, T., Thiele, J., Gisslinger, H., Finazzi, G., Vannucchi, A. M., & Tefferi, A. (2016). The 2016 revision of WHO classification of myeloproliferative neoplasms: Clinical and molecular advances. *Blood Review, 30*(6), 453–459.

Cervantes, F., Dupriez, B., Pereira, A., Passamonti, F., Reilly, J. T., Morra, E., & Tefferi, A. (2009). New prognostic scoring system for based on a study of the International Working Group for Myelofibrosis Research and Treatment. *Blood, 113*(13), 2895–2901.

Choi, C. W., Bang, S., Jang, S., Jung, C. W., Kim, H. J., Kim, H. Y., . . . Won, J. H. (2015). Guidelines for the management of myeloproliferative neoplasms. *Korean Journal of Internal Medicine, 30*(6), 771–788.

Mesa, R., Jamieson, C., Bhatia, R., Deininger, M. W., Gerds, A. T., Gojo, I., . . . Sundar, H. (2016). Myeloproliferative neoplasms. *Journal of the National Comprehensive Cancer Network, 14*(2), 1572–1611.

Passamonti, F., Cervantes, F., Vannucchi, A. M., Morra, E., Rumi, E., Pereira, A., . . . Tefferi, A. (2010). A dynamic prognostic model to predict survival in primary myelofibrosis: A study by the IWG-MRT. *Blood, 115*, 1703–1708.

Thiele, J., Kvasnicka, H. M., Facchetti, F., Franco, V., van der Walt, J., & Orazi, A. (2005). European consensus on grading bone marrow fibrosis and assessment of cellularity. *Haematologica, 90*(8), 1128–1132.

Vainchenker, W., & Constantinescu, S. N. (2013). JAK/STAT signaling in hematologic malignancies. *Oncogene, 32*, 2601–2613.

Vannucchi, A. M., Barbui, T., Cervantes, F., Harrison, C., Kiladjian, J. J., Kröger, N., . . . Buske, C. (2015). Philadelphia chromosome-negative chronic myeloproliferative neoplasms: ESMO clinical practice guidelines for diagnosis, treatment and follow-up. *Annals of Oncology, 26*(5), 85–99.

Lung Cancer

Courtney Robb

Definition

A. Lung cancer is the uncontrolled growth of abnormal cells that form in tissues of one or both lungs, usually in the cells lining air passages. These abnormal cells divide rapidly to form tumors.

B. The two main types are non-small cell lung cancer (NSCLC) and small cell lung cancer (SCLC).

   1. NSCLC.

      a. NSCLC is the most common type of lung cancer, comprising 85% of the lung cancer diagnoses.

      b. There are three histologic subtypes of NSCLC arising from different lung cells, which have similar prognosis and treatment.

         i. Adenocarcinoma.

            1) Most common subtype of NSCLC, making up roughly 40% of lung cancers, and it is the most common type of lung cancer found in nonsmokers.

            2) Originates in glandular cells that typically secrete mucus.

         ii. Squamous cell carcinoma.

            1) Typically linked to a history of smoking.

            2) Tumors are often located in the central area of the lungs near the main bronchus.

            3) Comprises 25% to 30% of lung cancer diagnoses.

            4) Originates in the flat cells that coat the inside of the airways called squamous cells.

         iii. Large cell (undifferentiated) carcinoma.

            1) Accounts for 10% to 15% of lung cancers.

            2) Can occur anywhere in the lung but often appears as a large peripheral mass on chest radiograph.

            3) Tends to grow and spread quickly.

            4) Due to its tendency for rapid growth and metastasis, it is more difficult to treat.

   2. SCLC.

      a. SCLC, previously known as oat cell lung cancer, accounts for 15% to 20% of all lung cancers.

      b. Associated with a poor prognosis due to the advanced stage (usually metastatic) at the time of diagnosis.

Incidence

A. Lung cancer is the second most common cancer among both women and men, accounting for approximately 14% of all new cancer diagnoses. However, it is the number one cause of cancer deaths among both women and men each year.

B. More individuals die annually from lung cancer than of breast, prostate, and colon cancer combined.

C. Lung cancer primarily occurs in people over the age of 65 with less than 2% being younger than age 45.

D. The average age at diagnosis is 70 years old.

E. The survival rate among individuals with lung cancer varies based on staging at the time of diagnosis. However, if diagnosed and treated early it can be cured.

F. Five-year overall survival rate is 17.7% for all patients or 55.2% for patients presenting with localized disease (i.e., early detection).

Pathogenesis

A. Lung cancer can be divided into two broad categories: Small cell and non-small cell carcinoma.

   1. Small cell carcinoma is almost exclusively caused by exposure to cigarette smoking.

   2. Non-small cell carcinoma (adenocarcinoma, squamous cell and large cell carcinoma) can be caused by other environmental factors such as:

      a. Smoking.

      b. Radon gas.

      c. Pollution.

      d. Asbestos.

      e. Radiation.

      f. Toxic dust.

      g. Coal.

      h. Diesel.

      i. Arsenic.

Predisposing Factors

A. History of smoking (cigarette/cigar/pipe/marijuana). This is dose dependent, meaning the increased quantity and duration of smoking increase the risk of lung cancer.

B. Exposure to radon or asbestos.

C. History of lung cancer in the immediate family.

D. Exposure to Agent Orange or other carcinogens.

E. Diagnosis of another respiratory disease such as chronic obstructive pulmonary disease (COPD), emphysema, chronic bronchitis, or pneumonia.

F. Contact with secondhand smoke.

Subjective Data

A. Common complaints/symptoms.

   1. Cough, especially if persistent (the most common).

   2. Shortness of breath.

   3. Hemoptysis.

   4. Pain in the chest, back, or shoulder unrelated to cough.

   5. Changes in voice or becoming hoarse.

   6. Recurrent lung problems, like bronchitis or pneumonia.

7. Wheezing.

8. Bone pain (with bone metastasis).

9. Headaches (with intracranial metastasis).

10. Unexplained weight loss.

11. Fatigue.

B. Common/typical scenario.

1. Patients are frequently asymptomatic with symptoms only developing once the disease is well advanced.

2. Often, lung cancer is discovered incidentally on chest imaging.

Physical Examination

A. Check vital signs including pulse oximetry.

B. Head and neck.

1. Evaluate pupils for symmetry and reaction to light. Tumor in the lung apex can cause compression of the cervical sympathetic plexus, which can cause Horner syndrome (ptosis, miosis, and anhidrosis).

2. Palpate the neck and supraclavicular area for adenopathy.

3. Evaluate the neck for facial edema, facial cyanosis, or jugular vein distention (JVD), which could indicate superior vena cava (SVC) syndrome if the tumor is obstructing the SVC.

C. Pulmonary system.

1. Observe for signs of dyspnea, increased work of breathing, or retractions.

2. Auscultate lung sounds in all lung fields. Lung tumor can lead to obstruction and collapse of a lobe or entire lung or postobstructive pneumonia. Pleural effusions may develop as well. All of these scenarios would lead to decreased breath sounds in those areas of the lung affected.

3. Percussion of the lung will be dull with collapsed lobes of the lung or pleural effusion.

D. Cardiovascular system.

1. Auscultate heart sounds, which should be normal. If the tumor has direct cardiac involvement, or pericardial effusion has developed, the heart sounds may be affected.

2. Assess for signs of cardiac tamponade, such as hypotension, distant/muffled heart sounds, pericardial rub, or JVD.

E. Gastrointestinal tract.

1. Auscultate for bowel sounds in all four quadrants.

2. Palpate for hepatomegaly. One of the most common sites of lung metastasis is the liver, which can manifest as tender hepatomegaly.

F. Musculoskeletal system.

1. Bone is another area of common metastasis.

2. Patients may report bone pain or tender spots on examination, including the spine.

3. Lung cancers that arise in the lung apex, called Pancoast tumors, can cause shoulder or scapula pain that radiates down the arm.

G. Central nervous system.

1. A neurological examination should be performed to evaluate for any focal neurological deficits that may be produced by intracranial metastases or spinal cord compression.

2. Evaluation for neuropathy, decreased sensation, or decreased strength should be performed.

Diagnostic Tests

A. Laboratory data.

1. Complete blood count (CBC).

2. Comprehensive metabolic panel (CMP).

3. Prothrombin time/international normalized ratio (PT/INR) and partial thromboplastin time (PTT).

B. Imaging and procedures.

1. Chest x-ray.

2. CT of the chest with contrast.

3. PET/CT scan to assess for metastatic disease.

4. Endobronchial ultrasound (EBUS) to evaluate mediastinal lymph nodes.

5. Brain MRI to complete staging.

C. Biopsy: Interventional radiology (IR) CT guided biopsy.

D. Ancillary tests prior to surgery.

1. EKG.

2. Pulmonary function test (PFT).

E. Diagnosis: Tissue sample or biopsy is required for diagnosis; these are typically obtained through a CT-guided biopsy of the lung nodule/mass.

1. Staging is one of the most important elements in determining therapeutic options and prognosis. The staging for NSCLC and SCLC differ as noted in the following.

    a. NSCLC.

      i. Like the majority of cancers, NSCLC is staged by the tumor, node, metastasis (TNM) system.

      ii. Higher numbers indicate more advanced lung cancer.

      iii. Staging determines the approach to treatment (i.e., surgery, chemotherapy, radiation, or combination of treatment modalities).

    b. SCLC: SCLC has a two-stage system: Limited versus extensive stage.

      i. Limited stage: Localized to one hemithorax. Lymph nodes may be involved but they too must be located in the ipsilateral hemithorax in relation to the primary tumor.

      ii. Extensive stage involves lung cancer in both hemithoraces and/or metastasis to other organs and/or contralateral nodal metastasis. Staging determines the approach to treatment (chemoradiation vs. chemotherapy alone).

Differential Diagnosis

A. Adenocarcinoma.

B. Squamous cell carcinoma.

C. Large cell carcinoma.

D. Small cell carcinoma.

E. Pulmonary nodule.

Evaluation and Management Plan

A. General plan.

1. Based on staging, patients will be offered chemotherapy +/− radiation, stereotactic body radiation therapy (SBRT), and/or surgery.

2. Targeted therapies.

B. Acute care issues in lung cancer.

1. Lung cancer patients are often only admitted for surgical resection.

    a. Pneumonectomy: Removal of the entire lung.

    b. Lobectomy: The most common surgical procedure in lung cancer patients, with removal of a single lobe of the lung.

    c. Segmental resection: Removal of a segment/portion of the involved lobe.

    d. Sleeve resection: Consider when the cancer is confined to the bronchus or pulmonary artery and requires bronchoplastic reconstruction.

e. Wedge resection: Removal of a small peripheral nodule; performed only on lung cancer patients with limited pulmonary reserve.

2. Postoperative lung surgery patients, without complications, will spend 3 to 5 days in the hospital after surgery.

3. The primary focus in the postoperative inpatient setting includes the following: Pain control, monitoring lab work, wound care, chest tube management, pulmonary toileting to avoid pneumonia, and early ambulation.

   a. Pain control.

      i. May be managed by epidural, intercostal nerve block, and/or PO/IV pain medications.

      ii. Optimizing pain control leads to faster recovery as pain control allows the patient to deep breathe, deep cough, and ambulate, thereby reducing the risk of pneumonia.

   b. Monitoring laboratory data: Routine blood work including CBC with differential, electrolyte panel, blood urea nitrogen (BUN), and creatinine must be monitored for anemia, infection, electrolyte imbalance/need for replacement, and kidney function.

   c. Infection.

      i. The incision site will be monitored daily for signs of infection and proper healing.

      ii. Pulmonary toileting with the incentive spirometer and acapella apparatuses are crucial to prevent pneumonia in the postoperative lung resection patient.

      iii. Early ambulation is also crucial for reducing the risk of postoperative pneumonia.

   d. Pneumothorax prevention/monitoring.

      i. The postlung surgery patient will have anywhere from one to two chest tubes placed in the operating room and managed in the recovery unit.

      ii. Chest tubes are placed on wall suction to help reinflate the lung and allow for fluid drainage.

      iii. The chest tube is a closed system that will need to be monitored for air leak and fluid drainage daily.

      iv. Daily chest x-rays should also be performed.

      v. Once there is evidence of no air leak and the chest x-ray shows an inflated lung, the chest tube may be removed.

Follow-Up

A. Five-year survival remains poor in this patient population.

B. Perform surveillance to manage complications and symptoms.

C. Follow-up visits recommended every 6 months for first 2 years.

D. In NSCLC: Perform CT chest every 6 months for first 2 years after resection and every year thereafter.

E. Assess for health-related quality of life at baseline and during follow-up visits.

Consultation/Referral

A. Most lung cancer patients are seen by:

   1. Medical oncologist, who orders chemotherapy.

   2. Radiation oncologist, who offers radiation therapy.

   3. Cardiothoracic surgeon to formulate a treatment plan based on clinical staging.

Special/Geriatric Considerations

A. Much evidence exists to suggest that elderly adults with good functional status can tolerate combination chemotherapy in the treatment of lung cancer.

B. Chronological age alone should not dictate treatment options.

C. Providers should work with patients to decide on the best alternatives of management.

Bibliography

National Cancer Institute. (2016, September 12). Surveillance, epidemiology, and end results program. Retrieved from https://seer.cancer.gov/faststats/selections.php?series=cancer

Lymphomas: Hodgkin Lymphoma

Melissa Timmons

Definition

A. Malignancies that develop from lymph nodes and lymphoid tissues are broadly classified into Hodgkin lymphoma (HL) and non-Hodgkin lymphoma (NHL).

B. HL, which originates in germinal center or postgerminal center B-lymphocytes, is characterized by the presence of a distinctive type of giant cell called a Reed–Sternberg cell in a background of reactive cells.

Incidence

A. HL accounts for approximately 10% of all lymphomas and approximately 0.6% of all cancers diagnosed annually in the developed world.

B. Median age at diagnosis is 39 years.

C. In 2016, an estimated 8,500 patients were diagnosed with HL, and an estimated 1,120 patients died of HL.

D. In the United States, the most common subtype of HL is classical HL, followed by mixed cellularity, lymphocyte-rich, and lymphocyte-depleted.

Pathogenesis

A. HL occurs due to the clonal proliferation of malignant Hodgkin/Reed–Sternberg cells in a background of reactive cells.

B. The proliferation of these malignant cells causes lymphadenopathy and enlargement of lymphoid tissue/organs (e.g., spleen).

C. Lymphoma generally spreads to contiguous lymph nodes following lymph vessels.

Predisposing Factors

A. Epstein–Barr virus (EBV) infection.

B. Immunosuppression (e.g., patients with HIV infection or long-term immunosuppressant use).

C. Family history of HL.

D. Most patients who develop HL have no identifiable risk factors.

Subjective Data

A. Common complaints/symptoms.

   1. Painless lymphadenopathy, most commonly in the neck, axilla, or groin, is the most common presenting complaint. Occasionally, lymph nodes can become painful after consuming alcohol.

2. B-symptoms: Unintentional weight loss, fever, and night sweats.
B. Common/typical scenario.
    1. Other signs and symptoms.
        a. Generalized pruritus.
        b. Fatigue.
        c. Lack of appetite.
        d. Cough, difficulty breathing, or chest pain secondary to large mediastinal mass or lymphadenopathy. Often a mediastinal mass will be discovered incidentally on a routine chest radiograph.
C. Family and social history.
    1. Elicit presence or absence and duration of symptoms.
    2. Ask about previous malignancy, prior treatment with chemotherapy or radiation therapy, history of immunosuppressive illnesses such as HIV, and family history of malignancy.
D. Review of systems: Determine the patient's performance status, as this can impact future treatment options.

Physical Examination

A. A complete physical examination, including vital signs, should be performed.
B. Special attention should be paid to the size and number of palpable peripheral lymph nodes and presence or absence of hepatosplenomegaly.
C. Comprehensive neurological examination should be performed to assess for central nervous system (CNS) involvement.

Diagnostic Tests

A. Definitive diagnosis is made by lymph node biopsy. An excisional biopsy is preferred for diagnosis but often core biopsy of an involved node is sufficient.
B. Complete workup should include complete blood count (CBC), erythrocyte sedimentation rate (ESR), comprehensive metabolic panel (CMP), lactate dehydrogenase (LDH), pregnancy test in women with childbearing potential, and HIV serology.
C. Clinical staging, including the following evaluations, should also be completed.
    1. Full-body PET/CT scan.
    2. Bilateral bone marrow biopsy/aspiration should be considered if the patient has pancytopenia.
    3. Lumbar puncture and/or dedicated brain imaging, only if CNS involvement is suspected.
D. HL is staged per the Ann Arbor Staging.
E. Other important tests to consider include pulmonary function tests and echocardiogram, as they will likely be needed for assessment prior to chemotherapy or radiation therapy.

Differential Diagnosis

A. HIV.
B. Other solid tumors.
C. NHL
D. Any disease with lymphadenopathy needs to be considered.

Evaluation and Management Plan

A. General plan.
    1. Treatment based on the stage of the disease at diagnosis, but can involve chemotherapy, radiation therapy, and immunotherapy, either alone or in combination.

2. Several chemotherapy regimens exist for the initial treatment of HL.
3. High-dose chemotherapy followed by autologous or allogeneic stem cell transplant may be indicated for refractory or recurrent disease.

Follow-Up

A. Based on individual needs and individual oncologists.
B. Basic schedule includes:
    1. Visits every 3 to 6 months for first 2 years, every 6 to 12 months in years 3 to 5, and annually after year 5.
    2. Usual tests are physical examination, blood work, imaging as indicated, and surveillance of symptom changes.

Consultation/Referral

A. Immediate referral to an oncologist should be made when HL is suspected or diagnosed.

Special/Geriatric Considerations

A. HL is one of the most curable malignancies in adults; however, survival rates in elderly patients are significantly lower than in younger patients.

Bibliography

Cheson, B. D., Fisher, R. I., Barrington, S. F., Cavalli, F., Schwartz, L. H., Zucca, E., & Lister, T. A. (2014). Recommendations for initial evaluation, staging, and response assessment of Hodgkin and non-Hodgkin lymphoma: The Lugano classification. *Journal of Clinical Oncology, 32*(27), 3059–3068.

National Cancer Institute. (2016, September 12). Surveillance, epidemiology, and end results program. Retrieved from https://seer.cancer.gov/faststats/selections.php?series=cancer

Siegel, R., Ma, J., Zou, Z., & Jemal, A. (2014). Cancer statistics, 2014. *CA: A Cancer Journal for Clinicians, 64*(1), 9–29.

Lymphomas: Non-Hodgkin Lymphoma

Megan Krug

Definition

A. Malignancies that develop from lymph nodes and lymphoid tissues are broadly classified into Hodgkin lymphoma (HL) and non-Hodgkin lymphoma (NHL).
B. NHL encompasses a diverse group of diseases with more than 50 distinct subtypes, which are further classified by histology and clinical presentation. These various subtypes are determined based on the cells from which they arise (B-cells, T-cells, natural killer cells) or by their degree of indolence versus aggressiveness.
C. Patients with indolent lymphomas typically survive for several years even without therapy. However, patients with aggressive lymphomas may only have months to live.

Incidence

A. NHL is relatively common in the United States with greater than 70,000 new cases each year (accounting for 4.3% of all cancer diagnoses), as compared to approximately 8,000 cases of HL each year.
B. The majority of NHL cases are B-cell neoplasms (85%), whereas T-cell/NK-cell neoplasms account for only 15% of NHLs.
C. The median age at diagnosis is 66, although it is seen in all age groups.

D. Between the years 2004 and 2013, rates of new cases have remained stable, though the rate of mortality has decreased an average of 2.4% each year.

Pathogenesis

A. Tumors associated with NHL originate from lymphoid tissues.

B. Most NHLs come from B-cell expansion.

Predisposing Factors

A. Immunodeficiency states.

B. Epstein–Barr virus (EBV) infection.

C. HIV infection.

D. Human T lymphotropic virus type 1 (HTLV-1) infection.

E. Autoimmune rheumatoid diseases (lupus, Sjögren's, rheumatoid arthritis).

F. Herbicide/pesticide exposure.

Subjective Data

A. Common complaints/symptoms.

  1. Rapidly enlarging lymph nodes (most commonly in neck or abdomen).

  2. *B Symptoms*: Fever greater than 38°C, drenching night sweats, unintentional weight loss of greater than 10% body weight.

B. Common/typical scenario.

  1. Other nonspecific symptoms: Malaise, fatigue, chronic pain, early satiety, cough/chest discomfort (seen with mediastinal involvement).

  2. Approximately 34% of all patients present with primary extranodal lymphoma at the time of diagnosis; the gastrointestinal (GI) tract is the most common site, followed by the skin.

Physical Examination

A. Vital signs.

B. Head and neck: Facial edema/jugular venous distention (JVD) can indicate superior vena cava syndrome (most commonly seen in primary mediastinal lymphoma).

C. Lymphatics: Cervical, axillary, inguinal, Waldeyer's ring (tonsils, base of tongue, nasopharynx).

D. Cardiopulmonary: Evaluate for signs of dyspnea/airway obstruction, evidence of malignant pleural effusion (decreased breath sounds/crackles), and signs of pericardial effusion/tamponade.

E. Abdomen: Evaluate for hepatomegaly/splenomegaly and ascites.

F. Neurological: Evaluate for signs of spinal cord compression, altered mental status, memory impairment, or cranial nerve dysfunction.

Diagnostic Tests

A. Laboratory data.

  1. Complete blood count (CBC) with differential.

  2. Comprehensive metabolic panel (CMP).

  3. Magnesium.

  4. Phosphorus.

  5. Lactate dehydrogenase (LDH).

  6. Uric acid.

  7. Coagulation studies: Prothrombin time/international normalized ratio (PT/INR) and partial thromboplastin time (PTT).

B. Lymph node biopsy.

C. PET/CT scan.

D. Bone marrow biopsy.

E. Lumbar puncture and brain/spine MRI if at risk for central nervous system (CNS) involvement.

F. Formal ophthalmologic examination if at risk for/confirmed CNS involvement (can also rarely be seen in mantle cell lymphoma and marginal zone lymphoma).

G. Hepatitis B and C serologies (risk of reactivation due to Rituxan).

H. HIV screen.

I. +/– serum protein electrophoresis (SPEP).

J. +/– echocardiogram (for patients who will receive an anthracycline).

K. Diagnosis/staging.

  1. Definitive diagnosis is confirmed with excisional or core needle biopsy (not fine needle aspiration [FNA]).

  2. The Lugano classification system, based on Ann Arbor Staging, is the most widely used classification system employed in NHL.

Differential Diagnosis

A. Solid tumors.

B. Hematological malignancies.

C. Hodgkin's lymphoma.

Evaluation and Management Plan

A. General plan/therapy.

  1. The indicated treatment varies greatly depending on the type of NHL, staging, and age/performance status/comorbidities.

  2. A majority of NHL is treated with chemotherapy alone, though there are variants of indolent lymphoma in which watchful waiting is appropriate.

  3. For some subtypes, radiation therapy is indicated as monotherapy.

  4. Infrequently, surgery is employed for excision of lymphoid tumors.

  5. Stem cell transplant (autologous or allogenic) is typically reserved for aggressive/late-stage disease, or for relapsed/refractory NHLs.

B. Acute care issues in lymphomas.

  1. Neutropenic fever (see sections on Leukemias).

  2. Tumor lysis syndrome (TLS; see sections on Leukemias).

  3. Superior vena cava (SVC) syndrome.

    a. The obstruction of blood flow through the SVC caused by external lymph node compression or by thrombus within the vena cava, and is most commonly seen associated with cases of primary mediastinal B-cell lymphoma.

    b. Clinical presentation most commonly reveals dyspnea, cough, facial swelling, upper extremity edema, or chest pain.

    c. Treatment should be initiated after the cause of the obstruction is clarified, so as not to confound accurate diagnosis; and is focused on treating the underlying cause with chemotherapy and/or radiation. Stent placement or surgical bypass are reserved for severe cases, and are rarely utilized.

  4. Spinal cord compression.

    a. Involvement of the spinal cord is not an unusual finding in patients with NHLs, and spinal cord compression typically manifests as severe back pain at the level of involvement, weakness (typically involving lower extremities), or paresthesia below the level of spinal involvement, bladder/bowel dysfunction (late finding).

b. Diagnosis is confirmed with MRI.

c. High-dose steroids and radiation therapy are the mainstays of treatment.

Follow-Up

A. Based on individual needs and individual oncologists.

B. Basic schedule includes:

1. Visits every 3 to 6 months for the first 2 years, every 6 to 12 months in years 3 to 5, and annually after year 5.

2. Usual tests are physical examination, blood work, imaging as indicated, and surveillance of symptom changes.

Consultation/Referral

A. Hematology oncology to manage patients with NHL.

B. Radiation oncology and surgery for placement of ports should be initiated.

C. Infectious disease is often consulted to manage neutropenic fevers.

Special/Geriatric Considerations

A. Elderly patients with NHL show similar features and prognostic factors as younger patients, suggesting similar treatment strategies should be offered to both groups.

B. Chronological age should not be the main determinant in treatment options, even in elderly patients older than 80 years.

Bibliography

National Cancer Institute. (2016, September 12). Surveillance, epidemiology, and end results program. Retrieved from https://seer.cancer.gov/faststats/selections.php?series=cancer

Krol, A. D. G., le Cessie, S., Snijder, S., Kluin-Nelemans, J. C., Kluin, P. M., & Noordijk, E. M. (2003). Primary extranodal non-Hodgkin's lymphoma (NHL): The impact of alternative definitions tested in the Comprehensive Cancer Centre West population-based NHL registry. *Annals of Oncology, 14*(1), 131–139. doi:10.1093/annonc/mdg004

Multiple Myeloma

Jerrad M. Stoddard

Definition

A. Plasma cell dyscrasias are a group of heterogeneous disorders that stem from the malignant proliferation of monoclonal plasma cells.

Incidence

A. Multiple myeloma (MM) is primarily a disease of the elderly, and the median age at diagnosis is 69.

B. MM represents approximately 1% of all cancers and approximately 10% of all hematologic malignancies.

Pathogenesis

A. Plasma cell dyscrasias arise from the monoclonal proliferation of plasma cells.

Predisposing Factors

A. Although not considered an inherited disease, the risk of developing MM is approximately 3.7-fold higher for persons with a first-degree relative with MM.

B. Twice as common in black persons.

C. Family history increases risk 2- to 4-fold.

D. Occupational exposures may contribute, such as:

1. Pesticides.

2. Petroleum workers.

3. Woodworkers.

4. Leather workers.

5. Ionizing radiation.

Subjective Data

A. Common complaints/symptoms.

1. The clinical presentation for plasma cell dyscrasias is quite variable.

2. Patients with MM often present with signs/symptoms related to plasma cell proliferation in the bone marrow and/or renal dysfunction.

a. Elevated total protein—due to hypersecretion of monoclonal immunoglobulin and light chains; often associated with decreased albumin.

b. Bone involvement—osteolytic lesions, pathologic fractures, hypercalcemia.

c. Anemia.

d. Renal failure.

e. Recurrent infections.

B. Common/typical scenario.

1. Patients may also present with an extramedullary plasmacytoma (soft tissue mass comprised of clonal plasma cells) that can cause spinal cord compression, cauda equina syndrome, severe back pain, paresthesia, and/or radiculopathy.

2. AL amyloidosis can lead to amyloid deposition in any organ, and patients can present with congestive heart failure, renal failure, skin changes, neuropathy, gastroparesis, or diarrhea depending on the organ system(s) involved.

Physical Examination

A. Head and neck: Conjunctival pallor due to anemia; macroglossia.

B. Musculoskeletal: Bone tenderness.

C. Lymphatics: Assess for lymphadenopathy.

D. Neurological: Vertebral compression fractures and/or plasmacytomas can cause neurological deficits if there is spinal cord or nerve compression.

Diagnostic Tests

A. Laboratory data.

1. Complete blood count (CBC) with differential.

2. Comprehensive metabolic panel (CMP) and calcium level.

3. Serum protein electrophoresis with immunofixation electrophoresis (SPEP/IFE).

4. 24-hour urine protein electrophoresis with immunofixation electrophoresis (UPEP/IFE)—Bence Jones proteinuria.

5. Serum free light chain assay (kappa and lambda).

6. Serum immunoglobulin levels (IgA, IgG, IgM, IgD).

7. β_2-microglobulin for staging and prognostication.

8. Lactate dehydrogenase (LDH) for staging and prognostication.

B. Imaging.

1. Bone survey with plain films to assess for axial and appendicular lytic bone lesions.

2. Consider PET/CT to assess for subtle bone lesions and/or plasmacytomas.

3. Consider MRI of the cervical, thoracic, and lumbar (C/T/L) spine if there is concern for spinal cord compression from extramedullary plasmacytoma or vertebral compression fracture.

C. Bone marrow aspiration and biopsy.

D. Diagnosis.

    1. CRAB criteria for symptomatic myeloma.

        a. **C**alcium (hypercalcemia)—serum calcium greater than 11 mg/dL.

        b. **R**enal insufficiency—serum creatinine greater than 2 mg/dL or CrCl less than 40 mL/min.

        c. **A**nemia—hemoglobin less than 10 g/dL.

        d. **B**one lesions—one or more osteolytic lesions on bone survey, MRI, CT, or PET/CT.

E. Staging.

    1. Staging systems for newly diagnosed myeloma patients.

        a. Revised International Staging System (R-ISS).

        b. Durie-Salmon staging (more subjective and less commonly utilized).

Differential Diagnosis

A. Non-Hodgkin lymphoma (NHL).

B. Amyloidosis.

C. Plasmacytoma.

Evaluation and Management Plan

A. General plan.

    1. Treatment depends on the plasma cell dyscrasia.

    2. Therapy options for MM and amyloidosis.

        a. Patients typically receive two to six cycles of induction systemic chemotherapy followed by autologous stem cell transplant (if eligible) or maintenance chemotherapy (if ineligible for transplant).

        b. Systemic chemotherapy.

        c. Autologous stem cell transplant.

        d. Allogeneic stem cell transplant.

            i. Not commonly utilized for MM.

            ii. Can be considered for patients with plasma cell leukemia, refractory myeloma, relapsed myeloma, or young patients with high-risk disease (based on fluorescent in situ hybridization [FISH] data).

        e. Maintenance chemotherapy.

        f. Radiation therapy.

        g. Surgical intervention.

            i. Vertebroplasty or kyphoplasty may be indicated for patients with vertebral compression fractures.

            ii. Excisional biopsy may be performed to confirm plasmacytomas.

B. Supportive care.

    1. Bone disease.

        a. All patients with osteolytic lesions and/or pathologic fractures should be initiated on IV bisphosphonates.

        b. Prior to initiation of bisphosphonate, patients must be evaluated by a dentist to assess for periodontal disease and risk for jaw osteonecrosis.

    2. Infectious prophylaxis.

    3. Thromboembolic prophylaxis.

    4. Pain management.

C. Emergencies and inpatient management.

    1. Pain management.

        a. Pain is primarily due to skeletal fractures and bone pain from lytic lesions.

        b. Pharmacologic therapy.

            i. Avoid nonsteroidal anti-inflammatory drugs (NSAIDs) due to nephrotoxicity.

            ii. Oral or IV analgesics.

        c. Surgical intervention for collapsed vertebral body.

            i. Vertebroplasty—injection of bone cement (methyl methacrylate) under fluoroscopy.

            ii. Kyphoplasty—placement of inflatable bone tamp prior to injection of bone cement.

    2. Hypercalcemia.

        a. Due to osteolysis and/or renal failure.

        b. Corrected calcium = serum calcium + 0.8 (normal albumin – serum albumin).

        c. Rule out other causes (e.g., hyperparathyroidism, thyrotoxicosis, medications, hypervitaminosis D).

        d. If asymptomatic and corrected calcium less than 12 mg/dL, patient may not require immediate treatment.

        e. Therapeutic intervention.

            i. Simultaneous administration of:

                1) Hydration—isotonic saline for volume expansion.

                2) Calcitonin—dose of 4 international units/kg (IU/kg).

                3) Bisphosphonates (e.g., zoledronic acid).

            ii. Consider dialysis for patients with severe hypercalcemia.

            iii. Repeat serum calcium.

    3. Renal failure.

        a. Due to light chain deposition in renal tubules (light chain cast nephropathy).

        b. Correct electrolyte abnormalities.

        c. Careful review of medications and discontinue or dose-adjust nephrotoxic agents.

        d. Consider kidney biopsy—stain for Congo red to rule out amyloidosis.

        e. IV hydration.

        f. Consider dialysis.

    4. Tumor lysis syndrome (see sections on Leukemias).

    5. Spinal cord compression.

        a. Due to vertebral compression fracture and/or plasmacytoma.

        b. Symptoms vary depending on the location of compression and may include:

            i. Back pain.

            ii. Motor deficits.

            iii. Paresthesia.

            iv. Bowel/bladder incontinence or dysfunction.

            v. Gait ataxia.

        c. Emergent evaluation with MRI of cervical, thoracic, and/or lumbar spine.

        d. If a mass is present, arrange biopsy of lesion for diagnosis.

        e. Requires emergent steroids, radiation therapy, and/or neurosurgical decompression.

    6. Hyperviscosity syndrome.

        a. Symptoms and signs include:

            i. Blurred vision.

            ii. Papilledema.

            iii. Headache.

            iv. Neurological symptoms.

            v. Oral/nasal bleeding.

            vi. Stupor/coma.

        b. Obtain IgM and serum viscosity levels.

        c. Requires emergent plasmapheresis if symptomatic (not based on serum viscosity level).

Follow-Up

A. Typically includes blood tests, radiologic testing, and bone marrow evaluation every 1 to 3 months.

B. Long-term surveillance varies on a case-by-case basis.

Consultation/Referral

A. Consult medical oncologists and surgical oncologists specializing in MM.

Special/Geriatric Considerations

A. Long-term and late effects of treatment can develop in survivors months or even years after treatment.

   1. These effects can be physical and/or emotional.

   2. Teach patients to identify and report them to their providers.

B. Elderly patients older than 70 years should not be denied chemotherapy based solely on age.

   1. Aggressive treatment should be discussed with the patient.

   2. Life expectancy, quality of life, and functional status should be taken into consideration.

Bibliography

Lynch, H. T., Sanger, W. G., Pirruccello, S., Quinn-Laquer, B., & Weisenburger, D. D. (2001). Familial multiple myeloma: A family study and review of the literature. *Journal of National Cancer Institute, 93*(19), 1479–1483.

National Cancer Institute. (2016, September 12). Surveillance, epidemiology, and end results program. Retrieved from https://seer.cancer.gov/faststats/selections.php?series=cancer

Palumbo, A., Avet-Loiseau, H., Oliva, S., Lokhorst, H. M., Goldschmidt, H., Rosinol, L., & Moreau, P. (2015). Group Revised International Staging System for Multiple Myeloma: A report from International Myeloma Working. *Journal of Clinical Oncology, 33*(26), 2863–2869.

Sarcoma

Siji Thomas

Definition

A. Sarcomas are divided into two broad categories.

   1. Soft tissue sarcoma.

   2. Bone sarcoma.

B. Soft tissues include adipose, muscle, tendinous, fibrous, and vascular tissues, and there are approximately 60 subtypes of soft tissue sarcoma. Examples include:

   1. Osteosarcoma.

   2. Ewing's sarcoma.

   3. Liposarcoma.

   4. Rhabdomyosarcoma.

   5. Leiomyosarcomas.

Incidence

A. In 2016, there was an estimated 12,310 new cases of soft tissue sarcomas and 4,990 patients died of the disease.

B. In 2016, there was an estimated 3,260 new cases of bone sarcomas and 1,550 patients died of the disease.

C. Although very rare in adults, sarcomas comprise ~15% of all pediatric cancers.

D. Males are affected more frequently than females.

Pathogenesis

A. Sarcomas, as with many cancers, are often associated with cytogenetic abnormalities or molecular mutations.

B. Sarcomas have a wide range of clinical behaviors and outcomes depending on the subtype and extent of disease.

C. Expert pathological review is necessary to determine the specific subtype. Differentiation patterns can be difficult to ascertain, as there are approximately 60 different histologic subtypes.

D. Classification of sarcomas depends on tissue appearance, histologic grade, and cell of origin.

Predisposing Factors

A. Genetic factors.

B. Exposure to radiation.

C. Exposure to chemical carcinogens (e.g., Agent Orange or polyvinyl chloride).

Subjective Data

A. Common complaints/symptoms.

   1. Sarcomas can occur in any anatomic area: About 46% occur in lower extremities, 18% occur in the torso, 13% occur in the upper extremities, 13% occur in the retroperitoneum, and 9% occur in the head and neck.

   2. The clinical presentation depends on the tumor's location.

   3. Patients often present with:

     a. Swelling.

     b. Palpable soft tissue or bone mass.

     c. Sometimes pain.

   4. Patients may present with:

     a. Constitutional symptoms such as fever, weight loss, and night sweats.

     b. Neurological symptoms if there is involved nerve compression.

   5. Patients with a mass increasing in size or a mass greater than 5 cm should undergo evaluation for possible sarcoma with imaging (x-rays, CT, and/or MRI).

Physical Examination

A. Vital signs.

B. Musculoskeletal: Evaluate location, size, and mobility of palpable mass.

C. Neurological: Assess for any sensory/motor deficits, gait abnormality, and strength.

D. Evaluate for metastatic disease.

   1. Lymphatics: Assess for adenopathy.

   2. Cough: Assess for metastatic spread to the lung.

   3. Ascites: Retroperitoneal sarcomas can metastasize to the liver producing fluid wave.

Diagnostic Tests

A. General plan.

   1. Imaging.

     a. CT or MRI for suspected soft tissue sarcoma.

     b. Conventional x-ray imaging should be performed for suspected bone sarcoma followed by CT and/or MRI.

     c. Consider PET scan.

   2. Biopsy.

     a. Definitive diagnosis is based on biopsy of the mass. Core needle biopsy is typically sufficient to make an accurate diagnosis.

     b. Fine needle aspiration (FNA) is not recommended.

   3. Molecular/cytogenetic markers.

4. Metastatic evaluation.

    a. May include MRI with gadolinium to evaluate for bone metastasis.

    b. CT of the chest and/or abdomen to assess for lung or liver metastasis.

    c. Consider whole body PET.

B. Staging.

    1. Complete staging includes chest x-ray, CT scan of the chest, and bone scan to assess for metastatic disease.

    2. For Ewing sarcoma, an MRI of the spine should be performed to assess for bone marrow metastases.

    3. Soft tissue sarcomas (except retroperitoneal sarcomas): The tumor, node, metastasis (TNM) staging system is used.

    4. Bone sarcomas: The Musculoskeletal Tumor Society (MSTS) staging system is used.

Differential Diagnosis

A. Lipoma.

B. Carcinoma.

C. Neuroma.

Evaluation and Management Plan

A. General plan.

    1. Treatment and prognosis vary depending on the subtype, location, and extent of disease.

    2. Therapy includes a combination of systemic therapy, radiation, surgery, and in some cases targeted therapy.

    3. For localized sarcomas, surgical excision is the mainstay of treatment.

    4. For metastatic disease, unresectable disease, large tumors (>5 cm), and tumors that are located in deeper tissues or have visceral involvement, systemic chemotherapy +/− radiation is often given followed by debulking surgery if indicated.

    5. Chemosensitivity and choice of treatment differs based on histologic subtype.

B. Acute care issues in sarcoma.

    1. Local surgical resections can be attempted as outpatient.

    2. Patients are usually admitted for extensive debulking or cytoreductive surgery or chemotherapy.

    3. Postoperative management usually focuses on pain control, wound care, pulmonary toileting, and early ambulation.

    4. Complex aggressive chemotherapy usually requires inpatient admission.

        a. High-dose chemotherapeutic combinations are employed depending on the type of sarcoma.

        b. Two-dimensional echocardiography.

        c. Routine blood work including electrolyte panel, blood urea nitrogen (BUN), and creatinine must be monitored for electrolyte imbalance/need for replacement and kidney function.

Follow-Up

A. Complete within first 6 weeks.

B. Surveillance in first year should occur at 3 months, 6 months, and then annually.

C. If patients have higher grade cancer, more frequent visits should be scheduled. An MRI of the primary site may be indicated.

Consultation/Referral

A. Referrals for patients with suspected sarcoma should be referred to a cancer center so they can be followed by a surgical oncologist, medical oncologist, and radiation oncologist.

B. Orthopedics should be consulted as well.

Special/Geriatric Considerations

A. Sarcomas are rare, but malignant tumors. Elderly patients are more often diagnosed with high stage sarcomas and have a higher mortality rate.

Bibliography

Lawrence, W., Jr., Donegan, W. L., Natarajan, N., Mettlin, C., Beart, R., & Winchester, D. (1987). Adult soft tissue sarcomas. A pattern of care survey of the American College of Surgeons. *Annals of Surgery, 205*(4), 349–359.

National Cancer Institute. (2016, September 12). Surveillance, epidemiology, and end results program. Retrieved from https://seer.cancer.gov/faststats/selections.php?series=cancer

Skin Cancer

Sijimol Mathew

Definition

A. Two main types.

    1. Melanoma (most aggressive).

    2. Nonmelanoma.

        a. Basal cell carcinoma (most common).

        b. Squamous cell carcinoma (second most common).

B. Other types of less common nonmelanoma skin cancers include Merkel cell carcinoma or trabecular cancer, Kaposi sarcoma (associated with HIV), cutaneous lymphoma, and skin adnexal tumors.

Incidence

A. Skin cancer is the most common cancer in the United States.

B. Each year there are more new cases of skin cancer than the combined incidence of cancers of the breast, prostate, lung, and colon.

C. Melanoma is one of only three cancers with an increasing mortality rate for men, along with liver cancer and esophageal cancer.

D. An estimated 76,380 new cases of melanoma were diagnosed in 2016 with 10,130 deaths.

E. Males are affected more than females, and non-Hispanic whites have higher incidence rates compared to other ethnicities.

F. The incidence and mortality rates in the United States are 19.9% and 2.7%, respectively.

G. The rates of new cases of melanoma have risen ~1.4% each year over the past 10 years.

Pathogenesis

A. Pathophysiology of skin cancer comes from damage to the DNA base.

B. Ultraviolet (UV) radiation from sunlight is an important risk factor for skin cancer.

C. UV sunlight appears to disable a tumor suppressor gene called p53.

Predisposing Factors

A. Male with age greater than 60 years.

B. Excess sun exposure and ultraviolet-based artificial tanning.

C. Family history of skin cancer.

D. Personal history of skin cancer.

E. History of sunburns, especially early in life.

F. History of indoor tanning.

G. Patients receiving immunosuppressive drugs.

H. Individuals with dysplastic or atypical nevi, with several large nondysplastic nevi, with many small nevi, or with moderate freckles.

I. Chemical exposure to arsenic, chromium, polycyclic aromatic hydrocarbons, or benzene.

J. Associated genetic syndromes; basal cell nevus syndrome, xeroderma pigmentosum, oculocutaneous albinism, epidermolysis bullosa, and Fanconi anemia are associated with an increased risk of skin cancer.

Subjective Data

A. Common complaints/symptoms.

  1. There are some general physical characteristics of malignant skin lesions but the appearance may vary with each skin cancer.

  2. The most common sign of skin cancer is a change in the skin including:

    a. A new growth.

    b. Nonhealing sore: Basal cell carcinomas often ulcerate and have an eczematous appearance.

    c. A change in appearance of a mole.

    d. Scar elevation (thickening or rising of a previously flat mole).

    e. Surface changes (scaling, erosion, oozing, bleeding, or crusting).

    f. Surrounding skin changes (redness, swelling, or small new patches of color around a larger lesion [satellite pigmentations]).

    g. Sensory changes (itching, tingling, or burning).

    h. Changes in consistency (friability).

  3. Metastatic melanoma signs and symptoms include:

    a. Unexplained weight loss or fatigue.

    b. Swollen or painful lymph nodes: This may be the first presenting sign in metastatic melanoma of unknown primary.

    c. Shortness of breath or persistent cough.

    d. Bone pain.

    e. Headaches, numbness, weakness, or decreased sensation.

    f. Seizures.

    g. Anorexia, abdominal pain, dysphagia, small bowel obstruction, hematemesis, and melena.

    h. Intraocular melanoma may present with altered vision.

Physical Examination

A. Integumentary system.

  1. Total body skin should be examined including scalp, dorsal feet, soles, toe webs, and nails.

  2. Assess the total number of nevi present on patient's skin and differentiate between typical and atypical lesions using the ABCDE criteria.

  3. Melanoma lesions are more likely to be asymmetrical, have irregular borders, appear very dark black or blue or have more variation in color than a benign mole and may be greater than 6 mm in diameter.

B. Lymphatic system.

  1. Melanoma may disseminate through the lymphatics.

  2. Palpate for hard and swollen lymph nodes.

C. Pulmonary system.

  1. Observe for tachypnea, dyspnea, or labored breathing.

  2. Auscultate all lung fields for lung sounds.

  3. Melanoma metastasis to lungs may cause persistent cough, shortness of breath, pain in the chest, or pleural effusion.

D. Cardiovascular system.

  1. Auscultate heart sounds for abnormal findings to evaluate the presence of a tumor that has direct cardiac involvement.

  2. Assess for signs of hypotension, jugular venous distension, or pericardial rub.

  3. Cardiac symptoms, pericardial effusion, and cardiac tamponade are associated with cardiac metastasis of melanoma.

E. Gastrointestinal tract.

  1. Auscultate bowel sounds in four quadrants.

  2. Palpate for hepatomegaly or tenderness to palpation.

  3. Liver metastases also may cause ascites.

F. Musculoskeletal system.

  1. Bone metastasis of melanoma can cause bone pain and discomfort.

  2. Examine for any tender area including spine.

G. Central nervous system.

  1. A neurological examination is essential to evaluate for any intracranial metastases.

  2. Evaluate for decreased strength, altered sensation, and/or neuropathy.

H. A complete eye examination is necessary to test the presence of intraocular melanoma.

  1. Uveal melanomas can arise in the iris or in the posterior uveal tract, and initially may be asymptomatic.

  2. Iris melanoma may cause distortion of the pupil; ciliary body melanoma may cause blurred vision.

  3. Choroidal melanoma may result in retinal detachment and decreased visual acuity.

Diagnostic Tests

A. Biopsy.

B. Nodal basin ultrasound and/or lymphoscintigraphy.

C. Imaging (if a sentinel lymph node is positive or symptoms warrant).

  1. CT of the chest/abdomen/pelvis with intravenous contrast.

  2. Consider whole body PET/CT.

  3. Consider brain MRI with IV contrast.

  4. If clinically indicated, perform a neck CT with IV contrast.

D. Staging.

  1. Staging for melanoma determines the degree of severity, treatment options, and prognosis.

  2. The American Joint Commission of Cancer staging system tumor, node, metastasis (TNM) classification of melanoma is similar to any other cancers.

Differential Diagnosis

A. Basal cell carcinoma.

B. Squamous cell carcinoma.

C. Malignant melanoma.

D. Benign lesions.

Evaluation and Management Plan

A. General plan.

1. Based on staging, the treatment options include surgery, immunotherapy, targeted therapy, and chemotherapy and/or radiation therapy (e.g., stereotactic radio surgery or whole brain radiation).

2. For metastatic and unresectable disease, systemic therapy is indicated.

3. Surgery.

4. Radiation therapy.

5. Immunotherapy and targeted therapy.

B. Acute care issues in skin cancers.

1. Most of the surgical procedures are done on an outpatient basis; however, hospitalization is indicated for complex surgeries and depends on reconstructive techniques.

2. Wound care, JP drain management and pain management, and monitoring for infection are the main areas of focus during postoperative management.

Follow-Up

A. Perform physical and skin examinations every 3 to 6 months for the first 2 to 3 years, then once a year after that.

B. Follow-up scans may be recommended.

Consultation/Referral

A. Patients with suspected skin cancer should be referred to dermatology, medical oncology, radiation oncology, and surgical oncology.

Special/Geriatric Considerations

A. The white skinned elderly population represents the largest patient group at risk for developing skin cancer.

B. Treatment of skin cancer in the elderly population should be based on life expectancy, quality of life, and patient functional status, and not solely on chronological age.

Bibliography

Aerts, B., Kock, M., Kofflard, M., & Plaisier, P. (2014). Cardiac metastasis of malignant melanoma: A case report. *Netherlands Heart Journal, 22*(1), 39–41.

National Cancer Institute. (2016, September 12). Surveillance, epidemiology, and end results program. Retrieved from https://seer.cancer.gov/faststats/selections.php?series=cancer

14 Immune System, Connective Tissue, and Joints Guidelines

Joanne Elaine Pechar

Back Pain

Joanne Elaine Pechar

Definition

A. Pain in the lower back region, which may, or may not, have a radicular component.

B. Low back pain (LBP) is categorized into three groups, based on duration of symptoms.

   1. Acute LBP: Pain that is 6 weeks or less in duration.

   2. Sub-acute LBP: Pain that continues between 6 and 12 weeks.

   3. Chronic LBP: Pain that is more than 3 months in duration.

C. Types of LBP.

   1. Benign back pain is a dull, aching pain that generally worsens with movement but improves with rest and lying.

   2. Tumor- or infection-related back pain typically presents with constant and dull pain. This pain is unrelieved by rest and is worse at night, therefore often awakening the patient.

   3. Disc herniation is worsened by coughing, valsalva maneuver, and sitting and is relieved by lying in the supine position.

   4. Spinal stenosis is associated with bilateral (and occasionally unilateral) sciatic pain that is worsened by activities such as walking, prolonged standing, and back extension. Pain is relieved by rest and forward flexion.

Incidence

A. The lifetime incidence of LBP is 70% and has an incidence of 5% per year.

B. The peak incidence of LBP is in the age range of 40s to 50s.

C. LBP is the second most common reason for physician visits in the United States.

D. For approximately 90% of the patients, the most common cause of LBP is related to disc degeneration.

Pathogenesis

A. LBP presents suddenly from an accident, fall, whiplash injury, or heavy lifting.

B. LBP develops gradually as a result of age-related changes to the spine.

C. Bony overgrowth (osteophytes) or disc herniation may directly impinge on spinal nerve roots or the spinal cord itself and can lead to instability and misalignment of the spine, which produces pain and neurological deficits.

D. Radiculopathy is caused by compression, inflammation, or injury to a spinal nerve root.

E. Sciatica is a form of radiculopathy caused by compression of the sciatic nerve, the large nerve that travels through the buttocks and extends down the back of the leg.

F. Spondylolisthesis is a condition in which a vertebra of the lower spine slips out of place, pinching the nerves exiting the spinal column.

G. Spinal stenosis is the narrowing of the spinal column, which then leads to pressure on the spinal cord and nerves.

   1. The spinal cord pressure can cause pain or numbness with walking and may, over time, lead to leg weakness and sensory loss.

   2. This is also known as neurogenic claudication.

Predisposing Factors

A. The first attack typically occurs between ages 30 and 40.

B. African American female.

C. Diet high in calories and fat.

D. Inactive lifestyle.

E. Obesity.

F. Cigarette smoking.

G. Occupation: Job that requires heavy lifting, pushing, pulling, or twisting.

Subjective Data

A. Common complaints/symptoms.

   1. LBP with radiation to buttocks, legs, or feet.

   2. Paraspinal muscle spasms.

   3. Muscle stiffness.

   4. Paresthesias.

   5. Gait disturbances.

   6. Numbness.

B. Common/typical scenario.

   1. Neurogenic claudication (low back, buttock, or leg pain, which may be relieved by sitting or with rest, induced by walking or standing).

   2. Fecal or urinary incontinence.

   3. Large post void residual greater than 100 mL and overflow incontinence.

   4. Perianal or perineal sensory loss.

   5. Dermatomal sensory loss.

   6. Focal leg weakness, paralysis, and hyporeflexia in the legs.

   7. Elevated erythrocyte sedimentation rate (ESR), C-reactive protein (CRP), and human leukocyte antigen (HLA), if infection is present.

   8. Fever.

C. Family and social history.
  1. Family history is typically noncontributory.
  2. Social history.
    a. Smoking, which is associated with LBP.
    b. Dietary and eating habits.
    c. Obesity is a major cause of LBP.
    d. Elicit drug use.
D. Review of systems.
  1. Elicit onset, frequency, duration, and location of symptoms.
  2. Inquire if pain is worse during activity, at rest, or at night.
  3. Inquire about exacerbating factors.
  4. Inquire if pain radiates to lower extremities.
  5. Inquire about associated symptoms, such as numbness, tingling, weakness, and sensory deficits.
  6. Determine if there is any recent loss or change in bowel or bladder function.
  7. Check if there is symptom improvement after taking pain medications.
  8. Determine whether patient has a history of trauma and chronic infection.
  9. Check for signs of systemic disease, which include history of cancer, age greater than 50 years, unexplained weight loss, duration of pain greater than 1 month, nighttime pain, and unresponsiveness to previous therapies.

Physical Examination

A. Check vital signs: Blood pressure, heart rate, respirations, and temperature.
B. Inspect.
  1. Examine the back for any warmth, erythema, swelling, purulent drainage, or abscess.
  2. Inspect the curvature of the spine.
  3. Observe for signs of previous surgery.
C. Check for tenderness or pain using palpation along the spine.
D. Check for radicular pain associated with straight-leg test.
  1. Straight-leg raise test is positive if test causes radicular pain of the affected leg radiating below the knee.
E. Complete neurological examination including:
  1. Motor strength.
  2. Sensation.
  3. Deep tendon reflexes.
F. Check back range of motion (ROM): Flexion, extension, side bending, and rotation.
G. Check hip ROM: Possible referred pain from hip pathology.
H. Assess gait.
I. Perform digital rectal examination to assess rectal sphincter tone or anal sphincter laxity.

Diagnostic Tests

A. Spine x-rays or films.
  1. Anteroposterior and lateral views.
  2. Demonstrates fractures, disc space narrowing, osteophyte formation, tumor, or instability.
B. MRI scan.
  1. Provides axial and sagittal views, which demonstrate normal and pathologic discs, ligaments, nerve roots, epidural fat, and shape and size of the spinal canal.
  2. Gold standard study in cases of suspected spinal infection, neoplasm, and epidural compression syndromes.
C. CT scan.
  1. Useful in evaluating vertebral fractures, facet joints, and posterior elements of the spine.

  2. When MRI scan is unavailable, CT myelography is the best substitute for conditions, such as epidural abscess or cord compression.
D. Nuclear medicine bone scan.
  1. Can also be used if infection and tumor are suspected.
E. Laboratory tests: ESR, CRP, complete blood count (CBC), blood cultures, and urinalysis.

Differential Diagnosis

A. Degenerative disc disease.
B. Spinal stenosis.
C. Spondylosis and spondylolisthesis.
D. Discitis.
E. Vertebral osteomyelitis.
F. Spinal cord or cauda equina compression.
G. Herniated intervertebral disc.
H. Spinal epidural abscess.
I. Ankylosing spondylitis.
J. Spine-related bone tumors.
K. Metastatic cancer.
L. Scoliosis and hyperkyphosis.
M. Vertebral compression fracture.
N. Myofascial pain syndrome.
O. Fibromyalgia pain syndrome.

Evaluation and Management Plan

A. General plan.
  1. General intervention.
    a. Bed rest for a few days. Limit bending, lifting, and twisting.
    b. Physical therapy and aerobic exercise.
    c. Local application of heat and ice.
    d. Brace is indicated for adolescents with spine curvature between 20°C and 40°C.
  2. Adjunct therapy.
    a. Transcutaneous electrical nerve stimulation (TENS).
    b. Biofeedback.
    c. Acupuncture.
  3. Red flags: Indications for imaging.
    a. Concern for malignancy: Age 50 or older, previous history of cancer, unexplained weight loss, pain unrelieved by bed rest, pain lasting more than a month, or LBP failure to improve in 1 month.
    b. Concern for infection: Elevated ESR greater than 20, intravenous drug abuse, urinary tract infection, skin infection, or fever.
    c. Concern for compression fracture: Corticosteroid use and/or age 50 or older.
    d. Concern for neurological problem: Sciatica.
    e. New fecal or urinary incontinence.
  4. Surgical intervention.
    a. Indications for surgery when <u>all three</u> criteria are met.
      i. Evidence of disc herniation as demonstrated by an imaging study.
      ii. Worsening clinical picture with neurological deficit.
      iii. Failed improvement after 4 to 6 weeks of conservative treatment.
      iv. NOTE: Cauda equina and spinal cord compression syndromes need urgent surgical decompression in 24 to 48 hours of symptom onset.
      v. Imaging demonstrates compressive abscess or epidural collection.

b. Types of spine surgery.

    i. Vertebroplasty and kyphoplasty are minimally invasive treatments to repair compression fractures of the vertebrae.

    ii. Spinal laminectomy or spinal decompression is used to treat spinal stenosis.

        1) Lamina or bony walls of the vertebrae and bone spurs are removed. The goal of the procedure is to open up the spinal column to remove pressure on the nerves.

    iii. Discectomy or microdiscectomy is recommended to remove herniated discs from pressing on nerve roots or the spinal cord.

    iv. Foraminotomy is an operation that enlarges the foramen, which is where a nerve root exits the spinal canal. The enlargement removes the blockage and relieves pressure, caused by bulging discs, on the nerve.

    v. Spinal fusion is used to treat degenerative disc disease and spondylolisthesis.

        1) The disc between two or more vertebrae is removed and the adjacent vertebrae are fused together by bone grafts or metal devices secured by screws.

        2) Spinal fusion can be performed through the abdomen with a procedure known as an anterior lumbar interbody fusion or it may be performed through the back in a procedure called posterior lumbar fusion.

B. Patient/family teaching points.

    1. Counsel in regards to exercise therapy.

    2. Counsel about smoking cessation and weight loss.

    3. Counsel about ergonomic interventions for prevention of occupational LBP.

C. Pharmacotherapy.

    1. First-line agents: Nonsteroidal anti-inflammatory drugs (NSAIDs) and Tylenol. Avoid NSAIDs after fusion.

    2. Muscle relaxants: Cyclobenzaprine, diazepam, or tizanidine.

    3. Opioids or narcotics.

    4. Antidepressants and anticonvulsants.

    5. Transforaminal or epidural steroid injections.

D. Discharge instructions.

    1. Patients should participate in physical therapy and start with first-line pharmacological agents for pain management.

    2. If the pain does not get better with treatment or it worsens, the patient should call the healthcare provider.

    3. Patients should also call if they suddenly feel something pop or snap in the back or if they have questions or concerns about their condition or care.

    4. Patients should seek urgent attention if change in bowel or bladder habits are observed.

Follow-Up

A. Patients who have not improved after 4 to 6 weeks of conservative therapy and who did not receive imaging during initial evaluations require follow-up.

B. Patients presenting with persistent and worsening symptoms should have an MRI for further evaluation.

Consultation/Referral

A. Patients without concerns for a particular etiology who have not improved after 12 weeks need imaging and referral to orthopedic spine surgery or neurosurgery specialists for further evaluation and treatment.

B. Patients with symptoms of spinal cord compression or severe neurological deficits should have immediate MRIs for further evaluation and also receive urgent specialist referrals.

Special/Geriatric Considerations

A. When performing a pain assessment in a cognitively impaired older adult, the American Geriatrics Society encourages the integration of the following six behavioral domains:

    1. Facial expressions.

    2. Verbalizations or vocalizations.

    3. Body movements.

    4. Changes in interpersonal interactions.

    5. Changes in activity patterns or routines.

    6. Mental status changes.

B. Clinicians should be mindful of older patients with dementia and chronic LBP and should accordingly adjust pain management.

    1. Dementia can alter pain reporting, pain behaviors, and pain coping.

    2. Older patients may not reliably communicate the need for analgesic medications.

C. Due to harmful side effects in older patients with non cancer pain, nonopioid medications are preferred to opioids.

D. Doses of opioid medications should be reduced in older adults and also titrated slowly.

    1. Decrease initial dose by 25% for a 60-year-old patient and by 50% for an 80-year-old patient.

Bibliography

Deyo, R. A., & Tsui-Wu, Y. (1987). Descriptive epidemiology of low-back pain and its related medical care in the United States. *Spine, 12*(3), 264–268. doi:10.1097/00007632-198704000-00013

Kasper, D. L., Fauci, A. S., Hauser, S. L., Longo, D. L., Jameson, J. L., & Loscalzo, J. (2015). *Harrison's principles of internal medicine* (19th ed.). New York, NY: McGraw-Hill.

Knight, C. Deyo, R., Staiger, T., & Wipf, J. (2017, December 6). Treatment of acute low back pain. In L. Kunins (Ed.), *UpToDate*. Retrieved from https://www.uptodate.com/contents/?source=search_result&search=acute%20low%20back%20pain&selectedTitle=1

Parvizi, J. (2010). *High yield orthopaedics*. Philadelphia, PA: Saunders/Elsevier.

Swiontkowski, M. F., & Stovitz, S. D. (2006). *Manual of orthopaedics* (6th ed.). Philadelphia, PA: Lippincott Williams & Wilkins.

Wheeler, S. G., Wipf, J. E., Staiger, T. O., Deyo, R. A., & Jarvik, J. G. (2018, July 12). Evaluation of low back pain in adults. In L. Kunins & S. I. Lee (Eds.), *UpToDate*. Retrieved from https://www.uptodate.com/contents/evaluation-of-low-back-pain-in-?source=search_result&search=acute%20low%20back%20pain&selectedTitle=2 26

Wright, R., Malec, M., Shega, J. W., Rodriguez, E., Kulas, J., Morrow, L., . . . Weiner, D. K. (2016). Deconstructing chronic low back pain in the older adult—Step by step evidence and expert-based recommendations for evaluation and treatment: Part XI: Dementia. *Pain Medicine, 17*(11), 1993–2002. doi:10.1093/pm/pnw247

Compartment Syndrome of the Lower Leg

Joanne Elaine Pechar

Definition

A. A surgical emergency, which refers to a build-up of pressure within a muscle compartment (surrounded by a closed fascia) leading to a decline in tissue perfusion in the injured extremity; causes permanent damage to muscle and nerves.

B. A serious complication typically resulting from a crush injury to a large bone. There is an increase in closed compartmental pressure causing ischemic changes and diminished microcirculation within the soft tissues.

Incidence

A. The average annual overall incidence of acute compartment syndrome (ACS) is 3.1 cases per 100,000 people.
B. Due to relatively larger muscle mass in men, ACS is more prevalent in men compared to women.
C. Tibial fractures caused by trauma account for approximately 75% of ACS cases; blunt soft tissue injury is the second-leading cause.
D. The most common sites of ACS are (in descending order of prevalence): Calf, forearm, thigh, upper arm, hand, and foot.

Pathogenesis

A. ACS develops when the intracompartmental pressure (ICP) exceeds venous capillary pressure.
B. Arteriovenous pressure gradient theory.
  1. Ischemia begins when local blood flow cannot meet the metabolic demands of surrounding affected tissue.
  2. As compartment pressure rises, venous outflow is reduced and venous pressure rises, leading to a decrease in the arteriovenous pressure gradient.
  3. Without intervention, due to arteriolar compression, microcirculation is compromised, and blood is shunted away from intracompartmental tissues, which ultimately reduces tissue perfusion.
  4. Inadequate tissue perfusion and oxygenation results in soft tissue ischemia, cellular necrosis, anoxia, and irreversible death of the cells.
C. Anatomy of the lower leg.
  1. There are four compartments in the lower leg: Anterior, lateral, superficial posterior, and deep posterior.
  2. Each individual compartment encloses specific muscles, nerves, arteries, veins, and bones.

Predisposing Factors

A. Trauma-related closed tibial shaft fracture is the major contributing factor to ACS and accounts for one-third of all ACS cases.
B. List of traumatic and nontraumatic ACS etiologies.
  1. Vascular: Reperfusion therapy, arterial puncture or injury, hemorrhage, and deep vein thrombosis.
  2. Soft tissue: Crush injury, contusion, fall, direct blow, burn, and snake bite.
  3. Iatrogenic: Drugs such as anticoagulants, bleeding disorders, circumferential wraps, casts or splints, constrictive dressings, tourniquets, long leg brace, extravasations of drugs and fluids, prolonged lithotomy positioning, viral myositis, and diabetic muscle infarction.

Subjective Data

A. Common complaints/symptoms.
  1. The cardinal symptom of ACS is pain out-of-proportion.
  2. Persistent burning pain at rest.
  3. Pain reproduced with passive stretch of the affected muscle compartment.
B. Common/typical scenario.
  1. Massive swelling of the limb with firm and tense feeling on deep palpation.
  2. Reduced two-point discrimination or vibration sense.
  3. Loss of light touch sensation.

C. Family and social history.
  1. Family and social history are noncontributory, as the cause of ACS is typically related to injury or surgery.
D. Review of systems.
  1. Pain out of proportion to injury is often an early and sensitive sign of ACS.
    a. Most patients at risk for ACS have sustained trauma, fracture, or injury to the nerve or soft tissue, which may be the source of pain.
    b. The injured extremity becomes swollen and tense as ACS develops. Increasing ICP builds up on nerve fibers and injured components within the compartment.
    c. Obtunded patients, patients emerging from anesthesia, or patients receiving nerve blocks may not accurately report pain.
    d. In the late stages of ACS, pain may not be a subjective clinical finding, as pain receptors and nerve fibers are at high risk of ischemic necrosis and death.
  2. Paresthesia.
    a. Onset, which suggests the first signs of ischemic nerve dysfunction, is within approximately 30 minutes to 2 hours following injury.

Physical Examination

A. Paralysis is found in the late stages of ACS.
  1. A higher ICP leads to ischemic neuronal tissues and nerve dysfunction and subsequent paresthesia, paresis, and, ultimately, complete paralysis.
  2. Motor function may deteriorate within 4 hours of muscle tissue ischemia.
  3. At 8 to 24 hours of ischemia, motor and sensory loss is irreversible.
B. Pulselessness is a late finding, which is a poor indicator of ACS.
  1. As ICP rises, a loss of limb pulses indicates a decline in arterial perfusion.
C. Pallor.
  1. Presence of pallor and longer capillary time in the injured limb indicates direct arterial injury.
D. Poikilothermia.
  1. Presence of coolness or a change in the temperature in the affected extremity.

Diagnostic Tests

A. High index of clinical suspicion and the "6 Ps" cardinal symptoms: Pain, pallor, poikilothermia, paresthesia, paralysis, and pulselessness.
B. Measuring limb ICP.
  1. Stryker pressure monitoring device: A hand-held digital monitor for single tissue fluid pressure readings. To measure, the clinician injects 0.3 mL of saline solution into each of the four leg compartments (see Figure 14.1).
  2. An ICP of 30 mmHg or above is considered a critical threshold for diagnosis of ACS, and, if ICP is elevated, emergent decompression should be considered.
  3. Normal pressure of a tissue compartment falls between 0 and 8 mmHg in resting stage.
  4. ICP should be measured in each compartment of interest but within 5 cm from the injured or fractured site.
C. Delta pressure.
  1. Delta pressure is the difference between the diastolic pressure and the measured ICP.
  2. Delta pressure of less than, or equal to, 30 mmHg is diagnostic of ACS.

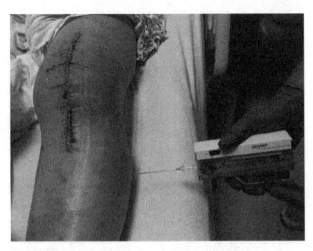

FIGURE 14.1 Advanced practice provider (APP) monitoring for compartment syndrome.

Differential Diagnosis

A. Deep vein thrombosis.
B. Thrombophlebitis.
C. Cellulitis.
D. Necrotizing fasciitis.
E. Peripheral vascular injury.
F. Rhabdomyolysis.
G. Shin splints.
H. Stress fractures.

Evaluation and Management Plan

A. General plan.
  1. Standard treatment: Emergent fasciotomy is a surgical limb-saving procedure to decompress the affected compartments and prevent critical limb ischemia.
    a. Two types of surgical technique: Single or double incision.
      i. Single-incision technique involves a single long incision made from the head of the fibula to the lateral malleolus.
      ii. Double-incision technique is the most common fasciotomy method: Four-compartment technique incorporating two longitudinal anterolateral and posteromedial incisions.
  2. In 48 to 72 hours, return to surgery is needed for reevaluation of muscle viability and wound debridement of nonviable tissues.
  3. Once ACS is completely resolved within 7 to 10 days, the fasciotomy wound is left open for delayed primary closure or skin grafting.
  4. To prevent bacterial colonization, improve circulation, and approximate wound edges, a negative pressure wound therapy is used for assisted closure of fasciotomy wounds.
  5. Nonoperative treatment measures.
    a. Loosening compression dressings, "bi-valving" casts, and complete removal of splints and casts.
    b. Elevation of the affected extremity to facilitate venous drainage, reduce edema, and maximize tissue perfusion.
B. Patient/family teaching points.
  1. ACS is a surgical emergency that can develop quickly.
  2. Permanent damage to muscles and nerves can occur within hours, which can necessitate amputation if not addressed immediately.
  3. Keep the affected limb propped up on pillows so the limb is level with the heart.
  4. Do not put any compressive bandages over the site.
C. Pharmacotherapy.
  1. There is no pharmacological treatment for ACS, only surgery will reduce the pressure in the compartment.
D. Discharge instructions.
  1. Seek care immediately if the pain or swelling does not improve, fever or rash develops, or the injured limb becomes cold or numb.
  2. Contact the provider with questions or concerns.

Follow-Up

A. Follow-up is needed in 1 to 2 weeks for neurovascular examination, control of swelling, and wound check to ensure complete wound healing.

Consultation/Referral

A. Early consultation and collaboration with orthopedic or vascular surgery is critical for limb salvage and to prevent possible devastating complications, such as the following.
  1. Wound infection.
  2. Paralysis.
  3. Permanent nerve damage.
  4. Contractures.
  5. Amputation.
  6. Rhabdomyolysis.
  7. Multiorgan failure.
  8. Sepsis.
  9. Death.

Special/Geriatric Considerations

A. Diagnosis of ACS may be delayed with older patients who received epidural anesthesia and who sustained neurovascular injuries following total knee arthroplasty (TKA).
  1. Continuous epidural analgesia can mask pain associated with passive stretching, therefore delaying diagnosis.
  2. Older patients may develop foot drop or peroneal nerve injury following TKA.

Bibliography

Asprey, D. P., & Dehn, R. W. (2013). *Essential clinical procedures*. Philadelphia, PA: Elsevier Health Sciences.

Azar, F. M., Canale, S. T., & Beaty, J. H. (2017). *Campbell's operative orthopaedics*. Philadelphia, PA: Elsevier.

Donaldson, J., Haddad, B., & Khan, W. S. (2014). The pathophysiology, diagnosis and current management of acute compartment syndrome. *The Open Orthopaedics Journal, 8*(1), 185–193. doi:10.2174/1874325001408010185

Gahtan, V., & Costanza, M. J. (Eds.). (2015). *Essentials of vascular surgery for the general surgeon*. New York, NY: Springer.

Murdock, M., & Murdoch, M. M. (2012). Compartment syndrome: A review of the literature. *Clinics in Podiatric Medicine and Surgery, 29*(2), 301–310. doi:10.1016/j.cpm.2012.02.001

Pechar, J., & Lyons, M. M. (2016). Acute compartment syndrome of the lower leg: A review. *The Journal for Nurse Practitioners, 12*(4), 265–270. doi:10.1016/j.nurpra.2015.10.013

Raza, H., & Mahapatra, A. (2015). Acute compartment syndrome in orthopedics: Causes, diagnosis, and management. *Advances in Orthopedics, 2005*, 1–8. doi:10.1155/2015/543412

Stahel, P. F., Mauser, N., Gissel, H., Henderson, C., Hao, J., & Mauffrey, C. (2013). Acute lower-leg compartment syndrome. *Orthopedics, 36*(8), 619–624. doi:10.3928/01477447-20130724-07

Vegari, D. N., Rangavajjula, A. V., Dilorio, T. M., & Parvizi, J. (2014). Fasciotomy following total knee arthroplasty: Beware of terrible outcome. *The Journal of Arthroplasty, 29*(2), 355–359. doi:10.1016/j.arth.2013.05.013

Joint Pain

Laura A. Santanna Lonergan

Definition

A. Joint pain can be discomfort, pain, or inflammation arising from any part of a joint including cartilage, bone, ligaments, tendons, or muscles.

B. Acute joint pain is defined as pain resolving within 6 weeks of onset.

C. Chronic joint pain extends past 6 weeks from onset of symptoms.

D. Many joint pain complaints stem from self-limiting conditions, but there are many causes that require immediate and ongoing care.

E. Osteoarthritis (OA) or degenerative joint disease (DJD), which presents with pain and swelling resulting in decreased joint mobility, is the most common form of joint disease. It may affect any joint in the body, notably the hips and knees.

F. OA can affect the cartilage that cushions the ends of bones and allows for easy movement of joints.

Incidence

A. It is estimated that approximately 5% of primary care office visits are for joint pain with OA being the most common diagnosis.

Pathogenesis

A. Sources of pain within the joint include the joint capsule, periosteum, ligaments, subchondral bone, and synovium, but not the articular cartilage, which lacks nerve endings.

B. The basic pathophysiologic types of joint disease and pain stem from synovitis, enthesopathy, crystal deposition, infection, and structural or mechanical derangements.

Predisposing Factors

A. A combination of clinical, laboratory, and imaging data can help to differentiate patients likely to have self-limited disease from those likely to have persistent arthritis.

B. Prediction models based upon patients with early arthritis have identified a number of features associated with persistent and/or erosive disease, including:

1. Duration of symptoms prior to presentation.
2. Older age.
3. Male gender.
4. High body mass index (BMI).
5. Duration of morning stiffness.
6. Number of tender or swollen joints.
7. Involvement of lower extremities.
8. Elevated acute phase reactants.
9. Rheumatoid factor.
10. Anti-cyclic citrullinated peptide (anti-CCP) antibody.
11. Erosive change on baseline radiograph.
12. Human leukocyte antigen (HLA)-DRB1 shared epitope alleles.

Subjective Data

A. Common complaints/symptoms.
1. Knee pain.
2. Shoulder pain.
3. Hip pain.
4. Hand pain.
5. Ankle and foot pain.
6. Soft tissue swelling or effusion.
7. Joint erythema and warmth.
8. Joint tenderness.
9. Joint contractures or deformity.
10. Joint stiffness.
11. Myalgias and muscle spasms.
12. Muscle weakness.

B. Common/typical scenario.
1. Rash.
2. Fever.
3. Crepitus.

C. Family and social history.
1. Family history may have a role in joint pain. Specific questions inquiring about autoimmune diseases in the family should be addressed.
2. Patient's daily routine may provide insight into causes of repetitive injuries.
3. Smoking can also contribute to joint pain.

D. Review of systems.
1. Specific symptoms to ask patients with joint pain.
   a. Fever.
   b. Weight loss.
   c. Night sweats.
   d. Rash.
   e. Nodules.
   f. Neuropathy.
   g. Joint swelling.
   h. Joint erythema.
   i. Tenderness.
   j. Warmth around joint.
   k. Inability to use joint.
   l. Eye pain.
   m. Eye dryness.
   n. Recent infection.
   o. Recent tick bite.
   p. Recent exposure to sexually transmitted infection (STI).
   q. Recent joint injection or surgery.
   r. History of immunosuppression.
2. Joint pain may represent a vast number of problems. The following questions can help direct clinical decision making and narrow down differential diagnosis.
   a. Is one joint affected or many joints affected?
      i. One joint = monoarticular.
      ii. Two to four joints = oligoarticular.
      iii. Greater than five joints = polyarticular.

E. Is inflammation present or absent?

F. What joints are involved?

G. Are there systemic symptoms?

Physical Examination

A. A complete history and physical examination is appropriate for all patients presenting with joint pain, since this symptom may be the initial manifestation of a systemic illness.

B. The following findings on physical examination could indicate a more serious pathogenesis of joint pain.
1. General survey: Level of patient's pain, ability to carry out activities of daily living (ADL).
2. Vital signs: Fever.
3. Eye: Keratoconjunctivitis sicca, uveitis, conjunctivitis, episcleritis.
4. Neck: Lymphadenopathy.
5. Mouth: Parotid enlargement, oral ulcerations.

6. Cardiovascular (CV): Murmur, pericardial, or pleural friction rubs.

7. Lungs: Fine inspiratory rales (secondary to interstitial lung disease).

8. Skin: Skin lesions may suggest that the joint symptoms are due to psoriatic arthritis, systemic lupus erythematosus (SLE), viral infection, or Still's disease.

9. Musculoskeletal: Swollen, erythematous, warm joints, joint deformities, range of motion of joints.

10. Neurovascular: Muscle tone, muscle strength, sensory perceptions, gait.

Diagnostic Tests

A. Arthrocentesis and examination of synovial fluid to include a cell count, gram stain, crystal analysis, and culture.
B. Laboratory tests.
   a. Complete blood count (CBC).
   b. Basic metabolic panel (BMP).
   c. Liver function test (LFTs).
   d. Erythrocyte sedimentation rate (ESR).
   e. C-reactive protein (CRP).
   f. Uric acid.
   g. Antinuclear antibody (ANA).
   h. Rheumatoid factor.
   i. Anti-CCP antibody.
C. Radiologic imaging of affected joint(s).
   a. X-rays.
   b. CT scan.
   c. MRI.
D. Tissue biopsy.

Differential Diagnosis

A. Adult Still's disease.
B. Ankylosing spondylitis.
C. Avascular necrosis.
D. Bone cancer.
E. Certain types of arthritis.
   1. OA.
   2. Juvenile rheumatoid arthritis.
   3. Psoriatic arthritis.
   4. Reactive arthritis.
   5. Rheumatoid arthritis.
   6. Septic arthritis.
F. Fractured bone.
G. Bursitis.
H. Complex regional pain syndrome.
I. Dislocation.
J. Gonococcal arthritis.
K. Gout.
L. Hypothyroidism.
M. Leukemia.
N. Lupus.
O. Lyme disease.
P. Osteomyelitis.
Q. Paget's disease of bone.
R. Polymyalgia rheumatica.
S. Pseudogout.
T. Rickets.
U. Sarcoidosis.
V. Sprains and strains.
W. Tendinitis.

Evaluation and Management Plan

A. General plan.
   1. Avoid using affected joint if doing so causes pain.

   2. Use ice to area 15 to 20 minutes of each hour.
   3. Specific treatment targeted to each individual diagnosis that may include but not be limited to:
      a. Physical therapy.
      b. Surgical management.
      c. Pharmacologic intervention (noted in the following section).
B. Patient/family teaching points.
   1. Exercise and weight loss are highly effective in relieving joint pain.
   2. Start with low-impact exercises that don't irritate the joint such as swimming or cycling.
   3. Short-term joint pain can be relieved with rest, ice, compressing with a wrap, and elevating the joint above the level of the heart.
C. Pharmacotherapy.
   1. Analgesic medications: Nonsteroidal anti-inflammatory drugs (NSAIDs), Tylenol.
   2. Steroids.
   3. COX-2 inhibitors.
   4. Disease-modifying antirheumatic drugs (DMARDs).
   5. Intra-articular injections.
D. Discharge instructions.
   1. Total hip arthroplasty (THA) and total knee arthroplasty (TKA) are highly effective elective procedures for patients who suffer from hip and knee pain, which is mainly due to joint deterioration from OA.
      a. THA and TKA can relieve pain, restore function, and improve quality of life by replacing the diseased articular surfaces with synthetic material.
      b. Discharge criteria.
         i. Stable vital signs and afebrile for more than 24 hours postoperatively.
         ii. Wound incision clean, dry, and intact.
         iii. Hip and knee pain well managed and controlled.
         iv. No signs and symptoms of infection, such as fever, hip erythema, and warmth.
         v. No signs and symptoms of blood clot, such as hip or leg swelling, and calf tenderness.
      c. Activity.
         i. Full weight-bearing status with physical therapy.
         ii. Walker and crutch training will be provided prior to hospital discharge.
         iii. Patient can resume most daily activities within a few weeks after surgery.
         iv. After a THA, patients may need to adhere to hip precautions for 6 weeks.
         v. Avoid bending and flexing hips greater than 90°C.
         vi. Avoid twisting leg in or out.
         vii. Avoid crossing legs at the knee or ankle.
         viii. Avoid allowing legs to cross midline.
         ix. Avoid raising knee higher than the hip.
         x. Avoid allowing toes to point inward (pigeon-toe) or to rotate outward (duck-walking).
         xi. Always lie on the back while resting in bed, and place a pillow between the thighs if laying on one's side.
         xii. Sit in chairs higher than knee height.
         xiii. Avoid low beds.
         xiv. Avoid pivoting on the operated leg, and take small steps when turning.
         xv. Before standing, scoot to the edges of beds and chairs.

xvi. After a TKA, the following measures are needed to protect a new knee joint.

  1) Place pillow between the thighs if laying on one's side.

  2) Avoid kneeling or squatting.

  3) Avoid twisting the new knee.

d. Diet.

  i. Patients are not able to eat or drink until fully recovered from anesthesia.

  ii. To avoid nausea after surgery, start patients slowly on a clear liquid diet.

  iii. Once clear liquid diets are tolerated, patients may be offered solid foods.

  iv. Since narcotics should not be mixed with alcohol, limit alcohol consumption.

  v. Eat healthy foods and watch weight.

  vi. Obesity can add more stress to the new joint.

e. Medications.

  i. Used for postoperative pain management, the multimodal perioperative pain protocol (MP3) consists of short- and long-acting opioids, oral nonsteroidal anti-inflammatory cyclooxygenase-2 inhibitor NSAIDs, intravenous NSAIDs, and anticonvulsants.

  ii. Percocet 5/325 mg 1 to 2 tablets every 4 to 6 hours as needed.

  iii. Gabapentin 100 mg twice a day for 2 weeks.

  iv. Celebrex 200 mg twice a day for 6 weeks.

  v. Toradol 7.5 mg intravenous every 6 hours as needed (do not exceed 5 days).

  vi. Morphine 2 mg intravenous every 2 hours as needed.

f. Wound care.

  i. Always keep the surgical wound clean and dry.

  ii. Unless instructed to do otherwise, do not apply any lotions, creams, oils, ointments, or powders to the surgical wound area.

  iii. Leave the dressing in place for 7 days postoperatively.

  iv. Dressing will be removed by a provider at rehab or by a home health nurse.

  v. Two weeks from the day of surgery, at the first orthopedic follow-up appointment, staples or sutures will be removed.

  vi. Patient may shower but the incision must be well covered. Do not scrub the incision.

g. Follow-up.

  i. Patients are instructed to follow-up with the surgeon in 6 weeks or immediately for any concerning signs or symptoms.

  ii. Discuss with patient.

  1) Concerning signs or symptoms to monitor.

  2) Difficulty breathing, shortness of breath, dyspnea, or pleuritic chest pain.

  3) Persistent nausea or vomiting.

  4) Persistent fever over 101°F, chills, and sweating.

  5) Signs of a blood clot.

  iii. Pain in the operative leg and calf tenderness.

  iv. Tenderness and erythema of the operative leg.

  v. Unexplained swelling, which does not dissipate with elevation, of the operative limb.

  1) Pain with rotation of the limb and worsening pain even after taking pain medicine.

  2) Unexplained limb shortening or extreme rotation.

  3) Wound drainage soaking through the bandage over the incision.

  4) Intermittent claudication, which is walking-based thigh pain that clears quickly with sitting.

  5) Signs of wound infection.

    a) Increased pain, swelling, warmth, or erythema around the incision.

    b) Pus fluid draining from the incision.

h. Intraoperative complications.

  i. Fracture.

  ii. Nerve injury.

  iii. Vascular injury.

i. Postoperative complications and readmission concerns.

  i. Deep vein thrombosis.

  ii. Pulmonary embolism.

  iii. Septic hip.

  iv. Cellulitis.

  v. Hematoma.

  vi. Hip dislocation.

  vii. Periprosthetic fracture.

  viii. Hip fractures.

  1) Femoral head fracture.

  2) Femoral neck fracture.

  3) Intertrochanteric fracture.

  4) Subtrochanteric fracture.

  5) Femoral shaft fracture.

  6) Distal femur fracture.

  ix. Knee fractures and tendon ruptures.

  1) Patella fracture.

  2) Quadriceps tendon rupture.

  3) Patella tendon rupture.

  4) Tibial plateau fracture.

  5) Tibia and fibula shaft fracture.

    a) Septic knee.

    b) Knee dislocation.

    c) Aseptic loosening.

    d) Heterotrophic ossification.

    e) Leg length discrepancy.

    f) Foot drop and peroneal nerve palsy.

Follow-Up

A. Follow-up with provider when joint pain begins. Do not wait until the pain is intense and the joint becomes stiff.

B. Physical therapy can assist patients in relieving joint pain with exercises.

Consultation/Referral

A. Based off of patient diagnosis, but may include:

  1. Primary care.

  2. Orthopedist.

  3. Rheumatologist.

  4. Infectious disease.

Special/Geriatric Considerations

A. Certain joint pain diagnoses are more frequent in older adults over age 60.

B. OA.

C. Gout and pseudogout.

D. Polymyalgia rheumatica.

E. Osteoporotic fracture.

F. Septic arthritis.

Bibliography

Baer, A. N. (2016, December 26). The approach to the painful joint. In H. S. Diamond (Ed.), *Medscape*. Retrieved from https://emedicine.medscape.com/article/336054-overview

Harrison, T. R., Kasper, D. L., Fauci, A. S., Hauser, S. L., Longo, D. L., Jameson, J. L., & Loscalzo, J. (2015). *Harrison's principles of internal medicine*. New York, NY: McGraw Hill Education.

Joint Pain. (2016, February 26). Mayo clinic. Retrieved from http://www.mayoclinic.org/symptoms/joint-pain/basics/definition/sym-20050668

Papadakis, M. A., McPhee, S. J., & Rabow, M. W. (Eds.). (2016). *Current medical diagnosis & treatment 2016*. New York, NY: McGraw-Hill.

Plamer, T., & Toombs, J. D. (2004). Managing joint pain in primary care. *Journal of the American Board of Family Medicine, 17*(Suppl. 1), 32–42. doi:10.3122/jabfm.17.suppl_1.S32

Shmerling, R. H. (2019, March 7). Evaluation of the adult with polyarticular pain. In M. Ramirez Curtis (Ed.), *UpToDate*. Retrieved from https://www.uptodate.com/contents/evaluation-of-the-adult-with-polyarticular-pain

Osteoarthritis

Joanne Elaine Pechar

Definition

A. Osteoarthritis (OA) is defined as evident cartilage loss without inflammatory or crystal arthropathy, irrespective of whether the patient has symptoms.

Incidence

A. OA is the most common type of joint disease, affecting more than 20 million individuals in the United States alone.
B. Ninety percent of all people have radiographic evidence of OA in weight-bearing joints by age 40.
C. Symptomatic disease increases with age.
D. Develops in women more frequently than in men.

Pathogenesis

A. OA is characterized by degeneration of cartilage and by hypertrophy of bone at the articular margins.
B. Cartilage, subchondral bone, and synovium have been found to all have key roles in disease pathogenesis.

Predisposing Factors

A. Hereditary and mechanical factors may be involved.
  1. Mechanical factors.
    a. Excessive weight, causing additional pressure.
    b. Repetitive movements or overuse, which causes damage to joints, tendons, and ligaments.
      i. Can break down cartilage over time.
B. Obesity is a risk factor for OA of the knee, hand, and hip.
C. Playing competitive contact sports increases the risk for developing OA.
D. Jobs requiring frequent bending and carrying increase the risk of knee OA.

Subjective Data

A. Common complaints/symptoms.
  1. The onset is insidious.
  2. The disease process may start with articular stiffness or deep aching joint pain lasting less than 30 minutes; may be most prominent upon awakening.
B. Common/typical scenario.
  1. Reduced range of motion and crepitus of affected joint is frequently present.
  2. There are no systemic manifestations.
C. Family and social history.
  1. May have genetic component.
  2. Repetitive use and jobs requiring heavy lifting and bending may contribute.
  3. Obesity.
D. Review of systems.
  1. Elicit onset, frequency, duration, and location of symptoms.
  2. Inquire if pain is worse during activity or at rest.
  3. Inquire about exacerbating factors.
  4. Inquire about presence and duration of morning stiffness.
  5. Determine if there are any systemic signs such as fever.

Physical Examination

A. Comprehensive musculoskeletal examination may reveal:
  1. Flexion contracture or varus deformity of the knee.
  2. Palpable osteophytes of the distal interphalangeal (DIP; Heberden nodes) and proximal interphalangeal (PIP; Bouchard) nodes.
  3. Limited range of motion of the affected joint or joints.
  4. Crepitus felt over the knee joint.
  5. Joint effusion and other articular signs of inflammation.

Diagnostic Tests

A. Laboratory test.
  1. Erythrocyte sedimentation rate (ESR)—OA does not cause elevation of the ESR or other laboratory signs of inflammation.
  2. Synovial fluid—tends to be noninflammatory.
B. Imaging.
  1. Plain film radiographs of the affected joint may reveal.
    a. Narrowing of the joint space.
    b. Osteophyte formation.
    c. Lipping of marginal bone.
    d. Thickened, dense subchondral bone.
    e. Bone cysts.

Differential Diagnosis

A. Gout.
B. Pseudogout.
C. Rheumatoid arthritis.
D. Psoriatic arthritis.
E. Reactive arthritis.
F. Septic arthritis.
G. Fibromyalgia.
H. Tendonitis.
I. Avascular necrosis.
J. Charcot joint.
K. Lyme disease.
L. Patellofemoral syndrome.
M. Prepatellar bursitis.

Evaluation and Management Plan

A. General plan.
  1. Nonpharmacologic.
    a. OA of the hand may benefit from assistive devices and instruction on techniques for joint protection.
  2. OA of the first carpometacarpal joint may benefit from splinting.
  3. OA of the knee or hip may benefit from a regular exercise program.
  4. If patient is overweight, he or she should be instructed to lose weight.

5. The use of assistive devices (e.g., a cane on the contralateral side) can improve functional status.

6. Surgical intervention.

    a. Total hip and knee replacements provide excellent symptomatic and functional improvement when involvement of that joint severely restricts walking or causes pain at rest.

    b. Arthroscopic surgery for knee OA is ineffective.

B. Patient/family teaching points.

1. General education of patients regarding benefits of exercise and weight loss.

2. Exercise can strengthen muscles and reduce pain and potentially help patients to avoid surgery.

3. Weight loss will reduce pressure on joints and slow down destruction of cartilage.

4. Avoid repetitive movements of an affected joint.

5. Use protective gear such as joint padding when playing sports to avoid injury.

C. Pharmacotherapy.

1. Acetaminophen is first-line analgesic therapy (2.6–4 g/day orally).

2. Nonsteroidal anti-inflammatory drugs (NSAIDs) provide more pain relief but have greater side effects of toxicity.

3. Chondroitin sulfate and glucosamine, alone or in combination, are no better than placebo in reducing pain in patients with knee or hip OA.

4. Intra-articular injections.

    a. Triamcinolone (20–40 mg) for patients with OA of the knee or hip may reduce the need for oral analgesics and can be repeated up to four times a year. The American College of Rheumatology does not recommend corticosteroid injections for OA of the hand.

    b. Sodium hyaluronate produces moderate reduction in symptoms in some patients with OA of the knee.

Follow-Up

A. Follow-up with your provider on a regular basis until your pain and mobility level are optimized.

B. The patient should call once joint pain starts for better management.

C. Follow-up at least once a year with your provider once your symptoms are controlled.

Consultation/Referral

A. Refer to an orthopedic surgeon when pain, loss of function, or both warrant consideration of hip or knee joint replacement surgery.

Special/Geriatric Considerations

A. OA may account for up to 70% of the geriatric population's joint pain.

B. This places geriatric patients at a higher risk for falls.

C. Nonsurgical candidates may be considered for physical reconditioning and pharmacologic pain control.

Bibliography

Egol, K. A., Koval, K. J., & Zuckerman, J. D. (2015). *Handbook of fractures*. Philadelphia, PA: Wolters Kluwer/Lippincott Williams & Wilkins Health.

Glyn-Jones, S., Palmer, A. J. R., Agricola, R., Price, A. J., Vincent, T. L., Weinans, H., & Carr, A. J. (2015). Osteoarthritis. *The Lancet, 368*(9991), 376–387. doi:10.1016/S0140-6736(14)60802-3

Lozada, C. J. (2016, November 30). Arthritis. *Medscape*. Retrieved from http://emedicine.medscape.com/article/330487

Maxey, L., & Magnusson, J. (2013). *Rehabilitation for the postsurgical orthopedic patient*. St. Louis, MO: Elsevier/Mosby.

Papadakis, M. A., McPhee, S. J., & Rabow, M. W. (2016). *Current medical diagnosis & treatment 2016*. New York, NY: McGraw Hill Education.

Peters, C. L., Shirley, B., & Erickson, J. (2006). The effect of a new multimodal perioperative anesthetic regimen on postoperative pain, side effects, rehabilitation, and length of hospital stay after total joint arthroplasty. *The Journal of Arthroplasty, 21*(6), 132–138. doi:10.1016/j.arth.2006.04.017

Scott, W. N. (2012). *Insall & Scott surgery of the knee* (5th ed.). Philadelphia, PA: Elsevier/Churchill Livingstone.

Rheumatoid Arthritis

Dana Cafaro

Definition

A. Rheumatoid arthritis (RA) is a chronic, inflammatory, symmetric polyarthritis that can have systemic effects on multiple organ systems with no clear etiology.

Incidence

A. Prevalence 1% with female to male ration of 3:1.

B. Peak onset for women is fourth to fifth decade.

C. Peak onset for men is sixth to eighth decade.

D. Annual incidence is 40 per 100,000.

E. Increased frequency of the disease in first-degree relatives and monozygotic twins.

Pathogenesis

A. No clear cause has been identified for RA; however, genetics and environment appear to contribute to the development of RA. The best characterized genetic risk factor is inheritance of the HLA DRB1 alleles encoding a "shared epitope."

B. Chronic synovitis and joint destruction are characteristic of RA.

C. Pannus, destructive vascular granulation tissue, is a distinctive feature of RA and destroys adjacent cartilage, bone, ligaments, and tendons.

Predisposing Factors

A. Gender-specific risk factors.

1. Women: Nulliparity and postpartum state can increase acute flare.

2. Men: Below normal testosterone levels.

B. Genetic predisposition.

C. Cigarette smoking, heavy caffeine consumption, and oral contraception, particularly in patients carrying the shared epitope.

D. Infection (both bacterial and viral) has been hypothesized to trigger RA but no specific bacterial or viral pathogens have been identified.

E. Autoantibody carriers, specifically rheumatoid factor (RF) and anti-citrullinated peptide/protein antibodies (ACPA), increase the risk for development of RA.

F. Occupational exposures including dust and silica.

Subjective Data

A. Common complaints/symptoms.

1. Insidious onset of polyarticular inflammation and complaints of joint pain and stiffness is the most common presentation but some patients may present with acute symptoms.

2. Joint stiffness will last more than 30 minutes and is prominent in the morning, after periods of inactivity and after strenuous activity.

3. Systemic manifestations can also be present.

4. Symptoms tend to be reported in the small joints of the hands, wrist, and forefoot. All joints of the extremities can be affected. Typically, the axial skeleton except for the cervical spine will not be involved.

B. Common/typical scenario.

1. Systemic symptoms include dryness of the eyes and mucous membranes, presence of rheumatoid nodules, pulmonary symptoms including cough and dyspnea, weight loss, fatigue, and depression.

2. Felty syndrome is seen in advanced disease and is characterized by splenomegaly and neutropenia. (C).

C. Family and social history.

1. Family history of RA.

2. Social history.

   a. Smoking.

   b. Caffeine intake.

   c. Occupational exposures.

D. Review of systems.

1. Joint pain and stiffness.

2. Swelling.

3. Presence of skin nodules.

4. Changes in skin color.

5. Dryness of mucous membranes.

6. Cough.

7. Dyspnea.

Physical Examination

A. Symmetrical, polyarticular swelling with pain, and tenderness is characteristic.

B. "Boggy" feeling over the affected joints due to synovial thickening or effusion.

C. Palmar erythema may be present in acute flares.

D. Deformities are common in late disease and may be asymmetrical.

E. Decreased grip strength is noted in disease affecting the hands and can be an early indicator of disease.

F. Ulnar deviation, swan neck deformities (flexion of the distal interphalangeal [DIP] joint with extension of the proximal interphalangeal [PIP] joint) and Boutonniere deformities (hyperextension of the DIP joint with flexion of the PIP joint) of the fingers are common in chronic RA.

G. Tendon ruptures can occur.

H. Rheumatoid nodules are subcutaneous nodules found over bony prominences (most commonly), bursae, and tendon sheaths and are found in 20% of patients.

I. Ocular findings include scleritis and episcleritis.

Diagnostic Tests

A. Radiographs (most specific testing): Early images may be normal or show evidence of soft tissue swelling and juxta-articular demineralization. Later images will reveal joint space narrowing and erosions.

B. Elevated erythrocyte sedimentation rate (ESR) and C-reactive protein levels: Elevated in acute phases.

C. Anti-cyclic citrullinated peptide (anti-CCP) antibodies and RF: present in about 3/4 of patients with RA.

D. Synovial fluid analysis: Inflammatory effusion often performed to rule out septic arthritis.

Differential Diagnosis

A. Fibromyalgia.

B. Lyme disease.

C. Myelodysplastic syndrome.

D. Osteoarthritis.

E. Sarcoidosis.

F. Systemic lupus erythematosus.

Evaluation and Management Plan

A. General plan.

1. Goals.

   a. Reduce pain and inflammation.

   b. Preserve function.

   c. Prevent deformity.

2. Nonpharmacologic.

   a. Physical and occupational therapy.

   b. Diet and exercise.

   c. Smoking cessation.

   d. Osteoporosis screening and treatment.

   e. Immunizations to reduce risk of immunosuppressive therapies.

B. Patient/family teaching points.

1. Similar to nonpharmacological management.

2. Diet.

3. Exercise.

4. Smoking cessation.

5. Physical and occupational therapy.

6. Routine screening and immunizations.

C. Pharmacotherapy.

1. Nonsteroidal anti-inflammatory drugs (NSAIDs): For symptomatic relief, but not to be used as monotherapy.

2. Corticosteroids.

   a. Used to bridge until disease-modifying antirheumatic drugs (DMARDs) are effective or during active disease.

   b. Will decrease inflammation and slow articular erosion.

   c. Recommended dose is prednisone 5 to 10 mg po daily.

     i. Higher doses may be needed to treat extra-articular manifestations and should be tapered when discontinuing.

   d. Intra-articular corticosteroids may be helpful to treat one to two symptomatic joints but may not be administered more than four times per year.

   e. Recommended dose is triamcinolone 10 to 40 mg based on size of joint being treated.

3. DMARDs.

   a. Begin as soon as RA is confirmed.

   b. More efficacious when used in combination than as a monotherapy.

   c. Most commonly used combination is methotrexate with a tumor necrosis factor (TNF) inhibitor.

     i. Methotrexate: Initial synthetic DMARD of choice (7.5 mg po weekly); can see improvement in 2 to 6 weeks.

     ii. TNF inhibitors: Added when patients do not respond to methotrexate.

Follow-Up

A. Patients should follow-up after starting or changes are made to medications.

Consultation/Referral

A. Rheumatology as early as possible to confirm diagnosis and manage disease.

Special/Geriatric Considerations

A. RA can be a debilitating disease that makes activities of daily living very difficult.

B. Geriatric patients may have increased risk associated with RA, such as:

1. Cognitive impairment.
2. Depression.
3. Falls.
4. Urinary incontinence.
5. Malnutrition.

Bibliography

Firestein, G. S. (2017, August 30). Pathogenesis of rheumatoid arthritis. In P. L. Romain (Ed.), *UpToDate*. Retrieved from https://www.uptodate.com/contents/pathogenesis-of-rheumatoid-arthritis

Hannon, R. A., & Porth, C. M. (Eds.). (2017). *Porth pathophysiology: Concepts of altered health states* (2nd ed.). Philadelphia, PA: Wolters Kluwer.

Moreland, L. W., & Cannella, A. (2018, May 31). General principles of management of rheumatoid arthritis in adults. In P. L. Romain (Ed.), *UpToDate*. Retrieved from https://www.uptodate.com/contents/general-principles-of-management-of-rheumatoid-arthritis-in-adults?source=search_result&search=treatment%20rheumatoid%20arthritis&selectedTitle=1

Papadakis, M. A. (2017). *Current medical diagnosis & treatment 2017* (56th ed.). New York, NY: McGraw-Hill Education/Medical.

Venables, P. J. W. (2017, October 12). Clinical manifestations of rheumatoid arthritis. In P. L. Romain (Ed.), *UpToDate*. Retrieved from https://www.uptodate.com/contents/clinical-manifestations-of-rheumatoid-arthritis?source=search_result&search=rheumatoid%20arthritis&selectedTitle=2

Spondyloarthropathies

Dana Cafaro

Definition

A. Spondyloarthropathies are a group of inflammatory conditions that affect the axial skeleton and also may have multisystem effects.

B. Inflammatory arthritis of the spine and sacroiliac joints, asymmetric oligoarthritis of the peripheral joints, and inflammation at sites where tendon and ligament insert into bone (enthesopathy) characterize spondyloarthropathies.

C. Spondyloarthropathies include ankylosing spondylitis, psoriatic arthritis, reactive arthritis, and arthritis associated with inflammatory bowel disease.

D. Also known as seronegative spondyloarthropathies.

E. Clinical presentation and diagnostic evaluation are similar for the seronegative spondyloarthropathies.

Incidence

A. Males are more often affected.

B. Onset is typically before age 40.

C. Ankylosing spondylitis is common to manifest in late teens and early 20s.

Pathogenesis

A. The cause of spondyloarthropathies is not well understood.

B. It appears to be a genetic relationship to human leukocyte antigen (HLA)-B27.

C. Some theories exist that attribute microbial exposure as a possible cause; for example, chlamydia-induced arthritis, psoriatic arthritis, and the development of arthritis in patients with Crohn's disease and ulcerative colitis.

Predisposing Factors

A. Male.

B. Genetic predisposition.

C. Bacterial infections.

Subjective Data

A. Common complaints/symptoms.

1. Low back pain more than 3 months' duration.
   a. Back pain may also have an "inflammatory pattern," which is insidious onset often before age 40. It improves with exercise, but not rest and nocturnal pain.
   b. Also characteristic can be relief of pain within 24 to 48 hours of taking nonsteroidal anti-inflammatory drugs (NSAIDs).
2. Peripheral arthritis will affect the knees and ankles predominantly, and will often be asymmetrical, affecting one to three joints.
3. Ocular complaints include redness, pain, and photophobia. These may be the first presenting symptoms of spondyloarthropathy.

B. Common/typical scenario.

1. Ankylosing spondylitis will progress in cephalad direction with limited chest expansion.
2. Heart disease characterized by atrioventricular conduction defects and aortic regurgitation will manifest in severe disease.
3. Constitutional symptoms are typically absent.
4. Psoriatic arthritis may present with symmetric polyarthritis similar to rheumatoid arthritis. Pitting of the nails and onycholysis is common.
5. Reactive arthritis (formerly Reiter syndrome) will present with oligoarthritis, conjunctivitis, urethritis, and mouth ulcers. Patients will often report a history of gastrointestinal (GI) or sexually transmitted infections. Systemic symptoms such as fever and weight loss are more common.

C. Family/social history.

1. Family history.
   a. Spondyloarthropathies.
   b. Inflammatory bowel disease.
2. Social history.
   a. Sexual activity.
   b. Exercise.

D. Review of systems.

1. Back pain.
2. Joint pain.
3. Swelling.
4. Eye pain.
5. Eye redness.
6. Mucosal ulcers.
7. Rashes.
8. Changes in nails.
9. Vomiting.
10. Bowel changes.
11. Diarrhea.
12. Dysuria.
13. Genital discharge.
14. Fever.
15. Weight loss.

Physical Examination

A. Musculoskeletal findings include the following.

1. Decreased range of motion in the back over time.
2. Edema in peripheral arthritis.
3. Enthesitis most commonly in the heel or Achilles tendon, but can be seen at the following.
   a. Iliac crests.
   b. Greater trochanters.
   c. Epicondyles, tibial plateaus.
   d. Costochondral junctions of the sternum.

e. Humeral tuberosities, manubrial-sternal joints.

f. Occiput.

g. Spinous processes.

4. Dactylitis is a characteristic feature of spondyloarthropathies, especially psoriatic arthritis and less frequently reactive arthritis. The physical finding is also known as "sausage toe or sausage finger" and is characterized by swelling of the entire digit without pain or tenderness.

5. Ocular findings include nonpurulent conjunctivitis and anterior uveitis.

6. Dermatologic findings include psoriasis and pitting nails, particularly in patients with peripheral joint manifestations.

Diagnostic Tests

A. No laboratory tests are specific for spondyloarthropathies.

B. HLA-B27: 90% of patients with ankylosing spondylitis and 50% to 70% of patients with other types of spondyloarthropathies will be positive.

C. Negative rheumatoid factor.

D. Elevated erythrocyte sedimentation rate (ESR) and C-reactive protein (CRP) are elevated in 35% to 50% of patients. They are also used to assess radiographic progression and response to therapy.

E. Uric acid levels may be high with psoriatic arthritis.

F. Synovial fluid cultures in reactive arthritis are negative.

G. Axial radiographs: Findings of sacroiliitis including erosions, ankylosis, changes in joint width, or sclerosis, are specific for spondyloarthropathies; however, it takes several years to be visible on radiograph. Syndesmophytes can develop on the spine.

H. MRI can be useful in patients with nonradiographic evidence of spondyloarthropathies.

I. Ultrasound has been used to confirm enthesitis.

Differential Diagnosis

A. Degenerative disc disease.

B. Kyphosis.

C. Spine fractures, dislocations.

D. Osteoarthritis.

E. Spinal stenosis.

Evaluation and Management Plan

A. General plan.

  1. Reduce swelling and pain.

  2. Treat infectious processes and skin disorders.

B. Patient/family teaching points.

  1. Encourage exercise.

C. Pharmacotherapy.

  1. NSAIDs (use in caution in patients with inflammatory bowel disease).

  2. Tumor necrosis factor (TNF) inhibitors have been used for NSAID refractory cases for ankylosing spondylitis and methotrexate refractory cases of psoriatic arthritis. Both may also be used for reactive arthritis.

  3. Methotrexate is used in psoriatic arthritis to treat both cutaneous and arthritic manifestations.

  4. Monoclonal antibody therapy has been used in psoriatic arthritis patients who do not respond to TNF inhibitors.

  5. Sulfasalazine for peripheral arthritis.

  6. Psoralen and ultraviolet A (PUVA) therapy for psoriasis skin lesions.

  7. Antibiotics may be needed to treat GI or genitourinary infections in patients with reactive arthritis.

Follow-Up

A. Interval follow-up is necessary to monitor medication safety and patient's response to therapy.

Consultation/Referral

A. Physical therapy for exercise regimens.

B. Dermatology for skin manifestations.

C. Gastroenterology for GI manifestations.

D. Ophthalmology for ocular manifestations.

E. Infectious disease for sexually transmitted infections or other infectious diseases.

Special/Geriatric Considerations

A. Markers of disease progression and treatment do not appear to be age-related.

B. Standard precautions in the elderly related to pharmacokinetics still apply.

Bibliography

Hannon, R. A., & Porth, C. M. (2017). *Porth pathophysiology: Concepts of altered health states* (2nd ed.). Philadelphia, PA: Wolters Kluwer.

Papadakis, M. A., McPhee, S. J., & Rabow, M. W. (2016). *Current medical diagnosis & treatment 2016.* New York, NY: McGraw Hill Education.

Yu, D. T., & van Tubergen, A. (2018, September 7). Overview of the clinical manifestations and classification of spondyloarthritis. In P. L. Romain (Ed.), *UpToDate.* Retrieved from https://www.uptodate.com/contents/overview-of-the-clinical-manifestations-and-classification-of-spondyloarthritis?source=search_result&search=spondyloarthropathy&selectedTitle=1

Yu, D. T., & van Tubergen, A. (2019, January 1). Pathogenesis of spondyloarthritis. In P. L. Romain (Ed.), *UpToDate.* Retrieved from https://www.uptodate.com/contents/pathogenesis-of-spondyloarthritis?source=search_result&

Systemic Lupus Erythematosus

Monica Richey

Definition

A. Systemic lupus erythematosus (SLE) is a chronic inflammatory disorder characterized by:

  1. Multisystem involvement.

  2. Presence of antinuclear antibodies.

B. It has a chronic relapsing nature.

C. The course of the disease is variable, alternating between periods of stable disease (remission) and/or flares with high disease activity.

Incidence

A. The incidence of SLE in the United States ranges from 2.0 to 7.6 cases per 100,000 persons per year.

B. Prevalence ranges from 14.6 to 68 cases per 100,000 persons.

Pathogenesis

A. SLE can be set off by a combination of predisposing genetic traits, hormonal and environmental factors, or infectious agents.

B. These result in an abnormal immune response with dysregulation of B and T cells, resulting in the following.

  1. Production and formation of autoantibodies.

  2. Complement fixing.

  3. Immune complexes that promote inflammation and tissue damage.

Predisposing Factors

A. Affects more females than males with a ratio of 9:1, with a higher incidence among women of childbearing age.

B. Disproportionately affects more black women with a three to four times higher prevalence than whites.

C. There is also a higher incidence of SLE among the Afro-Caribbean, Asian, American Indian, and Hispanic descent populations as compared to the white population.

Subjective Data

A. Common complaints/symptoms.
  1. Malar rash.
  2. Arthritis.
  3. Fatigue.
  4. Fever.
  5. Pleurisy.
  6. Edema.
  7. Anemia.
  8. Lymphadenopathy.
B. Common/typical scenario.
  1. Patients typically present with fever, joint pain, and rash in women of childbearing age.
C. Family and social history.
  1. Lupus may run in families.
  2. There is currently no screening or genetic tests available.
D. Review of systems.
  1. Common questions.
    a. Onset of symptoms.
    b. Length of symptoms.
    c. New onset or previously experienced.
    d. Any triggers.
    e. Recent infections.
  2. Constitutional.
    a. Fevers.
    b. Chills.
    c. Malaise.
    d. Weight loss.
    e. Photosensitivity.
  3. Skin.
    a. Rashes.
    b. Does the patient have a diagnosis of Raynaud's phenomenon, which is periodic cold and numbness to fingers and toes?
  4. Head, ear, eyes, nose, and throat (HEENT).
    a. Lymphadenopathy.
    b. Dry mouth/eye.
  5. Cardiovascular.
    a. Chest pain.
    b. Palpitations.
  6. Pulmonary.
    a. Shortness of breath.
    b. Pleuritic chest pain.
  7. Peripheral vascular.
    a. Edema.
    b. Raynaud's.
    c. Wounds.
  8. Musculoskeletal.
    a. Arthritis.
    b. Arthralgias.
    c. Joint deformities.
  9. Gastrointestinal.
    a. Nausea.
    b. Vomiting.
    c. Changes in stools.
    d. Abdominal pain.

Physical Examination

A. Physical examination for SLE requires a full head-to-toe examination.
B. Cutaneous manifestations.
  1. Cutaneous vasculitis: Palpable petechiae in dependent areas, cutaneous necrosis, ulceration, and gangrene.
  2. Raynaud's phenomenon: Red, white, and blue, independent of disease activity, ulceration, atrophy, and gangrene.
  3. Livedo reticularis: Antiphospholipid syndrome (APS), blanchable red-purple ring, lace like.
  4. Photosensitivity: Rashes, fever, malaise, adenopathy, arthritis.
  5. Malar rash: Erythematous, edematous, spares nasolabial folds.
  6. Mucocutaneous lesions: Upper palate, maybe painless, sharply marginated.
  7. Alopecia: Diffuse or patchy, reversible, or permanent.
C. Musculoskeletal manifestations.
  1. Arthralgias.
  2. Arthritis.
  3. Myalgia and myositis.
D. Pulmonary manifestations—add imaging as needed.
  1. Pleurisy.
  2. Acute lupus pneumonitis: 80% mortality rate.
  3. Interstitial lung disease ground glass or honeycomb.
  4. Pulmonary embolus.
  5. Pulmonary hemorrhage.
  6. Pulmonary hypertension.
  7. Shrinking lung syndrome.
E. Cardiac/peripheral vascular manifestations—add imaging as needed.
  1. Pericarditis (echo).
  2. Myocarditis and myocardial dysfunction.
  3. Myocardial infarction (MI).
  4. Deep vein thrombosis (DVT).
  5. Edema.
F. Central nervous system (CNS) manifestations (19 different manifestations).
  1. Central.
    a. Aseptic meningitis.
    b. Cardiovascular disease.
    c. Demyelinating syndrome.
    d. Headache.
    e. Movement disorder.
    f. Myelopathy.
    g. Seizure disorder.
    h. Acute confusional state.
    i. Anxiety disorder.
    j. Cognitive dysfunction.
    k. Mood disorder.
    l. Psychosis.
    m. CNS vasculitis: Fevers, seizures, meningismus, altered behavior patterns.
  2. Peripheral.
    a. Guillain–Barre syndrome, autonomic neuropathy.
    b. Mononeuropathy.
    c. Myasthenia gravis.
    d. Cranial neuropathy.
    e. Plexopathy.
    f. Polyneuropathy.
  3. Hematological manifestations.
    a. Anemia.
    b. Thrombocytopenia.
    c. Leukopenia.
    d. Pancytopenia.

Diagnostic Tests

A. The diagnosis of lupus is based on clinical presentation and laboratory analysis.

B. The clinician should suspect lupus if 2+ organ systems are involved.

    1. Positive laboratory workup only with no symptoms does not give the diagnosis and does not require treatment.

C. Drug-induced SLE should be ruled-out if there is a presence of the following medications.

    1. Anti-tumor necrosis factor (TNF).

    2. Hydralazine.

    3. Anticonvulsants.

    4. Isoniazid.

    5. Thorazine.

    6. Procainamide.

    7. Penicillamine.

    8. Minocycline.

D. Laboratory workup for diagnosis.

    1. Complete blood count (CBC)/comprehensive metabolic panel (CMP)/elevated erythrocyte sedimentation rate (ESR)/C-reactive protein (CRP)/antinuclear antibody (ANA).

    2. Anti-histone (if applicable).

    3. ANA.

    4. Anti-double-stranded deoxyribonucleic acid (DsDNA).

    5. C3.

    6. C4.

    7. Anti-Smith antibody.

    8. Ribonucleoprotein (RNP).

    9. Anti ro (SSa).

    10. Anti La (SSb).

    11. Urine with microscopy.

E. Laboratory workup for flares:

    1. CBC/CMP/ESR/CRP.

    2. C3.

    3. C4.

    4. DsDNA.

    5. Urine with microscopy.

F. Diagnostic criteria.

    1. The American College of Rheumatology (ACR) has established 11 criteria for classification of SLE.

    2. These criteria are used mostly in clinical trials and population studies rather than for diagnostic purposes.

    3. A minimum of four criteria out of 11 are necessary to participate in clinical trials. The 11 criteria are divided into four cutaneous, four systemic, and three lab components.

Differential Diagnosis

A. Malignancies.

B. Infectious processes (cytomegalovirus [CMV], Epstein–Barr virus (EBV), HIV, and hepatitis).

C. Rheumatoid arthritis.

D. Scleroderma.

E. Fibromyalgia.

F. Thrombotic thrombocytopenia purpura (TTP).

G. Multiple sclerosis.

H. Myositis/dermatomyositis.

Evaluation and Management Plan

A. General plan.

    1. If previously diagnosed with SLE.

        a. Assess and treat urgent symptoms (rashes, infections, arthritis, shortness of breath [SOB], chest pain)—will likely need corticosteroid and/or anti-inflammatory.

        b. Infectious process must be rule-out—antibiotics as needed.

        c. Pain medications as needed in a short course.

    2. If newly diagnosed.

        a. Start corticosteroids.

        b. Refer to specialist ASAP.

    3. Associated conditions.

        a. Lupus nephritis (LN).

            i. Persistent proteinuria of greater than 0.5g/day, measured by a spot urine protein/creatinine ratio and/or 24-hour protein urine collection.

            ii. Urine dipstick of 3+ and/or presence of active urinary sediment, such as:

                1) More than five red blood cells (RBCs) or more than five white blood cells (WBCs) in the absence of infection.

            iii. All patients with clinical evidence of active but previously untreated LN should undergo renal biopsy (unless contraindicated).

            iv. The indications for renal biopsy are:

                1) Increase in serum creatinine level without compelling causes (e.g., sepsis).

                2) Confirmed proteinuria (≥ 1.0 g per 24 hours [either 24-hour specimens or spot protein/creatinine ratio]).

                3) Combinations of the following, confirmed in at least two tests done in a short period of time and in the absence of alternative cause.

                    a) Proteinuria of 0.5 g or more per 24 hours plus hematuria.

                    b) Proteinuria of 0.5 g or more per 24 hours plus cellular cast.

        b. APS.

            i. Primary APS: Occurs in 1% to 6% of population; 8% of primary APS patients later develop SLE.

            ii. Secondary APS: 30% of SLE patients could develop APS (50% risk of thrombosis).

                1) Laboratory criteria.

                    a) Anticardiolipin antibody or IgG and/or IgM; medium or high titer on 2+ occasion at least 12 weeks apart.

                    b) Positive lupus anticoagulant test on 2+ occasions at least 12 weeks apart.

                2) Definite APS: One clinical + one laboratory criteria.

                3) Antiphospholipid antibodies (ApL): Only laboratory criteria—DO NOT TREAT.

                4) Catastrophic APS (CAPS).

                    a) Multiple organs over a short period of days. Multiple thrombosis of small and medium size vessel may occur despite anticoagulation. 50% mortality.

        c. Management of lupus flares.

            i. Glucocorticoids: Patients with organ disease require high doses of prednisone (1mg/kg—up to 60 mg daily) or equivalent for 4 to 6 weeks followed by taper of 10% per week.

            ii. Flares presenting with synovitis, fevers, rashes, or serositis are managed with lower doses (10–20mg daily) with quick taper.

            iii. Long-term therapy with corticosteroids can lead to myopathy, osteoporosis, hypertension, diabetes, cataracts, atherosclerotic vascular disease, avascular necrosis of the bone, and infections.

B. Patient/family teaching points.

1. Exercise and healthy lifestyle may be important factors in mitigating symptoms.

2. The disease is lifelong and the goal of care is to reduce flare-ups.

C. Pharmacotherapy.

1. Antimalarial drugs: Hydroxychloroquine, quinacrine for joint pain, rash, and fatigue.

2. Glucocorticoids: Prednisone, methylprednisolone, solumedrol.

3. Topical steroid: Hydrocortisone, triamcinolone, fluocinolone for rash, skin lesions.

4. Nonsteroidal anti-inflammatory drugs (NSAIDs): Many forms; arthralgias, polyarthritis, add proton pump inhibitor (PPI) as needed.

5. Immunosuppressive agents: Azathioprine, mycophenolate, belimumab, cyclophosphamide, methotrexate, rituximab, dapsone, thalidomide.

Follow-Up

A. Patient should always be referred to a rheumatologist as soon as possible for follow-up and further treatment decisions.

Consultation/Referral

A. Rheumatologist.

B. Other specialties as needed, including dermatology, nephrology, and cardiology.

C. Social work.

D. Physical/occupational therapy.

Special/Geriatric Considerations

A. Infections.

1. Patients with SLE/LN are at increased risk for infections.

2. They should be encouraged to receive all inactivated vaccines, following Centers for Disease Control and Prevention (CDC) recommendations for patients who are immunosuppressed.

B. Heart disease.

1. SLE patients have a 7.5-fold increase in coronary artery disease (CAD).

2. Routine care for patients with SLE should include:

a. Screening for cardiovascular risk factor.

b. Counseling for lifestyle modification, such as smoking cessation, encouraging physical activity, and weight loss.

c. Screening for symptoms suggestive of heart disease.

C. Contraception.

1. Contraceptive options and education should be offered to all women with SLE.

2. Intrauterine devices containing levonorgestrel are among the safest and most effective options.

3. Also, progesterone-only pills are effective in long-term contraception.

4. Intense screening of risk factors for thrombotic events in women with SLE is important when prescribing contraceptives.

D. Osteoporosis.

1. Recommendations for patients taking glucocorticoid for more than 3 months include smoking cessation, regular exercise, and the administration of calcium (1,200–1,500 mg) and vitamin D (800–1,000 international units).

2. All patients starting on chronic treatment with glucocorticoid for more than 5 mg/day should be started on a bisphosphonate if there are no contraindications.

E. Pregnancy concerns.

1. SLE patients have worse outcomes with increased rates of the following.

a. Preeclampsia.

b. Fetal loss.

c. Preterm delivery (higher rates of delivery <34 weeks).

d. Fetal growth retardation (fgr).

e. Infants small for gestational age.

2. Blood pressure control is of utmost importance in managing SLE/LN patients during pregnancy.

3. Angiotensin-converting enzyme (ACE) inhibitors and angiotensin receptor blockers (ARBs) are contraindicated during all three trimesters of pregnancy.

a. Switch patients to other agents safer to use (if the potential benefits justify the potential risk to the fetus), such as methyldopa, labetalol, or nifedipine.

4. Because of immunosuppressant's fetal toxicity, only glucocorticoids, azathioprine, and hydroxychloroquine can be used safely during pregnancy.

5. They should be managed by a high-risk obstetrician in a tertiary center with a multidisciplinary team approach.

Bibliography

American College of Rheumatology Ad Hoc Committee on Systemic Lupus Erythematosus Guidelines. (1999). Guidelines for referral and management of systemic lupus erythematosus in adults. *Arthritis and Rheumatology, 42*(9), 1785–1796.

Bailey, T., Rowley, K., & Bernknopf, A. (2011). A review of systemic lupus erythematosus and current treatment options. *Formulary, 46*, 178–194.

Bramham, K., Hunt, B. J., Bewley, S., Germain, S., Calatayud, I., Khamashta, M. A., & Nelson-Piercy, C. (2011). Pregnancy outcomes in systemic lupus erythematosus with and without previous nephritis. *The Journal of Rheumatology, 38*(9), 1906–1913.

Chakravarty, E. F. (2008). What we talk about when we talk about contraception. *Arthritis & Rheumatology, 59*(6), 760–761.

Faurschou, M., Mellemkjaer, L., Starklint, H., Kamper, A. L., Tarp, U., Voss, A., & Jacobsen, S. (2011). High risk of ischemic heart disease in patients with lupus nephritis. *The Journal of Rheumatology, 38*(11), 2400–2405.

Grossman, J. M., Gordon, R., Ranganath, V. K., Deal, C., Caplan, L., & Chen, W. (2010). American College of Rheumatology 2010 recommendations for the prevention and treatment of glucocorticoid-induced osteoporosis. *Arthritis Care & Research (Hoboken), 62*(11), 1515–1526.

Hahn, B. H., McMahon, M. A., Wilkinson, A., Wallace, W. D., Daikh, D. I., & Fitzgerald, J. D. (2012). American College of Rheumatology guidelines for screening, treatment, and management of lupus nephritis. *Arthritis Care & Research (Hoboken), 64*(6), 797–808.

Hahn, B. H., & Wallace, D. J. (Eds.). (2013). *Dubois' lupus erythematosus and related syndromes.* Philadelphia, PA: Elsevier/Saunders.

Hochberg, M. C. (1997). Updating the American College of Rheumatology revised criteria for the classification of systemic lupus erythematosus. *Arthritis and Rheumatism, 40*(9), 1725. doi:10.1002/art.1780400928

Märker-Hermann, E., & Fischer-Betz, R. (2010). Rheumatic diseases and pregnancy. *Current Opinion in Obstetrics & Gynecology, 22*(6), 458–465. doi:10.1097/GCO.0b013e3283404d67

Michalski, J. P., & Kodner, C. (2010). Systemic lupus erythematosus: Safe and effective management in primary care. *Primary Care, 37*(4), 767–778. doi:10.1016/j.pop.2010.07.006

Mosca, M., Tani, C., Aringer, M., Bombardieri, S., Boumpas, D., & Brey, R. (2010). European League against rheumatism recommendations for monitoring patients with systemic lupus erythematosus in clinical practice and in observational studies. *Annals of the Rheumatic Diseases, 69*(7), 1269–1274. doi:10.1136/ard.2009.117200

Podymow, T., August, P., & Akbari, A. (2010). Management of renal disease in pregnancy. *Obstetrics and Gynecology Clinics of North America, 37*(2), 195–210. doi:10.1016/j.ogc.2010.02.012

Rahman, A., & Isenberg, D. A. (2008). Systemic lupus erythematosus. *The New England Journal of Medicine, 358*(9), 929–939. doi:10.1056/NEJMra071297

Richey, M. (2014). The management of lupus nephritis. *The Nurse Practitioner, 39*(3), 1–6. doi:10.1097/01.NPR.0000443229.10476.61

Tan, E. M., Cohen, A. S., Fries, J. F., Masi, A. T., McShane, D. J., & Rothfield, N. F. (1982). The 1982 revised criteria for the classification of systemic lupus erythematosus. *Arthritis and Rheumatism, 25*(11), 1271–1277. doi:10.1002/art.1780251101

Tunnicliffe, D. J., Singh-Grewal, D., Kim, S., Craig, J. C., & Tong, A. (2015). Diagnosis, monitoring, and treatment of systemic lupus erythematosus: A systematic review of clinical practice guidelines. *Arthritis Care & Research, 67*(10), 1440–1452. doi:10.1002/acr.22591

Turano, L. (2013). Premature atherosclerotic cardiovascular disease in systemic lupus erythematosus: Understanding management strategies. *Journal of Cardiovascular Nursing, 28*(1), 48–53. doi:10.1097/JCN.0b013e3182363e3b

Wallace, D. J. (2008). *Lupus: The essential clinician's guide* (1st ed., pp. 78–80). New York, NY: Oxford University Press.

Vasculitis-Variable Vessel

Dana Cafaro

Definition

A. Part of a group of disorders that result from inflammatory changes to walls of veins and arteries, causing damage to the mural structures which ultimately may cause tissue ischemia and necrosis.

B. Nomenclature is changing for the specific forms of vasculitis based on the Chapel Hill Consensus Conference (CHCC).

C. Two main types.

  1. Behçet disease.

  2. Essential cryoglobulinemia.

Incidence

A. More common in patients of Asian, Turkish, and Middle Eastern descent.

B. Prevalence similar in men and women.

C. Commonly afflicts patients ages 20 to 40 years old.

D. Disease is more severe in young male patients from Middle East or Far Eastern Asia.

Pathogenesis

A. Vasculitis can be a primary pathology or can be secondary to another underlying disease process (Table 14.1).

B. Direct injury to the vessel, infectious agents, or immune processes are known to cause vasculitis.

C. Secondary vascular injury may occur from physical agents such as cold and irradiation, mechanical injuries, and toxins.

  1. Behçet disease.

    a. Affects both arteries and veins of all sizes.

  2. Essential cryoglobulinemia.

    a. Cold-precipitated, immune-complex mediated.

  b. Occurs in chronic underlying infection (hepatitis C most commonly), connective tissue disease, lymphoproliferative disorders.

Predisposing Factors

A. First degree relative with Behçet disease increases the risk for the disease.

B. Essential cryoglobulinemia is associated with chronic hepatitis C infection.

Subjective Data

A. Common complaints/symptoms.

  1. Constitutional symptoms are common with all size vessel vasculitis and include fever, weight loss, malaise, and arthralgias/arthritis.

  2. Behçet disease.

    a. Aphthous lesions of mouth and genitals.

    b. Tender, erythematous popular lesions which ulcerate.

    c. Knee and ankle arthritis.

    d. Posterior uveitis, hypopyon.

    e. Neurological conditions including sterile meningitis, cranial nerve palsies, seizures, encephalitis, mental status changes, and spinal cord lesions.

    f. Hypercoagulable states.

  3. Essential cryoglobulinemia.

    a. Palpable purpura.

    b. Peripheral neuropathy.

    c. Abdominal pain.

    d. Digital gangrene.

    e. Pulmonary disease.

    f. Glomerulonephritis.

B. Common/typical scenario.

  1. Essential cryoglobulinemia.

    a. Purpura.

    b. Weakness.

    c. Arthralgia.

  2. Behçet disease.

    a. Recurrent, painful ulcers of mouth and genitals.

    b. Follicular rash.

    c. Uveitis.

    d. Sterile pustules at needlestick sites.

    e. Arthritis.

C. Family and social history.

  1. Essential cryoglobulinemia.

    a. Sexual history.

    b. Intravenous (IV) drug use.

    c. Family history of Behçet disease.

D. Review of systems.

  1. Essential cryoglobulinemia.

    a. Abdominal pain.

TABLE 14.1 **Classification of Vasculitis**

Variable Vessel	Large Vessel	Medium Vessel	Small Vessel
Behçet disease Essential cryoglobulinemia	Takayasu arteritis Giant cell/temporal arteritis	Polyarteritis nodosa Kawasaki disease Buerger disease Primary angiitis of the central nervous system	Henöch Schonlein purpura ANCA associated disorders: • Granulomatosis with polyangiitis • Microscopic polyangiitis • Eosinophilic granulomatosis with polyangiitis

ANCA, antineutrophil cytoplasmic antibodies.

b. Sensitivity to cold.
c. Skin changes.
d. Paresthesias.
e. Weakness.
2. Behçet disease.
  a. Mucosal ulcers.
  b. Skin nodules.
  c. Skin rashes.
  d. Joint pain.
  e. Eye pain.
  f. Photophobia.
  g. Eye redness.
  h. Visual changes.
  i. Headache.
  j. Weakness.
  k. Mental status changes.
  l. Chest pain.
  m. Dyspnea.

Physical Examination

A. Behçet disease.
  1. Aphthous ulcers of mouth and genitals.
  2. Follicular rash.
  3. Erythema nodosum-like lesions.
  4. Hypopyon.
B. Essential cryoglobulinemia.
  1. Palpable purpura.
  2. Peripheral sensorimotor deficits.
  3. Raynaud's phenomenon.

Diagnostic Tests

A. Behçet disease.
  1. Elevated erythrocyte sedimentation rate (ESR) and C-reactive protein (CRP).
  2. No definitive tests.
  3. Positive pathergy test: At least a 2 mm papule will develop 24 to 48 hours after needle insertion to the skin.
B. Essential cryoglobulinemia.
  1. Elevated liver enzymes.
  2. Positive cryoglobulins.
  3. Low C4 level.

Differential Diagnosis

A. Hepatitis B.
B. Hepatitis C.
C. HIV.
D. Connective tissue disease.
E. Lymphoproliferative disorders.
F. Other types of vasculitis.

Evaluation and Management Plan

A. General plan.
  1. Based on cause and severity of the vasculitis.
  2. Alleviation of symptoms.
B. Patient/family teaching points.
  1. Regular follow-up is necessary to monitor condition.
  2. Patients should also be educated on side effects of medications used for treatment.
C. Pharmacotherapy.
  1. Behçet disease.
    a. Colchicine 0.6 mg 1 to 3 times per day and thalidomide 100 mg daily.
    b. Apremilast for oral ulcers.
    c. Corticosteroids or azathioprine for severe disease.

d. Infliximab, cyclosporine, or cyclophosphamide for ocular and neurological disease.
  2. Essential cryoglobulinemia.
    a. Corticosteroids and rituximab or cyclophosphamide for 2 to 4 months.
    b. Hepatitis C treatment.

Follow-Up

A. Regular follow-up determined based on severity and cause of vasculitis.

Consultation/Referral

A. Based on cause and course of disease.
B. Consider:
  1. Ophthalmology.
  2. Dermatology.
  3. Infectious disease.

Special/Geriatric Considerations

A. Progression of these diseases is unpredictable and can affect basically all body systems.
B. Treatment is symptomatic alleviation.

Bibliography

Hannon, R. A., & Porth, C. M. (2017). *Porth pathophysiology: Concepts of altered health states* (2nd ed.). Philadelphia, PA: Wolters Kluwer.
Merkel, P. A. (2019, March 1). Overview of and approach to the vasculitides in adults. In M. Ramirez Curtis (Ed.), *UpToDate*. Retrieved from https://www.uptodate.com/contents/overview-of-and-approach-to-the-vasculitides-in-adults/print
Papadakis, M. A., McPhee, S. J., & Rabow, M. W. (2016). *Current medical diagnosis & treatment 2016*. New York, NY: McGraw Hill Education.
Smith, E. L., & Yazici, Y. (2018, November 13). Clinical manifestations and diagnosis of Behçet syndrome. In M. Ramirez Curtis (Ed.), *UpToDate*. Retrieved from https://www.uptodate.com/contents/clinical-manifestations-and-diagnosis-of-behcets-syndrome

Vasculitis-Small Vessel

Dana Cafaro

Definition

A. Part of a group of disorders that result from inflammatory changes to walls of veins and arteries, causing damage to the mural structures that ultimately may cause tissue ischemia and necrosis.
B. Nomenclature is changing for the specific forms of vasculitis based on the Chapel Hill Consensus Conference (CHCC).
C. There are several main types of small vessel vasculitis.
  1. Henöch–Schonlein purpura (IgA vasculitis).
  2. Antineutrophil cytoplasmic antibodies (ANCA)-associated disorders.
    a. Granulomatosis with polyangiitis (formerly Wegener's granulomatosis).
    b. Microscopic polyangiitis.
      i. Most common cause of pulmonary-renal syndromes.
      ii. Does not cause chronic upper respiratory tract disease.
      iii. Does not have granulomatous inflammation on biopsy.
    c. Eosinophilic granulomatosis with polyangiitis (formerly Churg–Strauss syndrome).

Incidence

A. Henöch–Schonlein purpura (IgA vasculitis).
   1. 90% of cases occur in pediatric population.
B. ANCA-associated disorders.
   1. Granulomatosis with polyangiitis (formerly Wegener's granulomatosis).
      a. 12 cases in 1 million people annually.
      b. Not gender specific.
      c. Age of onset commonly fourth to fifth decades.
   2. Microscopic polyangiitis.
      a. Most common cause of pulmonary-renal syndromes.
   3. Eosinophilic granulomatosis with polyangiitis (formerly Churg–Strauss syndrome).
      a. Mean age of onset is 40.
      b. No gender specificity.
      c. Possibility of genetic predisposition.

Pathogenesis

A. Vasculitis can be a primary pathology or can be secondary to another underlying disease process.
B. Direct injury to the vessel, infectious agents, or immune processes are known to cause vasculitis.
C. Secondary vascular injury may occur from physical agents such as cold and irradiation, mechanical injuries, and toxins.
D. Small vessel vasculitis may also be associated with ANCA.
   1. Henöch–Schonlein purpura (IgA vasculitis): Associated with IgA subclass 1 deposition in vessel walls.
   2. ANCA-associated disorders.
      a. Granulomatosis with polyangiitis (formerly Wegener's granulomatosis).
         i. Characterized by upper and lower respiratory tract disease and glomerulonephritis.
         ii. Fatal if not treated.
      b. Microscopic polyangiitis: Caused by necrotizing vasculitis.
      c. Eosinophilic granulomatosis with polyangiitis (formerly Churg–Strauss syndrome): Idiopathic in patients with asthma.

Predisposing Factors

A. Henöch–Schonlein purpura (IgA vasculitis): Recent infection such as group A streptococcus.
B. ANCA-associated disorders: Systemic diseases such as systemic lupus erythematosus, rheumatoid conditions, and polychondritis can predispose patients.
   1. Granulomatosis with polyangiitis (formerly Wegener's granulomatosis).
   2. Microscopic polyangiitis.
   3. Eosinophilic granulomatosis with polyangiitis (formerly Churg–Strauss syndrome).

Subjective Data

A. Common complaints/symptoms.
   1. Small vessel vasculitis will often present with purpura, vesiculobullous lesions, urticaria, glomerulonephritis, alveolar hemorrhage, cutaneous extravascular necrotizing granulomas, splinter hemorrhages, uveitis, episcleritis, and scleritis.
      a. Henöch–Schonlein purpura (IgA vasculitis).
         i. Palpable purpura usually on lower extremities, arthralgias of knees and ankles, and hematuria.
      b. ANCA-associated disorders.
         i. Granulomatosis with polyangiitis (formerly Wegener's granulomatosis).
            1) Upper respiratory tract: Nasal congestion, crusting, ulceration, bleeding, septal perforation, "saddle nose," sinusitis, otitis media, mastoiditis, gingival edema, stridor, subglottic stenosis.
            2) Lower respiratory tract: Cough, dyspnea, hemoptysis.
            3) Renal system: Hematuria, often not evident until disease is advanced (UTD).
            4) Other systems: Arthritis, ocular manifestations such as proptosis, scleritis, episcleritis, conjunctivitis, skin lesions, neuropathy.
            5) Deep vein thrombosis (DVT)s and pulmonary embolism (PE)s are also common.
         ii. Microscopic polyangiitis.
            1) Palpable purpura.
            2) Ulcers.
            3) Splinter hemorrhages.
            4) Vesicular bullous lesions.
            5) Interstitial lung fibrosis.
            6) Pulmonary-renal syndromes.
         iii. Eosinophilic granulomatosis with polyangiitis (formerly Churg–Strauss syndrome).
            1) Allergic rhinitis.
            2) Asthma.
B. Review of systems.
   1. Fever.
   2. Fatigue.
   3. Weight loss.
   4. Arthralgias.
   5. Respiratory symptoms (rhinorrhea, cough).
   6. Skin changes.
   7. Eye pain.
   8. Eye redness.
   9. Hematuria.

Physical Examination

A. Henöch–Schonlein purpura (IgA vasculitis).
   1. Palpable purpura in lower extremities and buttock.
B. ANCA-associated disorders.
   1. Granulomatosis with polyangiitis (formerly Wegener's granulomatosis).
      a. Nasal examination will reveal the following.
         i. Congestion.
         ii. Crusting.
         iii. Ulceration.
         iv. Bleeding.
         v. Septal perforation.
      b. "Saddle nose" deformity is a late finding.
      c. Otitis media.
      d. Proptosis.
      e. Conjunctivitis.
      f. Scleritis.
      g. Episcleritis.
      h. Signs of DVT.
         i. Calf swelling.
         ii. Erythema.
         iii. Tenderness.
   2. Microscopic polyangiitis.
      a. Palpable purpura.
      b. Ulcers.
      c. Splinter hemorrhages.
      d. Vesiculobullous lesions.
      e. Pneumonitis.
   3. Eosinophilic granulomatosis with polyangiitis (formerly Churg–Strauss syndrome).

a. Skin and lung involvement.
  i. Wheezing.
  ii. Rhinitis.
  iii. Macular rash.
  iv. Urticaria.
  v. Palpable purpura.

Diagnostic Tests

A. Henöch–Schonlein purpura (IgA vasculitis).
  1. Biopsy will reveal leukocytoclastic vasculitis with IgA deposition.
B. ANCA-associated disorders.
  1. Granulomatosis with polyangiitis (formerly Wegener's granulomatosis).
    a. Leukocytosis, thrombocytosis, normocytic, normochromic anemia.
    b. Elevated creatinine.
    c. Elevated C-reactive protein (CRP) and elevated erythrocyte sedimentation rate (ESR).
    d. Positive ANCA.
    e. Red cell casts and proteinuria.
    f. Lung biopsy more likely to show granulomas.
    g. Chest CT.
  2. Microscopic polyangiitis.
    a. 75% will be positive.
    b. Microscopic hematuria, proteinuria, red blood cell casts.
    c. Renal biopsy for necrotizing glomerulonephritis.
  3. Eosinophilic granulomatosis with polyangiitis (formerly Churg–Strauss syndrome).
    a. Eosinophilia in peripheral blood smear.
    b. Positive ANCA.

Differential Diagnosis

A. Other types of vasculitis.
B. Infection.
C. Malignancy.
D. Atherosclerosis.
E. Thromboembolic disease.
F. Congenital/hereditary disorders.
G. Hypercoagulable states.
H. Inflammatory disorders (you may want to consider making this a general differential diagnosis for all forms of vasculitis).

Evaluation and Management Plan

A. General plan.
  1. Henöch–Schonlein purpura (IgA vasculitis).
    a. Corticosteroids have been controversial and have not demonstrated reduction in long-term complications.
  2. ANCA-associated disorders.
    a. The disease process involves multiple systems. Treatment is symptomatic.
B. Patient/family teaching points.
  1. Requires regular examinations and tests to monitor for complications of the disease process.
  2. Take medications as indicated.
C. Pharmacotherapy.
  1. Henöch–Schonlein purpura (IgA vasculitis).
    a. Nonsteroidal anti-inflammatory drugs (NSAIDs) and Tylenol for treatment of pain; corticosteroids are reserved for refractory pain.
  2. ANCA-associated disorders.
    a. Granulomatosis with polyangiitis (formerly Wegener's granulomatosis).

i. Induction of remission.
  1) Cyclophosphamide (2 mg/kg/day orally adjusted for renal disease and age >70) plus corticosteroids (1 mg/kg/day).
  2) Rituximab and corticosteroids.
  3) Bactrim for prophylaxis of opportunistic infections if using cyclophosphamide.
ii. Maintenance of remission.
  1) Azathioprine (up to 2 mg/kg/day orally) if no evidence of thiopurine methyltransferase deficiency is confirmed.
  2) Methotrexate (20–25 mg/week orally or IM) if no renal insufficiency.
  3) Rituximab (500 mg intravenous [IV]) at remission, repeat day 14 and then every 6 months three times.
b. Microscopic polyangiitis (treatment is the same as granulomatosis with polyangiitis [formerly Wegener's granulomatosis]).
c. Eosinophilic granulomatosis with polyangiitis (formerly Churg–Strauss syndrome).
  i. Prednisone 0.5 to 1.5 mg/kg/day.
  ii. Cyclophosphamide for severe disease.

Follow-Up

A. Interval follow-up based on severity of disease.

Consultation/Referral

A. Refer to rheumatology.
B. Consider consultation based on course of illness.
  1. Nephrology for renal disease.
  2. Pulmonology for pulmonary disease.

Special/Geriatric Considerations

A. The presence of comorbid diseases as commonly found in the geriatric population can impact care or obscure diagnosis.
B. Infection is a prominent cause of morbidity and mortality in vasculitis patients and particularly with geriatric patients whose immune system may be compromised by other conditions and age.
C. Influenza can be potentially life-threatening and there is no evidence that immunization has a negative impact on vasculitis patients.
D. Recommend all geriatric vasculitis patients receive annual influenza vaccination.
E. Use of glucocorticoids as a treatment for vasculitis can cause osteoporosis and may lead to increased risk of falls and fractures.

Bibliography

Dedeoglu, F., & Kim, S. (2017, October 16). IgA vasculitis (Henoch-Schönlein purpura): Management. In E. TePas (Ed.), *UpToDate*. Retrieved from https://www.uptodate.com/contents/henoch-schonlein-purpura-immunoglobulin-a-vasculitis-management

Falk, R. J., Merkel, P. A., & King, T. E., Jr. (2019, January 23). Granulomatosis with polyangiitis and microscopic polyangiitis: Clinical manifestations and diagnosis. In A. Q. Lam, & & M. Ramirez Curtis (Eds.), *UpToDate*. Retrieved from https://www.uptodate.com/contents/clinical-manifestations-and-diagnosis-of-granulomatosis-with-polyangiitis-and-microscopic-polyangiitis

Hannon, R. A., & Porth, C. M. (2017). *Porth pathophysiology: Concepts of altered health states* (2nd ed.). Philadelphia, PA: Wolters Kluwer.

King, T. E., Jr. (2018, November 29). Treatment and prognosis of eosinophilic granulomatosis with polyangiitis (Churg-Strauss). In H. Hollingsworth (Ed.), *UpToDate*. Retrieved from https://www.uptodate.com/contents/treatment-and-prognosis-of-eosinophilic-granulomatosis-with-polyangiitis-churg-strauss

Merkel, P. A. (2019, March 1). Overview of and approach to the vasculitides in adults. In M. Ramirez Curtis (Ed.), *UpToDate*. Retrieved from https://www.uptodate.com/contents/overview-of-and-approach-to-the-vasculitides-in-adults

Papadakis, M. A., McPhee, S. J., & Rabow, M. W. (2016). *Current medical diagnosis & treatment 2016*. New York, NY: McGraw Hill Education.

Vasculitis-Medium Vessel

Dana Cafaro

Definition

A. Part of a group of disorders that result from inflammatory changes to walls of veins and arteries, causing damage to the mural structures, which ultimately may cause tissue ischemia and necrosis.

B. Nomenclature is changing for the specific forms of vasculitis based on the Chapel Hill Consensus Conference (CHCC).

C. Several different types.

   1. Polyarteritis nodosa.

   2. Kawasaki disease (more common in peds).

   3. Buerger disease (thromboangiitis obliterans).

   4. Primary angiitis of the central nervous system.

Incidence

A. Polyarteritis nodosa.

   1. Not common: 30 cases per 1 million people.

   2. Males affected more than females; common age presentation is in sixth decade.

B. Buerger disease (thromboangiitis obliterans).

   1. Typical patient is a young, male smoker using raw tobacco.

C. Primary angiitis of the central nervous system.

   1. Rare disorder with male predominance.

   2. Can occur at any age, with median age being 50 years old.

Pathogenesis

A. Vasculitis can be a primary pathology or can be secondary to another underlying disease process.

B. Direct injury to the vessel, infectious agents, or immune processes are known to cause vasculitis.

C. Secondary vascular injury may occur from physical agents such as cold and irradiation, mechanical injuries, and toxins.

D. Polyarteritis nodosa.

   1. First form of vasculitis reported.

   2. Predilection for vessels of skin, peripheral nerves, mesenteric vessels, renal vessels, heart, and brain.

   3. 10% of cases caused by hepatitis B infection.

E. Buerger disease (thromboangiitis obliterans).

   1. Highly cellular and inflammatory occlusive thrombus affecting the extremities.

F. Primary angiitis of the central nervous system.

   1. Vasculitis affecting brain and spinal cord.

Predisposing Factors

A. Male gender.

B. Use of raw tobacco for Buerger disease.

Subjective Data

A. Common complaints/symptoms.

   1. Polyarteritis nodosa.

      a. Arthralgia, myalgia, and neuropathy.

      b. Skin manifestations include lower extremity malleoli skin ulcerations (most common), digital gangrene, livedo reticularis, and subcutaneous nodules.

      c. Acute abdomen presentation when abdominal vessels are affected including abdominal pain, nausea, and vomiting.

      d. Hypertension when renal vessels are affected.

   2. Buerger disease (thromboangiitis obliterans).

      a. Distal extremity ischemia, ischemic digit ulcers, digit gangrene, migratory phlebitis.

   3. Primary angiitis of the central nervous system.

      a. Weeks to months of headaches, encephalopathy, and multifocal strokes.

B. Common/typical scenario.

   1. Patients will complain of various symptoms upon presentation that may be mistaken for other diseases.

   2. In polyarteritis nodosa, patients commonly present with acute abdominal pain.

   3. In Buerger disease, patients present with pain in their extremities; in primary angiitis, patients may present with strokes.

C. Family and social history.

   1. Buerger disease: Use of raw tobacco.

D. Review of systems.

   1. Arthralgias.

   2. Myalgias.

   3. Paresthesias.

   4. Skin changes.

   5. Abdominal pain.

   6. Nausea, vomiting.

   7. Headaches.

   8. Ataxia.

Physical Examination

A. Polyarteritis nodosa.

   1. Ulcerations on malleoli.

   2. Motor and sensory deficits.

   3. Digital gangrene.

B. Kawasaki disease (more common in peds).

   1. Bilateral conjunctivitis without exudate.

   2. Lip and oral erythema.

   3. Cervical lymphadenopathy.

   4. Rash.

   5. Edema of hands and feet.

C. Buerger disease (thromboangiitis obliterans).

   1. Superficial phlebitis.

   2. Digit ischemia.

D. Primary angiitis of the central nervous system.

   1. Motor and sensory deficits.

Diagnostic Tests

A. Polyarteritis nodosa.

   1. Anemia and leukocytosis.

   2. Antineutrophil cytoplasmic antibodies (ANCA) negative.

   3. Elevated C-reactive protein (CRP) and elevated erythrocyte sedimentation rate (ESR).

   4. Hepatitis B screening.

   5. Biopsy and angiogram of vessels and organs.

B. Buerger disease (thromboangiitis obliterans).

   1. Normal CRP, ESR, immunologic panel, hypercoagulability screen, and toxicology screen.

   2. Positive anticardiolipin antibodies.

   3. Consider arteriogram of upper and lower extremities and aorta.

C. Primary angiitis of the central nervous system.
　1. Cerebrospinal fluid (CSF): Leukocytosis with increased protein.
　2. Angiograms: String of beads pattern.
　3. Positive brain biopsy.
　4. Clinical diagnosis made by ruling out infection, neoplasm, metabolic disorder, and cocaine use.

Differential Diagnosis

A. Other forms of vasculitis.
B. Thromboembolic events.

Evaluation and Management Plan

A. General plan.
　1. Symptom management.
　2. Exercise and healthy lifestyle changes.
　3. Buerger disease (thromboangiitis obliterans).
　　a. Smoking cessation is the cornerstone of treatment.
　　b. Local wound care.
　　c. Pneumatic compression and spinal cord stimulation for pain due to ischemia.
B. Patient/family teaching points.
　1. Treatment of vasculitis with corticosteroids or other immunocompromising medications causes an immunocompromised state.
　2. Corticosteroids can lead to complications with diabetes, weight gain, or osteoporosis.
C. Pharmacotherapy.
　1. Polyarteritis nodosa.
　　a. Prednisone 60 mg orally daily.
　　b. Methylprednisolone 1,000 mg intravenous (IV) daily for 3 days for the critically ill.
　　c. Immunosuppressive agents for moderate to severe disease.
　2. Buerger disease (thromboangiitis obliterans).
　　a. Calcium channel blockers for vasospasm.
　3. Primary angiitis of the central nervous system.
　　a. Corticosteroids and cyclophosphamide.

Follow-Up

A. Interval follow-up based on severity of disease.

Consultation/Referral

A. Refer to rheumatology.

Special/Geriatric Considerations

A. There are no specific age-related considerations in vasculitis-medium vessel.

Bibliography

Hajj-Ali, R. A., & Calabrese, L. H. (2017, July 3). Primary angiitis of the central nervous system in adults. In M. Ramirez Curtis (Ed.), Retrieved from https://www.uptodate.com/contents/primary-angiitis-of-the-central-nervous-system-in-adults

Hannon, R. A., & Porth, C. M. (2017). *Porth pathophysiology: Concepts of altered health states* (2nd ed.). Philadelphia, PA: Wolters Kluwer.

Merkel, P. A. (2019, March 1). Overview of and approach to the vasculitides in adults. In M Ramirez Curtis (Ed.), *UpToDate*. Retrieved from https://www.uptodate.com/contents/overview-of-and-approach-to-the-vasculitides-in-adults

Olin, J. W. (2018, September 20). Thromboangiitis obliterans (Buerger's disease). In K. A. Collins (Ed.), *UpToDate*. Retrieved from https://www.uptodate.com/contents/thromboangiitis-obliterans-buergers-disease

Papadakis, M. A., McPhee, S. J., & Rabow, M. W. (2016). *Current medical diagnosis & treatment 2016.* New York, NY: McGraw Hill Education.

Sundel, R. (2018, November 13). Kawasaki disease: Clinical features and diagnosis. In E. TePas (Ed.), *UpToDate*. Retrieved from https://https://www.uptodate.com/contents/kawasaki-disease-clinical-features-and-diagnosis

Vasculitis-Large Vessel

Dana Cafaro

Definition

A. Part of a group of disorders that result from inflammatory changes to walls of veins and arteries, causing damage to the mural structures which ultimately may cause tissue ischemia and necrosis.
B. Nomenclature is changing for the specific forms of vasculitis based on the Chapel Hill Consensus Conference (CHCC).
C. Two main types.
　1. Takayasu arteritis.
　2. Giant cell arteritis/temporal arteritis.

Incidence

A. Takayasu arteritis.
　1. Common in Asian descent.
　2. Women are typically more affected than men.
　3. Age of onset tends to be early adulthood.
B. Giant cell arteritis/temporal arteritis.
　1. Most common vasculitis (UTD).
　2. Afflicts more females than males; age greater than 50 with the most common presenting age between 70 and 79.
　3. Common in Scandinavian descent.

Pathogenesis

A. Vasculitis can be a primary pathology or can be secondary to another underlying disease process.
B. Direct injury to the vessel, infectious agents, or immune processes are known to cause vasculitis.
C. Secondary vascular injury may occur from physical agents such as cold and irradiation, mechanical injuries, and toxins (P).
D. Takayasu arteritis.
E. Granulomatous vasculitis of aorta and its major branches (C).
F. Possible immunogenetic predisposition (U).
G. Giant cell arteritis/temporal arteritis.
　1. Chronic inflammatory disease of cranial branches of carotid arteries.

Predisposing Factors

A. Female gender, age typically over 60 years old.
B. Some familial pattern.

Subjective Data

A. Common complaints/symptoms.
　1. Constitutional symptoms are common with all size vessel vasculitis and include fever, weight loss, malaise, and arthralgias/arthritis.
　2. Large vessel vasculitis will often present with limb claudication, asymmetric blood pressures, absence of pulses, bruits, and aortic dilatation.
　3. Takayasu arteritis.
　　a. Decreased pulses.
　　b. Unequal upper extremity blood pressures.
　　c. Carotid and subclavian artery bruits.
　　d. Limb claudication and hypertension.

4. Giant cell arteritis/temporal arteritis.
  a. Headache, scalp tenderness.
  b. Visual changes, such as amaurosis fugax.
  c. Jaw claudication.
  d. Throat pain.
  e. Temporal artery tenderness.
B. Common/typical scenario.
  1. See previous sections for common/typical scenario.
C. Family and social history.
  1. Inquire about family history of vasculitis.
D. Review of systems.
  1. See previous sections for review of systems.

Physical Examination

A. Cardiology.
  1. Decreased pulses.
  2. Unequal upper extremity blood pressures.
  3. Carotid and subclavian artery bruits.
B. Limb claudication and hypertension.
C. Headache, scalp tenderness.
D. Visual changes, such as amaurosis fugax.
E. Jaw claudication.
F. Throat pain.
G. Temporal artery tenderness.

Diagnostic Tests

A. Takayasu arteritis.
  1. Elevated C-reactive protein (CRP) and elevated erythrocyte sedimentation rate (ESR).
  2. MRI or CT angiography (CTA) of affected vessels.
B. Giant cell arteritis/temporal arteritis.
  1. Normochromic anemia, normal leukocytes, decreased serum albumin, elevated liver enzymes, and elevated CRP and ESR.
  2. Best diagnostic test to confirm is temporal artery biopsy (UTD).
  3. In patients with normal temporal artery biopsy, consider magnetic resonance angiography (MRA) or CTA for confirmation.

Differential Diagnosis

A. Other forms of vasculitis.
B. Nonarteritic anterior ischemic optic neuropathy (NAAION).

Evaluation and Management Plan

A. General plan.
  1. Giant cell arteritis: Early intervention is necessary to prevent blindness, which can become permanent.

B. Patient/family teaching points.
C. Pharmacotherapy.
  1. Takayasu arteritis.
    a. Prednisone 1 mg/kg orally for 1 month; then tapered over several months to 10 mg orally daily.
    b. Methotrexate and mycophenolate mofetil may also be helpful.
  2. Giant cell arteritis/temporal arteritis.
D. Must be initiated quickly to avoid permanent blindness; therefore, if clinically suspected begin treatment.
E. Visual loss present at time of diagnosis: Intravenous (IV) methylprednisone 1,000 mg IV daily for 3 days followed by oral steroids (UTD).
F. Prednisone 60 mg po daily × 1 month then taper dose.
G. Low dose aspirin—81 mg po daily.

Follow-Up

A. Giant cell arteritis.
  1. Follow-up should be monthly for 6 months if possible and then spaced accordingly.
  2. Consider ophthalmology consult for visual symptoms.
B. Takayasu arteritis.
  1. Requires regular monitoring.

Consultation/Referral

A. Refer to rheumatology.

Special/Geriatric Considerations

A. Chronic steroid use can cause osteoporosis, so consideration should be made to treat osteoporosis.

Bibliography

Docken, W. P. (2018, August 13). Treatment of giant cell arteritis. In M. Ramirez Curtis (Ed.), *UpToDate*. Retrieved from https://www.uptodate.com/contents/treatment-of-giant-cell-temporal-arteritis?source=see_link

Docken, W. P. (2018, October 5). Diagnosis of giant cell arteritis. In M. Ramirez Curtis (Ed.), *UpToDate*. Retrieved from https://www.uptodate.com/contents/diagnosis-of-giant-cell-arteritis?topicRef=8240&source=related_link#H18

Docken, W. P., & Rosenbaum, J. T. (2017, December 8). Clinical manifestations of giant cell arteritis. In M. Ramirez Curtis (Ed.), *UpToDate*. Retrieved from https://www.uptodate.com/contents/clinical-manifestations-of-giant-cell-temporal-arteritis

Hannon, R. A., & Porth, C. M. (2017). *Porth pathophysiology: Concepts of altered health states* (2nd ed.). Philadelphia, PA: Wolters Kluwer.

Merkel, P. A. (2019, March 1). Overview of and approach to the vasculitides in adults. In M Ramirez Curtis (Ed.), *UpToDate*. Retrieved from https://www.uptodate.com/contents/overview-of-and-approach-to-the-vasculitides-in-adults

Papadakis, M. A., McPhee, S. J., & Rabow, M. W. (2016). *Current medical diagnosis & treatment 2016*. New York, NY: McGraw Hill Education.

15 Dermatology Guidelines

Amber Tran

Atopic Dermatitis

Amber Tran

Definition

A. Dermatitis means inflammation of the skin. It is a broad description describing an abnormal finding of the skin. Causes may be mechanical, environmental, allergic, viral, bacterial, fungal, parasitic, inflammatory, autoimmune (drug, lupus, psoriasis), neoplastic, and occasionally a combination. Treatment requires removing the offending agent and decreasing the inflammation to allow the skin to repair.
B. The most important thing for the new acute care advanced practice provider (APP) is to differentiate and determine whether a skin finding is acute, chronic, and/or emergent. If it is emergent, decide whether it is a condition you can treat yourself or if it requires a consult for dermatology, or if other hospital team specialists are needed.
C. Chronic pruritic inflammatory skin disease is common on flexural areas; this is associated with allergic rhinoconjunctivitis, asthma, and food allergies.
D. Most develop rash after scratching.

Incidence

A. May occur at any age.
1. Typically starts in childhood and may continue through adulthood.
2. About 1% to 3% of adults.
B. In past few decades, it has increased to around 30% for most industrialized countries versus around 10% in other countries.
C. High latitude.
D. Peaks during cold dry weather.

Pathogenesis

A. Thought to be caused by defective skin barrier for healing and maintaining skin integrity, but true cause remains unknown.

Predisposing Factors

A. Family history of atopic dermatitis (AD).
B. Breakdown of skin.
1. Dry skin.
2. Abrasion or injury.
3. Contact dermatitis (allergies, irritants).
C. Seasonal, environmental, or food allergies.
D. Dry weather.
E. Heat.
F. Stress.

Subjective Data

A. Common complaints/symptoms.
1. Itch.
2. Dry skin patches.
3. Burning.
B. Common/typical scenario.
1. Chronic rash that comes and goes.
a. Worse in cooler months; better in summer.
b. Flares with different exposures and seasons.
C. Family and social history.
1. Family history of AD.
2. Frequent hand washer or bather.
D. Review of systems.
1. Usually negative except for cold hands/feet.
2. Seasonal allergies.

Physical Examination

A. Dry erythematous patches.
B. Lichenification of older lesions.
C. Crusting and oozing may happen with and without infection (may be impetiginized).
D. Excoriations (scratched areas).
E. Locations tend to be on face and flexural folds of neck, arms, trunk, legs, wrists, and ankles (see Figure 15.1A and 15.1B).

Diagnostic Tests

A. Potassium hydroxide (KOH) preparation should be negative.
B. Skin biopsy: New lesions are preferred over older lesions that have either been lichenified or "burnt out"; hyperpigmented macules and patches may represent postinflammatory hyperpigmentation and not active rash.

Differential Diagnosis

A. Tinea (corporis, gruris, versicolor, manis, pedis).
B. Seborrheic dermatitis.
C. Stasis dermatitis.
D. Scabies.
E. Psoriasis.
F. Contact dermatitis.
G. Molluscum contagiosum.
H. Mycosis fungoides/cutaneous T cell lymphoma.

Evaluation and Management Plan

A. General plan.
1. Avoid triggers.
2. Avoid exacerbations (dry heat, excessive washing/bathing, contact with irritants, or use of irritants).

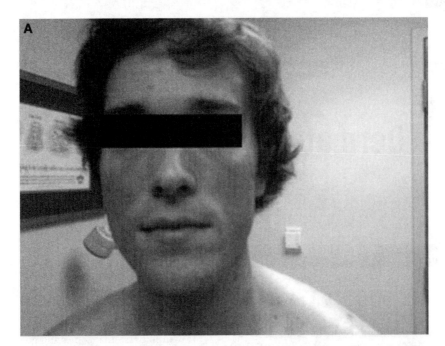

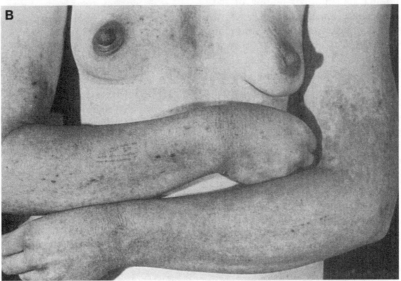

FIGURE 15.1 Examples of AD on the (A) face and (B) arms/trunk.
AD, atopic dermatitis.
Sources: (A) Lyons, F., & Ousley, L. (2015). *Dermatology for the advanced practice nurse.* New York, NY: Springer Publishing Company; (B) Courtesy of Centers for Disease Control and Prevention.

3. Maintain skin integrity through moisturization and decreasing inflammation.
B. Patient/family teaching points.
  1. Practice gentle skin care.
    a. Limit bathing to 5 minutes once daily at the most.
    b. Limit soap use.
    c. Use gentle nonsoap cleansers only.
    d. Do not use loofah or washcloth, only use hands to wash body.
    e. Only wash "dirty" areas: Face, axilla, genitalia, groin, hands, and feet.
    f. When drying after bathing pat skin dry gently; do not rub.
    g. For flares, apply topical medications within 5 minutes of leaving shower/bath.
    h. For nonflared areas and daily maintenance, apply moisturizer within 5 minutes of leaving shower/bath.
    i. Avoid wool clothing.
    j. Use hypoallergenic laundry detergents, hand soaps, body soaps, facial cleansers, and moisturizers.
    k. Use humidifier.
  2. Decrease stress.
  3. Avoid scratching.
  4. Treat early to help limit amount of topical/oral steroids needed.
C. Pharmacotherapy.
  1. Topical cream.
    a. Moisturizers.
      i. Lotions: Tend to not hold moisture in skin despite containing more water than creams and ointments.
      ii. Creams: Help lock in moisture better than lotions. Examples: Aveeno cream, Cetaphil cream, CeraVe cream, Eucerin cream, Lubriderm cream, Vanicream.
      iii. Ointments: Help lock in moisture better than creams. Examples: Vaseline, petroleum jelly.
      iv. Barrier creams: Zinc oxide.
  2. Topical steroid, typically twice daily for two consecutive weeks.

   a. Low potency for face, neck, groin, inner thighs, and buttocks.
   b. Medium potency for other areas.
   c. High potency for hands and feet.
 3. Oral steroid: Prednisone.
 4. Antihistamines.
   a. Low to medium strength: Claritin, Zyrtec, Benadryl.
   b. Medium to high strength: Hydroxyzine.
 5. Phototherapy: Refer to dermatology.
 6. Treat any secondary infections with oral therapy (viral, bacterial).

D. Discharge instructions (if standard accepted guidelines exist please use discharge template): If develops systemic signs of toxicity return to emergency department (ED).

Follow-Up

A. Primary care provider in 1 week.
B. Dermatology in 1 to 3 months depending on severity.

Consultation/Referral

A. If persists or worsens despite treatment, consult or refer to dermatology.
B. If diffuse, *always* refer to dermatology to rule out cutaneous lymphoma or another erythroderma. Cutaneous lymphoma is difficult to diagnosis and may take several skin biopsies before diagnosis is made.

Special/Geriatric Considerations

A. Controlling other allergies is essential.
B. Poor compliance and poor education will likely lead to longer duration of flares and worsening of them; consistent early treatment is best.
C. Elderly patients all develop drier and thinner skin with age, making it harder to clear and prevent flares.

Bibliography

Buttaro, T., Trybulski, J., Polgar Bailey, P., & Sandberg-Cook, J. (2013). *Primary care—E-book* (4th ed.). St. Louis, MO: Elsevier.
Fitzpatrick, J., & Morelli, J. (Eds.). (2011). *Dermatology secrets plus* (4th ed.) Philadelphia, PA: Elsevier.
Habif, T., Campbell, J. L., Jr., Chapman, M. S., Dinulos, J. G. H., & Zug, K. A. (2011). *Skin disease* (3rd ed.). Edinburgh, Scotland: Saunders/Elsevier.
Lyons, F., & Ousley, L. (2015). *Dermatology for the advanced practice nurse.* New York, NY: Springer Publishing Company.
Nutten, S. (2015). Atopic dermatitis: Global epidemiology and risk factors. *Annals of Nutrition and Metabolism, 66*(Suppl. 1), 8–16. doi:10.1159/000370220

Cellulitis

Amber Tran

Definition

A. Soft tissue infection primarily involving the skin that spreads and is frequently characterized by redness, warmth, swelling, and pain.
B. Cellulitis commonly occurs when there is a break in the skin.
C. An abscess may or may not be involved.

Incidence

A. May occur at any age.
B. More common in males.
C. May occur after an abrasion or surgical incision.
D. Typically in extremities, especially lower extremities.

E. Highly seasonal, more likely to occur during warmer summer months.
F. Costs \$3.74 billion annually; 30% of patients diagnosed with cellulitis are misdiagnosed, leading to unnecessary hospitalization and antibiotic use.

Pathogenesis

A. Most commonly caused by Group A beta-hemolytic streptococcus or methicillin-susceptible *Staphylococcus aureus* (MSSA).
B. Other less common causes.
 1. Other beta-hemolytic streptococcus.
 2. Methicillin-resistant *Staphylococcus aureus* (MRSA).
 3. *Streptococcus pyogenes* (presents with lymphangitis).
 4. *Pseudomonas aeruginosa.*
 5. *Erysipelothrix rhusiopathiae* from contact with raw meat (poultry, fish, other meat) typically seen in butchers or other handlers.
 6. Vibrio species from saltwater swimming, sea urchin impalement, or contact with raw seafood.
 7. *Aeromonas hydrophilia* from fresh water swimming.
 8. *Pasteurella multocida* from animal bite or injury.

Predisposing Factors

A. Injury or cut in affected area (abrasion, surgical incision, intravenous (IV) drug abuse, insect/animal bites, etc.).
B. Previous cellulitis.
C. Decreased mobility.
D. Impairment of vascular–lymphatic system.
 1. Venous insufficiency.
 2. Lymphedema due to impaired lymphatic drainage.
 3. Lymph node resection.
 4. Prior radiation treatments to affected area.
E. Chronic comorbidity conditions.
 1. Malnourishment, obesity, diabetes, chronic kidney disease, chronic liver disease, alcohol abuse.
 2. Immunosuppression (HIV, cancer, taking immunosuppressive agents).
 3. *Tinea pedis* or other dermatitis-affected skin integrity.

Subjective Data

A. Common complaints/symptoms.
 1. Elicit onset and duration of symptoms.
 2. Edema.
 3. Erythema.
 4. Tenderness or pain.
B. Common/typical scenario.
 1. Expanding sore erythematous edematous patch on lower extremity for 1 to 2 days, possibly near recent wound or injury.
C. Family and social history.
 1. Alcohol abuse.
 2. IV drug abuse.
 3. Any trauma to affected areas.
D. Review of systems.
 1. May have malaise.
 2. Fevers.
 3. Chills.
 4. Regional lymphadenopathy.
 5. Decreased mobility due to pain or swelling.

Physical Examination

A. One extremity (if bilateral it is very unlikely to be cellulitis. Stasis dermatitis is often bilateral and frequently misdiagnosed as cellulitis).

B. Usually a somewhat well-demarcated erythematous patch (a sharply demarcated indurated border increases likelihood of erysipelas; see Figure 15.2).

C. Tender.

D. Mild to moderate swelling.

E. Sometimes regional lymphadenitis (tender or enlarged) or lymphangitis.

F. Rarely blisters, necrosis.

G. If palpate warmth, need to rule out deep vein thrombosis (DVT).

H. If exquisite tenderness and rapid progression occurs, rule out necrotizing fasciitis.

I. Systemic signs of toxicity: Fever, hypotension, tachycardia.

Diagnostic Tests

A. Culture—when purulent discharge is present. Majority cannot be cultured unless abscess present for incision and drainage.

B. Biopsy—poor healing and low diagnostic yield.

C. Lab—elevated sedimentation rate and leukocytosis.

Differential Diagnosis

A. Stasis dermatitis.

B. Lipodermatosclerosis.

C. DVT.

D. Folliculitis.

E. Insect bite reaction.

F. Contact dermatitis.

G. Erysipelas.

H. Necrotizing fasciitis.

Evaluation and Management Plan

A. General plan.

   1. Antibiotics coverage for either gram-positive (most common), MRSA, or gram-negative (rare).

   2. Keep affected extremity raised.

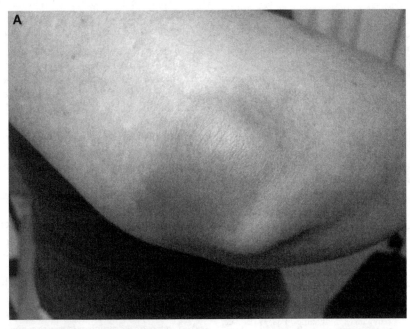

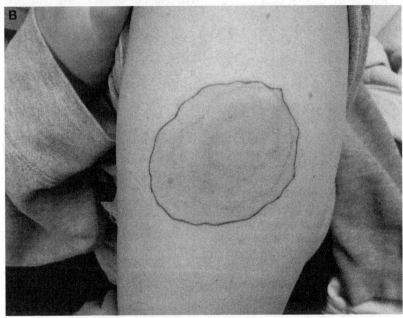

FIGURE 15.2   (A) An example of cellulitis. (B) Cellulitis resulting from a vaccination for varicella.
Source: Lyons, F., & Ousley, L. (2015). *Dermatology for the advanced practice nurse.* New York, NY: Springer Publishing Company.

3. Draw line on borders to monitor improvement or worsening.

4. If drainable abscess, incise and drain affected lesion.

5. If systemic symptoms present, check blood cultures first then initiate IV antibiotics.

6. Point of care ultrasound to differentiate abscess from cellulitis (which usually has cobblestone appearance).

B. Patient/family teaching points.

1. Keep affected extremity elevated.

2. Bathe once daily and clean area once daily with gentle soap and water.

3. Do not squeeze or irritate area.

4. If pain or rash is worsening, notify provider.

C. Pharmacotherapy.

1. Antibiotics for staphylococcus and streptococcus coverage: Dicloxacillin, azithromycin, clarithromycin, celphalexin, or cefazolin for 5 days.

2. Antibiotics for MRSA coverage: Clindamycin, trimethoprim-sulfamethoxazole, doxycycline, minocycline, linezolid, or tedizolid for 5 to 10 days.

3. Antibiotics for those with systemic signs of toxicity or who have extensive skin involvement, close proximity to indwelling medical device, inability to tolerate oral therapy, prior episode of MRSA or known colonization, or lack of response to antibiotic regimen that does not cover for MRSA.

  a. Empiric IV therapy for MRSA: Vancomycin or daptomycin.

  b. Once signs of infection are resolving, switch to oral regimen with coverage for MRSA and streptococcus.

4. Antibiotics for those with systemic signs of toxicity or who have extensive skin involvement with at least one of the following: Perioral/perirectal abscess, possible connection to pressure ulcer, or skin necrosis.

  a. Empiric IV therapy for MRSA.

  b. Start vancomycin or daptomycin with another antibiotic(s) to cover for gram-positive, gram-negative, and anaerobes.

D. Discharge instructions.

1. Complete course of antibiotics as directed by the provider.

2. Review with patient the common side effects of given antibiotic treatment (nausea, diarrhea, rash, and thrush/yeast infections).

3. Keep affected extremity elevated.

4. Warm compresses to affected area.

5. Avoid Neosporin to area as this can cause an allergic contact dermatitis.

6. If condition worsens, return to office.

Follow-Up

A. PCP in 1 to 2 days.

B. Dermatologist in 3 days.

C. If worsening or develops signs of systemic toxicity, patient should return to ED.

Consultation/Referral

A. If periorbital or orbital cellulitis, consult physician or infectious disease.

B. If no improvement within 24 to 48 hours of starting antibiotic therapy, consult infectious disease or dermatology.

C. If recurrent, consult/refer to dermatology and infectious disease.

Special/Geriatric Considerations

A. See section "Predisposing Factors." Many patients with cellulitis have comorbidities.

B. Immunosuppressed individuals have higher risk for complications such as necrotizing fasciitis, lymphangitis, gangrene, and severe sepsis.

C. Use extra caution with patients who have prosthetic joints or recent surgeries.

D. If patient has history of another known skin rash such as psoriasis, atopic dermatitis, or other, may be best to consult dermatology.

Bibliography

Cranendonk, D., van Vught, L., Wiewel, M., Cremer, O., Horn, J., Bonten, M., & Wiersinga, W. (2017). Clinical characteristics and outcomes of patients with cellulitis requiring intensive care. *Journal of the American Medical Association Dermatology, 153*(6), 578–582. doi:10.1001/jamadermatol.2017.0159

Dalal, A., Eskin-Schwartz, M., Mimouni, D., Ray, S., Days, W., Hodak, E., . . . Paul, M. (2017). Interventions for cellulitis and erysipelas: A summarised Cochrane review. *Cochrane Database System Review, 2017*(6), 227–228. doi:10.1002/14651858.CD009758.pub2

Lyons, F., & Ousley, L. (2015). *Dermatology for the advanced practice nurse.* New York, NY: Springer Publishing Company.

Marcelin, J., Challener, D., Tan, E., Lahr, B., & Baddour, L. (2017). Incidence and effects of seasonality on nonpurulent lower extremity cellulitis after the emergence of community-acquired methicillin-resistant *Staphylococcus aureus*. *Mayo Clinic Proceedings, 92*(8), 1227–1233. doi:10.1016/j.mayocp.2017.04.008

McCreary, E., Heim, M., Schulz, L., Hoffman, R., Pothof, J., & Fox, B. (2017). Top 10 myths regarding the diagnosis and treatment of cellulitis. *The Journal of Emergency Medicine, 53*, 485–492. doi:10.1016/j.jemermed.2017.05.007

Murphy-Lavoie, H., & LeGros, T. L. (2010). Emergent diagnosis of the unknown rash: An algorithmic approach. *Emergency Medicine, 42*(3), 6–17. Retrieved from https://www.mdedge.com/emergencymedicine/article/71662/dermatology/emergent-diagnosis-of-the-unknown-rash-algorithmic-approach

Peterson, R., Polgreen, L., Cavanaugh, J., & Polgreen, P. (2017). Increasing incidence, cost, and seasonality in patients hospitalized for cellulitis. *Open Forum Infectious Diseases, 4*(1), ofx008. doi:10.1093/ofid/ofx008

Santistevan, J., Long, B., & Koyfman, A. (2017). Rash decisions: An approach to dangerous rashes based on morphology. *The Journal of Emergency Medicine, 52*(4), 457–471. doi:10.1016/j.jemermed.2016.10.027

Spelman, D., & Baddour, L. (2017). Cellulitis and skin abscess in adults: Treatment. In E. L. Baron (Ed.), *UpToDate.* Retrieved from https://www.uptodate.com/contents/cellulitis-and-skin-abscess-in-adults-treatment

Weng, Q., Raff, A., Cohen, J., Gunasekera, N., Okhovat, J. P., Vedak, P., & Mostaghimi, A. (2017). Costs and consequences associated with misdiagnosed lower extremity cellulitis. *JAMA Dermatology, 153*(2), 141–146. doi:10.1001/jamadermatol.2016.3816

Seborrheic Dermatitis

Amber Tran

Definition

A. Chronic inflammatory superficial disease that mainly affects body oil baring surfaces such as scalp, brows, nasolabial folds, ears, chest, and groin.

Incidence

A. 3% to 5% of general population.

B. 40% to 80% of HIV population.

Pathogenesis

A. Caused by *Malassezia furfur*, lipophilic yeast that can overgrow in oily areas of the body.

Predisposing Factors

A. Stress.
B. Neurological disease (Parkinson's disease, stroke).
C. Rosacea or other oily skin.
D. Hormonal imbalance (diabetes, polycystic ovarian syndrome [PCOS]).
E. Immunosuppression (HIV common in diffuse and treatment-resistant forms).

Subjective Data

A. Common complaints/symptoms.
  1. Itch.
  2. Scale/flakes.
  3. Greasy hair.
B. Common/typical scenario.
  1. Chronic itchy flaky scalp for years.
  2. Better with more frequent hair washing.
  3. Worse in summer.
C. Family and social history.
  1. Typically negative.
  2. May have other family members with seborrheic dermatitis.
D. Review of systems.
  1. Typically negative.

Physical Examination

A. Yellow greasy scale on erythematous plaques; can be annular or polycyclic.
B. Mostly found on scalp (see Figure 15.3), brows, nasolabial folds, nasal alae, conchal bowls, and postauricular, sometimes on neck, chest, axillae, or groin folds.

Diagnostic Tests

A. KOH preparation should demonstrate hyphae.
B. Fungal culture—especially if suspicion for tinea is in differential diagnosis.
C. Skin biopsy—helpful for odd presentations that overlap with other dermatoses.

Differential Diagnosis

A. Tinea (capitis, corporis, cruris, versicolor).
B. Pityriasis rosacea.
C. Psoriasis.
D. Contact dermatitis.
E. Drug eruption.
F. Lupus erythematous.

Evaluation and Management Plan

A. General plan.
  1. Decrease oils on scalp and other affected areas.
  2. Decrease scale and itch.
B. Patient/family teaching points: Wash scalp more frequently, focus on scalp more than hair.
C. Pharmacotherapy.
  1. Topical antifungals.
    a. For face and body.
      i. Ketoconazole 2% cream once daily to affected areas for 2 weeks.
      ii. Ciclopirox 0.77% cream twice daily to affected areas for 2 to 4 weeks.
    b. For scalp.
      i. Ketoconazole 1% to 2% shampoo twice weekly; leave on damp scalp for 5 minutes, then rinse; repeat for 4 to 8 weeks.
      ii. Ciclopirox 1% shampoo twice weekly; leave on scalp damp for 5 minutes, then rinse; repeat for 2 to 4 weeks.
      iii. Selenium sulfide 1% to 2.5% shampoo or lotion twice weekly; leave on damp scalp for 5 minutes, then rinse; repeat for 2 to 4 weeks.
  2. Topical steroids for itch and irritation only.
    a. For face: Hydrocortisone 1% to 2.5% cream twice daily for 5 days.
    b. For scalp: Mometasone 0.1% solution nightly on affected areas of scalp after showers for 3 weeks.
D. Discharge instructions.

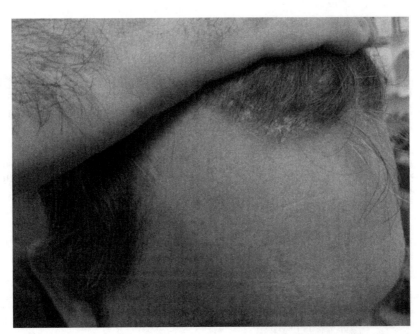

FIGURE 15.3 Seborrheic dermatitis.
Source: Lyons, F., & Ousley, L. (2015). *Dermatology for the advanced practice nurse.* New York, NY: Springer Publishing Company.

1. Discuss risks of prolonged topical steroid use: Atrophy of skin, hypopigmentation of skin, risk for glaucoma if use is near eyes or hands are not washed after use.
2. May take a few weeks to improve.

Follow-Up

A. Dermatology in next 1 to 3 months.

Consultation/Referral

A. If persists or worsens, consult/refer to dermatology.

Special/Geriatric Considerations

A. Nursing home patients may have a hard time adhering to washing regimen.

Bibliography

Buttaro, T., Trybulski, J., Polgar-Bailey, P., & Sandberg-Cook, J. (2013). *Primary care—E-book* (4th ed.). St. Louis, MO: Elsevier.

Fitzpatrick, J., & Morelli, J. (2011). *Dermatology secrets plus* (4th ed.). Philadelphia, PA: Elsevier.

Habif, T. (2011). *Skin disease*. Edinburgh, Scotland: Saunders/Elsevier.

Lyons, F., & Ousley, L. (2015). *Dermatology for the advanced practice nurse*. New York, NY: Springer Publishing Company.

Mameri, A., Carneiro, S., Mameri, L., Telles da Cunha, J., & Ramos-E-Silva, M. (2017). History of seborrheic dermatitis: Conceptual and clinico-pathologic evolution. *Skinmed, 15*(3), 187–194.

Yalçin, B., Tamer, E., Toy, G. G., Oztaş, P., Hayran, M., & Alli, N. (2006). The prevalence of skin diseases in the elderly: Analysis of 4099 geriatric patients. *International Journal of Dermatology, 45*(6), 672–676. doi:10.1111/j.1365-4632.2005.02607.x

Stasis Dermatitis

Amber Tran

Definition

A. Eczema-like inflammation of the lower extremities associated with impairment of the vascular–lymphatic system.

Incidence

A. Happens to 6.2% of people equal to or older than 65 years old.

Pathogenesis

A. Caused by back flow of veins with leaking hemosiderin from congested blood vessels.

Predisposing Factors

A. Decreased mobility.
B. Impairment of vascular–lymphatic system.
  1. Venous insufficiency.
  2. Lymphedema due to impaired lymphatic drainage.
  3. Lymph node resection.
  4. Prior radiation treatments to affected area.
C. Chronic comorbidity conditions.
  1. Malnourishment, obesity, diabetes, chronic kidney disease, chronic liver disease, alcohol abuse.
  2. Immunosuppression (HIV, cancer, taking immuno-suppressive agents).
  3. Tinea pedis or other dermatitis-affected skin integrity.

Subjective Data

A. Common complaints/symptoms.
  1. Itch, erythema.
  2. Dark patches.
  3. Dry skin.
  4. Sometimes swelling.
B. Common/typical scenario.
  1. Chronic rash that started on one lower leg at ankle and now is on both.
  2. Sometimes itchy.
  3. Happened over several weeks to months.
C. Family and social history.
  1. Smoker.
D. Review of systems.
  1. Usually negative.

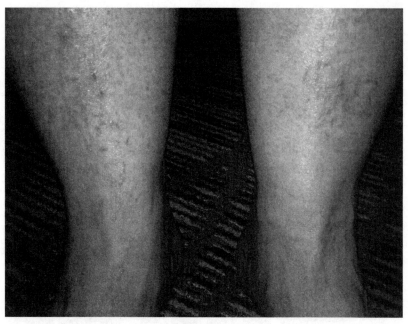

FIGURE 15.4 Example of stasis dermatitis.
Source: Lyons, F., & Ousley, L. (2015). *Dermatology for the advanced practice nurse*. New York, NY: Springer Publishing Company.

Physical Examination

A. Bronze to erythematous dry patch of skin with or without scale.

B. On bilateral extremities, worst on ankles (see Figure 15.4).

C. Mild to moderate swelling.

D. Rarely blisters, necrosis.

E. If palpate warmth, need to rule out deep vein thrombosis (DVT).

F. If exquisite tenderness and rapid progression occurs, rule out necrotizing fasciitis.

Diagnostic Tests

A. Culture: Usually negative, but can have secondary infection when purulent discharge is present. Majority cannot be cultured unless abscess present for incision and drainage.

B. Biopsy: Poor healing and low diagnostic yield.

C. Doppler ultrasound (if suspect DVT).

Differential Diagnosis

A. Cellulitis.

B. Lipodermatosclerosis.

C. DVT.

D. Venous ulcer.

E. Insect bite reaction.

F. Contact dermatitis.

G. Skin cancer (squamous cell carcinoma).

H. Erysipelas.

I. Necrotizing fasciitis.

Evaluation and Management Plan

A. General plan.
   1. Maintenance skin integrity.
   2. Increase venous return.

B. Patient/family teaching points.
   1. Elevate legs daily for 30 minutes four to five times daily.
   2. Compression stockings during daytime activities.

C. Pharmacotherapy.
   1. Topical steroids: Triamcinolone 0.05% cream/ointment twice daily for 2 weeks.

D. Discharge instructions (if standard accepted guidelines exist please use discharge template).

Follow-Up

A. Dermatology.

B. Follow-up in 1 to 3 months.

Consultation/Referral

A. If persists or worsens, consult/refer to dermatology.

Special/Geriatric Considerations

A. Elderly populations will have more difficulty with staying active to prevent blood and fluid from pooling in lower extremities.

Bibliography

Buttaro, T., Trybulski, J., Polgar-Bailey, P., & Sandberg-Cook, J. (2013). *Primary care—E-book* (4th ed.). St. Louis, MO: Elsevier.

Fitzpatrick, J., & Morelli, J. (2011). *Dermatology secrets plus* (4th ed.). Philadelphia, PA: Elsevier.

Habif, T. (2011). *Skin disease* (pp. 160–163). Edinburgh, Scotland: Saunders/Elsevier.

Lyons, F., & Ousley, L. (2015). *Dermatology for the advanced practice nurse.* New York, NY: Springer Publishing Company.

Yalçin, B., Tamer, E., Toy, G. G., Oztaş, P., Hayran, M., & Alli, N. (2006). The prevalence of skin diseases in the elderly: Analysis of 4099 geriatric patients. *International Journal of Dermatology, 45*(6), 672–676. doi:10.1111/j.1365-4632.2005.02607.x

16 Geriatric Guidelines

Frances M. Stokes and Karen Sheffield O'Brien

Delirium

Karen Sheffield O'Brien

Definition

A. Delirium includes five key characteristics as described in the *Diagnostic and Statistical Manual of Mental Disorders* (5th ed.; *DSM-5*; American Psychiatric Publishing; needed for diagnosis).
  1. Lack of attention and awareness.
  2. Developed over hours to days with a change in baseline functioning. May fluctuate with the time of day.
  3. Changes in cognition.
  4. Not influenced by an existing neurocognitive disorder or state of arousal (e.g., coma).
  5. Reasonable suspicion the change is caused by a medical condition, substance addiction or withdrawal, or medication side effect.
B. Additional features.
  1. Hyper- or hypoactivity with alterations in sleep.
  2. Emotional disturbance, some seeming psychotic, such as fear, euphoria, confusion, or depression.
  3. Extremes of mood including agitation.
  4. Sensory disturbances such as hallucinations.
  5. Motor alterations including tremors.
C. The terms *acute confusional state*, *delirium*, and *encephalopathy* are often used interchangeably.

Incidence

A. Age: More common in the aged, but can occur with any illness.
B. Incidence.
  1. Up to 50% of older surgical patients can experience delirium.
  2. Highest rates found among ICU patients, followed by ED and hospice.
C. Frequency: While once considered only a temporary condition common in ill patients, delirium is now associated with increased length of stay, rate of complications, and cost of hospitalization and, more importantly, in hospital mortality rates.

Pathogenesis

A. Multifactorial.
  1. Difficult to study in already ill patients.
  2. Affects arousal and attention.
    a. Arousal and attention are affected by the reticular activation system (RAS).
    b. The nondominant parietal and frontal lobes govern attention.

  c. Cortical functions are needed for insight and judgment.
  3. May be related to drug toxicity, inflammation from trauma, sepsis, surgery, neuronal injury, and environmental factors.

Predisposing Factors

A. Increase baseline vulnerability.
  1. Underlying brain disease.
  2. Advanced age.
  3. Sensory impairment.
  4. Use of restraints.
B. Precipitate the disturbance.
  1. Polypharmacy.
  2. Infection.
  3. Dehydration.
  4. Immobility.
  5. Malnutrition.
  6. Bladder catheters.

Subjective Data

A. Common complaints/symptoms.
  1. Feeling confused.
  2. Hallucinations.
  3. Difficulty maintaining attention.
B. Common/typical scenario.
  1. Patient with delirium is not able to give information or accurate details.
  2. Family or caregivers will often seek medical attention for the patient or the patient is brought in through emergency services.
C. Family and social history.
  1. Inquire if the patient uses drugs or drinks alcohol.
  2. Inquire about medications and recent travel.
D. Review of systems.
  1. Inquire about disturbances of consciousness.
    a. Change in level of awareness.
    b. Inability to focus.
    c. Loss of mental clarity.
    d. Family member may report "not acting like herself" or "not acting right."
    e. Distractible, usually noted in conversation.
    f. May have decreased level of consciousness (typical) or be hypervigilant (some situations like withdrawal).
    g. Day/night reversal.
  2. Inquire about altered cognition.
    a. Memory loss.
    b. Disorientation.
    c. Difficulty with language and speech.
    d. Perceptual disturbances.
      i. Delusions.

ii. Hallucinations: Visual, auditory, or somatosensory.
iii. Lack of insight.
3. Medications.
   a. Changes in medications, particularly any new medications, dose changes, or brand changes.
4. Changes in health status.
5. Note time of acute onset, fluctuation of symptoms, changes in consciousness, and decline.
6. Identify modifiable risk factors.
   a. Sensory impairment.
   b. Immobilization.
   c. Concurrent disease or illness.
   d. Metabolic derangements.
   e. Environment.
   f. Pain.
   g. Sleep deprivation.
7. Identify nonmodifiable risk factors.
   a. Dementia.
   b. Age older than 65.
   c. Multiple comorbidities.
   d. Renal or hepatic disease.

Physical Examination

A. Sometimes difficult with the delusional patient.
B. Be alert for signs that may point to a cause of the delirium.
1. Diaphoresis may be postfebrile, indicating some type of infection.
2. Jaundice indicating hepatic failure.
3. Stigmata of drug use.
4. Smell of alcohol.
5. Indication of postictal state.
6. Indication of sepsis.
C. Neurological examination is typically very difficult and can be misleading. Should assess:
1. Attention.
2. Arousal.
3. Motor function.
4. Senses.
5. Deep tendon reflexes.
6. Higher cognitive functioning.
7. Thought cohesiveness.

Diagnostic Tests

A. Confusion Assessment Method (CAM; see Exhibit 16.1).
1. Standard screen for delirium.
2. Takes 5 minutes.
3. Has a method especially for ICU patients, including vented patients, called the CAM-ICU.
B. Intensive care delirium screening checklist (ICDSC) is also used in the ICU setting (see Exhibit 16.2).
C. Mini Mental is not useful for this population.
D. Use the history and physical examination to guide additional diagnostic testing.
1. Labs for fluid/electrolyte disturbances, infections, toxicities, metabolic disorders, shock states, and postoperative status.
2. Arterial blood gas (ABGs).
3. Liver function test (LFT), thyroid, and B_{12} as with dementia.
4. EKG.
E. Medication review is very important as toxicities are culprits in 30% of all cases of delirium.
F. If no cause is found, further diagnostics are necessary.
1. CT/MRI head.
2. EEG.
3. Lumbar puncture.

Differential Diagnosis

A. Medical issues; determine if patient has a masked baseline dementia.
B. Treat sundowning as delirium until all medical issues are ruled out.
C. Wernicke's aphasia, bitemporal dysfunction, Anton's syndrome, tumors, or trauma in the frontal region.
D. Subacute brain lesions, stroke, or inflammation. Head injuries.
E. Nonconvulsive status epilepticus.
F. Dementia or primary psychiatric illness.

Evaluation and Management Plan

A. General plan.
1. Treat the underlying cause.
2. Supportive care.
B. Patient/family teaching points.
1. Treat pain issues.
2. Encourage movement.
3. Avoid overstimulation.
4. Manage behaviors.
5. Family might need a sitter to assist with care.
C. Pharmacotherapy.
1. Pharmacological treatment of delirium depends on cause.
   a. Removing medications may be the treatment.
   b. All medications should be evaluated for polypharmacy interactions.
2. Use BEERS criteria for prescribing medications for the elderly.
   a. Behavioral control.
      i. Haloperidol.
      ii. Risperidol.
      iii. Quetiapine.
   b. Agitation.
      i. Haloperidol (first line).
      ii. Olanzapine (oral only).
      iii. Risperidone.
   c. Anxiolytics-benzodiazepine, such as lorazepam.
   d. Cholinesterase inhibitor, such as donepezil.
D. Discharge instructions.
1. Behavioral management.
   a. Reorient patient frequently.
   b. Use large, visible clocks.
   c. An outside-facing window is preferable.
   d. Keep nighttime noise to a minimum.
   e. Try to provide uninterrupted sleep overnight.
   f. Limit napping during the day.
   g. Try to make the hospital room more like home.
   h. Allow family visits and support.
2. Safety.
   a. Consider a sitter to stay with the patient.

Follow-Up

A. Delirium usually subsides as the acute illness resolves.
B. If delirium persists, additional diagnostics should be considered.

Consultation/Referral

A. Geriatric psychiatry may be consulted if the patient has behavioral issues or is unusually aggressive.
B. Consult case management if placement outside the home will be required.
C. Consult social work if there is any concern for drugs or alcohol or evidence of abuse or neglect.

EXHIBIT 16.1   **Confusion Assessment Method**

Confusion Assessment Method for the ICU (CAM-ICU)
Worksheet
Instructions: To evaluate for the presence of delirium in your patient, complete this clinical assessment every shift (8–12 hours). CAM-ICU is a valid and reliable delirium assessment tool recommended by the Society of Critical Care Medicine (SCCM) in its 2013 Pain, Agitation, and Delirium (PAD) guidelines.

CAM-ICU	Criteria	✓ Present
FEATURE 1: Alteration/Fluctuation in Mental Status		
■ Is the patient's mental status different than his/her baseline? **OR** ■ Has the patient had any fluctuation in mental status in the past 24 hours as evidenced by fluctuation on a sedation scale (e.g., RASS, GCS), or previous delirium assessment?	If Yes for either question ▶	☐
FEATURE 2: Inattention 1: Alteration/Fluctuation in Mental Status		
Letters Attention Test:		
Tell the patient *"I am going to read to you a series of 10 letters. Whenever you hear the letter 'A,' squeeze my hand."*	If number of errors >2 ▶	☐
SAVEAHAART		
Count errors (each time patient fails to squeeze on the letter "A" and squeezes on a letter other than "A").		
FEATURE 3: Altered LOC		
■ Present if the RASS score is anything other than Alert and Calm (zero) OR ■ If SAS is anything other than Calm (4).	If RASS ≠ 0 **OR** SAS ≠ 4 ▶	☐
FEATURE 4: Disorganized Thinking		
Yes/No Questions: Ask the patient to respond: **1.** Will a stone float on water? **2.** Are there fish in the sea? **3.** Does 1 pound weigh more than 2 pounds? **4.** Can you use a hammer to pound a nail? Count errors (each time patient answers incorrectly). **Commands:** Ask the patient to follow your instructions: **a.** *"Hold up this many fingers."* (Hold two fingers up in front of the patient.) **b.** *"Now do the same thing with the other hand."* (Do **not** demonstrate the number of fingers this time.) ■ If unable to move both arms, for part "b" of command ask patient to "Hold up one more finger." **Count errors if patient is unable to complete the entire command.**	If combined number of errors >1 ▶	☐
If Features 1 and 2 are both present and either Features 3 or 4 are present:	**Delirium present**	☐
CAM-ICU is positive, delirium is present.	**Delirium absent**	☐

CAM-ICU, confusion assessment method for the ICU; GCS; Glasgow Coma Scale; LOC, level of consciousness.

Special/Geriatric Considerations

A. It may take geriatric patients 6 to 8 weeks to fully recover from a delirious event and they are at high risk of persistent delirium even if the cause is eliminated or treated.

Bibliography

American Psychiatric Association. (2013). *Diagnostic and statistical manual of mental disorders* (5th ed.). Arlington, VA: American Psychiatric Publishing.

Bergeron, N., Dubois, M. J., Dumont, M., Dial, S., & Skrobik, Y. (2001). Intensive care delirium screening checklist: Evaluation of a new screening tool. *Intensive Care Medicine, 27*, 859–864 .

Folstein, M. F., Folstein, S. E., & McHugh, P. R. (1975). "Mini-Mental state." A practical method for grading the cognitive state of patients for the clinician. *Journal of Psychiatric Research, 12*(3), 189.

Francis, J., Jr., & Young, G. B. (2014, August 22). Diagnosis of delirium and confusional states. In J. L. Wilterdink (Ed.), *UpToDate*. Retrieved from http://www.uptodate.com/contents/diagnosis-of-delirium-and-confusional-states

Ouimet, S., Riker, R., Bergeron, N., Cossette, M., Kavanagh, B., & Skrobik, Y. (2007). Subsyndromal delirium in the ICU: Evidence for a disease spectrum. *Intensive Care Medicine, 33*, 1007–1013.

Tullmann, D. F., Mion, L. C., Fletcher, K., & Foreman, M. D. (2012). Delirium. In M. Boltz, E. Capezuti, T. Fulmer, & D. Zwicker (Eds.), *Evidence-based geriatric nursing protocols for best practice* (4th ed., pp. 186–199). New York, NY: Springer Publishing Company.

EXHIBIT 16.2 Intensive Care Delirium Checklist for Screening

Intensive Care Delirium Screening Checklist (ICDSC)
Worksheet

■ Score your patient over the entire shift. Components don't all need to be present at the same time.

■ Components #1 through #4 require a focused bedside patient assessment. This cannot be completed when the patient is deeply sedated or comatose (i.e., SAS = 1 or 2; RASS = –4 or –5).

■ Components #5 through #8 are based on observations throughout the entire shift. Information from the prior 24 hr (i.e., from prior 1–2 nursing shifts) should be obtained for components #7 and #8.

1.	**Altered Level of Consciousness**		NO	0	1	Yes
	Deep sedation/coma over entire shift [SAS= 1, 2; RASS = –4, –5]	= Not assessable				
	Agitation [SAS = 5, 6, or 7; RASS= 1–4] at any point	= 1 point				
	Normal wakefulness [SAS = 4; RASS = 0] over the entire shift	= 0 points				
	Light sedation [SAS = 3; RASS = –1, –2, –3]	= 1 point (if no recent sedatives)				
		= 0 points (if recent sedatives)				
2.	**Inattention**		NO	0	1	Yes
	Difficulty following instructions or conversation; patient easily distracted by external stimuli. Will not reliably squeeze hands to spoken letter A: **SAVEAHAART**					
3.	**Disorientation**		NO	0	1	Yes
	In addition to name, place, and date, does the patient recognize ICU caregivers? Does patient know what kind of place he or she is in (list examples: Dentist's office, home, work, hospital)?					
4.	**Hallucination, delusion, or psychosis**		NO	0	1	Yes
	Ask the patient if he or she is having hallucinations or delusions (e.g., trying to catch an object that isn't there). Is the patient afraid of the people or things around him or her?					
5.	**Psychomotor agitation or retardation**		NO	0	1	Yes
	Either: (a) Hyperactivity requiring the use of sedative drugs or restraints in order to control potentially dangerous behavior (e.g., pulling IV lines out or hitting staff) OR (b) Hypoactive or clinically noticeable psychomotor slowing or retardation					
6.	**Inappropriate speech or mood**		NO	0	1	Yes
	Patient displays: Inappropriate emotion; disorganized or incoherent speech; sexual or inappropriate interactions; is either apathetic or overly demanding					
7.	**Sleep-wake cycle disturbance**		NO	0	1	Yes
	Either: Frequent awakening/< 4 hr sleep at night OR sleeping during much of the day					
8.	**Symptom fluctuation**		NO	0	1	Yes
	Fluctuation of any of the previous symptoms over a 24 hr period.					
	TOTAL SHIFT SCORE:		(0–8)			

	Score	Classification
	0	Normal
	1–3	Subsyndromal delirium
	4–8	Delirium

Source: Adapted from Bergeron, N., Dubois, M. J., Dumont, M., Dial, S., & Skrobik, Y. (2001). Intensive care delirium screening checklist: Evaluation of a new screening tool. *Intensive Care Medicine, 27,* 859–864; Ouimet, S., Riker, R., Bergeron, N., Cossette, M., Kavanagh, B., & Skrobik, Y. (2007). doi:10.1007/s001340100909
Subsyndromal delirium in the ICU: Evidence for a disease spectrum. *Intensive Care Medicine, 33,* 1007–1013. doi:10.1007/s00134-007-0618-y

Dementia

Karen Sheffield O'Brien

Definition

A. A major neurocognitive disorder in which the patient exhibits a significant cognitive decline in one or more of the areas described in the *Diagnostic and Statistical Manual of Mental Disorders* (5th ed.; *DSM-5*).

1. Complex attention.
2. Executive function.
3. Language.
4. Learning and memory.
5. Perceptual-motor function.
6. Social cognition.

B. The *DSM-5* also states the impairment should be acquired and a decline from the patient's normal functioning, inhibit independence and activities of daily living (ADLs), and not be occurring during bouts of delirium or as a function of another mental condition (e.g., depression or schizophrenia).

C. Alzheimer's disease (AD) accounts for most cases of dementia. While the term is often used interchangeably with dementia, AD only represents a single subtype of neurodegenerative dementia. Neurodegenerative dementias are progressive and exhibit an insidious onset.

Incidence

A. Age: Typically over the age of 65; however, early onset dementia accounts for 40 to 100 cases per 100,000 people in the developed world.

B. Incidence: Alzheimer's dementia affects more than 5 million individuals over the age of 65, accounting for 80% of dementia cases, with vascular dementia second.

Pathogenesis

A. Dementia can be influenced by multiple pathologies and is disease specific.

B. Types of dementia and selected pathophysiology.

   1. Neurodegenerative (Alzheimer's, dementia with Lewy bodies, Parkinson's disease).

   2. Vascular diseases (vascular, cerebral amyloid angiopathy, and angitis).

   3. Infectious diseases (prion disease such as Creutzfeldt–Jakob disease [CJD; mad cow], herpes encephalitis, neurosyphilis).

   4. Inflammatory and autoimmune (multiple sclerosis, para- and nonparaneoplastic, autoimmune diseases).

   5. Neurometabolic disorders.

   6. Other (traumatic encephalopathy, alcohol abuse, Wilson and Huntington diseases).

      a. Genetic.

      b. Malnutrition.

Predisposing Factors

A. Age (frequency increases with age).

B. Positive family history.

C. Female (could be related to life span).

D. History of head trauma or cerebrovascular accident (CVA).

E. Low education level.

F. Environmental factors: Aluminum, mercury, and viruses.

G. Physical condition and other medical factors (e.g., diabetes, hypertension, and hypercholesterolemia).

Subjective Data

A. Common complaints/symptoms.

   1. While memory is a problem, it is usually not mentioned by the patient, but by the significant other or family.

   2. Frequently cannot pinpoint the condition's onset; years may have passed with problems, but until a major change happens, such as needing to stop driving or a hospital admission, the patient may be mostly functional in his or her familiar environment.

   3. Signs and symptoms.

      a. Difficulty maintaining new information or task.

      b. Inability to manage complex task like balancing a checkbook.

      c. Lapses in reasoning.

      d. Becoming lost in familiar places.

      e. Word finding issues.

      f. Changes in behavior.

B. Common/typical scenario.

   1. Patients typically start with subtle short-term memory changes, frequent forgetfulness, difficulty finding the right words, or difficulty completing tasks.

   2. The patient may progress over months and years before coming to a provider.

C. Family and social history.

   1. Family history and first degree relatives may be important in AD.

   2. Obesity and chronic sedentary lifestyle may increase risk.

   3. Smoking, alcohol, and drug abuse increase risk of dementia.

D. Review of systems.

   1. Neurological: Ask about memory and any confusion or deficits in calculation and abstraction.

   2. Psychological: Ask about depressed mood, hopelessness, or suicide tendencies or changes in personality.

   3. Inquire about rate of onset of changes.

   4. History from a reliable source including medications.

Physical Examination

A. Assessment and physical examination change with the type of dementia present. Motor, somatosensory, and visual functions may remain intact until later in the disease process.

   1. Disorder of motion.

   2. Eye movement.

   3. Primary memory.

   4. Performance on cognitive assessments.

Diagnostic Tests

A. Cognitive function.

   1. Mini-Mental state examination (max score 30; less than 24 indicates possible dementia).

      a. Concentration.

      b. Language.

      c. Orientation.

      d. Memory.

      e. Attention.

   2. Montreal cognitive assessment (max score 30; lower than 25 indicates possible dementia).

   3. Clinical dementia rating (includes a caregiver).

   4. Mini-Cog (clock draw and recall test).

   5. Informant interview to ask caregivers about the patient's functioning.

      a. Issues with judgment.

      b. Lack of interest in usual activities.

      c. Repetition of questions, statements, stories.

      d. Difficulty learning new tools or household appliances.

      e. Inability to remember the month or year.

      f. Loss of ability to manage finances.

      g. Missing appointments.

      h. Persistent issues with thinking or memory.

B. Physical examination.

   1. Full neurological examination.

   2. General physical examination to identify any medical illness that could account for deficits.

   3. Motor examination to identify prior stroke or evidence of Parkinson disease or autoimmune issues.

   4. Evaluation of sleeping habits.

C. Lab studies (*as recommended by the American Academy of Neurology).

   1. Screen for B_{12} deficiency*.

   2. Hypothyroidism*.

   3. Rapid plasma reagin (RPR) screening*.

   4. Complete blood count (CBC).

   5. Comprehensive metabolic panel (CMP).

   6. LFT.

   7. Immune/autoimmune workup.

   8. Cerebrospinal fluid (CSF) analysis if infective cause is suspected.

D. Imaging: Neuroimaging (as recommended by the American Academy of Neurology) including CT or MRI and possibly electrophysiologic testing.

E. Brain biopsy not recommended unless in vasculitis, cancers, or infection.

F. Genetic testing is not recommended except for specific diseases in family history (e.g., Huntington disease).

Differential Diagnosis

A. Treatable: Thyroid, vitamin deficiencies, tumor, drug and medication intoxication, chronic infection, and severe depression. Once these are ruled out, the differential is among the types of dementia.

B. Structural: Cortical and hippocampus atrophy leads to AD.

C. Psychiatric history with pharmacological treatment may be drug related.

D. Associated: Gait disturbances could be vascular or Lewy body, including Parkinson, which may be based on time of onset.

E. Rapid onset could be CJD or frontotemporal dementia.

F. For early onset (under the age of 65): There is a much broader list of differentials and requires more extensive testing.

Evaluation and Management Plan

A. General plan.

  1. Includes finding and correcting any reversible causes.

    a. Vitamin or thyroid replacements.

    b. Stopping contributing medications or starting medications for contributing conditions such as depression.

    c. Treating any structural dysfunction such as neoplasms or increased intracranial pressure.

    d. Treating any infections contributing to mental status.

  2. When no correctable cause is found, supportive care for the patient and the caregiver is warranted.

  3. Diet.

    a. Patients with dementia often have decreased appetite for a variety of reasons.

    b. When possible, provide food to support adequate nutrition.

    c. Supplement any deficiencies.

    d. Adequate overall intake may be preferred over following a strict low cholesterol/glucose/fat/sodium diet.

  4. Other therapies/considerations.

    a. Provide utmost safety for the patient and caregivers while maintaining some form of independence for the patient.

    b. Modify environment.

    c. Maintain a routine.

    d. Treat occult conditions that could contribute to behavioral problems (like toothache or constipation).

    e. Provide simple physical activities.

    f. Provide caregiver respite as needed.

B. Patient/family teaching points.

  1. Patient teaching is more geared toward the caregiver.

  2. Many changes must be made in the patient's life, including relinquishing some independence for the sake of safety.

  3. When considering activities such as driving, safety for both the patient and public should be considered.

C. Pharmacotherapy.

  1. Food and Drug Administration (FDA) approved for AD: Cholinesterase inhibitors.

    a. Donepezil.

    b. Rivastigmine.

    c. Galantamine.

  2. FDA approved for AD: N-methyl-D-aspartate (NMDA) receptor antagonist.

    a. Memantine.

  3. Pharmaceutical therapy for symptom control.

    a. Phenothiazine.

    b. Benzodiazepines.

    c. Second-generation antipsychotics: Risperidone, quetiapine, olanzapine.

    d. Anticholinergics or sedatives.

    e. Antidepressants, especially selective serotonin reuptake inhibitors (SSRIs).

Follow-Up

A. Patient should be seen at regularly scheduled appointments dependent on several factors.

  1. Physical needs of the patient.

  2. Mental status and rate of decline.

  3. Emotional status.

  4. Ability of caregiver to maintain the safety and health of the patient.

B. Follow-up assessments include efficacy of medication, with changes, additions, and discontinuance as needed.

C. Monitor for correctable physical factors that may contribute to behavioral issues, both becoming withdrawn and outburst.

D. Assess for additional resources needed by the patient and caregiver, including ability of the patient to function with safety as the determining factor when discussing activity limitations.

Consultation/Referral

A. Neuropsychologist.

B. Social workers.

C. Cognitive rehab can help maintain memory and cognitive functioning while also providing some respite to caregiver.

D. Exercise programs.

E. Occupational therapy.

Special/Geriatric Considerations

A. Comorbid conditions.

B. Family support.

C. Daily care.

D. End of life plans.

Bibliography

Alzheimer's Association (n. d.). Know what to expect. Retrieved from https://www.alz.org/help-support/i-have-alz/know-what-to-expect

American Psychiatric Association. (2013). *Diagnostic and statistical manual of mental disorders (DSM-5)* (5th ed.) Arlington, TX: Author.

Brosch, J. R., & Farlow, M. R. (2018, June 8). Early-onset dementia in adults. In J. L. Wilterdink (Ed.), *UpToDate*. Retrieved from https://www.uptodate.com/contents/early-onset-dementia-in-adults

Cordell, C. B., Borson, S., Boustani, M., Chodosh, J., Reuben, D., Verghese, J., . . . Fried, L. B. (2013). Medicare detection of cognitive impairment workgroup. Alzheimer's Association recommendations for operationalizing the detection of cognitive impairment during the Medicare Annual Wellness Visit in a primary care setting. *Alzheimers Dementia, 9*(2), 141–150. doi:10.1016/j.jalz.2012.09.011

Folstein, M. F., Folstein, S. E., & McHugh, P. R. (1975). "Mini-Mental state." A practical method for grading the cognitive state of patients for the clinician. *Journal of Psychiatric Research, 12*(3), 189–198.

Galvin, J. E., Roe, C. M., Xiong, C., & Morris, J. C. (2006). Validity and reliability of the AD8 Informant interview in dementia. *Neurology, 67*(11), 1942–1948.

Falls

Frances M. Stokes

Definition

A. The clinician definition of a fall describes it as an inadvertent change in position and coming to rest on the ground, floor, or other lower level. This may include injury or noninjury as a result. There are a multitude of billing codes for falls within the ICD-10 coding system. These include falls on the same level, from an upper level, and other unspecified types of falls. This definition excludes an intentional change of position.

B. Categories.
   1. Accidental: This category is for the low risk patient. These patients fall for numbers of unplanned reasons: Tripping over an intravenous (IV) line or falling or sliding out of bed while reaching for something or another type of encounter with an environmental hazard, like a slippery floor, or other hazard such as the garbage can.
   2. Anticipated physiological: Patients with risk factors identified on admission or in advance secondary to a procedure or surgery such as an unsteady gait; use of walkers, canes, or medications; vision issues; urinary or fecal incontinence; delirium,; or dementia.
   3. Unanticipated physiological: Patients who are low risk who develop an event such as a seizure, stroke, arrhythmia, or syncopal episode. Falls that occur are unpredictable.
   4. Behavioral or intentional: Patients who purposely act out.

Incidence

A. Inpatient falls.
   1. In the United States, 700,000 to 1,000,000 patients fall yearly; two-thirds are elderly with 30% to 50% incurring injury overall.
   2. Length of stay may increase to as many as 6.7 additional inpatient hospital days.
   3. In the United States the cost of falls can exceed $34 billion annually.
   4. Elderly patients 65 years and older account for two-thirds of the total expenditures.
   5. Medical and surgical costs for a fall with injury can reach $14,000 per case.
   6. Costs incurred should also include postacute hospital needs, discharge to rehabilitation hospitals, and skilled nursing facilities.

B. Morbidity.
   1. Women are more likely to fall and sustain non-life-threatening injuries than men.
   2. Women are also 1.8% to 2.3% more likely to end up hospitalized and 2.2 times more likely to sustain a fracture after a fall than men.
   3. Falls are a contributing factor to admissions to rehabilitation centers, skilled nursing facilities, and ultimately nursing homes.

C. Mortality.
   1. Falls are the number one cause of death from unintentional injuries for those adults 65 years or older in the United States.
   2. Falls can also be associated with an indirect cause of death.

Pathogenesis

A. Intrinsic factors.
   1. Age-related decline.
   2. Chronic disease.
   3. Medications.
   4. Vitamin D.
B. Challenges to postural control.
   1. Environment.
   2. Changing positions.
   3. Normal activity.

C. Mediating factors.
   1. Risk-taking behaviors.
   2. Situational hazards.

Predisposing Factors

A. Medications.
   1. Anticholinergics.
   2. Antiarrhythmics.
   3. Antihypertensive medications.
   4. Narcotics.
   5. Muscle relaxants.
   6. Alcohol.
B. Incontinence: Urine and fecal incontinence.
C. Health conditions.
   1. Alzheimer's disease: Have two times the probability of falling than those of the same age without the disease.
   2. Parkinson disease: 38% to 68% of Parkinson disease fall due to gait disturbances.
   3. Diabetes: Women with diabetes are 1.6 times more likely to fall, and two times more likely to suffer fall-related injuries than women without diabetes.
   4. Depression: There is a 2.2-fold increase in the risk of falls in this population of elderly patients.
D. Physical impairments.
E. Past medical history.
   1. Previous falls.
   2. Diabetes.
   3. Chronic obstructive pulmonary disease (COPD).
   4. Coronary artery disease (CAD).
   5. Arrhythmias.
   6. Dementia-related diseases, Alzheimer's disease, vascular dementia (includes cerebrovascular accident [CVA]), Parkinson's dementia, and so forth.
   7. Osteoarthritis.
   8. Joint replacements (knee surgeries especially susceptible).
   9. Chronic pain.
   10. Blindness.
   11. Macular degeneration.
   12. Glaucoma.
   13. Chronic kidney disease.
   14. Vestibular disease.

Subjective Data

A. Common complaints/symptoms.
   1. Dizziness when bending over.
   2. Unsteady gait/balance.
   3. Poor vision.
   4. Fatigue, weakness.
   5. Other signs and symptoms.
      a. The need to use assistive equipment to ambulate.
      b. Walks along walls and uses furniture to maintain balance.
      c. Assistive devices or medications for visual or hearing impairments related to aging and other geriatric syndromes.
B. Family and social history.
   1. Noncontributory in most cases.
C. Review of systems.
   1. Review all medications.
   2. Use STRATIFY risk assessment tool to inquire about:
      a. History of falls.
      b. Mental status.
      c. Vision.
      d. Toileting.

    e. Transfer and mobility.
    f. Head, ear, eyes, nose, and throat (HEENT).
       i. Dizziness.
       ii. Poor vision.
       iii. Loss of peripheral vision.
       iv. Depth perception.
    g. Musculoskeletal.
       i. Unsteady gait.
       ii. Uses walls to maintain balance.
    h. Neurological.
       i. Neuropathy.
    i. General.
       i. Overall hazards in the home (rugs).

Physical Examination

A. Perform a head-to-toe physical examination.
  1. Neurological examination.
    a. Glasgow Coma Scale.
    b. National Institute of Health (NIH) stroke scale.
    c. Detailed neurological examination if indicated, cranial nerves, gait, and balance testing.
  2. Mentation status.
    a. Mini-Mental status examination.
    b. Confusion assessment method or other delirium screening tool.
    c. Thorough review of medications for offending medications.
  3. Cardiovascular examination.
    a. Murmurs/arrhythmias.
    b. Carotid bruits.
    c. Pulses weak/thready.
    d. Evaluate for edema.
  4. Orthostatic readings/pulmonary examination.
    a. SpO_2.
    b. Breath sounds.
    c. Accessory muscle use.
  5. Integumentary.
    a. Bruising, scrapes, and lacerations over knees, shoulders, forearms, shins, ankles, and toes. This indicates the patient is bumping into furniture or walls, which may indicate unaddressed balance issues or are defensive in nature.
    b. Excoriation in perianal area: This may indicate urinary (female) or fecal incontinence (male/female) related to diet, medications, or infection.
  6. Gastrointestinal.
    a. Abdominal bruits.
    b. Pain.
    c. Nodules or skin changes.
    d. Look for ecchymosis and signs of bleeding.
  7. Genitourinary.
    a. Incontinence, urgency, frequency.

Diagnostic Tests

A. Chiefly depends upon the etiology of the fall, past medical history, medications, and findings of physical examination.
B. CT of the head to rule out bleeding either from a stroke or as a result of the fall or a subdural or subarachnoid hemorrhage. Some cranial bleeds that are not related to a CVA can be spontaneous if a patient is on anticoagulation therapy or American Society of Anesthesiologists (ASA). CT Angiography (CTA) or MRI/magnetic resonance angiography (MRA) may be indicated.
C. X-rays of spinal column, ribs, long bones, and so forth, to rule out fractures in suspicious areas where there is evidence of impact from the fall.

D. Other diagnostics should be dependent upon patient history of present illness, past medical history, and physical examination.
  1. Basic chemistry with glucose.
  2. Carotid Doppler study.
  3. Complete blood count (CBC) w/differential.
  4. EKG.
  5. Echocardiogram (heart murmurs).
  6. Evaluate for vitamin deficiencies, B_{12}, Thiamine.
  7. Guaiac stools if indicated.
  8. MRA (suspect thrombus, hemorrhage).
  9. MRI (gait disturbances or neurological deficits).
  10. Serum 25-hydroxyvitamin D level.
  11. Tilt table test.
  12. Urinalysis to rule out infection.
E. Review diagnostic test results.
  1. Laboratory findings.
  2. Radiological examinations.

Differential Diagnosis

A. Anemia.
B. Arrhythmia.
C. Arthritis.
D. Carotid stenosis.
E. Dehydration.
F. Dementia.
G. Depression.
H. Electrolyte deficiencies (severe hyponatremia) and vitamin deficiencies.
I. Frailty.
J. Hypoglycemia/hyperglycemia.
K. Infection/sepsis.
L. Labyrinthitis.
M. Malnutrition.
N. Orthostatic/postural hypotension.
O. Peripheral neuropathy.
P. Peripheral vascular disease.
Q. Neurological disorders such as stroke, seizure, Parkinson disease, or vertigo.
R. Uncorrected farsightedness/nearsightedness or poor vision from macular degeneration, glaucoma, underlying infection, or diabetic retinopathy.
S. Medications can create a delirious state.
  1. Alcohol.
  2. Antiarrhythmics.
  3. Antidepressants.
  4. Antihypertensives.
  5. Antipsychotics.
  6. Diuretics.
  7. Hypnotics.
  8. Neuroleptics.
  9. Sedatives.

Evaluation and Management Plan

A. General plan.
  1. Perform a full medication review and use the BEERS criteria to determine medications that are contraindicated for older adults.
  2. Perform multidisciplinary rounds for patients at moderate and higher fall risk, all patients over 75 years of age, and those who are frail.
  3. Evaluate nutritional status, and order nutritional consult if indicated.
  4. Evaluate for safe discharge on admission utilizing case management and a social worker to collaborate with family and caregivers. Include nurses, advanced practice

nurses (APNs), prothrombin time (PT)/OT, a dietician, a pharmacist, and physicians.

5. Request fall risk alerts for patient safety to include an order for bed and chair alarms.

6. Correct underlying medical etiology or physical deficit if possible, which may include medication revisions, correction of vision/hearing with assist devices, and use of ambulatory devices to aid with balance.

7. Place on telemetry.

B. Patient/family teaching points.

  1. Discuss with patient/caregiver.

    a. Signs and symptoms to monitor.

    b. Common occurrences.

    c. Readmission concerns.

C. Discharge instructions.

  1. Evaluate for safe transfer of care from initiated unit, that is, ICU to floor, floor to home, or other institution.

  2. Accurate discharge summary of events including chief complaint and events leading up to admission and during hospitalization.

  3. Copy of discharge summary to the family or caregivers, primary care provider, and specialists to ensure communication and history of recent events are transferred to community providers. Inpatient providers should state patient's condition upon discharge and the patient's ability to transfer to the next level of care.

  4. Thorough medication reconciliation; ensure obsolete medications are removed from medication list.

  5. Separate education for medication reconciliation regarding discontinued medications, new medications, and administration.

  6. Education for signs and symptoms of worsening condition, what is expected to happen, and readmission concerns.

  7. Discharge education regarding physician follow-up; medications and instructions on medications; any medical treatments that require an explanation, including physical therapy or wound care therapy; and breathing treatment or injections, to name but a few.

  8. Use of any new assistive devices, walkers, canes, or braces.

  9. Education on making the patient's home safe from falls, such as removing scatter rugs and keeping lights on.

Follow-Up

A. Follow-up depends on the cause of the fall and the consequences of it.

B. For falls caused by cardiac disease, the patient should follow-up with cardiology.

C. If a patient has an injury due to the fall, the patient should follow-up with the appropriate services such as orthopedics for fractured bones or neurosurgery for head injury.

Consultation/Referral

A. Case management and social workers ensure safe discharge to appropriate level of care.

B. Arrange for delivery of any durable medical equipment to the patient's assisted living, adult living, group home, or home.

C. Considerations of insurance coverage and deductible amounts are important for elders on fixed budgets.

D. Financial resources and availability of social support through appropriate government resources are important for safe transition, especially to independent living and home.

1. Medications: Ensure insurance is available for medications and durable medical equipment necessary for safe patient discharge.

2. If possible, arrange for first follow-up medical appointments with appropriate physicians and/or specialists.

3. If home therapy is utilized for wound or physical/occupational therapy, ensure set-up and appointments for home visits are arranged.

4. If indicated, a home health visit can be set up to provide support and help arrange first appointments.

Special/Geriatric Considerations

A. Up to 50% of geriatric patients may not report history of falls to anyone for fear of being removed from the home.

Bibliography

Fauci, A. S. (2008). Nervous system dysfunction. In A. S. Fauci, E. Braunwald, D. L. Kasper, S. L. Hauser, D. L. Longo, J. L. Jameson, & J. Loscalzo (Eds.), *Harrison's principles of internal medicine* (pp. 139–180). New York, NY: McGraw-Hill Professional.

Fletcher, K. (2012). Dementia. In M. Boltz, E. Capezuti, T. Fulmer, & D. Zwicker (Eds.), *Evidence-based geriatric nursing protocols for best practice* (4th ed., pp. 163–185). New York, NY: Springer Publishing Company.

Fulmer, T., & Zwicker, D. (2012). *Evidence-based geriatric nursing protocols for best practice* (4th ed., pp. 186–199). New York, NY: Springer Publishing Company.

Stevens, J., Ballesteros, M., Mack, K., Rudd, R., DeCaro, E., & Adler, G. (2012). Gender differences in seeking care for falls in the aged Medicare population. *American Journal of Preventive Medicine, 43*(1), 59–62.

Urinary Incontinence

Frances M. Stokes

Definition

A. Urinary incontinence in men and women is defined as an involuntary leakage of urine. Incontinence is further broken down into types of urinary leakage as follows.

  1. Urgency is associated with a sense of an urgency to void. This may present suddenly. Precipitating factors include cold, the sound of running water, or washing hands, that is, putting hands in water.

  2. Stress incontinence occurs with strain, exertion, sneezing, or coughing.

  3. Mixed incontinence is the most common type of urinary incontinence for women. There is an urgency and exertion associated with it.

  4. Post void incontinence is associated with post void residual urine in the urethra which leaks out after voiding.

  5. Overactive bladder is associated with frequency, urgency, and nocturia. This may or may not have incontinence associated with it.

  6. Incomplete urinary emptying (overflow) incontinence relates to incomplete emptying of the bladder due to an impaired detrusor contractility or a bladder outlet obstruction.

  7. Functional/transient incontinence is usually self-limiting, transient, and potentially reversible due to treatable causes.

  8. Inability to reach bathroom secondary to functional ability .

  9. Reflex incontinence etiology is related to neurological dysfunction of the central nervous system.

Incidence

A. Globally, incidence affects 200 million people worldwide; in the United States, the number is 10 to 13 million.

   1. The percentage of elderly patients who reside in long-term care facilities is between 50% and 84%.

B. Prevalence in men increases with age.

C. Prevalence in females.

   1. 60 to 79 years is 23.3%.

   2. Over 80 years increases to 31.7%.

   3. Of the types of incontinence, stress is most commonly seen in women who are younger than 65 years old. However, urge incontinence and mixed are more common among women older than 65 years. Stress incontinence affects both young and older women at a rate of 15% to 60%; of these, 25% are nulliparous young college athletes.

Pathogenesis

A. Urgency can be related to an uninhibited detrusor activity. This is most common in men.

B. Stress incontinence is generally due to pressure on the bladder, which can happen with coughing, sneezing, laughing, heavy lifting, and so forth.

   1. Radical prostatectomy surgery is the most common cause in men due to damage to the prostatic apex. Transurethral resection of the bladder has less incidence of damage to the external sphincter and has a degree of less than 1%.

   2. In women, stress incontinence is due to lax perineal muscles.

C. Overflow incontinence is the least common cause of incontinence due to impaired detrusor contractility and/or a bladder outlet obstruction. Impaired detrusor contractility is usually related to neurogenic etiologies. These include neuropathies such as mitral stenosis (MS), diabetes mellitus, meningomyelocele, lumbosacral nerve disease from tumors, prolapsed intravertebral discs, and higher spinal cord injuries.

D. Mixed incontinence is a combination incontinence of stress and urge; this is most common in women. The bladder outlet is weak and the detrusor is overactive. This may also include urethral hypermobility coupled with detrusor instability.

E. Transient incontinence refers to a temporary loss of urine due to causes that could be reversible such as delirium, infection, atrophic vaginitis or urethritis, pharmaceuticals, or a psychological etiology related to excess fluid intake. Impaired mobility, endocrine disorders, medications, fecal impaction, atrophic urethritis or vaginitis, infections, and delirium are also included in etiologies of transient incontinence.

F. Reflex incontinence for specific neurological disease processes include, but are not limited to, MS and demyelinating plaques of the frontal lobe or lateral columns. Cerebrovascular accident (CVA) or vascular compromise of particular areas of the brain may result in lower urinary tract dysfunction.

Predisposing Factors

A. Advanced age.

B. Aging process.

   1. Atrophic vaginitis or urethritis.

   2. Enlarged prostate (urge/stress).

C. Problems with gastrointestinal system.

   1. Constipation.

   2. Fecal impaction.

D. Cancer.

   1. Pelvic organs.

   2. Pelvic radiation within 6 months.

   3. Prostate cancer (tumor status; urge/stress).

   4. Prostate surgery or radiation.

E. Central nervous system (CNS) or spinal cord disorders.

   1. Delirium or dementia.

   2. Normal pressure hydrocephalus.

   3. Neuropathies.

F. Connective tissue disorders.

G. Depression medications.

H. Obesity.

I. Pelvic organ prolapse (uterus/bladder).

J. Chronic obstructive pulmonary disease (COPD).

K. Mobility.

L. Sleep apnea.

M. Urinary tract stones or urinary tract infection (UTI), more than two episodes a year.

Subjective Data

A. Common complaints/symptoms.

   1. Sudden onset of the need to urinate.

   2. Urine leakage after emptying bladder.

   3. Unable to make it to the bathroom with the urge to urinate.

   4. Feeling of incomplete emptying of the bladder with urination.

   5. Burning with urination.

   6. Flu-like symptoms.

   7. Morbidity related to incontinence.

     a. Cellulitis.

     b. Constant skin irritation and sores.

     c. Falls and subsequent fractures.

     d. Perineal candida infections.

     e. Depression.

     f. Sleep deprivation.

   8. Psychological morbidity related to incontinence.

     a. Pressure sores.

     b. Poor self-esteem.

     c. Sexual dysfunction.

     d. Social withdrawal.

   9. Urine leakage.

   10. May complain of hygiene issues.

B. Common/typical scenario.

   1. Patients do not typically like to discuss incontinence, but will report varying degrees of urine urgency, frequency, or pain when urinating that may be minor, situational, or even debilitating.

C. Family and social history.

   1. Family and social history is noncontributory.

D. Review of systems.

   1. Dermatological: Ask about skin infections, itchiness, redness, and pressure sores.

   2. Psychological: Ask about social involvement, sexual functioning, mood, and sleep habits.

   3. Genitourinary: Ask about moisture felt in underwear, leakage issues, itching, burning during urination, frequency, urinating at night, perineal irritation.

   4. Gastrointestinal: What is the typical bowel pattern? Any there complaints of constipation or impaction?

Physical Examination

A. General.

   1. Appearance.

   2. Signs of depression.

   3. Any distress.

   4. Anxiety.

B. Gastrointestinal: Abdominal distention.
C. Musculoskeletal.
  1. Joint stiffness.
  2. Mobility.
  3. Range of motion (ROM).
  4. Use of assistive devices.
D. Neurological with emphasis on cognition, functional status, and pyramidal and extra-pyramidal symptoms. Integrity of sacral roots S2, S3, and S4; resting and follitional anal tone; and anal wink reflex. Evaluate for peripheral neuropathy.
E. Male.
  1. Visual examination of the penis, enlarged prostate, and scrotum.
  2. Review past medical history (PMH) for prostate issues.
F. Female.
  1. Review PMH for prolapse of pelvic organs and perineal irritation.

Diagnostic Tests

A. Laboratory.
  1. Chemistries with renal function and complete blood count (CBC).
  2. Prostate specific antigen (PSA) level.
  3. Urine analysis with cytology and microscopy.
B. Radiology.
  1. Post residual bladder scan.
  2. Renal ultrasound (US) if indicated by abnormal renal laboratory studies.
  3. CT of brain if hydrocephalus is suspected.

Differential Diagnosis

A. CNS or spinal cord disorders.
B. Connective tissue disorders.
C. Constipation or fecal impaction.
D. Medication induced.
E. Normal pressure hydrocephalus.
F. Neuropathy, diabetic neuropathy.
G. Obesity.
H. Pelvic organ prolapse (uterus/bladder).
I. Sleep apnea.
J. Urinary tract stones.
K. UTI.

Evaluation and Management Plan

A. General plan.
  1. Perform a full medication review and reconciliation.
  2. Perform multidisciplinary rounds for geriatric patients and include continence strategies for those who are incontinent, all patients over 75 years of age, and those who are frail. Include pharmacist, dietician, radiation therapy (RT), prothrombin time (PT)/OT, advanced practice provider, case management, social worker, and caregivers when indicated.
  3. Evaluate nutritional status; order nutritional consult if indicated.
  4. Patient safety.
    a. Modify inpatient environment; include toileting into hourly rounds, place call light within reach, use lights at night, and clear the walkway to bathroom/bedside commode.
    b. Patient/family caregiver education on use of the call light for assistance.
    c. Evaluate for safe discharge on admission utilizing case management and social worker to collaborate with

family and caregivers. Include nurses, APNs, PT/OT, dietician, pharmacist, and physicians.
    d. Request toileting rounds for patient safety to include an order for bed and chair alarms for those elderly patients with urgency and frequency.
    e. Urinals at bedside for male patients, bedpans for those unable to ambulate or get up to use a commode.
  5. Correct underlying medical etiology or physical deficit if possible, which may include medication revisions, correction of vision/hearing with assistive devices, and use of ambulatory devices.
B. Patient/family teaching points.
  1. Pelvic floor exercises.
  2. How to use absorbent products.
  3. Approaches to dealing with incontinence.
  4. Modifications to diet and lifestyle may help patient control incontinence to a certain degree.
C. Pharmacotherapy.
  1. Medications depend upon the type of urinary incontinence being treated.
  2. Medications may not be effective in stress incontinence.
  3. Anticholinergics (antimuscarinics) block cholinergic receptors of the bladder and decrease contractility.
  4. All antimuscarinics are contraindicated in narrow angle glaucoma, gastric retention, and if post void residual (PVR) is greater than 150 L. Educate for side effects. Costs vary.
  5. Benign prostatic hypertrophy (BPH)-related incontinence: Alpha blockers have extensive precautions for administration. Orthostatic hypotension, hypotension, bradycardia, vertigo, priapism, cautious administration, and lab surveillance in patients with hepatic impairment should be considered.
  6. UTI: Antibiotic-focused therapy, either oral or intravenous (IV), depending upon the severity and hemodynamic status of the patient.
  7. Other treatments.
    a. Barrier creams.
    b. Oral multivitamins with zinc.
    c. Absorbent undergarments.
    d. Pelvic floor exercises.
    e. Transient incontinence; treat the underlying cause, that is, infection, outlet obstruction, and so forth.
    f. Surgical interventions.
D. Discharge instructions.
  1. Evaluate for safe transfer of care from initiated unit, that is, ICU to floor, floor to home, or other institution.
  2. Doctor to doctor report or APN to doctor/APN report.
  3. Accurate discharge summary of events including chief complaint and events leading up to admission and medical nursing care during hospitalization.
  4. Copy of discharge summary to the family or caregivers, primary care provider, and specialists to ensure communication and history of recent events are transferred to community providers. Inpatient providers should state patient's condition upon discharge and the patient's ability to transfer to the next level of care.
  5. Thorough medication reconciliation; ensure obsolete medications are removed from medical admissions record (MAR) and home medication list.
  6. Separate education for medication reconciliation regarding discontinued medications, new medications, and administration.

7. Education for signs and symptoms of worsening condition, what is expected to happen, and readmission concerns.

8. Discharge education regarding physician follow-up; medications and instructions on medications; any medical treatments that require an explanation, including physical therapy or wound care therapy; and breathing treatment or injections, to name but a few.

9. Use of any new assistive devices, walkers, canes, braces, or hearing devices.

10. Education on making the incontinent patient's home safe from falls, such as removing scatter rugs and keeping lights on.

Follow-Up
A. Patient should follow-up with the provider in 2 weeks to assess progress in treatment plan.

Consultation/Referral
A. Urology.
B. Primary care provider/gerontologist.
C. Wound care if indicated.
D. Physiotherapist: Pelvic floor exercises, bladder training, and strategies to maintain continence.

Special/Geriatric Considerations
A. Case management and social worker are utilized to ensure safe discharge to appropriate level of care.
B. Arrange for delivery of any durable medical equipment to the patient's assisted living, adult living, group home, or home. Considerations of insurance coverage and deductible amounts are important for elders on fixed budgets. Financial resources and availability of social support through appropriate government resources is important for safe transition, especially to independent living and home.
  1. Medications: Ensure insurance is available for medications and durable medical equipment necessary for safe patient discharge, such as bedside commode, and so forth.
  2. If possible, arrange first follow-up medical appointments with appropriate physicians, and/or specialists (urologist).
  3. If home therapy is needed for wound therapy, ensure appointments for home visits are set up.
C. If indicated, set up home health visit to provide appropriate support in arranging first appointments.
D. Discuss with patient, caregiver, and/or family.
  1. Signs and symptoms to monitor.
  2. Common occurrences.
  3. Readmission concerns.

Bibliography
American Psychiatric Association. (2013). *Diagnostic and statistical manual of mental disorders (DSM-5)* (5th ed.). Arlington, VA: American Psychiatric Association.

Fauci, A . S. (2008). Nervous system dysfunction. In A. S. Fauci, E. Braunwald, D. L. Kasper, S. L. Hauser, D. L. Longo, J. L. Jameson, & J. Loscalzo (Eds.), *Harrison's principles of internal medicine* (17th ed., pp. 139–180). New York, NY: McGraw-Hill Professional.

Fletcher, K. (2012). Dementia. In M. Boltz, E. Capezuti, T. Fulmer, & D. Zwicker (Eds.), *Evidence-based geriatric nursing protocols for best practice* (4th ed., pp. 163–185). New York, NY: Springer Publishing Company.

Fulmer, T., & Zwicker, D. (2012). *Evidence-based geriatric nursing protocols for best practice* (4th ed., pp. 186–199). New York, NY: Springer Publishing Company.

17 Trauma Guidelines

Susan F. Galincyski

Chest Trauma

Susan F. Galincyski

Definition
A. Any mechanism that causes injury to the bony or soft tissue in the thorax.
B. Any of these injuries alone or in combination can be devastating and life-threatening to the patient, in a very short period of time.

Incidence
A. Account for up to 25% of all trauma-related deaths.
B. Approximately 80% to 85% of patients with chest trauma will experience at least one rib fracture.
C. Gunshot wounds to the chest tend to be more fatal.
D. Approximately 5% to 10% of chest trauma will involve sternal fractures.

Pathogenesis
A. Related to mechanism of injury.
B. Common mechanisms: Blunt chest trauma, penetrating trauma (gunshot wounds, stab wounds, impalements, acceleration–deceleration shearing forces, and compressive forces).

Predisposing Factors
A. Chest trauma can occur in anyone, but there is a higher incidence in younger males who may engage in high risk behaviors.

Subjective Data
A. Common complaints/symptoms.
  1. Chest wall and back pain, worse with movement, coughing, breathing.
  2. Shortness of breath.
  3. Increased pain with palpation.
B. Common/typical scenario.
  1. Other signs and symptoms.
    a. Crepitus in the presence of fractures.
    b. Splinting or shallow breathing.
    c. Decreased breath sounds on the affected side (pneumothorax).
    d. Beck's triad: Muffled, distant heart sounds (cardiac tamponade), jugular venous distention, and narrowed pulse pressures.
C. Subjective data/review of systems.

  1. Ask the patient about the events surrounding the injury. With falls, ask if the patient tripped or passed out. Determine if syncope needs to be ruled out.
  2. If motor vehicle collisions (MVC) occur, ask the patient about restraints. Was there a steering wheel deformity?
  3. Assess for chest pain. Location? Characteristics? Reproducible?

Physical Examination
A. Aimed at identifying the most life-threatening injury first.
B. Advanced trauma life support (ATLS) guidelines provide a quick but thorough approach to patient assessment.

Diagnostic Tests
A. FAST examination: May show cardiac tamponade and can be used to determine the presence of a pneumothorax without the use of chest x-ray.
B. Plain radiograph of the chest to identify fractures, atelectasis, pneumothorax, or widened mediastinum (possible aorta injury).
C. CT and CT angiogram help to identify specific bony, organ, and vascular injuries.
D. ECG.
E. Arterial blood gas: May show respiratory acidosis related to hypoventilation as a result of pain and splinting.
F. Cardiac enzymes.

Differential Diagnosis
A. Common traumatic chest injuries.
  1. Bony injuries.
    a. Rib fractures.
      i. Definition: Fractures of one or more ribs. Can be located bilaterally, or may be displaced and can stand alone or result in injury to underlying structures such as the lungs, subclavian vessels, or organs such as the spleen and liver.
        1) Flail chest: Occurs when at least two adjacent ribs are broken in multiple places, creating a free moving segment allowing that segment of the chest wall to move independently. If fractures are near the sternum, there can be a free-floating segment of the sternum, as well as rib. This can be a life-threatening condition.
    b. Sternal fractures.
      i. Definition: Fractures of the manubrium or sternal body. Persons older than 65 years will have increased risk of death (10%–12%) with one rib

fracture. The rate increases by 5% with each additional rib fracture.

  ii. Management.
    1) Rule out underlying injury to other tissues or organs.
    2) Cardiac echo will determine if there is a cardiac contusion or other heart-related injury.
    3) Pain management.
    4) Aggressive pulmonary hygiene. Encourage incentive spirometer.
    5) Supplemental oxygen.
    6) Displaced rib fractures or flail segments may require operative intervention for stabilization.

2. Lung injuries.
  a. Pulmonary contusion.
    i. Definition.
      1) Bruising to the lung parenchyma.
      2) Clinical course: Tend to worsen in the first 24 to 48 hours. Can lead to atelectasis, infiltrate, effusions, or empyema.
      3) Frequently associated with rib fractures.
    ii. Management.
      1) Supplemental oxygen.
      2) May require intubation and supported ventilation.
      3) Analgesia.
      4) Chest physiotherapy.
  b. Pneumothorax.
    i. Definition.
      1) Accumulation of air in the pleural space, resulting in partial or complete collapse of the lung.
      2) Tension pneumothorax: Life-threatening condition. As air accumulates in the pleural space, it exerts an increased pressure on the heart; mediastinal shift to the unaffected side can lead to circulatory collapse.
  c. Hemothorax.
    i. Definition.
      1) Blood accumulates in the pleural space.
      2) Considered "massive hemothorax" when drainage exceeds 1.5 L in less than 2 hours after injury, necessitating emergent thoracotomy.
    ii. Physical examination findings of pneumothorax or hemothorax.
      1) Decreased breath sounds on the affected side.
      2) Deviated trachea is a late sign.
      3) Respiratory distress, hypoxia, tachycardia, or hypotension may be present.
    iii. Other physical findings.
      1) Cyanosis.
      2) Diaphoresis.
      3) Chest pain.
      4) Altered mental status.
    iv. Management.
      1) Small pneumothorax or hemothorax can be managed conservatively by observation and repeat chest x-ray (CXR).
      2) Pneumothorax greater than 20% requires thoracostomy tube (chest tube) insertion.
      3) Massive hemothorax with drainage of more than 1.5 L in 2 hours may require thoracotomy and repair of lung injury.

  d. Cardiac tamponade.
    i. Definition: Accumulation of blood or fluid in the pericardial sac, causing a compression of the heart muscles. This leads to decreased cardiac output, which is life-threatening.
    ii. Physical examination findings.
      1) Beck's triad: A constellation of findings suggestive of tamponade.
        a) Jugular vein distention.
        b) Hypotension with narrowing pulse pressures.
        c) Distant or muffled heart sounds.
    iii. Other physical findings.
      1) Tachycardia.
      2) Pulsus paradoxus.
      3) Altered mentation.
      4) Oliguria.
      5) Signs of impending shock.
    iv. Management.
      1) Pericardiocentesis.
      2) Management of shock.
  e. Great vessel injuries.
    i. Definition.
      1) Interruption of the wall of any of the great vessels is a life-threatening event. Injuries to the aorta, internal vena cava, or subclavian vessels can be the result of laceration from bony segments or shearing or compressive forces. These require operative intervention.
      2) Physical findings.
        a) Chest or back pain, shortness of breath, weakness.
        b) Hypotension.
        c) Variations in blood pressure (BP) in both upper extremities.
        d) Shock.
      3) Management.
        a) Thoracotomy with repair to affected vessels; may require cardiopulmonary bypass.
        b) Mechanical ventilation.
        c) Replacement of blood volume with transfusion, may require massive transfusion protocols.
        d) May require hemodynamic support with vasopressors and volume resuscitation.

Evaluation and Management Plan

A. General plan.
  1. Identify specific injuries and treat accordingly.
  2. Primary goals of therapy.
    a. Pain management.
    b. Prevention of atelectasis and pneumonia.
    c. Supplemental oxygen.
  3. Explain expectant course with patient and family.
  4. Consider adding cardiac enzymes to workup to rule out underlying stress to heart.
  5. May require multiple radiographs to evaluate course of healing.
  6. For patients with chest tubes, document the output and consistency of drainage and whether or not an air leak is present.
B. Patient/family teaching points.
  1. Cough and deep breathing exercises.

2. Incentive spirometry or other airway clearance devices.
3. Incisional wound care.
C. Pharmacotherapy.
1. When indicated, vasopressors to support hemodynamics.
2. Multimodal pain management using opioids only when indicated.
a. Nonsteroidal anti-inflammatory drugs (NSAIDs) and Tylenol, mild pain.
b. Lidocaine patch for localized pain.
c. Intravenous (IV) Toradol and Tylenol with supplemental opioid for moderate pain.
d. For severe pain, consider:
i. Epidural pain medication.
ii. Intercostal nerve block.
iii. Patient-controlled analgesia (PCA) pain management.
3. Bronchodilator treatments when indicated.

Follow-Up

A. Follow-up should be dictated by the level of injury and hospital course.
B. For minor injuries, patients may follow-up with the primary care provider in 1 to 2 weeks.
C. Postsurgical follow-up may be indicated in a 7- to 14-day period for wound checks, repeat imaging, or suture/staple removal.

Consultation/Referral

A. Patients with severe injury should always be referred to a high level of care if the institution does not have the resources to treat the patient.
B. Refer any additional injuries requiring specialist consultation.

Special/Geriatric Considerations

A. Morbidity associated with rib fractures increases with age and is the highest in elderly patients.

Bibliography

Alisha, C., Gajanan, G., & Jyothi, H. (2015). Risk factors affecting the prognosis in patients with pulmonary contusion following chest trauma. *Journal of Clinical Diagnostic Research, 9*(8), OC17–OC19. doi:10.7860/JCDR/2015/13285.6375
Sawa, J., Green, R., Thoma, B., Erdogan, M., & Davis, P. (2017, August 11). Risk factors for adverse outcomes in older adults with blunt chest trauma: A systematic review. *Canadian Journal of Emergency Medicine, 20*(4), 1–9. doi:10.1017/cem.2017.377
Senn-Reeves, J. N., & Stafileno, B. A. (2013). Long term outcomes after blunt injury to the boney thorax. *Journal of Trauma Nursing, 20*(1), 56–64. doi:10.1097/JTN.0b013e318286629b
Stewart, D. J. (2014). Blunt chest trauma. *Journal of Trauma Nursing, 21*(6), 282–286. doi:10.1097/JTN.0000000000000079

Penetrating Chest Injuries

Susan F. Galincyski

Definition

A. A penetrating chest injury is one in which the projectile enters the thorax in any area below the level of the clavicle to the diaphragm.
B. Organs at risk for injury include: Chest wall, ribs, lungs and pleura, esophagus, trachea, diaphragm, thoracic blood vessels, the heart, and mediastinal structures.

C. As stated previously, gunshot wounds carry a higher mortality than blunt trauma.

Incidence

A. Thoracic injuries account for approximately 20% to 25% of all traumatic deaths.
B. Approximately 16,000 deaths annually in the United States can be attributed to thoracic injury.
C. Increase in number with the increase in the number of violent crimes.
D. Much of the research in thoracic trauma comes from military experiences.

Pathogenesis

A. A bullet or projectile object can enter the body at any location but if it travels into the thoracic cavity, any of the structures there are at risk for injury.

Predisposing Factors

A. Males are more prone than females.
B. Males older than 65 years of age.
C. Single people are more prone than married people.
D. Inner city resident.
E. Lower income individuals.
F. Members of ethnic minority groups.
G. Drug and alcohol use.
H. History of depression.
I. History of previous suicide attempts.

Subjective Data

A. Common complaints/symptoms.
1. Most patients with penetrating chest wounds will be brought into the ED via emergency medical services.
2. These patients complain of chest pain and shortness of breath. If the patient is in a state of shock, he or she may be minimally responsive to answering questions.
B. Common/typical scenario.
1. Common scenario occurs from low velocity injuries such as an impalement by a structure like a knife, medium velocity injuries from hand guns, or high velocity injuries from rifles and military weapons.
C. Family and social history.
1. Family history is noncontributory. Penetrating chest injuries occur more frequently in violent areas, large metropolitan areas, and areas of conflict.
D. Review of systems.
1. Neuro: Ask about dizziness, lightheadedness.
2. Cardiac: Heart racing, palpitations, lightheadedness.
3. Respiratory: Shortness of breath, breathing difficulties, airway obstructions.
4. Dermatology: Areas of bleeding or bruising.

Physical Examination

A. Assess chest, back, and abdomen for additional wounds.
B. Dermatology—The physical examination requires a thorough investigation of the skin for breaks in the skin, redness, or discoloration with particular attention to the chest, back, and abdomen.
C. Neurology—Assess cognition and responsiveness.
D. Cardiology—Monitor blood pressure (BP) and heart rate (HR).
E. Respiratory—Assess quality of breath sounds and respiratory rate.

Diagnostic Tests

A. CT.
B. Supine chest film can help to identify foreign bodies, that is, bullets and pneumothorax.

Differential Diagnosis

A. There is typically no need for a differential diagnosis. An inspection will provide the diagnosis in this case.

Evaluation and Management Plan

A. General plan.
  1. The primary approach to penetrating trauma to the thorax is to answer the question of whether or not the patient needs operative intervention.
  2. Criteria for operative intervention.
    a. Hemodynamic instability: BP less than 90 or HR greater than 120.
    b. Hypotension despite fluid resuscitation.
    c. Altered mental status without obvious head injury.
    d. Metabolic acidosis.
    e. Significant findings on diagnostic studies.
  3. Goals of treatment are aimed at controlling hemorrhage and maintaining perfusion, promptly addressing airway compromise, and maintaining adequate perfusion.
B. Patient/family teaching points.
  1. Patient and family education should be geared toward anticipated patient needs as discharge nears.
  2. Some examples include wound care, tracheotomy care, physical medicine, and rehab goals.
C. Pharmacotherapy.
  1. In the acute phase of care, interventions may include:
    a. Hemodynamic support: Blood transfusions and vasopressors may be necessary to reduce risks of hypotension related to hypovolemia and shock states.
    b. Sedation and pain management with continuous infusions to keep the patient comfortable.
    c. Prophylactic antibiotic treatment for operative care and for any ICU-related infections.

Follow-Up

A. Many of these patients have a long critical care and hospital course and will become deconditioned. Preparing the patient and family for potential rehabilitation needs is key.
B. If the patient has multiple injuries not related to just one organ system, education about follow-up with those injury-specific specialty groups is recommended.
C. Physical medicine and rehab may have a very active role in postdischarge care.

Consultation/Referral

A. Trauma.
B. Cardiothoracic surgery.
C. Other necessary consultants, based on injury.
D. Physical medicine and rehab services.
E. Psychiatry for self-inflicted wounds/suicide attempts.

Special/Geriatric Considerations

A. Indicators of poor outcomes/higher mortality include:
  1. Lower Glasgow Coma Score (GCS) on arrival.
  2. Increased age.
  3. Suicide attempt (self-inflicted).
  4. Coagulopathy.

Bibliography

Berg, R. J., Karamanos, E., Inaba, K., Okoye, O., Teixeira, P. G., & Demetriades, D. (2014, February). The persistent diagnostic challenge of thoracoabdominal stab wounds. *Journal of Trauma and Acute Care Surgery, 76*(2), 418–423. doi:10.1097/TA.0000000000000120

Davis, J. S., Satahoo, S. S., Butler, F. K., Dermer, H., Naranjo, D., Julien, K., . . . Schulman, C. I. (2014, August). An analysis of prehospital deaths: Who can we save? *Journal of Trauma and Acute Care Surgery, 77*(2), 213–218. doi:10.1097/TA.0000000000000292

Kamarova, M., & Kendall, R. (2017, December). 13 Prophylactic antibiotics for penetrating injury: A review of practice at a major trauma centre, literature review and recommendations. *Emergency Medicine Journal, 34*(12), A869. doi:10.1136/emermed-2017-207308.13

Madden, B. P. (2017, January). Evolutional trends in the management of tracheal and bronchial injuries. *Journal of Thoracic Disease, 9*(1), E67–E70. doi:10.21037/jtd.2017.01.43

Mollberg, N. M., Tabachnik, D., Farjah, F., Lin, F. J., Vafa, A., Abdelhady, K., . . . Massad, M. G. (2013, August). Utilization of cardiothoracic surgeons for operative penetrating thoracic trauma and its impact on clinical outcomes. *Annals of Thoracic Surgery, 96*(2), 445–450. doi:10.1016/j.athoracsur.2013.04.033

Seamon, M. J., Haut, E. R., VanArendonk, K., Barbosa, R. R., Chiu, W. C., Dente, C. J., . . . Rhee, P. (2015, July). An evidence-based approach to patient selection for emergency department thoracotomy: A practice management guideline from the Eastern Association for the Surgery of Trauma. *Journal of Trauma and Acute Care Surgery, 79*(1), 159–173. doi:10.1097/TA.0000000000000648

Penetrating Intracranial Injuries

Susan F. Galincyski

Definition

A. A penetrating intracranial injury is one in which the projectile enters the cranium.
B. Penetrating injuries, more specifically gunshot wounds (GSW), are high energy, high velocity injuries that can cause extensive damage as the object enters the body.
C. Gunshot wounds carry a higher mortality than other penetrating wounds. They are almost always fatal if the bullet crosses the mid-line, crosses both hemispheres, or lodges in the brain.
D. The blast energy of a bullet can be as high as 30 to 40 times the diameter of the bullet and can cause increased tissue damage as the bullet travels and displaces surrounding tissue. In contrast, stab wounds are considered low impact and the focus is more on the immediate tissue injury.

Incidence

A. Death rates have increased over the past 20 years.
B. Affects almost 2 million people annually.
C. Stab wounds are considered low velocity and are localized to the area of impact.

Pathogenesis

A. A bullet or projectile object crosses the skull barrier and enters the brain parenchyma.

Predisposing Factors

A. Males are more prone than females.
B. Males older than 65 years of age.
C. Single people are more prone than married people.
D. Inner city resident.
E. Lower income individuals.
F. Members of ethnic minority groups.
G. Drug and alcohol use.
H. History of depression.
I. History of previous suicide attempts.

Subjective Data

A. Common complaints/symptoms.

1. Patients will typically come in via emergency services, but will occasionally walk in or be driven by friends or family with a foreign object that has penetrated the skull.

B. Family and social history (pertinent findings—positive/negative).

1. Family history is noncontributory. Penetrating head injuries occur more frequently in violent areas, large metropolitan areas, and areas of conflict.

C. Review of systems (pertinent findings—positive/negative).

1. Neuro—ask about headaches, dizziness, vertigo.

2. Head, ear, eyes, nose, and throat (HEENT)—blurry vision, double vision, loss of vision, changes in smell, bleeding from anywhere on the head.

3. Musculoskeletal—any weakness in the arms or legs or numbness/tingling.

Physical Examination

A. Perform a Glasgow Coma Score (GCS; see Table 17.1). The score ranges from 3 to 15. If the patient is intubated, that is notated by the use of the letter "T" after the number, such as 8T to indicate GCS of 8 in an intubated patient.

B. Assess for signs of other injuries by completely undressing the patient. Axillae and groin are areas that require inspection—as stab wounds and GSW wounds are often found in those locations.

C. Assess the head, scalp, and face for contusions, lacerations, or hematoma.

D. A detailed neuro examination is performed when possible to determine baseline neurological function.

Diagnostic Tests

A. CT—noncontrast of head and cervical spine as indicated.

B. Flat plate of skull can be done to identify foreign bodies (i.e., bullets).

TABLE 17.1	**Glasgow Coma Score (GCS)**

Eye Opening (E)
Spontaneous 4
To voice 3
To pain 2
No response 1
Verbal Response (V)
Oriented conversation 5
Confused/disoriented 4
Incomprehensible words 3
Incomprehensible sounds 2
No response 1
Motor Response (M)
Moves all extremities 6
Localizes to pain 5
Withdraws to pain 4
Decorticate posture 3
Decerebrate posture 2
No response 1
Total GCS = E+V+M

GCS, Glasgow Coma Score.

Differential Diagnosis

A. There is typically no need for a differential diagnosis. An inspection will provide the diagnosis in this case.

Evaluation and Management Plan

A. General plan.

1. These patients are often critically ill and have a higher mortality.

2. Goals of treatment are geared toward preventing secondary brain injury by maintaining adequate perfusion and oxygenation to the brain.

B. Patient/family teaching points.

1. Patient and family education should be geared toward anticipated patient needs as discharge nears.

2. Some examples include wound care, tracheotomy care, physical medicine, and rehab goals.

C. Pharmacotherapy.

1. In the acute phase of care, interventions may include:

a. Hemodynamic support: Blood transfusions and vasopressors may be necessary to reduce risks of hypotension related to hypovolemia and shock states.

b. Seizure prophylaxis is indicated for severe brain injury and may include Keppra, Dilantin, or fosphenytoin.

c. Sedation and pain management with continuous infusions are used to keep the patient comfortable and avoid elevations in increased intracranial pressure (ICP).

d. Antibiotic treatments that cross the blood–brain barrier such as ceftriaxone are warranted for open fractures and for any ICU-related infections.

e. Osmotic diuretics such as mannitol and hypertonic saline help to reduce ICP.

Follow-Up

A. If the patient survives, follow-up with neurosurgeon in 10 to 14 days post discharge is recommended.

B. If the patient had any additional injuries (multiple GSW often do), follow-up with those injury-specific specialty groups is recommended.

C. Physical medicine and rehab may have a very active role in postdischarge care. Most head trauma will require rehabilitative care and potentially neurological cognitive testing, evaluation, and management.

Consultation/Referral

A. Trauma is consulted on all trauma cases.

B. Neurosurgery will be consulted on penetrating injuries to the brain.

C. Other necessary consultants are selected based on the type and extent of injury.

D. Physical medicine and rehab services are needed.

E. Refer to psychiatry for self-inflicted wounds/suicide attempts.

Special/Geriatric Considerations

A. Indicators of poor outcomes/higher mortality include:

1. Lower GCS on arrival.

2. Increased age.

3. Suicide attempt (self-inflicted).

4. Transcranial injury.

5. Perforated brain injury (entrance and exit wounds).

6. Coagulopathy.

7. Any episode of hypoxia prehospital or during hospitalization.

Bibliography

Aarabi, B., Tofighi, B., Kufera, J. A., Hadley, J., Ahn, E. S., Cooper, C., . . . Uscinski, R. H. (2014, May). Predictors of outcome in civilian gunshot wounds to the head. *Journal of Neurosurgery, 120*(5), 1138–1146. doi:10.3171/2014.1.JNS131869

Burgess, P., Sullivent, E., Sasser, S., Wald, M., Ossmann, E., & Kapil, V. (2010). Managing traumatic brain injury secondary to explosions. *Journal of Emergencies, Trauma and Shock, 3*(2), 164–172. doi:10.4103/0974-2700.62120

Folio, L., Solomon, J., Biassou, N., Fischer, T., Dworzak, J., Raymont, V., . . . Grafman, J. (2013, March). Semi-automated trajectory analysis of deep ballistic penetrating brain injury. *Military Medicine, 178*(3), 338–345. doi:10.7205/MILMED-D-12-00353

Mac Donald, C. L., Johnson, A. M., Cooper, D., Nelson, E. C., Werner, N. J., Shimony, J. S., . . . Brody, D. L. (2011, June 2). Detection of blast-related traumatic brain injury in U.S. military personnel. *The New England Journal of Medicine, 364*(22), 2091–2100. doi:10.1056/NEJMoa1008069

Paiva, W. S., de Andrade, A. F., Amorim, R. L., Figueiredo, E. G., & Teixeira, M. J. (2012, October). Brainstem injury by penetrating head trauma with a knife. *British Journal of Neurosurgery, 26*(5), 779–781. doi:10.3109/02688697.2012.655809

Saito, N., Hito, R., Burke, P. A., & Sakai, O. (2014). Imaging of penetrating injuries of the head and neck: Current practice at a level I trauma center in the United States. *The Keio Journal of Medicine, 63*(2), 23–33. doi:10.2302/kjm.2013-0009-RE

Shock

Heather H. Meissen and Alison M. Kelley

Definition

A. Impaired tissue oxygenation or inadequate cell utilization of oxygen.

B. Shock is a condition that occurs due to inadequate oxygen delivery for aerobic cellular respiration, therefore leading to inadequate perfusion of tissue, irreversible cellular damage, and subsequently leading to death.

C. Shock is not defined as hypotension; however, hypotension can be a clinical indicator.

D. Types of shock (see Table 17.2).
  1. Hypovolemic: Intravascular volume depletion.
  2. Cardiogenic: Pump failure.
  3. Distributive: Loss of peripheral vascular tone.
  4. Obstructive: Impedance of adequate cardiac filling.

Incidence

A. 16% of shock states are hypovolemic.

B. 16% of shock states are cardiogenic.

C. Incidence—62% of shock states are distributive in nature and due to sepsis and 4% are distributive in nature from causes other than sepsis (Angus & van der Poll, 2013).

D. Incidence—2% of shock states are obstructive (NEJM, 2013).

Pathogenesis

A. Inadequate oxygen delivery changes cell metabolism from aerobic to anaerobic.

B. This leads to inadequate energy production and metabolic failure.

C. Anaerobic metabolism leads to lactic acid production, causing the cell to cease function and swell. Once the cell swells, the membrane becomes permeable, allowing electrolytes and fluids to seep in. This causes the sodium and potassium pumps to fail, leading to mitochondrial damage and cell death.

Predisposing Factors

A. Hemodynamic.
  1. Hemorrhage.
  2. Vomiting.
  3. Diarrhea.
  4. Poor oral intake.

B. Cardiogenic.
  1. Myopathic: Myocardial ischemia.
  2. Valvular/mechanical failure.
  3. Drug overdose.

C. Distributive.
  1. Sepsis.
  2. Anaphylaxis.
  3. Adrenal insufficiency.
  4. Neurogenic.
  5. Liver failure.

D. Obstructive.
  1. Cardiac tamponade.
  2. Pulmonary embolism.
  3. Tension pneumothorax.
  4. Constrictive pericarditis.

Subjective Data

A. Common complaints/symptoms.
  1. Blood pressure.
    a. Systolic blood pressure (SBP) less than 90 mmHg.
    b. Mean arterial pressure (MAP) less than 60 mmHg.
    c. Change is SBP greater than 40 mmHg.
  2. Altered mental status.
  3. Oliguria.
  4. Lactic acidosis (anion gap acidosis).

B. Common/typical scenario.
  1. Noted hypotension.
    a. Chronic—absence of tissue hypoperfusion.
    b. Acute—presence of tissue hypoperfusion (↓ urine output [UOP], altered mental status [AMS]).
      i. Start workup to determine type of shock while treating patient so as to not to allow circulatory collapse to occur.

TABLE 17.2 **Hemodynamic Profile of Shock**

Types of Shock	HR	CO	Ventricular Filling Pressure	SVR	Pulse Pressure	SVO2
Cardiogenic	↑	↓	↑	↑	↓	↓
Hypovolemic	↑	↓	↓	↑	↓	↓
Distributive	↑	↑ or ↓	↓	↓	↑	↑
Obstructive	↑	↓	↑ or normal	↑	↓	↓

CO, cardiac output; HR, heart rate; SVO2, Mixed venous oxygen saturation; SVR, systemic vascular resistance.
Source: Information was taken from Bergeron, N., Dubois, M.J., Dumont, M., Dial, S., Skrobik, Y. (2001). Intensive care delirium screening checklist: evaluation of a new screening tool. Intensive Care Medicine, 27, pp. 859-864. doi:10.1007/s001340100909

C. Family/social history.

1. Further history needs to be obtained as well as a more thorough assessment.

2. Does the patient have a history that is significant for cardiac problems?

3. Does the patient have a history that is significant for exposure to infectious sources?

Physical Examination

A. Does the patient's skin feel cool and clammy, warm, or normal?

B. If the patient has cool and clammy skin, significant cardiac history, or new chest pain, avoid fluids and start workup by obtaining a stat ECHO.

C. Is skin warm or normal to touch? 62% of patients in shock will be distributive/septic in nature. Start treatment for presumed sepsis until otherwise noted.

1. Fluid bolus of 30 mL/kg of isotonic fluids within the first 3 hours.

Diagnostic Tests

A. For all forms of shock, obtain labwork and additional data points as quickly as possible.

B. Complete blood count (CBC).

C. Arterial blood gas (ABG).

D. Lactate.

E. Comprehensive metabolic panel (CMP).

F. ScVO2 (if central access is in place).

G. Central venous pressure (CVP) can be monitored with minimally invasive monitoring through the arterial line.

H. Obtaining additional parameters such as passive leg raise, fluid challenges against stroke volume measurements, or variations in systolic pressures, pulse pressure, or stroke volume changes while on mechanical ventilation should be considered when applicable.

I. Start vasopressors if patient is unresponsive to fluid for all forms of shock.

1. If patient is unresponsive to vasopressor support and history is suggestive, consider obstructive shock and implement treatment quickly. This is often referred to as pressor refractory shock.

J. Once data points are back—identify correct diagnosis and treat appropriately (see Table 17.2).

Differential Diagnosis

A. Myocardial infarction.

B. Thyroid storm.

C. Acute pancreatitis.

D. Pulmonary embolism.

E. Sepsis.

F. Toxic/metabolic syndrome.

G. Coagulopathy.

H. Poisoning.

Evaluation and Management Plan

A. General plan.

1. Correct underlying process.

2. Fluids.

   a. Bolus.

     i. 10 to 30 mL/kg depending on the type of shock encountered.

     ii. The Surviving Sepsis Campaign recommends 30 mL/kg intravenous (IV) fluids within the first 3 hours of diagnosis of septic shock.

   b. Types of fluids.

     i. Isotonic fluids.

       1) Lactated Ringers.

       2) Normal saline.

       3) Plasma-lyte A.

     ii. Blood products: Replacement of blood products should be based on the individual patient's laboratory values. Advanced trauma life support guidelines recommend massive transfusion protocol with universal red blood cells (RBCs) and plasma platelet pool for each six units of RBCs.

3. Vasopressor support.

   a. Terminology.

     i. Chronotropic: To change heart rate.

     ii. Inotropic: To change the force of the heart contraction. Positive inotropes increase the force of the contraction and negative inotropes weaken the force of contraction—otherwise known as squeeze.

   b. Norepinephrine.

     i. Endogenous catecholamine.

     ii. Acts as an excitatory neurotransmitter.

     iii. Alpha receptor-mediated peripheral vasoconstriction.

     iv. Weak β_1 receptor agonist.

     v. Dose: 0.01 to 1 mcq/kg/min and titrate to effect.

     vi. Side effects: Local tissue necrosis.

     vii. First line pressor for septic shock.

   c. Epinephrine.

     i. Endogenous catecholamine.

     ii. Most potent β_1 agonist.

     iii. Both alpha and beta properties.

     iv. Potent inotropic and chronotropic.

     v. Dose: 0.01 to 1 mcq/kg/min.

     vi. Second pressor choice in septic shock.

   d. Phenylephrine.

     i. Pure alpha receptor agonist.

     ii. Produces widespread vasoconstriction.

     iii. Dose: 0.1 to 5 mcq/kg/min.

     iv. Side effects.

       1) Bradycardia.

       2) Low cardiac output.

       3) Hypoperfusion to kidneys and bowel.

     v. Not recommended in septic shock.

   e. Vasopressin.

     i. Antidiuretic hormone (ADH)/osmoregulatory hormone.

     ii. Acts through v1 receptors to produce vasoconstriction.

     iii. Dose: 0.03 units/min.

     iv. Typically not titratable.

     v. Not recommended as single agent.

     vi. Use with norepinephrine to decrease dose or to improve perfusion by increasing mean arterial pressure (MAP).

B. Treatment of specific shock states.

1. Hypovolemic.

   a. Fluids.

   b. Vasopressor support.

   c. Control cause of fluid loss.

     i. Stop ongoing bleeding.

     ii. Stop ongoing emesis or diarrhea.

2. Cardiogenic.

   a. Improve myocardial function—percutaneous coronary intervention (PCI).

   b. Treat arrhythmias.

   c. Vasopressors plus inotropes.

3. Obstructive.
    a. Relief of obstruction.
4. Distributive.
    a. Fluids.
    b. Vasopressors.
    c. Treatment of cause.
        i. Antibiotics.
        ii. Removal of source of infection.

Follow-Up

A. Resolution of hypotension.
B. Increased urine output.
C. Decreased heart rate.
D. Lactic acid—trend until the level falls below 2.

Consultation/Referral

A. Consult critical care team for management of shock.
B. Consult appropriate service for type of shock.
    1. Cardiac surgery for cardiogenic shock or interventional radiology for obstructive shock, that is, pulmonary embolism or infectious diseases when sepsis is the cause of shock.
    2. General surgery may need to be consulted if an abdominal source of sepsis is suspected.

Special/Geriatric Considerations

A. Consider age-related changes in geriatric patients.
B. Response to treatment may occur much more slowly than in younger patients.
C. Signs of shock may go unrecognized early on in geriatric patients due to loss of compensatory mechanisms that are common with aging.
D. Also medications such as beta-blockers may diminish the body's ability to compensate.

Bibliography

Angus, D., & van der Poll, T. (2013). Severe sepsis and septic shock. *The New England Journal of Medicine, 369*, 840–851. doi:10.1056/NEJMra1208623

Beck, V., Chateau, D., & Bryson, G. L. (2014). Timing of vasopressor initiation and mortality in septic shock: A cohort study. *Critical Care, 18*(3), R97. doi:10.1186/cc13868

Bisschop, M., & Bellou, A. (2012). Anaphylaxis. *Current Opinion in Critical Care, 18*, 308–317. doi: 10.1097/MCC.0b013e3283557a63

Dalton, T., Rushing, M., Escott, M., & Monroe, B. (2015, November 2). Complexities of geriatric trauma patients. *Journal of Emergency Medical Services, 40*. Retrieved from http://www.jems.com/articles/print/volume-40/issue-11/features/complexities-of-geriatric-trauma-patients.html?c=1

Dellinger, R., Levy, M., Rhodes, A., Annane, D., Gerlach, H., Opal, S., . . . Moreno, R. (2013). Surviving Sepsis Campaign: International guidelines for management of severe sepsis and septic shock: 2012. *Critical Care Medicine, 41*(2), 580–637. doi:10.1097/CCM.0b013e31827e83af

Gutierrez, G., Reines, H., & Wulf-Gutierrez, M. (2004). Clinical review: Hemorrhagic stroke. *Critical Care, 8*, 373–381. doi:10.1186/cc2851

Kadri, S., Rhee, C., Strich, J., Morales, M., Hohmann, S., Menchaca, J., . . . Klompas, M. (2017). Estimating ten year trends in septic shock incidence and mortality in United States Academic Medical Centers using clinical data. *Chest, 151*(2), 278–285. doi:10.1016/j.chest.2016.07.010

Klein, T., & Ramani, G. (2012). Assessment and management of cardiogenic shock in the emergency department. *Cardiology Clinics, 30*, 651–664. doi:10.1016/j.ccl.2012.07.004

Maier, R. V. (2001). Approach to the patient with shock. In J. Jameson, A. S. Fauci, D. L. Kasper, S. L. Hauser, D. L. Longo, & J. Loscalzo (Eds.), *Harrison's principles of internal medicine* (20th ed.). New York, NY: McGraw-Hill.

Moranville, M., Mieure, K., & Santayana, E. (2011). Evaluation and management of shock states: Hypovolemic, distributive and cardiogenic. *Journal of Pharmacy Practice, 24*(1), 44–60. doi:10.1177/0897190010388150

Pandit, V., Rhee, P., Hashmi, A., Kulvatunyou, N., Tang, A., Khalil, M., . . . Joseph, B. (2014). Shock index predicts mortality in geriatric trauma patients: An analysis of the National Trauma Data Bank. *Journal of Trauma and Acute Care Surgery, 76*(4), 1111–1115. doi:10.1097/TA.0000000000000160

Pauler, P., Newell, M., Hildebrandt, D., & Kirkland, L. (2017). Incidence, etiology and implications of shock in therapeutic hypothermia. *Journal of the Minneapolis Heart Institute Foundation, 1*, 19–23. doi:10.21925/2475-0204-1.1.19

Reynolds, H., & Hochman, J. (2008). Cardiogenic shock: Current concepts and improving outcomes. *Circulation, 117*, 686–697. doi:10.1161/CIRCULATIONAHA.106.613596

Rhee, C., Murphy, M. V., & Li, L. (2015). Lactate testing in suspected sepsis: Trends and predictors of failure to measure levels. *Critical Care Medicine, 43*(8), 1669–1676. doi:10.1097/CCM.0000000000001087

Richards, J., & Wilcox, S. (2014). Diagnosis and management of shock in the emergency department. *Emergency Medicine Practice, 16*(3), 1–22.

Silva, J., Concalves, L., & Sousa, P. (2018). Fluid therapy and shock: An integrative review. *British Journal of Nursing, 27*(8), 449–454. doi:10.12968/bjon.2018.27.8.449

Spinal Cord Injuries

Susan F. Galincyski

Definition

A. Spinal cord injury (SCI) is any damage to the spinal cord that causes temporary or permanent changes that disrupt normal function. This includes changes to motor, sensory, or autonomic function in the body below the level of the SCI.
B. It is a challenging medical condition due to the limited therapeutic options available to treating physicians. There is a significant economic and social burden of SCI patients as well as society.

Incidence

A. Can affect up to 750 per million annually.
B. In the United States, there are approximately 10,000 to 12,000 new traumatic SCIs per year.
C. Approximately 280,000 people are presently living with SCI in North America.
D. Up to 60% of injuries include the cervical spine.
E. For the geriatric population, a majority of injuries are incomplete.
F. For the geriatric patient, mortality and morbidity are significantly higher.
G. Higher incidence of central cord injuries occurs in the geriatric population.

Pathogenesis

A. Spinal cord injuries are considered high impact injuries, often resulting from high speed motor vehicle crashes or falls from significant height.
B. Other mechanisms may include:
    1. Hyperextension injury with or without longitudinal ligament tear.
    2. Vertical column loading (axial load) compression.
    3. Distraction injuries (seen with hangings).
    4. Penetrating injuries.
    5. Pathological fractures (seen more commonly in the elderly).

Predisposing Factors

A. Male.
B. Persons between 15 and 24 years of age.
C. Increasing occurrence in elderly.

Subjective Data

A. Common complaints/symptoms.

1. Neck or back pain.
2. Numbness.
3. Loss of limb function.
4. Paresthesia.
B. Common/typical scenario.
   1. Other signs and symptoms.
     a. Bowel and bladder dysfunction.
     b. Priapism.
     c. Hyperparesthesia/pain.
C. Family and social history.
   1. Emergency medical support (EMS) report may give you significant information regarding the scene and how the patient was found.
   2. If possible, ask the patient about the history of events: Mechanism? Motor vehicle collisions (MVC)? Location in car? Restrained? Ejected? Mechanical fall or syncope? Fall from height? How far?
   3. Blunt versus penetrating.
   4. Distraction injury to spine? Hyperextension, hyperflexion, hyperrotation?
   5. Ask the patient about pain and the ability to move extremities after injury (see Figure 17.1).
   6. Assess for drug or alcohol use as this may impact your examination.

Physical Examination

A. Primary survey (advanced trauma life support [ATLS]) to assess for life-threatening injuries.
B. Pay particular attention to respiratory status as level of injury can impact spontaneous breathing.
   1. Injuries above C3 result in respiratory arrest.
   2. Injuries at C5 to C6 spare the diaphragm and diaphragm breathing is seen.
   3. Injuries below T1 to the level of L2 can affect the intercostals.
C. Motor and sensory assessment to assess level of injury.

D. Cardiovascular changes seen with SCI: SCI can impact the sympathetic pathways leading to alterations in blood pressure, heart rate, and temperature regulation.
E. Gastrointestinal changes associated with SCI may include loss of bowel function, development of an ileus, or obstruction.
F. GU: urinary incontinence and retention.
G. Always have a heightened suspicion for other injuries.

Diagnostic Tests

A. CT.
B. MRI.
C. Plain films (x-rays) can help identify fractures.

Differential Diagnosis

A. Central cord syndrome.
B. Anterior cord syndrome.
C. Posterior cord syndrome.
D. Brown-Sequard syndrome (often seen with penetrating trauma).

Evaluation and Management Plan

A. General plan.
   1. Interventions in SCI are aimed at preventing secondary injury.
   2. Earlier surgical intervention, when indicated, has been shown to improve neurological recovery.
   3. Maintain adequate airway and respirations.
   4. Cervical spine immobilization.
   5. Thoracic and lumbar bracing if necessary.
   6. Maintain adequate circulation.
   7. Ongoing neurological assessment.
   8. Assess for signs of neurogenic shock and support hemodynamics.

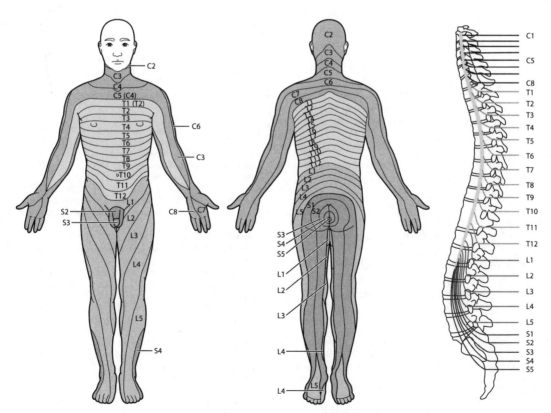

FIGURE 17.1 Dermatome map.

9. Aggressive bowel regimen to prevent constipation.

10. Monitor urine with either a Foley catheter or self-catheterization as needed.

B. Patient/family teaching points.

1. Patients need to be taught how to monitor and assess their skin for any breakdown.

2. Depending on the level of the ACI, patients may have bowel, bladder, and sexual dysfunction.

3. Teach patients and caregivers to recognize a life-threatening condition called autonomic dysreflexia, which can be caused by bladder spasms, urinary tract infections, or even external factors such as too tight clothing, belts, or shoes.

4. Physical and occupational therapy will be necessary for reducing muscle contractures and atrophy.

C. Pharmacotherapy.

1. Use of glucocorticoids, specifically methylprednisone, after acute traumatic SCI has been a controversial concept. The recommendations were to use methylprednisone for either 24 or 48 hours, depending on whether it was started 3 or 8 hours after injury, respectively.

    a. Many studies are showing early surgical intervention with decompression is preferable to steroid use.

2. Other pharmacological agents used in human clinical trials include: Tirilazad, naloxone, GM ganglioside, and riluzole. Recent neuroprotection agents involved in clinical trial include BA-120 (Cethrin) and minocycline.

3. Antibiotics for penetrating injuries.

4. Gastrointestinal (GI) prophylaxis and bowel regimen.

Follow-Up

A. SCI patients have a long course of physical medicine and rehabilitation.

B. Neurosurgery, orthopedics, and any other specialty group needed is involved in care.

Consultation/Referral

A. Neurosurgery/orthopedics (bony injuries) for management and possible fixation/fusion.

B. Prompt transfer to a Level I trauma center needs to be prioritized.

Special/Geriatric Considerations

A. SCI is an ever-increasing challenge with annual incidence of 750 per million in the developed world and even higher incidence in the developing world.

B. Pathophysiology of SCI involves primary and secondary injury mechanisms with future treatment strategies and emphasis on preventing or reversing secondary injury.

C. Medical management of SCI patients is in accordance with Advanced Trauma Life Support guidelines. Surgery for acute SCI within 24 hours of injury as a treatment option is not associated with any increased risk of complications and may provide a neurological benefit.

D. Patients with an unstable spinal column with incomplete SCI should be considered for acute stabilization as soon as possible after obtaining necessary imaging studies.

Bibliography

Bracken, M. B., Shepard, M. J., Collins, W. F., Jr., Holford, T. R., Baskin, D. S., Eisenberg, H. M., . . . Marshall, L. F. (1992). Methylprednisolone or naloxone treatment after acute spinal cord injury: 1-year follow-up data. Results of the Second National Acute Spinal Cord Injury Study. *Journal of Neurosurgery, 76*(1), 23–31. doi:10.3171/jns.1992.76.1.0023

Bracken, M. B., Shepard, M. J., Collins, W. F., Holford, T. R., Young, W., Baskin, D. S., . . . Maroon, J. (1990). A randomized, controlled trial of methylprednisolone or naloxone in the treatment of acute spinal-cord injury. Results of the Second National Acute Spinal Cord Injury Study. *The New England Journal of Medicine, 322*(20), 1405–1411. doi:10.1056/NEJM199005173222001

Bracken, M. B., Shepard, M. J., Holford, T. R., Leo-Summers, L., Aldrich, E. F., Fazl, M., & Young, W. (1997). Administration of methylprednisolone for 24 or 48 hours or tirilazad mesylate for 48 hours in the treatment of acute spinal cord injury: Results of the Third National Acute Spinal Cord Injury Randomized Controlled Trial. *Journal of the American Medical Association, 277*(20), 1597–1604. doi:10.1001/jama.1997.03540440031029

Cengiz, S. L., Kalkan, E., Bayir, A., Ilik, K., & Basefer, A. (2008). Timing of thoracolomber spine stabilization in trauma patients; impact on neurological outcome and clinical course. A real prospective (rct) randomized controlled study. *Archives of Orthopaedic and Trauma Surgery, 128*(9), 959–966. doi:10.1007/s00402-007-0518-1

Cheung, V., Hoshide, R., Bansal, V., Kasper, E., & Chen, C. (2015). Methylprednisolone in the management of spinal cord injuries: Lessons from randomized, controlled trials. *Surgical Neurology International, 6*, 142. doi:10.4103/2152-7806.163452

Conrad, B. P., Horodyski, M., Wright, J., Ruetz, P., & Rechtine, G. R., 2nd. (2007). Log-rolling technique producing unacceptable motion during body position changes in patients with traumatic spinal cord injury. *Journal of Neurosurgery Spine, 6*(6), 540–543. doi:10.3171/spi.2007.6.6.4

DeVivo, M. J. (1997). Causes and costs of spinal cord injury in the United States. *Spinal Cord, 35*(12), 809–813. doi:10.1038/sj.sc.3100501

Fassett, D. R., Harrop, J. S., Maltenfort, M., Jeyamohan, S. B., Ratliff, J. D., Anderson, D. G., . . . Sharan, A. D. (2007). Mortality rates in geriatric patients with spinal cord injuries. *Journal of Neurosurgery Spine, 7*(3), 277–281. doi:10.3171/SPI-07/09/277

Fehlings, M. G., & Perrin, R. G. (2006). The timing of surgical intervention in the treatment of spinal cord injury: A systematic review of recent clinical evidence. *Spine (Phila Pa 1976), 31*(11 Suppl.), S28–S35. doi:10.1371/journal.pone.0032037

Fehlings, M. G., & Sekhon, L. (2000). Cellular, ionic, and biomolecular mechanisms of the injury process. In C. H. Tator & E. Benzel (Eds.), *Contemporary management of spinal cord injury: From impact to rehabilitation* (pp. 33–50). Chicago, IL: American Association of Neurological Surgeons . doi:10.1097/01.brs.0000217973.11402.7f

Fehlings, M. G., Vaccaro, A., Wilson, J. R., Singh, A., Cadotte, W. D., Harrop, J. S., . . . Rampersaud, R. (2012). Early versus delayed decompression for traumatic cervical spinal cord injury: Results of the surgical timing in acute spinal cord injury study (STASCIS). *PLOS ONE, 7*(2), e32037. doi:10.1371/journal.pone.0032037

Hadley, M. N., Walters, B. C., Grabb, P. A., Oyesiku, N. M., Przybylski, G. J., Resnick, D. K., & Ryken, T. C. (2002a). Blood pressure management after acute spinal cord injury. *Neurosurgery, 50*(Suppl. 3), S58–S62. doi:10.1097/00006123-200203001-00012

Hadley, M. N., Walters, B. C., Grabb, P. A., Oyesiku, N. M., Przybylski, G. J., Resnick, D. K., & Ryken, T. C. (2002b). Treatment of subaxial cervical spinal injuries. *Neurosurgery, 50*(Suppl. 3), S156–S165. doi:10.1097/00006123-200203001-00024

Hagen, S. (1999). *CBO memorandum: Projections of expenditures for long-term care services for the elderly.* Washington, DC: Congressional Budget Office.

Hamamoto, Y., Ogata, T., Morino, T., Hino, M., & Yamamoto, H. (2007). Real-time direct measurement of spinal cord blood flow at the site of compression: Relationship between blood flow recovery and motor deficiency in spinal cord injury. *Spine, 32*(18), 1955–1962. doi:10.1097/BRS.0b013e3181316310

Katoh, S., el Masry, W. S., Jaffray, D., McCall, I. W., Eisenstein, S. M., Pringle, R. G., & Ikata, T. (1996). Neurologic outcome in conservatively treated patients with incomplete closed traumatic cervical spinal cord injuries. *Spine, 21*(20), 2345–2351. doi:10.1097/00007632-199610150-00008

La Rosa, G., Conti, A., Cardali, S., Cacciola, F., & Tomasello, F. (2004). Does early decompression improve neurological outcome of spinal cord injured patients? Appraisal of the literature using a meta-analytical approach. *Spinal Cord, 42*(9), 503–512. doi:10.1038/sj.sc.3101627

Levi, L., Wolf, A., & Belzberg, H. (1993). Hemodynamic parameters in patients with acute cervical cord trauma: Description, intervention, and prediction of outcome. *Neurosurgery, 33*(6), 1007–1016. doi:10.1227/00006123-199312000-00008

Liverman, T. C., Altevogt, B. M., Joy, E. J., & Johnson, T. R. (Eds.). (2005). *Spinal cord injury: Progress, promise, and priorities.* Washington, DC: National Academy of Sciences.

McKinley, W., Meade, M. A., Kirshblum, S., & Barnard, B. (2004). Outcomes of early surgical management versus late or no surgical intervention after acute spinal cord injury. *Archives of Physical Medicine and Rehabilitation, 85*(11), 1818–1825. doi:10.1016/j.apmr.2004.04.032

Oyinbo, C. A. (2011). Secondary injury mechanisms in traumatic spinal cord injury: A nugget of this multiply cascade. *Acta Neurobiologiae Experimentalis, 71*(2), 281–299.

Pointillart, V., Petitjean, M. E., Wiart, L., Vital, J. M., Lassié, P., Thicoipé, M., & Dabadie, P. (2000). Pharmacological therapy of spinal cord injury during the acute phase. *Spinal Cord, 38*(2), 71–76. doi:10.1038/sj.sc.3100962

Pollard, M. E., & Apple, D. F. (2003). Factors associated with improved neurologic outcomes in patients with incomplete tetraplegia. *Spine, 28*(1), 33–39. doi:10.1097/00007632-200301010-00009

Rahimi-Movaghar, V. (2005). Efficacy of surgical decompression in the setting of complete thoracic spinal cord injury. *Journal of Spinal Cord Medicine, 28*(5), 415–420. doi:10.1080/10790268.2005.11753841

Rowland, J. W., Hawryluk, G. W., Kwon, B., & Fehlings, M. G. (2008). Current status of acute spinal cord injury pathophysiology and emerging therapies: Promise on the horizon. *Neurosurgical Focus, 25*(5), E2. doi:10.3171/FOC.2008.25.11.E2

Sapkas, G. S., & Papadakis, S. A. (2007). Neurological outcome following early versus delayed lower cervical spine surgery. *Journal of Orthopaedic Surgery, 15*(2), 183–186. doi:10.1177/230949900701500212

Sekhon, L. H., & Fehlings, M. G. (2001). Epidemiology, demographics, and pathophysiology of acute spinal cord injury. *Spine, 26*(24 Suppl.), S2–S12. doi:10.1097/00007632-200112151-00002

Tanhoffer, R. A., Yamazaki, R. K., Nunes, E. A., Pchevozniki, A. I., Pchevozniki, A. M., Nogata, C., . . . Fernandes, L. C. (2007). Glutamine concentration and immune response of spinal cord-injured rats. *Journal of Spinal Cord Medicine, 30*(2), 140–146. doi:10.1080/10790268.2007.11753925

Tator, C. H., Duncan, E. G., Edmonds, V. E., Lapczak, L. I., & Andrews, D. F. (1987). Comparison of surgical and conservative management in 208 patients with acute spinal cord injury. *The Canadian Journal of Neurological Sciences, 14*(1), 60–69. doi:10.1017/S0317167100026858

Velmahos, G. C., Toutouzas, K., Chan, L., Tillou, A., Rhee, P., Murray, J., & Demetriades, D. (2003). Intubation after cervical spinal cord injury: To be done selectively or routinely? *The American Surgeon, 69*(10), 891–894.

Waters, R. L., Meyer, P. R., Jr., Adkins, R. H., & Felton, D. (1999). Emergency, acute, and surgical management of spine trauma. *Archives of Physical Medicine and Rehabilitation, 80*(11), 1383–1390. doi:10.1016/S0003-9993(99)90248-4

Wyndaele, M., & Wyndaele, J. J. (2006). Incidence, prevalence and epidemiology of spinal cord injury: What learns a worldwide literature survey? *Spinal Cord, 44*(9), 523–529. doi:10.1038/sj.sc.3101893

Xu, K., Chen, Q.-X., Li, F.-C., Chen, W.-S., Lin, M., & Wu, Q. (2009). Spinal cord decompression reduces rat neural cell apoptosis secondary to spinal cord injury. *Journal of Zhejiang University Science B, 10*(3), 180–187. doi:10.1631/jzus.B0820161

Traumatic Brain Injury

Susan F. Galincyski

Definition

A. Traumatic brain injury (TBI) is an insult to the brain caused by direct physical force causing a physical force that may produce a diminished or altered state of consciousness, which may result in an impairment of cognitive abilities or physical functioning.

B. These impairments may be temporary or permanent, depending on the degree of injury.

Incidence

A. Leading cause of trauma-related death in persons under age 45.

B. Often occurs during the most productive years.

C. Represents approximately 200 cases per 100,000 injuries annually in the United States.

D. Responsible for approximately 12% to 30% of all traumatic deaths.

E. Motor vehicle collisions (MVC) are the leading cause of TBI.

F. Penetrating head trauma is the leading cause of brain injury deaths.

Pathogenesis

A. According to the Centers for Disease Control and Prevention, more than 130,000 unintentional deaths were documented in 2013. Although there are many mechanisms that can result in traumatic injury, these injuries can be primarily divided into two categories: Blunt or penetrating injuries. Blunt injuries are those that result from a blunt force and do not break the skin. Injuries are usually localized to the area of impact. Mechanisms of injury described as blunt injury can be motor vehicle accidents, assaults, falls, and sports-related injuries.

B. Two main forces are associated with TBI.

    1. Impact loading is the direct force against the skull, causing disruption of brain tissue, vascular, and nerve structures.

    2. Impulsive loading is sudden movement without direct impact as seen with acceleration–deceleration injury.

Predisposing Factors

A. Males are more prone than femalea.

B. Ages 15 to 25; over 65 years of age.

C. Single people are more prone than married people.

D. Inner city residents.

E. Lower income individuals.

F. Members of ethnic minority groups.

G. Drug and alcohol use.

H. History of previous TBI.

Subjective Data

A. Common complaints/symptoms.

    1. ± loss of consciousness.

    2. Nausea and/or vomiting.

    3. Headache.

    4. Amnesia to events surrounding trauma.

B. Common/typical scenario.

    1. Other signs and symptoms.

        a. Altered mentation.

        b. Increased lethargy.

        c. Slurred speech.

        d. Combative behavior.

        e. History of seizures.

C. Family and social history.

    1. Ask patient to describe events leading up to trauma. What is the last thing the patient remembers? What symptoms is he or she experiencing? Nausea? Vomiting? Headache? Dizziness? Photophobia? Does the patient have pain? Location? Characteristics?

    2. Ask the patient about recent drug and alcohol use.

    3. Ask the patient about past medical history. Seizures? Concussions?

    4. Determine if the patient is on any anticoagulants or antiplatelet medications.

Physical Examination

A. The American College of Surgeons has developed the Advanced Trauma Life Support guidelines to provide a quick but systematic approach to assessment to help identify those injuries that can be life-threatening as soon as possible. Using the mnemonic A-B-C-D-E, the primary survey must be completed before the secondary survey can be started and a plan of care established (see Table 17.3).

System	Assessment Points
TABLE 17.3	**Primary Survey**
A- Airway	Is it patent? Is patient talking? Normal voice? Hoarse? Is airway occluded by debris? Blood? Vomit? Teeth? Could there be an airway injury given the mechanism? Is the cervical spine immobilized?
B- Breathing	Is the patient breathing? Are there breath sounds bilaterally? Are lungs clear?
C- Circulation	Does the patient have pulses? Is there active hemorrhage?
D- Disability	What is the GCS? Is the patient awake and following commands? Is the patient confused? Is the patient conscious?
E- Exposure	Undress the patient completely. Look for any holes, lacerations, unusual bruising, or marks.

GCS, Glasgow Coma score.

B. If any potentially life-threatening issue is identified during the primary survey, it needs to be addressed before moving onto the next assessment. For example, if the patient has decreased breath sounds (B) on the right side and has sustained chest trauma, a pneumothorax should be suspected. A chest tube should be placed before moving on with assessment to circulation (C).

The secondary survey is a complete head-to-toe evaluation of the patient, looking for other potential injuries, once it is determined that the patient is stable at the end of the primary survey.

C. Perform a Glasgow Coma Score (GCS; see Table 17.1).

D. Assess for signs of other injuries by completely undressing the patient.

E. Assess head, scalp, and face for contusions, lacerations, or hematoma.

Diagnostic Tests

A. CT head, cervical spine, thoracic spine, lumbar spine, chest, abdomen, and pelvis. CT head and cervical, thoracic, and lumbar spine are noncontrast. CT chest, abdomen, and pelvis are with contrast.

Differential Diagnosis

A. Concussion.

B. Cerebral contusion.

C. Coup-contrecoup injuries.

D. Epidural hematoma.

E. Subdural hematoma.

F. Subarachnoid hematoma.

G. Mass lesion (may have prompted fall).

Evaluation and Management Plan

A. General plan.

  1. For concussion, treatment is symptom based.

  2. Consult neurosurgery for more severe injuries.

  3. Prevent hypotension and hypoxemia.

B. Patient/family teaching points.

  1. Monitoring for postconcussive syndrome is important.

  2. Follow-up with concussion clinic may be advised based on the degree of concussion and residual symptoms.

  3. Neuropsychology depending on severity of symptoms.

C. Pharmacotherapy.

  1. Try to avoid opioids.

  2. For more severe head injury, seizure prophylaxis may be indicated for up to 10 days. Length depends on whether the patient presents with a seizure or has any seizure activity during hospitalization.

  3. For severe head injury, osmotic diuretics may be used to reduce edema.

Follow-Up

A. No contact sports for minimum of 6 weeks.

B. Prothrombin time (PT)/OT/speech consults.

C. Neurosurgical evaluation 10 to 14 days post discharge. May need repeat CT head.

Consultation/Referral

A. Inpatient referrals: Trauma and neurosurgery.

B. May need rehab referral.

C. Outpatient concussion follow-up for post concussive syndrome.

Special/Geriatric Considerations

A. For persons with repeated concussion, a discussion regarding cessation of sports is imperative. Repeated concussions have been shown to have a residual effect.

B. For patient on anticoagulation or antiplatelet therapy, risk of injury and complications need to be discussed.

C. If the GCS is less than 8, intubation should be considered as the patient may not be awake enough to maintain a patent airway.

Bibliography

Carney, N., Totten, A., O'Reilly, C., Ullman, J., Hawryluk, G., Bell, M., & Ghajar, J. (2016). Guidelines for the management of severe traumatic brain injury, fourth edition. *Neurosurgery, 80,* 1–10. doi:10.1227/NEU.0000000000001432

Esterov, D., & Greenwald, B. D. (2017, August 11). Autonomic dysfunction after mild traumatic brain injury. *Brain Sciences, 7*(8), e100. doi:10.3390/brainsci7080100

Haring, R. S., Narang, K., Canner, J. K., Asemota, A. O., George, B. P., Selvarajah, S., & Schneider, E. B. (2015, January 15). Traumatic brain injury in the elderly: Morbidity and mortality trends and risk factors. *The Journal of Surgical Research, 195,* 1–9. doi:10.1016/j.jss.2015.01.017

Steyerberg, E. W., Mushkudiani, N., Perel, P., Butcher, I., Lu, J., McHugh, G. S., & Maas, A. I. (2008, August 5). Predicting outcome after traumatic brain injury: Development and international validation of prognostic scores based on admission characteristics. *PLOS Medicine, 5*(8), e165. doi:10.1371/journal.pmed.0050165

Teasdale, G., & Jennett, B. (1974). Assessment of coma and impaired consciousness. *Lancet, 2,* 81–84. doi:10.1016/S0140-6736(74)91639-0

Teasdale, G., & Jennett, B. (1976). Assessment and prognosis of coma after head injury. *Acta Neurochirurgica, 34,* 45–55. doi:10.1007/BF01405862

Thompson, D. O., Hurtado, T. R., Liao, M. M., Byyny, R. L., Gravitz, C., & Haukoos, J. S. (2011, November). Validation of the simplified motor score in the out-of-hospital setting for the prediction of outcomes after traumatic brain injury. *Annals of Emergency Medicine, 58*(5), 417–425. doi:10.1016/j.annemergmed.2011.05.033

Tian, H. L., Geng, Z., Cui, Y. H., Hu, J., Xu, T., Cao, H. L., & Chen, H. (2008, August, 14). Risk factors for posttraumatic cerebral infarction in patients with moderate or severe head trauma. *Neurosurgical Review, 31,* 431–436. doi:10.1007/s10143-008-0153-5

II Perioperative Considerations

18 Preoperative Evaluation and Management

Kristopher R. Maday

Scope of Chapter

The advanced practice provider (APP) frequently evaluates a patient prior to surgery. The APP must be aware of risk factors, appropriate testing, and the American Society of Anesthesiologists (ASA) classification of risk and medications in order to make an informed decision of a patient's readiness for surgery. This chapter explores what the APP needs to know to make these decisions.

Considerations

Kristopher R. Maday

Risk Factors

A. Age: There is a linear increase in surgical risk with age as a result of an increasing number of comorbidities.

B. Exercise capacity.

    1. Ability to perform four or more metabolic equivalents (METs) reduces the risk of cardiovascular complications associated with surgery. Examples include:

        a. Walking up a flight of stairs.

        b. Mowing the lawn.

        c. Walking at ground level at 4 miles per hour.

        d. Performing heavy work around the house.

    2. Inability to perform four or more METs is associated with increased length of stay and perioperative complications.

        a. Preoperative evaluation by physical therapy for prehabilitation, or cardiology for cardiac testing, can be beneficial in higher risk patients.

C. Nutritional.

    1. Obesity is a risk factor for pulmonary thromboembolism, and presents increased rate of wound infections, pneumonia, and others.

    2. Malnutrition prior to surgery is associated with:

        a. Increased infection risk.

        b. Poor wound healing.

        c. Intestinal bacterial overgrowth.

        d. Increased hospital length of stay.

    It increases postoperative complications; for example, anastomotic leak can result in enterocutaneous fistula formation.

D. Pulmonary.

    1. Obstructive sleep apnea: Increases risk of postoperative hypoxemia, reintubation, and ICU admission.

    2. Smoking: Increased risk of wound complications, infections, and ICU admissions.

E. Alcohol: Screen for the possibility of developing withdrawal and/or delirium tremens in the postoperative period.

F. Illicit drug use and prescription drug abuse: Screen for opioid narcotics, benzodiazepines, or amphetamines as perioperative and postoperative pain control may prove to be difficult. Withdrawal may also occur and needs to be assessed.

G. Endocrine disorders: Diabetes increases risk of surgical site infection, as well as perioperative cardiac events.

H. Medication use.

    1. A full medication reconciliation should be obtained before surgery, including the use of over-the-counter medications, such as aspirin, ibuprofen, and other nonsteroidal anti-inflammatory drugs (NSAIDs), which are associated with an increased risk of perioperative bleeding.

    2. Alternative, herbal, and natural supplement use should also be documented due to drug interactions and risk of bleeding.

    3. Anticoagulants.

I. Personal/family history of anesthetic complications such as malignant hypertension (HTN) or postoperative nausea and vomiting.

Calculating Risk of Perioperative Complications

A. American College of Surgeons Surgical Risk Calculator: riskcalculator.facs.org/RiskCalculator/.

    1. Factors that can affect surgical risk.

        a. Age.

        b. Gender.

        c. Functional status.

        d. American Society of Anesthesiologists classification.

        e. Diabetes, HTN, and/or congestive heart failure (CHF).

        f. Smoking and/or history of chronic obstructive pulmonary disease (COPD).

        g. Renal disease and/or on dialysis.

        h. Steroid use for chronic conditions.

        i. Presence of ascites.

        j. Disseminated cancer.

        k. Emergency surgery.

Bibliography

Cohen, M. E., Liu, Y., Ko, C. Y., & Hall, B. L. (2017). An examination of American College of Surgeons NSQIP surgical risk calculator accuracy. *Journal of the American College of Surgeons, 224*(5), 787–795. doi:10.1016/j.jamcollsurg.2016.12.057

Dindo, D., Muller, M. K., Weber, M., & Clavien, P. A. (2003). Obesity in general elective surgery. *Lancet, 361*(9374), 2032–2035. doi:10.1016/S0140-6736(03)13640-9

Fleisher, L. A., Fleischmann, K. E., & Auerbach, A. D. (2014). 2014 ACC/AHA guideline on perioperative cardiovascular evaluation and management of patients undergoing noncardiac surgery: A report of the American College of Cardiology/American Heart Association Task Force on Practice Guidelines. *Journal of the American College of Cardiology, 64*(22), e77–e137. doi:10.1016/j.jacc.2014.07.945

Grønkjær, M., Eliasen, M., & Skov-Ettrup, L. S. (2014). Preoperative smoking status and postoperative complications: A systematic review and meta-analysis. *Annals of Surgery, 259*(1), 52–71. doi:10.1097/SLA .0b013e3182911913

Kaw, R., Pasupuleti, V., Walker, E., Ramaswamy, A., & Foldvary-Schafer, N. (2012). Postoperative complications in patients with obstructive sleep apnea. *Chest, 141*(2), 436–441. doi:10.1378/chest.11-0283

Kleinwächter, R., Kork, F., & Weiss-Gerlach, E. (2010). Improving the detection of illicit substance use in preoperative anesthesiological assessment. *Minerva Anestesiologica, 76*(1), 29–37.

Oresanya, L. B., Lyons, W. L., & Finlayson, E. (2014). Preoperative assessment of the older patient: A narrative review. *Journal of the American Medical Association, 311*(20), 2110–2120. doi:10.1001/jama.2014. 4573

Sidney, M. J. K., & Blumchen, G. (1990). Metabolic equivalents (METs) in exercise testing, exercise prescription, and evaluation of functional capacity. *Clinical Cardiology, 13*, 555–565. doi:10.1002/clc.4960130809

Tønnesen, H., Nielsen, P. R., Lauritzen, J. B., & Møller, A. M. (2009). Smoking and alcohol intervention before surgery: Evidence for best practice. *British Journal of Anaesthesia, 102*(3), 297–306. doi:10.1093/bja/ aen401

Care Principles

Kristopher R. Maday

Testing in the Perioperative Setting

A. The American Society of Anesthesiologists (ASA) recommends against routine preoperative laboratory testing in the absence of clinical indications.

1. Testing should occur depending on the patient's medical history, underlying disease, increased perioperative risk, or high risk surgery. Common testing includes:

a. Complete blood count (CBC).

i. Hemoglobin/hematocrit.

1) Cardiac surgery patients should have a hemoglobin greater than 7 g/dL to reduce cardiac complications as a result of surgery. Patients may require transfusion for hemoglobin of 7 or less.

2) Patients with anemia or thrombocytopenia prior to major surgery may need to be seen and cleared by hematology.

ii. Platelet count.

1) Greater than 50,000/μL for most major surgery.

2) Greater than 100,00/μL for neurosurgery/ocular surgery.

3) Greater than 80,000/μL for epidural anesthesia.

4) 20,000 to 50,000/μL for endoscopy.

b. Coagulation studies.

i. Only perform if clinically indicated by history or physical examination.

ii. Tests include prothrombin time (PT) or partial thromboplastin time (PTT).

iii. International Ratio (INR) may be variable. If less than 2.0, there is no indication that the patient will have more than normal tissue oozing.

1) If the patient is taking warfarin, the medication should be stopped and the level should predictably drop to less than 1.5 within 4 to 5 days.

2) In elderly patients, the reversal of warfarin may be longer and presents with increased risk

of a thromboembolic event. Patients may need to be covered with therapeutic low molecular weight heparin or unfractionated heparin in these cases.

c. Basic metabolic profile (BMP).

i. It is recommended to obtain routine screening BMP.

ii. Patients with type 2 diabetes mellitus taking oral antihypoglycemic agents should be converted to sliding scale insulin until oral medications can be resumed postoperatively.

iii. Patients with a history of type 1 diabetes mellitus should have a perioperative insulin plan depending on the type of insulin they are using and the type of surgical procedure they are undergoing.

iv. Due to the risk of diabetic ketoacidosis, patients with type 1 diabetes mellitus must have basal insulin supplied at all times.

v. Renal function: Obtain serum creatinine in patients over the age of 50 if undergoing intermediate or higher surgery.

d. Urine pregnancy test for all women of childbearing years.

e. EKG.

i. Routine screening in asymptomatic patients undergoing low-risk surgery is not recommended.

ii. Intermediate or high risk surgery, patients with known coronary disease, peripheral vascular disease, cerebrovascular disease, dysrhythmias, or other structural heart disease should have at least a preoperative 12-lead ECG performed. Consultation with anesthesiology or cardiology for further testing recommendations (such as cardiac stress testing or echocardiogram) may be needed depending on underlying cardiac conditions and the type of surgery the patient is undergoing.

f. Chest radiography.

i. Unless the type of surgery warrants preoperative radiograph, routine screening is not indicated.

g. Pulmonary function testing.

i. May be required for lung surgery, if patient has underlying history of chronic obstructive pulmonary disease (COPD), or if surgery is dependent on lung volume measurements.

ii. Not indicated for routine screening.

ASA Classifications

A. Physical status classification system.

1. Simple classification system to predict preoperative risk of increased mortality and morbidity associated with anesthesia and surgery.

2. Six-tiered system.

a. ASA 1: Healthy patient.

b. ASA 2: Mild systemic disease.

c. ASA 3: Severe systemic disease.

d. ASA 4: Severe systemic disease that is a constant threat to life.

e. ASA 5: Moribund patient who is not expected to survive without the operation.

f. ASA 6: Declared brain-dead patient who is undergoing organ procurement.

B. Mallampati classification.

1. Used to predict ease of intubation.

2. May help predict obstructive sleep apnea.

3. Simple test done during physical examination.

a. Patient should sit upright with head in neutral position.

b. Ask patient to open mouth and extend tongue without speaking or making noise.

4. Scoring.

    a. Class I—complete visualization of soft palate.

    b. Class II—complete visualization of uvula (see Figure 18.1).

    c. Class III—visualization of base of uvula.

    d. Class IV—soft palate not visible at all.

Nutrition and Fluids

A. Preoperative nutritional considerations.

  1. Preoperative nutritional assessment.

    a. Nutritional Risk Screening (NRS 2002) tool.

      i. This score is calculated from two variables.

        1) Impaired nutritional status: Recent weight loss, decreased food intake, body mass index (BMI) $\leq$ 18.5.

        2) *Severity of illness.*

      ii. A score 3 or more would indicate need for nutritional supplementation/support prior to surgery.

    b. Protein status.

      i. Serum albumin, transferrin, and prealbumin have all been studied, but there is conflicting data on utility.

      ii. Only a serum albumin less than 2.2 g/dL has shown to be the most predictive.

    c. Patient with severe preoperative malnutrition may benefit from nutritional support prior to surgery.

      i. Options include oral supplementation with high-protein shakes, tube feedings with indwelling feeding tube, and/or total parenteral nutrition (TPN).

    d. ASA fasting guidelines.

      i. Lowest risk for aspiration.

      ii. 2 hours after clear liquids.

      iii. 4 hours after breast milk.

      iv. 6 hours after light meal.

      v. 8 hours after regular meal.

B. Fluid considerations.

  1. Patients may be *nil per os* (NPO) for up to 12 hours before surgery.

  2. Inpatient.

    a. Dextrose-containing fluids should be started when NPO to prevent lean muscle catabolism.

  3. Outpatient.

    a. Fluid status should be assessed and intravenous fluid administered accordingly.

Bibliography

American Society of Anesthesiologists. (2014). *ASA Physical Status Classification System.* Retrieved from https://www.asahq.org/resources/clinical-information/asa-physical-status-classification-system

American Society of Anesthesiologists Committee. (2011). Practice guidelines for preoperative fasting and the use of pharmacologic agents to reduce the risk of pulmonary aspiration: Application to healthy patients undergoing elective procedures: An updated report by the American Society of Anesthesiologists Committee on Standards and Practice Parameters. *Anesthesiology, 114*(3), 495–511. doi:10.1097/ALN.0b013e3181fcbfd9

Apfelbaum, J. L., & Connis, R. T. (2012). Practice advisory for preanesthesia evaluation: An updated report by the American Society of Anesthesiologists Task Force on Preanesthesia Evaluation. *Anesthesiology, 116*(3), 522–538. doi:10.1097/ALN.0b013e31823c1067

Chee, Y. L., Crawford, J. C., Watson, H. G., & Greaves, M. (2008). Guidelines on the assessment of bleeding risk prior to surgery or invasive procedures. British Committee for Standards in Haematology. *British Journal of Haematology, 140*(5), 496–504. doi:10.1111/j.1365-2141.2007.06968.x

Fleisher, L. A., Fleischmann, K. E., & Auerbach, A. D. (2014). 2014 ACC/AHA guideline on perioperative cardiovascular evaluation and management of patients undergoing noncardiac surgery: A report of the American College of Cardiology/American Heart Association Task Force on Practice Guidelines. *Journal of the American College of Cardiology, 64*(22), e77–e137. doi:10.1016/j.jacc.2014.07.945

García-Miguel, F. J., Serrano-Aguilar, P. G., & López-Bastida, J. (2003). Preoperative assessment. *Lancet, 362*(9397), 1749–1757. doi:10.1016/S0140-6736(03)14857-X

Kaplan, E. B., Sheiner, L. B., & Boeckmann, A. J. (1985). The usefulness of preoperative laboratory screening. *Journal of the American Medical Association, 253*(24), 3576–3581. doi:10.1001/jama.1985.03350480084025

Kondrup, J., Rasmussen, H. H., Hamberg, O., & Stanga, Z. (2003). Nutritional risk screening (NRS 2002): A new method based on an analysis of controlled clinical trials. *Clinical Nutrition, 22*(3), 321–336. doi:10.1016/S0261-5614(02)00214-5

Kumar, A., Mhaskar, R., & Grossman, B. J. (2015). Platelet transfusion: A systematic review of the clinical evidence. *Transfusion, 55*(5), 1116–1127. doi:10.1111/trf.12943

Lawrence, V. A., Dhanda, R., Hilsenbeck, S. G., & Page, C. P. (1111). Risk of pulmonary complications after elective abdominal surgery. *Chest, 110*(3), 744–750. doi:10.1378/chest.110.3.744

Macpherson, D. S. (1993). Preoperative laboratory testing: Should any tests be "routine" before surgery? *The Medical Clinics of North America, 77*(2), 289–308. doi:10.1016/S0025-7125(16)30252-8

Mallampait, S. R. (1985). A clinical sign to predict difficult tracheal intubation: A prospective study. *Canadian Anaesthetists' Society Journal, 32*(4), 429–434. doi:10.1007/BF03011357

McClave, S. A., Kozar, R., Martindale, R. G., Heyland, D. K., Braga, M., Carli, F., . . . Wischmeyer, P. E. (2013). Summary points and consensus recommendations from the North American Surgical Nutrition Summit. *Journal of Parenteral and Enteral Nutrition, 37*(5 Suppl. 1), 99S–105S. doi:10.1177/0148607113495892

O'Neill, F., Carter, E., Pink, N., & Smith, I. (2016). Routine preoperative tests for elective surgery: Summary of updated NICE guidance. *British Medical Journal, 354*, i3292. doi:10.1136/bmj.i3292

van Stijn, M. F., Korkic-Halilovic, I., Bakker, M. S., van der Ploeg, T., van Leeuwen, P. A., & Houdijk, A. P. (2013). Preoperative nutrition status and postoperative outcome in elderly general surgery patients: A systematic review. *Journal of Parenteral and Enteral Nutrition, 37*(1), 37–43. doi:10.1177/0148607112445900

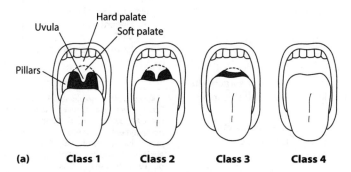

FIGURE 18.1 Mallampati classification. Visualization used to predict ease of intubation.

Medication Management

Kristopher R. Maday

Preoperative Medication Management

A. Anticoagulation.
  1. Risk of bleeding versus risk of thromboembolism must be assessed when deciding to stop anticoagulation.
    a. Estimation of risk for a thromboembolic event.
      i. Atrial fibrillation 0.2% to 1.2% based on three major studies.
        1) RE-LY.
        2) Rocket AF.
        3) ARISTOTLE.
      ii. Prosthetic heart valves—increase the risk of a thromboembolic event of anticoagulation by 3.7-fold.
      iii. Recent thromboembolic event (venous or arterial) within last 3 months.
        1) Elective surgery should be delayed if possible.
        2) Venous thromboembolism risk of anticoagulation.
          a) Within first month of occurrence is 50%.
          b) Between first month and third month of occurrence decreases to 8% to 10%.
          c) After 3 months, the risk decreases to 4% to 5%.
        3) Arterial embolism risk of anticoagulation.
          a) 0.5% per day first month after occurrence.
          b) Estimate risk of bleeding.
      iv. High bleeding risk 2% to 4%.
        1) Coronary bypass surgery.
        2) Procedures greater than 45 minutes.
        3) Procedures in compartments that can increase the severity of bleeding complications such as intracranial or pericardial.
      v. Low bleeding risk 0% to 2%.
        1) Carpal tunnel surgery.
        2) Hysterectomy.
  2. Determine timing of anticoagulation cessation.
    a. Low bleeding risk surgeries may not require anticoagulation cessation.
      i. Cutaneous procedures such as skin biopsy.
      ii. Cardiac implantable device.
      iii. Endovascular procedures.
      iv. Certain dental procedures.
    b. For surgeries with a moderate to high risk of bleeding, consider the following.
      i. Warfarin.
        1) Stop 5 days prior to surgery.
        2) Check the international ratio (INR) the day before.
          a) If greater than 1.5 administer 1 to 2 mg oral vitamin K.
          b) OK for surgery if 1.4 or less.
        3) Resume 12 to 24 hours after surgery due to prolonged action of onset. Full therapeutic effect may take up to 5 days.
      ii. Direct thrombin inhibitor—dabigatran.
        1) Stop 2 to 3 days prior to surgery.
        2) May need longer if:
          a) Patient has renal insufficiency.
          b) Surgery has high risk for bleeding.
        3) Rapid onset of action.
          a) Delay restarting for 1 day after surgery with procedures that are low risk for bleeding.
          b) Delay restarting for 2 to 3 days after surgery with procedures that are high risk for bleeding.
      iii. Direct Factor Xa inhibitors—rivaroxaban, apixaban, edoxaban.
        1) Stop 2 to 3 days prior to surgery.
        2) May need longer if:
          a) Patient has renal insufficiency.
          b) Surgery has high risk for bleeding.
        3) Rapid onset of action.
          a) Delay restarting for 1 day after surgery with procedures that are low risk for bleeding.
          b) Delay restarting for 2 to 3 days after surgery with procedures that are high risk for bleeding.
  3. Determine if bridge needed.
    a. Used mainly in patients with high risk of thromboembolic event due to atrial fibrillation, mechanical heart valve, or history of thromboembolic event.
    b. When to consider bridging (see Table 18.1).
    c. Bridging preoperatively versus postoperatively or both.
      i. Use Thrombosis Canada Tool to determine if bridging is required preoperatively, postoperatively, or both.

TABLE 18.1   **Perioperative Bridging: When It Is Appropriate to Bridge in the Perioperative Period**

High Risk (consider bridging)	Moderate Risk (case by case)
Atrial fibrillation • Recent (<3 months) stroke/TIA • CHADS$_2$ 5–6 • Rheumatic heart	**Atrial fibrillation** • CHADS$_2$ = 3–4 Mechanical heart valve • Bileaflet aortic valve + risk factor
Mechanical heart valve • Ball or tilting disc valve • Mitral valve • Recent (<3 month) stroke/TIA	**Venous thromboembolism** • VTE 3–12 months prior cancer
	Low Risk (consider NOT bridging)
Venous thromboembolism • Recent (<3 months) VTE • Severe thrombophilia	**Atrial fibrillation** • CHADS$_2$ 0–2 Mechanical heart valve • Bileaflet aortic valve + risk factor
	Venous thromboembolism • VTE > 12 month ago

TIA, transient ischemic attack; VTE, venous thromboembolism.
Source: Data from Douketis, J. D., Spyropoulos, A. C., Spencer, F. A., Mayr, M., Jaffer, A. K., Eckman, M. H., . . . Kunz, R. (2012). Perioperative management of antithrombotic therapy: Antithrombotic therapy and prevention of thrombosis, 9th ed: American College of Chest Physicians evidence-based clinical practice guidelines. *Chest, 141,* e326. doi:10.1378/chest.11-2298.

ii. Url: thrombosiscanada.ca/tools/?calc=perioperative AnticoagulantAlgorithm

d. Inferior vena cava filter (IVC).

i. Consider temporary IVC filter if patient is unable to restart anticoagulation for 3 to 4 weeks after surgery.

4. Case example: 74-year-old man, with nonvalvular atrial fibrillation and ischemic stroke, on warfarin who needs a total knee replacement.

a. Stop warfarin 5 days before surgery.

b. Preoperative bridging with low-molecular weight (LMW) heparin starting 3 days before surgery and stopped the day of surgery.

c. Resume warfarin within 24 hours of surgery.

d. Resume LMW heparin within 24 hours of surgery and continue until INR is therapeutic.

B. Antiplatelet medications.

1. Common examples include:

a. Aspirin: Can be continued through most surgeries.

b. Clopidogrel and ticagrelor: Should be discontinued at least 5 days before surgery.

c. Prasugrel: Should be discontinued at least 7 days before surgery.

d. Ticlopidine: Should be discontinued at least 10 days before surgery.

e. Cilostazol: Discontinued 3 to 5 days before surgery.

2. Nonsteroidal anti-inflammatory drugs (NSAIDs) can cause decreased platelet function and should be discontinued 3 days before surgery.

C. Diabetic medications.

1. Diabetes type 1.

a. Patients with type 1 diabetes are prone to ketosis and acidosis and extremes of blood glucose during surgery.

b. Extreme caution in regulating fluid and electrolyte balance and blood sugar levels must be taken.

c. Goal blood sugar is 110 to 180 mg/dL.

d. Start dextrose containing solution during case at 75 to 125 cc/hr.

e. Check blood sugar every hour.

f. Short procedures less than 2 hours.

i. Discontinue short or rapid acting insulin on the morning of surgery.

ii. If patient takes two types of insulin only in the morning, give one-half to two-thirds of intermediate or long acting insulin on day of surgery to prevent complications with ketosis.

iii. If patients take insulin multiple times per day, give one-third to one-half total morning dose of intermediate or long acting insulin.

g. Long procedures.

i. Start intravenous (IV) insulin infusion.

2. Diabetes type 2.

a. In patients who manage their diabetes with diet alone, no additional therapy is required.

b. Oral hypoglycemics and non-insulin injectables.

i. Should be held the morning of surgery.

ii. Sliding scale insulin regimen can be used to manage postoperative hyperglycemia if needed.

c. Insulin: Should give one-third to one-half the regular morning dose on the day of surgery. Recommendations are to keep the same dose the night before.

D. Glucocorticoid.

1. No need for perioperative stress dose corticosteroids if:

a. Any dosing less than 3 weeks.

b. Less than 5 mg daily, or less than 10 mg every other day.

2. Stress dose corticosteroids indicated if:

a. Greater than 20 mg daily for more than 3 weeks.

b. Cushingoid appearance.

c. Adrenocorticotropic hormone (ACTH) stimulation testing should be performed for any patient with a question of hypothalamic–pituitary–adrenal (HPA) axis suppression.

E. Cardiovascular medications.

1. Most commonly prescribed medications should be continued perioperatively and include:

a. Beta blockers.

b. Angiotensin-converting enzyme (ACE) inhibitors and angiotensin receptor blockers (ARBs).

c. Calcium channel blockers.

d. Statins.

Preoperative Checklist

Preoperative Checklist	
Risk factors	1. 2. 3.
American College of Surgeons risk score	(score)
Preoperative testing	1. Test—Result 2. Test—Result
ASA classification	(class)
Nutritional considerations	(NRS2002 score). Nutritional support type
Medications	1. Drug—why on—when to stop—plan 2. Drug—why on—when to stop—plan

ASA, American Society of Anesthesiologists.
Source: Data from DeLamar, L. M. (2005). Preparing your patient for surgery. *Topics in Advanced Practice Nursing eJournal, 5*(1). Retrieved from https://www.medscape.com/viewarticle/500887_2

Bibliography

DeLamar, L. M. (2005). Preparing your patient for surgery. *Topics in Advanced Practice Nursing eJournal, 5*(1). Retrieved from https://www.medscape.com/viewarticle/500887_2

Douketis, J. D., Spyropoulos, A. C., Spencer, F. A., Mayr, M., Jaffer, A. K., Eckman, M. H., & Kunz, R. (2012). Perioperative management of antithrombotic therapy: Antithrombotic therapy and prevention of thrombosis, 9th ed: American College of Chest Physicians evidence-based clinical practice guidelines. *Chest, 141*, e326. doi:10.1378/chest.11-2298

Douketis, J. D., Woods, K., Foster, G. A., & Crowther, M. A. (2005). Bridging anticoagulation with low-molecular-weight heparin after interruption of warfarin therapy is associated with a residual anticoagulant effect prior to surgery. *Thrombosis and Haemostasis, 94*, 528. doi:10.1160/TH05-01-0064

Dunn, A. S., Spyropoulos, A. C., & Turpie, A. G. (2007). Bridging therapy in patients on long-term oral anticoagulants who require surgery: The Prospective Peri-operative Enoxaparin Cohort Trial (PROSPECT). *Journal of Thrombosis and Haemostasis, 5*(11), 2211–2218. doi:10.1111/j.1538-7836.2007.02729.x

Fleisher, L. A., Fleischmann, K. E., Auerbach, A. D., Barnason, S. A., Beckman, J. A., & Bozkurt, B. (2014). 2014 ACC/AHA guideline on perioperative cardiovascular evaluation and management of patients undergoing noncardiac surgery: A report of the American College of Cardiology/American Heart Association Task Force on Practice Guidelines. *Circulation, 130*, e278. doi:10.1161/CIR.0000000000000105

Garcia, D., Alexander, J. H., Wallentin, L., Wojdyla, D. M., Thomas, L., Hanna, M., & Lopes, R. D. (2014). Management and clinical outcomes in patients treated with apixaban vs warfarin undergoing procedures. *Blood, 124*(25), 3692–3698. doi:10.1182/blood-2014-08-595496

Healey, J. S., Eikelboom, J., Douketis, J., Wallentin, L., Oldgren, J., Yang, S., . . . Ezekowitz, M. (2012). Periprocedural bleeding and thromboembolic events with dabigatran compared with warfarin: Results from the Randomized Evaluation of Long-Term Anticoagulation Therapy (RE-LY) randomized trial. *Circulation, 126*(3), 343. doi:10.1161/CIRCULATIONAHA.111.090464

Marik, P. E., & Varon, J. (2008). Requirement of perioperative stress doses of corticosteroids: A systematic review of the literature. *Archives of Surgery, 143*(12), 1222–1226.

Sherwood, M. W., Douketis, J. D., Patel, M. R., Piccini, J. P., Hellkamp, A. S., Lokhnygina, Y., . . . ROCKET AF. Investigators (2014). Outcomes of temporary interruption of rivaroxaban compared with warfarin in patients with nonvalvular atrial fibrillation: Results from the rivaroxaban once daily, oral, direct Factor Xa inhibition compared with vitamin K antagonism for prevention of stroke and embolism trial in atrial fibrillation. *Circulation, 129*(18), 1850. doi:10.1161/CIRCULATIONAHA.113.005754

Thrombosis Canada (n. d.). Retrieved from http://thrombosiscanada.ca/tools/?calc=perioperativeAnticoagulantAlgorithm

Umpierrez, G. E., Smiley, D., Jacobs, S., Peng, L., Temponi, A., Mulligan, P., & Rizzo, M. (2011). Randomized study of basal-bolus insulin therapy in the inpatient management of patients with type 2 diabetes undergoing general surgery (RABBIT 2 surgery). *Diabetes Care, 34*, 256. doi:10.2337/dc10-1407

Van den Berghe, G., Wilmer, A., Hermans, G., Meersseman, W., Wouters, P. J., Milants, I., . . . Bouillon, R. (2006). Intensive insulin therapy in the medical ICU. *The New England Journal of Medicine, 354*, 449–461. doi:10.1056/NEJMoa052521

Van den Berghe, G., Wouters, P., Weekers, F., Verwaest, C., Bruyninckx, F., Schetz, M., & Bouillon, R. (2001). Intensive insulin therapy in critically ill patients. *The New England Journal of Medicine, 345*, 1359–1367. doi:10.1056/NEJMoa011300

19 Perioperative and Intraoperative Management

Kristopher R. Maday

Kristopher R. Maday

This section is not meant to be exhaustive in teaching the advanced practice provider (APP) how to function in the intraoperative setting. Rather, this section is included to provide an overview of the process that occurs to patients while they are in surgery, as well as to help the APP in the postoperative period understand why certain complications occur. For instance, patient positioning may impact postoperative atelectasis or a difficult airway may delay extubation. By understanding the general concepts of anesthesia, the APP will be knowledgeable about how to optimize physiologic parameters.

Considerations

Kristopher R. Maday

Goals of Anesthesia

A. Primary.
  1. Maintain homeostasis and optimize physiologic response to surgical insult.
B. Secondary.
  1. Amnesia and anxiolysis.
    a. Minimizing the memory of the operative and perioperative experience.
    b. Data shows one patient per 14,560 will have recall of the surgical experience.
    c. Commonly used medications include:
      i. Benzodiazepines.
      ii. Propofol.
      iii. Ketamine.
  2. Analgesia.
    a. Multimodal approach should be used to limit adverse effects of opioids and include:
      i. Opioid/narcotic medications.
      ii. Nonsteroidal anti-inflammatory drugs (such as Toradol).
      iii. Local anesthetics.
      iv. Regional blockade.
  3. Monitored anesthesia care (MAC).
    a. Local anesthesia with sedation and analgesia.
      i. Patient-controlled sedation may be used.
      ii. Continuous intravenous (IV) infusion.
      iii. Target-controlled infusion.
    b. First choice in many types of surgery.
      i. Colonoscopy.
      ii. Bronchoscopy.
      iii. Outpatient procedures.
    c. Patients able to answer questions and protect airway.
      i. Use bispectral index (BIS) to monitor patient consciousness.
    d. Goal of MAC.
      i. Safe sedation.
      ii. Control of patient anxiety.
      iii. Pain control.
    e. Medications.
      i. Midazolam—short acting benzodiazepine without analgesic effect, can cause respiratory depression especially in conjunction with other sedatives or opioids.
      ii. Propofol—rapidly acting sedative without analgesic effects, can transition to general anesthesia if needed.
      iii. Opioids.
        1) Fentanyl—short acting opioid.
        2) Remifentanil—ultrashort acting opioid typically given as an infusion.
      iv. Dexmedetomidine—infusion with sedative, anxiolytic, and analgesic effects. Does not produce respiratory depression.
      v. Ketamine—heavy analgesic effect with minimal respiratory depression. Can reduce the need for opioids.
  4. Neuromuscular blockade.
    a. Optimal operative conditions may require the patient to be still during surgery.
    b. Common medications include:
      i. Depolarizing agents.
        1) Succinylcholine.
          a) Faster onset, shorter acting.
          b) Good for induction.
          c) Side effects include bradycardia, hyperkalemia, fasciculations, rhabdomyolysis.
      ii. Nondepolarizing agents.
        1) Longer acting, available in drip.
        2) Good for surgical procedures or sustained blockade.
        3) Examples.
      iii. Rocuronium.
      iv. Vecuronium.
      v. Cisatracurium.
        1) Side effects include increased peripheral vascular resistance, tachycardia, and hypertension.

5. Maintenance of hemodynamic stability and hemostasis.

    a. Fluids—goal of fluids during surgery is normovolemia; avoid liberal or fixed volume approaches to fluid replacement.

        i. Crystalloid—such as Ringer's lactate or PlasmaLyte—used instead of normal saline. Goal is to maintain volume with balanced electrolytes.

            1) Most commonly used.

            2) Avoid large volume of fluid.

            3) Typically 1 to 2 L balanced electrolyte solution is adequate hydration.

        ii. Colloid—such as human albumin or hydroxyethyl starch (HES)—may expand microvascular volume without edema; it is not superior to use of crystalloids and should be reserved for unique situations.

        iii. Blood products—replace intraoperative blood loss.

        iv. Follow hemodynamic parameters and anticipated blood loss (>500 mL) to guide fluid replacement.

    b. Vasopressors.

        i. Phenylephrine.

        ii. Norepinephrine.

        iii. Epinephrine.

        iv. Ephedrine.

        v. Dobutamine.

    c. Transfusions.

        i. Packed red blood cells (PRBCs)—transfusion should be considered at hemoglobin concentrations of 7 g/dL or less.

        ii. Fresh frozen or thawed plasma—given to correct coagulopathy, reversal of warfarin, or correction of known coagulation factor deficiencies.

        iii. Platelets—may be given if suspected platelet dysfunction such as in the presence of antiplatelet agents and bleeding. Indicated if platelet count falls below the accepted threshold of $50 \times 10^9/L$ in the presence of excessive bleeding.

        iv. Cryoprecipitate—used when fibrinogen is less than 80 to 100 mg/dL in the presence of excessive bleeding, in the presence of fibrinolysis.

        v. Indications for autotransfusion—same as PRBC, but use patient's own supply. A person can donate his or her own blood weekly up to 5 days prior to surgery. Most hospitals can only hold autologous blood for a limited period of time such as 35 to 40 days.

        vi. Pharmacologic treatments.

            1) Desmopressin—promotes platelet adhesion and aggregation.

            2) Tranexamic acid—used as prophylaxis of excessive bleeding before and/or during a procedure.

            3) Coagulation factor concentrates—can be beneficial in cardiac surgery for emergency reversal of novel oral anticoagulants (NOAC) therapy. Off label use for microvascular bleeding attributed to coagulation factor deficiencies. Can increase risk of thromboembolic event.

            4) Thrombin gel—used for hemostasis intraoperatively.

6. Antiemetics to prevent postoperative nausea and vomiting (PONV).

    a. Highest risk in the 24 hours after surgery and also after laparoscopic gastrointestinal (GI) and GYN surgeries.

    b. Prevention.

        i. Scopolamine patch 2 hours prior to induction.

        ii. Dexamethasone 4 to 8 mg IV after induction.

        iii. Ondansetron 4 mg IV at the conclusion of surgery.

    c. Other alternative treatments.

        i. Promethazine 6.25 to 12.5 mg IV at induction.

        ii. Prochlorperazine 5 to 10 mg IV at the conclusion of surgery.

7. Reversal agents.

    a. Most inhaled and IV anesthetics are turned off in advance of emergence at the end of the case. These volatile substances clear quite quickly from the system without the need for reversal.

    b. Neuromuscular blockade.

        i. Neostigmine.

        ii. Sugammadex.

Anesthetic Considerations

A. Local.

  1. Indications: Used at incision site.

  2. Most common medications used are as follows.

    a. Lidocaine (0.5%, 1%, 2%).

        i. Onset: 2 to 5 minutes, but typically faster.

        ii. Duration: 30 to 120 minutes (180 minutes with epinephrine).

        iii. Maximum dose.

            1) With epinephrine: 7 mg/kg.

            2) Without epinephrine: 4 mg/kg.

    b. Bupivacaine (0.125%, 0.25%).

        i. Onset: 5 to 10 minutes.

        ii. Duration: Up to 6 hours.

        iii. Maximum dose.

            1) With epinephrine: 3 mg/kg.

            2) Without epinephrine: 2 mg/kg.

  3. Complications.

    a. Toxicity.

        i. Cardiac.

            1) Lidocaine is a Class I antiarrhythmic medication and can cause cardiac disturbances such as:

                a) Bradycardia.

                b) Decreased inotropy.

                c) Atrioventricular block.

                d) Vasodilation.

                e) Dysrhythmias.

                f) Cardiac arrest.

        ii. Central nervous system.

            1) Seizures.

            2) Paresthesias.

            3) Tinnitus.

            4) Neuraxial anesthesia.

B. Regional blocks.

  1. Types.

    a. Upper extremity.

        i. Brachial plexus.

            1) Interscalene.

            2) Supraclavicular.

            3) Infraclavicular.

            4) Axillary.

b. Lower extremity.
  i. Sciatic.
  ii. Femoral.
  iii. Fascia iliaca.
  iv. Lumbar plexus.

2. Contraindications and complications.
  a. Body habitus may make regional blockade difficult due to equipment limitations.
  b. Active infection at the site of injection.
  c. Coagulopathy and noncompressible site of injection.
  d. Preexisting neural deficits in the distribution of the block.
  e. Hemidiaphragm paralysis.
  f. Laryngeal nerve paralysis.
  g. Horner's syndrome can be caused by upper extremity blocks.

C. Spinal.

1. Indications.
  a. Lower extremity procedures (total hip/knee replacement, knee arthroscopy, etc.) in patients with high risk for general anesthesia.
  b. Shorter, known duration of surgery.
  c. Patients who cannot withstand general anesthesia for a procedure.

D. Epidural.

1. Indications.
  a. Longer surgical procedures.
  b. Unknown duration of surgery.
  c. Help with postoperative pain management.
  d. Extremity surgery in patients who are poor surgical candidates due to American Society of Anesthesiologists (ASA) class or other comorbidities.

2. Contraindications and complications.
  a. Hypovolemia: May cause spinal shock.
  b. Coagulopathy: May cause spinal hematoma.
  c. Increased intracranial pressure.
  d. Abscess.

3. Procedure.
  a. Ultrasound has increased the safety and efficacy of regional blockade as the operator can identify the structures directly and inject at the site of the nerve.

4. Three phases of general anesthesia.
  a. Induction.
    i. Often achieved with a combination of IV and inhaled medications; however, may be done with either alone as well.
    ii. Rapid instillation (<2 minutes) of medications to prepare patient for intubation and surgery.
    iii. IV medications.
      1) Propofol.
      2) Etomidate.
      3) Ketamine.
      4) Midazolam.
      5) Opioid narcotics: Fentanyl.
      6) Neuromuscular blockade.
    iv. Inhalational medications.
      1) Adult patients.
        a) Commonly used for quick induction.
        b) May have an unpleasant taste.
        c) May have increased postoperative nausea/vomiting.
        d) May be considered in higher risk patient who is spontaneously breathing.

2) Pediatric patients.
  a) May be preferred due to fear and pain of needle stick.

b. Maintenance of general anesthesia.
  i. Inhalational.
    1) Sevoflurane.
    2) Desflurane.
    3) Nitrous oxide.
  ii. IV.
    1) Propofol.
    2) Neuromuscular blockade.
    3) Opioids.
      a) Fentanyl.
      b) Sufentanil.
      c) Remifentanil.

c. Emergence.
  i. Returning the patient to a state of consciousness.
  ii. Many variables; depends on IV versus inhaled, type used, and patient physiology. The overall steps are to stop these and allow the patient to slowly metabolize and emerge.
  iii. Timing is critical and occurs in a stepwise approach.
    1) Discontinue anesthetic agents.
    2) Administer antiemetic.
    3) Assess adequacy of analgesia: Elevations in blood pressure, heart rate, and respiratory rate indicate inadequate pain control.
    4) Assess adequacy of tidal volume and minute ventilation of spontaneous respiration by arterial blood gas analysis.
    5) Assess level of wakefulness.
      a) Patient following commands.
      b) Coughing with airway in place.
    6) Extubation or removal of supraglottic airway.

d. Complications of general anesthetics.
  i. Malignant hyperthermia.
    1) Hallmark sign is temperature greater than 40°C and muscle rigidity.
  ii. Laryngospasm/bronchospasm.
    1) Hallmark sign is inspiratory stridor.
  iii. Nausea/vomiting.
  iv. Agitation/delirium.
  v. Urinary retention.

Bibliography

Berde, C. B. (1993). Toxicity of local anesthetics in infants and children. *The Journal of Pediatrics, 122*(5 Pt. 2), S14–S20. doi:10.1016/S0022-3476(11)80004-1

Borgeat, A., Ekatodramis, G., Kalberer, F., & Benz, C. (2001). Acute and nonacute complications associated with interscalene block and shoulder surgery: A prospective study. *Anesthesiology, 95*(4), 875–880. doi:10.1097/00000542-200110000-00015

New York School of Regional Anesthesia. (n.d.). *Spinal anesthesia*. Retrieved from http://www.nysora.com/techniques/neuraxial-and-perineuraxial-techniques/landmark-based/3423-spinal-anesthesia

Pollard, R. J., Coyle, J. P., Gilbert, R. L., & Beck, J. E. (2007). Intraoperative awareness in a regional medical system: A review of 3 years' data. *Anesthesiology, 106*(2), 269–274. doi:10.1097/00000542-200702000-00014

Thwaites, A., Edmends, S., & Smith, I. (1997). Inhalation induction with sevoflurane: A double-blind comparison with propofol. *British Journal of Anaesthesia, 78*(4), 356–361. doi:10.1093/bja/78.4.356

White, P. F., Kehlet, H., & Neal, J. M. (2007). The role of the anesthesiologist in fast-track surgery: From multimodal analgesia to perioperative medical care. *Anesthesia and Analgesia, 104*(6), 1380–1396. doi:10.1213/01.ane.0000263034.96885.e1

Care Principles

Kristopher R. Maday

Positioning
A. Goals of proper patient positioning.
    1. Maintain airway.
    2. Provide adequate surgical exposure.
    3. Allow for proper patient monitoring.
    4. Prevent vascular compression and ischemia.
    5. Prevent nerve damage.
    6. Keep patient comfortable.
B. Each surgical specialty has specific considerations for each surgery.
C. Four basic positions.
    1. Supine (see Figure 19.1).
    2. Prone.
    3. Lateral.
    4. Lithotomy (see Figure 19.2).
D. Special positions.
    1. Trendelenburg (see Figure 19.3).
    2. Reverse Trendelenburg (see Figure 19.4).
    3. Fowler's (see Figure 19.5).
    4. Jackknife (see Figure 19.6).
E. Complications.
    1. Compression nerve injuries: Specific nerve compression is dependent on the position used and the adequacy of the padding.
    2. Pressure sores: May start to occur in as little as 60 minutes if not positioned/padded appropriately.
    3. Cerebral perfusion: Head positioning can cause decreased perfusion and can result in anoxic brain injuries if not properly monitored.

4. Upper airway edema: Particularly for patients in steep Trendelenburg.

Principles of Aseptic Technique
A. Surgical scrub.
    1. Length.
        a. 3 to 5 minutes.
        b. Stroke count method.
    2. Area: 5 cm above the elbow to the fingertips.
    3. Procedure.
        a. Remove all jewelry from hands.
        b. Use nail file to clean under the nails.
        c. Always keep hands higher than elbow to prevent contamination.
        d. Lather entire area with soap.
            i. Commonly accepted soaps for scrub: Chlorhexidine or povidone-iodine-containing soaps.
        e. Use warm water. Hot water can destroy a healthy layer of protective skin.
        f. Start the scrub with fingertips and work to the elbows.
            i. Rinse from fingers to elbow in one direction only.
            ii. Scrub each side of the finger and back/front of the hand for 2 minutes.
            iii. Scrub from wrist to elbow on each arm for 1 minute.
            iv. Repeat the process on the other hand and arm.
            v. Rinse hands and arms by passing them through the water in one direction only.
        g. Proceed to the operating room with hands up and above the elbows.

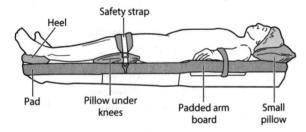

FIGURE 19.1 Supine position.
Source: Goodman, T., & Spry, C. (2017). Essentials of perioperative nursing (6th ed.). Burlington, MA: Jones & Bartlett.

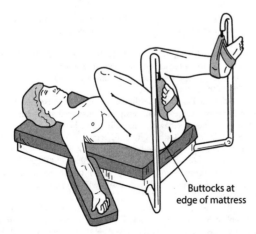

FIGURE 19.2 Lithotomy position.
Source: Goodman, T., & Spry, C. (2017). Essentials of perioperative nursing (6th ed.). Burlington, MA: Jones & Bartlett.

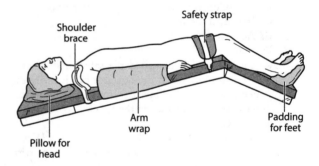

FIGURE 19.3 Trendelenburg position.
Source: Goodman, T., & Spry, C. (2017). Essentials of perioperative nursing (6th ed.). Burlington, MA: Jones & Bartlett.

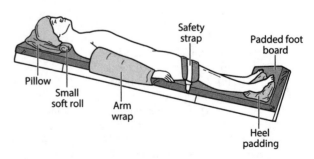

FIGURE 19.4 Reverse Trendelenburg.
Source: Goodman, T., & Spry, C. (2017). Essentials of perioperative nursing (6th ed.). Burlington, MA: Jones & Bartlett.

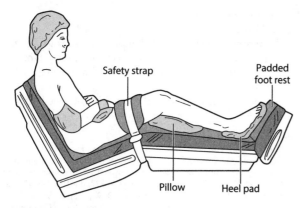

FIGURE 19.5 Fowler's position.
Source: Goodman, T., & Spry, C. (2017). Essentials of perioperative nursing (6th ed.). Burlington, MA: Jones & Bartlett.

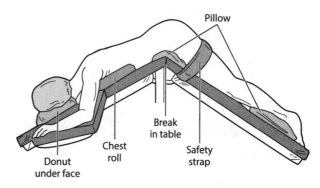

FIGURE 19.6 Jackknife position.
Source: Goodman, T., & Spry, C. (2017). Essentials of perioperative nursing (6th ed.). Burlington, MA: Jones & Bartlett.

h. Once in the operating room, hands and arms should be dried with a sterile towel and aseptic technique prior to placing on the gown and gloves.
B. Sterile field in operating room.
  1. From nipple area to waist.
  2. Only in the front.
  3. Neck can be contaminated by mask and is not considered a sterile part of the field.
C. Prepping the surgical patient.
  1. Skin antisepsis.
    a. Decrease the burden of skin flora and reduce the rate of surgical site infections.
    b. Common examples.
      i. Chlorhexidine—alcohol is the preferred scrub prep for surgeons and assistants.
      ii. Povidone-iodine—must be used when prepping an open wound or mucous membrane, such as the vagina or rectum.
      iii. Iodine and isopropyl alcohol.
      iv. Iodine-impregnated adhesive covering.
  2. Draping.
    a. Sterile draping of the surgical field is performed by the surgical assistants in order to:
      i. Provide a sterile field.
      ii. Provide adequate surgical area exposure.
      iii. Cover all nonsterile area in the operative field.

Wound Classifications

A. Clean: Uninfected wounds without inflammation.
B. Clean-contaminated: Controlled entering of viscus entered during sterile operation.
C. Contaminated.
  1. Open, fresh accidental wounds.
  2. Major breaks in sterile techniques.
  3. Gross spillage of viscous contents.
D. Dirty: Old, traumatic wounds with retained devitalized tissue, foreign bodies, or fecal contamination.

Wound Healing

A. Primary intention.
  1. Used for clean incisions.
  2. Suturing is performed early.
  3. Minor cosmetic scar.
B. Secondary intention.
  1. Used for wider wounds.
  2. Allow granulation tissue to fill the base of the wound with no suturing.

    a. The key to healing is through granulation of the tissue.
  3. Larger cosmetic scar.
C. Tertiary intention.
  1. Used for irregular wounds.
  2. Allow granulation tissue to fill the base of the wound with delayed primary closure.
  3. Usually used for larger cosmetic scars.

Role of the First Assistant

A. The main role of a surgical first assistant is to provide support for the primary surgeon during a surgical procedure.
B. The first assistant's scope of practice will vary from state-to-state and by hospital. These roles can be dictated by the surgeon and/or the institution and can include any of the following.
  1. Providing exposure.
  2. Hemostasis.
  3. Surgical tying and suturing.
  4. Suctioning.
C. First assistants are generally positioned opposite of the surgeon's preferred side or based on the procedure being performed.

Documentation Requirements

A. What to include in brief operative notes.
  1. Procedure—state what procedure was done.
  2. Complications—indicate any complications that occurred during surgery.
  3. Intake/output—list how much fluid was given and what the urinary output was.
  4. Estimated blood loss (EBL)—indicate the amount of EBL during the case. In some surgeries, this amount may be minuscule. The EBL can be very subjective.
  5. Postoperative vital signs—the vital signs at the end of the case.
  6. Discuss postoperative checks—indicate if any specific physical examination was completed. For instance, after a spine case, motor function would be assessed.

Bibliography

Anderson, K., & Hamm, R. (2012). Factors that impair wound healing. *Journal of the American College of Clinical Wound Specialists, 4*(4), 84–91. doi:10.1016/j.jccw.2014.03.001

Berríos-Torres, S. I., Umscheid, C. A., Bratzler, D. W., Leas, B., Stone, E. C., Kelz, R. R., . . . Schecter, W. P. (2017). Centers for disease control and prevention guideline for the prevention of surgical site infection. *JAMA Surgery, 152*(8), 784–791. doi:10.1001/jamasurg.2017.0904

Gardner, D., & Anderson-Manz, E. (2001). *How to perform surgical hand scrub*. Retrieved from http://www.infectioncontroltoday.com/articles/2001/05/how-to-perform-surgical-hand-scrubs.aspx

Goodman, T., & Spry, C. (2017). Essentials of perioperative nursing. (6th ed.). Burlington, MA: Jones & Bartlett.

Leaper, D. J. (2006). Traumatic and surgical wounds. *British Medical Journal, 332*(7540), 532–535. doi:10.1136/bmj.332.7540.532

Medication Management

Kristopher R. Maday

Preoperative Antibiotics

A. Antimicrobial prophylaxis to prevent surgical site infections depends on several factors.
  1. Cost.
  2. Safety.
  3. Pharmacokinetic profile.
  4. Bactericidal activity.
  5. Type of surgical specialty and/or specific operation.
B. Given within 60 minutes of surgical incision to have optimal tissue concentration.

C. Common examples.
  1. First generation cephalosporin: Cefazolin.
  2. Second generation cephalosporin (broader gram-negative coverage): Cefuroxime, cefoxitin, cefotetan.
  3. Penicillin-allergy alternatives: Vancomycin, clindamycin.
  4. Metronidazole is typically added in colorectal cases.

Bibliography

Anderson, D. J., Podgorny, K., Berríos-Torres, S. I., Bratzler, D. W., Dellinger, E. P., Greene, L., . . . Kaye, K. S. (2014). Strategies to prevent surgical site infections in acute care hospitals: 2014 update. *Infection Control & Hospital Epidemiology, 35*(6), 605–627. doi:10.1086/676022

Berríos-Torres, S. I., Umscheid, C. A., Bratzler, D. W., Leas, B., Stone, E. C., Kelz, R. R., . . . Schecter, W. P. (2017). Centers for Disease Control and Prevention guideline for the prevention of surgical site infection, 2017. *JAMA Surgery, 152*(8), 784–791. doi:10.1001/jamasurg.2017.0904

Bratzler, D. W., Dellinger, E. P., Olsen, K. M., Perl, T. M., Auwaerter, P. G., Bolon, M. K., . . . Weinstein, R. A. (2013). Clinical practice guidelines for antimicrobial prophylaxis in surgery. *Surgical Infections, 14*(1), 73–156. doi:10.1089/sur.2013.9999

Spruce, L., & Van Wicklin, S. (2014). Back to basics: Positioning the patient. *AORN Journal, 100*, 299–303. doi:10.1016/j.aorn.2014.06.004

20 Postoperative Evaluation and Management

John Hurt and Catherine Harris

Scope of Chapter

John Hurt and Catherine Harris

The postoperative period is a vulnerable time for the patient. The advanced practice provider (APP) must perform a timely physical assessment, anticipate postoperative complications, manage surgical wounds, and treat pain. This section provides an overview on managing patients during this time frame.

Outcomes

John Hurt & Catherine Harris

A. Patient assessment.
B. Postoperative complications.
C. Wound healing.
D. Pain management.

Patient Assessment

A. Patient assessment.
    1. Physical examination.
    2. Vital signs.
    3. Skin integrity.
    4. Pain management.
B. Two phases of the postanesthesia care unit (PACU).
    1. Phase I: Patient assessment ensuring that a patient recovers fully from anesthesia and has return of normal vital signs; includes pain management and monitoring for postoperative complications.
    2. Phase II: Focuses on wound assessment, patient comfort, review of medications, and hand-off to the nurse from the inpatient unit.
C. Hand-off communication.
    1. Communication between the OR and PACU is critical and should contain the following elements at minimum.
        a. Type of anesthesia used during case.
        b. Type of procedure performed and duration.
        c. Medications given in the OR.
        d. Positioning of patient.
        e. Intake and output including amount of estimated blood loss.
        f. Complications or unusual events during the case.
        g. Wound closure.
        h. Types of dressings, lines, and monitoring devices.
D. Postoperative orders for inpatient stays.
    1. Admit to team, physician, type of unit.
    2. Diagnosis and procedure done.
    3. Condition postoperatively.

    4. Allergies.
    5. Vital signs and frequency.
    6. Activity.
    7. Any specific nursing procedures such as wound care, when to notify house officer, or incentive spirometry.
    8. Deep vein thrombosis (DVT) prophylaxis.
    9. Intake and output, intravenous (IV) fluids, and drains.
    10. Medications.
    11. Any special laboratory tests and when they should be drawn.
    12. Radiology per surgeon for postoperative evaluation of procedure.
    13. Pain management.
    14. Enhanced recovery after surgery (ERAS) guidelines.
        a. Diet—patients should be advanced to oral nutrition within the first 24 hours of uncomplicated surgery. Consider oral supplements with meals if unable to tolerate food.
        b. Early intake of oral fluids—offer day of surgery.
        c. Early removal of urinary catheters and discontinuing IV fluids.
        d. Early ambulation—ambulate patient day of surgery as tolerated.
        e. Multimodal approach to opioid—sparing pain control and mitigate nausea and vomiting.
        f. Early discharge when possible.
    15. Oxygen requirements.
    16. Consults such as physical therapy, social work, dietician.

Common Postoperative Complications

A. Pulmonary.
    1. Tachypnea (respiratory rate >30 breaths/minute).
        a. Inadequate pain control.
            i. Supplemental analgesia if inadequate pain control.
        b. Laryngospasm.
            i. Jaw thrust/chin lift to promote airflow.
        c. Airway edema.
            i. May need to be reintubated for airway protection.
        d. Negative pressure pulmonary edema.
            i. Provide positive pressure ventilation.
        e. Pulmonary embolism.
            i. Management depends on cardiopulmonary compromise.
        f. Fever.
            i. Add fluids and antipyretics as needed.
    2. Bradypnea (respiratory rate <8 breaths/minute).
        a. Oversedated from anesthesia or narcotic use; typically seen in PACU setting.

i. Consider adding anesthesia reversal agents if oversedated.

B. Cardiovascular.

1. Hypotension (systolic blood pressure <90 mmHg).

  a. Most often due to volume depletion, anesthetic medications (opioids, benzodiazepines, propofol), regional anesthesia techniques, and drug reactions to antibiotics.

  b. Management: Give crystalloid bolus, may start with 250 to 500 mL and reassess blood pressure. Repeat as needed to maintain adequate blood pressure and urine output. May need to add vasopressors if nonresponsive. Review anesthesia record for accurate reflection of intake and output.

2. Hypertension.

  a. Most commonly due to inadequate pain control and agitation emerging from anesthesia.

  b. Management: Provide analgesia to maintain blood pressure within defined parameters.

3. Dysrhythmias.

  a. Tachycardia (heart rate >100 beats/minute).

    1. Typically due to pain, hypovolemia, or anemia from blood loss.

  b. Bradycardia (heart rate <40 beats/minute).

    1. Usually due to reversal agents for neuromuscular blockade such as neostigmine or regional anesthesia techniques.

    2. Hypoxemia and myocardial infarction can also cause bradycardia.

  c. Atrial fibrillation, atrial flutter, and ventricular tachycardia should be managed by Advanced Cardiac Life Support algorithms. For more information, refer to Chapter 3.

C. Gastrointestinal.

1. Nausea/vomiting.

  a. Most common postoperative complication.

  b. Often rated worse than pain by patients.

  c. Management.

2. Elevate head of bed.

3. Antiemetic medication options.

  a. Serotonin receptor agonists: Ondansetron 4 mg IV.

  b. Glucocorticoids: Dexamethasone 4 to 8 mg IV.

  c. Anticholinergics: Scopolamine patch.

  d. Phenothiazines: Promethazine 5 to 10 mg IV.

  e. Butyrophenones: Droperidol 0.625 mg IV or haldol 1 mg IV.

D. Genitourinary.

1. Acute renal failure.

  a. Persistent oliguria and elevated creatinine.

  b. Management.

    i. May need diuretics if overloaded.

    ii. Need to balance effective circulating volume with output.

    iii. Avoid nephrotoxic agents.

    iv. Avoid contrast agents.

2. Urinary infection.

  a. Management.

    i. Early removal of urinary catheter.

    ii. Maintain adequate hydration.

    iii. Early ambulation.

3. Postoperative urinary retention (POUR).

  a. Risk greater in patients who:

    i. Have neuropathy or neurological damage.

    ii. Have chronic constipation.

    iii. Take anticholinergic medications.

    iv. Had bladder or anorectal procedures.

    v. Had long duration of anesthesia.

    vi. Use of opioid medications.

  b. Strategies to reduce risk.

    i. Adequate hydration perioperatively.

    ii. Early mobilization.

    iii. Use of commode.

4. Metabolic derangements.

  a. Monitor and replace electrolytes to maintain normal values.

    i. Potassium.

    ii. Magnesium.

    iii. Phosphorous.

  b. Maintain acid base balance.

E. Postoperative pain control.

1. Early intervention and better pain management essential.

2. Untreated surgical pain can limit cough and deep breathing, which contributes to a decrease in alveolar ventilation.

3. Inadequate relief may result in psychological changes such as:

  a. Minor depression.

  b. Pain-related catastrophizing.

  c. Chronic postsurgical pain.

F. Neuropsychiatric.

1. Transient ischemic attack or stroke.

  a. Avoid ischemia.

  b. Avoid hypotension or hypertension.

2. Delirium during emergence is highest during the first hour postanesthesia.

  a. Management.

    i. Reassurance with familiar family/friends at the bedside.

    ii. Assess for signs of uncontrolled pain and treat.

    iii. Consider low-dose benzodiazepine for sedation.

3. Discharge from PACU.

  a. Postanesthetic Discharge Scoring System (PADSS): Score of 9 or greater can be safely discharged to the accepting unit.

Vital Signs

0 = *Blood pressure and pulse ≥40% preoperative baseline.*

1 = *Blood pressure and pulse 20%–40% preoperative baseline.*

2 = *Blood pressure and pulse <20% preoperative baseline.*

Activity

0 = *Unable to ambulate.*

1 = *Requires assistance.*

2 = *Ambulates without assistance, no dizziness.*

Nausea and Vomiting

0 = *Severe/continuous despite treatment.*

1 = *Moderate/treated with parenteral medications.*

2 = *Minimal/treated with oral medications.*

Pain Controlled with Oral Analgesics and Acceptable by Patient

1 = *No.*

2 = *Yes.*

Surgical Bleeding

0 = Severe, or ≥3 dressing changes.
1 = Moderate, or up to 2 dressing changes.
2 = Minimal, or no dressing changes.

Source: Reproduced with permission from Chung, F., Ghan, V. W. S., & Ong, D. (1995). A post-anesthetic discharge scoring system for home readiness after ambulatory surgery. *Journal of Clinical Anesthesia, 7,* 500–506. doi:10.1016/0952-8180(95)00130-A

G. Fever.

1. Fever is a common complication after surgery that can be attributed to many different causes. Always consider the following.

a. Fever immediately after surgery.

i. Atelectasis ("Wind").

ii. Medication reactions ("Wonder Drugs").

iii. Endocrine emergencies ("Wonky Glands").

b. Fever 48 to 72 hours after surgery.

i. Urinary tract infection ("Water").

ii. Wound infection ("Wound").

iii. DVT ("Walking").

iv. Alcohol or drug reactions ("Withdrawal").

H. DVT.

1. Patients should be encouraged to ambulate as early and as often as safely possible.

a. Improves pulmonary function, prevents atelectasis, prevents DVT.

2. Optimal timing for pharmacological thromboprophylaxis in nonorthopedic patients is unknown and should be individualized.

3. If risk of bleeding is low, pharmacological agents can begin 2 to 12 hours preoperatively.

4. Initiate pharmacological treatment for DVT prevention in patients not considered suitable for preoperative pharmacological thromboprophylaxis or who have a high risk of bleeding 2 to 72 hours postoperatively.

a. Low-dose unfractionated heparin.

b. Low molecular weight heparin.

c. Factor Xa inhibitors and direct thrombin inhibitors are used less commonly for DVT prophylaxis and more frequently in patients with allergy to heparin or in some vascular patients for full treatment.

5. The Modified Caprini Risk Assessment Score provides an individualized risk assessment for DVT prevention (see Table 20.1).

Bibliography

Aarts, M. A., Okrainec, A., Glicksman, A., Pearsall, E., Victor, J. C., & McLeod, R. S. (2012). Adoption of enhanced recovery after surgery (ERAS) strategies for colorectal surgery at academic teaching hospitals and impact on total length of hospital stay. *Surgical Endoscopy, 26*(2), 442–450. doi:10.1007/s00464-011-1897-5

Apfel, C. C., Korttila, K., & Abdalla, M. (2004). A factorial trial of six interventions for the prevention of postoperative nausea and vomiting. *The New England Journal of Medicine, 350*(24), 2441–2451. doi:10.1056/NEJMoa032196

Apfelbaum, J. L., Silverstein, J. H., & Chung, F. F. (2013). Practice guidelines for postanesthetic care: An updated report by the American Society of Anesthesiologists task force on postanesthetic care. *Anesthesiology, 118*(2), 291–307. doi:10.1097/ALN.0b013e31827773e9

Caprini, J. A. (2005). Thrombosis risk assessment as a guide to quality patient care. *Disease-a-Month, 51,* 70–78. doi:10.1016/j.disamonth.2005.02.003

Caprini, J. A. (2010). Risk assessment as a guide for the prevention of the many faces of venous thromboembolism. *American Journal of Surgery, 199*(Suppl. 1), S3–S10. doi:10.1016/j.amjsurg.2009.10.006

Chung, F., Ghan, V. W. S., & Ong, D. (1995). A post-anesthetic discharge scoring system for home readiness after ambulatory surgery. *Journal of Clinical Anesthesia, 7,* 500–506. doi:10.1016/0952-8180(95)00130-A

Gould, M. K., Garcia, D. A., Wren, S. M., Karanicolas, P. J., Arcelus, J. I., Heit, J. A., . . . Samama, C. M. (2012). Prevention of VTE in non-orthopedic surgical patients antithrombotic therapy and prevention of thrombosis, 9th ed: American College of Chest Physicians evidence-based clinical practice guidelines. *Chest, 141*(2), e227S–e277S. doi:10.1378/chest.11-2297

Kearon, C., Akl, E., Ornelas, J., Blaivas, A., Jimenez, D., Bounameaux, H., . . . Moores, L. (2016). Antithrombotic therapy for VTE disease. CHESTGuideline and expert panel report. *Chest, 149,* 315–352. doi: 10.1.16/j.chest.2015.11.026

Macario, A., Weinger, M., Carney, S., & Kim, A. (1999). Which clinical anesthesia outcomes are important to avoid? The perspective of patients. *Anesthesia and Analgesia, 89*(3), 652–658.

Maday, K. R., Hurt, J. B., Harrelson, P., & Porterfield, J. (2016). Evaluating postoperative fever. *Journal of the American Academy of PAs, 29*(10), 23–28. doi:10.1097/01.JAA.0000496951.72463.de

Whitlock, E. L., Vannucci, A., & Avidan, M. S. (2011). Postoperative delirium. *Minerva Anesesiologica, 7*(4), 448–456.

Wound Management

John Hurt and Catherine Harris

Infection Prevention

A. Surgical site infections (SSI).

1. Can be superficial (skin/subcutaneous tissue), deep (muscle/fascia), or organ and surrounding space specific.

2. Occurs within 30 days of surgery.

3. Majority of cases of SSI superficial infections (83%), deep infections (7%), and the rest were organ-specific infections.

4. Factors associated with SSI.

a. Previous surgery.

b. Prolonged surgery time.

c. Hypoalbuminemia.

d. History of chronic obstructive pulmonary disease (COPD).

e. Obesity.

f. Diabetes.

g. American Society of Anesthesiologists (ASA) score.

h. Wounds classified as "dirty."

i. Type of surgical procedure such as bowel surgery may increase risk of infection.

5. Organisms associated with SSI.

a. Staphylococci.

b. Streptococci.

c. Enteric bacilli; enterococci.

d. Pseudomonas.

e. Clostridia.

f. Mycobacterium tuberculosis.

g. Multidrug-resistant organisms.

6. Prevention strategies.

a. Standard precautions.

b. Perioperative antibiotics.

i. Administer 1 hour before skin incision.

ii. Discontinue within 24 hours.

c. Clip operative site, but avoid shaving.

d. Control of perioperative glucose values less than 180 mg/dL.

e. Aseptic technique.

B. Classification of surgical wounds.

1. Class I: Clean—uninfected operative wound.

TABLE 20.1	Modified Caprini Risk Assessment Score		
1 Point	**2 Points**	**3 Points**	**4 Points**
Age 41–60 years	Age 61–74 years	Age ≥75 years	Stroke within 1 month
Minor surgery	Arthroscopic surgery	History of VTE	Elective arthroplasty
BMI ≥25	Major open surgery	Family history of VTE	Pelvis, hip, or leg fracture
Swollen legs	Laparoscopic surgery	Genetic clotting disorder	Acute spinal cord injury
Varicose veins	Malignancy		
Pregnancy/postpartum	Confined to bed >72 hr		
History of spontaneous abortion	Lower extremity immobilization		
Oral hormone medication	Central venous access		
History of sepsis <1 month			
Underlying lung disease			
Abnormal pulmonary function			
History of AMI			
CHF			
History of IBD			
Score	**Surgical Risk**	**Intervention for DVT Prevention**	
0	Very low	*Early mobilization*	
1–2	Low	*Early mobilization + mechanical compression devices*	
3–4	Moderate	*Pharmacologic prophylaxis*	
≥5	High		

AMI, acute myocardial infarction; CHF, congestive heart failure; DVT, deep vein thrombosis; IBD, inflammatory bowel disease; VTE, venous thromboembolism.
Sources: Caprini, J. A. (2005). Thrombosis risk assessment as a guide to quality patient care. *Disease-a-Month, 51*, 70–78. doi:10.1016/j.disamonth.2005.02.003; Kearon, C., Akl, E., Ornelas, J., Blaivas, A., Jimenez, D., Bounameaux, H., . . . Moores, L. (2016). Antithrombotic therapy for VTE disease. CHEST Guideline and expert panel report. *Chest, 149*, 315–352. doi:10.1016/j.chest.2015.11.026

2. Class II: Clean-contaminated—operative wound in which respiratory, alimentary, genital, or urinary tracts are entered under controlled conditions.

3. Class III: Contaminated—open, fresh, accidental wounds; major breaks in sterile technique; gross spillage from gastrointestinal tract; incisions in acute nonpurulent inflammation is encountered.

4. Class IV: Dirty/infected—old traumatic wounds with retained devitalized tissue and those that involve existing clinical infection or perforated viscera; organisms present before procedure.

C. Wound healing.
  1. Classified by etiology.
    a. Surgical.
    b. Traumatic.
  2. Classified by initial presentation.
    a. Closed wound (preferred).
    b. Open wound (based on amount of tissue lost).
  3. Types of wound healing.
    a. Primary intention—wound is clean, little loss of tissue.
      i. Preferred technique.
      ii. Heals quickly with minimal scarring.
    b. Secondary intention—occurs in open wounds due to difficulty of reapproximating edges secondary to amount of tissue loss.
      i. Granulation tissue fills defect.
      ii. Healing takes longer.
      iii. Results in more scarring.

      1) May inhibit normal physiologic function in that area.
    c. Tertiary intention.
      i. Delayed primary closure.
      ii. Cannot close wound due to concern for infection.
      iii. Wound remains open until resolution of infection.
      iv. Increased granulation and inflammatory reaction compared to primary intention.
  4. Factors that delay wound healing.
    a. Age.
    b. Immunosuppressed states.
      i. HIV/AIDS.
      ii. Diabetes.
      iii. Cancer.
    c. Autoimmune disorders.
    d. Altered nutritional status.
    e. Smoking.
    f. Anemia.
    g. Inadequate oxygenation (i.e., COPD).
    h. Vascular disease.
  5. Medications that impair wound healing.
    a. Anticoagulants.
    b. Anti-inflammatory agents (aspirin, nonsteroidal anti-inflammatory drugs [NSAIDs]).
    c. Steroids.
    d. Colchicine.

6. Herbal medicines that may impair wound healing.
   a. Ephedra—increases heart rate and blood pressure.
   b. Feverfew—inhibits platelet activity.
   c. Garlic—inhibits platelet aggregation.
   d. Gingko—inhibits platelet activation.
   e. Nicotine—impairs oxygen delivery.

D. Wound assessment.
   1. Dressings.
      a. Applied under sterile conditions in the OR.
      b. Prevent contamination of wound.
      c. Protect wound from further trauma.
      d. Absorb exudate.
      e. Provide physical support.
   2. High risk patients may require wound care consult.
   3. Compressive wraps must not impair blood flow.
      a. Assess for:
         i. Pulses.
         ii. Cyanosis.
         iii. Capillary refill.
         iv. Temperature of body around dressing.
   4. Types of dressings.
      a. Primary intention closure.
         i. Transparent polyurethane dressings.
            1) Protect wound.
            2) Check incision site without disturbing dressing.
            3) Can be left in place for 3 to 5 days.
         ii. Semipermeable films.
            1) Provides a barrier against bacteria.
         iii. Surgical glue.
      b. Secondary intention closure.
         i. Alginates.
            1) Maintains moist wound surface.
            2) Removal of cellular debris.
         ii. Polyurethane foams.
            1) Absorbent.
            2) Maintains optimum healing environment.
            3) Reduces trauma during dressing changes.
         iii. Hydrocolloids.
            1) Absorbent.
            2) Maintains moist wound surface.
         iv. Hydrogels.
            1) Rehydration of tissues.
            2) Some absorbency.
         v. Low-adherent wound contact layers.
            1) Minimizes risk of trauma at wound surface.
            2) Decreases pain during dressing change.
         vi. Antimicrobial carrying dressings.
            1) Stimulates immune system for wound healing.

Bibliography

Anderson, K., & Hamm, R. (2012). Factors that impair wound healing. *Journal of the American College of Clinical Wound Specialists, 4*(4), 84–91. doi:10.1016/j.jccw.2014.03.001

Berríos-Torres, S. I., Umscheid, C. A., Bratzler, D. W., Leas, B., Stone, E. C., Kelz, R. R., . . . Schecter, W. P. (2017). Centers for Disease Control and Prevention guideline for the prevention of surgical site infection. *JAMA Surgery, 152*(8), 784–791. doi:10.1001/jamasurg.2017.0904

Dumville, J., Gray, T., Walter, C., Sharp, C., Page, T., Macefield, R., & . . . Blazeby, J. (2016). Dressings for the prevention of surgical site infection. *Cochrane Database of Systematic Reviews, 2016*(12). doi:10.1002/14651858.CD003091.pub4

Maver, T., Maver, U., Kleinschek, S., Smrke, D., & Kreft, S. (2015). A review of herbal medicines in wound healing. *International Journal of Dermatology, 54*(7), 740–751. doi:10.1111/ijd.12766

Mu, Y., Edwards, J. R., Horan, T. C., Berrios-Torres, S. I., & Fridkin, S. K. (2011). Improving risk-adjusted measures of surgical site infection for the National Healthcare Safety Network. *Infection Control & Hospital Epidemiology, 32*(10), 970–986. doi:10.1086/662016

National Collaborating Centre for Women's and Children's Health (UK). (2008). Surgical site infection: Prevention and treatment of surgical site infection. London, UK: RCOG Press.

National Healthcare Safety Network, Centers for Disease Control and Prevention. (2019, January). *Surgical site infection (SSI) event.* Retrieved from http://www.cdc.gov/nhsn/pdfs/pscmanual/9pscssicurrent.pdf

Medication Management

John Hurt and Catherine Harris

Pain Management

A. Should be a multimodal approach.
B. Types of pain.
   1. Nociceptive pain.
      a. Somatic pain—associated mostly with surgery, results from damage to connective tissue, muscle, bone, and skin.
      b. Visceral pain—associated with pain in internal organs.
   2. Can be described as aching, pressure, or sharp.
   3. Associated with periosteum, joints, muscle injury, colic, and muscle spasm.
   4. Can have effects on various systems such as:
      a. Cardiovascular—increased heart rate and blood pressure.
      b. Pulmonary—decreased deep breathing.
      c. Endocrine—decrease in insulin production, fluid retention.
      d. Metabolic—increased blood sugar.
      e. Gastrointestinal—delayed gastric emptying, nausea, decreased motility, and potential for ileus.
   5. Neuropathic pain—may result from injury to nerves during surgery.
   6. Psychogenic pain—may be due to psychological factors that exaggerate pain problem.
C. Assessment of pain.
   1. Wong–Baker Visual Analog Scale—uses pictures to help the patients express how much pain they are in.
   2. Numerical rating scale—rating scale that rates pain from 0 to 10 with 0 being no pain and 10 being the worst pain imaginable.
   3. Verbal rating scale—patient reports pain on four possible points: No pain, mild pain, moderate pain, severe pain.
   4. Elements of pain assessment.
      a. Onset and pattern of pain.
      b. Location.
      c. Quality of pain.
      d. Intensity of pain.
      e. Aggravating or relieving factors.
      f. Previous treatment.
      g. Effect on physical function, emotional distress.
      h. Consider barriers that might affect reliability of pain assessment.
D. Nonpharmacological management of pain.
   1. Relaxation therapy.
   2. Hypnosis.
   3. Cold or heat.
   4. Splinting of wounds.
   5. Compression binders.
   6. Teach patient about benefits of transcutaneous electrical nerve stimulation (TENS unit) and acupuncture in the outpatient setting.

E. Pharmacological management of pain.

  1. World Health Organization (WHO) analgesic ladder.

    a. Mild pain—nonopioids.

    b. Moderate pain—use weak opioids with or without nonopioids.

    c. Severe pain—use strong opioids with or without nonopioids.

  2. Pain medication options.

    a. Nonopioids.

      i. Nonsteroidal anti-inflammatory drugs (NSAIDs): Use cautiously due to their antiplatelet effect and concern for delayed bone healing and acute renal failure. Caution in elderly, may need to adjust doses.

      ii. NSAIDs such as ketorolac are commonly used after major orthopedic surgery and spine surgery. They are highly effective, but carry the perceived risk of increased bleeding. To date there are NO human studies that exist to support this belief, only animal studies. NSAID use remains controversial after surgery.

        1) Ketorolac: 15 to 30 mg every 6 × 48 hours.

        2) Ibuprofen: 800 mg every 8 hours.

        3) Diclofenac: 50 mg every 8 hours.

      iii. Acetaminophen: 1,000 mg every 6 hours—maximum dosage per day is 4 g in a patient without liver dysfunction.

      iv. Adjuvant medications.

        1) Steroids such as dexamethasone.

        2) Antidepressants such as nortriptyline, desipramine, and amitriptyline.

        3) Anticonvulsants—gabapentin, pregabalin, and carbamazepine.

        4) N-methyl-D-aspartate (NMDA) receptor antagonists for neuropathic pain—ketamine infusion.

        5) Cannabinoids.

        6) Lidocaine patch.

        7) Lidocaine infusion.

    b. Opioids—weak.

      i. Codeine oral 30 mg every 4 to 6 hours.

      ii. Tramadol oral 50 to 100 mg every 4 to 6 hours.

      iii. Propoxyphene oral 100 mg every 4 hours.

      iv. Oxycodone low dose oral 5 mg every 4 to 6 hours.

      v. Hydrocodone oral 5 to 10 mg every 4 to 6 hours.

        1) Contains acetaminophen and needs to be calculated in 4 g/day limit.

    c. Opioids—strong.

      i. Morphine intravenous (IV) 5 to 10 mg q3 hours.

      ii. Fentanyl IV 25 mg per hour for breakthrough.

      iii. Hydromorphone IV 1 to 2 mg q3 hours.

        1) Elderly patients consider starting with 0.25 to 0.5 mg.

      iv. Oxycodone high dose oral—10 to 15 mg every 4 hours.

    d. Special considerations of opioid use in the elderly.

      i. Start with low doses.

      ii. Consider longer dosing intervals.

      iii. Slow titration to find optimal dose.

    e. Interventional therapy.

      i. Nerve blocks.

      ii. Epidural analgesia with or without opioids.

      iii. Spinal analgesia (intrathecal opioid).

F. Delivery of pain medications.

  1. Oral is preferred route of delivery for patients who can take oral medications.

    a. Scheduled.

    b. PRN.

  2. Subcutaneous.

    a. Good absorption.

    b. Onset more rapid.

    c. Can have longer duration of action.

    d. Be aware that absorption may be unpredictable, especially if the peripheries are poorly perfused.

  3. Intravenous push.

    a. Scheduled.

    b. PRN.

  4. Patient-controlled analgesia (PCA) pumps.

    a. Used when parenteral route is needed for systemic analgesia for more than a few hours.

    b. Avoid basal rate in opioid naïve adults.

    c. Dosed until pain relief, or patient becomes symptomatic—increased somnolence, hypoxemia, or hypotension.

Bibliography

American Society of Anesthesiologists Task Force on Acute Pain Management. (2012). Practice guidelines for acute pain management in the perioperative setting: An updated report by the American Society of Anesthesiologists task force on acute pain management anesthesiology. *Anesthesiology, 116*(2), 248–273. doi:10.1097/ALN.0b013e31823c1030

Buvanedran, A., & Kroin, J. S. (2009). Multimodal analgesia for controlling acute postoperative pain. *Current Opinion Anesthesiology, 22*(5), 588–593. doi:10.1097/ACO.0b013e328330373a

Dahl, J. B., Nielsen, R. V., Nikolajsen, L., Hamunen, K., Kontinen, V. K., Hansen, M. S., . . . Mathiesen, O. (2014). Postoperative analgesic effects of paracetamol, NSAID's, glucocorticoids, gabapentinoids and their combination: A topical review. *Acta Anaesthesiologica Scandinavica, 58*(10), 1165–1181. doi:10.1111/aas.12382

DeCosmo, G. (2015). The use of NSAIDs in the postoperative period: Advantages and disadvantages. *Journal of Anesthesia & Critical Care, 3*(4), 00107. doi:10.15406/jaccoa.2015.03.00107

Garimella, V., & Cellini, C. (2013). Postoperative pain control. *Clinics Colon Rectal Surgery, 26*(3), 191–196. doi:10.1055/s-0033-1351138

Roden, A., & Sturman, E. (2009). Assessment & management of patients with wound-related pain. *Nursing Standard, 23*(45), 53–62. doi:10.7748/ns.23.45.53.s52

World Health Organization. (2009). *WHO's pain relief ladder.* Retrieved from http://www.who.int/cancer/palliative/painladder/en

World Union of Wound Healing Societies. (2007). *Principles of best practice: Minimizing pain at wound dressing-related procedures. A consensus document.* Toronto: WoundPedia.

III Procedures

- Ankle-Brachial Index Measurement
- Arterial Lines
- Bone Marrow Aspiration and Biopsy
- Bronchoscopy
- Central Venous Access
- Chest Tube Insertion
- Chest Tube Removal
- Digital Nerve Blocks
- Extracorporeal Membrane Oxygenation
- Endotracheal Intubation
- Endotracheal Extubation
- External Ventricular Drain
- Intraosseous Vascular Access
- Long Leg Casting
- Lumbar Puncture
- Peripherally Inserted Central Catheter Placement
- Reduction of the Ankles
- Reduction of the Fingers
- Reduction of the Hip
- Reduction of the Patella
- Reduction of the Shoulder
- Splinting
- Synovial Fluid Aspiration
- Thoracentesis
- Transpyloric Feeding Tube Placement

ANKLE-BRACHIAL INDEX MEASUREMENT

Kelly Cimino

DESCRIPTION

A. A tool used to objectively detect the presence of lower-extremity peripheral arterial disease (PAD).

B. Compares the blood pressure measured in the ankles with that of the arms.

INDICATIONS

A. Primary care setting.
 1. Used in a symptomatic patient, to diagnose PAD.
 2. Used in an asymptomatic patient, to assess the vascular risk for PAD.

B. Emergency or trauma setting.
 1. Useful to evaluate patients at risk for lower-extremity arterial injury, as follows.
 2. An ankle-brachial index (ABI) less than 0.90 suggests a need for further vascular imaging: Angiography in a stable patient, and operative exploration in an unstable patient.
 3. An ABI greater than 0.90 decreased the likelihood of an arterial injury; thus, the patient may be observed with serial ABI assessments or may undergo a vascular study on a delayed basis.

PRECAUTIONS

A. ABI measurement is contraindicated in the following patients.
 1. Patients with the presence of deep vein thrombosis. Obtaining an ABI measurement could lead to a thrombus dislodgement.
 2. Patients with excruciating pain in their legs.

EQUIPMENT REQUIRED

A. Blood pressure cuff—appropriate size for upper and lower extremities.

B. Sphygmomanometer.

C. Doppler device.

D. Ultrasound transmission gel.

E. Examination table.

PROCEDURE

A. Place the patient in the supine position, with the arms and legs at the same level as the heart, for a minimum of 10 minutes before measurement.

B. Obtain brachial systolic pressures of both arms using the Doppler device.

C. Choose the higher of the two values as the "brachial systolic pressure."

D. Obtain the posterior tibial and dorsalis pedis systolic pressures of the extremity in question, and choose the higher of the two values as the "ankle pressure measurement" (see Figure 1).

E. Divide the ankle pressure by the brachial artery pressure; the result is the ABI.

EVALUATION AND RESULTS

A. Values obtained for the ABI are interpreted in Table 1.

CLINICAL PEARLS

A. Patients who are unable to remain supine for the duration of the examination are not candidates for an adequate ABI.

B. Any form of sedative or anesthetic may affect the accuracy of the examination because of the effect on blood pressure.

C. Patients with an ABI less than 0.90 have a higher risk of coronary artery disease, stroke, and death, and therefore should be referred to a credentialed vascular laboratory for further testing.

D. Claudication is a specific, but not a sensitive, finding in patients with PAD.
 1. One study reports that up to 90% of patients with a documented ABI of less than 0.90 did not report claudication as a symptom.

(continued)

ANKLE-BRACHIAL INDEX MEASUREMENT *(continued)*

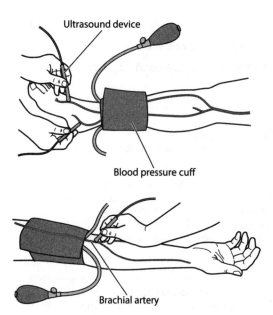

FIGURE 1 Ankle-brachial index test.

TABLE 1	Interpretation of Values Obtained for the ABI
ABI Reading	**Interpretation of the ABI for PAD**
1.00–1.29	Normal
0.91–0.99	Borderline
0.41–0.90	Mild to moderate disease—sufficient to cause claudication
≤0.40	Severe disease—sufficient to cause resting pain or gangrene
≥1.30	Noncompressible disease—severely calcified vessel

Source: Data from Rooke, T. W., Hirsch, A. T., Misra, S., Sidawy, A. N., Beckman, J. A., Findeiss, L. K., . . . Zierler, R. E. (2011, November 1). 2011 ACCF/AHA focused update of the guideline for the management of patients with peripheral artery disease (updating the 2005 guideline): A report of the American College of Cardiology Foundation/American Heart Association Task Force on Practice Guidelines. *Journal of the American College of Cardiology, 58*(19), 2020–2045. doi:10.1016/j.jacc.2011.08.023

E. An ABI of 0.91 to 0.99 is borderline.
   1. The patient may be asymptomatic at rest, but may experience symptoms related to the compromised vascular flow when ambulating.
   2. Exercise test may help evaluate a patient who has borderline ABI results.

F. Heavily calcified vessels may falsely elevate ankle pressure measurements, providing a false positive.

BIBLIOGRAPHY

Bailey, M. A., Griffin, K. J., & Scott, D. J. (2014, December). Clinical assessment of patients with peripheral arterial disease. *Seminars in Interventional Radiology, 31*(4), 292–299. doi:10.1055/s-0034-1393964

Davies, J. H., Kenkre, J., & Williams, E. M. (2014, April 17). Current utility of the ankle-brachial index (ABI) in general practice: Implications for its use in cardiovascular disease screening. *BMC Family Practice, 15*, 69. doi:10.1186/1471-2296-15-69

Ferket, B. S., Spronk, S., Colkesen, E. B., & Hunink, M. G. (2012). Systematic review of guidelines on peripheral artery disease screening. *The American Journal of Medicine, 125*(2), 198. doi:10.1016/j.amjmed.2011.06.027

Rooke, T. W., Hirsch, A. T., Misra, S., Sidawy, A. N., Beckman, J. A., Findeiss, L. K., . . . Zierler, R. E. (2011, November 1). 2011 ACCF/AHA focused update of the guideline for the management of patients with peripheral artery disease (updating the 2005 guideline): A report of the American College of Cardiology Foundation/American Heart Association Task Force on Practice Guidelines. *Journal of the American College of Cardiology, 58*(19), 2020–2045. doi:10.1016/j.jacc.2011.08.023

ARTERIAL LINES

Heather Warren Cook

DESCRIPTION

A. Insertion of arterial catheter.
   1. Radial.
   2. Brachial.
   3. Femoral.
   4. Dorsalis pedis.
   5. Axillary.

INDICATIONS

A. Frequent blood gas monitoring: Patient in respiratory distress or metabolic derangements.

B. Continuous blood pressure monitoring.
   1. Sepsis.
   2. Patient on vasopressors.

C. Continuous monitoring of cardiac output and stroke volume.

PRECAUTIONS

A. When inserting an arterial line there are a few precautions to be aware of.

B. Pain at the insertion site may cause the patient to pull away or move the arm.

C. Bleeding can occur with arterial punctures and multiple attempts, especially if the patient is on anticoagulants or antiplatelet agents; holding pressure with the arm elevated may help hemostasis to occur.

D. Any puncture through the skin can provide access for potential infection.

E. Hematomas can occur at the insertion site.
   1. Nerves run laterally along arteries and can be injured during insertion; make sure to palpate the pulse when inserting the arterial catheter (see Figures 1 and 2).

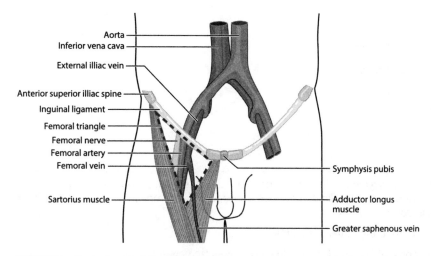

FIGURE 1 Illustration depicting femoral anatomy.

EQUIPMENT REQUIRED

A. Sterile gloves.

B. Sterile gauze/towels.

C. Sterile drape.

D. Sterile clear adhesive dressing.

E. Chlorhexidine/Betadine for skin preparation.

F. Appropriate catheter size for cannulation of the artery.

G. Sutures.

(continued)

ARTERIAL LINES (*continued*)

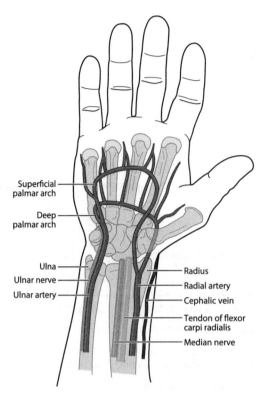

FIGURE 2 Illustration depicting radial anatomy.

H. Adhesive tape.

I. Arm-board.

J. Pressure tubing.

K. 500 to 1,000 mL 0.9 NSS bag.

L. Pressure bag for 0.9 NSS bag.

M. 1% Lidocaine 5 mL vial.

N. Pressure tubing.

O. Transducer.

PROCEDURE

A. Arterial line placement is typically done at the bedside while the patient is in a supine position. Any arterial line placement collateral blood flow to the limb should be checked. For example: Perform the Allen test on the wrist prior to radial artery cannulation.

B. Explain the procedure to the patient and family.

C. Obtain informed consent unless the procedure is an urgent/emergent need.

D. Wash hands/perform hand hygiene.

E. Perform a procedural "time out" with the nursing staff.

F. Perform Allen test/check pulses.

G. R/L extremity is supinated.

H. Position patient with tape and arm-board (if using radial).

I. Sterilize area with chlorhexidine/Betadine as per protocol.

J. Place sterile drape over the extremity.

K. Open all equipment needed for cannulation.

L. Have pressure bag/saline/transducer cord prepared by RN for monitoring.

(*continued*)

ARTERIAL LINES *(continued)*

M. Don sterile gloves, personal protective equipment, and goggles/face shield.

N. Palpate pulse and visualize with bedside ultrasound.

O. Inject around the site with 1% lidocaine to numb the area.

P. Using the appropriate catheter with introducer needle, hold with dominant hand (like a pencil) at a 35° angle to the extremity.

Q. Insert needle below area of palpation and view window of catheter for a flash of blood.

R. Simultaneously, visualize needle advancement into vessel lumen with bedside ultrasound (see Figure 3).

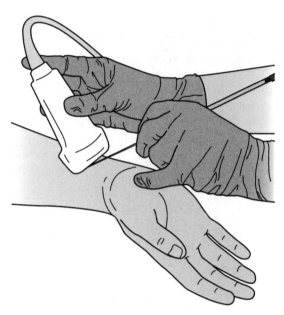

FIGURE 3   Ultrasound-guided insertion of a radial arterial catheter.

S. After obtaining flash, using the nondominant hand advance the wire to secure the position of the catheter (the wire should advance smoothly).

T. Slowly advance the catheter over the wire/needle into the vessel.

U. Hold pressure above the catheter insertion site and remove the wire/needle.

V. Attach pressure tubing and view monitor for an appropriate waveform.

W. Once this is confirmed, suture line in place and cover insertion site with sterile clear adhesive dressing.

X. Remove sterile drape and dispose of all sharps in sharps container.

Y. Document procedure, number of attempts, and any complications in the patient's record.

EVALUATION AND RESULTS

A. Have the nurse level, zero, and flush the arterial line showing the square wave test and adequate whip.

B. Assess the arterial waveform for the systolic upstroke, dicrotic notch, and diastolic runoff.

C. The line is now useful for closer blood pressure monitoring, trending arterial blood gasses, and drawing frequent labs in the critically ill patient.

(continued)

ARTERIAL LINES (*continued*)

CLINICAL PEARLS

A. Notify the nurse prior to performing procedure.

B. Always perform "time out" prior to any procedure.

C. Have all of the equipment needed for the procedure set up and opened before donning sterile gloves.

D. Hold firm pressure or cover catheter opening with thumb, preventing pulsatile blood from coming out of the catheter before attaching pressure tubing.

E. If hematoma occurs, hold firm pressure and apply pressure dressing.

F. Always start at the most distal place on the extremity if possible.

BIBLIOGRAPHY

Koyfman, A., Radwine, Z., & Sawyer, J. L. (2018, March 16). Arterial line placement. In V. Lopez Rowe (Ed.), *Medscape*. Retrieved from https://emedicine.medscape.com/article/1999586-overview

Tegtmeyer, K., Brady, G., Lai, S., Hodo, R., & Braner, D. (2006). Placement of an arterial line. *The New England Journal of Medicine, 354*, e13. doi:10.1056/NEJMvcm044149

BONE MARROW ASPIRATION AND BIOPSY

Jerrad M. Stoddard

DESCRIPTION

A. Bone marrow.
   1. Consists of hematopoietic stem cells, which produce red blood cells, white blood cells, and platelets.
   2. Found in axial bones including the sternum, ribs, vertebral bodies, skull, and pelvis.

B. Used for the diagnosis and staging of hematologic conditions/malignancies, such as aplastic anemia, multiple myeloma, leukemias, and lymphomas.

C. Bone marrow examination includes the assessment of bone marrow cellularity (age dependent), cellular morphology, and maturation.

D. Ancillary tests are often performed on a bone marrow specimen.
   1. Cytogenetics.
   2. Fluorescent in situ hybridization (FISH).
   3. Molecular testing.

INDICATIONS

A. Evaluation of unexplained abnormal peripheral blood counts or suspected hematologic disease.

B. Diagnosis and staging of lymphoma or solid tumors.

C. Evaluation of fever of unknown origin.

PRECAUTIONS

A. Primary risks of the procedure are bleeding or infection.

B. Absolute contraindications include uncorrected coagulopathies or thrombocytopenia.
   1. Disseminated intravascular coagulopathy.
   2. Severe hemophilia.
   3. Severe thrombocytopenia (platelet count <10,000/µL).

C. The only relative contraindication is anticoagulation.
   1. Consider holding anticoagulation (if clinically appropriate) prior to procedure.
   2. Anticoagulants can be resumed the day after the bone marrow procedure.
   3. MD Anderson guidelines for holding common anticoagulants are listed in Table 1.

D. Patients with suspected multiple myeloma should *NEVER* undergo sternal aspiration due to bone fragility and risk of sternal perforation.

E. Assess for allergies to anesthetics (e.g., lidocaine).

EQUIPMENT REQUIRED

A. Bone marrow aspiration/biopsy kits contain all required materials, as noted in steps C and D in the text that follows.

B. Anxiolytics (e.g., midazolam or alprazolam) if patient is anxious.

C. Equipment required for procedure.
   1. Sterile gloves.
   2. Drape for sterile field.
   3. Iodine or chlorhexidine solution.
   4. Buffered lidocaine (1% or 2%) ± epinephrine solution.
   5. Luer lock syringes.
      a. 5 mL syringe for local anesthesia.
      b. 20 mL syringe for aspiration.
   6. Needles for local anesthesia.
      a. ~25 ga × 5/8² needle for subcutaneous administration.
      b. ~20 ga × 1–1/2² needle for deep administration.
   7. Sterile gauze and bandages.
   8. Bone marrow needle with stylet for aspiration.
   9. Jamshidi biopsy needle with stylet.

D. Equipment required for obtained specimens.
   1. All tubes and slides should be labeled with patient information.
   2. Labeled collection tubes.
   3. Labeled glass slides and coverslips.
   4. Petri dish and pipette.

(continued)

BONE MARROW ASPIRATION AND BIOPSY (continued)

| TABLE 1 | Guidelines for Holding Anticoagulation Prior to Bone Marrow Procedure |

Medication	When to Hold
Aspirin or NSAIDs	No need to hold
Heparin products • Heparin • Enoxaparin (Lovenox) • Dalteparin (Fragmin)	Morning of procedure
Factor Xa inhibitors • Apixaban (Eliquis) • Rivaroxaban (Xarelto) • Fondaparinux (Arixtra)	2 days prior to procedure
Direct thrombin inhibitors (univalent) • Argatroban (Acova) • Dabigatran (Pradaxa)	2 days prior to procedure
Warfarin (Coumadin)	3 days prior to procedure (and INR <2.0)
Platelet inhibitors • Prasugrel (Effient) • Clopidogrel (Plavix)	5 days prior to procedure

INR, international normalized ratio; NSAIDs, nonsteroidal anti-inflammatory drugs.
Sources: Patel, I. J., Davidson, J. C., Nikolic, B., Salazar, G. M., Schwartzberg, M. S., Walker, T. G., . . . Saad, W. A. (2012). Consensus guidelines for periprocedural management of coagulation status and hemostasis risk in percutaneous image-guided interventions. *Journal of Vascular and Interventional Radiology, 23*(6), 727–736. doi:10.1016/ j.jvir.2012.02.012; Pudusseri, A., & Spyropoulos, A. C. (2014). Management of anticoagulants in the periprocedural period for patients with cancer. *Journal of the National Comprehensive Cancer Network, 12*(12), 1713–1720. doi: https://doi.org/10.6004/ jnccn.2014.0173. Spyropoulos, A. C., & Douketis, J. D. (2012). How I treat anticoagulated patients undergoing an elective procedure or surgery. *Blood, 120*(15), 2954–2962. doi:10.1182/blood-2012-06-415943.

PROCEDURE

A. Can be performed on posterior iliac crest (most common), anterior iliac crest, sternum, or tibia. As bone marrow aspiration and biopsy on sites other than the posterior iliac crest are not commonly performed, the focus of this procedure will be on the preferred site of the posterior iliac crest.

B. Sternal biopsies are contraindicated, and only aspiration can be performed.

C. Some facilities use ultrasound or CT guided aspirations/biopsies; however, the procedure is commonly done with palpation alone.

D. The procedure.
1. Explain the procedure to the patient and family and obtain informed consent.
2. Wash hands/perform hand hygiene.
3. Perform a proper time out. All present in the room must identify the patient and agree on the correct procedure and correct site of the procedure.
4. Administer premedications (e.g., alprazolam) if needed.
5. Position patient in prone (recommended) or lateral decubitus position.
6. Palpate for posterior iliac crest.
7. Select and mark site.
   a. Approximately three finger widths from the midline and two finger widths (see Figure 1A, B) inferior to the posterior iliac crest.
   b. Avoid areas concerning for skin or soft tissue infection (e.g., erythema or induration).
8. Using sterile technique, open the bone marrow tray and inspect all components.
9. Cleanse the marked area with povidone-iodine solution or chlorhexidine and drape the sterile field.
10. Anesthetize the skin and subcutaneous tissue of the marked site with 1% or 2% lidocaine solution using a 23-gauge needle.
    a. Perform aspiration.

(continued)

BONE MARROW ASPIRATION AND BIOPSY *(continued)*

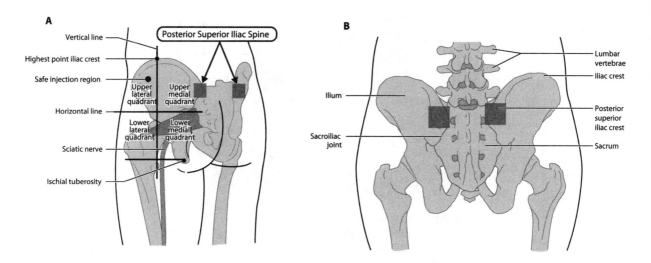

FIGURE 1 (A) Pelvic anatomy for bone marrow procedures. (B) The posterior superior iliac crest is a bony prominence located superolateral to the coccyx (indicated by the gray box)

    i. Place middle finger and index finger on either side of the marked site.
    ii. Insert a 21-gauge needle into the marked site between the fingers and advance to the periosteum at a perpendicular angle.
    iii. Anesthetize the periosteum by continually injecting small amounts of lidocaine on the bone surface (approximately a quarter-sized area).
    iv. Make note of the angle of the needle and the landscape of the bone (particularly flat areas).
    v. Allow 2 to 3 minutes for local anesthesia to take effect. In the meantime, prepare the bone marrow tray.
    vi. Insert the bone marrow needle with stylet in place perpendicular to the marked site (see Figure 2) with the same approach and angle as the anesthetic needle.
    vii. Gently approach the periosteum and ensure that area is anesthetized (patients should only experience dull sensations).
    viii. Steadily rotate the needle back and forth in a twisting motion to advance through the bone cortex.
    ix. Once the needle enters the marrow space, a "give" is felt, and the patient may note discomfort.
    x. Ensure the needle is anchored in the bone and remove the stylet.
    xi. Attach a 10 to 20 mL syringe to the aspiration needle.
    xii. Aspirate 1 mL of marrow initially and aliquot for the clot section.
    xiii. Additional aspirates will be required for smears and ancillary testing (e.g., flow cytometry, cytogenetics, molecular testing). An assistant should handle the smears while the proceduralist continues to aspirate.
    xiv. In general, it is not recommended to aspirate greater than 5 mL at a time as the contents may clot.
  b. Perform biopsy (if required).
    i. Using the same site, advance a Jamshidi needle into the cortical bone with a steady twisting motion until the needle is firmly lodged (see Figure 2).
    ii. Remove the stylet.
    iii. Advise the patient that he or she should anticipate a dull, aching pressure.
    iv. Advance the needle 1 to 2 cm with a rotating motion applying pressure.
    v. Once an adequate core biopsy depth is attained, rotate the needle 360° in both directions several times to separate the biopsy from surrounding tissue.
    vi. Slowly remove the biopsy specimen by gently pulling and rotating the needle.
    vii. Insert the stylet into the distal end of the needle after it has been removed from the body to expel the biopsy specimen onto a slide.
    viii. Inspect the biopsy specimen for adequate size (1–2 cm). A second attempt may be required to obtain a complete specimen.
    ix. Send specimen to pathology with the equipment used to collect it.
  c. Apply dressing.
    i. Hold pressure over the site for hemostasis.
    ii. Use alcohol prep pads to cleanse the area.
    iii. Apply sterile gauze and affix a pressure bandage.
    iv. Advise patient to leave dressing intact and dry (no bathing/swimming) for 24 or 48 hours (if biopsy performed).

(continued)

BONE MARROW ASPIRATION AND BIOPSY (*continued*)

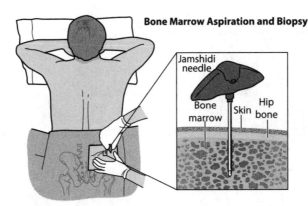

FIGURE 2 Bone marrow aspiration and biopsy. The Jamshidi needle is perpendicularly inserted into the posterior iliac crest through the outer bony cortex and into the spongy bone marrow.

EVALUATION AND RESULTS

A. Evaluation of the bone marrow aspiration and biopsy includes the following.
  1. Microscopic evaluation.
  2. Immunohistochemical staining.
  3. Flow cytometry, cytogenetics.
  4. FISH.
  5. Molecular testing, and/or cultures.

CLINICAL PEARLS

A. Maintain dialog with the patient throughout the procedure and guide him or her through the process so the patient anticipates needles, aspiration, and so on.

B. Once the periosteum is anesthetized, the patient should only experience a dull, aching sensation.
  1. If the patient experiences sharp pain during the procedure, consider repositioning the needle to the anesthetized area or giving additional local anesthetic.

C. If the initial aspirate does not yield any contents, replace the stylet and advance the needle further.
  1. If multiple attempts are unsuccessful, consider another site.

D. Disease-specific issues.
  1. Use caution when advancing the aspirate or biopsy needle through the bony cortex in elderly patients or patients with multiple myeloma. Osteoporotic bone is weak, and the needle can penetrate the bone with little pressure.
  2. Aspiration for patients with myeloproliferative disorders (e.g., myelofibrosis) may result in a "dry tap" due to increased marrow fibrosis. Consider repositioning the needle to another anesthetized site.

BIBLIOGRAPHY

Bain, B. J. (2001, September). Bone marrow aspiration. *Journal Clinical Pathology, 54*(9), 657–663.
Patel, I. J., Davidson, J. C., Nikolic, B., Salazar, G. M., Schwartzberg, M. S., Walker, T. G., . . . Saad, W. A. (2012). Consensus guidelines for periprocedural management of coagulation status and hemostasis risk in percutaneous image-guided interventions. *Journal of Vascular and Interventional Radiology, 23*(6), 727–736. doi:10.1016/ j.jvir.2012.02.012
Pudusseri, A., & Spyropoulos, A. C. (2014). Management of anticoagulants in the periprocedural period for patients with cancer. *Journal of the National Comprehensive Cancer Network, 12*(12), 1713–1720. doi: https://doi.org/10.6004/jnccn.2014.0173.
Radhakrishnan, N. (2017). Bone marrow aspiration and biopsy. In E. C. Besa (Ed.), *Medscape*. Retrieved from https://emedicine .medscape.com/article/207575-overview
Spyropoulos, A. C., & Douketis, J. D. (2012). How I treat anticoagulated patients undergoing an elective procedure or surgery. *Blood, 120*(15), 2954–2962. doi:10.1182/blood-2012-06-415943

BRONCHOSCOPY

E. Moneé Carter-Griffin

DESCRIPTION

A. Direct visualization of the lower airways (e.g., trachea, bronchi, and bronchioles) with a scope containing a camera.

B. Most institutions have a bronchoscopy cart with all the required equipment, including a video screen to allow for visualization.

C. Typically, a respiratory therapist and/or a nurse will assist with the procedure.

INDICATIONS

A. Identifying the cause of hemoptysis or other symptoms that indicate endobronchial disease.

B. Obtaining samples for pathology of abnormal spots or lesions noted on imaging.

C. Diagnosis and staging of lung carcinomas.

D. Removal of excessive secretions, mucus plugs, polyps, and so on.

E. Removal of foreign objects.

F. Assistance with difficult intubations and to verify endotracheal tube placement.

G. Use during and postprocedural (e.g., dilation of tracheal stenosis).

H. Postoperative assessment of lung transplants.

PRECAUTIONS

A. Patients with coagulopathies: Aggressive suctioning or endobronchial interventions can cause bleeding.

B. Avoid in patients with severe hypoxemia and/or those requiring increased ventilatory support (e.g., acute respiratory distress syndrome [ARDS]), if possible.

C. Can cause irritation to the vocal cords and airways leading to laryngospasm and bronchospasm, respectively.

EQUIPMENT REQUIRED

A. Bronchoscopy cart.

B. Bronchoscope with light source.

C. Bite block (only placed in intubated patient prior to bronchoscope insertion).

D. Swivel adapter for the bronchoscope.

E. Water-soluble lubricant.

F. Gauze (used to wipe secretions from the bronchoscope).

G. Suction tubing and suction device (e.g., wall suction unit or device on bronchoscopy cart).

H. Sterile bowl.

I. 10 to 20 mL syringes (2–3).

J. Saline (nonbacteriostatic).

K. Sputum trap if collecting a specimen.

L. Gloves, mask, and eye protection.

M. Moderate sedation medications.

PROCEDURE

A. Explain the procedure to the patient and family.

B. Always identify the patient and obtain informed consent.

C. Ensure the patient has intravenous (IV) access and hemodynamic monitoring (e.g., blood pressure, O_2 saturations, etc.) throughout the entirety of the procedure.

(continued)

BRONCHOSCOPY (*continued*)

D. Assemble all equipment prior to procedure.

E. Ensure the light source is working on the bronchoscope.

F. Connect suction tubing to the bronchoscope and a suction device.

G. Add saline to the sterile bowl.

H. Fill the syringes with saline prior to starting the procedure. The saline can be used to help with secretion clearance and for collection of a bronchoalveolar lavage (BAL).

I. Determine the entry route for the bronchoscope.
   1. Nonintubated patient: Nose is preferred entry site.
   2. Intubated patient: Bronchoscope will enter through the existing endotracheal tube.

J. If the patient has a preexisting endotracheal tube, adjust the ventilator settings by increasing the fraction of inspired oxygen to 100% and placing the patient on assist control. Connect the swivel adapter to the endotracheal tube.

K. If the patient is not receiving mechanical ventilation, then an oxygen source is typically applied (e.g., nasal cannula).

L. Prior to procedure initiation, don a gown, gloves, mask, and eye protection.

M. Instruct the assistant to administer moderate sedation to assist with comfort and tolerance of the procedure.

N. Apply the water-soluble lubricant to the bronchoscope.

O. In a nonintubated patient: Insert the bronchoscope through the nose. In an intubated patient: Insert the bronchoscope through the swivel adapter connected to the endotracheal tube (see Figure 1).

P. Advance the bronchoscope through the trachea and into the lungs.
   1. The indications for performing bronchoscopy will determine what interventions are completed (e.g., aspiration of secretions, biopsy of a lesion, removal of foreign objects, etc.).
   2. Prior to removing the bronchoscope, inspect the lungs for hemostasis or evidence of possible complications from the procedure.

Q. Once the procedure is complete, remove the bronchoscope.

R. Send a specimen collected in sputum trap to pathology and/or microbiology.

S. Obtain a chest x-ray postprocedure to assess lungs.

T. Document the procedure, indication, diagnostics sent, any complications, and the patient's tolerance of the procedure.

EVALUATION AND RESULTS

A. Results will vary on the rationale for performing the procedure.

B. Results could include clearance of secretions and mucus plugs, resulting in better oxygenation, identification of lesions for appropriate treatment, and so on.

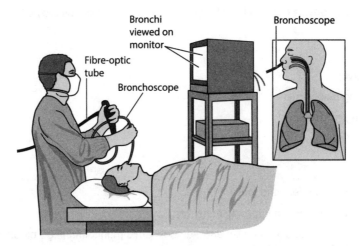

FIGURE 1 Illustration depicting bronchoscopy procedure.

(*continued*)

BRONCHOSCOPY *(continued)*

CLINICAL PEARLS

A. If using a traditional bronchoscope, the patient will need at least a 7.5 size endotracheal tube to pass the bronchoscope into the lungs.

B. The use of saline can help remove thick secretions from the airway.

BIBLIOGRAPHY

Du Rand, I. A., Blaikley, J., Booton, R., Chaudhuri, N., Gupta, V., Khalid, S., . . . Munavvar, M. (2013, August). British Thoracic Society guideline for diagnostic flexible bronchoscopy in adults: Accredited by NICE. *Thorax, 68*(Suppl. 1), i1–i44. doi:10.1136/thoraxjnl-2013-203618

Lessnau, K.-D., & Lazo, K. (2017, March 23). Transbronchial biopsy techniques. , In Z. Mosenifar (Ed.), *Medscape*. Retrieved from https://emedicine.medscape.com/article/1894323-technique

CENTRAL VENOUS ACCESS

Alison M. Kelley and Heather Meissen

DESCRIPTION

A. A central venous catheter (CVC), also called a central line, is a thin, flexible catheter which is percutaneously placed and whose tip sits in the central circulation (see Figure 1).

B. Ideal location of the tip is the superior vena cava (SVC).

INDICATIONS

A. Rapid administration of intravenous (IV) fluids (in the setting of sepsis, trauma, shock, burns) or blood products.

B. Inadequate peripheral access.

C. Emergent venous access.

D. Administration of medications more likely to cause vascular damage when administered peripherally, including:
  1. Vasopressors.
  2. Inotropes.
  3. Chemotherapy.
  4. Total parenteral nutrition.
  5. Hypertonic solutions such as 3%, 7.5%, and 23.4% saline.

E. Administration of incompatible drugs.

F. Access for placement of pulmonary artery catheters (PACs), hemodialysis catheters, and plasmapheresis catheters.

G. Hemodynamic monitoring, including central venous pressure (CVP).

H. Measurement of central venous oxygen saturation (SVO_2).

I. Cardiac pressures via PAC including CVP, pulmonary artery systolic and diastolic pressures, and pulmonary artery wedge pressure.

J. Measurement of mixed venous oxygen saturation, SVO_2, from a PAC.

K. Frequent blood draws (in patients without arterial lines).

L. Transvenous cardiac pacing.

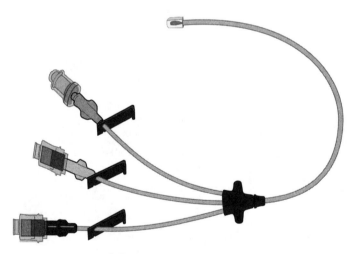

FIGURE 1   Illustration of a CVC.
CVC, central venous catheter.

(continued)

CENTRAL VENOUS ACCESS (*continued*)

PRECAUTIONS

A. In order to help prevent complications, the following precautions, taken by an experienced provider, should be utilized when inserting a CVC.

B. Ultrasound (US) guidance.
   1. Use of US guidance for placement of internal jugular (IJ) CVCs is now considered gold standard (see Figure 2).
      a. US guidance has been proven to decrease complications, especially arterial cannulation.
      b. US guidance for insertion of central venous access in subclavian and femoral veins has less evidence and requires further research.

C. Manometry is one of three ways of measuring pressure during CVC insertion in order to ensure venous rather than arterial puncture.
   1. Once the operator has inserted the needle into a vessel and has blood return, a sterile tube is connected to the hub of the needle or catheter.
   2. Tubing should then be filled with blood. This is done by lowering the sterile tubing below the level of the vein.
   3. The tubing is then held vertically over the patient. This allows for the blood level to equilibrate with venous pressure.
      a. If the needle is in an artery, the blood will continue to rise up the tube.
      b. If the needle is in the vein, the blood will begin to travel back down the column.

D. Operators should choose US guidance and pressure manometry (see Figure 3) as techniques to reduce complications. While dynamic US guidance helps reduce the risk of arterial sticks, pressure manometry reduces the risk of arterial cannulation.

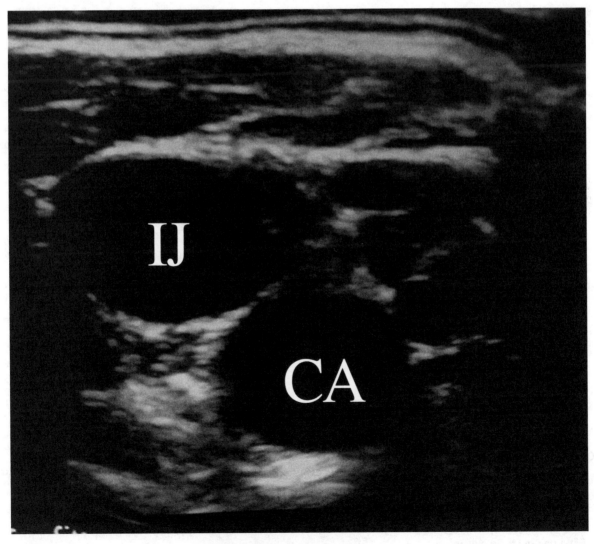

FIGURE 2 US showing IJ and CA.
CA, carotid artery; IJ, internal jugular; US, ultrasound.

(*continued*)

CENTRAL VENOUS ACCESS *(continued)*

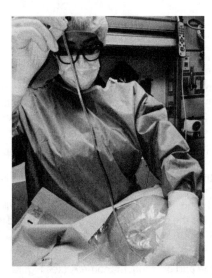

FIGURE 3 Image of a advanced practice provider demonstrating pressure manometry on a mannequin.

E. Additional precautions.
   1. The nurse must be present during all portions of the procedure.
   2. The provider must confirm correct catheter tip location via chest x-ray prior to use.
   3. Antibiotic impregnated CVCs are sometimes used when available; the provider should check institutional policies.
   4. The Pronovost Checklist has been shown to reduce CVC-related bloodstream infections when utilized together.
   5. Prior to donning sterile gloves, the practitioner should use an antimicrobial soap or alcohol sanitizer.
   6. Chlorhexidine.
      a. Prior to draping a patient, a sterile solution of chlorhexidine or Betadine should be applied to the site by scrubbing for 30 seconds.
      b. The site should then be allowed to air dry for at least 2 minutes.
   7. Maximal barrier precautions.
      a. A full body drape should be placed over the patient.
      b. All those performing the procedures should wear a mask, cap, sterile gown, and sterile gloves.
      c. Any additional persons present in the room should wear a mask and cap.
   8. Timely removal of CVC is desired when deemed no longer necessary.
   9. Avoid femoral vein insertion, which is associated with greater risk of infection as compared to the subclavian vein or jugular vein.

F. Multiple complications are associated with CVC placement, including but not limited to:
   1. Catheter-related infection.
   2. Catheter-related thrombosis.
   3. Arterial puncture.
   4. Arterial cannulation.
   5. Vascular injury.
   6. Arrhythmia.
   7. Bleeding.
   8. Venous air embolism.
   9. Pneumothorax.
   10. Hemothorax.

EQUIPMENT REQUIRED

A. CVC kit.

B. Caps and mask for everyone present in the room.

C. Sterile gown for all operators.

D. Extra pair of sterile gloves.

(continued)

CENTRAL VENOUS ACCESS *(continued)*

E. Sterile full body drape.

F. Sterile US probe cover.

G. Chlorhexidine.

H. Sterile saline.

I. Pressure tubing for manometry.

J. Central line dressing.

K. If provider does not have access to an US, consider using smaller gauge needles as a finder needle.

PROCEDURE

A. Placement of IJ CVC.
1. Explain the procedure to the patient and family.
2. Obtain consent for CVC placement based on the institution's policy.
3. Wash hands/perform hand hygiene.
4. Perform a proper time out. All present in the room must identify the patient and agree on the correct procedure and correct site of the procedure.
5. US patient anatomy prior to positioning of patient.
6. Place the patient in the Trendelenburg position. If the patient cannot tolerate the Trendelenburg, place the patient as flat as possible or consider placing a femoral line.
7. Have the patient turn his or her head 45° in the opposite direction of the side where the operator is placing the catheter (see Figure 4).
8. Prior to beginning procedure, use the US to identify the IJ vein and the carotid artery. The IJ is compressible when gentle pressure is applied. The artery is not (see Figure 5).
9. If not using an US, please see section on anatomical landmarks.
10. Ensure that everyone who will remain present in the room has on a surgical cap and mask.
11. Place a cap on the patient.
12. Open up the CVC tray.
13. Don sterile gown and sterile gloves.
14. Prepare the skin with chlorhexidine, per Centers for Disease Control and Prevention (CDC) guidelines.
15. Remove the sterile full body drape from the central line kit and drape it over the patient. There will be a hole, which should be placed over the site previously identified.
16. Set up a sterile kit in an orderly fashion. Ensure that all equipment is within arm's reach.

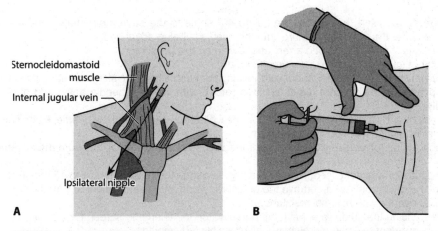

FIGURE 4 Landmarks for accessing the IJ vein. (A) Aim the needle toward the ipsilateral nipple. (B) Insert the needle at the apex of the SCM.
IJ, internal jugular; SCM, sternocleidomastoid muscle.

(continued)

CENTRAL VENOUS ACCESS (*continued*)

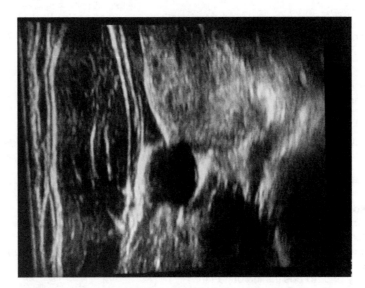

FIGURE 5 The IJ is being compressed with gentle pressure as evidenced by the oblong shape that is formed from the previous circular shape in Figure 2. The muscles around the CA make it much more difficult to compress the CA; therefore, it maintains its shape. Compression allows the practitioner to easily differentiate the two vessels.
CA, carotid artery; IJ, internal jugular.

17. Flush all ports of the catheter with sterile saline to ensure they are functioning properly.
18. Place a sterile US probe cover on the US probe.
19. Most kits provide 2% lidocaine without epinephrine.
    a. Draw up the desired amount of lidocaine in an available syringe.
    b. Replace the needle used to draw up lidocaine with a subcutaneous needle.
    c. Using the US, identify the IJ vein and center it in the middle of the US screen.
    d. While watching the US screen to identify the needle, make an initial stick with the needle.
    e. Prior to injecting lidocaine, draw back to ensure you do not have blood return.
    f. Inject lidocaine into the subcutaneous tissue.
20. Maintain visualization of the IJ in the center of the US field.
21. Continue to hold the US probe in the nondominant hand while picking up the introducer needle with the dominant hand.
22. With the bevel up, insert the needle at a 30° to 45° angle to the patient directed at the ipsilateral needle (see Figure 6). Aspirate the syringe the entire time the needle is being advanced.
23. Maintain visualization of the carotid artery and IJ vein on the US screen.
24. If one does not immediately aspirate venous blood.
    a. Slightly withdraw the needle, without withdrawing the needle from the skin, and attempt to angle more laterally.
    b. If this position also does not result in blood return, withdraw the needle again and attempt to angle more medially.
25. Once venous blood is aspirated, remove the syringe while securely holding the needle. Place finger over the needle hub in order to reduce the risk of air embolism.
26. Now, attach tubing for pressure measurement as discussed earlier. Other pressure measurements may also be used.
27. If the carotid artery was accessed, remove the needle and hold pressure for 10 to 15 minutes.
28. After venous entry is confirmed, remove the pressure tubing and insert the guide wire through the needle.
    a. It should advance with minimal resistance.
    b. While advancing the guide wire, have the nurse watch the telemetry screen for ectopy.
    c. It is also important to listen for telemetry alarms while advancing.
    d. Patients may experience some PVCs.
    e. If the patient goes into ventricular tachycardia (VT), completely remove the wire.
29. While holding the guide wire, remove the introducer needle. Never let go of the guide wire while it is in the patient.

(*continued*)

CENTRAL VENOUS ACCESS *(continued)*

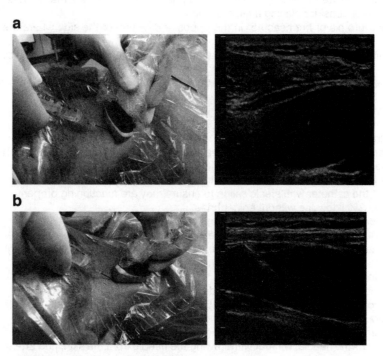

FIGURE 6 Accessing the IJ with US. (A) Direct the needle toward the center of the US probe. (B) Advance the needle forward and look for penetration of the needle into the vessel.

IJ, internal jugular; US, ultrasound.

Source: Reproduced with permission from Saugel, B., Scheeren, T. W. L., & Teboul, J.-L. (2017). Ultrasound-guided central venous catheter placement: A structured review and recommendations for clinical practice. *Critical Care, 21*, 225. doi:10.1186/s13054-017-1814-y

30. An additional confirmation of venous entry can be performed by obtaining a transverse view via US of the IJ vein and following the guide wire down to the vein.
31. Once the introducer needle has been removed, make a small nick in the skin at the site of entry while continuing to hold the guide wire. The nick should be made with the scalpel facing away from the operator and should be a small in-out stabbing motion.
32. Now, pass the dilator over the guide wire while continuing to hold the guide wire.
33. Dilate and retract the dilator while continuing to hold the guide wire.
34. Make sure the distal port does not have a cap on it so the guide wire can pass through.
35. Pass the catheter over the guide wire. The guide wire will come out the distal port.
36. Continue advancing the catheter while holding the guide wire.
    a. Once the guide wire can be seen coming out of the distal port of the catheter, grasp the guide wire.
    b. Finish advancing the catheter until the appropriate depth is reached.
37. While holding the catheter in place, pull out the guide wire. It should remove without any resistance.
38. Aspirate and flush each port to confirm blood return.
39. Suture the central line into place at the insertion site.
40. Clean the area again with the antiseptic of choice, most often chlorhexidine or Betadine.
41. Place a sterile dressing over the insertion site.
42. Obtain a chest x-ray for radiograph placement and to rule out a pneumothorax.
43. Proper placement on chest x-ray will demonstrate the tip of the catheter in the SVC.
44. Document the procedure appropriately in the patient's record.

B. Placement of subclavian CVC.
    1. Explain the procedure to the patient and family.
    2. Obtain consent for CVC placement based on the institution's policy.
    3. Wash hands/perform hand hygiene.
    4. Perform a proper time out. All present in the room must identify the patient and agree on the correct procedure and correct site of the procedure.
    5. US guidance is not able to be used in subclavian procedures due to the obstruction of the view of the vein by the clavicle.

(continued)

CENTRAL VENOUS ACCESS (*continued*)

6. Place the patient in the Trendelenburg position. If the patient cannot tolerate the Trendelenburg, place the patient as flat as possible or consider placing a femoral line.
7. Have the patient turn his or her head 45° in the opposite direction of the side where the operator is placing the catheter.
8. Prior to beginning the procedure, identify the landmarks—the sternal notch and the curve of the clavicle (see Figure 7).
9. Ensure that everyone who will remain present in the room has on a surgical cap and mask.
10. Place a cap on the patient.
11. Open up the CVC tray.
12. Don a sterile gown and sterile gloves.
13. Prepare the skin with chlorhexidine.
14. Remove the sterile full body drape from the central line kit and drape it over the patient. There will be a hole, which should be placed over the site previously identified.
15. Set up a sterile kit in an orderly fashion. Ensure that all equipment is within arm's reach.
16. Flush all ports of the catheter with sterile saline to ensure they are functioning properly.
17. Most kits provide 2% lidocaine without epinephrine.
    a. Draw up the desired amount of lidocaine in an available syringe.
    b. Replace the needle used to draw up lidocaine with a subcutaneous needle.
    c. Advance the subcutaneous needle into the subcutaneous tissue at the clavicular angle.
    d. Prior to injecting lidocaine, draw back to ensure you do not have blood return.
    e. Inject with lidocaine.
18. To access the subclavian vein, pick up the introducer needle with the dominant hand.
19. With the bevel up, insert the needle at a 30° to 45° angle to the patient directed at the sternal notch. Aspirate the syringe the entire time the needle is being advanced.
20. If one does not immediately aspirate venous blood.
    a. Slightly withdraw the needle, without withdrawing the needle from the skin, and attempt to angle more cephalad.
    b. If this position also does not result in blood return, withdraw the needle again and attempt to angle more caudal.
21. Once venous blood is aspirated, remove the syringe while securely holding the needle. Place a finger over the needle hub in order to reduce the risk of air embolism.
22. Now, attach tubing for pressure measurement as discussed earlier. Other pressure measurements may also be used.

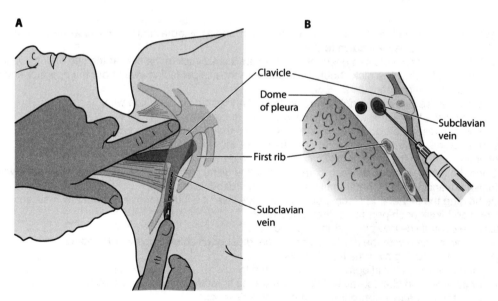

FIGURE 7 Advancing the needle in subclavian access. Direct the tip of the needle toward the sternal notch.
Source: Reichman, E. F. (Ed.). (2013). *Emergency medicine procedures* (2nd ed.). New York, NY: McGraw-Hill/Medical. Retrieved from https://accessemergencymedicine.mhmedical.com/content.aspx?bookid=683&sectionid=45343634.

(*continued*)

CENTRAL VENOUS ACCESS (*continued*)

23. If the subclavian artery was accessed, remove the needle and hold pressure for 10 to 15 minutes. The clavicle may make it difficult or impossible to hold direct pressure over the subclavian artery. Call a stat vascular consult if bleeding cannot be controlled.
24. After venous entry is confirmed, remove the pressure tubing and insert the guide wire through the needle.
    a. It should advance with minimal resistance.
    b. While advancing the guide wire, have the nurse watch the telemetry screen for ectopy.
    c. It is also important to listen for telemetry alarms while advancing.
    d. Patients may experience some PVCs.
    e. If the patient goes into VT, completely remove the wire.
25. While holding the guide wire, remove the introducer needle. Never let go of the guide wire while it is in the patient.
26. Once the introducer needle has been removed, make a small nick in the skin at the site entry while continuing to hold the guide wire. The nick should be made with the scalpel facing away from the operator and should be a small in-out stabbing motion.
27. Now, pass the dilator over the guide wire while continuing to hold the guide wire.
28. Dilate and retract the dilator while continuing to hold the guide wire.
29. Make sure the distal port does not have a cap on it so the guide wire can pass through.
30. Pass the catheter over the guide wire. The guide wire will come out the distal port. Continue advancing the catheter while holding the guide wire.
    a. Once the guide wire can be seen coming out of the distal port of the catheter, grasp the guide wire.
    b. Finish advancing the catheter until the appropriate depth is reached.
31. While holding the catheter in place, pull out the guide wire. It should remove without any resistance.
32. Aspirate and flush each port to confirm blood return.
33. Suture the central line into place at the insertion site.
34. Clean the area again with the antiseptic of choice, most often chlorhexidine or Betadine.
35. Place a sterile dressing over the insertion site.
36. Obtain a chest x-ray for radiograph placement and to rule out a pneumothorax.
37. Proper placement on a chest x-ray will demonstrate the tip of the catheter in the SVC.
38. Document the procedure appropriately in the patient's record.

C. Anatomical landmarks for CVC placement without US guidance.
   1. US guidance for placement of IJ CVCs is considered the gold standard. However, not all hospitals have access to bedside US.
   2. When US is not readily available for CVC insertion, it is important that an experienced operator use the following anatomical markings.
      a. IJ landmarks.
         i. Identify the triangle formed by the sternum and two heads of the sternocleidomastoid muscle (SCM). After identifying this triangle, palpate the carotid pulse.
         ii. While maintaining palpation of the carotid pulse, pull the carotid medially and insert your needle lateral to the carotid.
      b. Subclavian vein landmarks.
         i. Identify the sternal notch.
         ii. Find the curve of the clavicle, which is generally two-thirds of the distal length of the clavicle from the sternal notch (see Figure 8).
         iii. Palpation of the subclavian artery is not possible and visualization with US is not possible due to the clavicle obstructing the view.
         iv. While maintaining the landmarks with the nondominant hand, use the dominant hand to insert the introducer needle at a 45° angle to the curve of the clavicle, then walk the needle down the height of the clavicle until the needle is easily able to pass under the clavicle.
      c. Femoral vein.
         i. Identify the femoral triangle created by the inguinal ligament, sartorius muscle, and adductor longus muscle in the inguinal femoral area (see Figure 9). Whenever possible, use US to access the vein using these landmarks.
         ii. Palpate the femoral artery.
         iii. The femoral vein will be medial to the femoral artery, and the bladder is in the pelvis medial to the vein. Use the femoral artery as a guide to avoid being too medial and inserting the needle into the bladder.
         iv. Insert the needle with a 20° to 30° angle with the skin toward the umbilicus.

EVALUATION AND RESULTS

A. Maintain all ports flushed and patent.

B. Aspiration of blood from the ports should be nonpulsatile.

(*continued*)

CENTRAL VENOUS ACCESS (*continued*)

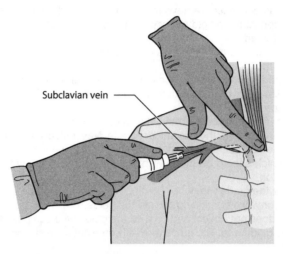

Subclavian vein

FIGURE 8   Accessing the subclavian vein.

Femoral Triangle

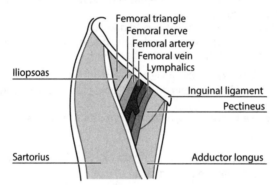

Femoral triangle
Femoral nerve
Femoral artery
Femoral vein
Lymphalics

Iliopsoas

Inguinal ligament
Pectineus

Sartorius

Adductor longus

FIGURE 9   Anatomy of the femoral triangle.

C. Connect to pressure tubing if uncertain to ascertain if a waveform is present. A catheter in the vein will produce a single nonpulsatile wave on the monitor, whereas a catheter in the artery will produce a waveform consistent with a peak and dicrotic notch.

D. If arterial access is achieved with placement of the catheter, consult vascular surgery immediately.

E. Confirm placement with abdominal x-ray.

F. Tip of catheter should be located above the confluence of the iliac vein.

CLINICAL PEARLS

A. Always maintain sterile technique; having nursing presence will help ensure sterility is maintained.

B. Always use US guidance if available.

C. Choose a method of pressure measurement and use it along with US guidance.

D. Always confirm line placement with a chest x-ray for IJ and subclavian lines, and abdominal x-ray for femoral lines.

E. Never hesitate to ask for help or supervision when first learning to perform central lines.

(*continued*)

CENTRAL VENOUS ACCESS (*continued*)

BIBLIOGRAPHY

CAE Healthcare. (n. d.) Gen I Central Venous Access Ultrasound Training Model Tissue Insert. Retrieved from http://www.bluephantom .com/product/Gen-I-Central-Venous-Access-Ultrasound-Training-Model-Tissue-Insert.aspx?cid=562

Institute of Healthcare Improvement. (n. d.) Central line insertion team checklist. Retrieved from http://www.ihi.org/resources/Pages/ Tools/CentralLineInsertionCareTeamChecklist.aspx

Marino, P. L., & Sutin, K. M. (2006). *The ICU book* (3rd ed., pp. 107–128). New York, NY: Lippincott Williams & Wilkins.

Reichman, E. F. (Ed.). (2013). *Emergency medicine procedures* (2nd ed.). New York, NY: McGraw-Hill/Medical. Retrieved from https://accessemergencymedicine.mhmedical.com/content.aspx?bookid=683&sectionid=45343634

Rupp, S. M., Apfelbaum, J. L., Blitt, C., Caplan, R. A., Connis, R. T., Domino, K. B., . . . Tung, A. (2012). Practice guidelines for central venous access: A report by the American Society of Anesthesiologists Task Force on Central Venous Access. *Anesthesiology, 116*(3), 539–573. doi:10.1097/ALN.0b013e31823c9569

Saugel, B., Scheeren, T. W. L., & Teboul, J. L. (2017). Ultrasound-guided central venous catheter placement: A structured review and recommendations for clinical practice. *Critical Care, 21*, 225. doi:10.1186/s13054-017-1814-y

PROCEDURE

CHEST TUBE INSERTION

E. Moneé Carter-Griffin

DESCRIPTION

A. The insertion of a chest tube into the pleural space to drain collected fluid or air.

INDICATIONS

A. Any fluid collection in the pleural space.
   1. Pleural effusion.
   2. Hemothorax (blood collection).
   3. Empyema (pus collection).
   4. Hydrothorax (serous fluid collection).
   5. Chylothorax (lymphatic fluid collection).

B. Pneumothorax (air collection).

C. Postoperative drainage of the thoracic cavity.

PRECAUTIONS

A. Assess coagulation profile. A patient with a coagulopathy may have excessive bleeding during and post insertion.

B. Avoid areas with adhesions or lung adherence to the pleura.

C. Careful consideration should be given to differentiate between pulmonary bullae versus a pneumothorax.

EQUIPMENT REQUIRED

A. Personal protective equipment.
   1. Sterile gloves, gown, and drape.
   2. Cap, mask, and protective eyewear.

B. Chest tube drainage system with a water seal.

C. Suction tubing and connector.

D. Various thoracostomy tube sizes: Size used depends on collection being drained.

E. Antiseptic solution with chlorhexidine or povidone-iodine.

F. Lidocaine 1% with or without epinephrine for local anesthesia.

G. A 5 and 10 mL syringe.

H. 25-gauge, 5/8–1 inch needle.

I. 20 to 23 gauge, 1-½ inch needle.

J. Chest tube insertion tray.
   1. 4 × 4 sterile gauze.
   2. Hemostats (2).
   3. Kelly clamps (2—large and medium).
   4. No.10 scalpel.
   5. Suture scissors.
   6. Needle driver.
   7. Nylon or silk suture.

K. Occlusive dressing: Vaseline gauze, 4 × 4s, and tape.

L. Surgical marker: Not required but helpful in identifying the point of entry.

PROCEDURE

A. Explain procedure to patient and family.

B. Always identify the patient and obtain informed consent.

C. Ensure patient has intravenous (IV) access and hemodynamic monitoring (e.g., blood pressure, O_2 saturations, etc.).

D. Choose a chest tube size. A smaller chest tube, less than 24 Fr, can typically be used for pneumothoraces and a larger chest tube, greater than 24 Fr, is indicated for fluid collections.

E. Wash hands/perform hand hygiene.

F. Place patient in the supine position with the ipsilateral arm raised above the head (see Figure 1).

(continued)

CHEST TUBE INSERTION (*continued*)

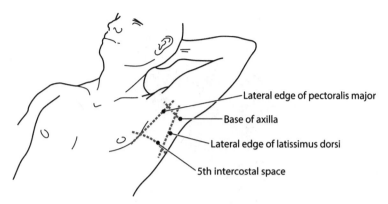

Lateral edge of pectoralis major

Base of axilla

Lateral edge of latissimus dorsi

5th intercostal space

FIGURE 1   Patient positioning for chest tube insertion.

G. Verify location for chest tube placement.
   1. Use a marker to identify location/point of entry.
   2. Locate the fifth intercostal space and midaxillary line.
   3. The incision is typically made in between the anterior and midaxillary lines.

H. Don sterile attire and prepare sterile field prior to initiating the procedure: Can also be completed with help of an assistant after provider has donned sterile attire.
   1. Ensure all equipment is available in the chest tube insertion tray.
   2. The chest tube may be added during set up or the assistant can add it to the sterile field.

 I. Administer moderate sedation.

 J. Cleanse area with chlorhexidine or a povidone-iodine solution. Allow to passively dry.

K. Use the larger Kelly clamp to grasp the proximal end of the chest tube and place it to the side within the sterile field.

L. Perform a time out.

M. Cleanse the area again with chlorhexidine or a povidone-iodine solution.

N. Drape the identified area with the sterile drape.

O. Use the 25 gauge, 5/8 inch needle and the 5 mL syringe to inject a small wheal of lidocaine.

P. Use the 20 gauge, 1½ inch needle and the 10 mL syringe to infiltrate lidocaine into a wide area of subcutaneous tissue, periosteum, and pleura.

Q. Make an incision with a No. 10 scalpel in the same direction as the rib and below the desired entry level. The incision should be slightly larger than the chest tube size.

R. Insert the medium Kelly clamp downward through the incision, creating a tunnel by opening and closing the clamp (blunt tissue dissection). Create the tunnel tack over the fifth rib. Aim toward superior aspect until the pleura of the fourth intercostal space is reached.

S. Once the pleura is reached, close the clamp, advance through the parietal pleura into the pleural space, then open/close the clamp to widen the hole.

T. Insert a finger into the tract to ensure it ends at the upper border of the rib above the incision (see Figure 2).

U. Grasp the other Kelly clamp with the chest tube connected.
   1. Advance proximal end into the pleural space, remove Kelly clamp, and guide tube further into the pleural space.
   2. Air and/or fluid may be in the space.

V. Connect chest tube to drainage system and have the assistant connect to suction. Typical suction setting is −40 cm H₂O, but the provider will indicate the desired amount of suction.

W. Suture chest tube in place to the chest wall using a purse string technique and wrap additional suture around the chest tube.

(*continued*)

CHEST TUBE INSERTION (continued)

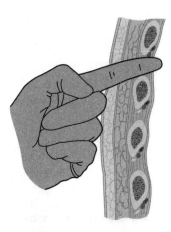

FIGURE 2 Illustration demonstrating index finger inserted into the tract.

X. Place petroleum gauze around the test tube, add 4 × 4, and secure with tape.

Y. Dispose of all equipment.

Z. Obtain a chest x-ray immediately following placement.

AA. Document the procedure, indication, complications, and postprocedure imaging.

EVALUATION AND RESULTS

A. Depending on indication for placement, expect air or fluid removal.

B. Reexpansion of the lung tissue should occur.

CLINICAL PEARLS

A. The insertion site for chest tube placement depends on the indication for chest tube insertion.

B. In order for thoracostomy tubes to function properly, all of the fenestrations in the tube must be within the thoracic cavity. The last side-hole in a thoracostomy tube is indicated by a gap in the radiopaque line; if it is not within the thoracic cavity or there is evidence of subcutaneous air, the tube may not have been completely inserted.

C. Ultrasound guidance is beneficial for identification of fluid accumulation and may reduce risk of complications.

D. Continuous bubbles indicate there is a leak within the patient or the chest tube system. Small fluctuations during inspiration and expiration are normal and expected.

BIBLIOGRAPHY

Roberts, J. R., Custalow, C. B., & Thomsen, T. W. (Eds.). (2013). *Roberts and Hedges' clinical procedures in emergency medicine* (6th ed.) Philadelphia, PA: WB Saunders.

Sethuraman, K. N., Duong, D., Mehta, S., Director, T., Crawford, D., St George, J., . . . Rathlev, N. K. (2011, January). Complications of tube thoracostomy placement in the emergency department. *The Journal Emergency Medicine, 40*(1), 14–20. doi:10.1016/j.jemermed.2008.06.033

CHEST TUBE REMOVAL

E. Moneé Carter-Griffin

DESCRIPTION

A. Removal of a chest tube from the pleural space when it is no longer needed for drainage of air or fluids.

INDICATIONS

A. Reexpansion of the lung tissue.

B. Resolution of air leaks (continuous bubbling) for at least 24 hours.

C. Pleural effusions: Tubes should have output less than 200 mL for greater than 24 hours prior to removal.

D. Cardiac surgery: Tubes can be removed once the fluid has changed from sanguineous to serosanguineous, no air leak is present, and less than 100 mL of fluid observed in the preceding 8 hours.

PRECAUTIONS

A. Avoid the introduction of air or contaminants during the removal to minimize further complications.

EQUIPMENT REQUIRED

A. Gloves, gown, mask, and eye protection.

B. Waterproof pad(s) to place under the removal site/area.

C. Suture removal kit.

D. Chlorhexidine or povidone-iodine antiseptic swabs/solution.

E. Kelly clamps (2).

F. Petrolatum gauze.

G. 4 × 4 gauzes.

H. Steri-Strips or some other form of elastic closure device.

I. Tape.

PROCEDURE

A. Prior to removal, verify there is no air leak and/or chest tube output.

B. Review imaging and assess respiratory status.

C. Explain procedure to patient and family.

D. Always identify the patient and obtain informed consent.

E. Ensure patient has intravenous (IV) access and hemodynamic monitoring (e.g., blood pressure, O_2 saturations).

F. Wash hands/perform hand hygiene.

G. Don clean gloves.

H. Place patient in semi-Fowler's position with waterproof pads directly under patient and chest tube site.

I. Gather all supplies. Open the suture removal kit, petrolatum gauze, and 4 × 4 gauzes.

J. Remove the suction from the drainage system. Assess for an air leak.

K. Remove dressing/tape and cleanse area with chlorhexidine.

L. Clip and remove the sutures. Ensure chest tube is free from sutures.

M. Pleural chest tubes: Cover insertion site with the petrolatum gauze and the mediastinal chest tube site with 4 × 4 gauzes.

N. Clamp chest tube with Kelly clamps.

O. Instruct patient to take a deep breath, hold it, and perform the Valsalva maneuver for removal of each chest tube.

P. Remove chest tube quickly and smoothly in one rapid motion while patient is performing the Valsalva maneuver. Immediately apply pressure once tube is removed.

(continued)

CHEST TUBE REMOVAL *(continued)*

Q. Secure the dressing in place.

R. Assess patient's respiratory and hemodynamic status immediately following procedure.

S. Dispose of all equipment.

T. Obtain a chest x-ray 1 to 2 hours following removal.

U. Document procedure, indications, complications, and patient tolerance.

EVALUATION AND RESULTS

A. Lung tissue should remain expanded post tube removal.

B. Chest tube insertion site should remain infection free.

C. Patient should have no signs and symptoms of respiratory distress postremoval.

CLINICAL PEARLS

A. Patients on invasive mechanical ventilation should have chest tube removed during peak inspiration.

B. Examine each chest tube postremoval to ensure the tube is intact.

BIBLIOGRAPHY

Bell, R. L., Ovadia, P., Abdullah, F., Spector, S., & Rabinovici, R. J. (2001). Chest tube removal: End-inspiration or end-expiration? *Trauma, 50*(4): 674-677.

DIGITAL NERVE BLOCKS

Frank O. Amanze

DESCRIPTION

A. A method of providing anesthesia to digit (finger or toe).

B. Performed by injecting a prescribed amount of anesthetic into the subcutaneous space forming a ring around the proximal portion of the affected digit.

C. Anesthetic can be:
1. A short-acting drug, such as lidocaine 2%.
2. A long-acting drug, such as bupivacaine 0.5%.
3. A 50:50 mixture of both to provide both short and longer action.

D. Differs from standard local anesthetic of a wound, as it avoids the difficulty of distorting a laceration site with large amounts of infiltration.

INDICATIONS

A. Need for local anesthetic to the distal portion of a digit in order to perform a short, painful procedure, such as suturing.

PRECAUTIONS

A. Inject no more than 4 mL into any digit to avoid risk of compartment syndrome.

B. As with all blind injections, aspirate syringe prior to instillation to avoid injecting anesthetic into a blood vessel.

EQUIPMENT REQUIRED

A. Povidone iodine or chlorhexidine prep for cleansing site.

B. 22 to 30 gauge needle for injection.

C. Separate 18 to 20 gauge needle/blunt for drawing up anesthetic.

D. 2 to 3 mL syringes.

E. Vial of selected anesthetic (lidocaine/bupivacaine).

F. Sterile gloves.

PROCEDURE

A. Goal is to surround nerves in a bath of anesthetic (not reach nerves directly).

B. Wash hands/perform hand hygiene.

C. Don clean gloves.

D. Prepare the skin with antibacterial solution.

E. Using a blunt or 18 to 22 gauge needle and syringe, draw up anesthetic.

F. Change needle to smaller gauge for injection of anesthetic into the affected digits.

G. Make one to three punctures on palmer surface of base of digit (see Figure 1).
1. Fan punctures out in a circumferential manner.
2. Instill maximum total of 4 mL into the space around the proximal phalange.

H. Make two punctures from the dorsal surface: One into the web spacing on each side of the phalange/phalanx (see Figure 2).

EVALUATION AND RESULTS

A. Test areas of effectiveness prior to beginning the intended painful procedure.

B. If needed, administer additional blocking agent (maximum 4 mL total per digit).

CLINICAL PEARLS

A. If using one puncture, try to withdraw the needle almost to the base of the skin before redirecting toward the other side of the bone to get the most coverage from one puncture.

(continued)

DIGITAL NERVE BLOCKS *(continued)*

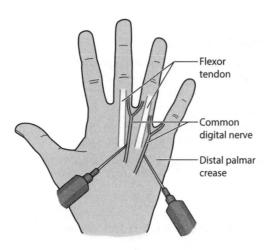

Flexor tendon

Common digital nerve

Distal palmar crease

FIGURE 1   Illustration showing the digital nerve block.

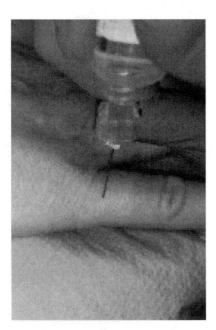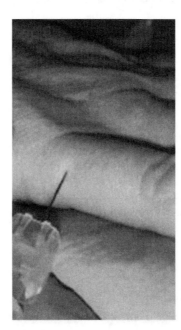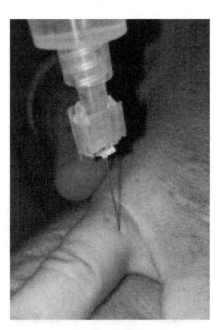

FIGURE 2   Digital block around nerves.
Source: Campo, T. M., & Lafferty, K. A. (Eds.). (2016). *Essential procedures for emergency, urgent, and primary care settings* (2nd Ed.). New York, NY: Springer Publishing Company.

B. If using two puncture sites, when instilling blocking agents to the opposite surface, try to numb the intended site of the second puncture to minimize pain of the second puncture.

C. If the intended procedure will be performed immediately (e.g., suturing), then lidocaine alone is sufficient.

D. If the patient will be anesthetized and then sent for radiologic imaging for an extended period, then a 50:50 mixture of lidocaine/bupivacaine will be advantageous due to a much longer duration.

BIBLIOGRAPHY

Baldor, R., & Mathes, B. (2017, June 19). Digital nerve block. In J. Grayzel (Ed.), *UpToDate*. Retrieved from https://www.uptodate.com/contents/digital-nerve-block

Okur, O. M., Şener, A., Kavakli, H. Ş., Çelik, G. K., Doğan, N. Ö., Içme, F., . . . Günaydin, G. P. (2017). Two injection digital block versus single subcutaneous palmar injection block for finger lacerations. *European Journal Trauma and Emergency Surgery, 43*, 863. doi:10.1007/s00068-016-0727-9

EXTRACORPOREAL MEMBRANE OXYGENATION

Heather H. Meissen and Alison M. Kelley

DESCRIPTION

A. Extracorporeal membrane oxygenation (ECMO) was created as an adaptation to conventional cardiopulmonary bypass.

B. ECMO can be divided into veno-venous (VV) ECMO and veno-arterial (VA) ECMO.
   1. VV ECMO is used for oxygenation in patients with severe acute respiratory distress syndrome (ARDS) and does not provide hemodynamic support.
   2. VA ECMO supports cardiac output in addition to providing oxygenation.

C. This chapter will primarily discuss VV ECMO in the adult population. Although use of VA ECMO has grown in recent years, the incidence of VA ECMO is still less than VV ECMO.

D. Although this procedure is outside the scope of practice for an advanced practice provider (APP), the APP is often involved in the procedure and in managing the system after the line is placed.

INDICATIONS

A. Hypoxemic respiratory failure.

B. Pneumonia.

C. ARDS.

D. Pulmonary contusions.

E. Smoke inhalation.

F. Status asthmaticus.

G. Aspiration.

H. Bridge to lung transplant.

PRECAUTIONS

A. ECMO cannulation is considered a surgical procedure and is to be performed only by a cardiovascular or thoracic surgeon with the assistance of an experienced surgical team. The presence of an ECMO-trained surgical team and a multidisciplinary team trained in management of ECMO following cannulation reduces the risks of complications. The surgical team includes:
   1. Cardiovascular or thoracic surgeon.
   2. ECMO-trained physician.
   3. Cardiac anesthesiologist.
   4. Respiratory therapist to manage ventilator settings.
   5. ECMO-trained critical care nurse.
   6. Cardiovascular perfusionist.
   7. Surgical scrub tech/nurse.
   8. Circulating nurse.
   9. ECMO-trained acute care nurse practitioner or physician assistant may or may not be present during cannulation. However, APPs play a vital role in the management of the critically ill ECMO patient after cannulation.

B. After a proper time out has been completed, the patient should be sedated and paralyzed prior to placement of the venous cannula.

C. Patient should be typed and crossmatched for blood products.
   1. Whether cannulation is taking place at bedside or in the operating room, continuous vital signs, telemetry, and pulse oximetry must be continuously monitored.
   2. Equipment and medications are needed for treatment of arrhythmias and bradycardia.
   3. Aortic dissection (during VA ECMO) or vessel rupture will result in the need for emergent sternotomy. Proper equipment and personnel should be available.
   (Modified from *ECMO Specialist Training Manual*, third edition).

D. Complications of ECMO.
   1. Aortic dissection 2/2 to arterial cannulation.
   2. Venous rupture.
   3. Acute anemia 2/2 blood loss.
   4. Venous spasm: Prevented by avoiding excessive manipulation.
   5. Arrhythmias.
   6. Bradycardia 2/2 to stimulation of vagus nerve.
   7. Distal extremity thrombosis and ischemia.

(continued)

EXTRACORPOREAL MEMBRANE OXYGENATION (*continued*)

EQUIPMENT REQUIRED

A. Sterile gowns and gloves.

B. Sterile saline.

C. Syringes and needles.

D. Povidone-iodine solution.

E. Povidone-iodine ointment.

F. Semipermeable transparent membrane type dressing.

G. Absorbable gelatin sponge.

H. Surgical lubricant.

I. Blood.
   1. Emergency situation: Uncrossmatched blood should be available.
   2. Difficult cannulation: 10 to 20 mL/kg of blood is often required for appropriate resuscitation.

J. Surgical caps and masks.

K. Electrocautery.

L. Wall suction.

M. Tubing clamps.

N. Pump (roller or centrifugal).

O. Membrane oxygenator.

P. Venous catheters.
   1. Patient's oxygenation is directly related to blood flow.
   2. To allow for maximal blood flow, largest possible internal diameter should be utilized.

PROCEDURE

A. Discuss procedure with patient and/or family.

B. Select cannula (decided by primary operator: Cardiovascular or thoracic surgeon); cannula size and selection directly affect the support patient is receiving from ECMO circuit.

C. Perform a time out.

D. Sedate patient; may also be paralyzed depending on surgeon preference.

E. Prime ECMO circuit with albumin (12.5 g) and CaCl (1 g).

F. Venous access obtained with introducer/sheath. In emergency cannulation situations, the APP may be the first provider on scene and can initiate this step.

G. Two main percutaneous techniques performed for VV ECMO by a trained cardiovascular or cardiothoracic surgeon.
   1. Placement of two cannulae; internal jugular and femoral vein, or bilateral femoral veins (see Figure 1).
      a. Cannula (23–29 French) placed for drainage of blood from inferior vena cava (IVC) via femoral vein.
      b. Cannula (21–23 French) placed for reinfusion of blood through jugular vein.
   2. Double lumen cannula is used to allow blood to drain from both the IVC and superior vena cava (SVC). The cannula's internal membrane directs blood across the tricuspid valve to minimize recirculation, avoiding femoral vein cannulation, and allowing patients to be more mobile while on ECMO.

H. Following cannulation, management of the patient on VV ECMO includes managing flow and ventilator settings, sedation, gas exchange, and anticoagulation, as well as SaO_2 and SvO_2 monitoring.

EVALUATION AND RESULTS

A. ECMO circuit.
   1. Primary purpose is exchange of both carbon dioxide (CO_2) and oxygen.
   2. Oxygenator is responsible for oxygenation and CO_2 elimination; has semipermeable membrane to allow diffusion by blood and gas flow in countercurrent directions.

(*continued*)

EXTRACORPOREAL MEMBRANE OXYGENATION (*continued*)

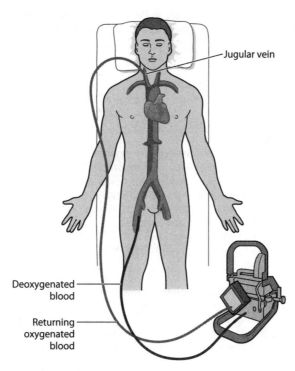

Jugular vein

Deoxygenated blood

Returning oxygenated blood

FIGURE 1   Illustration showing ECMO connectors.
ECMO, extracorporeal membrane oxygenation; VV, veno-venous.

3. Determine rate diffusion occurs by adjusting gas sweep rate and blood flow rate.
    a. Gas sweep is the primary factor in CO_2 clearance.
        i. Other factors affecting CO_2 removal: Blood flow, total body surface area.
        ii. Sweep gas flow rate is measured in liters per minute.
        iii. Initial cannulation: Set at 2 to 4 L/min.
        iv. As rate of gas sweep increases, so does rate of decarboxylation.
    b. Blood flow rate is rate at which blood flows through ECMO circuit's oxygenator; one of the primary determinants of oxygenation.
        i. Other factors influencing oxygenation include fraction of inspired oxygen (FiO_2) and hemoglobin.
        ii. Measured in liters per minute and recommended that blood flow rates be 3 mL/kg/min.

B. Ventilator management for patient on ECMO.
    1. Varies from institution. Further research is needed to understand which ventilator settings in ECMO patients have the best outcomes.
    2. Many centers practice ultraprotective ventilation for patients on ECMO to allow for lung rest; targets low tidal volumes, often 3 to 4 mL/kg/ideal body weight, and positive end-expiratory pressure (PEEP) of 10 to 15 cmH$_2$O while maintaining peak pressure less than 20 to 25 cmH$_2$O.
    3. Respiratory rates often set anywhere from 4 to 10 breaths per minute. Patients on ECMO are able to tolerate such low respiratory rates due to the high rate of CO_2 clearance provided by the ECMO circuit. As the ECMO circuit is responsible for fully oxygenated blood, FiO_2 settings on the ventilator can be minimal, often set to less than 30%.

C. Continuous management and monitoring.
    1. Required monitoring.
        a. Daily chest x-ray (CXR).
        b. Daily labs including:
            i. Complete blood count (CBC).
            ii. Lactate dehydrogenase (LDH).
            iii. D-Dimer.
            iv. Comprehensive metabolic panel (CMP).
            v. Erythrocyte sedimentation rate (ESR).
            vi. Prothrombin time/international normalized ratio (PT/INR).
            vii. Fibrinogen level.
        c. Plasma free hemoglobin when concern for hemolysis.

(*continued*)

EXTRACORPOREAL MEMBRANE OXYGENATION (*continued*)

    d. Heparin is gold standard anticoagulant to use while a patient is on ECMO. Based on institution, monitoring of heparin may vary and include activated partial thromboplastin time (APTT), activated clotting time (ACT), or heparin assays. These labs should be checked every 6 hours.

    e. Blood cultures as indicated.

    f. Electrolyte monitoring and repletion.

    g. Thorough inspection of entire circuit every shift.

    h. Frequent pulse checks.

    i. Monitoring of hematuria.

    j. Maintain minimal ventilator settings.

2. Suggested monitoring and management.

    a. Avoiding percutaneous procedures due to bleeding concerns.

    b. Avoiding subcutaneous injections due to bleeding concerns.

    c. Limiting invasive procedures to those that can be performed with a bovie.

    d. Removing any excessive lines, which may lead to bleeding.

    e. Gentle suctioning and gentle placement of nasogastric (NG) and orogastric (OG) tubes.

    f. Passive range of motion exercises to avoid contractures.

    g. Provide full nutritional support as soon as possible.

    h. Minimizing sedation while maintaining adequate pain control.

    i. Daily SvO_2 or $ScvO_2$ monitoring.

3. Weaning ECMO.

    a. Weaning trial should be performed often once there has been significant clinical improvement while on ECMO, as evidenced by sufficient oxygenation with gas flow rate 0 L/min. Note that the ECMO blood flow cannot be decreased to 0 due to risk of thrombosis; only the gas flow is decreased to 0 L/min.

    b. Increase ventilator settings to ensure adequate CO_2 removal during trial.

    c. Once ventilator settings have been increased, slowly decrease gas flow rate until reaching 0 L/min; decrease rate is at discretion of attending physician.

    d. While gas flow rate is maintained at 0 L/min, blood gases should be drawn and evaluated for a goal PaO_2 of greater than 60 mmHg and a goal $PaCO_2$ of 30 to 45 mmHg.

    e. Each institution has varying requirements for weaning trials. Ensuring a patient is stable for anywhere from 4 to 24 hours with a gas flow rate of 0 L/min is desired prior to decannulation.

    f. Turn heparin off at least 2 hours prior to cannula removal once a patient has passed the designated weaning trial.

    g. Decannulation should be performed by experienced ECMO-trained medical staff due to significant bleeding risk and potential need for vascular repair.

CLINICAL PEARLS

A. Watch ECMO lines for clotting or cannula movement, which could indicate hypovolemia or anemia.

B. Follow arterial blood gases (ABGs) and coagulation frequently.

C. Success of patient on ECMO is dependent on teamwork and collaboration among a multidisciplinary team of skilled providers.

D. Pay attention to details of patient's care including nutrition, daily diuresis, skin integrity, and pain management/sedation.

BIBLIOGRAPHY

Allen, S., Holena, D., McCunn, M., Kohl, B., & Sarani, B. (2011). A review of the fundamental principles and evidence base in the use of extracorporeal membrane oxygenation (ECMO) in critically ill adult patients. *Journal of Intensive Care Medicine, 26*(1), 13–26. doi:10.1177/0885066610384061

Marasco, S. F., Lukas, G., McDonald, M., McMillan, J., & Ihle, B. (2008). Review of ECMO (extra corporeal membrane oxygenation) support in critically ill adult patients. *Heart, Lung and Circulation, 17*(Suppl. 4), S41–S47. doi:10.1016/j.hlc.2008.08.009

Short, B. L., & Williams, L., (eds.). (2010). *ECMO specialist training manual* (3rd ed.). Ann Arbor, MI: Extracorporeal Life Support Organization.

ENDOTRACHEAL INTUBATION

E. Moneé Carter-Griffin

DESCRIPTION

A. Insertion of an endotracheal tube (ETT) into the airway to maintain patency, protection, delivery of oxygen, and/or ventilate a patient.

INDICATIONS

A. Inability to protect the airway (e.g., altered level or loss of consciousness).

B. Inadequate ventilation (e.g., hypercapnic respiratory failure).

C. Inadequate oxygenation (e.g., acute respiratory distress syndrome [ARDS], pneumonia).

D. Anticipated clinical decline/impending respiratory failure (e.g., septic shock).

E. Airway obstruction (e.g., facial trauma, burns, angioedema).

F. Ineffective ability or inability to clear secretions with high risk for aspiration.

G. Cardiac/respiratory arrest.

PRECAUTIONS

A. Surgical intervention is warranted in patients with total airway obstruction or loss of oropharyngeal landmarks.

EQUIPMENT REQUIRED

A. Ambu bag, mask, and oxygen source.

B. Sedatives and paralytics.

C. Laryngoscope handle and blade.
   1. Ensure light source works prior to intubation.
   2. Have more than one blade available.
   3. Standard blade sizes for adults are a three and four.
   4. Know the differences between blades.
      a. A Macintosh is a curved blade.
      b. A Miller is a straight blade.

D. Use videolaryngoscope as alternative to allow for direct visualization of oropharynx via camera (see Figure 1).

E. ETT.
   1. Varies in size: The size refers to the internal diameter of the tube.
   2. Size 7 to 7.5 mm for an average-sized female; a size 8 mm is usually adequate for an average-sized male.

F. Stylet.

G. 10-mL syringe.

H. Water-soluble lubricant.

I. Suction catheter and source.

J. Oral airways.

K. End-tidal CO_2 detector.

L. Bougie may be needed for difficult airways; keep at bedside.

M. ETT securing device/holder or tape postintubation.

N. Mask, eye protection, gloves, gown.

PROCEDURE

A. Preparation.
   1. Explain the procedure to patient and family.
   2. Obtain informed consent from patient if possible or family if more appropriate.
   3. Inquire if patient has a history of a difficult airway or prior upper airway or neck injuries, disorders, or surgeries that may make intubation difficult.

(continued)

ENDOTRACHEAL INTUBATION (*continued*)

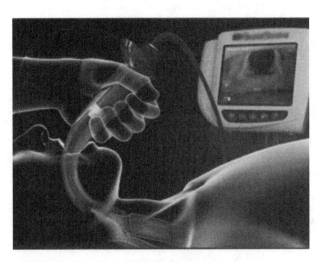

FIGURE 1   GlideScope video-assisted laryngoscopy.
Source: Campo, T. M., & Lafferty, K. (Eds.). (2016). *Essential procedures for emergency, urgent, and primary care settings: A clinical companion* (2nd ed.). New York, NY: Springer Publishing Company.

4. Wash hands/perform hand hygiene.
5. Don clean gloves.
6. Assess oral cavity for oropharyngeal landmarks, dentures, missing teeth, or other potential obstructions.
7. Ensure patient has a functional intravenous (IV) line.
8. Patient should have telemetry, blood pressure, respiratory, and O_2 saturation monitoring.
9. Vital signs should be visible and checked frequently.
10. Ensure all equipment is available.

B. Procedure.
   1. Choose appropriate size ETT.
   2. Check ETT cuff by attaching 10-mL syringe and inflating cuff.
   3. Ensure there are no leaks and cuff is inflating appropriately.
   4. Remove air from cuff until it is completely deflated.
   5. Insert stylet into ETT ensuring it does not pass beyond the tip of the ETT. Lubricate deflated balloon with water-soluble lubricant.
   6. Choose blade size and attach it to laryngoscope handle or select blade size for videolaryngoscope.
   7. Ensure light is working on traditional laryngoscope and camera on videolaryngoscope.
   8. Prior to performing the procedure, the provider should obtain gloves, a mask, and eye protection. If there is a concern for vomiting, copious secretions, or bleeding, then the provider may need a gown.
   9. Position patient with head extended and neck flexing forward ("sniffing position").
   10. Assess patient's mouth and remove any dentures.
   11. Suction mouth as needed for a clear view of oropharynx.
   12. Preoxygenate patient for 3 to 5 minutes with 100% oxygen.
       a. If breathing: Passive oxygenation with a mask is sufficient.
       b. If inadequate respirations or apnea, bagging is needed.
   13. Administer ordered sedative first.
   14. Administer ordered paralytic second.
   15. Use scissor-like motion to open mouth with the right hand.
   16. Using the left hand, insert the laryngoscope at the right side of the mouth, moving midline while pushing the tongue to the left.
   17. Advance blade into oropharynx past base of tongue, toward epiglottis using a "lift up and away" movement of the left hand until vocal cords are visible (see Figure 2).
   18. Use the right hand to take ETT and insert it into the right side of the mouth; under direct visualization, advance ETT into the oropharynx until the cuff passes through the cords. Advance an additional 1 to 2 cm.
   19. Remove stylet and inflate cuff on ETT.

(*continued*)

ENDOTRACHEAL INTUBATION *(continued)*

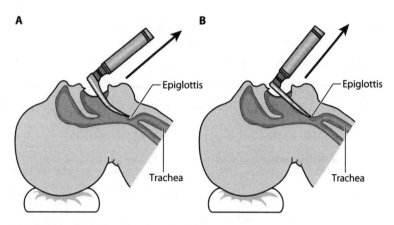

FIGURE 2   Illustration showing use of laryngoscope.

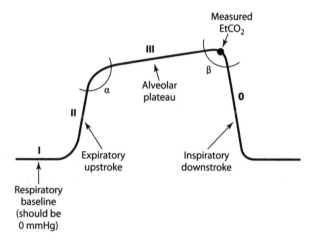

FIGURE 3   The point of measured end-tidal CO_2.

20. If the patient is observed to have a difficult airway, the provider may insert a bougie into the right side of the mouth and advance it through the cords. The ETT will be inserted over the bougie until it passes through the vocal cords. Once the ETT is through the vocal cords, the bougie is removed and the cuff inflated. The provider will continue the process with steps 21 to 23.
21. Attach CO_2 detector or capnography and observe for color change (gold indicates correct placement) or end-tidal CO_2 reading (a plateaued waveform, as shown in Figure 3, with a value of at least 35 mmHg). Auscultate breath sounds over the stomach and over the lungs bilaterally.
22. Hold ETT carefully in place until securement device or tape has been applied.
23. Attach patient to ventilator and immediately obtain chest x-ray to confirm placement.

EVALUATION AND RESULTS

A. Correct and secure placement of the ETT.

B. Adequate ventilation and oxygenation.

C. Secretion clearance.

(continued)

ENDOTRACHEAL INTUBATION (*continued*)

CLINICAL PEARLS

A. If unable to get an adequate "sniffing position," place a roll under the patient's shoulders.

B. Ensure a patent airway prior to administering any paralytic.

C. Laryngoscope handle should always lift up and away from the provider doing the procedure.

D. Never lever laryngoscope back in the oropharynx because it can cause trauma/damage to the teeth.

BIBLIOGRAPHY

Al-Shaikh, B., & Stacey, S. (2013). *Essentials of anaesthetic equipment* (4th ed.). London, England: Churchill Livingstone/Elsevier.

Bennett, L., & Cohen, F. M. (2017). Endotracheal intubation. In N. Multak (Ed.), *Clinical procedures for health professionals* (pp. 169–172). Burlington, MA: Jones & Bartlett.

Campo, T. M., & Lafferty, K. (Eds.). (2016). *Essential procedures for emergency, urgent, and primary care settings: A clinical companion* (2nd ed.). New York, NY: Springer Publishing Company.

O'Connor, M. F., & Glick, D. B. (2015). Airway management. In J. B. Hall, G. A. Schmidt, & J. P. Kress (Eds.), *Principles of critical care* (4th ed., pp. 384–395). New York, NY: McGraw-Hill.

Salhi, B. A., Taylor, T. A., & Ander, D. S. (2017). Intubation and airway support. In S. C. McKean, J. J. Ross, D. D. Dressler, & D. B. Scheurer (Eds.), *Principles and practice of hospital medicine* (2nd ed., pp. 895–899). New York, NY: McGraw-Hill.

ENDOTRACHEAL EXTUBATION

E. Moneé Carter-Griffin

DESCRIPTION

A. Removal of an endotracheal tube, allowing the patient to breathe using his or her own upper airway.

INDICATIONS

A. Initial condition that led to the need for invasive mechanical ventilation has improved or resolved.

B. Hemodynamic stability has been obtained.

C. Patient can adequately protect his or her airway, clear secretions, and/or maintain minimal risk for aspiration.

PRECAUTIONS

A. Ensure patient has met parameters usually outlined in a protocol or by provider prior to extubation to avoid need for reintubation.

EQUIPMENT REQUIRED

A. Gloves, eye protection, and mask.

B. Oxygen delivery device (e.g., nasal cannula, face mask) and source.

C. Suction catheter and source.

D. 10-mL syringe.

E. Scissors for patients with an endotracheal tube secured with tape.

F. Ambu bag and mask connected to oxygen source.

G. Supplies for endotracheal intubation in case emergent reintubation is required.

PROCEDURE

A. Explain the procedure to the patient and/or family and obtain informed consent.

B. Assess the patient's readiness for extubation, hemodynamic status, and ability to cough.

C. Ensure the patient has a functional intravenous (IV) line.

D. Patient should have telemetry, blood pressure, respiratory, and O_2 saturation monitoring.

E. Wash hands/perform hand hygiene.

F. Don clean gloves.

G. Place patient in semi- or high Fowler's position prior to extubation.

H. Hyperoxygenate and suction through the endotracheal tube.

I. If the patient has tape, then use scissors to cut. If the patient has a securement device, then disconnect and remove.

J. Suction oral cavity.

K. Attach 10-mL syringe to pilot balloon and deflate cuff.

L. Instruct the patient to take a deep breath in and remove the endotracheal tube.

M. Once the tube has been removed, instruct the patient to take a deep breath and cough.

N. Suction mouth and apply supplemental oxygen.

O. Discard used supplies and equipment.

P. Document procedure, indication, postextubation physical assessment, complications, and patient tolerance.

EVALUATION AND RESULTS

A. Stable respiratory status and oxygenation.

B. Atraumatic extubation.

(continued)

ENDOTRACHEAL EXTUBATION *(continued)*

CLINICAL PEARLS

A. Assessment of an air leak may be indicated in patients suspected of having ongoing upper airway edema.

B. A decreased air leak does not always suggest patient will fail postextubation.

BIBLIOGRAPHY

Hyzy, R. (2019, February 6). Extubation management in the adult intensive care unit. In G. Finlay (Ed.), *UpToDate*. Retrieved from https://www.uptodate.com/contents/extubation-management

EXTERNAL VENTRICULAR DRAIN

Catherine Harris

DESCRIPTION

A. External ventricular drains are tubes that are used to drain and monitor cerebrospinal fluid in the brain.

INDICATIONS

A. Reduce intracranial pressure by allowing cerebrospinal fluid to be removed from the lateral ventricles.

B. Monitor and measure cerebrospinal fluid chemistry and cytology.

C. Monitor intracranial pressure in the perioperative setting.

PRECAUTIONS

A. Any opening created in the skull increases chances of infection; strict sterile technique is mandatory.

B. Aggressive drilling can cause intracranial bleeding at the site; exercise caution past the second layer of compact bone.

EQUIPMENT REQUIRED

A. Ventriculostomy kit.

B. Cranial access kit: Drill, drill bit, scalp retractor, needles/syringes, forceps, trochar.

C. Sterile gown, gloves, drapes, mask, hat.

D. Betadine.

E. Hair clippers.

F. Lidocaine with epinephrine.

G. External ventricular setup.

PROCEDURE

A. Explain procedure to patient and/or family and obtain informed consent.

B. Wash hands/perform hand hygiene.

C. Place patient supine with head elevated 30°.

D. Perform a proper time out. All present in the room must identify the patient and agree on the correct procedure and correct site of the procedure.

E. Clip hair around site of drain insertion.

F. Pre-prep site with betadine.

G. Mark superficial landmarks for the planned incision. Kocher's point: Found 10 to 11 cm back from nasion, as shown in Figure 1A and B, and 2.5 to 3 cm lateral to middle (midpupillary point).

H. Set up sterile field: Prep and drape site.

I. Infiltrate marked skin incision with 1% lidocaine with epinephrine.

J. Make a straight sagittal 1-inch incision with a #11 blade down to the bone.

K. Use self-retaining clamps to hold skin back.

L. Use a handheld twist drill with a quarter inch bit to create a burr hole down to the dura.

M. Once the dura has been exposed, puncture with a sharp spinal needle.

N. Advance ventricular catheter about 5 cm into the lateral ventricle.

O. After catheter placement, remove the stylet and assess for cerebrospinal fluid.
   1. If present, record opening pressure.
   2. If not present, remove catheter, then reintroduce stylet and attempt a second pass.

P. Attach a trochar to the distal end of the catheter and tunnel it under the scalp about 3 cm away from the burr hole. *Do not move the intracranial catheter.*

Q. Once in place, confirm catheter position with flow of cerebrospinal spinal.

(continued)

EXTERNAL VENTRICULAR DRAIN (*continued*)

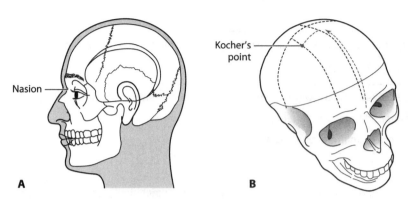

FIGURE 1 (A) Location of the nasion and (B) Kocher's point.

R. Attach plastic connector from external drain system and secure with 3-0 silk tie.

S. Anchor catheter to scalp with 3-0 nylon to prevent dislodgement.

T. Confirm catheter still drips cerebrospinal fluid.

U. Return to initial incision, irrigate with saline, and achieve hemostasis.

V. Close scalp wound with running 3-0 monocryl suture. *Do not puncture underlying catheter*.

W. Follow institution's policy for dressing drain site.

EVALUATION AND RESULTS

A. Confirmation of proper placement evidenced by return of cerebrospinal fluid.

CLINICAL PEARLS

A. If there is a lot of blood in the ventricle, clots may get into holes of the catheter and impede spontaneous flow; catheter may need to be repositioned, or another catheter may need to be placed.

B. Positioning catheter toward landmarks is critical, but watch trajectory of placement. If ventricle is not entered after a couple passes, seek expert guidance.

C. Do not go further than 7 cm deep. Critical brain structures may be damaged.

BIBLIOGRAPHY

Muirhead, W. R., & Basu, S. (2012). Trajectories for frontal external ventricular drain placement: Virtual cannulation of adults with acute hydrocephalus. *British Journal of Neurosurgery, 26*, 710–716. doi:10.3109/02688697.2012.671973

Toma, A. K., Camp, S., Watkins, L. D., Grieve, J., & Kitchen, N. D. (2009). External ventricular drain insertion accuracy: Is there a need for change in practice? *Neurosurgery, 65*, 1197–1200. doi:10.1227/01.NEU.0000356973.39913.0B

INTRAOSSEOUS VASCULAR ACCESS

Laura A. Santanna Lonergan

DESCRIPTION

A. Method for utilizing noncollapsible venous plexuses through the bone marrow cavity to achieve systemic circulation for fluid and medication administration.

B. Intraosseous (IO) access and infusion is possible because of the presence of veins that drain the medullary sinuses in the bone marrow of long bones.

C. Any intravenous (IV) drug or routine resuscitation fluid can be administered safely by the IO route.

INDICATIONS

A. In patients of all ages when venous access cannot be quickly and reliably established during circulatory collapse.

PRECAUTIONS

A. Proximal ipsilateral fracture.

B. Ipsilateral vascular injury.

C. Severe osteoporosis.

D. Osteogenesis imperfecta.

EQUIPMENT REQUIRED

A. Commercially available and approved rapid IO drill device.

B. Standard bone aspiration needle or specialized IO infusion needle.

C. Standard precautions and safety equipment.

PROCEDURE

A. Explain the procedure to the patient and/or family and obtain informed consent.

B. Wash hands/perform hand hygiene.

C. Select site.
  1. Primary site in all age groups should be proximal tibia, unless otherwise contraindicated. Landmark for proximal tibia.
     a. Aim for insertion two finger breadths below the patella and 1 to 2 cm medial to the tibial tuberosity in adults.
  2. Other sites indicated with landmarks.
     a. Distal femur (under 12 months of age).
        i. Aim for the anterolateral surface, 3 cm above the lateral condyle.
     b. Distal tibia or fibula (over 12 months of age).
        i. Aim for 3 cm proximal to the most prominent aspect of the medial malleolus.
     c. Proximal humerus (over 18 years of age).
        i. Aim for approximately 1 cm above the surgical neck on the anterior shaft of the humerus, which is the greater tubercle.
     d. Manubrium (over 12 years of age).
        i. Superior one third of the sternum may be accessed.
        ii. Requires a specialized device and training for insertion.

D. Establish the patient in a comfortable position.

E. Don sterile gloves.

F. Ensure sterile preparation of the site using chlorhexidine solution or povidone iodine.

G. Infiltrate site to include skin and periosteum with 1% to 2% lidocaine if patient is conscious.

H. Stabilize leg with nondominant hand.

I. Hold IO needle in dominant hand (see Figure 1).

J. Direct needle perpendicular to bone and away from joint spaces.

K. Twist and apply constant pressure until sudden loss of resistance.

L. Remove stylet.

(continued)

INTRAOSSEOUS VASCULAR ACCESS *(continued)*

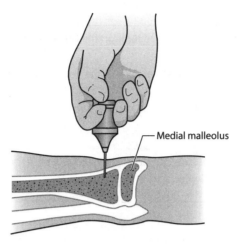

Medial malleolus

FIGURE 1 Illustration depicting IO needle insertion.
IO, intraosseous.

M. Confirm placement by aspiration or infusion.

N. Secure placement with dressing.

EVALUATION AND RESULTS

A. Confirm placement and rule out procedure-induced fracture with x-ray.

B. Complications: Cellulitis, osteomyelitis, iatrogenic fracture, physeal plate injury, fat embolism.

CLINICAL PEARL

A. The 2005 American Heart Association (AHA) Guidelines for CPR and Emergency Cardiovascular Care recommend for the first time IO access over endotracheal drug administration during resuscitation.

BIBLIOGRAPHY

ECC Committee, Subcommittees and Task Forces of the American Heart Association. (2005). 2005 American Heart Association guidelines for cardiopulmonary resuscitation and emergency cardiovascular care. *Circulation, 112*(24 Suppl), IV-1–IV-203.
Ngo, A., Oh, J., Chen, Y., Yong, D., & Ong, M. (2009). Intraosseous vascular access in adults using the EZ-IO in an emergency department. *International Journal of Emergency Medicine, 2*(3), 155. doi:10.1007/s12245-009-0116-9

LONG LEG CASTING

Joanne Elaine Pechar

DESCRIPTION

A. Long leg cast is an immobilization device that covers and encases the entire circumference of the leg and foot.

B. Long leg cast is used to stabilize and hold anatomical structures in place until healing is achieved.

INDICATIONS

A. Immobilize and treat acute nondisplaced fractures, dislocations, and injured ligaments.

B. Allow earlier ambulation by stabilizing fractures of the lower extremity.

C. Improve function by stabilizing or positioning a joint.

D. Correct and treat congenital deformities, such as clubfoot and joint contractures.

E. Manage chronic foot and ankle ulcers.

PRECAUTIONS

A. Ensure sufficient gauze or other dressing material is applied to absorb blood if cast is applied over a wound.

EQUIPMENT REQUIRED

A. Stockinette.
   1. Stretchable, sock-like material in varying widths.
   2. Acts as a barrier between skin and cast padding.
   3. Pulled over rough edges of cast to provide comfortable padded cast borders.

B. Fiberglass casting material.
   1. Comes in rolls of varying widths.
   2. Commonly used (as opposed to plaster) because of its strength, durability, light weight, and ease of application.
   3. Begins to harden in 3 to 4 minutes. Fully hardens in 1 to 2 hours. Must be kept in its airtight foil package before application.
   4. Due to its sticky resin content, gloves should be worn when handling fiberglass.

C. Webril (cotton) or synthetic undercast padding.
   1. Available in 2-, 3-, 4-, 5-, and 6-inch widths, packaged in individual rolls.
   2. 3- or 4-inch padding is used on lower leg; 5- or 6-inch padding is used on upper leg.

D. Basin full of cool or room temperature water.
   1. Avoid lukewarm water: Can increase probability of exothermic reaction of cast materials, which can increase risk of thermal injury to the skin.

E. Bandage scissors.

F. Cast cutter and spreader.

G. Gloves and gown.

PROCEDURE

A. Position the patient.
   1. Supine, with the ankle over the edge of the table.
   2. Knee flexed to approximately 20° to 35° to relax the gastrocnemius muscle and reduce possible hyperextension.

B. Apply stockinette.
   1. Support the leg (an assistant should support the leg to be casted).
   2. Measure the length of stockinette (see Figure 1). Cut stockinette to appropriate length with an extra 4 inches of stockinette on each end of the cast.
   3. Apply stockinette, which is placed beyond the anticipated cast border.
   4. Proximal edge of cast should lie below the greater trochanter on the lateral side, and just below the groin on the medial side. Distal edge of cast will be located at the level of metatarsal heads, while toes should remain free.
   5. Important positioning of foot: Plantigrade with toes pointing up (see Figure 2).

(continued)

LONG LEG CASTING (*continued*)

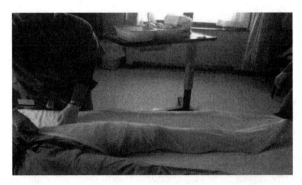

FIGURE 1 A nurse measuring the length of stockinette.

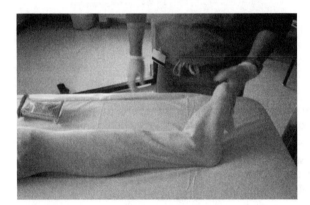

FIGURE 2 Foot should be plantigrade with toes pointing up.

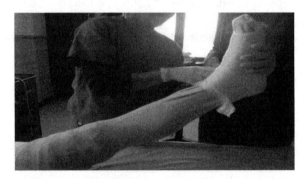

FIGURE 3 Provide two to three padding layers before applying cast.

C. Apply Webril or synthetic undercast padding.
1. Select appropriate cast padding size. Starting at distal border, gently roll and wind the padding, smoothly overlapping each time about 50% around the foot. Two to three padding layers is usually sufficient (see Figure 3).
2. To protect pressure points against pressure ulcers, apply additional webril padding over the patella, malleoli, and heel.
3. When rolling padding, keep the roll in continuous contact with the extremity to avoid undesirable wrinkles that occur when the roll is lifted during application.
4. Wind cast padding toward knee with an overlap of 50%, creating a double layer of padding.
5. Cast padding should extend slightly beyond the planned length of the cast, so that when the end of the stockinette is folded over, the end of the cast will be well-padded.

(continued)

LONG LEG CASTING *(continued)*

6. Extend padding about 2 inches beyond intended proximal and distal cast borders, and add an additional two layers of padding at proximal and distal borders of cast (see Figure 4).

D. Apply fiberglass bandage.
1. Use 3- to 6-inch bandage rolls to provide sufficient time for molding.
2. Two or three layers of fiberglass are usually adequate, and construct a cast with uniform thickness.
3. Completely soak and immerse the roll of fiberglass bandage in a basin of cool water for 10 seconds, gently squeeze the bandage to remove excess moisture and water, and remove fiberglass bandages from water as soon as bubbling stops.
4. Starting with the bottom of the foot, roll fiberglass bandage on smoothly around ankle, overlapping each time by 50%.
5. In the same manner as webril padding, pass fiberglass bandage over heel and then toward knee with 50% overlap.
6. Where the first bandage ends, apply a second fiberglass bandage, continuing proximally toward planned upper edge of cast and then returning toward foot.
7. As additional fiberglass bandages are required, they should begin at the end of the previous bandage to ensure even thickness of cast.
8. Avoid wrinkling by folding or tucking fiberglass roll.

E. Form the proximal end of the cast.
1. Fold loose end of the stockinette over the proximal edge of the cast.
2. Starting below the proximal edge, add another fiberglass bandage to secure the loose end of the stockinette and fiberglass (see Figure 5).

F. Form the distal end of the cast.
1. To create a padded and rolled edge border, pull the stockinette and cast padding over the distal end of the cast edge prior to rolling and securing the final layer of the fiberglass bandage.

G. Final molding.
1. While the fiberglass is still soft, mold the cast to the contour of the extremity by gently, but firmly, rubbing the cast between the palm of gloved hands.
2. To ensure the foot is plantigrade, apply gentle pressure to the sole of the forefoot.

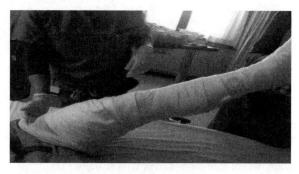

FIGURE 4   Padding extends beyond cast.

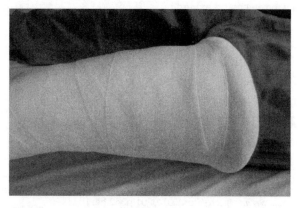

FIGURE 5   Secure loose ends of stockinette and fiberglass.

(continued)

LONG LEG CASTING (*continued*)

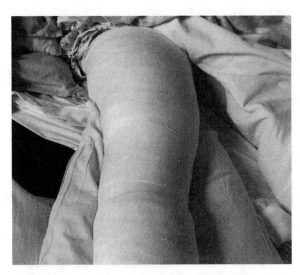

FIGURE 6   Long leg cast completed.

3. Apply liquid soap for fiberglass to harden.
4. Application of gentle pressure should be continued until fiberglass hardens.

H. Completed cast.
1. Application of the long leg circular cast is now complete (see Figure 6).
2. Place a small pillow under ankle until cast is fully hard and dry.
3. Weight bearing is restricted for 1 to 2 hours until cast has fully hardened to avoid denting and cracking.
4. If cast is to be used for walking, apply extra layers of padding and fiberglass bandage to sole and heel areas. Finally, place a cast shoe for ambulation.

EVALUATION AND RESULTS

A. Ask patient if cast feels loose or tight to ensure comfortable fit.

B. Check if cast extends to proper boundaries while not interfering with range of motion.

C. Check for any cast indentations or sharp edges. Trim sharp edges using a cast saw or bandage scissors.

D. Instruct patients regarding:
1. Signs and symptoms of compression, such as swelling within the cast.
2. Required elevation of injured extremity for 2 to 3 days.
3. Timing for being able to walk on cast.
4. Weight bearing and ambulation, which include crutch or walker training.
5. Avoidance of insertion of any objects under cast in an attempt to relieve itching.
6. Return to office for a cast check in 5 to 7 days.
7. Prompt notification for any tingling, numbness, weakness, skin ulcerations or discoloration, pallor, paresthesias, paralysis, or worsening pain in the casted extremity.

CLINICAL PEARLS

A. In order to sufficiently protect the injured limb, the ideal cast must be thick and rigid.

B. During the setting process, do not place the patient at risk for thermal injury.

C. When supporting the extremity, be careful not to indent the cast with fingertips.

D. "Bivalve" (split) the cast immediately if unexpected swelling occurs in a long leg cast to avoid risk of acute compartment syndrome.

BIBLIOGRAPHY

Gravlee, J. R., & Van Durme, D. J. (2007, February 1). Braces and splints for musculoskeletal conditions. *American Family Physician, 75*(3), 342–348. Retrieved from https://www.aafp.org/afp/2007/0201/p342.html

Halanski, M., & Noonan, K. J. (2008, January). Cast and splint immobilization: Complications. *Journal of the American Academy of Orthopaedic Surgeons, 16*(1), 30–40. doi:10.5435/00124635-200801000-00005

LUMBAR PUNCTURE

Courtney Connolley

DESCRIPTION

A. Also known as a spinal tap.

B. Performed in the lower back to remove a sample of cerebrospinal fluid (CSF).

INDICATIONS

A. To obtain analysis of CSF for diagnostic purposes.
1. Meningitis/encephalitis.
2. Subarachnoid hemorrhage.
3. Demyelinating diseases.
4. Carcinomatous diseases.

B. To evaluate and treat various neurological conditions.
1. Guillain-Barre syndrome.
2. Normal pressure hydrocephalus.
3. Pseudotumor cerebri.

C. To instill substances into the subarachnoid space.
1. Chemotherapy.
2. Contrast media.

PRECAUTIONS

A. Stay in L4–L5 region to avoid puncturing spinal cord (ends around L1). Identify highest point of iliac crest bilaterally with palpation to site of L4 (see Figure 1).

B. Maintain sterile field to prevent infection.

C. Do not drain too much CSF to avoid risk of cerebral herniation (20–40 mL of CSF can be safely removed).

D. Bleeding at level of lumbar puncture could cause nerve irritation and damage to surrounding structures.

EQUIPMENT REQUIRED

A. Sterile gown, mask, gloves.

B. Lumbar puncture needle.

C. Lumbar puncture kit.
1. 3-mL Luer lock syringe.
2. 25G 5/8 inch needle.
3. Lidocaine 1%.
4. Four specimen tubes with caps; tubes should be numbered 1 through 4.
5. Sponge applicators.
6. Three gauze pads.
7. Fenestrated drape.
8. Band-Aid.
9. One stopcock—three way.
10. Two piece manometer.
11. 22G 1-½ inch needle.
12. Infiltration with 20G × 3 ½ inch needle.

D. Sterile prep with chlorhexidine or povidone iodine solution.

PROCEDURE

A. Explain the procedure to the patient and/or family and obtain informed consent.

B. Wash hands/perform hand hygiene.

C. Position the patient in the lateral decubitus position with knees flexed.

D. Perform a proper time out. All present in the room must identify the patient and agree on the correct procedure and correct site of the procedure.

E. Palpate the highest level of iliac crests bilaterally to assess level of L3–L4, or L4–L5 interspace. Palpate midline, in space between spinous processes (see Figure 2).

(continued)

LUMBAR PUNCTURE (*continued*)

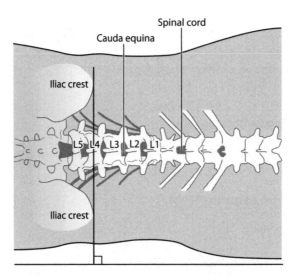

FIGURE 1 Anatomical landmarks for lumbar puncture.

Lumbar puncture

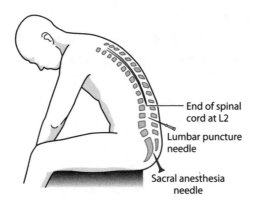

FIGURE 2 Illustration depicting placement of lumbar puncture needle.
Source: http://blogs.brown.edu/emergency-medicine-residency/lumbar-puncture-part-2-pearls-pitfalls-and-troubleshooting/

F. Mark point of entry.

G. Prepare sterile field; drape the area.

H. Prepare the skin in usual sterile fashion.

I. Skin and fascia of marked interspace should be infiltrated with 2% lidocaine with a 25-gauge needle.

J. Introduce spinal needle (including stylet) with bevel parallel to spine to dissect the fibers longitudinally; avoids trauma to tissues.

K. Advance needle parallel to floor and perpendicular to back of patient, aiming toward head with a 20° to 30° angle.
   1. Bone should be felt superiorly and needle redirected in caudal direction.
   2. Slight resistance should be felt as needle is advanced into ligamentum flavum.
   3. Smooth pop should be felt as needle penetrates dural sac.
   4. Stop advancing needle.

L. Rotate bevel toward the head of the patient.

(*continued*)

LUMBAR PUNCTURE (*continued*)

M. Remove stylet and assess for drainage of CSF.

N. If CSF comes out, then use the manometer to measure the pressure of the subarachnoid space and record.

O. Use the collection tubes in the lumbar puncture kit to collect CSF. Fill in numerical order. The amount collected in each tube will vary depending on the purpose of the lumbar puncture.

P. After CSF collection is completed, reinsert the stylet and remove the needle.

Q. Hold pressure at the site and then place a Band-Aid over the site.

R. Recommend the patient lay flat for 1 to 2 hours after the procedure.

EVALUATION AND RESULTS

A. Observe color of CSF.

B. Apply a manometer promptly to the needle.

C. Record an opening pressure.

D. State volume of CSF collected and sent to the laboratory.

CLINICAL PEARLS

A. Lumbar puncture is a blind stick.
1. It is possible to hit one of the nerves of the cauda equina.
2. If patient complains of pain down left leg, reposition needle right to stay central, and vice versa.

B. Positioning is the most important part of a successful lumbar puncture.
1. If interspace of spinal processes is difficult to palpate, have patient pull both knees up toward chest.
2. The more the knees are pulled up, the more the spinous processes will open up, making them easier to palpate.

C. A traumatic tap will be evidenced by blood in the CSF that diminishes in quantity collected in the specimen tubes. In subarachnoid hemorrhage, the amount of blood will not vary significantly.

D. As blood breaks down it creates xanthochromia, which is seen as a yellow tinge in CSF. This is indicative of blood being present for several hours. It is very important to get the specimen tubes to the laboratory as quickly as possible to distinguish between a traumatic tap (which will have no xanthochromia) and bleeding in the subarachnoid space, which may be caused by the rupture of a vessel such as an aneurysm.

BIBLIOGRAPHY

Burke-Doe, A. *Ventricles and coverings of the brain*. Retrieved from https://accessphysiotherapy.mhmedical.com/data/Multimedia/grandRounds/ventricles/media/ventricles_print.html

Doherty, C., & Forbes, R. (2014). Diagnostic lumbar puncture. *Ulster Medical Journal, 83*(2), 93–102. Retrieved from https://www.ums.ac.uk/umj083/083(2)093.pdf

Fastle, R., & Bothner, J. (2018). Lumbar puncture: Indications, contraindications, technique and complications in children. In J. F. Wiley, 2nd. (Ed.), *UpToDate*. Retrieved from https://www.uptodate.com/contents/lumbar-puncture-indications-contraindications-technique-and-complications-in-children

PERIPHERALLY INSERTED CENTRAL CATHETER PLACEMENT

Jingyi Deng

DESCRIPTION

A. A 3 French to 6 French catheter is inserted into the upper arm via the basilic or brachial vessel until the tip reaches the superior vena cava junction.

INDICATIONS

A. According to the Centers for Disease Control and Prevention (CDC), the peripherally inserted central catheter (PICC) line is the safest central vascular catheter (CVC) capable of remaining indwelling for over a year.

B. Long-term antibiotics, total parenteral nutrition (TPN), vasopressors, and multiple incompatible medications.

PRECAUTIONS

A. Chronic kidney disease/end-stage renal disease (CKD/ESRD).
   1. Extended PICC line dwell time in peripheral vasculature can lead to stenosis of brachial or basilic vessel due to intima hypertrophy/scarring; can complicate future fistula formation or graft placement.
   2. If renal replacement therapy (RRT) is imminent, nephrology should be consulted to decide if PICC would be suitable for the patient.
   3. Patient should receive tunneled jugular line placed by intervention radiology (IR) instead.

B. Bacteremia: Can result in central line-associated bloodstream infection (CLABSI). If cultures are pending, 48 hours of negative cultures or infectious disease approval is needed for PICC placement.

C. Permanent pacemaker: PICC lines should never occupy the same vessel as pacemaker wires as this could potentially lead to wire displacement.

D. Coagulopathy: Cut off for platelets, international normalized ratio (INR), partial thromboplastin time (PTT), and so forth, will differ based on facility. Determine if static parameters should delay an intervention (e.g., a patient with disseminated intravascular coagulopathy will not improve and this could prohibit placement of PICC).

EQUIPMENT REQUIRED

A. Ultrasound.

B. Insertion kit with PICC line.
   1. One bag, bedside white 6⅗″ × 3½″ × 11¾″.
   2. One bag, poly, 7″ × 10″ × 2 Mil.
   3. One band bag, 36″ × 28″ clear.
   4. One basin, emesis, 700 mL.
   5. Two cups, 2 oz each.
   6. One drape, 53″ × 77¾″.
   7. One dressing, 4¾″ × 4.
   8. One forcep.
   9. 10 gauze 4 × 4″.
   10. One gown.
   11. One needle 18 G × 1½″ length.
   12. One pouch 17¼″ × 22¾.
   13. One scalpel #11.
   14. One scissor.
   15. One skin marker.
   16. Two syringes 10 mL.
   17. One table cover, 44″ × 76″ × 3 Mil.
   18. Seven towels.

C. Probe cover.

D. Chlorhexidine solution.

E. Lidocaine 2%.

F. Extra wire.

(continued)

PERIPHERALLY INSERTED CENTRAL CATHETER PLACEMENT (*continued*)

PROCEDURE

A. Explain the procedure to the patient and/or family and obtain informed consent.

B. Perform a proper time out. All present in the room must identify the patient and agree on the correct procedure and correct site of the procedure.

C. Abduct patient's arm to 90° and proceed to identify vessel.

D. Measure from insertion site to right supraclavicular notch, then add 6 cm to the measurement.

E. Wash hands and open insertion tray.

F. Apply tourniquet to procedure arm.

G. Don sterile gown and gloves.

H. Drape patient's body with whole body drape.

I. Drape patient's arm with window dressing.

J. Prepare site with chlorhexidine for 30 seconds and allow 1 minute for dry time.

K. Flush all lumens of PICC line.

L. Apply probe cover to ultrasound probe.

M. Inject lidocaine to desired insertion site and wait 60 seconds.

N. Use ultrasound to identify target vessel and access vessel with needle or angiocatheter.

O. Upon seeing flashback, proceed to walk needle into the vessel.

P. Slide wire into the needle, then remove the needle or angiocatheter.

Q. Undo tourniquet.

R. Slide peelaway introducer onto wire, then remove wire. The peelaway introducer allows the introducer to be peeled away and removed, leaving the catheter in place.

S. Confirm insertion site is the same as measured in step C, then cut catheter to that length.

T. Remove introducer from sheath, then insert PICC into sheath.

U. Continue to advance catheter until PICC is at the hub of the sheath.

V. Proceed to peel away the sheath.

W. Confirm blood return and flush all ports.

X. Place probe on the jugular of the procedure side and flush the catheter. Ensure no sparkles appear on screen to confirm PICC is not in jugular.

Y. Apply occlusive dressing and discard sharps in appropriate container.

Z. Return patient room to preprocedure state.

AA. Page for x-ray for radiographic confirmation.

AB. Document procedure in the patient's record.

CLINICAL PEARLS

A. In a difficult catheter advancement, additional wire could increase stiffness and increase success.

B. A j looped wire could potentiate success as this can maneuver around difficult anatomy.

C. Larger French equates to higher risk of upper extremity deep vein thrombosis (DVT). Catheter-associated DVTs are more likely to originate from the fibrin sheath that forms from decreased blood flow around the catheter due to decreased lumen size.

D. Using an angiocatheter for initial pads allows for catheter threading and decreased risk for unintentional posterior wall puncture.

(continued)

PERIPHERALLY INSERTED CENTRAL CATHETER PLACEMENT (*continued*)

BIBLIOGRAPHY

Kelly, L. (2013). A practical guide to safe PICC placement. *British Journal of Nursing, 22*(Suppl. 5), S13–S19. doi:10.12968/bjon.2013.22. Sup5.S13

O'Grady, N. P., Alexander, M., Dellinger, E. P., Gerberding, J. L., Heard, S. O., Maki, D. G., & Weinstein, R. A. (2002). Guidelines for the prevention of intravascular catheter-related infections. *MMWR Recommendations and Reports, 51*(RR-10), 1–26. Retrieved from https://www.cdc.gov/mmwr/preview/mmwrhtml/rr5110a1.htm?vm=r

Sansivero, G. E. (2000). The microintroducer technique for peripherally inserted central catheter placement. *Journal of Intravenous Nursing, 23*, 345–351.

Wallace, B. A., & Taylor, T. (n.d.). Ultrasound-guided venous access. Retrieved from https://saem.org/cdem/education/online-education/m3-curriculum/bedside-ultrasonagraphy/venous-access

REDUCTION OF THE ANKLES

Laura A. Santanna Lonergan

DESCRIPTION

A. Ankle dislocations seen after a traumatic injury.

B. May be associated with fracture/ligamentous injury.

INDICATIONS

A. Prompt reduction of ankle fractures reduces tension on skin and prevents soft tissue swelling.

B. Most ankle fractures that require reduction will also require surgical intervention.

C. Goal of reduction is restoration of the ankle mortise.

EQUIPMENT REQUIRED

A. 18 g needle.

B. 10 mL syringe.

C. 1% Lidocaine.

D. Facility approved conscious sedation protocol.

E. Sugar-tong splint.

F. Assistive device as needed.

PROCEDURE

A. Explain the procedure to the patient and/or family and obtain informed consent.

B. Position the patient in the supine position with the affected limb flexed at the knee over the end of the bed.
   1. May perform intra-articular joint block of affected ankle for pain control.
   2. Conscious sedation may be necessary to perform adequate reduction.

C. Perform a proper time out. All present in the room must identify the patient and agree on the correct procedure and correct site of the procedure.

D. Internally rotate and supinate or pronate while giving limb distal traction until audible or palpable reduction is achieved (see Figure 1).

E. Splint patient with lower extremity sugar-tong splint with proper molding around ankle joint for added stability.

EVALUATION AND RESULTS

A. Postreduction imaging to evaluate success of reduction and ensure no procedural injuries.

B. Perform postreduction neurovascular examination of bilateral lower extremities.

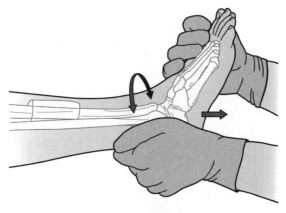

FIGURE 1 Illustration demonstrating manual traction of ankle.

(continued)

REDUCTION OF THE ANKLES *(continued)*

C. Provide patient with appropriate assistive device (crutches, cane, walker) and instruct no weight bearing on limb.

D. Follow-up with orthopedics for surgical evaluation of fracture/dislocation.

CLINICAL PEARLS

A. Repeated forceful attempts at reduction can cause additional injury.

B. Failure of reduction after two to three attempts may warrant surgical intervention.

C. If a closed injury converts to an open injury, tetanus prophylaxis and antibiotic coverage should be administered.

BIBLIOGRAPHY

Arnold, C., Fayos, Z., Bruner, D., & Arnold, D. (2017, December). Managing dislocations of the hip, knee, and ankle in the emergency department. *Emergency Medicine Practice, 19*(12), 1–28.

Melenevsky, Y., Mackey, R. A., Abrahams, R. B., & Thomson, N. B., 3rd. (2015, May-June). Talar fractures and dislocations: A radiologist's guide to timely diagnosis and classification. *Radiographics, 35*(3), 765–779. doi:10.1148/rg.2015140156

Rammelt, S., & Goronzy, J. (2015, June). Subtalar dislocations. *Foot and Ankle Clinics, 20*(2), 253–264. doi:10.1016/j.fcl.2015.02.008

Wight, L., Owen, D., Goldbloom, D., & Knupp, M. (2017, October). Pure ankle dislocation: A systematic review of the literature and estimation of incidence. *Injury, 48*(10), 2027–2034. doi:10.1016/j.injury.2017.08.011

REDUCTION OF THE FINGERS

Laura A. Santanna Lonergan

DESCRIPTION

A. Loss of alignment of a digit joint: Distal interphalangeal (DIP), proximal interphalangeal (PIP), and metacarpophalangeal (MCP) joint.

INDICATIONS

A. Finger reduction is indicated when diagnosis of dislocation has been determined and likelihood of fracture has been eliminated.

PRECAUTIONS

A. Prior to reduction, obtain imaging to rule out associated fracture.

EQUIPMENT REQUIRED

A. Lidocaine 1% or 2% without epinephrine for digital block (optional).

B. Finger splint.

C. Tape.

PROCEDURE

A. Explain the procedure to the patient and family and obtain informed consent.

B. Wash hands/perform hand hygiene.

C. Perform a proper time out. All present in the room must identify the patient and agree on the correct procedure and correct site of the procedure.

D. Administer digital block in the proximal aspect of the affected finger.
   1. Reduction of dorsal dislocation.
      a. Apply axial traction with simultaneous flexion of joint (see Figure 1).
      b. If unsuccessful, try again but first hyperextend the distal portion to "unlock" the joint. Continue with axial traction and flexion.
      c. DIP dorsal dislocation splint in full extension while allowing full range of motion of the PIP joint.
      d. PIP dorsal dislocation splint with PIP in 20° to 30° of flexion.

E. Reduction of volar dislocation.
   1. Gently hyperflex while pushing the base of the dislocated phalanx into place (see Figure 2).
   2. Splint the PIP in 20° to 30° of flexion.

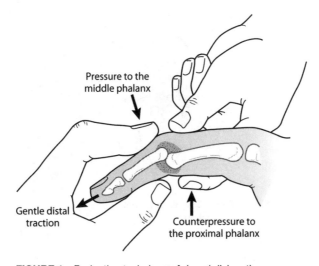

Pressure to the middle phalanx

Gentle distal traction

Counterpressure to the proximal phalanx

FIGURE 1   Reduction technique of dorsal dislocation.

(continued)

REDUCTION OF THE FINGERS *(continued)*

F. Reduction of lateral joint dislocation.
   1. Gently hyperextend the joint while correcting the ulnar or radial deformity (see Figure 3).
   2. DIP lateral dislocation splint in full extension.
   3. PIP lateral dislocation; apply dorsal splint with the PIP 20° to 30° of flexion.

EVALUATION AND RESULTS

A. Perform postreduction imaging to evaluate the success of reduction and to ensure no procedural injuries.

B. Refer to orthopedic or hand surgeon if:
   1. Joint cannot be reduced (may require open reduction).
   2. Patient has fracture dislocations.
   3. Patient has open-fracture dislocations.

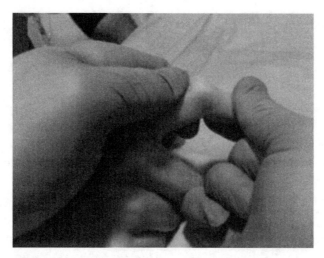

FIGURE 2 Closed reduction of PIP joint dislocation.
PIP, proximal interphalangeal.
Source: Campo, T. M., & Lafferty, K. (Eds.). (2016). *Essential procedures for emergency, urgent, and primary care settings: A clinical companion* (2nd ed.). New York, NY: Springer Publishing Company.

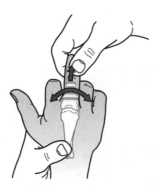

FIGURE 3 Lateral joint dislocation.

(continued)

REDUCTION OF THE FINGERS (*continued*)

CLINICAL PEARLS

A. An aggressive attempt at reducing fingers can cause a fracture of the joint being reduced.

B. Infection is a concern if there is an open fracture.

C. Inadequate mobilization can lead to redislocation.

BIBLIOGRAPHY

Campo, T. M., & Lafferty, K. (Eds.). (2016). *Essential procedures for emergency, urgent, and primary care settings: A clinical companion* (2nd ed.). New York, NY: Springer Publishing Company.

Leggit, J. C., & Meko, C. J. (2006). Acute finger injuries: Part II. Fractures, dislocations, and thumb injuries. *American Family Physician, 73*, 827.

Muelleman, R. L., & Wadman, M. C. (2004). Injuries to the hand and digits. In J. E. Tintinalli, G. D. Kelen, & J. S. Stapczynski (Eds.), *Emergency medicine: A comprehensive study guide* (6th ed., pp. 1665–1673). New York, NY: McGraw-Hill.

REDUCTION OF THE HIP

Laura A. Santanna Lonergan

DESCRIPTION

A. The displacement of the femoral head from the acetabulum.

B. Posterior dislocation more common than anterior dislocation.

INDICATIONS

A. Needed in all hip dislocations.

B. Less emergent in patients status post hip arthroplasty, as risk of osteonecrosis of femoral head is not present.

PRECAUTIONS

A. Contraindicated in patients with associated femoral neck fracture.

EQUIPMENT REQUIRED

A. Facility approved conscious sedation protocol.

B. Second provider/assistant for traction.

C. Abduction pillow.

PROCEDURE

A. Explain the procedure to the patient and/or family and obtain informed consent.

B. Position the patient supine in bed.

C. Perform a proper time out. All present in the room must identify the patient and agree on the correct procedure and correct site of the procedure.

D. Place sheet around the proximal thigh of the affected limb.

E. Administer conscious sedation per facility protocol.

F. Stand on the patient's bed, straddling lower extremities.

G. Use Allis method for posterior dislocations.
   1. Have a provider or assistant stabilize the pelvis by applying direct, downward (see Figure 1) pressure on patient's bilateral anterior superior iliac spines (ASISs).

H. Apply traction in-line with femur.

I. While traction is maintained, slowly flex hip to 70° (see Figure 2).

J. If necessary, gently rotate the hip as well as having second provider/assistant pull laterally on the sheet around the thigh.

K. Continue traction and manipulation until palpable reduction is felt.

L. Place abduction pillow between the patient's legs.

EVALUATION AND RESULTS

A. Postreduction imaging to evaluate success of reduction and ensure no procedural injuries.

B. Postreduction CT scan of the hip recommended to verify concentric reduction as well as evaluate for intra-articular bony fragments.

C. Follow-up with orthopedics for continued evaluation.

CLINICAL PEARLS

A. Another option for positioning the patient for a hip reduction is to place the patient on a backboard using a strap across the pelvis. This may work better than having an assistant apply pressure or may provide extra stabilization.

B. Make sure to use a steady sustained force during reduction.

C. If there is not any movement of the joint, try rocking back and forth with internal and external rotation at the hip.

(continued)

REDUCTION OF THE HIP (*continued*)

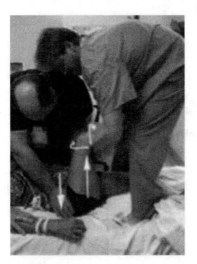

FIGURE 1 Nurses performing the Allis technique on a patient.
Source: Campo, T. M., & Lafferty, K. (Eds.). (2016). *Essential procedures for emergency, urgent, and primary care settings: A clinical companion* (2nd ed.). New York, NY: Springer Publishing Company.

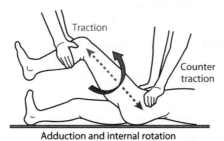

Adduction and internal rotation

FIGURE 2 Adduction and internal rotation of hip.

BIBLIOGRAPHY

Campo, T. M. & Lafferty, K. (Eds.). (2016). *Essential procedures for emergency, urgent, and primary care settings: A clinical companion* (2nd ed.). New York, NY: Springer Publishing Company.

Hendey, G. W., & Avila, A. (2011). The Captain Morgan technique for the reduction of the dislocated hip. *Annals of Emergency Medicine, 58*, 536–540. doi:10.1016/j.annemergmed.2011.07.010

Nordt, W. E., 3rd., (1999). Maneuvers for reducing dislocated hips: A new technique and literature review. *Clinical Orthopedic and Related Research, 360*, 260–264. doi:10.1097/00003086-199903000-00032

Waddell, B., Mohamed, S., Glomset, J., & Meyer, M. (2016). A detailed review of hip reduction maneuvers: A focus on physician safety and introduction of the Waddell technique. *Orthopedic Reviews, 8*(1), 6253. doi:10.4081/or.2016.6253

REDUCTION OF THE PATELLA

Laura A. Santanna Lonergan

DESCRIPTION

A. Loss of patellar alignment.

B. Most typical is lateral dislocation.

INDICATIONS

A. First-time dislocations can be treated with reduction and immobilization.

B. Recurrent dislocations or those dislocations unable to be reduced need operative open reduction.

PRECAUTIONS

A. Do not attempt closed reduction if there are associated injuries to dislocation.

EQUIPMENT REQUIRED

A. 18 g needle.

B. 20 mL syringe.

C. 5 to 10 mL lidocaine.

D. Knee immobilizer brace.

PROCEDURE

A. Explain the procedure to the patient and/or family and obtain informed consent.

B. Traumatic hematoma present: Instill lidocaine at insertion site of needle if performing aspiration to decompress hematoma, allowing patella to sit within the trochlear groove.

C. Extend affected knee (see Figure 1).

D. If extension alone does not relocate the patella, apply medially directed force to the laterally dislocated patella.

E. Brace with knee immobilizer.

EVALUATION AND RESULTS

A. Postreduction imaging to evaluate success of reduction and to ensure no procedural injuries.

B. Follow-up with orthopedics and/or physical therapy.

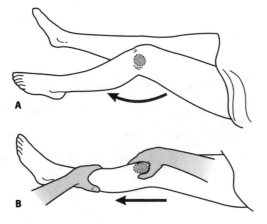

FIGURE 1   Illustration showing reduction of the patella.

(continued)

REDUCTION OF THE PATELLA (*continued*)

CLINICAL PEARLS

A. Patellar dislocations are a common musculoskeletal injury.

B. Reductions of the patella typically do not require imaging or procedural sedation.

C. Recurrent dislocations should be followed up with rehabilitation.

BIBLIOGRAPHY

Davenport, M. (2017, April 13). Reduction of patellar dislocation technique. In E. Schraga (Ed.), *Medscape*. Retrieved from https://emedicine.medscape.com/article/109263-technique

Mehta, V. M., Inoue, M., Nomura, E., & Fithian, D. C. (2007, June). An algorithm guiding the evaluation and treatment of acute primary patellar dislocations. *Sports Medicine and Arthroscopy Review, 15*(2), 78–81. doi:10.1097/JSA.0b013e318042b695

Stefancin, J. J., & Parker, R. D. (2007, February). First-time traumatic patellar dislocation: A systematic review. *Clinical Orthopedics Related Research, 455*, 93–101. doi:10.1097/BLO.0b013e31802eb40a

REDUCTION OF THE SHOULDER

Laura A. Santanna Lonergan

DESCRIPTION

A. A shoulder joint is considered dislocated or subluxed when the articular surfaces of the joint have lost all contact through displacement.

B. The head of the humerus becomes displaced from the glenoid fossa.

INDICATIONS

A. Joint is displaced.

B. Determined by imaging studies.

C. Palpable or visual shoulder deformity with a mechanism of injury suggestive of dislocation.

PRECAUTIONS

A. Obtain imaging of shoulder prior to reduction to rule out evidence of fracture.

EQUIPMENT REQUIRED

A. Stretcher.

B. Weights.

C. Analgesia.

D. Shoulder immobilizer.

PROCEDURE

A. Stimson technique (gravity-assisted reduction).

B. Explain the procedure to the patient and/or family and obtain informed consent.

C. Perform a proper time out. All present in the room must identify the patient and agree on the correct procedure and correct site of the procedure.

D. Administer analgesia as indicated.

E. Perform neurological examination of the bilateral upper extremities to include, but not limited to, function of axillary, musculocutaneous, median, radial, and ulnar nerves.

F. Place the patient prone on a stretcher with the dislocated extremity hanging off the side edge of the stretcher.

G. Have the assistant sit on the floor and apply gentle downward traction to the arm OR attach 5 to 15 pounds of weight to the patient's arm (Stimson maneuver; see Figure 3.44).

H. While traction is performed, place the left thumb on the patient's acromion and left fingers on the front of the humeral head (see Figure 3.45).

I. Gently push the humeral head downward until it reduces into the glenoid fossa.

J. Brace shoulder using immobilizer.

EVALUATION AND RESULTS

A. Postreduction imaging to complete reduction with no procedural injuries.

B. Perform postreduction bilateral upper extremity neurovascular examination and document findings.

C. Follow-up with orthopedic surgeon for continued evaluation.

D. Perform physical therapy/exercises for strength building and return of preinjury function.

CLINICAL PEARLS

A. Many shoulder dislocations can easily be reduced by medical professionals after injury in many cases before muscles go into spasm.

B. Recurrences of shoulder dislocations are common after the first injury.

(continued)

REDUCTION OF THE SHOULDER (*continued*)

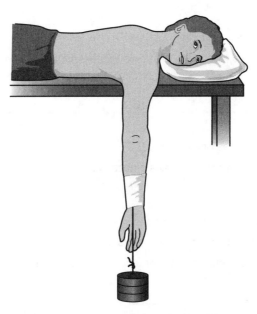

FIGURE 1 Illustration depicting the Stimson maneuver. Patient should lie prone on the table. A 5- to 15-pound weight should be attached to the affected arm, hanging off of the edge of the table as shown.

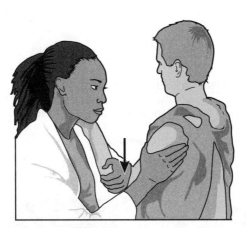

FIGURE 2 The Cunningham technique. Face the patient diagonally and instruct him or her to relax and pull back his or her shoulders.

BIBLIOGRAPHY

DeLee, J., Drez, D., & Miller, M. D. (Eds.). (2003). *DeLee and Drez's orthopaedic sports medicine* (2nd ed., pp. 1038–1040). Philadelphia, PA: Elsevier Science.

Marinelli, M., & de Palma, L. (2009, March). The external rotation method for reduction of acute anterior shoulder dislocations. *Journal of Orthopedics and Traumatology, 10*(1), 17–20. doi:10.1007/s10195-008-0040-4

Westin, C. D., Gill, E. A., Noyes, M. E., & Hubbard, M. (1995, May-June). Anterior shoulder dislocation. A simple and rapid method for reduction. *American Journal of Sports Medicine, 23*(3), 369–371. doi:10.1177/036354659502300322

SPLINTING

Laura A. Santanna Lonergan

DESCRIPTION

A. Mechanism used to immobilize an injured extremity.

B. A splint is similar to a cast in that its function is to immobilize, but its main advantage allows for soft tissue swelling during the acute phase of an injury.

INDICATIONS

A. Immobilization of acute fractures.

B. Immobilization of dislocation after it has been reduced.

C. Treatment of soft tissue injuries not limited to sprains and strains.

PRECAUTIONS

A. Do not place over broken, undressed skin/lacerations.

B. Ensure proper splint padding and placement to defer pressure sore.

C. Ensure patient's proper position of function while splinted to avoid further injury to the patient.

EQUIPMENT REQUIRED

A. Length- and width-appropriate prefabricated splint.

B. Additional padding.

C. Bucket of cool water.

D. Dry towel.

E. Elastic bandage wraps.

PROCEDURE

A. Short arm ulnar gutter (see Figure 1).
   1. To treat fractures of the fourth and fifth metacarpals and phalanges.
   2. Apply splint on ulnar aspect of upper extremity, from the tip of the little finger to just distal to the elbow.
   3. Place wrist in 20° extension, metacarpophalangeals (MCPs) flexed to 50°, and distal interphalangeal (DIP) and proximal interphalangeal (PIP) joints in slight flexion.
   4. Pad upper extremity as indicated per patient presentation.
   5. Immerse splint in bucket of cool water.
   6. Remove excess water from splint with towel.

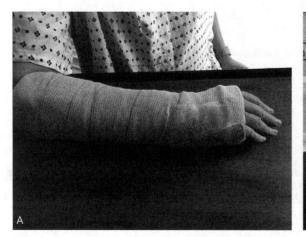 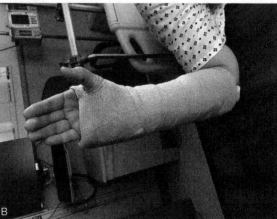

FIGURE 1 Short arm ulnar gutter: (A) supine view; (B) prone view.

(continued)

SPLINTING *(continued)*

7. Apply splint with patient holding position of function, securing with angiotensin-converting enzyme (ACE) bandages.
8. Perform postsplint application neurovascular examination to bilateral upper extremities.

B. Long arm posterior splint (see Figure 2).
1. Used for acute immobilization of midforearm or proximal forearm fractures.
    a. It can also be used for fractures of the distal humerus.
2. Place elbow in 90° flexion, with forearm in neutral pronation or supination.
3. Apply splint to the ulnar aspect of the forearm, extending from the palmer crease to several inches above the elbow.
4. Pad the upper extremity as indicated per patient presentation.
5. Immerse the splint in a bucket of cool water.
6. Remove excess water from the splint with a towel.
7. Apply the splint with the patient holding the position of function, securing with ACE bandages.
8. Perform a postsplint application neurovascular examination to the bilateral upper extremities.

C. Upper extremity sugar-tong splint (Figure 3).
1. Can be used for acute splinting of forearm fractures.
    a. May provide more stability than a volar splint.
2. Splint begins at the palmar crease, moves along the volar forearm, moves around the elbow joint, and ends at the dorsal aspect of the MCP joints.
3. Pad the upper extremity as indicated per patient presentation.

Long arm posterior splint

• Indications

- Distal humerus #

- Both-bone forearm #

- Unstable proximal radius or ulna # (sugar-tong better)

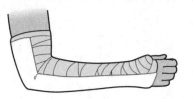

FIGURE 2 Long arm posterior splint.

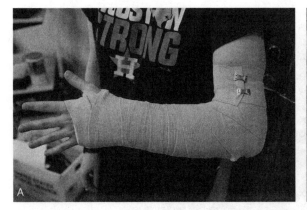
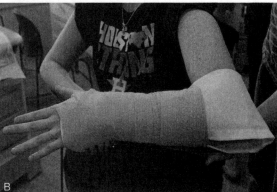

FIGURE 3 Upper extremity sugar-tong splint: (A) completed wrapping; (B) wrap around underlying pad.

(continued)

SPLINTING *(continued)*

4. Immerse the splint in a bucket of cool water.
5. Remove excess water from the splint with a towel.
6. Apply the splint with the patient holding the position of function, securing with ACE bandages.
7. Perform a postsplint application neurovascular examination to the bilateral upper extremities.

D. Volar wrist splint (Figure 4).
1. Can be used for sprains of the wrist or for stable fractures of the distal radius and/or ulna.
2. Splint extends from the volar surface of the MCP joints to the proximal forearm.
3. Pad the upper extremity as indicated per patient presentation.
4. Immerse the splint in a bucket of cool water.
5. Remove excess water from the splint with a towel.
6. Apply the splint with the patient holding the position of function, securing with ACE bandages.
7. Perform a postsplint application neurovascular examination to the bilateral upper extremities.

E. Thumb spica splint (Figure 5).
1. Used for sprains or fractures of the scaphoid, first metacarpal, or thumb proximal phalanx.
2. Splint runs along the thumb from above the interphalangeal (IP) joint, along the radial aspect of the wrist to the forearm.
3. Wrist is splinted in the neutral position while the thumb is splinted slightly flexed: Have the patient oppose the thumb toward the index finger as if to make the "OK" sign.
4. Pad the upper extremity as indicated per patient presentation.
5. Immerse the splint in a bucket of cool water.
6. Remove excess water from the splint with a towel.
7. Apply the splint with the patient holding the position of function, securing with ACE bandages.
8. Perform a postsplint application neurovascular examination to the bilateral upper extremities.

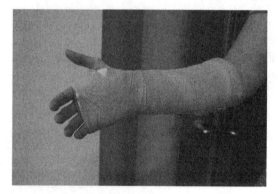

FIGURE 4   Volar wrist splint.

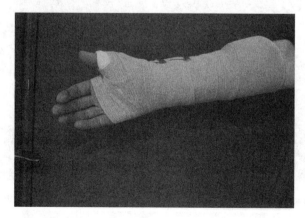

FIGURE 5   Thumb spica splint.

(continued)

SPLINTING (*continued*)

F. Short leg posterior splint (Figure 6).
   1. Used for acute immobilization of severe ankle sprains and fractures of the distal leg, ankle, and foot.
   2. Splint is applied along the posterior aspect of the lower leg from 1 inch distal to the popliteal fossa to the distal ends of the toes.
   3. Pad the lower extremity as indicated per patient presentation.
   4. Immerse the splint in a bucket of cool water.
   5. Remove excess water from the splint with a towel.
   6. Apply the splint with the patient holding the position of function, securing with ACE bandages.
   7. Perform a postsplint application neurovascular examination to the bilateral lower extremities.

G. Lower leg sugar-tong splint.
   1. Can be used as an alternative to the short leg posterior splint when more stability is desired.
   2. It is a "U"-shaped splint starting at the lateral aspect of the knee, which goes under the proximal foot and heel and moves upward, stopping at the medial aspect of the knee (see Figure 7).
   3. Pad the lower extremity as indicated per patient presentation.
   4. Immerse the splint in a bucket of cool water.
   5. Remove excess water from the splint with a towel.
   6. Apply the splint with the patient holding the position of function, securing with an elastic bandage wrap.
   7. Perform a postsplint application neurovascular examination to the bilateral lower extremities.

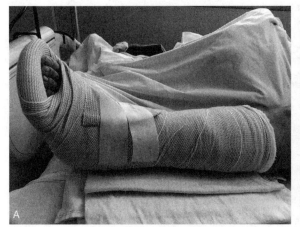 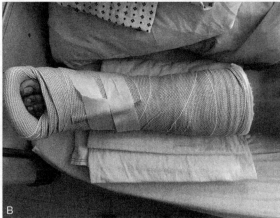

FIGURE 6　Short leg posterior splint: (A) lateral view; (B) supine view.

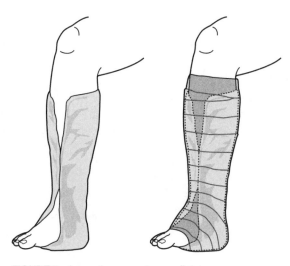

FIGURE 7　Lower leg sugar-tong splint.

(*continued*)

SPLINTING (*continued*)

EVALUATION AND RESULTS

A. After splint placement, carefully assess to ensure the splint:
   1. Is in extension (not flexed).
   2. Does not interfere with range of motion of necessary joints.
   3. Does not have finger indentations or sharp edges puncturing the patient's skin.

B. The splint is never to be removed by the patient; only by a professional after follow-up with the specified specialist.

C. If the splint is on the lower extremity, go over weight-bearing status with the patient and make sure he or she has sufficient and safe means of mobility (crutches, cane, walker, etc.).

D. The splint is to stay dry at all times. If the splint gets wet, a new splint needs to be placed.

E. Educate the patient that splints are usually temporary and he or she will most likely need to follow-up with a specialist for continued care and treatment of the injury.

CLINICAL PEARLS

A. Extremities should be splinted in their correct anatomical position unless there is resistance or loss of circulation.

B. A poorly immobilized fracture can be more harmful than no splint at all.

C. When in doubt, splint an extremity even if it is not clear if there is a fracture.

BIBLIOGRAPHY

Do, T. (2017). Splinting. In E. D. Schraga (Ed.), *Medscape*. Retrieved from https://emedicine.medscape.com/article/1997864-overview

Egol, K. A., Koval, K. J., & Zuckerman, J. D. (2015). *Handbook of fractures* (5th ed., pp. 1–72). Philadelphia, PA: Wolters Kluwer.

Nackenson, J., Baez, A. A., & Meizoso, J. P. (2017). A descriptive analysis of traction splint utilization and IV analgesia by emergency medical services. *Prehospital and Disaster Medicine, 32*(6), 631–635. doi:10.1017/S1049023X17006859

SYNOVIAL FLUID ASPIRATION

Joanne Elaine Pechar

DESCRIPTION

A. Joint aspiration, also known as joint arthrocentesis, is a procedure to drain and remove fluid from the joint space using a needle and syringe.

B. Joint aspiration, commonly done under local anesthesia, offers both therapeutic and diagnostic benefits and is commonly done to relieve swelling or to obtain fluid for analysis.

INDICATIONS

A. Therapeutic.
    1. Hemarthrosis or bleeding into joint space.
    2. Symptomatic relief of joint effusion.

B. Diagnostic.
    1. Septic joint.
    2. Crystal-induced joint disease.
    3. Unexplained joint effusion.

PRECAUTIONS

A. Infection of overlying tissues is considered a relative contraindication.

B. In some cases, joint aspiration is still performed as it provides critical diagnostic information.

EQUIPMENT REQUIRED

A. Betadine swab.

B. Alcohol swab.

C. Ethyl chloride or cold anesthetic spray.

D. One pair of hemostats.

E. 16 or 18 gauge needle.

F. 10 to 60 mL syringe.

G. Gauze.

H. Tape.

I. Pen marker.

J. Three vacutainer lab tubes for joint fluid analysis (gram stain, cell count, culture, and crystals).

K. Gloves.

PROCEDURE

A. Explain the procedure to the patient and/or family and obtain informed consent.

B. Use standard precautions to prep for procedure.

C. Perform a proper time out. All present in the room must identify the patient and agree on the correct procedure and correct site of the procedure.

D. Assess for any evidence of infection or inflammation.

E. Place the patient supine with knee in extension.

F. Use medial approach when effusion is small and lateral approach with larger effusions.

G. Identify bony landmarks, namely the superior pole and lateral edge of the patella and the soft spot approximately 1 to 2 cm below the lateral edge of the patella.

H. Mark entry site.

I. Prep site with Betadine and alcohol swab.

J. Ethyl chloride spray can be used to anesthetize the site.

(continued)

SYNOVIAL FLUID ASPIRATION *(continued)*

K. Lightly hold patella between thumb and index finger.

L. Using an anteromedial or anterolateral approach, insert the needle into the joint space (see Figure 1).

M. Once the needle enters the joint space, aspirate fluid. Advance needle until synovial fluid is obtained (see Figure 2).

N. Resistance to the flow of synovial fluid can be met at the level of the joint capsule.

O. To "milk" additional fluid, have the assistant apply manual pressure to the opposite side of the joint.

P. In order to maximize extraction of effusion or blood, directing the needle in multiple angles inside the joint space may be needed.

Q. If the syringe becomes full of fluid, empty it by removing the syringe from the hub of the needle and replace it with an empty syringe. Repeat aspiration until synovial fluid can no longer be aspirated or until knee effusion is no longer visible.

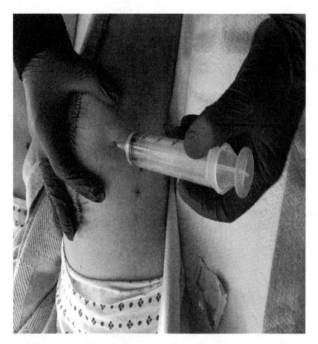

FIGURE 1   Insertion of needle into the joint space.

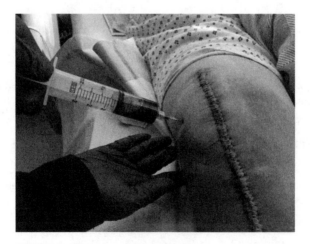

FIGURE 2   Extraction of synovial fluid.

(continued)

SYNOVIAL FLUID ASPIRATION (*continued*)

R. When procedure is completed, hold direct pressure for at least 5 minutes.

S. Apply dressing.

T. Send fluid to the laboratory for analysis. If infection is suspected, obtain gram stain, cell counts, and cultures.

U. Instruct patients to avoid use of the joint for at least 1 day.

EVALUATION AND RESULTS

A. Review the results of the synovial fluid (see Table 1).

TABLE 1   Synovial Fluid Findings

Findings	Normal Joint	Noninflammatory	Inflammatory	Septic	Hemorrhagic
Clarity	Transparent	Transparent	Translucent or cloudy	Opaque or turbid	Bloody
Color	Clear	Straw to yellow	Yellow	Yellow, green, purulent	Red
Fluid cell count: WBC	<200	<2,000	2,000–50,000	>50,000	200–2,000
Segmented neutrophils or PMNs	<25%	<25%	>70%	>90%	50%–75%
Fluid culture	Negative	Negative	Negative	Positive	Negative

PMN, polymorphonuclear leukocyte; WBC, white blood cell.

B. Most purulent synovial fluid or effusions are due to septic arthritis.

C. Noninflammatory conditions include degenerative joint disease (DJD), osteochondritis dissecans, and neuropathic arthropathy.

D. Inflammatory conditions include rheumatoid arthritis (RA), gout, pseudogout, reactive arthritis, ankylosing spondylitis, and rheumatic fever.

E. Hemorrhagic conditions include hemarthrosis, hemophilia or other hemorrhagic diathesis, and trauma with or without fracture.

CLINICAL PEARLS

A. If there is a suspicion of joint infection, cell count, culture, and gram stain should be urgently sent for lab analysis.

B. Patients receiving anticoagulation at therapeutic levels can generally undergo arthrocentesis safely, but bleeding is to be expected.

BIBLIOGRAPHY

Shlamovitz, G. (2019, February 28). Knee arthrocentesis technique. In E. D. Schraga (Ed.), *Medscape*. Retrieved from https://emedicine.medscape.com/article/79994-technique

Zhang, Q., Zhang, T., Lv, H., Xie, L., Wu, W., Wu, J., & Wu, X. (2012, July). Comparison of two positions of knee arthrocentesis: How to obtain complete drainage. *American Journal of Physical Medicine & Rehabilitation, 91*(7), 611–615. doi:10.1097/PHM.0b013e31825a13f0

Zuber, T. J. (2002, October 15). Knee joint aspiration and injection. *American Family Physician, 66*(8), 1497–1501. Retrieved from https://www.aafp.org/afp/2002/1015/p1497.html

THORACENTESIS

E. Moneé Carter-Griffin

DESCRIPTION

A. Needle insertion into the pleural space to remove excess fluid.

INDICATIONS

A. Therapeutic drainage of symptomatic pleural effusions.

B. Diagnostic evaluation of pleural fluid.

PRECAUTIONS

A. Patients with coagulopathies.

B. Avoid areas of skin infections on the chest wall.

C. Increased risk of pneumothorax in patients receiving positive pressure ventilation.

D. Patient's habitus or anatomy may hinder identifying landmarks.

EQUIPMENT REQUIRED

A. Sterile gloves, drape, and towels.

B. Antiseptic solution with chlorhexidine or povidone-iodine.

C. Lidocaine 1% with or without epinephrine for local anesthesia.

D. Keep atropine at the bedside for potential emergency administration.

E. 25-gauge, 5/8 to 1 inch needle.

F. 20 to 23 gauge, 1½ inch needle.

G. 14 to 18 gauge needle.

H. 12 to 16 gauge catheter.

I. Pressure tubing.

J. Three-way stopcock.

K. 5 mL syringe.

L. 20 mL syringe.

M. 60 mL syringe.

N. Specimen vials and tubes, aerobic/anaerobic media bottles.

O. Vacutainers, evacuated bottles, or drainage bag.

P. Pressure/connector tubing.

Q. Sterile 4 × 4 gauze.

R. Adhesive dressing.

S. Keep a thoracostomy tray with supplies available in case of a pneumothorax.
   1. Chlorhexidine solution.
   2. Drapes.
   3. Gauze.
   4. Curved hemostat.
   5. Curved Kelly clamp.
   6. Scissors.
   7. Needle holder.
   8. Sterile thoracotomy tube.
   9. Scalpel.
   10. 4-0 silk suture on cutting needle.
   11. Petroleum-soaked gauze.
   12. Underwater sealed drainage system.

(continued)

THORACENTESIS *(continued)*

PROCEDURE

A. Explain the procedure to the patient and family and obtain informed consent.

B. Always identify patient.

C. Wash hands/perform hand hygiene.

D. Ensure intravenous (IV) access and hemodynamic monitoring (e.g., blood pressure, O_2 saturations).

E. Position patient (help of an assistant may be needed).
1. Position patient on edge of bed with feet on a solid surface (e.g., ground, stool).
2. The assistant will stand in front of the patient or patient will lean on a bedside table directly in front with the head on his or her arms.

F. Verify location for pleural drainage with ultrasound.
1. If ultrasound is unavailable, utilize physical examination to locate area of effusion.
2. Optimal site for needle insertion is posterolateral (midaxillary and midline) between seventh and ninth intercostal space, 6 to 8 cm lateral to spine (see Figure 1).

G. Don sterile attire.

H. Assemble all equipment and set up sterile field.

I. Perform a proper time out. All present in the room must identify the patient and agree on the correct procedure and correct site of the procedure.

J. Cleanse area again with chlorhexidine or a povidone-iodine solution.

K. Drape identified area.

L. Use 25 gauge 5/8 inch needle and 5 mL syringe to inject small wheal of lidocaine.

M. Use 20 gauge 1½ inch needle and 10 mL syringe to infiltrate lidocaine into a wide area of subcutaneous tissue, periosteum, and pleura.

N. For therapeutic thoracentesis, insert 14 or 18 gauge needle with a 20 mL syringe attached into anesthetized area until pleural fluid is obtained.

O. Remove syringe and occlude needle with a finger.

P. Insert 16 or 12 gauge catheter through gauged needle, positioned downward toward the diaphragm into the pleural space.

Q. Once the catheter is in place, remove the needle and attach the three-way stopcock and 60 mL syringe.

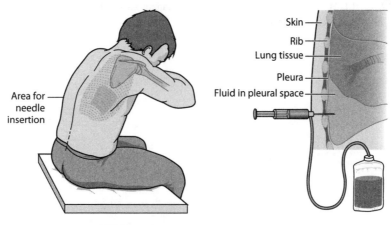

Area for needle insertion

Skin
Rib
Lung tissue
Pleura
Fluid in pleural space

FIGURE 1 Illustration showing insertion site.

(continued)

THORACENTESIS (*continued*)

R. Fill 60 mL syringe with pleural fluid, turn stopcock off to catheter, and remove syringe. Fill each specimen vial with pleural fluid.

S. Attach pressure tubing to three-way stopcock and vacutainer.

T. Open stopcock to vacutainer and allow pleural fluid to flow into vacutainer. Limit drainage to 1 to 1.5 L to reduce risk of reexpansion pulmonary edema.

U. Remove catheter and apply pressure to puncture site.

V. Apply adhesive bandage and aid patient back into bed.

W. Dispose of all equipment.

X. Obtain chest x-ray to evaluate for improvement in pleural effusion and to assess for complications (e.g., pneumothorax).

Y. Document procedure, indication, amount of fluid removal, diagnostics sent, and patient's tolerance of the procedure.

EVALUATION AND RESULTS

A. Resolution of pleural effusion and reexpansion of lung tissue.

B. Resolution of respiratory distress in patients with excess pleural fluid.

C. Etiology of pleural effusion determined based on pleural fluid analysis.

CLINICAL PEARLS

A. Ultrasound guidance to reduce complications and drainage location.

B. Some institutions may have prepackaged thoracentesis kits.

C. If the patient is unable to sit up, have him or her lay in the lateral recumbent position on the unaffected side.

D. Cease procedure if patient develops a cough.

E. Emergency medications such as atropine for symptomatic bradycardia should be placed at bedside.

F. Keep thoracostomy supplies available in case patient develops a pneumothorax.

BIBLIOGRAPHY

Dimov, V., & Altaqi, B. (2005). *Thoracentesis: A step-by-step procedure guide with photos* [Blog post]. Retrieved from http://note3.blogspot.com/2004/02/thoracentesis-procedure-guide.html

Schildhouse, R., Lai, A., Barsuk, J. H., Mourad, M., & Chopra, V. (2017, April). Safe and effective bedside thoracentesis: A review of the evidence for practicing clinicians. *Journal of Hospital Medicine, 12*(4), 266–276. doi:10.12788/jhm.2716

Seneff, M. G., Corwin, R. W., Gold, L. H., & Irwin, R. S. (1986, July). Complications associated with thoracocentesis. *Chest, 90*(1), 97–100. doi:10.1378/chest.90.1.97

TRANSPYLORIC FEEDING TUBE PLACEMENT

Catherine Harris

DESCRIPTION

A. Dobhoff tubes are flexible, nasogastric tubes used to administer nutrition and medications to patients unable to receive them by mouth.

B. The tube is inserted into the stomach via the nasal passages.

INDICATIONS

A. Sedated or mechanically ventilated patients who need to receive nutrition and/or medications.

B. Critical illness.

C. Severe malnutrition.

D. Prolonged anorexia.

E. Difficulty swallowing.

F. High risk aspiration.

PRECAUTIONS

A. Improper setup and placement may result in placing tube in lung, causing pneumothorax.

B. In patients with a basilar skull fracture, placement should be done with a clear visual pathway, typically performed with a scope by a member of the ear, nose, and throat (ENT) service. In very rare cases, a tube can circumnavigate to the brain without direct visualization.

C. Spinal cord fractures.
   1. Patient is typically encouraged to bend his/her neck forward for placement.
   2. Avoid this movement in patients with confirmed or suspected cervical spine fractures.
   3. Direct placement may be required.

D. Patients on a ventilator or who are sedated may have a decreased or absent cough reflex: Pay special attention to ANY changes in tidal volume, decrease in oxygen saturation, or persistent coughing.

EQUIPMENT REQUIRED

A. 10 Fr feeding tube with guidewire (see Figure 1).

B. Water-soluble lubricant.

C. 60 mL syringe.

D. Nasal strip tape to hold feeding tube in place.

E. Gloves.

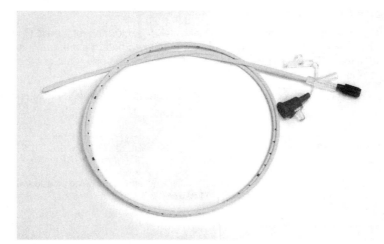

FIGURE 1 Photograph of a 10 Fr feeding tube with guidewire.

(continued)

TRANSPYLORIC FEEDING TUBE PLACEMENT (*continued*)

PROCEDURE

A. Measure tube from tip of nose to subxyphoid process (about 30–35 cm in most patients).

B. Have patient sit upright and lean head forward.

C. Remove the feeding tube from the package and place some water-soluble lubricant on the tip to help facilitate passage of the tube through the nasal passages.

D. Place tube through one nare and ask the patient to swallow as the tube passes down the oropharynx. Patients may gag but should not start coughing: Persistent coughing may be a warning sign that the tube is in the airway rather than the esophagus.

E. At 35 cm, STOP and confirm with chest x-ray that the tube is in the esophagus and not the mainstem bronchus.
   1. Confirmation is made if feeding tube follows path of trachea straight below carina.
   2. If placement is in airway, the tube will curve into either the right or left mainstem bronchus; remove feeding tube and start again.

F. Once x-ray confirms the feeding tube is in the esophagus, advance into stomach.

G. Check placement by insufflating with air.

H. Advance feeding tube to about 80 to 100 cm.

I. Leave guidewire in place and obtain an abdominal x-ray (not chest).

J. If tube is postpylorus, secure it and remove wire; start feeds.

K. If tube is not postpylorus, advance it further and obtain another abdominal x-ray.

EVALUATION AND RESULTS

A. Verify placement of feeding tube with chest x-ray first to establish that tube is below carina and not in right or left mainstem bronchus.

B. Verify placement of feeding tube with abdominal x-ray once tube is advanced and expected to be postpylorus.

C. Once visual placement is made, remove wire and start tube feeds.

CLINICAL PEARLS

A. Positioning and setup are essential for success.

B. If patient is awake, have the patient bend his or her neck as far forward as possible.

C. Aim the tip of the feeding tube toward the very back of the nasal passage and allow the natural curvature of the tube to guide itself.

D. If there is significant resistance, try another naris.
   1. Strictures, polyps, and dried mucus may cause obstruction.
   2. After a couple unsuccessful attempts, consult an ENT for the direct visual approach.

E. When placing feeding tubes in patients on a ventilator, remember an endotracheal tube (ETT) cuff balloon will prevent placing the feeding tube in the lung, but not always. Never force the catheter past the balloon.
   1. Sometimes after hitting the ETT cuff balloon, the tube will curl back and come out of the patient's mouth.
   2. After a couple unsuccessful tries, consult an ENT for the direct visual approach.

F. Do NOT rely on air insufflation to check correct position; always get an x-ray before beginning any tube feeds.

BIBLIOGRAPHY

Powers, J., Chance, R., Bortenschlager, L., Hottenstein, J., Bobel, K., Gervasio, J., & McNees, T. (2003). Bedside placement of small-bowel feeding tubes in the intensive care unit. *Critical Care Nurse, 23*(1), 16–24. Retrieved from http://ccn.aacnjournals.org/content/23/1/16.long

Simons, S. R., & Abdallah, L. M. (2012). Bedside assessment of enteral tube placement: Aligning practice with evidence. *The American Journal of Nursing, 112*(2), 40–46. doi:10.1097/01.NAJ.0000411178.07179.68

IV Special Topics

END-OF-LIFE CONSIDERATIONS

Jennifer Coates

INTRODUCTION

With life, comes death. The dying process is not only an inevitable part of the life cycle, but it is also an important aspect of healthcare. Although discussions surrounding death and dying can be difficult for patients, caregivers, and even healthcare providers, such discussions are essential to ensure supportive and compassionate end-of-life care aligns with the patient's and his or her family's desires.

Advances in healthcare treatment mean that people are living longer. Currently, life expectancy in the United States is 78.8 years. Annually, there are 823.7 deaths per 100,000 people. Increased life expectancy means that people are not only living longer in general, but also that people are living longer with chronic diseases. Nearly 75% of all deaths in the United States are from the following 10 causes.

A. Heart disease.

B. Cancer.

C. Chronic lower respiratory diseases.

D. Unintentional injuries.

E. Stroke.

F. Alzheimer's disease.

G. Diabetes.

H. Influenza and pneumonia.

I. Kidney disease.

J. Suicide.

Of these conditions, seven are chronic conditions. Of further note, two of these diseases (heart disease and cancer) together accounted for nearly 48% of all deaths. This information helps the advance practice provider (APP) consider important aspects of discussing and providing end-of-life care, including the role of institutions and acute care during the death experience.

DISCUSSING THE DEATH EXPERIENCE

Discussing the death experience requires a shift in the healthcare provider's mind-set. In tertiary care, the overall goal of care is to extend the patient's life in an attempt to delay death. However, the first step in planning and providing end-of-life care is acceptance that death is the likely outcome. Specifically, the goal in acute care should be that the dying patient and his or her family are supported as the patient completes his or her life cycle.

Understanding the overall goal of end-of-life care prepares the APP to discuss the patient's and the family's preferences for end-of-life care and the dying experience. When entering into this discussion with a patient and his or her family, the APP should remember that when a patient will die is only one factor in that patient's death experience. Where the patient will die and how he or she will die are also important aspects of the death experience that need to be discussed. In general, where a patient dies has changed over time. In the early part of the 20th century, most people died at home; however, today most people will die in an institution. The increased number of patients who experience cognitive impairment and dementia is one possible reason for this change. Some people have preferences about where they would like to die, so it is important to discuss this with the patient and his or her family.

DEFINING A "GOOD DEATH"

Another important factor to discuss is how the patient prefers to die. Every patient's experience with death is unique. To help the patient complete his or her life cycle in a way aligned with his or her preferences and beliefs, healthcare providers need to have a firm grasp on what a "good" death means for each patient. Defining a "good" death requires the APP to engage in an honest, open discussion that is focused on several important themes.

PREFERENCES FOR THE DYING PROCESS

Each patient has different preferences regarding where he or she prefers to die, the manner in which he or she will die, and who will be present when the patient completes his or her life cycle. In order to respect the patient's preferences, the APP should encourage the patient to express these preferences, both verbally in conversation and in written form via an advance directive.

(continued)

END-OF-LIFE CONSIDERATIONS (*continued*)

PAIN

Assessing and effectively managing pain is an important part of providing compassionate and comprehensive end-of-life care. Conversations about pain assessment, pain management, and side effect management will vary based on the patient's diagnosis. However, these discussions should center on how the patient's comfort level will be assessed, and which interventions will be used to manage pain and side effects.

EMOTIONAL WELL-BEING AND SUPPORT SYSTEM

Another important part of completing one's life cycle includes having the opportunity to discuss the meaning of death and to identify the role of a support system in death. The APP should be sure to allow the patient to discuss his or her personal wishes and ensure that an emotional support system is in place. People and organizations that are included in a patient's emotional support system vary, but may include church, family, friends, a community, and/or beloved pets. In addition to identifying an emotional support system, the APP should also help the patient determine the role of his or her support system as the patient completes the life cycle. For example, how will family and friends be involved in the process?

The APP plays an important role in emotionally supporting and preparing the patient's friends and family for the patient's death. The APP should help the patient's family and friends accept and prepare for the patient's death. This may include facilitating discussions, being available to answer questions, and providing resources as needed.

DIGNITY

Respecting all patients as individuals is central to providing end-of-life care. The APP can achieve this by empowering the patient to be independent and in control of his or her care. Dignity in death can take on many forms and it is highly individualized. Asking the patient open-ended questions about what he or she feels is important will help the APP provide appropriate and respectful care during the patient's final months and days of life.

LIFE COMPLETION AND SPIRITUALITY

Saying goodbye and receiving religious/spiritual comfort are important aspects of life completion. When discussing this theme with patients, the APP should be sure to inquire about the role of religion and spiritual comfort in the patient's life completion. During this discussion, the APP also should ask how he or she can help facilitate the opportunity for the patient to meet with clergy, if he or she desires, and how he or she can help the patient see friends and family at life's completion.

TREATMENT PREFERENCES

As previously noted, the focus of treatments and interventions provided during end-of-life care shift from prolonging the patient's life to supporting the patient and his or her family as the patient's life completes. During this time, the APP should take care to answer any questions the patient and his or her family may have. Often, the patient and his or her family want to know if all available treatments were offered, and that they have control over treatment decisions.

QUALITY OF LIFE

The APP should be sure to discuss how he or she could help the patient maintain hope, pleasure, and gratitude as the patient completes his or her life cycle. Discussion should focus on how the disease is affecting the patient's physical mobility, emotional well-being, and social well-being. Conversation with the patient should center on strategies to help the patient feel that he or she has a life that is worth living.

RELATIONSHIP WITH TREATMENT TEAM

Building a strong relationship between the patient and the healthcare team is essential to providing supportive and comprehensive end-of-life care. The patient needs to trust as well as feel supported and comforted by the healthcare team. This relationship may be garnered in a variety of ways, but stems from the healthcare provider being comfortable with death and dying. Such a relationship will enable the patient to be at ease, which will, in turn, allow the patient to freely discuss his or her preferences, spiritual beliefs, and fears with the healthcare provider.

PORTABLE ORDERS FOR LIFE-SUSTAINING TREATMENT

As part of the ongoing discussion surrounding the type of death experience the patient desires, it is important that the APP also discusses the role of Portable Orders for Life-Sustaining Treatment (POLST) in ensuring the patient's desires are upheld. Sometimes called Physician Orders for Life-Sustaining Treatment, the POLST is a form that provides standing medical orders that healthcare providers can act on immediately when the patient is in an acute situation. It outlines the type of care a patient wishes to receive, or does not wish to receive, during end of life. POLST topics include the patient's preferences concerning CPR, antibiotics, mechanical ventilation, and artificial nutrition. The POLST form is intended

END-OF-LIFE CONSIDERATIONS (*continued*)

to help healthcare providers, including first responders, provide the type of treatment the patient wants, even if the patient is unable to communicate at the time care is provided. It has been shown to be more effective than traditional advance directives at limiting unwanted life-sustaining treatments.

The APP should initiate discussion about a POLST form with any patient with a serious or chronic illness who may not be expected to live past 1 year. Without a POLST form (see Table 1), emergency responders will provide all appropriate medical interventions.

| **TABLE 1** | **POLST Form** |

POLST	Medical Order
Who completes POLST?	Healthcare professional such as MD, NP, PA, but will vary from state to state who can sign the order
What does it communicate?	Code status
Would the patient want CPR? Check one	• Attempt resuscitation/CPR • Do not attempt resuscitation/DNR
What type of medical interventions are available? Check one	• Full treatment—No limitation in aggressive treatment options • Limited treatment—use medical treatment such as antibiotics, IV fluids, and cardiac monitor. No intubation, advanced airway interventions, or mechanical ventilation • Comfort measures only—Comfort through symptom management
Artificially administered nutrition? Check one	• Long-term artificial nutrition by tube • Defined period of artificial nutrition by tube • No artificial nutrition by tube
Review	By health-care professionals

DNR, do not resuscitate; IV, intravenous; POLST, Portable Orders for Life-Sustaining Treatment.

PALLIATIVE CARE

As end-of-life approaches, palliative care may be offered to the patient. Palliative care focuses on symptom assessment and treatment, and it may be offered simultaneously with life-prolonging and curative therapies. During end of life, palliative care typically focuses on assessing and treating pain, dyspnea, anxiety, fatigue, depression, constipation, and delirium.

PAIN

Pain is the most common symptom a patient experiences at end of life. Effective pain control can be achieved by using a combination of several treatments. Nonpharmacologic treatments are those interventions that do not require the use of medications. This may include imagery, aromatherapy, relaxation, music therapy, massage, and distraction techniques. Pharmacologic treatments, or those that involve medications, may include the use of opioids and nonsteroidal anti-inflammatory agents, and acetaminophen. Ideal pain management in end of life can be achieved through a long acting agent with the addition of an immediate release agent for breakthrough pain.

DYSPNEA

Dyspnea is another common symptom during the end-of-life phase. The APP should aim to treat reversible causes, if possible. Nonpharmacologic interventions can also be especially helpful. These interventions can include providing reassurance, offering distraction techniques, and encouraging relaxation exercises.

ANXIETY

When a patient in an end-of-life situation experiences anxiety, it is important for the APP to first assess the cause of anxiety, identifying both physical and psychological contributors. After the cause or causes are identified, the APP should find ways to modify any anxiety contributors, if possible. Nonpharmacologic interventions include supportive counseling and reassurance. When considering pharmacologic intervention, the APP should use benzodiazepines cautiously, as they may increase delirium in older adults.

(*continued*)

END-OF-LIFE CONSIDERATIONS *(continued)*

FATIGUE

Fatigue may be caused by a number of medical problems. When considering the best intervention for fatigue, the APP should address any contributing medical problems. These may include anemia, electrolyte imbalances, infection, or hypoxemia. Depending on the cause of fatigue, nonpharmacologic and/or pharmacologic therapies may be indicated. Nonpharmacologic therapy may include energy conservation, frequent naps, occupational therapy, and physical therapy. Pharmacologic therapy may include considering corticosteroids and psychostimulants on a case-by-case basis.

DEPRESSION

Many patients will experience some degree of depression at the end of their life cycle. Some patients who experience depression in end of life may benefit from supportive psychotherapy. Pharmacologic therapy may be considered depending on the patient's life expectancy, since many antidepressants need several weeks to take effect.

CONSTIPATION

The APP should be sure to assess the end-of-life patient for constipation. Preventive treatment for constipation should be given to all patients taking opioid pain medicine. Stool softeners may be given; the patient may also benefit from increased consumption of prune juice as well as taking a pharmacologic stimulant or osmotic laxative.

DELIRIUM

The APP should identify underlying and reversible causes of delirium to determine the most appropriate interventions. Nonpharmacologic intervention primarily focuses on ensuring a calm environment with family, friends, or caregivers at the bedside. Pharmacologic interventions may be warranted if delirium is severe. Benzodiazepines should be avoided, as they may worsen delirium.

HOSPICE CARE

Hospice care provides support and services to a patient with a terminal illness and focuses on providing comfort for the patient in the final weeks and months of his or her life, not curing the patient's illness. Hospice referral occurs when patients are entering their final weeks and months of life and when patients and their families choose to focus on the patients' comfort. In many cases, hospice occurs in the home, but it may also occur in other settings, such as the hospital, a nursing home, or a resident living facility.

U.S. MEDICARE HOSPICE ELIGIBILITY

Hospice care is delivered by a multidisciplinary team and it is covered under Medicare, Medicaid, and many private insurance plans. Those eligible for Medicare Part A include U.S. citizens or legal residents who are:

A. Eligible for Social Security or railroad retirement benefits and are over age 65.

B. Under age 65 and eligible for Medicare because of a long-term disability.

To be covered, a referral must be made to a hospice that is Medicare certified by the Centers for Medicare and Medicaid Services. Certification from the healthcare provider should state that the patient has a terminal diagnosis and most likely has less than 6 months to live. If patients outlive their estimated 6-month prognosis while on hospice, the benefit can be renewed indefinitely as long as there is clinical evidence of continued decline consistent with disease progression. Some examples of end-stage disease that would make patients candidates for hospice referral include cancer, dementia due to Alzheimer's disease, heart disease, liver disease, pulmonary disease, renal disease, stroke, and amyotrophic lateral sclerosis.

DELIVERING BAD NEWS

When and How to Deliver Bad News

Caring for patients in the end of life may require the APP to communicate bad news to patients and their families. *Bad news* is any information that will have a significant negative impact on an individual's view of the future. Sharing bad news is a complex communication task that requires more than just stating the words; it requires responding to a patient's emotions. The APP can achieve this by:

A. Identifying the important information.

B. Talking honestly and in a straightforward way.

(continued)

END-OF-LIFE CONSIDERATIONS *(continued)*

C. Being willing to talk about death/dying.

D. Delivering bad news in a sensitive way.

E. Listening.

F. Encouraging questions.

G. Being sensitive to patients when they want to talk about difficult issues.

SPIKES

SPIKES refers to a method for delivering bad news. It is comprised of six steps, which are outlined in the following sections.

Step 1: Setting Up the Interview

It is important to consider the setting where the news will be delivered as well as what will be said. Arrange for a place that will provide some privacy, and involve significant others in the interview. It is also helpful to engage in a mental rehearsal of what will be said. During the interview, the APP should sit down with the patient, maintain eye contact, and effectively manage time constraints and interruptions.

Step 2: Assess the Patient's Perception

During the interview, use open-ended questions to ask the patient what he or she understands about the disease process. Listen to the patient's level of comprehension, and be sure to correct any misinformation.

Step 3: Obtain the Patient's Invitation

It is important to assess how much or how little information the patient would like to have. Some people want to know detailed information, while other patients prefer not to know. Accept the patient's right not to know, and offer to answer questions later, if needed.

Step 4: Giving Knowledge

When speaking to patients, use vocabulary words and terminology that are aligned with the comprehension level of the patient. Giving information in small chunks, and pausing in between each chunk, can help increase the patient's understanding. It is also helpful to check in with the patient as you are giving information to ensure the patient understood what you said.

Step 5: Address the Patient's Emotions

When receiving difficult news, patients often feel shock, isolation, and grief. It is important for the APP to acknowledge these feelings and to offer support. Give the patient time to express his or her feelings.

Step 6: Strategy and Summary

After speaking with the patient and answering any questions, it is important to close the meeting by discussing plans for the future or next steps.

FINAL DAYS AND HOURS OF LIFE

In the final days and hours of life, patients may experience several symptoms, including:

A. Loss of appetite.

B. Excessive fatigue and sleep.

C. Increased physical weakness.

D. Mental confusion or disorientation.

E. Labored breathing.

F. Social withdrawal.

G. Changes in urination (oliguria or anuria).

(continued)

END-OF-LIFE CONSIDERATIONS (*continued*)

H. Swelling in the feet and ankles.

I. "Death rattle," which refers to a gurgling sound created by air moving through uncleared secretions in the trachea and vocal cords.

During this time, the APP should continue to provide compassionate care aligned with the patient's and family's preferences. The patient and family may ask questions about food and water intake, express fears of the unknown, and have concerns about symptom management. The APP should answer any questions the family and the patient have, and provide continued support.

DEATH PRONOUNCEMENT

The following medical procedures should be followed during the clinical examination for pronouncing death.

A. Properly identify the patient using the ID bracelet.

B. Check the pupils for position and response to light.

C. Check response to tactile stimuli—examine respectfully, refraining from sternal rubs or nipple pinches.

D. Check for spontaneous respiration for 1 minute.

E. Check for apical heart tones and pulses for 1 minute.

F. Record the time of death.

The following items should be included in the death note.

A. Date and time of death.

B. Name of provider pronouncing death.

C. Brief statement of cause of death.

D. Documentation of the absence of a pulse, respiration, and pupil response.

E. Notation of family presence at the death and/or family notification of the death.

F. Document notification of attending physician, pastoral care staff, social work staff, or other staff as appropriate.

A death certificate needs to be filled out, with all marked sections completed using black ink. This is often the duty of the attending healthcare provider.

SUMMARY

It is important to remember that death is a natural part of life. When providing end-of-life care, the APP should remember that his or her primary role is to support the patient and the patient's family and to empower the patient to articulate the type of death he or she would like. This is achieved by facilitating open and honest communication, asking and answering questions, and eliciting information about the patient's specific priorities and goals.

BIBLIOGRAPHY

Baile, W. F., Buckman, R., Lenzi, R., Glober, G., Beale, E. A., & Kudelka, A. P. (2000). SPIKES—A six-step protocol for delivering bad news: Application to the patient with cancer. *The Oncologist, 5*, 302–311. doi:10.1634/theoncologist.5-4-302

Bailey, F. A., & Williams, B. R. O. S. A. (2005). Preparation of residents for death pronouncement: A sensitive and supportive method. *Palliative & Supportive Care, 3*, 107–114. doi:10.1017/S1478951505050182

Bloomer, M. J., Moss, C., & Cross, W. M. (2011). End-of-life care in acute hospitals: An integrative literature review. *Journal of Nursing and Healthcare of Chronic Illness, 3*, 165–173. doi:10.1111/j.1752-9824.2011.01094.x

Buck, H. G., & Fahlberg, B. (2014). Using POLST to ensure patients' treatment preferences. *Nursing, 44*, 16–17. doi:10.1097/01.NURSE. 0000443322.11726.91

Buckman, R. (1992). *How to breakbad news: A guide for health care professionals* (p. 15). Baltimore, MD: Johns Hopkins University Press.

Byock, I. (2004). *The four things that matter most: Essential wisdom for transforming your relationships and your life,* (c.240p). Free Pr: S. & S.

Chronic Disease Overview. (n. d.). Retrieved from https://www.cdc.gov/chronicdisease/pdf/nccdphp-overview-508.pd

Electronic Code of Federal Regulation. (2017, March 15). U.S. government publishing office. Retrieved from https://www.ecfr.gov/cgi-bin/ECFR?page=browse

Halter, J. B., Ouslander, J. G., Studenski, S., High, K. P., Asthana, S., Supaino, M. A., & Ritchie, C. S. (Eds.). (2017). *Hazzard's geriatric medicine and gerontology* (7th ed.). New York, NY: McGraw-Hill.

Meier, E. A., Gallegos, J. V., Thomas, L. P. M., & Depp, C. A. (2016). Defining a good death (successful dying): Literature review and a call for research and public dialogue. *The American Journal of Geriatric Psychiatry, 24*, 261–271. doi:10.1016/j.jagp.2016.01.135

National Health Center for Statistics. (n. d.). Retrieved from https://www.cdc.gov/nchs/data/factsheets/nchs_overview.pdf

HEALTH PREVENTION AND SCREENING

Michele DeCastro

INTRODUCTION

Prevention and screening are important parts of providing comprehensive acute care. Appropriate prevention and screening can help keep diseases from occurring, detect diseases in their earliest stages, and improve healthcare outcomes. As such, it is of vital importance that the advanced practice provider (APP) in the acute care setting be familiar with the different levels of prevention and the different types of prevention. It is also important to understand common vaccinations and screening recommendations.

LEVELS OF PREVENTION

There are three main levels of prevention dispensed by the APP: Primary prevention, secondary prevention, and tertiary prevention. Primary prevention refers to interventions that focus on preventing disease from occurring. Examples of primary prevention include recommending smoking cessation to a patient to reduce his or her risk of lung cancer, administering influenza immunizations, and recommending a mastectomy for the breast cancer 1 (BRCA) positive patient.

Secondary prevention focuses on interventions that detect disease early and prior to when symptoms and effects present. Examples of secondary prevention include performing regular PAP smears on female patients to detect precancerous lesions and testing for HIV in at-risk populations even in the absence of symptoms. Tertiary prevention refers to anything that prevents diseases from becoming worse or decreases the complications from a particular disease process. Examples may include recommending that a patient use a beta-blocker after having a myocardial infarction (MI), or treating hypertension (HTN) and hyperlipidemia in diabetic patients. Ophthalmology examinations in patients with diabetes mellitus (DM) may also be considered a form of tertiary prevention.

TYPES OF PREVENTION

As mentioned previously, prevention can be provided in different ways. Common types of prevention include screening, immunization, and recommending lifestyle modifications to prevent disease.

For APPs in the acute care setting, understanding screening and immunizations is especially important, as many patients will present without access to these preventive measures. Knowing which high-risk conditions they are most at-risk for developing can help with diagnosis, inpatient treatment, and posthospital care planning.

SCREENING

For APPs in the acute care setting, understanding screening guidelines is essential to practice. It is important to know which common conditions the patient should have been screened for based upon his or her age and risk factors. Most screening recommendations used by healthcare providers in the United States are created by one of several expert groups. The U.S. Preventive Services Task Force (USPSTF) is the leading creator of screening recommendations. The USPSTF is an independent panel of nonfederal experts who specialize in prevention and evidence-based medicine and who come from a variety of fields. They complete thorough reviews of current research and make recommendations for primary care screening and prevention. In their review, the USPSTF assigns a letter grade to each of their recommendations based on the strength of evidence to support the recommendation and the balance of benefits against harms of the recommendation. The benefits of a recommendation must outweigh risks, and the USPSTF's focus is on overall health and quality of life of patients, not just on the identification of disease. Other expert bodies make prevention and screening recommendations on their clinical area of expertise. Some of these organizations include the American College of Cardiology (ACC), the American Heart Association (AHA), the American Cancer Society (ACS), and the American College of Physicians (ACP). Screening and prevention of the two leading causes of death in the United States, cardiovascular disease (CVD) and cancer, are discussed in further detail later in this section.

IMMUNIZATIONS

Another form of prevention is immunization. Immunizations may be indicated based on the patient's age, lifestyle, health factors, or risk factors. It is important for the APP to know immunization status and immunization needs in order to make an appropriate diagnostic assessment, create an inpatient plan, and to coordinate and recommend any appropriate follow-up care. Age-appropriate immunization schedules are provided in Tables IV.1 and IV.2. The following sections outline other common immunizations that may be indicated for adult patients.

Haemophilus influenzae Type B

Haemophilus influenzae type B vaccine is administered to patients with anatomical or functional asplenia (including sickle cell disease). These patients, if immunized as children, are vaccinated by giving one dose of the immunization in adulthood. Patients undergoing hematopoietic stem cell transplant should also receive vaccination. Regardless of Hib vaccination history, the patient receives three doses (at least 4 weeks apart) beginning 6 to 12 months after transplant. Evidence of immunity occurs with documented vaccination.

(continued)

HEALTH PREVENTION AND SCREENING (*continued*)

Hepatitis A

Hepatitis A immunization is indicated for patients who use illicit substances, for men who have sex with men (MSM), for patients with chronic liver disease and/or receive clotting factor concentrates, and for patients who work in or travel to areas of high endemic disease. For adults, two separate 1 mL vaccinations are done 6 to 12 months apart.

Hepatitis B

Immunization against hepatitis B may be indicated based on the patient's age or lifestyle. The following factors indicate immunization is recommended.

A. Sexually active persons who are not in a long-term, mutually monogamous relationship.

B. Persons seeking evaluation or treatment for a sexually transmitted disease (STD).

C. Current or recent injection drug users.

D. MSM.

E. Healthcare personnel and public safety workers who are potentially exposed to blood or other infectious body fluids.

F. Persons with diabetes who are younger than age 60 years as soon as feasible after diagnosis.

G. Persons with end-stage renal disease.

H. Persons with HIV infection.

I. Persons with chronic liver disease.

J. Household contacts and sex partners of hepatitis B surface antigen–positive persons.

K. Healthcare workers.

L. Persons working in institutional settings.

M. Persons with DM who are older than 60 years.

Primary vaccination consists of three intramuscular doses of hepatitis B vaccine given at months 0, 1, and 6. An alternative regimen consists of a combined Hep A and Hep B vaccine (Twinrix) given in the same dosing schedule for patients with risk factors for both diseases. Evidence of immunity occurs with documented administration of the vaccine for most patients. However, serologic testing for immunity is recommended for persons whose subsequent clinical management depends on knowledge of their immune status, certain healthcare and public safety workers, chronic hemodialysis patients, HIV-infected persons, and sex or needle-sharing partners of hepatitis B positive patients.

Influenza

Although most adults in general good health will recover from influenza, certain populations, such as the very young, the very old, and those with immunocompromising conditions, may be especially susceptible to more severe infections with influenza. As such, the Centers for Disease Control and Prevention (CDC) recommend that all adults receive the influenza vaccination annually. Influenza vaccination is contraindicated in adults with a history of egg allergy more severe than hives, including difficulty breathing, respiratory distress, or angioedema. Patients who have only hives after exposure to egg should receive age-appropriate vaccine.

Measles, Mumps, and Rubella

Adult patients are immune to measles, mumps, and rubella (MMR) if:

1. They were born before 1957.

2. There is documentation of receipt of MMR

3. There is laboratory evidence of immunity.

This immunization is contraindicated for patients who are pregnant and immunocompromised adults. The CDC recommends adult immunization to students in postsecondary education, those who work in healthcare, and patients who travel internationally. Patients should receive second immunizations, 28 days after the first.

(*continued*)

TABLE 1 Vaccines for Teenagers 13–18 Years

Age	Flu (Influenza)	Tdap (Tetanus, Diphtheria, Pertussis)	HPV	Meningococcal MenACWY	Meningococcal MenB	Pneumococcal	Hepatitis B	Hepatitis A	Polio	MMR	Chickenpox (Varicella)
11–12 years	Yearly[a]	Vaccine recommended x1	Vaccine recommended x1	Vaccine recommended x1	Vaccine for high risk recommended x1[c]	Vaccine for high risk recommended x1[c]	Catch up/missed dose[d]	Catch up/missed dose	Catch up/missed dose	Catch up/missed dose	Catch up/missed dose
13–15 years	Yearly	Catch up/missed dose[a]	Catch up/missed dose	Catch up/missed dose	Vaccine for high risk recommended x1[c]	Vaccine for high risk recommended x1[c]	Catch up/missed dose	Catch up/missed dose	Catch up/missed dose	Catch up/missed dose	Catch up/missed dose
16–18 years	Yearly	Catch up/missed dose	Catch up/missed dose	Booster at age 16	Optional vaccine[d]	Vaccine for high risk recommended x1[c]	Catch up/missed dose	Catch up/missed dose	Catch up/missed dose	Catch up/missed dose	Catch up/missed dose

Note: [a]Yearly means that the vaccine is recommended every year.

[b]Catch up/missed dose indicates that the vaccine should be given if the patient is catching up on missed doses.

[c]Vaccine recommended for patients with certain health or lifestyle conditions that put them at risk for serious diseases.

[d]Optional vaccine is for patients who are not at increased risk, but wish to be vaccinated after speaking with a healthcare provider.

HPV, human papillomavirus; MMR, measles, mumps, rubella.

TABLE 2 **Vaccines for Adults by Age: 19+ Years**

	Flu (Influenza)	Td/Tdap (Tetanus, Diphtheria, Pertussis)	Shingles (Zoster)	Pneumococcal		Meningococcal	
				PCV13	PPSV23	MenACWY or MPSV4	MenB
Age							
19–21 years	Yearly	Recommended		May be recommended[a]	May be recommended[a]	May be recommended[a]	May be recommended[a]
22–26 years	Yearly	Recommended		May be recommended[a]	May be recommended[a]	May be recommended[a]	May be recommended[a]
27–59 years	Yearly	Recommended		May be recommended[a]	May be recommended[a]	May be recommended[a]	May be recommended[a]
60–64 years	Yearly	Recommended	Recommended	May be recommended[a]	May be recommended[a]	May be recommended[a]	May be recommended[a]
65+ years	Yearly	Recommended	Recommended	Recommended	Recommended	May be recommended[a]	May be recommended[a]
	Get flu vaccine every year	Get Td booster every 10 years. You also need 1 dose of Tdap vaccine. Women should get Tdap vaccine during EVERY pregnancy	You should get shingles vaccine if you are 60+ years even if you have previously had shingles	You should get 1 dose of PCV13 and at least 1 dose of PPSV23 depending on your age and health condition			

(continued)

(continued)

TABLE 2 Vaccines for Adults by Age: 19+ Years

Vaccines for Adults by Health Condition

	Flu (Influenza)	Td/Tdap (Tetanus, Diphtheria, Pertussis)	Shingles (Zoster)	Pneumococcal — PCV13	Pneumococcal — PPSV23	Meningococcal — MenACWY or MPSV4	Meningococcal — MenB
Pregnancy	Yearly	Recommended	DO NOT GET VACCINE		May be recommended[a]	May be recommended[a]	
Weakend immune system	Yearly	Recommended	DO NOT GET VACCINE	Recommended	Recommended	May be recommended[a]	May be recommended[a]
HIV: CD4 Count less than 200	Yearly	Recommended	DO NOT GET VACCINE	Recommended	Recommended	Recommended	May be recommended[a]
HIV: CD4 Count 200+	Yearly	Recommended	Recommended	Recommended	Recommended	Recommended	May be recommended[a]
Kidney disease	Yearly	Recommended	Recommended	Recommended	Recommended	May be recommended[a]	May be recommended[a]
Asplenia	Yearly	Recommended	Recommended	Recommended	Recommended	Recommended	Recommended
Heart disease/chronic lung disease/alcoholism	Yearly	Recommended	Recommended	Recommended	Recommended	May be recommended[a]	May be recommended[a]
Diabetes (Type 1 and 2)	Yearly	Recommended	Recommended	Recommended	Recommended	May be recommended[a]	May be recommended[a]
Chronic liver disease	Yearly	Recommended	Recommended	May be recommended[a]	Recommended	May be recommended[a]	May be recommended[a]
	Get flu vaccine every year	Get Td booster every 10 years. You also need 1 dose of Tdap vaccine. Women should get Tdap vaccine during EVERY pregnancy	You should get shingles vaccine if you are 60+ years even if you have previously had shingles	You should get 1 dose of PCV13 and at least 1 dose of PPSV23 depending on your age and health condition			

	HPV — For Women	HPV — For Men	Chickenpox (Varicella)	Hepatitis A	Hepatitis B	Hib	MMR
	Recommended	Recommended	Recommended	May be recommended[a]	May be recommended[a]	May be recommended[a]	Recommended
	Recommended	May be recommended[a]	Recommended	May be recommended[a]	May be recommended[a]	May be recommended[a]	Recommended
	Recommended		Recommended	May be recommended[a]	May be recommended[a]	May be recommended[a]	Recommended
			Recommended		Recommended	May be recommended[a]	
			Recommended		May be recommended[a]	May be recommended[a]	

MMR/HPV/Chickenpox/Hep A/Hep B: You should get this vaccine if you did not get it when you were a child. HPV: You should get HPV vaccine if you are a woman through the age of 26 or a man through the age of 21 and did not already complete the series.

(continued)

TABLE 2   Vaccines for Adults by Age: 19+ Years

Vaccines for Adults by Health Condition

MMR	HPV For Women	HPV For Men	Chickenpox (Varicella)	Hepatitis A	Hepatitis B	Hib
DO NOT GET VACCINE			DO NOT GET VACCINE	May be recommended[a]	May be recommended[a]	May be recommended[a]
DO NOT GET VACCINE	Recommended	Recommended	DO NOT GET VACCINE	May be recommended[a]	May be recommended[a]	Recommended
DO NOT GET VACCINE	Recommended	Recommended	DO NOT GET VACCINE	May be recommended[a]	Recommended	May be recommended[a]
Recommended	Recommended	Recommended	Recommended	May be recommended[a]	Recommended	May be recommended[a]
Recommended	Recommended	Recommended	Recommended	May be recommended[a]	Recommended	May be recommended[a]
Recommended	Recommended	Recommended	Recommended	May be recommended[a]	May be recommended[a]	
Recommended	Recommended	Recommended	Recommended	May be recommended[a]	May be recommended[a]	May be recommended[a]
Recommended	Recommended	Recommended	Recommended	May be recommended[a]	Recommended	May be recommended[a]
Recommended	Recommended	Recommended	Recommended	Recommended	Recommended	May be recommended[a]
MMR/HPV/Chickenpox/Hep A/Hep B: You should get this vaccine if you did not get it when you were a child. HPV, You should get HPV vaccine if you are a woman through the age of 26 or a man through the age of 221 and did not already complete the series.						You should get Hib vaccine if you have sickle cell disease, had a bone marrow transplant, or you do not have a spleen

Note: Recommended—This is recommended unless a healthcare provider tells you that you do not need it or should not get it.

[a]May be recommended—This vaccine may be for you if you have certain risk factors such as age, health condition, or other. Discuss with your healthcare provider.

Hib, haemophilus influenzae type b; HPV, human papillomavirus; MenACWY, serogroups A, C, W, and Y meningococcal vaccine; MenB, serogroup B meningococcal vaccine; MMR, measles, mumps, rubella; PCV13, 13-valent pneumococcal conjugate vaccine; PPSV23, 23-valent pneumococcal polysaccharide vaccine.

HEALTH PREVENTION AND SCREENING (continued)

Meningococcal

There are two meningococcal vaccines that immunize against serogroups A, C, W, and Y meningococcal vaccine (MenACWY) and serogroup B meningococcal vaccine (MenB). MenACWY is given in either one or two doses and is indicated for patients who have:

A. Anatomical or functional asplenia (including sickle cell disease and other hemoglobinopathies).

B. HIV infection.

C. Persistent complement component deficiency.

D. Eculizumab use.

E. Travel to or live in countries where meningococcal disease is hyperendemic or epidemic.

F. At-risk from a meningococcal disease outbreak attributed to serogroup A, C, W, or Y.

G. Microbiologists routinely exposed to Neisseria meningitides.

H. Military recruits.

I. First-year college students who live in residential housing.

MenB can be given in a two or three dose series, depending on manufacturer, and is indicated for patients with the following characteristics.

A. Anatomical or functional asplenia (including sickle cell disease).

B. Persistent complement component deficiency.

C. Eculizumab use.

D. At-risk from a meningococcal disease outbreak attributed to serogroup B.

E. Microbiologists routinely exposed to Neisseria meningitidis.

Evidence of immunity occurs with documented administration of the vaccine for most patients.

Tetanus

The Td (tetanus and diphtheria toxoids)/Tdap (tetanus toxoid, reduced diphtheria toxoid, and acellular pertussis vaccine) vaccinations should be given once every 10 years to all patients 19 years and older. Tdap is generally recommended for all patients at approximately 11 years of age. If this was not completed, or status is unknown, all adults should receive Tdap once in adulthood, followed by Td immunization every 10 years. Adults with an unknown or incomplete history of a three-dose primary series with tetanus and diphtheria toxoid-containing vaccines should complete the primary series that includes one dose of Tdap. All pregnant women should receive one dose of Tdap regardless of previous immunization.

PNEUMONIA

There are two different types of immunizations used to help prevent pneumonia: PPSV23 and PCV13. The APP should consider the patient's age, lifestyle, and any medical conditions the patient has to determine which vaccination to administer.

PPSV23 vaccine is typically administered to all adults older than 65 years. These adults should receive 13-valent pneumococcal conjugate vaccine (PCV13) followed by 23-valent pneumococcal polysaccharide vaccine (PPSV23) at least 1 year after PCV13. If PPSV23 was previously administered but not PCV13, administer PCV13 at least 1 year after PPSV23. When both are indicated, PCV13 should be given before PPSV23 whenever possible. Administering PPSV23 may be indicated in patients younger than 65 years if the patient has the following conditions or lifestyle factors.

A. Chronic heart or lung disease.

B. DM.

C. Alcoholism.

D. Chronic liver disease.

E. Adults who smoke cigarettes.

(continued)

HEALTH PREVENTION AND SCREENING (*continued*)

The previously noted patients should receive PPSV23 at the age of onset of the earlier conditions. Then, administer one dose of PCV13 at **65 years or older**. This dose should be given at least 1 year after PPSV23. Administer one more dose (the final dose) of PPSV23 at 65 years or older. This dose should be given at least 1 year after PCV13 and at least 5 years after the most recent dose of PPSV23.

Both PPSV23 and PCV13 may be indicated before the age of 65 for adults with the following conditions.

A. Cerebrospinal fluid (CSF) leaks.

B. Cochlear implants.

C. Sickle cell disease or other hemoglobinopathies.

D. Congenital or acquired asplenia.

E. Congenital or acquired immunodeficiencies.

F. HIV infection.

G. Chronic renal failure.

H. Nephrotic syndrome.

I. Leukemia.

J. Lymphoma.

K. Hodgkin disease.

L. Generalized malignancy.

M. Iatrogenic immunosuppression.

N. Solid organ transplant.

O. Multiple myeloma.

For those who have not received any pneumococcal vaccines, or those with unknown vaccination history, the APP should administer one dose of PCV13, and then administer one dose of PPSV23 at least 8 weeks later. Administer a second dose of PPSV23 at least 5 years after the previous dose. Please note, a second dose is not indicated for those with CSF leaks or cochlear implants. The APP also should administer one final dose of PPSV23 at 65 years or older. This dose should be given at least 5 years after the most recent dose of PPSV23. Evidence of immunity occurs with documented administration of the vaccine.

Varicella

All adults without evidence of immunity should receive two doses of the varicella vaccine, 4 weeks apart. Vaccination should be especially emphasized for those with high-risk contacts, such as healthcare workers, childcare workers, and workers in an institutional setting. This vaccination is contraindicated in pregnancy. Evidence of immunity includes the following.

A. Documentation of four doses at least 4 weeks apart.

B. U.S. born before 1980; except healthcare workers and pregnant women.

C. History of herpes zoster.

D. Laboratory evidence of immunity.

Zoster

As of October 2017, recombinant zoster vaccine (RZV) is recommended for the prevention of herpes zoster and related complications for immunocompetent adults aged ≥50 years. RZV is a two-dose vaccine given 2 to 6 months apart. Prior to this variation of the vaccine, zoster vaccine live (ZVL) was the only vaccine available to prevent herpes zoster in adults over 50 years. It is recommended to administer two doses of RZV 2 to 6 months apart to adults who previously received ZVL at least 2 months after ZVL. CDC guidelines state that RZV is preferred over ZVL for the prevention of herpes zoster and related complications. Both vaccines are contraindicated in patients who are pregnant or in patients with severe immunodeficiency, such as patients with AIDS or who are undergoing cancer treatment. Evidence of immunity occurs with documented administration of the vaccine.

(continued)

HEALTH PREVENTION AND SCREENING (*continued*)

SCREENING AND PREVENTION FOR CVD

The CDC reports that 633,842 deaths were attributed to heart disease, making it the leading cause of death in the United States. There are many screening and prevention methods that the APP should consider when assessing and caring for patients who exhibit risk factors for CVD.

USE OF CV RISK CALCULATOR

An appropriate initial step in screening patients for CVD is to use a CV risk calculator. The CV risk calculator that is based on the ACC/AHA 2013 Cholesterol Guidelines is the most commonly used, and it is available on the ACC's website. It is a form of pooled risk assessment that considers a patient's risk factors, including age, race, weight, cholesterol levels, and blood pressure. The calculator was based on multiple community-based population studies and considers stroke risk as well as risk of MI.

HYPERTENSION

There is clear evidence that controlling HTN will decrease one's risk for developing CVD. As such, it is vital to screen all adults who are 18 years and older for high blood pressure. The APP should recommend annual screening for those deemed at-risk based on results of the CVD risk calculator. Readings of blood pressure should be obtained outside of the clinic setting prior to definitive diagnosis. Please refer to Chapter 3 in this book for more information on diagnosis and management of HTN.

CAROTID ARTERY STENOSIS

Approximately 15% of strokes are caused by large artery atherothrombotic disease, which includes carotid artery stenosis (CAS). The presence of asymptomatic CAS (>70% stenosis) in the population is estimated to be 1.7%. However, most ischemic strokes are not caused by CAS. Therefore, the burden of CAS causing stroke among the general population is low. The risks of intervention through performing a carotid endarterectomy (CEA) or carotid angioplasty and stenting (CAAS) are high, and include stroke, MI, pulmonary embolus, and death. Typically, screening for this occurs in patients by performing a carotid duplex ultrasonography. According to the USPSTF, the AHA, and the American Stroke Association, there is no clear benefit for screening via ultrasound or auscultation in asymptomatic patients. Patients who are at high risk for the disease include: Patients with a carotid bruit heard on auscultation, those with confirmed atherosclerotic disease, and those age 65 years or older with a history of one or more of the following atherosclerotic risk factors: Coronary artery disease, smoking, or hypercholesterolemia. For these patients it is a reasonable expectation to consider screening. However, for many of these patients, optimal medical therapy has already been initiated to treat their known atherosclerotic disease.

LIPIDS

Evidence has linked high cholesterol levels with increased risk of CVD. As such, the USPSTF recommends that all men older than 35 years and all women older than 45 years be screened with a serum lipid profile. Men 20 to 35 years and women 20 to 45 years with increased risk should also be screened for elevated lipid levels (total cholesterol, low-density lipoprotein [LDL], high-density lipoprotein [HDL], and triglycerides). For patients with no history of CV events, there is no clear end date for when to END screening.

ECG

There is no clear evidence that resting ECG is helpful for low- or high-risk patients in looking for coronary heart disease in asymptomatic patients. Therefore, the USPSTF does not recommend using an ECG as a method to screen for CVD for patients with no symptoms.

DIABETES

The APP should screen for diabetes as a part of a cardiovascular risk assessment in all adults aged 40 to 70 years who are overweight or obese. All patients with abnormal blood glucose results should be offered intensive behavioral counseling on diet and exercise.

ABDOMINAL AORTIC ANEURYSM

It is recommended that men aged 65 to 75 years who have ever smoked should undergo one-time screening for abdominal aortic aneurysm. Evidence seems to show a small benefit exists for screening men aged 65 to 75 years who have never smoked; however, evidence is inconclusive regarding screening for women aged 65 to 75 years who have ever smoked. It is not necessary to screen women aged 65 to 75 years who have never smoked as there is a very low possibility of diagnosis.

(*continued*)

HEALTH PREVENTION AND SCREENING (*continued*)

TOBACCO USE

The U.S. Surgeon General reports that one-third of deaths from CVD are caused by smoking. It is important that the APP ask all adult patients about nicotine and tobacco use. All adult tobacco users and all pregnant women who use tobacco should be advised to stop. These patients should also be offered both pharmacologic and nonpharmacologic/behavioral interventions for tobacco cessation.

OBESITY

All adults should be screened for obesity. Clinicians should offer or refer patients with a body mass index (BMI) of 30 kg/m^2 or higher to intensive, multicomponent behavioral interventions. Weight loss can improve blood pressure, glycemic control, and decrease overall cardiovascular risk.

CANCER SCREENING AND PREVENTION

Cancer is attributed as the cause of 595,930 deaths annually, making it the second-leading cause of death in the United States. The highest rates of cancer are cancer of the female breast, prostate cancer, lung and bronchus cancer, colon and rectal cancer, and corpus and uterine cancer. The greatest number of deaths from cancer is due to lung, colorectal, breast, and pancreatic cancers, respectively. Of these, pancreatic cancer has the highest mortality rate (6% survival rate in 5 years). The United States has not met goals for screening for breast, cervical, prostate, and colorectal cancer as set by *Healthy People 2020*.

Cancer prevention includes measures such as tobacco cessation counseling for all patients due to its association with multiple cancers. The following sections outline leading prevention and screening recommendations from the USPSTF, the ACS, and other expert recommendations for each type of the most common forms of cancer.

BREAST

When considering which screening and prevention recommendation is appropriate, it is important for the clinician to determine the patient's risk of breast cancer. There are multiple models used to determine risk of developing breast cancer. One of the most commonly accepted and used tools for determining risk is the Breast Cancer Risk Assessment Tool as developed by the National Cancer Institute. Factors considered in this model include:

A. Family history.

B. Age.

C. Ethnicity.

D. Previous history of abnormal breast biopsy.

E. Obstetric history.

Women with family or personal history of breast, ovarian, or peritoneal cancer, genetic predisposition, and women with a history of radiation to the chest are all considered higher risk.

USPSTF Recommendation

The USPSTF recommends that in women 40 to 49 years, the decision to screen should be an individual one. Screening should be considered in higher risk women. In women 50 to 74 years, screening reduces mortality and should be performed every 1 to 2 years. In women older than 75 years, evidence is insufficient to make a definitive screening recommendation.

ACS Recommendation

The ACS recommends that women aged 40 to 44 years should have the opportunity to begin annual screening if they chose to and in discussion with a healthcare provider. Women with an average risk of breast cancer should undergo regular screening mammography starting at age 45 years. Annual screening should continue in women until they are 54 years old. Women aged 55 years and older should transition to biennial screening or have the opportunity to continue screening annually. Women who have a life expectancy greater than 10 years and are in good health may continue screening with mammography. Women who are at high risk should undergo annual screening mammography and MRI starting at age 30 years. High-risk women are those with a known BRCA mutation; women who are untested, but have a first-degree relative with a BRCA mutation; or women with an approximately 20% to 25% or greater lifetime risk of breast cancer based upon risk-estimation models.

(*continued*)

HEALTH PREVENTION AND SCREENING (*continued*)

Other Expert Recommendation

The ACP has the following age-specific recommendations for women of average risk.

A. 40 to 49 years: Discuss risks/benefits; biennial mammogram if informed woman requests.

B. 50 to 74 years: Biennial mammogram.

C. Younger than 40 years or older than 75 years **OR** life expectancy less than 10 years: No screening.

The American Congress of Obstetricians and Gynecologists (ACOG) recommends that women 40 years and older receive annual screening with mammogram.

Prevention

Mastectomy may be indicated as a preventive measure for very high-risk patients.

CERVICAL

USPSTF Recommendation

The USPSTF recommends that women who are younger than 21 years do not need to be screened for cervical cancer, and women younger than 30 years do not need to have human papillomavirus (HPV) testing. Women 21 to 65 years receive screening every 3 years with cytology (PAP). Women aged 30 to 65 years should be screened every 5 years with cytology (PAP) in combination with HPV testing. Women who are 65 years of age and have had adequate screening need no further testing. The APP should not screen women with hysterectomy who do not have a history of cervical cancer or high grade precancerous lesion.

ACS Recommendation

The ACS recommends that women who are 21 to 29 years should have a PAP test every 3 years. Women who are 30 to 64 years should have a PAP test with HPV every 5 years, or every 3 years with PAP alone. Women who are older than 65 years should no longer be screened for cervical cancer if they have had three consecutive negative cytology results **or** two consecutive negative cytology with negative HPV test results within 10 years, with the most recent test done within 5 years.

Other Expert Recommendation

The American College of Physicians (ACP) does not recommend screening average-risk women younger than 21 years. Average-risk women should be screened for cervical cancer beginning at age 21 years, and once every 3 years with cytology (PAP tests without HPV tests). Average-risk women should not be screened for cervical cancer with cytology more often than once every 3 years. Clinicians may choose to use a combination of PAP testing and HPV testing once every 5 years in average-risk women who are 30 years or older. However, clinicians should not perform HPV testing in average-risk women younger than 30 years.

The ACP recommendations are largely in line with the ACS recommendation: Women older than 65 years who have had three consecutive negative cytology results or two consecutive negative cytology plus HPV test results within 10 years, with the most recent test done within 5 years, should no longer be screened for cervical cancer. They do not recommend screening average-risk women of any age who have had a hysterectomy with removal of the cervix. Also, clinicians should not perform cervical cancer screening with a bimanual pelvic examination.

Prevention

The leading cause of cervical cancer is HPV. As such, preventing HPV infection is a primary form of prevention for cervical cancer. Interventions to prevent HPV infection may include:

A. Vaccinating against HPV (see Tables IV.1 and IV.2 for age-appropriate vaccination recommendations).

B. Encouraging the patient to use a barrier method during sexual intercourse.

Treatment and/or assessment of abnormal cells on cytology and treatment and/or assessment of HPV are also important preventive measures.

(*continued*)

HEALTH PREVENTION AND SCREENING (continued)

COLORECTAL

USPSTF Recommendation

Patients age 50 to 75 years with an average risk should be screened for colorectal cancer. The test for screening chosen will determine the frequency of screening. Screening may begin earlier for patients with increased risk. Patients with a personal or family history of colon cancer are considered at increased risk. The APP should make an individualized decision in whether to screen patients older than 75 years. The overall health of the patient should be considered as well as the patient's ability to tolerate treatment, if diagnosed, and if previously screened. There is no superior test; however, if less invasive tests are positive, then direct visualization with colonoscopy is necessary.

Tests may also be indicated. Tests that detect cancer and colorectal polyps are as follows.

A. Flex sig: Perform every 5 years. If abnormal, proceed to colonoscopy.

B. Colonoscopy: Perform every 10 years.

C. Double contrast barium enema: Perform every 5 years. If abnormal, proceed to colonoscopy.

D. CT colonography: Perform every 5 years. If abnormal, proceed to colonoscopy.

Tests that detect cancer are as follows.

A. Guaiac-based fecal occult testing: Perform annually. If abnormal, proceed to colonoscopy.

B. Fecal immunochemical test: Perform annually. If abnormal, proceed to colonoscopy

C. Stool DNA test: Perform at uncertain interval. If abnormal, proceed to colonoscopy.

ACS Recommendation

The ACS recommends that both men and women with average risk who are older than 50 years should start cancer screening. Refer to the USPSTF for type of testing recommendations.

Prevention

It is recommended that the APP perform early screening for abnormal tissue that could become cancer.

LUNG

USPSTF Recommendation

Current or former smokers with a history of smoking 30 packs per year should be screened for lung cancer from 50 to 74 years of age. Screening includes a low dose/helical CT (LDCT) scan of the lung. Informed and shared decision-making discussion should occur between the patient and provider. Screening should stop once the patient is no longer willing to undergo treatment with curative lung surgery. Experts have not agreed about the frequency of screening. Providers should use their own clinical judgment to determine the frequency of screening with LDCT.

ACS Recommendation

Current or former smokers with a history of smoking 30 packs per year should be screened annually from age 50 to 74 years. Screening should include an LDCT scan of the lung. An informed and shared decision-making discussion should occur between patient and provider.

Other Expert Recommendation

The American Association for Thoracic Surgery recommends that patients who are 55 to 79 years old and who have a history of smoking 30 packs per year should be screened with LDCT. Lung cancer survivors should be screened with LDCT starting 5 years after treatment. Patients who are younger than 50 years and who have a 20 pack per year smoking history should be screened if they have an additional risk factor that produces a 5% risk of developing a lung cancer over the next 5 years.

Prevention

Since cigarette smoking is the leading cause of lung cancer, smoking cessation is the primary form of prevention.

(continued)

HEALTH PREVENTION AND SCREENING (*continued*)

PROSTATE

USPSTF Recommendation

The USPSTF recommends that the decision to screen for prostate cancer should be an individual one. The main modality for screening is a serum prostate-specific antigen (PSA) test. Before undergoing screening, men should have the chance to discuss the benefits of screening as well as weighing the risks of diagnosis and treatment. Complications of diagnosis and treatment include infection, erectile dysfunction, and incontinence. Prostate cancer is common. Many men have no symptoms of the disease, and are only diagnosed through screening. Risk factors for the disease include men of older age, men who are African American, and men with a family history of prostate cancer. Only men who have been counseled on their own risk for the disease, and the risks and benefits of screening and treatment, should be offered testing.

ACS Recommendation

Informed decision making with a healthcare provider about whether to be screened for prostate cancer is indicated for patients considered to have average risk, are older than 50 years of age, and have at least a 10-year life expectancy. The APP should provide information to the patient about the potential benefits, risks, and uncertainties associated with prostate cancer screening. Screening should not happen in the absence of an informed decision-making process. Screening may be indicated for men who are 45 years and older who are at higher risk, including African American men and men with a first-degree family member (father or brother) who was diagnosed with prostate cancer before age 65 years.

Men who are 40 years and older should consider screening if they are at appreciably higher risk. This may include men who have had multiple family members diagnosed with prostate cancer before age 65 years.

Other Expert Recommendation

The American Urological Association recommends against PSA screening for men younger than 40 years, and also does not recommend screening for patients who are 40 to 54 years old.

They recommend that patients who are 55 to 69 years engage in the shared decision-making process (see also the Affordable Care Act [ACA] recommendation for this age range). For those men who do elect screening after a shared decision-making process with their providers, screening should only occur at an interval of every 2 years or longer in between screenings. The American Urological Association does not recommend screening for patients who are older than 70 years or for any man with less than a 10- to 15-year life expectancy.

The ACP recommends that clinicians should have a one-time discussion (more if the patient requests them) with average-risk patients aged 50 to 69 years that inquire about PSA-based prostate cancer screening. This discussion should inform the patient about the limited potential benefits and substantial harms of screening for prostate cancer using the PSA test. For men who have average risk and are aged 50 to 69 years who have not had an informed discussion and do not express a clear preference for screenings, no screening should be performed. Clinicians should not screen for prostate cancer using the PSA test in average-risk men younger than 50 years, those older than 69 years, or people whose life expectancy is less than 10 years.

SEXUALLY TRANSMITTED INFECTION SCREENING AND PREVENTION

The CDC and USPSTF have provided specific guidance on sexually transmitted infection (STI) screenings for adults based upon risk and specific STIs. Understanding STI risk and prevention is especially important in caring for any patients that may present in the acute care setting with a new STI, be unaware of the source of infection, or have a complication from an STI. All STI prevention includes counseling patients on having protected intercourse with a condom, and avoiding high-risk behaviors, such as sharing injection drug paraphernalia. The act of screening is also considered a prevention method as identifying asymptomatic patients and treating their infection will prevent the spread of disease to other persons.

HIV

Patients can present in the acute phase of HIV infection. However, they also may present with an opportunistic infection or complication of HIV, and HIV screening would be warranted. All adults between the ages of 13 to 65 should be screened for HIV at least once. Anyone who has unprotected intercourse and/or shares injection drug equipment should be screened for HIV annually. Sexually active gay and bisexual men should be screened for HIV more frequently (every 3–6 months).

All pregnant women should also be screened for HIV. Also, sex partners of persons who are HIV positive or are injection drug users should be screened.

(*continued*)

HEALTH PREVENTION AND SCREENING (*continued*)

CHLAMYDIA AND GONORRHEA

All sexually active women under the age of 25 should be screened for chlamydia and gonorrhea. Women over age 25 who are higher risk should also be routinely screened. At-risk women are those who have a new sex partner, more than one sex partner, a sex partner with concurrent partners, or a sex partner who has a STI. Young men (younger than 25 years) who are presenting in a high-prevalence clinical setting should also be screened. MSM should be screened annually, or every 3 to 6 months, for higher risk MSM. MSM are considered high risk if they or their partners have multiple partners.

HEPATITIS B

High-risk and women should be screened annually. Those who are high risk include:

A. MSM.

B. Persons born in areas of high occurrence (>2% population).

C. Persons on immunosuppressant medications.

D. Patients on hemodialysis.

E. Patients who are HIV positive.

F. Patients who are injection drug users.

Pregnant women should also be screened at their first prenatal visit.

HEPATITIS C

All men and women born between 1945 and 1965 should have a one-time screening for hepatitis C. Higher risk MSM should also be screened for hepatitis C. All patients with HIV should also be screened for hepatitis C annually.

SUMMARY

The APP in acute care may not always be the clinician who is offering prevention and screening initiatives to his or her patients. However, many patients treated in the acute care setting will have limited access to healthcare and may not have been offered important screening and prevention measures. While the acute care environment is not the setting to offer many of these interventions, the clinicians working in these settings need to know which of these measures these patients have missed. This may help when both diagnosing current conditions and planning for any appropriate outpatient follow-up.

BIBLIOGRAPHY

American Diabetes Association. (2017). 3. Comprehensive medical evaluation and assessment of comorbidities. *Diabetes Care, 40*(Suppl. 1), S25–S32. doi:10.2337/dc17-S006

The American Heart Association & American College of Cardiology. (n.d.). 2013 prevention guidelines tools—CV risk calculator. Retrieved from http://professional.heart.org/professional/GuidelinesStatements/PreventionGuidelines/UCM_457698_Prevention-Guidelines.jsp

Carter, H. B., Albertsen, P. C., Barry, M. J., Etzioni, R., Freedland, S., Greene, K., & Zietman, A. (2013). Early detection of prostate cancer: AUA guideline. Retrieved from https://www.auanet.org/education/guidelines/prostate-cancer-detection.cfm

Centers for Disease Control and Prevention. (n.d.). What are the risk factors for lung cancer? Retrieved from https://www.cdc.gov/cancer/lung/basic_info/risk_factors.htm

Centers for Disease Control and Prevention. (2015). Screening recommendations and considerations referenced in treatment guidelines and original sources. Retrieved from https://www.cdc.gov/std/tg2015/screening-recommendations.htm

Centers for Disease Control and Prevention. (2019). Table 1. Recommended adult immunization schedule for ages 19 years or older, United States, 2019. Retrieved from https://www.cdc.gov/vaccines/schedules/hcp/adult.html

Eckel, R. H., Jakicic, J. M., Ard, J. D., de Jesus, J. M., Houston Miller, N., Hubbard, V. S., . . . Yanovski, S. Z. (2014). 2013 AHA/ACC guideline on lifestyle management to reduce cardiovascular risk: A report of the American College of Cardiology/American Heart Association task force on practice guidelines. *Circulation, 129*(25 Suppl. 2), S76–S99. doi:10.1161/01.cir.0000437740.48606.d1

Goff, D. C., Lloyd-Jones, D. M., Bennett, G., Coady, S., D'Agostino, R. B., Gibbons, R., . . . Wilson, P. W. F. (2014). 2013 ACC/AHA guideline on the assessment of cardiovascular risk: A report of the American College of Cardiology/American Heart Association Task Force on Practice guidelines. *Circulation, 129*(25 Suppl. 2), S49–S73. doi:10.1161/01.cir.0000437741.48606.98

Hesse, B. W., & Gaysynsky, A., Ottenbacher, A., Moser, R. P., Blake, K. D., Chou, W. -Y. S., . . . Beckjord, E. (2014). Meeting the Healthy People 2020 goals: Using the Health Information National Trends Survey to monitor progress on health communication objectives. *Journal of Health Communication, 19*, 1497–1509. doi:10.1080/10810730.2014.954084

(*continued*)

HEALTH PREVENTION AND SCREENING (continued)

Jaklitsch, M. T., Jacobson, F. L., Austin, J. H., Field, J. K., Jett, J. R., Keshavjee, S., . . . Sugarbaker, D. J. (2012). The American Association for Thoracic Surgery guidelines for lung cancer screening using low-dose computed tomography scans for lung cancer survivors and other high-risk groups. *The Journal of Thoracic and Cardiovascular Surgery, 144*(1), 33–38 . doi:10.1016/j.jtcvs.2012.05.060

Jensen, M. D., Ryan, D. H., Apovian, C. M., Ard, J. D., Comuzzie, A. G., Donato, K. A., . . . Yanovski, S. Z. (2014). 2013 AHA/ACC/TOS guideline for the management of overweight and obesity in adults: A report of the American College of Cardiology/American Heart Association Task Force on Practice Guidelines and the Obesity Society. *Circulation, 129*(25 Suppl. 2), S102–S138. doi:10.1161/01.cir.0000437739.71477.ee

Jonas, D. E., Feltner, C., Amick, H. R., Sheridan, S., Zheng, Z.-J., Watford, D. J., . . . Harris, R. (2014). Screening for asymptomatic carotid artery stenosis: A systematic review and meta-analysis for the U.S. Preventive Services Task Force. Retrieved from https://www.ncbi.nlm.nih.gov/books/NBK223227/#__NBK223227_dtls__

National Cancer Institute. (n.d.). *The breast cancer risk assessment tool.* Retrieved from https://www.cancer.gov/bcrisktool

National Center for Health Statistics. (2017). Leading causes of death. Retrieved from https://www.cdc.gov/nchs/fastats/leading-causes-of-death.htm

National Cancer Institute. (2019, March 1). *HPV and cancer.* Retrieved from https://www.cancer.gov/about-cancer/causes-prevention/risk/infectious-agents/hpv-fact-sheet#q2

Oeffinger, K. C., Fontham, E. T. H., Etzioni, R., Herzig, A., Michaelson, J. S., Shih, Y. -C. T., . . . Wender, R. (2015). Breast cancer screening for women at average risk: 2015 guideline update from the American Cancer Society. *Journal of the American Medical Association, 314*(15), 1599–1614. doi:10.1001/jama.2015.12783

Office of the Surgeon General. (2014). *The health consequences of smoking—50 years of progress: A report of the surgeon general.* Rockville, MD: U.S. Department of Health and Human Services. Retrieved from https://www.surgeongeneral.gov/library/reports/50-years-of-progress/full-report.pdf

Qaseem, A., Snow, V., Sherif, K., Aronson, M., Weiss, K. B., & Owens, D. K. (2007, April 3). Screening mammography for women 40 to 49 years of age: A clinical practice guideline from the American College of Physicians. *Annals of Internal Medicine, 146*(7), 511–515. doi:10.7326/0003-4819-146-7-200704030-00007

Scarinci, I. C., Garcia, F. A. R., Kobetz, E., Partridge, E. E., Brandt, H. M., Bell, M. C., & Castle, P. E. (2010). Cervical cancer prevention: New tools and old barriers. *Cancer, 116*(11), 2531–2542. doi:10.1002/cncr.25065

Smith, R. A., Andrews, K., Brooks, D., DeSantis, C. E., Fedewa, S. A., Lortet-Tieulent, J., . . . Wender, R. C. (2016). Cancer screening in the United States, 2016: A review of current American Cancer Society guidelines and current issues in cancer screening. *CA: A Cancer Journal for Clinicians, 66*, 95–114.

U.S. Cancer Statistics Working Group. (2016). *United States cancer statistics: 1999–2013 incidence and mortality web-based report.* Atlanta, GA: U.S. Department of Health and Human Services, Centers for Disease Control and Prevention and National Cancer Institute. Retrieved from https://www.cdc.gov/cancer/npcr/pdf/uscs_factsheet.pdf

U.S. Preventive Services Task Force. (2013). Final update summary: Human immunodeficiency virus (HIV) infection: Screening. Retrieved from https://www.uspreventiveservicestaskforce.org/Page/Document/UpdateSummaryFinal/human-immunodeficiency-virus-hiv-infection-screening?ds=1&s=hiv

U.S. Preventive Services Task Force. (2015). Final update summary: Coronary heart disease: Screening using non-traditional risk factors. Retrieved from https://www.uspreventiveservicestaskforce.org/Page/Document/UpdateSummaryFinal/coronary-heart-disease-screening-using-non-traditional-risk-factors

U.S. Preventive Services Task Force. (2016a). Final recommendation statement: Lung cancer: Screening. Retrieved from https://www.uspreventiveservicestaskforce.org/Page/Document/RecommendationStatementFinal/lung-cancer-screening

U.S. Preventive Services Task Force. (2016b). Final update summary: Abdominal aortic aneurysm. Retrieved from https://www.uspreventiveservicestaskforce.org/Page/Document/UpdateSummaryFinal/abdominal-aortic-aneurysm-screening

U.S. Preventive Services Task Force. (2016c). Final update summary: Breast cancer: Screening. Retrieved from https://www.uspreventiveservicestaskforce.org/Page/Document/UpdateSummaryFinal/breast-cancer-screening1

U.S. Preventive Services Task Force. (2016d). Final update summary: Breast cancer: Screening. Retrieved from https://www.uspreventiveservicestaskforce.org/Page/Document/UpdateSummaryFinal/breast-cancer-screening1?ds=1&s=breast

U.S. Preventive Services Task Force. (2016e). Final update summary: Cervical cancer: Screening. Retrieved from https://www.uspreventiveservicestaskforce.org/Page/Document/UpdateSummaryFinal/cervical-cancer-screening?ds=1&s=cervical

U.S. Preventive Services Task Force. (2016f). Final update summary: Colorectal cancer: Screening. Retrieved from https://www.uspreventiveservicestaskforce.org/Page/Document/UpdateSummaryFinal/colorectal-cancer-screening2?ds=1&s=colorec

U.S. Preventive Services Task Force. (2016g). Final update summary: Coronary heart disease: Screening with electrocardiography. Retrieved from https://www.uspreventiveservicestaskforce.org/Page/Document/UpdateSummaryFinal/coronary-heart-disease-screening-with-electrocardiography

U.S. Preventive Services Task Force. (2016h). Final update summary: High blood pressure in adults: Screening. Retrieved from https://www.uspreventiveservicestaskforce.org/Page/Document/UpdateSummaryFinal/high-blood-pressure-in-adults-screening

U.S. Preventive Services Task Force. (2016i). Final update summary: Obesity in adults: Screening and management. Retrieved from https://www.uspreventiveservicestaskforce.org/Page/Document/UpdateSummaryFinal/obesity-in-adults-screening-and-management

U.S. Preventive Services Task Force. (2017). Final update summary: Abnormal blood glucose and type 2 diabetes mellitus: Screening. Retrieved from https://www.uspreventiveservicestaskforce.org/Page/Document/UpdateSummaryFinal/screening-for-abnormal-blood-glucose-and-type-2-diabetes?ds=1&s=diabetes

Wender, R., Fontham, E. T., Barrera, E., Colditz, G. A., Church, T. R., Ettinger, D. S., , . . . Smith, R. A. (2013). American Cancer Society lung cancer screening guidelines. *CA: A Cancer Journal for Clinicians, 63*(2), 106–117. doi:10.3322/caac.21172

Wilt, T. J., Harris, R. P., & Qaseem, A. (2015). Screening for cancer: Advice for high-value care from the American College of Physicians. *Annals of Internal Medicine, 162*(10), 718–725. doi:10.7326/M14-2326

Wolf, A., Wender, R., Etzioni, R., Thompson, I., D'Amico, A., Volk, R., , . . . Smith, R. (2010). American Cancer Society guideline for the early detection of prostate cancer: Update 2010. *CA: A Cancer Journal for Clinicians, 60*, 70–98. doi:10.3322/caac.20066

HEMODYNAMIC MONITORING DEVICES

Heather Meissen and Alison M. Kelley

Disclosure: Healthcare equipment is continuously developing. It is the responsibility of the provider to stay abreast to new products and evolving technology. The provider must ensure that the products they choose are validated with sufficient, unbiased evidence, and are safe for patient care. This author does not promote or recommend any particular product. This chapter is strictly an overview of current technology at the time of this writing.

OVERVIEW OF CONDITION

Hemodynamic instability is one of the leading causes of admission to the ICU. Hemodynamic collapse, considered to be any instability in a patient's blood pressure (BP), can lead to inadequate arterial blood flow to organs. It often results from the mismatch between oxygen demand and oxygen consumption, which leads to tissue hypoxia and cell death. Patients who experience hemodynamic instability are at risk for organ damage and possibly death.

Hemodynamic instability requires physiological and mechanical support to ensure there is adequate cardiac input and output, or BP. The goal of the critical care provider is to quickly identify the type of hemodynamic collapse present and to treat the condition appropriately to improve survival. See Box 1 for a list of definitions and abbreviations commonly use in reference to hemodynamic monitoring equipment.

BOX 1: EQUIPMENT DEFINITIONS AND ABBREVIATIONS

■ **Calibration:** Refers to the process of modifying equipment to ensure optimal precision and accuracy of measurements.
  - **Calibrated devices** perform continuous measurements and should be recalibrated at frequent intervals to ensure accuracy.
  - **Noncalibrated devices** use patient demographics, such as age and ideal body weight, to derive and determine measurements.
  Note: When using noncalibrated devices, the provider is responsible for understanding that the accuracy of these products diminishes when preload, afterload, or contractility are significantly altered, such as in cases of high vasopressor support or significant cardiovascular collapse.

■ Commonly used abbreviations.
  - CO: Cardiac output.
  - CI: Cardiac index.
  - SV: Stroke volume.
  - SVV: Stroke volume variance.
  - PPV: Pulse pressure variance.
  - CVP: Central venous pressure.
  - SVR: Systemic vascular resistance.

INDICATIONS

In the past, providers have followed vital signs, such as heart rate (HR), BP, and decreased urine output (UOP), to determine if shock is present. Unfortunately, these symptoms develop late in the disease process, and alterations in these vital signs can occur due to a myriad of causes. This makes diagnosis difficult and delayed.

Many providers are now searching for new technologies to aid the diagnosis of cardiovascular collapse. This chapter will outline many devices that will assist the provider in identifying specific parameters related to hemodynamic instability.

NONINVASIVE MONITORING

Noninvasive hemodynamic monitoring may be indicated for patients who are stable but still require monitoring, patients who are prone to infections, or patients and their families who do not desire invasive lines. There are no inherent precautions for noninvasive monitoring. There are several different types of noninvasive hemodynamic monitoring devices that may be used.

TRANSTHORACIC ECHOCARDIOGRAPHY

Transthoracic echocardiography (TTE) provides information on:

A. Left ventricular function.

B. Right ventricular function.

C. Inferior vena cava (IVC) dimensions.

Measurements that can be obtained through this type of monitoring include: Preload, cardiac output (CO), ejection fraction, and IVC compressibility, which can be calculated as a measurement determining fluid status.

(continued)

HEMODYNAMIC MONITORING DEVICES (*continued*)

NONINVASIVE PULSE CONTOUR ANALYSIS

Noninvasive pulse contour analysis is performed through the use of devices that calculate stroke volume (SV) and/or CO from analysis of the arterial pressure waveform. This analysis of the arterial pressure waveform is completely noninvasive. It may be achieved through noninvasive finger pressure that tracks changes in the intra-arterial wall.

DEVICES

Several different devices can be used to achieve noninvasive pulse contour analysis. Many of these devices use photoplethysmography via a finger probe. Once in use, the devices can estimate CO/cardiac index (CI), SV, stroke volume variance (SVV), systemic vascular resistance (SVR), and pulse pressure variance (PPV), and can provide continuous BP monitoring. Although these devices have variable accuracy, they are sometimes indicated for use in patients undergoing moderate to high risk surgeries who may not have an arterial line and in patients where determining fluid responsiveness is informative.

THORACIC BIOIMPEDANCE AND THORACIC BIOREACTANCE

Thoracic bioimpedance is a noninvasive form of monitoring that uses skin electrodes to send a high frequency current across the thorax and measures the amplitude of that current against the returning current. This form of monitoring estimates ventricular ejection fraction, SV, HR, and CO.

Thoracic bioreactance is an advancement on bioimpedance. This form of monitoring measures the phase shift in voltage through four electrodes that send alternating voltage of known frequency through the thorax. Sensors then calculate time delay, referred to as phase shift. Thoracic bioreactance devices can measure SV, SVI, CO/CI, and total peripheral resistive index.

ESTIMATED CONTINUOUS CO MONITORING

Estimated continuous CO monitoring determines CO by pulse oximetry and pulse wave transit time, and can also incorporate pulse oximetry and ECG signals. This is a noncalibrated system.

PASSIVE LEG RAISE

Fluid responsiveness can also be determined using a passive leg raise. This simple bedside test involves a leg raise that, by way of gravity, will return an estimated 150 to 300 mL of blood back to the heart. Changes in BP and HR should be analyzed by the healthcare provider to determine if the patient would respond to fluid administration.

ULTRASONOGRAPHY

Ultrasonography is another form of noninvasive monitoring that can be used to evaluate volume status. To assess the IVC, the probe in ultrasound is held in the subcostal longitudinal view (see Figure 1). An average IVC is approximately 1.5 to 2.5 cm in diameter. If the IVC diameter is less than 1.5 cm, this may indicate volume depletion. In trauma, a diameter less than 1.0 cm is likely related to hemorrhage. If the IVC is greater than 2.5 cm, then the patient likely will not respond to more fluids as this diameter suggests fluid overload.

It is also important to be aware of IVC compressibility. The IVC typically collapses 50% during inspiration. A collapse less than 50% typically suggests fluid overload. A collapse greater than 50% typically suggests intravascular volume depletion.

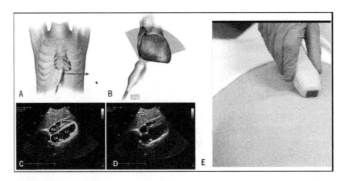

FIGURE 1   Subcostal window to visualize IVC.
IVC, inferior vena cava.
Source: Reproduced with permission from Mayo Foundation for Medical Education and Research.

(*continued*)

HEMODYNAMIC MONITORING DEVICES (*continued*)

ULTRASONIC CO MONITORING

Ultrasonic CO monitoring can be used to calculate the aortic and pulmonary outflow tracts to estimate CO. It is important to note that patients with structural heart disease may provide false values. Clinical correlation is warranted and more invasive testing may be indicated for further evaluation. Values obtained in this form of monitoring are:

A. CO/CI.

B. SV.

C. SVR.

D. HR.

MINIMALLY INVASIVE MONITORING

Forms of minimally invasive monitoring use some combination of noninvasive and invasive monitoring to provide the most accurate information about the patient's hemodynamic status with the most minimal use of invasive devices possible. For example, the pulmonary artery catheter (PAC), an invasive centrally placed catheter, was used to provide critical information. It has been replaced largely by waveform analysis using an arterial catheter, which is considered minimally invasive. Minimally invasive monitoring is preferred over invasive monitoring whenever appropriate.

ESOPHAGEAL DOPPLER (TRANSESOPHAGEAL ECHOCARDIOGRAM)

Esophageal Doppler (transesophageal echocardiogram [TEE]) is a Doppler device that is placed into the mid-esophagus to obtain ultrasound views of the heart from within the body. Some TEE devices allow for frequent or continuous monitoring and allow the provider to visualize heart chambers, valves, blood flow, and any abnormalities that may exist. These abnormalities may include pericardial effusion or wall motion abnormalities. TEE also allows the provider to measure blood flow velocity, CO, and ejection fraction.

DEVICES

Several devices can be used for TEE that calculate the SV, and subsequently the CO, from measuring the arterial pulse pressure via an indwelling arterial catheter. Values obtained are:

A. CO/CI.

B. HR.

C. SV.

D. SVR.

E. SVV.

Using an indwelling arterial catheter for TEE allows for providers to obtain measurements by estimating the SV by measuring the area under the curve of the systolic phase. This is a noncalibrated measurement that obtains the following.

A. CO/CI.

B. SV.

C. HR.

D. PPV.

E. SVV.

Other devices determine SV, and subsequently CO, by measuring the area under the curve of the entire cardiac cycle, both systolic and diastolic. These are calibrated devices that deliver predetermined amounts of lithium chloride to the patient through a central or peripheral line. The remaining concentration of lithium is then measured at the arterial catheter site. Values obtained using these devices are:

A. CO/CI.

B. SV.

(continued)

HEMODYNAMIC MONITORING DEVICES (*continued*)

C. HR.

D. SVR.

E. SVV.

MINIMALLY INVASIVE PULSE CONTOUR ANALYSIS

Several types of minimally invasive devices can calculate SV and/or CO from analysis of the arterial pressure waveform. The devices use proprietary algorithms to calculate pressure–volume relationships based on SVR, arterial compliance, and/or aortic impedance from the arterial line waveform (see Figure 2). Most of these devices provide loose accuracy when patients become significantly unstable.

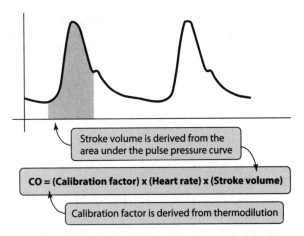

FIGURE 2 Example of minimally invasive pulse contour analysis.

TRANSPULMONARY THERMODILUTION

Transpulmonary thermodilution is the method of injecting cold saline into a central access point and measuring the change in temperature at the arterial access point. Calculations used in this method are derived from the thermodilution equation, which is:

$$CO = \frac{\{(Tb-Ti) \times K\}}{\{\int_0^\infty \Delta Tb(t)dt\}}$$

Tb = Blood temperature
Ti = Injectate temperature
K = Computed constant

(1)

DEVICES

Several devices can be used to achieve transpulmonary thermodilution to obtain the following values.

A. CO/CI.

B. HR.

C. SV.

D. SVR.

(*continued*)

HEMODYNAMIC MONITORING DEVICES (*continued*)

   E. SVV.

   F. PPV.

   G. Global end diastolic volume (GEDV), which can estimate preload.

   H. Intrathoracic blood volume (ITBV).

   I. Pulmonary vascular permeability index (PVPI).

   J. Global ejection fraction (GEF).

ULTRASOUND FLOW DILUTION

The final minimally invasive form of monitoring is ultrasound flow dilution, which can be used to measure CO. This can be achieved using a machine that calculates CO via transpulmonary ultrasound dilution technology by measuring changes in blood ultrasound velocity and blood flow after saline injection. The device requires a central line and arterial line as well as an extracorporeal arteriovenous (AV loop) tube set. This calibrated device obtains the following values.

   A. CO/CI.

   B. SV/SVI.

   C. Total ejection fraction.

   D. SVR/SVRI.

   E. Total end diastolic volume index.

   F. Central blood volume index.

INVASIVE MONITORING

Invasive monitoring is a relative term that typically includes central vein access and arterial monitoring, but can also refer to devices on a continuum. For instance, a radial arterial line is technically an invasive procedure, but is considered minimally invasive when compared to the placement of a brachial arterial line. Central lines are invasive, but less invasive than PACs when used with noninvasive cardiac monitoring devices. Patients who require invasive monitoring are typically hemodynamically unstable with indications that the use of minimally invasive or noninvasive methods would be unreliable or ineffective. Precautions vary based on the form of monitoring. Arterial monitoring precautions include:

   A. Hemorrhage.

   B. Thrombosis.

   C. Pseudoaneurysm formation.

   D. Infection.

Central monitoring precautions include:

   A. Infection.

   B. Damage to surrounding structures.

   C. Thrombosis.

   D. Arterial puncture.

CENTRAL VENOUS PRESSURE MONITORING

Central venous pressure (CVP) is the measurement of the pressure of the right atrium. In this form of monitoring, CVP is obtained from a central venous catheter that is placed in the subclavian or internal jugular vein and terminates in the superior vena cava at the right atrium. Although CVP is commonly used as a marker of fluid status, many studies have shown that CVP does not correlate to circulating blood volume, and that CVP cannot predict fluid responsiveness in many clinical scenarios. Therefore, CVP monitoring is not useful in guiding fluid management in most cases; however, it should be noted that CVP monitoring could guide management of the right ventricle and prove beneficial in patients who have right ventricular dysfunction from either myocardial infarct or pulmonary embolism.

(*continued*)

HEMODYNAMIC MONITORING DEVICES (*continued*)

PULMONARY ARTERY CATHETER

A PAC is a flow-directed catheter that is fed through a central venous introducer. The catheter is guided through the introducer to the right atrium, through the right ventricle, and to the pulmonary artery. At one point, this device was the gold standard tool for measurement of fluid status, but its use has recently fallen out of favor. Many studies have found no mortality benefits with the use of PAC, and some studies even show a risk of increasing mortality. Many reports have shown misinterpretation of data and user error as leading to the inaccuracy of the values obtained. For these reasons, less invasive tools are now being utilized more frequently. However, PAC can still be a beneficial measurement tool in right ventricular heart failure or pulmonary hypertension. Values obtained with this form of monitoring are:

A. CVP.

B. Pulmonary artery pressure (PAP).

C. Pulmonary artery occlusion pressure (PAOP).

EVALUATION AND RESULTS

Use of hemodynamic monitoring should be tailored and interpreted carefully for each patient. Critically ill patients may have confounding factors that make absolute interpretations difficult. Noninvasive monitoring may be limited by patient cooperation or body habitus. Invasive monitoring may be limited by poor circulation or misplacement of lines. It is essential that the healthcare provider provide careful interpretation in each individual case.

CLINICAL PEARLS

When using hemodynamic monitoring devices, the advanced practice provider (APP) should keep the following in mind.

A. Positioning is the key to optimal visualization in noninvasive monitoring using echocardiography.

B. Arterial lines may become dampened if the BP is very low. However, this may also be caused by air pockets in the transducer. Flushing the lines may resolve this issue.

C. Always use optimal view on the monitor.

D. Invasive monitoring can provide significant information about the patient's condition, but information must be interpreted with caution.

BIBLIOGRAPHY

Bender, J. S., Smith-Meek, M. A., & Jones, C. E. (1997). Routine pulmonary artery catheterization does not reduce morbidity and mortality of elective vascular surgery: Results of a prospective, randomized trial. *Annals of Surgery, 226*, 229–237. doi:10.1097/00000658-199709000-00002

CNSystems Medizintechnik. (n.d.). *CNAP monitor 500 HD*. Retrieved from http://www.cnsystems.com/products/cnap-monitor-500

Hadian, M., & Pinsky, M. (2006). Evidence-based review of the use of the pulmonary artery catheter: Impact data and complications. *Critical Care, 10*(Suppl. 3), S8. doi:10.1186/cc4834

Ilies, C., Bauer, M., Berg, P., Rosenberg, J., Hedderich, J., Bein, B., . . . Hanss, R. (2012). Investigation of the agreement of a continuous non-invasive arterial pressure device in comparison with invasive radial artery measurement. *British Journal of Anaesthesia, 108*, 202–210. doi:10.1093/bja/aer394

Marik, P. E. (2013). Noninvasive cardiac output monitors: A state-of the-art review. *Journal of Cardiothoracic Vascular Anesthesia, 27*, 121–134. doi:10.1053/j.jvca.2012.03.022

Marik, P. E., Baram, M., & Vahid, B. (2008). Does central venous pressure predict fluid responsiveness?: A systematic review of the literature and the tale of seven mares. *Chest, 134*(1), 172–178. Retrieved from http://www.sciencedirect.com/science/article/pii/S0012369208601634

Mimoz, O., Rauss, A., Rekik, N., Brun-Buisson, C., Lemaire, F., & Brochard, L. (1994). Pulmonary artery catheterization in critically ill patients: A prospective analysis of outcome changes associated with catheter-prompted changes in therapy. *Critical Care Medicine, 22*, 573–579. doi:10.1097/00003246-199404000-00011

Monnet, X., & Teboul, J. L. (2015). Minimally invasive monitoring. *Critical Care Clinics, 31*, 25–42. doi:10.1016/j.ccc.2014.08.002

Murdoch, S. D., Cohen, A. T., & Bellamy, M. C. (2000). Pulmonary artery catheterization and mortality in critically ill patients. *British Journal of Anaesthesia, 85*, 611–615. doi:10.1093/bja/85.4.611

Rajaram, S. S., Desai, N. K., Kalra, A., Gajera, M., Cavanaugh, S. K., Brampton, W., & Rowan, K. (2013). Pulmonary artery catheters for adult patients in intensive care. *Cochrane Database of Systematic Reviews, 2013*(2), CD003408. doi:10.1002/14651858.CD003408.pub3

Renner, J., Grünewald, M., & Bein, B. (2016). Monitoring high-risk patients: Minimally invasive and non-invasive possibilities. *Best Practice & Research Clinical Anaesthesiology, 30*, 201–216. doi:10.1016/j.bpa.2016.04.006

Richard, C., Warszawski, J., Anguel, N., Deye, N., Combes, A., Barnoud, D., & Teboul, J.-L. (2003). Early use of the pulmonary artery catheter and outcomes in patients with shock and acute respiratory distress syndrome. *Journal of the American Medical Association, 290*, 2713–2720. doi:10.1001/jama.290.20.2713

(continued)

HEMODYNAMIC MONITORING DEVICES *(continued)*

Roth, S., Fox, H., Fuchs, U., Schulz, U., Costard-Jäckle, A., Gummert, J., . . . Bitter, T. (2018). Noninvasive pulse contour analysis for determination of cardiac output in patients with chronic heart failure. *Clinical Research in Cardiology, 107*, 395–404. doi:10.1007/s00392-017-1198-7

Sangkum, L., Liu, G. L., Yu, L., Yan, H., Kaye, A. D., & Liu, H. (2016). Minimally invasive or noninvasive cardiac output measurement: An update. *Journal of Anesthesia, 30*, 461–480. doi:10.1007/s00540-016-2154-9

Saugel, B., Cecconi, M., Wagner, J. Y., & Reuter, D. A. (2015). Noninvasive continuous cardiac output monitoring in perioperative and intensive care medicine. *British Journal of Anaesthesia, 114*, 562–575. doi:10.1093/bja/aeu447

Shah, M. R., Hasselblad, V., Stevenson, L. W., Binanay, C., O'Connor, C. M., Sopko, G., & & Califf, R. M. (2005). Impact of the pulmonary artery catheter in critically ill patients. *Journal of the American Medical Association, 294*, 1664–1670. doi:10.1001/jama.294.13.1664

Vincent, J. L., Rhodes, A., Perel, A., Martin, G. S., Della Rocca, G., Vallet, B., & Singer, M. (2011). Clinical review: Update on hemodynamic monitoring—a consensus of 16. *Critical Care, 15*, 229. doi:10.1186/cc10291

TELEMEDICINE IN ACUTE CARE

RuthAnne Skinner

INTRODUCTION

As technology evolves, so does its role in the provision of healthcare. For centuries, technology has helped enable healthcare providers to streamline patient care and improve health outcomes. In more recent years, technology has also helped providers expand the care they provide as well as helped providers reach medically underserved populations through the use of telemedicine. Telemedicine refers to the process of providing medical care, such as diagnosis and treatment, remotely through technology. Telemedicine continues to rapidly grow, become more widely used, and helps healthcare providers provide care to more and more people. Although guidelines for appropriate uses of telemedicine are not yet standardized for advanced practice providers (APPs), it is important for the APP to have a firm grasp on challenges this evolving specialty poses, such as patient security and privacy. Consideration of such challenges will help APPs to create guidelines as the field of telemedicine progresses.

HISTORY

The invention of the telephone was the first step toward connecting individuals to a healthcare provider remotely. After its invention, obstetric calls were one of the most common sources of early telemedicine usage. These calls usually included giving direction to midwives who were helping mothers laboring at home.

Later in April 1924, *Radio News* magazine created an article called, "The Radio Doctor, maybe." In the article, the writer notes the next step in telemedicine—using television to provide healthcare. The article described an attachment to a television screen that enabled communication and assessment techniques, such a hearing a heartbeat. The first television transmission did not occur until 1927, so this article was a visionary approach to treating remote patients. This marked the first conceptual idea of telemedicine as we know it today.

Although the *Radio News* article introduced the idea of remote treatment and assessment in 1924, it was not until roughly two decades later that the University of Nebraska was credited for actually performing the first telemedicine consult. In 1959, experts at the University of Nebraska used two-way, closed-circuit, microwave television for medical treatment and education. During this exchange, they successfully completed a neurological examination remotely with the accuracy of an assessment done in person.

Over the next few decades, healthcare providers continued to find new ways to use technology to expand how they delivered medicine. In the 1970s, a project named the Space Technology Applied to Rural Papago Advanced Health Care (STARPAHC) was first introduced. This program, run by the National Aeronautics and Space Administration (NASA) with the support of Lockheed Missiles and Space Corporation (LMSC) and Indian Health Services (IHS), increased the availability of healthcare to Papago Indians, who were located on an Indian reservation in southwest Arizona. The Papago Reservation lacked the medical resources to diagnose and manage patients. Additionally, NASA wanted to ensure that they could adequately respond to medical concerns for their astronauts in space. This unique partnership reinforced the importance of advance planning, clear objectives, and active community involvement. In the 1990s, radiology began using and interpreting digital reports on a regular basis. Teleradiologists, who were often called "nighthawks," originally provided this form of medicine for emergencies or night coverage.

THE INTERNET AND MODERN TELEMEDICINE

Although each of the aforementioned technological advances played an important role in furthering telemedicine technology, few advancements parallel the enduring effect of the Internet. The Internet provides a global network of information and communication, which has revolutionized how APPs deliver healthcare. The linked communication has created more opportunities for telemedicine than any other technology to date, and has improved availability of healthcare to remote patients. For example, patients can now use at-home monitoring devices that send data to a clinical decision support database. Furthermore, providers in dermatology can review uploaded images and case scenarios, allowing them to treat double their current patient load. Phone applications (apps) are also being created and used to remind patients when to take their medications. The Internet, along with other medical technologies, enables healthcare providers to engage in many different types of telemedicine, including TeleICU, TelePsych, and Telemonitoring.

TeleICU

TeleICU refers to the remote management and monitoring of patients in the ICU. Using TeleICU monitoring, healthcare providers can remotely monitor changes in patient conditions. This care approach improves patient outcomes, especially in remote areas that do not have access to an intensivist.

TelePsych

TelePsych refers to the remote management and consultation for psychological disorders. Care provided in this setting may include consultation, cognitive behavioral therapy, and emergency psychiatric care. In addition to expanding the number of patients served, TelePysch can reduce the burden of EDs waiting for inpatient psychiatric rooms. TelePsych has reduced emergency holding time for patients with behavioral health concerns who are waiting for an available psychiatrist.

(continued)

TELEMEDICINE IN ACUTE CARE *(continued)*

Telemonitoring

Telemonitoring refers to any form of monitoring patients remotely. This can include monitoring a patient's heart rate, blood pressure, glucose level, or other vital indicators. This form of telemedicine may be used to prevent readmission of certain patients. For example, healthcare providers may remotely monitor patients with congestive heart failure (CHF) who were recently discharged from the hospital to evaluate and treat exacerbations as an outpatient.

TELEMEDICINE IN ACUTE CARE

Various forms of telemedicine have a significant effect on improving acute care delivery as well as improved quality of acute care. For example, healthcare providers may help prevent readmission by remotely monitoring patients. One example of this is remotely monitoring patients in skilled nursing facilities (SNFs) to manage concerns typically sent to the ED at night. Telemedicine may also be used to enhance performance initiatives. An example of this is providers who perform ventilator rounding to optimize ventilator settings and complete ventilator bundle order sets. Providers remotely round on patients to ensure quality measures, like deep vein thrombosis prophylaxis and stress ulcer prophylaxis, are met.

Telemedicine may also help increase the number of available providers. Telemedicine providers take call and can assess patients overnight when nocturnal providers are limited. Furthermore, remote hospitals may not always have an intensivist to manage the intensive care patients. Telemedicine intensivist providers can offer expert advice and management no matter where they are located.

It can also be used to decrease ED visits. Urgent care consults can be conducted via smartphone application or other Internet application. After hours telemedicine consults can be conducted to treat and manage patients. When appropriate, patients can be encouraged to go to the brick and mortar ED.

PRIVACY AND SECURITY

As technology evolves and telemedicine practice expands, new challenges emerge with regard to maintaining patient confidentiality and privacy. These challenges often require solutions that involve legislative action as well as adopting certain technology use and information sharing practices.

Health Insurance Portability and Accountability Act

Likely the most recognizable legislative measure in effect is the Health Insurance Portability and Accountability Act (HIPAA) Security Rule (SR). HIPAA protects the patient and his or her **electronic protected health (ePHI) record**. An ePHI is any protected health information that can be produced or saved in electronic form. There are 16 HIPAA identifiers that require special care and protection. They include the following.

A. Names.

B. Phone numbers.

C. Fax numbers.

D. Email addresses.

E. Social Security numbers.

F. Medical records.

G. Health plan beneficiaries.

H. Account numbers.

I. License numbers.

J. Vehicle identifiers.

K. Device identifiers.

L. Universal resource locators (URLs).

M. Internet protocol (IP) addresses.

N. Biometrics.

O. Photographic images.

P. Any other unique identifying number or characteristic.

Currently, there is no regulatory body for HIPAA compliance. HIPAA compliance is regulated by self-governance, third-party audits, or by using software that is built into your processes that ensure compliance.

(continued)

TELEMEDICINE IN ACUTE CARE *(continued)*

Store and Forward

Store and forward is a telecommunications technique in which information is stored prior to being forward to the final destination. This allows information to meet regulatory standards. Email is not considered HIPAA compliant, so store and forward is the method of choice for electronic communication. Some states allow email and text with expressed written consent on file.

Legislative Regulations

Telemedicine legislation and regulations vary from state to state. For example, some states differ in the services that may be reimbursed, such as:

A. Medicaid reimbursed services.

B. Services provided via live video.

C. Remote patient monitoring (RPM) services.

Other differences in telemedicine legislation may relate to store and forward services. Not all state regulators have granted unrestricted licensure. Several state medical boards even require special telemedicine licenses or certification. Specifically, nurse practitioners providing telemedicine are subjected to the state board of nursing for which the patient resides. Nurse practitioners must be licensed in the state where the patient resides. Therefore, there has been an additional push for the creation of the COMPACT APRN license, which would allow APRNs to hold a single multistate license. The scope of practice, licensure, and regulatory restrictions for other APPs also depends on the current state where the patient resides. All APPs should review each state's specific laws.

TELEMEDICINE AND HEALTHCARE QUALITY

In addition to making healthcare more widely available to underserved populations, telemedicine also has the ability to improve the quality of healthcare provided. The Health and Medicine Division (HMD) of the National Academies of Science, formerly called the Institute of Medicine (IOM), is a nonprofit organization that has published a series of evidence-based research recommendations on quality and safety in healthcare. In 1996, before the general knowledge and acceptance of telemedicine, the HMD published a report encouraging the use of telemedicine to increase availability of care and improve patient outcomes. Since that time, telemedicine has become an important part of measuring and improving healthcare quality.

This acknowledgment of the importance of telemedicine in improving healthcare is evident in the Department of Health and Human Service's *Healthy People 2020* initiative. *Healthy People 2020* sets several national health goals, which are to:

A. Improve preventable disease.

B. Eliminate health disparities.

C. Create environments to promote good health.

D. Promote quality of life.

One specific goal of *Healthy People 2020* is to use health information strategies to improve patient outcomes, quality, and equity.

Those who practice telemedicine are not only concerned with improving access to healthcare, but also to maintaining and improving the quality of healthcare provided through telemedicine. Specifically, those who provide telemedicine often refer to the National Quality Measures Clearinghouse (NQMC). The NQMC is a public database for healthcare providers that contains summaries of evidence-based research guidelines and measures. Telemedicine operation centers use NQMC measures to round on patients in the hospital and optimize treatment plans.

LOOKING AHEAD

Electronic Medical Record

Electronic medical records provide easy access to records remotely. Remote access to medical records expands the ability of an interprofessional team of healthcare providers to seamlessly manage and treat patients. Electronic medical records work hand-in-hand with electronic health information exchanges (HIEs), which improve the efficiency of patient information sharing to ensure more thorough telemedicine consults due to the increase in patient past medical history.

(continued)

TELEMEDICINE IN ACUTE CARE (*continued*)

Health Information Technology for Economic and Clinical Health

The Health Information Technology for Economic and Clinical Health (HITECH) Act, created under the Recovery and Reinvestment Act of 2009, funds the expansion of health information technology. It established meaningful use of electronic medical records to encourage adoption. Meaningful use provides incentives for adoption of electronic medical records and associated improvements in care. Adoption prior to 2015 was voluntary, and a 1% penalty was applied after that to eligible providers and eligible hospitals. After 2017, a 3% penalty was applied. Additional meaningful use components include the following.

A. Electronic prescribing.

B. Electronic exchange of health information.

C. Clinical quality improvements, such as clinical decision support system (CDSS).

Continual Improvement and Key Factors Moving Forward in Telemedicine Reimbursement

Currently, telemedicine is a risk-based reimbursement, which rewards providers for improved patient outcomes. In the future, it is anticipated that there will be more opportunities for reimbursement.

Similarly, Medicare and Medicaid continue to increase items that can be reimbursed. This is made possible through the standardization of how healthcare services are documented. The U.S. Centers for Medicare and Medicaid Services (CMS) funded the Current Procedural Terminology (CPT) and the *International Classification of Diseases* 10th revision (*ICD-10*). *ICD-10* included telemedicine, and telemedicine services codes are continually added to the CPT database.

BIBLIOGRAPHY

Bashshur, R. (1980). Technology serves the people: The story of a co-operative telemedicine project by NASA, the Indian health service and the Papago people. Washington, DC: U.S. Government Printing Office.

Field, M. (1996). *Telemedicine: A guide to assessing telecommunications in health care*. Washington, DC: National Academies Press.

Freiburger, G., Holcomb, M., & Piper, D. (2007). The STARPAHC collection: Part of an archive of the history of telemedicine. *Journal of Telemedicine Telecare, 13*(5), 221–223. doi:10.1258/135763307781458949

Goran, S. (2010). A second set of eyes: An introduction to Tele-ICU. *Critical Care Nurse, 30*, 46–55. doi:10.4037/ccn2010283

Lyuboslavsky, V. (2015). *Telemedicine and telehealth 2.0: A practical guide for medical providers and patients*. Chicago, IL: NCSBN.

National Council of State Boards of Nursing. (2015). *APRN compact*. Retrieved from https://www.ncsbn.org/aprn-compact.htm

U.S. Department of Health and Human Services. (2014). *Healthy People 2020*. Retrieved from https://www.healthypeople.gov/

TRANSITIONAL CARE

Amy Blake

INTRODUCTION

Care transitions are receiving widespread focus in academia, clinical practice, and executive and regulatory forums. The Hospital Readmissions Reduction Program, created under the Affordable Care Act (ACA) in 2012, has imposed financial penalties for higher-than-expected readmissions for acute myocardial infarction, heart failure, pneumonia, chronic obstructive pulmonary disease, and total hip and knee arthroplasties. Higher-than-expected readmissions come with additional costs and can be associated with increased mortality and poor outcomes. This has inspired institutions to focus on the development of programs dedicated to improving a patient's transition from one setting to another.

Healthcare can appear to be fast paced, fragmented, and confusing to both the lay observer and to those who participate in healthcare delivery. Understanding how the various branches of healthcare situate themselves among the kaleidoscope of options available to a consumer can be a challenge for anyone. Navigating a patient's healthcare path is a complex process that is becoming a specialty unto itself. Finding the safest, most cost-effective continuum is currently one of healthcare's hottest topics.

CARE TRANSITIONS DEFINED

Efforts to define transitional care have focused on determining a set of actions to minimize known risks, such as fragmentation, poor communication, and poor coordination, that can lead to unfavorable outcomes. Fragmentation of care has been associated with increased hospital readmissions. The 2003 position statement from the American Geriatrics Society defined transitional care as a set of actions designed to ensure the coordination and continuity of healthcare as patients transfer between different locations or between different levels of care within the same location. Representative locations include (but are not limited to) the following.

A. Hospitals.

B. Subacute and postacute nursing facilities.

C. The patient's home.

D. Primary and specialty care offices.

E. Long-term care (LTC) facilities.

In this definition, transitional care is based on several factors that encompass both the sending and receiving aspects of care, including:

A. A comprehensive plan of care.

B. The availability of healthcare practitioners who are well-trained in chronic care and have current, clearly communicated information about the patient's problems, goals, preferences, and clinical status.

C. Defined logistical arrangements, education of the patient and family, and coordination among all health professionals involved in the transition.

Naylor and Keating (2008) note that transitional care encompasses a broad range of time-limited services designed to:

A. Ensure healthcare continuity.

B. Avoid preventable poor outcomes.

C. Ensure timely transfer of patients from one level of care to another or from one type of setting to another.

Communication as Cornerstone

It is important to remember that no matter the exact definition, the cornerstone to effective transitional care is communication. Communication must be embedded in an easily accessible platform throughout each phase of the continuum to allow for effective coordination and delivery of appropriate care. Lack of communication leads to poor understanding of priorities, fragmentation, unnecessary duplication of tests, and, at times, omission of important follow-up. The Society for Post-Acute and Long-Term Care Medicine (AMDA) stresses that communication is key to improving care transitions between nursing facilities and acute care hospital settings. Specific recommendations include the following.

A. Information about the patient, including medication and care plans, should be collected through the hospital stay and be available well in advance of any transfer.

(continued)

TRANSITIONAL CARE (*continued*)

B. Professionals involved in the care of LTC patients and other frail, at-risk patients should actively work with other relevant professionals and each site of care to create and improve policies and procedures that assure timely and accurate communication.

C. When possible, information about transfers should be communicated from professional to professional in different sites of care.

D. The sending and receiving professionals should have reliable contact information for each other.

When considering transitional care, it is also important to remember that transitions occur not only from setting to setting, but also from provider to provider. For example, an elderly patient with a history of chronic obstructive pulmonary disease and congestive heart failure could be hospitalized after a fall for an acute hip fracture. The patient may undergo repair, have his or her diuretic held for mild kidney injury, experience elevated blood pressure due to pain, and transition to a skilled rehab center to focus on strength and mobility. In the new setting, the patient will be at risk should a chronic comorbidity decompensate, thus potentially shifting the balance and priorities of care. This shifting continuum will recur in a dynamic fashion among all settings from hospital to postacute care to home, and back again as a different condition demands priority.

INTERIM RISKS IN TRANSITIONAL CARE

Multiple transitions through different settings with different providers and managing shifting priorities caused by dynamic comorbidities leaves a multitude of avenues for fragmentation and care breakdown. Interim risks include several different factors.

Medication Changes and Errors

Medication errors are a common area of communication breakdown. Medication lists are reconciled numerous times from setting to setting, and new changes and formulary substitutions are accommodated. Forster et al. (2003) estimates that approximately one in five patients experience adverse drug events in the weeks following hospitalization, and up to one-third of these adverse events are considered to be preventable or ameliorable. Medications with higher rates of adverse effects include:

A. Antibiotics.

B. Corticosteroids.

C. Cardiovascular medications.

D. Anticoagulants.

E. Antiepileptics.

F. Analgesic medications, including narcotics.

New, changed, and discontinued medications should be clearly noted in the discharge summary along with important reasons for the change, such as an adverse reaction or complication that prompted the change.

Unclear Follow-Up Instructions

Unclear follow-up instructions are another common area of risk in transitional care. Incompletely communicated instructions for follow-up care and pending or incomplete diagnostic and laboratory studies leave abundant space for important aspects of care to fall through the cracks. A higher margin for miscommunication exists in patients with long hospitalizations, during which multiple specialists see the patient and order multiple diagnostic tests. Strategies to increase communication of follow-up instructions include the following.

A. Important diagnostic studies, procedures, and lab values should be clearly documented in discharge instructions along with and pending results that require follow-up.

B. Providers that a patient should follow-up with should also be clearly documented along with contact information.

C. Information regarding durable medical equipment (DME) required at discharge such as noninvasive ventilators (continuous positive airway pressure [C-pap], bilevel positive airway pressure [biPap], average volume assure pressure support [AVAP]) should be included along with settings and the equipment provider's name and contact number. It is helpful to include whether the equipment is rented or if the patient requires a qualification process or further testing in order to have the equipment at home.

   1. Example: If a patient with respiratory failure requires BiPap or AVAP at home, he or she requires special qualification processes in order to have a home machine. A skilled nursing facility may rent an interim machine for the patient, but

TRANSITIONAL CARE (continued)

if care is not taken to qualify and attain approval for the equipment, a patient could ultimately end up at home without a crucial noninvasive ventilator, rendering him or her at high risk for readmission from hypercapnic respiratory failure.

Poorly Communicated or Unaddressed Advance Directives

Poorly communicated or unaddressed advance directives and code status put a patient at risk for treatments and resuscitation he or she may have decided for or against. It is important for the advanced practice provider (APP) to take the following actions.

A. Ensure a discussion has taken place regarding advance directives and the identification of a healthcare proxy or durable power of attorney for healthcare.

B. Ensure that each patient is asked about a living will or similar document. This document describes in detail the patient's wishes with regard to resuscitation, hospitalization, treatment goals and limits, and a healthcare proxy.

C. The goal of advance directives is to provide the patient autonomy in decisions regarding his or her manner and location of death as well as **relieving family burden and conflict** while the older individual is **mentally competent** to do so.
   1. The Five Wishes Form is useful to guide choices. The Five Wishes Form is a document that assists individuals in making preferences and care wishes in the case of an emergency or incapacity. This form will help the designated decision maker to make informed choices on the patient's behalf. The form asks the patient to indicate the following.
      a. The person I want to make care decisions for me when I cannot.
      b. The kind of medical treatment I want or do not want.
      c. How comfortable I want to be.
      d. How I want people to treat me.
      e. What I want my loved ones to know.
   2. Many states have a MOST form (**m**edical **o**rders for **s**cope of **t**reatment) or POLST form (**p**hysician **o**rder for **l**ife **s**ustaining **t**reatment). The exact type of form varies from state to state. The APP should become familiar with the form used in his or her own state. This is a legal document that specifies the type of care a person would like in his or her final year of life and provides orders, signed by a provider, whereas the advance directive provides general wishes.

D. Clearly communicate a patient's advance directive desires and code status in the discharge summary and ensure the appropriate MOST or POLST forms are completed before transfers take place.

Complex Problem Lists

Problem lists are specified in the discharge summary by priority. Recall that priorities remain dynamic and can shift unexpectedly. Clearly delineate primary and secondary problem lists with the associated plan, if helpful. Consider the following notes that may appear in the chart of the aforementioned patient.

Primary Dx.

A. Acute hip fx or if continue PT/OT.

B. AKI—mild: Home doses of Lasix and lisinopril held for create bump in creatinine to 2.0 from baseline 1.3. Monitor creatinine closely and restart when closer to baseline.

C. HTN stable on beta-blocker, note ACE inhibitor and diuretic on hold secondary to #2.

D. Pain management: Vicodin every 4 to 6 hours as needed.

E. Chronic biventricular heart failure with EF 30% and diastolic dysfunction. Stable. Continue beta-blocker. Restart loop diuretic and ACE inhibitor when able. Monitor daily weight and fluid balance closely.

AKI, acute kidney injury; EF, ejection fraction; fx, fracture; HTN, hypertension; OT, occupational therapy; PT, physical therapy.

Consider the scenario that a receiving facility is out of Vicodin, and no one is immediately available to substitute a pain medication. The patient's blood pressure elevates from pain over the next 24 to 48 hours in the setting of biventricular heart failure. The information regarding the patient's heart failure was not communicated since it was "stable." The patient's family is happy she is finally out of the hospital and brings her all of her favorite drinks and a nice ham dinner. The information pertaining to the temporary cessation of her diuretic and angiotensin-converting enzyme (ACE) inhibitor was not clearly communicated. She is at risk for decompensated heart failure, hypertensive urgency, and pulmonary edema. Clear communication is key. Ideally, a clear, well-constructed problem list might appear as the following.

(continued)

TRANSITIONAL CARE (*continued*)

Current Problem	Diagnosis	Tracking
Heart failure	Heart failure biventricular with EF 30%	Ongoing
Cardiac disease	Old myocardial infarction	Ongoing
Hypertension	Hypertension	Ongoing

EF, ejection fraction.

Varying Medical Record Systems

Different providers have privileges allowing access to different medical record systems, whether they are electronic medical records (EMRs) or paper based. Different facilities and offices can have many different brands of EMRs. Unless there is a functional unifying accessible electronic medical system that is capable of pulling from all of these varied systems and documents, chances are limited that a provider will view a complete, up-to-date picture of a patient's plan of care. This makes communication an ongoing challenge.

Geriatric Needs

Frail, elderly patients are routinely transferred from setting to setting multiple times, often with a sense of urgency. This vulnerable population may have limited ability to communicate their needs, expectations, complex comorbidities, and recent circumstances, let alone navigate the overwhelming continuum of healthcare they are experiencing. They remain at risk for poor outcomes and decompensation from a variety of transitional risk perspectives. It is of vital importance for the APP to consider these challenges when providing transitional care to geriatric patients, and to consider the special communication needs of these patients to ensure continuity of care.

ACTIONS TO MITIGATE RISKS IN TRANSITIONAL CARE

It cannot be stated enough: Good communication is the cornerstone to improving care transitions. However, communication in a fast-paced world is often more difficult in reality than postulated. Phone calls can go unanswered or result in return calls that arrive outside of a crucial evaluation window. Messages logged and passed via computer can be brief and lackluster in clarifying complexity, and messages passed via word of mouth may not ultimately reach the assessing provider. Such messages may not even contain the originally communicated content. Faxes may not transmit. Routine texting is not Health Insurance Portability and Accountability Act (HIPAA) compliant. Complete medical records may not arrive with a patient or in a timely manner. EMR systems may not communicate with each other. Many states have made progress in this area by implementing statewide EMR housing systems. Secure texting platforms are now available; however, they may not be uniformly utilized by all systems, organizations, or providers in a community.

Bridging Gaps

Specific actions have been recommended to bridge the known gaps in transitional care. Strategies focused on population health are being trialed, such as placing a hospitalist in postacute and LTC settings. Specialists, such as cardiologists, pulmonologists, and wound care experts, are being deployed to postacute settings to enhance and direct the care of patients with congestive heart failure, chronic obstructive pulmonary disease, and complex wounds.

The Care Transitions Intervention

Another approach is referred to as the Care Transitions Intervention. This nationally recognized program is led by Eric Coleman from the University of Colorado. Within this program, Coleman developed four pillars, also called *domains*, of transitional care interventions. These pillars are:

A. Medication self-management.

B. Maintenance of a personal health record.

C. Close follow-up with a primary care provider.

D. The identification of red flags that should prompt evaluation.

When implemented, the program is led by a transitions coach who oversees the transition of the patient from hospitalization to home. The coach identifies patient goals and assists in the development of self-management skills. In summary, key components of a successful transitional care plan involve the following.

(*continued*)

TRANSITIONAL CARE (continued)

A. Firming up the pitfalls that can lead to poor outcomes.

B. Providing uniformity across the continuum of settings.

C. Paying close attention to medication reconciliation and delineating any medication changes or substitutions.

D. Developing clear, legible discharge templates that identify important features of the hospitalization, including:
   1. Pertinent diagnostic and laboratory tests.
   2. Pending diagnostic and laboratory tests.
   3. Future plan of care.
   4. Providers involved in the hospitalization and the providers that are needed for follow-up.

E. Clearly defining and continuously reviewing goals of care, advance directives, and code status in every setting.

This approach implements evidence-based practices that utilize dedicated, focused transitional providers to improve outcomes and reduce hospitalizations. Providers armed with evidence-based strategies can do the following.

A. Bridge the information and communication gap between settings.

B. Set goals among patients and the healthcare team.

C. Educate patients and families to self-manage.

D. Simultaneously provide complex monitoring, evaluation, and early intervention for decompensating dynamic comorbidities.

MOVING FORWARD

Future efforts in transitional care should seek to integrate and improve care across continuums instead of in isolated circumstances and settings. Such efforts will reduce stress and increase the health and well-being of our society as a whole. Population health strategies that focus on medical home models and transitional care management are exciting alternatives to fragmented traditional care. Medical homes without walls and telemedicine also provide promising alternatives by bringing advanced care providers and technology into the patient's home. Advances in unified, accessible health information databases will also improve care and reduce unnecessary duplication and overuse of health services. Advanced practice studies should include focus on the broadened responsibility and complex communication skills required to advance transitional care and, in doing so, increase the satisfaction of patients and providers alike.

BIBLIOGRAPHY

Aging With Dignity. (2011). *Five wishes*. Retrieved from https://fivewishes.org/docs/default-source/default-document-library/product-samples/fwsample.pdf?sfvrsn=2

American Medical Directors Association. (2010). *Transitions of care in the long-term care continuum clinical practice guideline*. Columbia, MD: Author. Retrieved from https://www.nhqualitycampaign.org/files/Transitions_of_Care_in_LTC.pdf

Bixby, M. B., & Naylor, M. D. (2010). The transitional care model (TCM): Hospital discharge screening criteria for high risk older adults. *Medsurg Nursing, 19*(1), 62–63.

Cohen-Mekelburg, S., Rosenblatt, R., Gold, S., Scherl, E., Burakoff, R., Steinlauf, A., & Unruh, M. (2018). Fragmented care is prevalent among IBD hospitalizations and is associated with worse outcome. *Gastroenterology, 154*(1 Suppl.), S101. doi:10.1053/j.gastro.2017.11.239

Coleman, E. A. (2001, November 2). *Infusing true person centered care into improving the quality of transitional care*. Paper presented at Transitions of Care: Improving Care Across Settings, Cincinnati, OH: Greater Cincinnati Health Council.

Coleman, E. A. (2003). Falling through the cracks: Challenges and opportunities for improving transitional care for persons with continuous complex care needs. *Journal of the American Geriatrics Society, 51*(4), 549–555. doi:10.1046/j.1532-5415.2003.51185.x

Forster, A. J., Murff, H. J., Peterson, J. F., Gandhi, T. K., & Bates, D. W. (2003). The incidence and severity of adverse events affecting patients after discharge from the hospital. *Annals of Internal Medicine, 138*(3), 161–167. doi:10.7326/0003-4819-138-3-200302040-00007

Jencks, S. F., Williams, M. V., & Coleman, E. A. (2009). Rehospitalizations among patients in the Medicare fee-for-service program. *The New England Journal of Medicine, 360*(14), 1418–1428. doi:10.1056/NEJMsa0803563

Jha, A. K., Joynt, K. E., Orav, E. J., & Epstein, A. M. (2012). The long-term effect of premier pay for performance on patient outcomes. *The New England Journal of Medicine, 366*(17), 1606–1615. doi:10.1056/NEJMsa1112351

Joynt, K. E., & Jha, A. K. (2012). Thirty-day readmissions—truth and consequences. *The New England Journal of Medicine, 366*(15), 1366–1369. doi:10.1056/NEJMp1201598

Naylor, M. D., Aiken, L. H., Kurtzman, E. T., Olds, D. M., & Hirschman, K. B. (2011). The importance of transitional care in achieving health reform. *Health Affairs, 30*(4), 746–754. doi:10.1377/hlthaff.2011.0041

Naylor, M. D., & Keating, S. A. (2008). Transitional care. *American Journal of Nursing, 108*(Suppl. 9), 58–63. doi:10.1097/01.NAJ.0000336420.34946.3adoi:10.1097/01.NAJ.0000336420.34946.3a

Nelson, J., & Pulley, A. (2015). Transitional care can reduce hospital readmissions. *American Nurse Today, 10*(4). Retrieved from https://www.americannursetoday.com/transitional-care-can-reduce-hospital-readmissions

Transitional Care Model. (n.d.) Retrieved from http://www.nursing.upenn.edu/ncth/transitional-care-model/index.php

V | Appendix

Normal Laboratory Values

Appendix: Normal Laboratory Values

ABIM Laboratory Test Reference Ranges—January 2019

Laboratory Tests	Reference Ranges
1,25-Dihydroxyvitamin D (1,25-Dihydroxycholecalciferol), serum	See vitamin D metabolites
17-Hydroxyprogesterone, serum	
Female, follicular	<80 ng/dL
Female, luteal	<285 ng/dL
Female, postmenopausal	<51 ng/dL
Male (adult)	<220 ng/dL
5-Hydroxyindoleacetic acid, urine	2–9 mg/24 hr
6-Thioguanine, whole blood	230–400 pmol/8 × 10^8 RBCs
ANC	2,000–8,250/μL
25-Hydroxyvitamin D (25-Hydroxycholecalciferol), serum	See vitamin D metabolites
ACE, serum	8–53 U/L
Acid phosphatase, serum	
Prostatic fraction	0.1–0.4 unit/mL
Total	0.5–2.0 (Bodansky) units/mL
ACTH, plasma	10–60 pg/mL
aPTT	25–35 sec
ADAMTS13 activity	>60%
ACTH, plasma	10–60 pg/mL
Albumin, serum	3.5–5.5 g/dL
Albumin, urine	<25 mg/24 hr
Albumin-to-creatinine ratio, urine	<30 mg/g
Aldolase, serum	0.8–3.0 IU/mL
Aldosterone, plasma	
Supine or seated	Up to 10 ng/dL
Standing	<21 ng/dL
Low sodium diet (supine)	Up to 30 ng/dL
Aldosterone, urine	5–19 mcg/24 hr
Alkaline phosphatase, bone specific	5.6–18.0 mcg/L for premenopausal women
Alkaline phosphatase, serum	30–120 U/L
AAT, serum	150–350 mg/dL
Alpha$_2$-antiplasmin activity, plasma	75%–115%
Alpha-amino nitrogen, urine	100–290 mg/24 hr

(continued)

ABIM Laboratory Test Reference Ranges—January 2019 (*continued*)

Alpha-fetoprotein, serum	<10 ng/mL
Amino acids, urine	200–400 mg/24 hr
Aminotransferase, serum alanine (ALT, SGPT)	10–40 U/L
Aminotransferase, serum aspartate (AST, SGOT)	10–40 U/L
Ammonia, blood	40–70 mcg/dL
Amylase, serum	25–125 U/L (80–180 [Somogyi] units/dL)
Amylase, urine	1–17 U/hr
Androstenedione, serum	Female: 30–200 ng/dL; male: 40–150 ng/dL
Anion gap, serum	7–13 mEq/L
Antibodies to double-stranded DNA	0–7 IU/mL
Anticardiolipin antibodies	
IgG	<20 GPL
IgM	<20 MPL
Anti-cyclic citrullinated peptide, antibodies to	<20 units
Antideoxyribonuclease B	<280 units
Anti-F-actin antibodies, serum	1:80 or less
Antihistone antibodies	<1:16
Anti-LKM antibodies	<1:20
Antimitochondrial antibodies	1:5 or less
Anti-myelin associated glycoprotein antibody	<1:1,600
Antimyeloperoxidase antibodies	<1 U
Antinuclear antibodies	1:40 or less
Anti-smooth muscle antibodies	1:80 or less
Antistreptolysin O titer	<200 Todd units
Antithrombin activity	80%–120%
Antithyroglobulin antibodies	<20 U/mL
Antithyroid peroxidase antibodies	<2.0 U/mL
Anti-tissue transglutaminase antibodies	See tissue transglutaminase antibody
Arterial blood gas studies (patient breathing room air):	
pH	7.38–7.44
$PaCO_2$	38–42 mmHg
PaO_2	75–100 mmHg
Bicarbonate	23–26 mEq/L
Oxygen saturation	95% or greater
Methemoglobin	0.5%–3.0%
Ascorbic acid (vitamin C), blood	0.4–1.5 mg/dL
Ascorbic acid, leukocyte	16.5 ± 5.1 mg/dL of leukocytes
(1,3)-Beta-D-glucan, serum	<60 pg/mL
Beta subunit chorionic gonadotropin, urine	<2 mIU/24 hr
$Beta_2$-glycoprotein I antibodies:	
IgG	<21 SGU
IgM	<21 SMU
Beta-hydroxybutyrate, serum	<0.4 mmol/L
$Beta_2$-microglobulin, serum	0.54–2.75 mg/L
Bicarbonate, serum	23–28 mEq/L

(*continued*)

ABIM Laboratory Test Reference Ranges—January 2019 (*continued*)

Bilirubin, serum	
Total	0.3–1.0 mg/dL
Direct	0.1–0.3 mg/dL
Indirect	0.2–0.7 mg/dL
Bleeding time (template)	<8 min
BUN, serum or plasma	8–20 mg/dL
B-type natriuretic peptide, plasma	<100 pg/mL
C peptide, serum	0.8–3.1 ng/mL
Calcitonin, serum	Female: 5 pg/mL or less; male: 10 pg/mL or less
Calcium, ionized, serum	1.12–1.23 mmol/L
Calcium, serum	8.6–10.2 mg/dL
Calcium, urine	Female: <250 mg/24 hr; male: <300 mg/24 hr
Carbohydrate antigens, serum	
CA 19–9	0–37 U/mL
CA 27–29	<38.0 U/mL
CA 125	<35 U/mL
Carbon dioxide content, serum	23–30 mEq/L
Carboxyhemoglobin, blood	<5%
Carcinoembryonic antigen, plasma	<2.5 ng/mL
Carotene, serum	75–300 mcg/dL
Catecholamines, plasma	
Dopamine	<30 pg/mL
Epinephrine	
Supine	<50 pg/mL
Standing	<95 pg/mL
Norepinephrine	
Supine	112–658 pg/mL
Standing	217–1,109 pg/mL
Catecholamines, urine	
Dopamine	65–400 mcg/24 hr
Epinephrine	2–24 mcg/24 hr
Norepinephrine	15–100 mcg/24 hr
Total	26–121 mcg/24 hr
CD4 T-lymphocyte count	530–1,570/μL
Cell count, CSF:	
Leukocytes (WBCs)	0–5 cells/μL
Ceruloplasmin, serum (plasma)	25–43 mg/dL
Chloride, CSF	120–130 mEq/L
Chloride, serum	98–106 mEq/L
Chloride, urine	
Spot	mEq/L; varies
24-hr measurement	mEq/24 hr; varies with intake
Cholesterol, serum	

(*continued*)

ABIM Laboratory Test Reference Ranges—January 2019 (*continued*)

Total	
Desirable	<200 mg/dL
Borderline-high	200–239 mg/dL
High	>239 mg/dL
High-density lipoprotein	
Low	Female: <50 mg/dL;
	male: <40 mg/dL
Low-density lipoprotein	
Optimal	<100 mg/dL
Near-optimal	100–129 mg/dL
Borderline-high	130–159 mg/dL
High	160–189 mg/dL
Very high	>189 mg/dL
Cholinesterase, serum (pseudocholinesterase)	0.5 or more pH units/hr
Packed cells	0.7 or more pH units/hr
Chorionic gonadotropin, beta-human (beta-hCG), serum	Female, premenopausal nonpregnant: <1.0 U/L; female, postmenopausal: <7.0 U/L; male: <1.4 U/L
Chromogranin A, serum	<93 ng/mL
Citrate, urine	250–1,000 mg/24 hr
Clotting time (Lee-White)	5–15 min
Coagulation factors, plasma	
Factor I (fibrinogen)	200–400 mg/dL
Factor II (prothrombin)	60%–130%
Factor V (accelerator globulin)	60%–130%
Factor VII (proconvertin)	60%–130%
Factor VIII (antihemophilic globulin)	50%–150%
Factor IX (plasma thromboplastin component)	50%–150%
Factor X (Stuart factor)	60%–130%
Factor XI (plasma thromboplastin antecedent)	60%–130%
Factor XII (Hageman factor)	60%–130%
Factor XIII	57%–192%
Cold agglutinin titer	>1:64 positive
Complement components, serum	
C3	100–233 mg/dL
C4	14–48 mg/dL
CH50	110–190 units/mL
Copper, serum	100–200 mcg/dL
Copper, urine	0–100 mcg/24 hr
Coproporphyrin, urine	50–250 mcg/24 hr
Cortisol, free, urine	4–50 mcg/24 hr
Cortisol, plasma	
8:00 a.m.	5–25 mcg/dL
4:00 p.m.	<10 mcg/dL
1 hr after cosyntropin	18 mcg/dL or greater
Overnight suppression test (1-mg)	<1.8 mcg/dL

(*continued*)

ABIM Laboratory Test Reference Ranges—January 2019 (*continued*)

Overnight suppression test (8-mg)	>50% reduction in cortisol
Cortisol, saliva, 11 p.m.— midnight	<0.09 mcg/dL
C-reactive protein, serum	0.8 mg/dL or less
C-reactive protein (high sensitivity), serum	Low risk = <1.0 mg/L; average risk = 1.0–3.0 mg/L; high risk = more than 3.0 mg/L
Creatine kinase, serum	
Total	Female: 30–135 U/L; male: 55–170 U/L
MB isoenzymes	<5% of total
Creatine, urine	Female: 0–100 mg/24 hr; male: 0–40 mg/24 hr
Creatinine clearance, urine	90–140 mL/min
Creatinine, serum	Female: 0.50–1.10 mg/dL; male: 0.70–1.30 mg/dL
Creatinine, urine	
Spot	mg/dL; varies
24-hr measurement	15–25 mg/kg body weight/24 hr
Cyclosporine, whole blood (trough)	
Therapeutic	100–200 ng/mL
0–3 mo posttransplantation	150–250 ng/mL
More than 3 mo posttransplantation	75–125 ng/mL
D-dimer, plasma	<0.5 mcg/mL
DHEA-S, serum	Female: 44–332 mcg/dL; male: 89–457 mcg/dL
Delta-aminolevulinic acid, serum	<20 mcg/dL
Digoxin, serum	Therapeutic: 1.0–2.0 ng/mL (<1.2 ng/mL for patients with heart failure)
Dihydrotestosterone, serum	Adult male: 25–80 ng/dL
Dopamine, plasma	<30 pg/mL
Dopamine, urine	65–400 mcg/24 hr
D-Xylose absorption	
(after ingestion of 25 g of D-xylose)	
Serum	25–40 mg/dL
Urinary excretion	4.5–7.5 g during a 5-hr period
Electrolytes, serum	
Sodium	136–145 mEq/L
Potassium	3.5–5.0 mEq/L
Chloride	98–106 mEq/L
Bicarbonate	23–28 mEq/L
Epinephrine, plasma	
Supine	<110 pg/mL
Standing	<140 pg/mL
Epinephrine, urine	<20 mcg/24 hr
Erythrocyte count	4.2–5.9 million/μL
Erythrocyte sedimentation rate (Westergren)	Female: 0–20 mm/hr; male: 0–15 mm/hr
Erythrocyte survival rate (^{51}Cr)	T½ = 28 d
Erythropoietin, serum	4–26 mU/mL

(continued)

ABIM Laboratory Test Reference Ranges—January 2019 (continued)

Estradiol, serum	
Female, follicular	10–180 pg/mL
Mid-cycle peak	100–300 pg/mL
Luteal	40–200 pg/mL
Postmenopausal	<10 pg/mL
Male	20–50 pg/mL
Estriol, urine	>12 mg/24 hr
Estrogen receptor protein	Negative: <10 fmol/mg protein
Estrone, serum	10–60 pg/mL
Ethanol, blood	<0.005% (< 5 mg/dL)
Coma level	More than 0.5% (more than 500 mg/dL)
Intoxication	0.08%–0.1% or greater (80–100 mg/dL or greater)
Euglobulin clot lysis time	2–4 hr at 37.0 C
Everolimus, whole blood (trough)	Therapeutic: 3.0–8.0 ng/mL
Factor XIII, B subunit, plasma	60–130 U/dL
Fecal fat	<7 g/24 hr
Fecal nitrogen	<2 g/24 hr
Fecal pH	7.0–7.5
Fecal potassium	<10 mEq/L
Fecal sodium	<10 mEq/L
Fecal urobilinogen	40–280 mg/24 hr
Fecal weight	<250 g/24 hr
Ferritin, serum	Female: 11–307 ng/mL; male: 24–336 ng/mL
Fibrin(ogen) degradation products	<10 mcg/mL
Fibrinogen, plasma	200–400 mg/dL
Fibroblast growth factor-23, serum	30–80 RU/mL
Flecainide, serum	Therapeutic: 0.2–1.0 mcg/mL
Folate, red cell	150–450 ng/mL of packed cells
Folate, serum	1.8–9.0 ng/mL
Follicle-stimulating hormone, serum	
Female, follicular/luteal	2–9 mIU/mL (2–9 U/L)
Female, mid-cycle peak	4–22 mIU/mL (4–22 U/L)
Female, postmenopausal	>30 mIU/mL (>30 U/L)
Male (adult)	1–7 mIU/mL (1–7 U/L)
Children, Tanner stages 1, 2	0.5–8.0 mIU/mL (0.5–8.0 U/L)
Children, Tanner stages 3, 4, 5	1–12 mIU/mL (1–12 U/L)
Free kappa light chain, serum	3.3–19.4 mg/L
Free kappa-to-free lambda light chain ratio, serum	0.26–1.65
Free lambda light chain, serum	5.7–26.3 mg/L
Fructosamine, serum	175–280 mmol/L
Gamma globulin, CSF	6.1–8.3 mg/dL
Gamma-glutamyl transpeptidase, serum	Female: 8–40 U/L; male: 9–50 U/L
Gastric secretion	
Basal acid analysis	10–30 units of free acid
Basal acid output	Female: 2.0 ± 1.8 mEq of HCl/hr; male: 3.0 ± 2.0 mEq of HCl/hr

(continued)

ABIM Laboratory Test Reference Ranges—January 2019 (*continued*)

Maximal output after pentagastrin stimulation	23 ± 5 mEq of HCl/hr
Gastrin, serum	<100 pg/mL
Gentamicin, serum	Therapeutic: peak 5.0–10.0 mcg/mL; trough: <2.0 mcg/mL
Glucose, CSF	50–75 mg/dL
Glucose, plasma (fasting)	70–99 mg/dL
Glucose-6-phosphate dehydrogenase, blood	5–15 units/g of hemoglobin
Glycoprotein α-subunit, serum	<1 ng/mL
Growth hormone, serum	
At rest	<5 ng/mL
Response to provocative stimuli	>7 ng/mL
Haptoglobin, serum	83–267 mg/dL
Hematocrit, blood	Female: 37%–47%; male: 42%–50%
Hemoglobin A$_{1C}$	4.0%–5.6%
Hemoglobin, blood	Female: 12–16 g/dL; male: 14–18 g/dL
Hemoglobin fractionation	
Hb A	96%–98%
Hb A$_2$	1.5%–3.5%
Hb F	<1%
Hemoglobin, plasma	<5.0 mg/dL
Heparin–anti-factor Xa assay, plasma	0.3–0.7 IU/mL (therapeutic range for standard [unfractionated] heparin therapy)
Heparin–platelet factor 4 antibody, serum	Positive: >0.4 optical density units
Hepatic copper	25–40 mcg/g dry weight
Hepatic iron index	<1.0
Histamine excretion, urine	20–50 mcg/24 hr
Homocysteine, plasma	5–15 μmol/L
Beta-hCG, serum	Female, premenopausal nonpregnant: <1.0 U/L; female, postmenopausal: <7.0 U/L; male: <1.4 U/L
Hydroxyproline, urine	10–30 mg/m^2 of body surface/24 hr
Immature platelet fraction	1%–5% of platelet count
Immune complexes, serum	0–50 mcg/dL
Immunoglobulins, serum	
IgA	90–325 mg/dL
IgE	<380 IU/mL
IgG	800–1,500 mg/dL
IgM	45–150 mg/dL
Immunoglobulin free light chains, serum	
Kappa	3.3–19.4 mg/L
Lambda	5.7–26.3 mg/L
Kappa-to-lambda ratio	0.26–1.65
Insulin, serum (fasting)	<20 μU/mL
IGF-1 (somatomedin-C), serum	
Ages 16–24	182–780 ng/mL
Ages 25–39	114–492 ng/mL
Ages 40–54	90–360 ng/mL
Ages 55 and older	71–290 ng/mL

(*continued*)

ABIM Laboratory Test Reference Ranges—January 2019 (continued)

Iodine, urine	
Spot	mcg/L; varies
Iron, serum	50–150 mcg/dL
Iron-binding capacity, serum (total)	250–310 mcg/dL
Lactate, arterial blood	<1.3 mmol/L (<1.3 mEq/L)
Lactate, serum or plasma	0.7–2.1 mmol/L
Lactate, venous blood	0.6–1.8 mEq/L; 6–16 mg/dL
Lactate dehydrogenase, serum	80–225 U/L
Lactic acid, serum	6–19 mg/dL (0.7–2.1 mmol/L)
Lactose tolerance test, GI	Increase in plasma glucose: >15 mg/dL
Lead, blood	15–40 mcg/dL
Lead, urine	<80 mcg/24 hr
Leukocyte count	4,000–11,000/μL
Segmented neutrophils	50%–70%
Band forms	0%–5%
Lymphocytes	30%–45%
Monocytes	0%–6%
Basophils	0%–1%
Eosinophils	0%–3%
Lipase, serum	10–140 U/L
Lipoprotein(a), serum	Desirable: <30 mg/dL
Lithium, plasma	
Therapeutic	0.6–1.2 mEq/L
Toxic level	>2 mEq/L
LH, serum	
Female, follicular/luteal	1–12 mIU/mL (1–12 U/L)
Female, mid-cycle peak	9–80 mIU/mL (9–80 U/L)
Female, postmenopausal	>30 mIU/mL (>30 U/L)
Male (adult)	2–9 mIU/mL (2–9 U/L)
Children, Tanner stages 1, 2, 3	<9.0 mIU/mL (< 9.0 U/L)
Children, Tanner stages 4, 5	1–15 mIU/mL (1–15 U/L)
Lymphocyte subsets	
CD3	900–3,245/μL
CD4	530–1,570/μL
CD8	430–1,060/μL
CD19	208–590/μL
Magnesium, serum	1.6–2.6 mEq/L
Magnesium, urine	14–290 mg/24 hr
Mean corpuscular hemoglobin	28–32 pg
Mean corpuscular hemoglobin concentration	33–36 g/dL
Mean corpuscular volume	80–98 fL
Mean platelet volume	7–9 fL
Metanephrines, fractionated, plasma	
Metanephrine	<0.5 nmol/L
Normetanephrine	<0.9 nmol/L

(continued)

ABIM Laboratory Test Reference Ranges—January 2019 (*continued*)

Metanephrines, fractionated, 24-hr urine	
Metanephrine	<400 mcg/24 hr
Normetanephrine	<900 mcg/24 hr
Myoglobin, serum	<100 mcg/L
Norepinephrine, plasma	
Supine	70–750 pg/mL
Standing	200–1,700 pg/mL
Norepinephrine, urine	0–100 mcg/24 hr
Normetanephrine, fractionated, plasma	<0.9 nmol/L
Normetanephrine, fractionated, 24-hr urine	<900 mcg
N-telopeptide, urine	Female: 11–48 nmol BCE/mmol creatinine; male: 7–68 nmol BCE/mmol creatinine
NT-pro-BNP, serum or plasma	If eGFR >60 mL/min/1.73 m^2

	18–49 y of age
	  Heart failure unlikely: 300 pg/mL or less
	  High probability of heart failure: 450 pg/mL or greater
	
	50–75 y of age
	  Heart failure unlikely: 300 pg/mL or less
	  High probability of heart failure: 900 pg/mL or greater
	
	Older than 75 y of age
	  Heart failure unlikely: 300 pg/mL or less
	  High probability of heart failure: 1,800 pg/mL or greater
	
	If eGFR <60 mL/min/1.73 m^2
	
	18 y of age or older
	  High probability of heart failure: 1,200 pg/mL or greater

Osmolality, serum	275–295 mOsm/kg H$_2$O
Osmolality, urine	38–1,400 mOsm/kg H$_2$O
Osmotic fragility of erythrocytes	Increased if hemolysis occurs in over 0.5% NaCl; decreased if hemolysis is incomplete in 0.3% NaCl
Osteocalcin, serum	Male: 11.3–35.4 ng/mL; female: 7.2–27.9 ng/mL
Oxalate, urine	<40 mg/24 hr
Oxygen consumption	225–275 mL/min
Oxygen saturation, arterial blood	95% or greater
Parathyroid hormone, serum	
C-terminal	150–350 pg/mL
Intact	10–65 pg/mL
Intact (dialysis patients only)	Target: 130–585 pg/mL
Parathyroid hormone-related protein, serum	<1.5 pmol/L
Partial thromboplastin time (activated)	25–35 sec
pH, urine	4.5–8.0
Phenolsulfonphthalein, urine	At least 25% excreted by 15 min; 40% by 30 min; 60% by 120 min
Phenytoin, serum	Therapeutic: 10–20 mcg/mL
Phosphatase (acid), serum	
Total	0.5–2.0 (Bodansky) units/mL
Prostatic fraction	0.1–0.4 unit/mL

(continued)

ABIM Laboratory Test Reference Ranges—January 2019 (*continued*)

Phosphatase (alkaline), serum	30–120 U/L
Phospholipids, serum (total)	200–300 mg/dL
Phosphorus, serum	3.0–4.5 mg/dL
Phosphorus, urine	500–1,200 mg/24 hr
Platelet count	150,000–450,000/μL
PFA-100:	
Collagen–epiephrine closure time	60–143 sec
Collagen–ADP closure time	58–123 sec
Platelet survival rate (^{51}Cr)	10 d
Potassium, serum	3.5–5.0 mEq/L
Potassium, urine	
Spot	mEq/L; varies
24-hr measurement	mEq/24 hr; varies with intake
Prealbumin, serum	16–30 mg/dL
Pregnanetriol, urine	0.2–3.5 mg/24 hr
Pressure (opening; initial), CSF	70–180 mm CSF (70–180 mm H_2O)
Procalcitonin, serum	Less than or equal to 0.10 ng/mL
Progesterone, serum	
Female, follicular	0.02–0.9 ng/mL
Female, luteal	2–30 ng/mL
Male (adult)	0.12–0.3 ng/mL
Proinsulin, serum	3–20 pmol/L
Prolactin, serum	<20 ng/mL
Prostate-specific antigen, serum	ng/mL; no specific normal or abnormal level
Protein C activity, plasma	65%–150%
Protein C antigen, plasma	70%–140%
Protein catabolic rate, urine	Goal: 1.0–1.2 g/kg/24 hr
Protein S activity, plasma	57%–131%
Protein S antigen, plasma	
Total	60%–140%
Free	60%–130%
Protein, urine	
Spot	mg/dL; varies
24-hr measurement	<100 mg/24 hr
Proteins, CSF total	15–45 mg/dL
Proteins, serum	
Total	5.5–9.0 g/dL
Albumin	3.5–5.5 g/dL
Globulin	2.0–3.5 g/dL
Alpha1	0.2–0.4 g/dL
Alpha2	0.5–0.9 g/dL
Beta	0.6–1.1 g/dL
Gamma	0.7–1.7 g/dL
Protein-to-creatinine ratio, urine	<0.2 mg/mg
Prothrombin time, plasma	11–13 sec
Pyruvic acid, blood	0.08–0.16 mmol/L

(*continued*)

ABIM Laboratory Test Reference Ranges—January 2019 (*continued*)

Quinidine, serum	Therapeutic: 2–5 mcg/mL
Red cell distribution width (RDW)	9.0–14.5
Red cell mass	Female: 22.7–27.9 mL/kg; male: 24.9–32.5 mL/kg
Renin activity (angiotensin-I radioimmunoassay)	
Peripheral plasma	
Normal diet	
Supine	0.3–2.5 ng/mL/hr
Upright	0.2–3.6 ng/mL/hr
Low sodium diet	
Supine	0.9–4.5 ng/mL/hr
Upright	4.1–9.1 ng/mL/hr
Diuretics + low sodium diet	6.3–13.7 ng/mL/hr
Renal vein concentration	Normal ratio (high:low): <1.5
Reptilase time	10–12 sec
Reticulocyte count	0.5%–1.5% of red cells
Reticulocyte count, absolute	25,000–100,000/μL
Rheumatoid factor (nephelometry)	<24 IU/mL
Rheumatoid factor, latex test for	1:80 or less
Ristocetin cofactor activity of plasma	50%–150%
Russell viper venom time, dilute	33–44 sec
Salicylate, plasma	Therapeutic: 20–30 mg/dL
Sex hormone-binding globulin	Female, nonpregnant: 18–144 nmol/L; male: 10–57 nmol/L
Sodium, serum	136–145 mEq/L
Sodium, urine	
Spot	mEq/L; varies
24-hr measurement	mEq/24 hr; varies with intake
Specific gravity, urine	1.002–1.030
Sperm density	10–150 million/mL
Sweat test for sodium and chloride	<60 mEq/L
T3 resin uptake	25%–35%
T-lymphocyte count, CD4	530–1,570/μL
Tacrolimus, whole blood (trough)	Therapeutic: 5–15 ng/mL (For transplant patients: 10.0–15.0 ng/mL [0–3 mo posttransplantation]; 5.0–10.0 ng/mL [more than 3 mo posttransplantation])
Testosterone, bioavailable, serum	Female, age 18–69 y: 0.5–8.5 ng/dL
Testosterone, free, serum	Male: 70–300 pg/mL
Testosterone, serum	Female: 18–54 ng/dL; male: 291–1,100 ng/dL
Theophylline, serum	Therapeutic: 8–20 mcg/mL
Thrombin time	17–23 sec
Thyroid function studies	
T3 resin uptake	25%–35%
Thyroglobulin, serum	<20 ng/mL
Thyroidal iodine (^{123}I) uptake	5%–30% of administered dose at 24 hr
TSH, serum	0.5–4.0 μU/mL (0.5–4.0 mU/L)
TSI	<130%
Thyroxine-binding globulin, serum	12–27 mcg/mL

(continued)

ABIM Laboratory Test Reference Ranges—January 2019 (*continued*)

Thyroxine index, free (estimate)	5–12
Thyroxine (T_4), serum	
Total	5–12 mcg/dL
Free	0.8–1.8 ng/dL
Triiodothyronine (T_3), serum	
Total	80–180 ng/dL
Reverse	20–40 ng/dL
Free	2.3–4.2 pg/mL
Tissue transglutaminase antibody, IgA (by chemiluminescence method)	<20 AU
Tissue transglutaminase antibody, IgA (by ELISA)	<4.0 U/mL
Tissue transglutaminase antibody, IgG (by chemiluminescence method)	<20 AU
Tissue transglutaminase antibody, IgG (by ELISA)	<6.0 U/mL
Total proteins, CSF	15–45 mg/dL
Transaminase, serum glutamic oxaloacetic (SGOT)	See aminotransferase, serum aspartate (AST, SGOT)
Transaminase, serum glutamic pyruvic (SGPT)	See aminotransferase, serum alanine (ALT, SGPT)
Transferrin saturation	20%–50%
Transferrin, serum	200–400 mg/dL
Triglycerides, serum (fasting)	
Optimal	<100 mg/dL
Normal	<150 mg/dL
Borderline-high	150–199 mg/dL
High	200–499 mg/dL
Very high	>499 mg/dL
Troponin I, cardiac, serum	0.04 ng/mL or less
Troponin T, cardiac, serum	0.01 ng/mL or less
Tryptase, serum	<11.5 ng/mL
Urea clearance, urine	
Standard	40–60 mL/min
Maximal	60–100 mL/min
Urea nitrogen, blood	8–20 mg/dL
Urea nitrogen, urine	12–20 g/24 hr
Uric acid, serum	3.0–7.0 mg/dL
Uric acid, urine	250–750 mg/24 hr
Uroporphyrin, urine	10–30 mcg/24 hr
Vanillylmandelic acid, urine	<9 mg/24 hr
Venous oxygen content, mixed	14–16 mL/dL
Venous studies, mixed, blood	
pH	7.32–7.41
PCO_2	42–53 mmHg
PO_2	35–42 mmHg
Bicarbonate	24–28 mEq/L
Oxygen saturation (SvO_2)	65%–75%
Viscosity, serum	1.4–1.8 cp

(*continued*)

ABIM Laboratory Test Reference Ranges—January 2019 (*continued*)

Vitamin A, serum:	
Adult	32.5–78.0 mcg/dL
Pediatric, age 1–2 y (retinol)	20–43 mcg/dL
Vitamin B₁₂, serum	200–800 pg/mL
Vitamin D metabolites, serum	
1, 25-Dihydroxyvitamin D (1, 25-Dihydroxycholecalciferol)	15–60 pg/mL
25-Hydroxyvitamin D (25-Hydroxycholecalciferol)	30–60 ng/mL
Vitamin E, serum:	
Adult	5.5–17.0 mg/L
Pediatric, age 1–2 y (alpha-tocopherol)	2.9–16.6 mg/L
Volume, blood	
Plasma	Female: 43 mL/kg body weight; male: 44 mL/kg body weight
Red cell	Female: 20–30 mL/kg body weight; male: 25–35 mL/kg body weight
von Willebrand factor antigen, plasma	50%–150%
Zinc, serum	75–140 mcg/dL

AAT, alpha₁-antitrypsin; ABIM, American Board of Internal Medicine; ACE, angiotensin-converting enzyme; ALT, alanine aminotransferase; ANC, absolute neutrophil count; anti-LKM, anti-liver-kidney microsomal; aPTT, activated partial thromboplastin time; AST, aspartate aminotransferase; beta-hCG, beta-human chorionic gonadotropin; BUN, blood urea nitrogen; CSF, cerebrospinal fluid; DHEA-S, dehydroepiandrosterone sulfate; GFR, glomerular filtration rate; GI, gastrointestinal; IGF-1, insulin-like growth factor 1; LH, luteinizing hormone; NT-pro-BNP, N-terminal-pro-B-type natriuretic peptide; PFA, platelet function analysis; RBC, red blood cell; RDW, red cell distribution width; SGOT, serum glutamic oxaloacetic transaminase; SGPT, serum glutamic pyruvic transaminase; TSH, thyroid-stimulating hormone; TSI, thyroid-stimulating immunoglobulin.

Source: Reproduced with permission from the American Board of Internal Medicine. Retrieved from https://www.abim.org/~/media/ABIM%20Public/Files/pdf/exam/laboratory-reference-ranges.pdf

Index